CURRENT
PSYCHIATRIC
THERAPY

DAVID L. DUNNER, M.D.

Outpatient Psychiatry Center
for Anxiety and Depression;
Professor, Department of Psychiatry
Director, Outpatient Psychiatry
Co-Director, Center for Anxiety and Depression
Vice-Chairman for Clinical Services
University of Washington
Seattle, Washington

W. B. SAUNDERS COMPANY

Harcourt Brace Jovanovich, Inc.

Philadelphia, London, Toronto, Montreal, Sydney, Tokyo

W. B. SAUNDERS COMPANY
Harcourt Brace Jovanovich, Inc.

The Curtis Center
Independence Square West
Philadelphia, Pennsylvania 19106

Library of Congress Cataloging-in-Publication Data

Current psychiatric therapy / [edited by] David L. Dunner.
   p.   cm.
Includes bibliographical references.
ISBN 0-7216-3973-9
   1. Psychiatry. I. Dunner, David L.
   [DNLM: 1. Mental Disorders—therapy. WM 400 C9756]
RC480.C86 1993
616.89'1—dc20
DNLM/DLC   92-3812

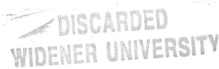

Current Psychiatric Therapy   ISBN   0-7216-3973-9

CONTRIBUTORS

MICHAEL E. ADDIS, B.A.

Pre-doctoral candidate in Clinical Psychology, University of Washington, Seattle, Washington

Brief Psychotherapies

ANNE MARIE ALBANO, Ph.D.

Research Scientist, Department of Psychology, State University of New York at Albany, Albany, New York

Review of Psychosocial Treatments for Anxiety Disorders

LAWRENCE J. ALBERS, M.D.

Department of Psychiatry and Behavioral Sciences, University of California, Orange, California

Schizophrenia: An Overview of Pharmacological Treatment

HUBERT E. ARMSTRONG, Ph.D.

Associate Professor, University of Washington, Seattle, Washington

Review of Psychosocial Treatments for Schizophrenia

DAVID H. AVERY, M.D.

Associate Professor, University of Washington School of Medicine, Seattle, Washington

Electroconvulsive Therapy

LORI A. BAKER, M.A.

Senior Technical Writer, Department of Psychiatry and Human Behavior, Brown University Medical School, Providence, Rhode Island

Classification and Treatment of Dysthymia

DAVID H. BARLOW, Ph.D.

Distinguished Professor, Department of Psychology, State University of New York, Albany, New York

Review of Psychosocial Treatments for Anxiety Disorders

LEWIS R. BAXTER, M.D.

Associate Professor, Psychiatry and Biobehavioral Sciences, UCLA School of Medicine, Los Angeles, California

Neuro Imaging: Uses in Psychiatry

CONTRIBUTORS

ELIZABETH S. BOWMAN, M.D.

Associate Professor of Psychiatry, Indiana University School of Medicine, Indianapolis, Indiana

Genetics of Psychiatric Diagnosis and Treatment

WILLIAM F. BOYER, M.D.

Assistant Professor, University of California San Diego; and Feighner Research Institute, San Diego, California

Future Antidepressants

ALAN BREIER, M.D.

Research Associate Professor, Department of Psychiatry, University of Maryland School of Medicine, Baltimore, Maryland

Paranoid Disorder: Clinical Features and Treatment

TIMOTHY A. BROWN, Psy.D.

Associate Director, Phobia and Anxiety Disorders Clinic, Center for Stress and Anxiety Disorders, State University of New York, Albany, New York

Review of Psychosocial Treatments for Anxiety Disorders

DANIEL J. BUYSSE, M.D.

Assistant Professor of Psychiatry, University of Pittsburgh, Pittsburgh, Pennsylvania

Classification of Sleep Disorders: A Preview of the DSM-IV; Parasomnias

ENOCH CALLAWAY, M.D.

Professor Emeritus, University of California, San Francisco, California

Electroencephalograms and Event-Related Potentials in Clinical Psychiatry

MAGDA CAMPBELL, M.D.

Professor of Psychiatry, New York University School of Medicine, New York, New York

Proposed Changes in the DMS-IV Criteria for Child Psychiatry

GABRIELLE A. CARLSON, M.D.

Professor of Psychiatry and Pediatrics, State University of New York at Stony Brook, Stony Brook, New York

Psychosis and Mania in Adolescents

JOHN E. CARR, Ph.D.

Professor of Psychiatry and Behavioral Sciences and Psychology, University of Washington, Seattle, Washington

Simple and Social Phobia

DANIEL E. CASEY, M.D.

Professor of Psychiatry and Associate Professor of Neurology, Oregon Health Sciences University, Portland, Oregon

Tardive Dyskinesia

JOHN A. CHILES, M.D.

Professor, Department of Psychiatry, The University of Texas Health Sciences Center, San Antonio, Texas
The Suicidal Patient: Assessment, Crisis Management, and Treatment

ROLAND D. CIARANELLO, M.D.

Nancy Friend Pritzker Professor of Psychiatry and Behavioral Science, Stanford University School of Medicine, Stanford, California
Structural Foundations of Illness and Treatment: Receptors

C. ROBERT CLONINGER, M.D.

Psychiatrist-in-Chief, Washington University Medical School, St. Louis, Missouri
Somatoform and Dissociative Disorders: A Summary of Changes for DSM-IV

JONATHAN O. COLE, M.D.

Professor of Psychiatry, Harvard Medical School, Boston, Massachusetts
Psychotropic-Induced Sexual Dysfunction

LIRIO S. COVEY, Ph.D.

Associate Research Scientist, Department of Psychiatry, College of Physicians and Surgeons, Columbia University, New York, New York
Nicotine Use

DEBORAH S. COWLEY, M.D.

Associate Professor, Department of Psychiatry and Behavioral Sciences, University of Washington, Seattle, Washington
Generalized Anxiety Disorder

JAMES W. CROAKE, Ph.D

Professor, Department of Psychiatry, University of South Alabama College of Medicine, Mobile, Alabama
Group Therapy and Marital/Family Treatment

CHRISTOS S. DAGADAKIS, M.D., M.P.H.

Lecturer, Department of Psychiatry and Behavioral Sciences, University of Washington, Seattle, Washington
Psychiatric Emergencies

STEPHEN R. DAGER, M.D.

Associate Professor, Department of Psychiatry and Behavioral Sciences and Bioengineering, University of Washington School of Medicine, Seattle, Washington
Alzheimer's Diseases

CONTRIBUTORS

GREGORY W. DALACK, M.D.

Assistant in Clinical Psychiatry, College of Physicians and Surgeons, Columbia University, New York, New York

Nicotine Use

DAVID DAVIS, M.D., F.R.C.Psych., D.P.M.

Professor of Psychiatry, Department of Psychiatry and Behavioral Sciences, University of Texas Medical School, Galveston, Texas; Professor Emeritus of Psychiatry, University of Missouri, Columbia, Missouri

Multiple Personality, Fugue, and Amnesia

JOHN M. DAVIS, M.D.

Gilman Professor of Psychiatry, University of Illinois, Chicago, Illinois

Neuroleptic Malignant Syndrome

ROBIN R. DEAN, Ph.D.

Research Associate, Department of Psychiatry, Stanford University School of Medicine, Stanford, California

Structural Foundations of Illness and Treatment: Receptors

EDWARD F. DOMINO, M.D.

Professor of Pharmacology, University of Michigan School of Medicine, Ann Arbor, Michigan

Treatment of Psychedelic Drug-Induced Psychoses

REBECCA A. DULIT, M.D.

Assistant Professor of Psychiatry, Cornell University Medical College, New York, New York

Cluster B Personality Disorders

CURTISS DuRAND, M.D.

Clinical Instructor in Psychology, Harvard Medical School, Boston, Massachusetts

An Overview of the Treatment of Geriatric Disorders

SAMUEL F. DWORKIN, D.D.S., Ph.D.

Professor, Department of Psychiatry; Professor, Department of Dentistry, University of Washington, Seattle, Washington

Somatoform Pain Disorder and Its Treatment

EVERETT H. ELLINWOOD, M.D.

Department of Psychiatry and Pharmacology, Duke University Medical Center, Durham, North Carolina

Stimulant Abuse: Cocaine and Amphetamine

MONIQUE ERNST, M.D., Ph.D.

Clinical Instructor in Psychiatry, Research Fellow, New York University School of Medicine, New York, New York

Proposed Changes in the DMS-IV Criteria for Child Psychiatry

GARY A. FAST, M.D.

Assistant Professor, Department of Psychiatry, University of Kansas School of Medicine, Wichita, Kansas

Therapeutic Drug Monitoring

GEORGE FEIN, Ph.D.

Professor of Medical Psychology, University of California, San Francisco, California

Electroencephalograms and Event-Related Potentials in Clinical Psychiatry

JOHN P. FEIGHNER, M.D.

Associate Professor, University of California San Diego; and Director, Feighner Research Institute, San Diego, California

Future Antidepressants

MARIE LOURDES FILS-AIME, M.D.

Clinical Associate, National Institute on Alcoholism and Alcohol Abuse, Bethesda, Maryland

Sedative-Hypnotic Abuse

ALLEN J. FRANCES, M.D.

Professor and Chairman, Department of Psychiatry, Duke University Medical College, Durham, North Carolina

Cluster B Personality Disorders

ROBERT H. GERNER, M.D.

Associate Clinical Professor, Department of Psychiatry, UCLA: Director, Center for Mood Disorders, Los Angeles, California

Psychiatric Effects of Nonpsychiatric Medications

DONNA E. GILES, Ph.D.

Associate Professor, University of Pittsburgh Medical Center, Pittsburgh, Pennsylvania

Parasomnias

J. CHRISTIAN GILLIN, M.D.

Professor of Psychiatry, University of California, San Diego, School of Medicine, La Jolla, California

Clinical Sleep-Wake Disorders in Psychiatric Practice: Dyssomnias

ALEXANDER H. GLASSMAN, M.D.

Professor of Clinical Psychiatry, College of Physicians and Surgeons, Columbia University, New York, New York

Nicotine Use

TANA A. GRADY, M.D.

Medical Staff Fellow, National Institute of Mental Health/Laboratory of Clinical Science, Bethesda, Maryland

Obsessive-Compulsive Disorder and Trichotillomania

JOHN F. GREDEN, M.D.

Professor and Chairman, Department of Psychiatry, Research Scientist, Mental Health Research Institute, University of Michigan Medical Center, Ann Arbor, Michigan
The Laboratory in Psychiatry

BARRY H. GUZE, M.D.

Assistant Clinical Professor of Psychiatry and Biobehavioral Sciences, UCLA School of Medicine, Los Angeles, California
Neuro Imaging: Uses in Psychiatry

COLLEEN M. HADIGAN, B.A.

Department of Psychiatry, College of Physicians and Surgeons, Columbia, University, New York, New York
Proposed DSM-IV Criteria for Eating Disorders

JAMES A. HALIKAS, M.D.

Professor, Department of Psychiatry, University of Minnesota; Director of Chemical Dependence Treatment Program, Minneapolis, Minnesota
Opioid Dependence

KATHERINE A. HALMI, M.D.

Professor in Psychiatry, Cornell University Medical Center, White Plains, New York
Treatment of Anorexia Nervosa

KENRIC W. HAMMOND, M.D.

Assistant Professor of Psychiatry and Behavioral Science, University of Washington School of Medicine, Seattle, Washington
Post-traumatic Stress Disorder

JULIA R. HEIMAN, Ph.D.

Professor of Psychiatry and Behavioral Sciences, University of Washington School of Medicine, Seattle, Washington
Sexual Dysfunctions

MARK R. HELLER, Ph.D.

Research Associate, Department of Psychiatry, Stanford University School of Medicine, Stanford, California
Structural Foundations of Illness and Treatment: Receptors

ROBERT M. HERTZ, M.D.

Adjunct Professor of Psychiatry, SUNY; Clinical Instructor in Psychiatry, Albany Medical College, Albany, New York
Review of Psychosocial Treatments for Anxiety Disorders

LYNNE HOFFMAN, M.D.

Instructor in Psychiatry, Cornell University Medical Center, White Plains, New York
Treatment of Anorexia Nervosa

STEVEN D. HOLLON, Ph.D

Professor of Psychology, Vanderbilt University, Nashville, Tennessee
Review of Psychosocial Treatments for Mood Disorders

THOMAS M. HYDE, M.D., Ph.D.

Director, Neurology Consultation Clinics, Neuroscience Center at St. Elizabeths Hospital, National Institute of Mental Health, Washington, D.C.
Structural Foundations of Mental Illness and Treatment: Neuroanatomy

PHILIP G. JANICAK, M.D.

Professor of Psychiatry, University of Illinois, Chicago, Illinois
Neuroleptic Malignant Syndrome

JAMES W. JEFFERSON, M.D.

Professor of Psychiatry, University of Wisconsin Medical School, Madison, Wisconsin
Mood Stabilizers: A Review

MICHAEL R. JOHNSON, M.D.

Instructor, Department of Psychiatry and Behavioral Sciences, Medical University of South Carolina, Charleston, South Carolina
Future Trends in the Psychopharmacology of Anxiety Disorders

RICARDO JORGE, M.D.

Fellow Associate, Department of Psychiatry, University of Iowa, Iowa City, Iowa
Organic Mood, Delusional, and Anxiety Disorders

WAYNE KATON, M.D.

Professor of Psychiatry, Chief of Division of Consultation-Liaison Psychiatry, University of Washington School of Medicine, Seattle, Washington
Somatization Disorder, Hypochondriasis, and Conversion Disorder

IRA R. KATZ, M.D., Ph.D.

Professor of Psychiatry, Medical College of Pennsylvania, Philadelphia, Pennsylvania
Delirium

PAUL E. KECK, Jr., M.D.

Associate Professor of Psychiatry, University of Cincinnati College of Medicine, Cincinnati, Ohio
Rapid Cycling

SAMUEL J. KEITH, M.D.

Clinical Professor of Psychiatry, Georgetown University, School of Medicine, Washington, D.C.
The Implication of Criteria Changes for DSM-IV Schizophrenia

CONTRIBUTORS

MARTIN B. KELLER, M.D.

Professor and Chairman, Department of Psychiatry and Human Behavior, Brown University Medical School, Providence, Rhode Island

Classification and Treatment of Dysthymia

JEFFREY E. KELSEY, M.D., Pн.D.

Psychiatry Resident, Department of Psychiatry, Stanford University School of Medicine, Stanford, California

Structural Foundations of Illness and Treatment: Receptors

ARIFULLA KHAN, M.D.

Associate Professor, Department of Psychiatry and Behavioral Sciences, University of Washington, Seattle, Washington

Neuroleptic Malignant Syndrome

MARGARET A. KITCHELL, M.D.

Clinical Assistant Professor, Department of Psychiatry and Behavioral Sciences, University of Washington School of Medicine, Seattle, Washington

Alzheimer's Disease

DONALD F. KLEIN, M.D.

Professor of Psychiatry, College of Physicians and Surgeons, Columbia University, New York, New York

Atypical Depression

JOEL E. KLEINMAN, M.D., Pн.D.

Chief, Neuropathology Section, Clinical Brain Disorders Branch, Intramural Research Program, National Institute of Mental Health, Washington, D.C.

Structural Foundations of Mental Illness and Treatment: Neuroanatomy

KELLY KOERNER, B.A.

Pre-doctoral candidate in Clinical Psychology, University of Washington, Seattle, Washington

Brief Psychotherapies

K. RANGA R. KRISHNAN, M.D.

Associate Professor of Psychiatry, Duke University Medical Center, Durham, North Carolina

Hormonal Regulation of Behavior

KENNETH KUHN, M.D.

Senior Resident in Psychiatry, former Chemical Dependency Fellow, University of Minnesota, Minneapolis, Minnesota

Opioid Dependence

CONTRIBUTORS

DAVID J. KUPFER, M.D.

Professor and Chairman, Department of Psychiatry, University of Pittsburgh School of Medicine, Pittsburgh, Pennsylvania

Classification of Sleep Disorders: A Preview of the DSM-IV

ALFRED J. LEWY, M.D., Ph.D.

Professor of Psychiatry, Ophthalmology and Pharmacology, Oregon Health Sciences University, Portland, Oregon

Seasonal Mood Disorders

MICHAEL R. LIEBOWITZ, M.D.

Professor of Clinical Psychiatry, College of Physicians and Surgeons, Columbia University, New York, New York

Proposed Changes in DSM-IV for Anxiety Disorders

J. PIERRE LOEBEL, M.D.

Clinical Professor, Department of Psychiatry and Behavioral Sciences, University of Washington School of Medicine, Seattle, Washington

Alzheimer's Diseases

JOSEPH LoPICCOLO, Ph.D.

Professor of Psychology, University of Missouri, Columbia, Missouri

Paraphilias

R. BRUCE LYDIARD, M.D., Ph.D.

Associate Professor, Department of Psychiatry and Behavioral Sciences, Medical University of South Carolina, Charleston, South Carolina

Future Trends in the Psychopharmacology of Anxiety Disorders

ROLAND D. MAIURO, Ph.D.

Associate Professor, Department of Psychiatry and Behavioral Sciences, University of Washington School of Medicine, Seattle, Washington

Intermittent Explosive Disorder

STEPHEN R. MARDER, M.D.

Professor of Psychiatry and Biobehavioral Sciences, UCLA Medical School, Los Angeles, California

Future Directions in Antipsychotic Drug Treatment

DEBORAH B. MARIN, M.D.

Assistant Professor, Mount Sinai School of Medicine, New York, New York

Cluster B Personality Disorders

SUSAN M. MATTHEWS, B.A.

National Institute of Mental Health, Rockville, Maryland

The Implication of Criteria Changes for DSM-IV Schizophrenia

PETER E. MAXIM, M.D., Ph.D.

Associate Professor, Department of Psychiatry and Behavioral Sciences, University of Washington School of Medicine, Seattle, Washington

Brief Dynamic Therapy

ELIZABETH McCAULEY, Ph.D.

Associate Professor, Department of Psychiatry and Behavioral Sciences, University of Washington, Seattle, Washington

Treatment of Depressive Disorders in Adolescents

JOSEPH M. McCREERY, M.D.

Chief, Inpatient Services, Addictions Treatment Center, VA Medical Center, Seattle, Washington

Alcohol Problems

SUSAN L. McELROY, M.D.

Associate Professor of Psychiatry, University of Cincinnati College of Medicine, Cincinnati, Ohio

Rapid Cycling

PATRICK J. McGRATH, M.D.

Associate Professor of Clinical Psychiatry, College of Physicians and Surgeons, Columbia University, New York, New York

Atypical Depression

NORMAN S. MILLER, M.D.

The New York Hospital—Cornell Medical Center, White Plains, New York

Dual Diagnosis: Concept, Diagnosis, and Treatment

JAMES E. MITCHELL, M.D.

Professor, Department of Psychiatry; Director, Division of Adult Psychiatry, University of Minnesota, Minneapolis, Minnesota

Bulimia Nervosa

KATHLEEN MYERS, M.D., M.S., M.P.H.

Assistant Professor, Department of Psychiatry and Behavioral Sciences, University of Washington, Seattle, Washington

Treatment of Depressive Disorders in Adolescents

CATHERINE A. NAGEOTTE, M.D.

Assistant Professor, Research, University of Illinois, Chicago, Illinois

Disorders in Children: Autistic Disorder, Psychosis, Attention-Deficit Hyperactivity Disorder, Anxiety Disorders, and Depression

CHARLES B. NEMEROFF, M.D., Ph.D.

Professor and Chairman, Department of Psychiatry, Emory University School of Medicine, Atlanta, Georgia

Hormonal Regulation of Behavior

NANCY C. NITENSON, M.D.

Instructor in Psychiatry, Harvard Medical School, Boston, Massachusetts
Psychotropic-Induced Sexual Dysfunction

JOHN I. NURNBERGER, Jr., M.D., Ph.D.

Professor of Psychiatry and Medical Neurobiology, Indiana University School of Medicine, Indianapolis, Indiana
Genetics of Psychiatric Diagnosis and Treatment

MADELEINE M. O'BRIEN, M.D.

Department of Psychiatry, Bronx VA Medical Center, Bronx, New York
Cluster A Personality Disorders

ELSA O'CONNOR, Ed.D

Lecturer, Department of Psychiatry and Behavioral Sciences, University of Washington, Seattle, Washington
Group Therapy and Marital/Family Treatment

SAMUEL PERRY, M.D.

Professor of Psychiatry, Cornell University Medical College, New York, New York
Psychiatric Treatment of Adults with Human Immunodeficiency Virus Infection

BRUCE PFOHL, M.D.

Associate Professor, University of Iowa College of Medicine, Iowa City, Iowa
Proposed DSM-IV Criteria for Personality Disorders

TERESA A. PIGOTT, M.D.

Assistant Professor of Psychiatry, Director of Psychopharmacology Research, Georgetown University Medical Center, Washington, D.C.; Assistant Professor of Psychiatry, Uniformed Services University of the Health Sciences, Bethesda, Maryland
Obsessive-Compulsive Disorder and Trichotillomania

ROBERT M. POST, M.D.

Chief, Biological Psychiatry Branch, National Institute of Mental Health, Bethesda, Maryland
Mood Disorders: Acute Mania

STEVEN G. POTKIN, M.D.

Professor and Director of Research, Department of Psychiatry and Behavioral Sciences, University of California, Orange, California
Schizophrenia: An Overview of Pharmacological Treatment

WILLIAM Z. POTTER, M.D., Ph.D.

National Institute of Mental Health, Rockville, Maryland
Maintenance Treatment for Mood Disorders

CONTRIBUTORS

SHELDON H. PRESKORN, M.D.

Professor and Vice Chairman, Department of Psychiatry, University of Kansas School of Medicine, Wichita, Kansas

Therapeutic Drug Monitoring

ROBERT F. PRIEN, Ph.D.

National Institute of Mental Health, Rockville, Maryland

Maintenance Treatment for Mood Disorders

FREDERIC M. QUITKIN, M.D.

Professor of Clinical Psychiatry, College of Physicians and Surgeons, Columbia University, New York, New York

Atypical Depression

JUDITH G. RABKIN, Ph.D., M.P.H.

Professor of Clinical Psychology in Psychiatry, College of Physicians and Surgeons, Columbia University, New York, New York

Atypical Depression

B. ASHOK RAJ, M.D.

Associate Professor of Psychiatry, University of South Florida College of Medicine, Tampa, Florida

Panic Disorder

JEFFREY L. RAUSCH, M.D.

Professor and Vice Chairman, Department of Psychiatry and Health Behavior, Medical College of Georgia, Augusta, Georgia

Premenstrual Syndrome

CHARLES A. REYNOLDS, Pharm. D.

Senior Pharmacist, UCLA Neuropsychiatric Hospital, Los Angeles, California

Neuro Imaging: Uses in Psychiatry

CHARLES F. REYNOLDS III, M.D.

Professor of Psychiatry and Neurology. University of Pittsburgh School of Medicine, Pittsburgh, Pennsylvania

Classification of Sleep Disorders: A Preview of the DSM-IV

ELLIOTT RICHELSON, M.D.

Professor of Psychiatry and Professor of Pharmacology, Mayo Medical School, Rochester, Minnesota

Review of Antidepressants in the Treatment of Mood Disorders

GLENN RICHMOND, M.D.

Department of Psychiatry and Behavioral Sciences, University of California Irvine Medical Center, Orange, California

Schizophrenia: An Overview of Pharmacological Treatment

RICHARD K. RIES, M.D.

Associate Professor, Department of Psychiatry and Behavioral Sciences, University of Washington Medical School, Seattle, Washington

Dual Diagnosis: Concept, Diagnosis, and Treatment

STEVEN C. RISSE, M.D.

Associate Professor, Department of Psychiatry and Behavioral Sciences, University of Washington School of Medicine, Seattle, Washington

Post-traumatic Stress Disorder

ROBERT G. ROBINSON, M.D.

Professor and Head, Department of Psychiatry, University of Iowa, College of Medicine, Iowa City, Iowa

Organic Mood, Delusional, and Anxiety Disorders

ROGER A. ROFFMAN, D.S.W.

Associate Professor, University of Washington School of Social Work, Seattle, Washington

Cannabis Dependence

PETER P. ROY-BYRNE, M.D.

Professor of Psychiatry, Director, Anxiety Disorder Programs, University of Washington School of Medicine, Seattle, Washington

Review of Anxiolytic Drugs

CHERYL S. RUBENSTEIN, M.A.

Doctoral Candidate in Clinical Psychology, The American University, Washington, D.C.

Obsessive-Compulsive Disorder and Trichotillomania

A. JOHN RUSH, M.D.

Psychiatry Staff, St. Paul Hospital, Presbyterian Hospital, Parkland Hospital, Zale Lipshy University Hospital, Dallas, Texas

Mood Disorders in DSM-IV

CORDELIA WARD RUSSELL, B.A.

Senior Research Assistant, Department of Psychiatry and Human Behavior, Brown University Medical School, Providence, Rhode Island

Classification and Treatment of Dysthymia

MARTHA SAJATOVIC, M.D.

Assistant Professor, Department of Psychiatry, Case Western Reserve University, Cleveland, Ohio

Typical Antipsychotic Medication: Clinical Practice

CARL SALZMAN, M.D.

Associate Professor of Psychiatry, Harvard Medical School, Boston, Massachusetts

An Overview of the Treatment of Geriatric Disorders

ALAN F. SCHATZBERG, M.D.

Kenneth T. Norris, Jr. Professor of Psychiatry and Behavioral Sciences, and Chairman, Stanford University School of Medicine, Stanford, California

Future Psychopharmacology for the Aging Patient: Treatment of Alzheimer's Disease

CHESTER W. SCHMIDT, Jr., M.D.

Associate Professor, Department of Psychiatry, The Johns Hopkins School of Medicine, Baltimore, Maryland

Report of DSM-IV Work Group on Sexual Disorders

MARC ALAN SCHUCKIT, M.D.

Professor of Psychiatry and Director, Alcohol Research Center, San Diego VA Hosptial, and UCSD Medical School, San Diego, California

Keeping Current with the DSMs and Substance Use Disorders

S. CHARLES SCHULZ, M.D.

Professor and chairman, Department of Psychiatry, Case Western Reserve University, Cleveland, Ohio

Typical Antipsychotic Medication: Clinical Practice

RAYMOND M. SCURFIELD, D.S.W.

Director, Post Traumatic Stress Treatment Program; Clinical Instructor, School of Social Work, University of Washington, Seattle, Washington

Post-traumatic Stress Disorder

STEPHEN R. SETTERBERG, M.D.

Assistant Professor of Clinical Psychiatry, College of Physicians and Surgeons, Columbia University, New York, New York

Proposed Changes in the DSM-IV Criteria for Child Psychiatry

DAVID SHAFFER, M.D.

Irving Philips Professor of Child Psychiatry; Director, Division of Child and Adolescent Psychiatry, College of Physicians and Surgeons, Columbia, University, New York, New York

Proposed Changes in the DSM-IV Criteria for Child Psychiatry

DAVID V. SHEEHAN, M.D.

Professor of Psychiatry, University of South Florida College of Medicine, Tampa, Florida

Panic Disorder

LARRY J. SIEVER, M.D.

Director, OPT Psychiatry, Department of Psychiatry, Bronx VA Medical Center, Bronx, New York

Cluster A Personality Disorders

SAMUEL G. SIRIS, M.D.

Professor of Psychiatry, Albert Einstein College of Medicine, New York, New York

The Treatment of Schizoaffective Disorder

DAVID SPIEGEL, M.D.

Department of Psychiatry and Behavioral Sciences, Stanford University Medical School, Stanford, California

Hypnosis for Psychiatric Disorders

JAMES SPIRA, Ph.D., M.P.H.

Department of Psychiatry and Behavioral Sciences, Stanford University Medical School, Stanford, California

Hypnosis for Psychiatric Disorders

ROY M. STEIN, M.D.

Associate Professor, Department of Psychiatry, Duke University Medical Center, Durham, North Carolina

Stimulant Abuse: Cocaine and Amphetamine

ROBERT S. STEPHENS, Ph.D.

Assistant Professor, Virginia Polytechnic Institute, Blacksburg, Virginia

Cannabis Dependence

JONATHAN W. STEWART, M.D.

Associate Professor of Clinical Psychiatry, College of Physicians and Surgeons, Columbia University, New York, New York

Atypical Depression

MICHAEL H. STONE, M.D.

Professor of Clinical Psychiatry, College of Physicians and Surgeons, Columbia University, New York, New York

Cluster C Personality Disorders

KIRK STROSAHL, Ph.D.

Clinical Adjunct Professor, Department of Psychiatry and Behavioral Sciences, University of Washington Medical Center, Seattle, Washington

The Suicidal Patient: Assessment, Crisis Management, and Treatment

CARRIE SYLVESTER, M.D., M.P.H.

Assistant Professor, Department of Psychiatry, University of Illinois, Chicago, Illinois

Disorders in Children: Autistic Disorder, Psychosis, Attention-Deficit Hyperactivity Disorder, Anxiety Disorders, and Depression

GARY D. TOLLEFSON, M.D., Ph.D.

Associate Professor of Psychiatry, University of Minnesota, Minneapolis, Minnesota; Chairman, Department of Psychiatry, St. Paul-Ramsey Medical Center, St. Paul, Minnesota

Major Depression

ROBERT L. TRESTMAN, Ph.D., M.D.

Assistant Professor, Department of Psychiatry, Bronx VA Medical Center, Bronx, New York

Cluster A Personality Disorders

GARY J. TUCKER, M.D.

Professor and Chairman, Department of Psychiatry and Behavioral Sciences, University of Washington, Seattle, Washington

DSM-IV: Organic Disorders

ALAN S. UNIS, M.D.

Assistant Professor, Department of Psychiatry and Behavioral Sciences, University of Washington, Seattle, Washington

Safety of Psychotropic Agents in the Treatment of Child and Adolescent Disorders

THEODORE VAN PUTTEN, M.D.

Professor of Psychiatry and Biobehavioral Sciences, UCLA Medical School, Los Angeles, California

Future Directions in Antipsychotic Drug Treatment

R. DALE WALKER, M.D.

Chief, Addictions Treatment Center, VA Medical Center, Seattle, Washington

Alcohol Problems

B. TIMOTHY WALSH, M.D.

Professor of Clinical Psychiatry, College of Physicians and Surgeons, Columbia University, New York, New York

Proposed DSM-IV Criteria for Eating Disorders

PAUL H. WENDER, M.D.

Distinguished Professor of Psychiatry, University of Utah School of Medicine, Salt Lake City, Utah

The Diagnosis and Treatment of Attention-Deficit Hyperactivity Disorder in Adults

LAWRENCE G. WILSON, M.D.

Associate Professor, Department of Psychiatry and Behavioral Sciences, University of Washington, Seattle, Washington

Consultation-Liaison Psychiatry

LEANNE WILSON, Ph.D.

Research Assistant Professor, Department of Oral Medicine, University of Washington, Seattle, Washington

Somatoform Pain Disorder and Its Treatment

DANE WINGERSON, M.D.

Research Fellow, University of Washington School of Medicine, Seattle, Washington
Review of Anxiolytic Drugs

WILLIAM C. WIRSHING, M.D.

Assistant Professor, Department of Psychiatry and Behavioral Sciences, UCLA Medical School, Los Angeles, California
Future Directions in Antipsychotic Drug Treatment

SEAN YUTZY, M.D.

Instructor in Psychiatry, Washington University Medical School, St. Louis, Missouri
Somatoform and Dissociative Disorders: A Summary of Changes for DSM-IV

MARTINA de ZWAAN, M.D.

Research Fellow, Eating Disorders Program, Department of Psychiatry, University of Minnesota, Minneapolis, Minnesota
Bulimia Nervosa

PREFACE

Treatment of psychiatric disorders, or for that matter any medical disorder, is an evolving process and changes over time. Thus, a text on treatment should really serve two purposes: first to summarize the current available knowledge regarding treatment and second to indicate potential changes for the future.

Determining the proper treatment for a psychiatric condition involves a number of steps, but primary among these is the assessment of the correct diagnosis for the condition to be treated. For this reason, we have incorporated information regarding diagnostic criteria for each of the disorders and conditions discussed in this volume. The authors were instructed to describe the clinical characteristics of each condition, its epidemiology, longitudinal course and differential diagnosis. Furthermore, each author was asked to briefly summarize the familial factors of each condition, any pertinent laboratory data, and to give a sense of the inclusion and exclusion criteria for the syndrome or condition under discussion. The treatment of the condition would follow using treatment approaches appropriate for the specific disorder.

In planning this book, we recognize that the present diagnostic criteria (DSM-III-R) are about to change. Thus, we have requested an introductory chapter for the major conditions to review briefly the diagnostic changes under consideration for DSM-IV. We realize that many of these options will be further refined prior to the publication of DSM-IV; however, having these changes in mind is meant to assist the user of this volume in determining the most appropriate treatment options for the patient.

There are other sections of this book that have been added to help round out the reader's thinking about treatment and to enable the reader to understand advances in treatments during the next few years. The introductory section outlines the basis for psychopathology and treatment approaches that might be applied interms of structure, biological testing, neurochemistry and application of familial factors. There are a number of treatments that are not specific to particular conditions but apply to a number of psychiatric disorders. Thus, we believed it appropriate to discuss these treatments—such as brief psychotherapy or electroconvulsive treatment—as chapters independent of the conditions to which they are applied. The section, "Future Psychopharmacology," was designed to give the reader some idea of the drugs that may be released for prescriptive use over the next few years as well as a sense of where the psychopharmacological field is headed. Child and adolescent psychiatric conditions are increasingly coming to the attention of practitioners. We are pleased to include chapters regarding treatment of children and adolescents who have psychiatric problems.

Although each chapter was edited, we attempted to keep intact the writing style of the individual authors as much as possible. Thus, treatment approaches reflect the interests of the individual authors. Of course, the treatment of an individual patient may have complexities related to that particular patient, and the material in this book should be used as a guide to treatment approaches but not necessarily applied to every patient within a particular diagnostic category.

We hope that this book will be useful to people involved in the treatment of patients with mental disorders: psychiatrists, psychologists, social workers and other therapists. This book was also designed to be of use to family physicians and internists who frequently encounter psychiatric conditions in their everyday practice.

In terms of my role as editor, I have tried to maintain the integrity of the contributions without being too intrusive. I wish to thank the contributors whose efforts have resulted in this book. Indeed, I learned a lot from reading their chapters. I am also most appreciative of the assistance received from Ann Carr.

DAVID L. DUNNER, M.D.

CONTENTS

PART I

FOUNDATION
of
ILLNESS
and
TREATMENT

STRUCTURAL FOUNDATIONS OF MENTAL ILLNESS AND TREATMENT: Neuroanatomy

JOEL E. KLEINMAN, M.D., Ph.D. and THOMAS M. HYDE, M.D., Ph.D.

The elucidation of a neuroanatomy relevant to major mental illnesses is an attractive but unrealized goal. To a certain extent the failure to elucidate the anatomy and pathology has separated mental illnesses from neurologic disorders, where the neuropathology or genetics or both are more clear-cut. It is in neurological disorders that the advantages of defining the neuroanatomy has yielded its most noteworthy accomplishments. For example, the discovery that there was a loss of dopamine in the nigrostriatal pathway in Parkinson's disease[1] led to the development of a replacement strategy with L-dopa.[2] This accomplishment was greatly aided in Parkinson's disease by the observation that there was a loss of pigment from the substantia nigra. The hope is that a similar understanding of the neuroanatomy of schizophrenia or affective disorders could lead to new and improved treatments. In order to accomplish this goal, it would be useful to know where to look in the brain, a strategy which has received a significant boost through advances in neuroimaging, neurochemistry, neuropsychology, and neuropharmacology. This chapter will attempt to highlight some of these advances in schizophrenia and affective disorders.

SCHIZOPHRENIA

Two of the major hypotheses regarding the pathophysiology of schizophrenia are the dopamine hypothesis and the notion that there are structural abnormalities in the brains of schizophrenic patients. Each of these has helped to narrow the search for relevant brain structures in this syndrome.

Dopamine Hypothesis

The dopamine hypothesis of schizophrenia is more properly a hypothesis with regard to psychosis. As such, schizophrenia is one of the several psychoses that can make use of a series of pharmacological findings that have implicated excess dopaminergic activity in the development of psychotic symptoms.

Dopamine agonists (L-dopa and amphetamine) can cause or exacerbate psychotic symptoms in nonpsychotic or psychotic subjects.[3] These pharmacologic findings have gained support and refinement from studies that have shown that dopamine receptor-type II (D_2) blockers are clinically effective antipsychotic agents in proportion to the extent of the D_2 blockade.[4]

Studies of the brain distribution of D_2 receptors serves as a clue to the neuroanatomy of psychosis in general and schizophrenia in particular. The bulk of postmortem D_2 receptor studies in human brains have focused on the basal ganglia (caudate, putamen, and nucleus accumbens) where the largest concentrations of D_2 receptors are found.[5] These three loci appear to have the highest concentrations of D_2 receptors in in vivo neuroimaging studies as well.[5] Although there are D_2 receptors in other brain structures, they are substantially less in the globus pallidus, substantia nigra, and cerebral cortex.[5] Although localization of psychotic symptoms is not necessarily a question of the number of receptors, the presence of D_2 receptors in structures with connections to the limbic system and neocortex, such as the nucleus accumbens, is attractive for its potential to explain the emotional and cognitive aspects of schizophrenia. The nucleus accumbens receives a significant input from the ventral tegmentum[6] as well as from the hippocampus–amygdala complex and the entorhinal cortex. Although entorhinal cortex (part of the parahippocampal gyrus) has similar connections,[6] its D_2 receptors are significantly fewer than in the accumbens.

In addition to their importance for neuroanatomy, the study of these D_2 receptors in schizophrenia has been a major focus of neuropathology and, more recently, neuroimaging. The bulk of postmortem studies have found increases in D_2 receptors in schizophrenics in caudate, putamen, and nucleus accumbens.[5] It is unclear, however, whether this is a result of prior antipsychotic treatment with D_2 blockers or whether this is primary to the syndrome. Attempts to unravel this issue by in vivo neuroimaging (positron emission tomography) of drug-naive patients has led to conflicting results.[5] Further studies may determine the relevance of these D_2 receptors to the neuropathology of schizophrenia. At this time, however, D_2 receptors are, at the least, a valuable clue to the relevant neuroanatomy.

Structural Abnormalities

A second major hypothesis of schizophrenia is that there are structural abnormalities in the brains of patients with this syndrome. Support for this idea from pneumoencephalography[7] was largely discounted until a series of computed tomographic (CT) brain studies showed ventriculomegaly and widened sulci and fissures in schizophrenics relative to controls.[8] This has been replicated in over 100 studies to date, including several studies of first-break patients,[8] suggesting that this abnormality is present at least from the onset of symptoms and is not a result of the treatment. Attempts to understand the relevance of these findings have focused on cognitive deficits and negative symptoms,[8] some of which can help to focus on particular brain regions. In general, however, the degree of anatomical resolution on CT scans does not lend itself to the type of neuroanatomical localization one would hope to achieve.

Magnetic resonance imaging (MRI) does have the resolving power necessary to visualize neuroanatomical structures thought to be relevant to schizophrenia (i.e., hippocampus, amygdala, and nucleus accumbens). Magnetic resonance imaging (MRI) studies have implicated the temporal cortex as being reduced in size in schizophrenics relative to controls.[5,9] One should bear in mind that these are group differences between schizophrenics and controls in MRI studies. They are not diagnostic, nor are they clearly present in every case. Moreover, they give ample warning of the problems of variability in both schizophrenics and controls that could lead to a type II statistical error (i.e. not finding an abnormality that is present).

In an attempt to reduce the effect of the wide range of normal variability in the size of structures in the brain, twins discordant for schizophrenia have been studied with MRI.[9] Even when the ventricles appear to be normal in size, the ventricles of the schizophrenic twin are larger than the nonschizophrenic almost every time.[9] This approach has also confirmed the involvement of the temporal cortex and extended the neuroanatomy to include the hippocampus.[9] It should be pointed out, moreover, that these structures—temporal cortex, (especially parahippocampal or entorhinal cortex), amygdala, and hippocampus—have been the subject of the most consistent structural abnormalities in postmortem studies.[5]

The most consistent postmortem findings involve the width or volume or both of the parahippocampal gyrus.[5] One of these studies[10] has also been cited as supporting a predominately left-sided abnormality.

In that study, there is an apparent reduction in size of the left parahippocampal gyrus of schizophrenics relative to controls, but no difference between schizophrenics and controls on the right. Interestingly enough, there is no difference between the parahippocampal gyrus on the left and right in the schizophrenics, but the left side of the controls is larger than the right side of the controls and both sides of the schizophrenics.

Two assumptions are necessary in order to conclude from these data that schizophrenia is a left-hemisphere problem. The first is that there is a normal asymmetry of the parahippocampal gyrus with the left being larger than the right. Second, the data from the controls must accurately represent normal neuroanatomy. As it turns out, the normals from this study were affective-disorder patients who came to autopsy. The assumption that their asymmetry is normal remains to be proven.

In an attempt to study this same area with brains from schizophrenics, nonpsychotic suicides (comparable to the previous study's affective patients), and normals, the findings in schizophrenics and affective patients were replicated.[11] However, the normal control brains did not appear to be asymmetric and were essentially the same size as the left side of nonpsychotic suicides. The correct interpretation of these data is that schizophrenics have a bilateral reduction in the size of the parahippocampal gyrus relative to normal controls. If any group has lateralized findings, it is the affective-disorder patients, with a reduction in the size of the parahippocampal gyrus on the right.

Lastly, the nature of the pathology appears to involve the fundamental macroscopic and microscopic organization of the cortex. The apparent lack of gliosis[8] raises the possibility of an early development abnormality. The lack of progression of structural abnormalities in follow-up studies of schizophrenics with CT scans[12] is consistent with a nonprogressive lesion, not atrophy as this has sometimes been described. How this pathology relates to the clinical aspects of schizophrenia remains to be determined. Memory deficits, as one might expect from abnormalities in the hippocampal–parahippocampal region are not the most prominent neuropsychological abnormality in schizophrenia. However, schizophrenic patients do have some memory deficits as measured by neuropsychological testing.[13]

Neuropsychological testing has provided a number of insights into the neuroanatomy of schizophrenia. Problems in performance of the Wisconsin Card Sort Task (WCST)[14] has implicated the dorsolateral prefrontal cortex (DLPFC) in schizophrenics. This finding has been explored further in studies using measures of cerebral blood flow. Whereas normals increase blood flow in the DLPFC as they perform the WCST, many schizophrenic patients cannot do this task and do not increase their blood flow in the DLPFC.[15,16] This does not appear to be a result of improper effort, since they perform adequately on other neuropsychological tests administered at that time. Moreover, when this study has been done using a discordant schizophrenic identical twin paradigm, the schizophrenic patient was identified properly in every pair as having reduced blood flow in the DLPFC while doing the WCST.[17]

Attempts to study the neurochemistry of the structures implicated in schizophrenia are in their infancy. The most consistent findings in the prefrontal cortex and temporal cortex to date involve increases in glutamate receptors[5] and decreases in serotonin (5-HT$_2$) receptors[5,18,19] in schizophrenics compared to controls. One study failed to find reductions in 5-HT$_2$ receptors in prefrontal cortex of schizophrenics.[18] This may be related to the increase in this receptor associated with suicide,[19] which could be a confounding variable, or the failure to perform a full Scatchard analysis. The relationship between alterations in glutamate or serotonin neurotransmission and neuropsychological abnormalities such as the WCST is problematic, as primate models have to date only implicated dopamine type-I neurotransmission.[20]

Despite many problems, the neuroanatomy of schizophrenia has made major advances in the last two decades, with substantial evidence implicating the prefrontal cortex, the parahippocampal-hippocampal–amygdala complex, and the nucleus accumbens. That is not to say that thalamus, ventral tegmentum, or other structures are not involved. They may very well be, but they are not the prime suspects at this point in time.

AFFECTIVE DISORDERS

The neuroanatomy of affective disorders presents a variety of problems different from those in the syndrome of schizophrenia. Since the treatment and genetics vary enormously in bipolar and unipolar illness, this should not be surprising.

If one focuses on unipolar depression, the task may be somewhat easier, since the neuroanatomy as elucidated by antidepressant treatment may yield more clues than pharmacological treatment for mania (i.e., lithium). This may be helpful for the pharmacological approach, but unfortunately, affective disorders per se have not been the focus of many postmortem studies. In large part, most studies of unipolar depression have been studies of suicide, many of which are significantly composed of patients with unipolar depression. Nevertheless, it is probably worthwhile to see where the clues from neuropharmacology, neuroimaging, neuropsychology, and neuropathology lead us in considering affective disorders as they present in unipolar depression and suicide.

Starting with a pharmacological approach, the common theme in the treatment of unipolar depression appears to be the enhancement of serotoninergic (5-HT) or nonadrenergic (NE) activity or both. Monoamine oxidase inhibitors, agonists such as amphetamines, and 5-HT or NE reuptake blockers share the common property of acute enhancement of 5-HT or NE neurotransmission or both. This clue suggests that the neuroanatomy of affective disorders probably should focus on 5-HT and NE neuronal networks. Cell bodies of 5-HT and NE neurons originate in the brainstem in a number of nuclei, the best known of which are the raphe neurons (5-HT) and the locus coeruleus (NE).[21,22] These neurons project via the medial forebrain bundle to a host of forebrain structures including the amygdala, hippocampus, hypothalamus, mammillary bodies, nucleus accumbens, and cerebral cortex.[21,22] These disseminated projections allow us to "explain" almost any affective symptom, including loss of appetite, insomnia, depressed affect, loss of interest and pleasure, decreased concentration, and suicide.

Unfortunately, many of the other clues to unipolar depression are also lacking in specificity. There are no specific neuropsychological tests that identify the majority of unipolar depressions. Patients may have a "pseudodementia," but this resolves with treatment. Some affective-disorder patients have persistent abnormalities on neuropsychological testing.[23] Although the previously mentioned parahippocampal gyrus studies[10,11] could provide a neuroanatomical locus for these abnormalities in affective disorders and suicide, this is highly speculative. Moreover, ventriculomegaly has been reported on CT scans,[24] but its significance is unclear.

Two rather consistent findings may help us understand the significance of the lack of neuroanatomical localization in affective disorders. Poststroke depression appears to be more than just a reaction to a loss of function.[25] An alternative explanation for poststroke depression is that cortical strokes interrupt NE and 5-HT projections at the point of the infarct, and this damage produces the increased incidence of depression. In Parkinson's disease and Alzheimer's disease, where there is an increased evidence of depression, there are significant pathological changes in brainstem NE and 5-HT cell groups.[26,27] A second major finding in depression is the increased number of subcortical white matter abnormalities seen on MRI scans of elderly depressed patients.[28] They do not seem to have a particular localization other than their potential for interrupting the diffuse NE/5-HT neuronal projections to the cortex.

Is there other evidence to support the hypothesis of alterations in NE/5-HT brain systems in affective disorders? The strongest current evidence involves postmortem findings of reduced imipramine/paroxetine binding (5-HT reuptake sites) in suicides.[19,29] These 5-HT reuptake findings are most prominent in frontal pole, hypothalamus, and hippocampus.[29] Several studies have failed to replicate the 5-HT reuptake findings,[29,30] but again, the potential for type II errors is probably quite high in this area of research. In addition, there are apparent increases in ketanserin binding (postsynaptic 5-HT$_2$ receptors) in frontal pole of suicides.[19,31] Again, there have been several failures to replicate.[29–32] Nevertheless, if these 5-HT receptor and reuptake findings are correct, they are consistent with studies that have found reductions in the 5-HT metabolite, 5-hydroxyindoleacetic acid, in cerebrospinal fluid following violent suicide attempts.[33]

The neuroanatomy of unipolar depression/suicide time is suggestive of a loss of 5-HT or NE cell bodies or both or reuptake mechanisms leading to reduced 5-HT or NE function. Since there is little evidence for the former except in Alzheimer's and Parkinson's disease and some direct evidence against it (normal α_2-receptor numbers in locus coeruleus of suicides[34]) the weight of the hypothesis rests on the release and reuptake mechanisms for NE and 5-HT. This puts us back in the forebrain, in the cerebral cortex and limbic structures.

CONCLUSION

At the current time, there is increasing scientific evidence for a neuroanatomy of mental illness. Technological advancements in neuroimaging, neurochemistry, and neuropathology make it possible that remaining areas of conjecture will be replaced by fact that could lead to improved understanding and treatment of mental illness in this, the Decade of the Brain.

REFERENCES

1. Ehringer H, Hornykiewicz O: Verteilung von noradrenalin und dopamin (3-hydroxytyramine) im gehim des menschen und ihr verhalten bei erkrankungen des extrapyramidalen systems. Wien Klin Wochenschr 72:1236, 1960.
2. Cotzias GC, Van Woert MH, Schiffer LM: Aromatic amino acids and modification of parkinsonism. N Engl J Med 276:374, 1967.
3. Griffith JD, Cavanaugh JH, Held J: In Costa E, Garattini S, eds. Amphetamines and Related Compounds. New York: Raven Press, 1969:897.
4. Creese L, Burt DR, Snyder S: Dopamine receptor binding predicts clinical and pharmacological potencies of antischizophrenic drugs. Science 192:481, 1976.
5. Hyde TM, Casanova MF, Kleinman JE, et al: Neuroanatomical and neurochemical pathology in schizophrenia. In Tasman A, Goldfinger SM eds. Review of Psychiatry. Vol. 10. Washington, DC: American Psychiatric Press, 1991:7–23.
6. Csernansky JG, Greer MM, Faustman WO: Limbic/mesolimbic connections and the pathogenesis of schizophrenia. Biol Psychiatry 30:383, 1991.
7. Huag JO: Pneumoencephalographic studies in mental disease. Acta Psychiatr Scand 38(suppl 165):1, 1962.
8. Shelton RC, Weinberger DR: X-ray computerized tomography studies in schizophrenia: A review and synthesis. In Nasrallah HA, Weinberger DR, eds. Handbook of Schizophrenia. Vol. 1. The Neurology of Schizophrenia. Amsterdam. Elsevier Press, 1986:207–250.
9. Suddath RL, Christison GW, Torrey EF, et al: Anatomical abnormalities in the brains of monozygotic twins discordant for schizophrenia. N Engl J Med 322:789, 1990.
10. Brown R, Colter N, Corsellis JAN et al: Postmortem evidence of structural brain changes in schizophrenia. Arch Gene Psychiatry 43:36, 1986.
11. Altshuler L, Casanova MF, Goldberg TE, et al: The hippocampus and parahippocampus in schizophrenic, suicide and control brains. Arch Gen Psychiatry 47:1029, 1990.
12. Illowsky BK, Juliano DM, Bigelow LB, et al: Stability of CT scan findings in schizophrenia: Results of an eight year follow-up study. J Neurol Neurosurg Psychiatry 51:209, 1988.
13. Levin S, Yurgelun-Todd D, Craft S: Contributions of clinical neuropsychology to the study of schizophrenia. J Abnorm Psychology 98:341, 1989.
14. Goldberg TE, Weinberger DR: Probing prefrontal function in schizophrenia with neuropsychological paradigms. Schizophr Bull 14:179, 1988.
15. Berman KF, Zec RF, Weinberger DR: Physiological dysfunction of dorsolateral prefrontal cortex in schizophrenia. II. Role of neuroleptic treatment, attention, and mental effort. Arch Gen Psychiatry 43:126, 1986.
16. Berman KF, Illowsky BK, Weinberger DR: Physiological dysfunction of dorsolateral prefrontal cortex in schizophrenia. IV. Further evidence for regional and behavioral specificity. Arch Gen Psychiatry 45:616, 1988.
17. Berman KF, Torrey EF, Daniel DG, et al: Prefrontal cortical blood flow in monozygotic twins concordant and discordant for schizophrenia. Schizophr Res 2:129, 1989.
18. Arora RC, Meltzer HY: Serotonin-2 (5HT-2) receptor binding in the frontal cortex of schizophrenic patients. J Neural Transm 85:19, 1991.
19. Laruelle M, Abi-Dargham A, Casanova MF et al: Selective abnormalities of prefrontal serotonergic receptors in schizophrenia: A postmortem study. Arch Gen Psychiatry. (in press.)
20. Sawaguchi T, Goldman-Rakic PS: D1 dopamine receptors in prefrontal cortex: Involvement in working memory. Science 251:947, 1991.
21. Ungerstedt U: Stereotaxic mapping of the monoamine pathways in the rat brain. Acta Physiol Scand 64(suppl 247):37, 1971.
22. Moore RY, Bloom FE: Central catecholamine systems: Anatomy and physiology of norepinephrine and epinephrine systems. Ann Rev Neurosci 2:113, 1979.
23. Gold JM, Goldberg TE, Kleinman JE, et al: The impact of symptomatic state and pharmacological treatment on cognitive functioning of patients with schizophrenia and mood disorders. In Mohr E, Brouwers P, eds. Handbook of Clinical Trials: The Neurobehavioral Approach. Amsterdam: Swets and Zeitlinger, 1991:185–216.
24. Targum SD, Rosen LN, DeLisi LE et al: Cerebral ventricular size in major depressive disorder: Association with delusional symptoms. Biol Psychiatry 18:329, 1983.
25. Robinson RG, Szetela P: Mood change following left hemisphere brain injury. Ann Neurol 9:447, 1981.
26. Mann DMA, Yates PO, Hawkes J: The pathology of the human locus coeruleus. Clin Neuropathol 2:1, 1983.
27. Javoy-Agid F, Rubert M, Taquer H, et al: Biochemical neuropathology of Parkinson's disease. Adv Neurol 40:189, 1984.
28. Coffey CE, Figiel GS, Djang WT et al: Leukoencephalopathy in elderly depressed patients referred for ECT. Biol Psychiatry 24:143, 1988.
29. Ferrier IN, McKeith IG, Cross AJ, et al: Postmortem neurochemical studies in depression. In Mann JJ, Stanley M, eds. Psychobiology of Suicidal Behavior. Ann NY Acad Science 487:128, 1986.
30. Arora RC, Meltzer HY: 3H-Imipramine binding in the frontal cortex of suicides. Psychiatry Res 30:125, 1989.
31. Arango V, Ernsberger P, Marzuk PM, et al: Autoradiographic demonstration of increased 5-HT2 and β-adrenergic receptor binding sites in the brain of suicide victims. Arch Gen Psychiatry 47:1038, 1990.

32. Gross-Isseroff R, Salama D, Israeli M, et al: Autoradiographic analysis of 3H-ketanserin binding in the human postmortem brain: Effect of suicide. Brain Res 507:208, 1990.
33. Asberg M, Nördstrom P, Träskman-Bendz AL: Cerebrospinal fluid studies in suicide: An overview. In Mann JJ, Stanley M, eds. Psychobiology of Suicidal Behavior. Ann NY Acad Sciences 487:243, 1986.
34. Ko G, Unnerstall JR, Kuhar MJ et al: Alpha-2 agonist binding in schizophrenic brains. Psychopharmacol Bull 22:1011, 1986.

2

STRUCTURAL FOUNDATIONS OF ILLNESS AND TREATMENT: Receptors

ROBIN R. DEAN, Ph.D., JEFFREY E. KELSEY, M.D., Ph.D., MARK R. HELLER, Ph.D., and ROLAND D. CIARANELLO, M.D.

The idea that drugs, neurotransmitters, and hormones produced their biological effect by interacting with a specific "receptor" was proposed by Langely and Erlich at the turn of the century. Since then, the work of many investigators has contributed to our present-day concept of receptors. The first receptors to be identified and characterized were those for the classical neurotransmitters: acetylcholine (ACh), dopamine (DA), norepinephrine (NE), epinephrine, and serotonin (5-HT). Receptors for a variety of endogenous peptide neurotransmitters or neuromodulators such as β-endorphin, enkephalins, dynorphin, vasoactive intestinal peptide (VIP), somatostatin, substance P, tachykinins, cholecystokinin (CCK), thyrotropin-releasing hormone (TRH), as well as others have also been identified in the brain. Similarly, the amino acid neurotransmitters, gamma-aminobutyric acid (GABA), glycine, glutamate, and aspartate, have also been found to have specific receptors in the central nervous system (CNS). More recently, the application of molecular biological methods to the study and identification of receptors has made significant contributions to our understanding of mechanisms underlying receptor-activated signal transduction, receptor structure, and receptor involvement in various behavioral states and psychoactive drug effects.

The study of drug interactions with a specific neurotransmitter receptor (i.e., Dale's studies of nicotine and muscarine interactions with the ACh receptor in 1914), and the ability of a single neurotransmitter or drug to elicit different physiological responses in different tissues (i.e., morphine effects in guinea pig ilium and rat vas deferens), revealed the existence of multiple receptor types and subtypes for most of the neurotransmitters. These findings demonstrated that the early concept of one receptor for each neurotransmitter or hormone was too simplistic. The proliferation of known receptor types and subtypes continues today; each neurotransmitter is thought to act at multiple receptor subtypes. Serotonin receptors, for example, are divided into four distinct receptor types, $5\text{-}HT_1$, $5\text{-}HT_2$, $5\text{-}HT_3$, and $5\text{-}HT_4$; and the $5\text{-}HT_1$ type is further subdivided into $5\text{-}HT_{1A}$, $5\text{-}HT_{1B}$, $5\text{-}HT_{1C}$, and $5\text{-}HT_{1D}$, subtypes according to their affinity for serotonin and other drugs.

Binding of a ligand (a drug, hormone, neurotransmitter, or any molecule which binds to a protein) does not, by itself, define a receptor molecule. Functional receptors bind appropriate specific ligands with high affinity and stereochemical specificity; the binding is saturable, since there are a finite number of receptors; and the binding is reversible (mass-action equilibrium reaction). In addition, binding should modulate transmembrane signaling, which will transduce information into a biological response. Compounds that bind specifically to receptors act as agonists, antagonists, or as mixed (agonist/antagonist) agents. An agonist is a compound which activates a receptor, typically mimicking the action of the endogenous neurotransmitter. An antagonist binds to the receptor, thereby preventing the endogenous neurotransmitter from acting at that receptor, but has no effect of its own. A mixed agonist/antagonist shows some characteristics of each.

Drugs acting at specific neurotransmitter receptors appear to be very effective in treating certain types of psychiatric diseases, thereby implicating involvement of those receptors in the disease process. For example, the potency of neuroleptics in treating schizophrenia parallels their dopamine receptor antagonist affinity.[1] Similarly, drugs acting to increase the level of monoamine neurotransmitters at the synapse have a long history in the treatment of depression. Monoamine oxidase inhibitors (MAOI), which decrease the degradation of NE and 5-HT, were first developed for the treatment of tuberculosis (TB), and were found to have mood-elevating effects in TB patients. Tricyclic antidepressants (TCA), originally developed as phenothiazine analogs, were found to be ineffective at quieting agitated psychotic patients, but were beneficial in the treatment of depression.[2] Tricyclic antidepressants inhibit the reuptake of NE or 5-HT or both and presumably increase the synaptic concentration of these neurotransmitters. Benzodiazepines, which are widely used as anxiolytics, produce a facilitation of the GABA$_A$-linked chloride channel conductance. The fact that unrelated compounds (influencing different neurotransmitters and interacting with different receptors) are frequently used to treat the same disease suggests that the mechanisms underlying psychiatric disorders are complex. It is not yet clear what role receptors play in the etiology or pathogenesis of psychiatric syndromes.

The purpose of this chapter is to provide an overview of the biology of receptors. Four topics will be discussed: receptor distribution, structure, signal transduction, and receptor regulation. *Receptor distribution* is most commonly mapped by radioligand binding methods, but the development of receptor-specific antibodies should add valuable new information. In situ hybridization of receptor-specific messenger ribonucleic acid (mRNA) localizes the cell bodies that synthesize receptor proteins.[3] Knowledge of *receptor structure* and its corresponding function has been greatly advanced by the application of molecular biological techniques, which have demonstrated that many of the neurotransmitter receptors belong to one of two gene superfamilies: the G protein-linked receptors, or the ligand-gated ion channels. *Transduction* of the signal following receptor activation is accomplished by multiple mechanisms. These include the opening or closing of ion channels, enzymatic amplification by second messengers such as cyclic adenosine monophosphate (cAMP), inositol-trisphosphate (IP$_3$), diacylglycerol (DAG), or combinations of the above. Second messenger systems involved in transduction of the signal impinge on the biochemical milieu of the cell by altering enzyme activity, ion channels, release of neurotransmitters, and transcriptional activity of genes, to name but a few effector mechanisms. Finally, *receptor regulation* brings together a wide range of biochemical processes involving multiple steps along the signal transduction pathway that will undoubtedly prove increasingly important in the pharmacological treatment of psychiatric illness.

RECEPTOR LOCALIZATION

Principles

Receptors were initially studied using bioassays which involved isolated tissue preparations used to test the response to applied agents. Despite the apparent "crudeness" of these assays, the sensitivity approached that of some radioimmunoassays (RIA). The study of receptors and receptor binding became widespread with the development of radioligand binding methods in the 1970s. These methods aided in the discovery of CNS opioid receptors and their endogenous ligands, β-endorphin, leu-enkephalin, met-enkephalin, and dynorphin. Subsequently, brain receptors for other drugs were identified.

The primary determinants of the sites of drug/neurotransmitter action are the location and concentration of the receptors for that drug or neurotransmitter. Today, in vitro receptor autoradiography is the method of choice for mapping receptor distribution and concentration. Prior to the development of in vitro receptor autoradiography,[4] binding studies were performed on isolated homogenized brain regions, or in vivo by injecting the whole animal with a radiolabeled compound. Thus, resolution of receptor locations and densities was limited by the dissecting ability of the investigator or the chemical characteristics of the labeled ligand, respectively. As more selective drugs became available, a number of receptor subtypes were defined on the basis of their binding affinities for those compounds.

In vitro autoradiography affords an order-of-magnitude-better resolution than homogenate-binding by localizing the receptors in situ in slide-mounted thin tissue sections (10 to 30 μm thick). Because the labeling is done in vitro, problems with diffusion and drug metabolism are eliminated. In this technique, sections are incubated in pM–nM concentrations of [^{3}H] or [^{125}I]-labeled ligands until equilibrium is reached. This is followed by a series of washes to remove label that is not specifically bound to the receptor. Nonspecific binding is defined by incubating alternate sections in the presence of μM concentrations of an unlabeled compound with high affinity for the receptor. The labeled slide-mounted sections are then dried and apposed to [^{3}H]/[^{125}I]-sensitive film. Following an appropriate exposure time, which varies from hours to weeks, the film is developed and the resulting autoradiograms are analyzed using computer-aided microdensitometry and image analysis. The areas of high receptor density appear black on the autoradiogram (Fig. 2–1). The use of radioactive standards on each film allows the construction of a standard curve which can be used to quantify the density of receptors present. The total number of receptors present in a given area, binding

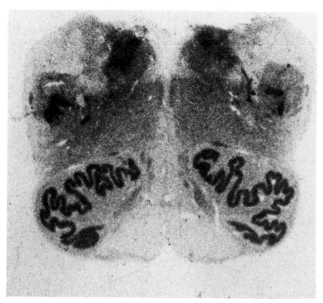

Figure 2–1. Autoradiogram of opioid receptors in the human medulla labeled with [³H]-dihydromorphine.

maximum (B_{max}) and the dissociation constant (K_D), which reflects ligand-receptor affinity, can also be determined. Computer enhancements can be added to the image; colors are assigned to the different optical density ranges, resulting in a "pseudocolor" image of the black and white autoradiogram. The widespread use of in vitro autoradiography has contributed greatly to our knowledge of the distribution of most of the neurotransmitter receptors and expanded our understanding of sites and mechanisms of drug action (therapeutic effects as well as undesirable side effects).

Clinical Importance of Receptor Localization

When a drug acts at a receptor that is widely distributed in the brain, there are numerous side effects in addition to the desired therapeutic goal. In contrast, a drug acting at a receptor with a very limited distribution is likely to have fewer side effects. A clinically relevant example is that of antipsychotic drugs. Their clinical potency correlates with their ability to antagonize the effects of dopamine at the D_2 receptor.[1] Antagonism of dopamine actions within the basal ganglia, notably the caudate, putamen, and globus pallidus, is thought to produce the extrapyramidal side effects frequently associated with antipsychotic treatment. Recently, a new dopamine receptor, the D_3 receptor, was cloned. Its expression appears to be limited to brain areas within the limbic system (i.e., amygdala, hippocampus, septal nuclei). Pharmacological analysis of the D_3 gene expressed in a heterologous cell system was used to compare binding affinities of a number of neuroleptics for the D_2 and D_3 receptors.[5] Typical neuroleptic drugs, such as haloperidol and spiperone, have a 10–20-fold higher affinity for the D_2 relative to the D_3 receptor. Since the basal ganglia possess a high density of D_2 receptors, typical neuroleptics have a high potential for causing extrapyramidal side effects. In contrast, some of the atypical neuroleptics such as raclopride and clozapine, which are less frequently associated with extrapyramidal effects, have only a two- to threefold higher affinity for the D_2 receptor. Putative autoreceptor-selective agents appear to be more potent at the D_3 than D_2 receptor. These data suggest that D_3-selective drugs might be very useful as antipsychotics and have a lower potential for producing extrapyramidal side effects.

While neurotransmitters are selective for their respective receptors, exogenous drugs are frequently more promiscuous. This lack of specificity contributes to a number of unwanted side effects. A clinical example of this phenomenon is the tricyclic antidepressants. Their primary mechanism of action is thought to be inhibition of serotonin or norepinephrine reuptake, effectively increasing the concentration of transmitter at the synapse. In addition to this therapeutic effect, the tricyclics act as antagonists at muscarinic cholinergic receptors,[6] α_1-adrenergic receptors,[7] as well as H_1 and H_2 histamine receptors.[8] These actions are responsible for side effects such as sedation, cognitive impairment, and postural hypotension.

The synthesis of new drugs with higher selectivity and their use in radioligand binding studies has led to the identification of many new neurotransmitter receptor types and subtypes. Each receptor subtype is differentiated on the basis of various affinities for a variety of agonists and antagonists and exhibits a characteristic rank order of potencies for these compounds. Autoradiographic studies typically reveal heterogeneous binding distributions of the receptor/subtypes in the brain, which provides another level of anatomical specificity. For example, 5-HT$_{1A}$ receptors are most dense in the raphe nuclei and hippocampal CA1 region. 5-HT$_2$ receptors are most dense in lamina Va[9] of the cortex and are thought to mediate the hallucinations produced by many 5-HT$_2$–acting drugs (a significant correlation exists between 5-HT$_2$ binding affinities and human hallucinogenic potencies, particularly d-LSD[10]). A 5-HT$_{1A}$–specific drug, therefore, is less likely to produce hallucinations than a compound that selectively activates 5-HT$_2$ receptors.

STRUCTURE

The addition of molecular biological methods to the arsenal of techniques used to study receptors has yielded a wealth of new knowledge and contributed significantly to our understanding of receptor-activated signal transduction in the CNS, its relationship to behavior, and the biology of psychoactive drugs. Cloning and characterization of complementary DNA (cDNA) for many neurotransmitter receptors has shown that most receptors fall into one of two classes of gene superfamilies: the first is ligand-gated channels. These receptors are directly associated with ion channels and include the nicotinic acetylcholine, $GABA_A$, 5-HT_3, and glycine receptors. The second class is G protein-linked receptors. This family of receptors includes many of the neurotransmitter receptors studied to date, such as α- and β-adrenergic, dopaminergic, muscarinic cholinergic, adenosinergic, histaminergic, a glutaminergic, many serotonergic, as well as a number of the hormone and peptide receptors.[11,12] One notable feature of these receptors is that they transduce signals via linkage to second-messenger cascades, thereby amplifying the ligand-receptor binding signal.

G Protein-Linked Receptors

The G protein-linked receptors couple agonist-occupation of the receptor to signal amplification and transduction events in the cell by activating a GTP-binding regulatory protein (G protein). This receptor family is highly conserved across the evolutionary spectrum: its members include bacteriorhodopsin, yeast mating pheromone receptors, the chemotactic cAMP signaling system in *Dictyostelium discoidium*, visual opsins, as well as G protein receptors in the mammalian CNS. The agonist-occupied receptor activates a G protein (another highly conserved gene superfamily), which transduces the sig-

nal by direct interaction with an ion channel, or by activation of an effector enzyme leading to the production of intracellular second messengers (see Figs. 2–4 and 2–5 later in chapter).

Structure of G Protein-Linked Receptors

G protein-coupled receptors share some common structural features. All consist of a single polypeptide chain containing seven putative membrane-spanning α helices, an extracellular amino (NH_2)-terminus and an intracellular carboxy (COOH)-terminal end (Fig. 2–2). The receptor plays several roles in the G protein-linked signal transduction scheme: It binds stereospecifically to a neurotransmitter/ligand; if this compound is an agonist, the activated receptor links to the appropriate G protein, initiating signal amplification and transduction. G proteins are divided into several types including G_i (adenylyl cyclase inhibitory); G_s (adenylyl cyclase stimulatory); G_t (transducin); and putative "G_p" (phospholipase C-linked). Amino acid sequences of cloned receptors have been compared to identify structural motifs required for ligand-binding specificities, coupling to G proteins, and potential sites of modification by phosphorylation or palmitoylation or both.

Significant progress has been made toward understanding the structural elements necessary and sufficient to determine the ligand-binding and G protein-

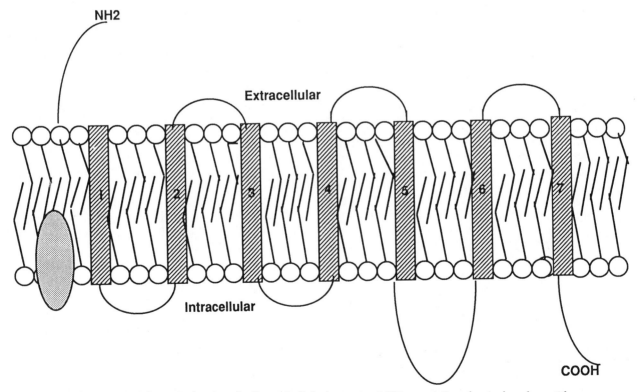

Figure 2–2. Schematic drawing of a G protein-linked receptor, 5-HT_2, consisting of a single polypeptide chain with seven membrane-spanning domains, an extracellular aminoterminal end, an intracellular carboxyterminal end, and the longer third intracellular loop associated with G protein binding.

binding domains of G protein-linked receptors. Some of the results of structure/function, biochemical, and genetic analyses of cloned receptors are summarized below. The following is a collation of data from cloning, transfection, and pharmacological studies:

1. Mutation studies with the β-adrenergic receptor[13] and structural studies of the rhodopsin receptor indicate that the receptor-binding pocket is within the plane of the cell membrane and is formed by the interaction of most or all of the seven transmembrane α helices. Thus, determinants for the ligand-binding domain itself, or determinants which help form the framework for the binding domain, are distributed throughout much of the primary structure of the protein, but physically are in close proximity to one another when the receptor is in its native configuration in the cell membrane. Pharmacological analyses of chimeric adrenergic receptors in which domains from G_s-coupled β_2- and G_i-coupled α_2-adrenergic receptors were mixed in a number of combinations indicate that the sixth and seventh transmembrane domains appear to be important in determining the ligand-binding specificity.[14] The close sequence homology between the serotonin 5-HT_{1A} and the β-adrenergic receptors in this region might account for the lack of specificity of some agents for these different receptors.

2. An aspartate (Asp) residue is invariant in the third transmembrane domain of all catecholamine and serotonin G protein-linked receptors. This finding suggests that binding involves an ionic interaction between the carboxylate side chain of the Asp and the neurotransmitter amino group. A conserved proline residue is present in each of transmembrane domains four through seven. These prolines may introduce bends in the α helices important for receptor structure.

3. The various receptor types show great diversity in the length and sequence of the third cytoplasmic loop and COOH-terminal domains. Receptors which inhibit adenylyl cyclase through G_i have long cytoplasmic loops and short COOH-terminal tails, while receptors which stimulate adenylyl cyclase through G_s have short C3 loops and long tails. The third cytoplasmic loop and the adjacent membrane proximal amino acids are believed to physically interact with G proteins. Consistent with this, adaptation/desensitization of rhodopsin, β-adrenergic, yeast pheromone, and the chemoattractant cAMP receptors has been correlated with phosphorylation of serine and threonine residues in both the third cytoplasmic loop and the intracellular COOH-terminal domain of the receptors.

4. A cysteine residue is highly conserved at roughly equivalent positions in the COOH-terminal cytoplasmic tail in a large number of G protein-linked receptors (β_1-, β_2-, α_1-, α_2-adrenergic; M_{1-5}-cholinergic; D_2-dopaminergic; 5-HT_{1A}, 5-HT_{1C}, and 5-HT_2-serotonergic; substance K, and rhodopsin).

Thioesterification of this cysteine residue has been found necessary for expression of the guanylyl cyclase-sensitive high-affinity binding component of the receptor. Studies of retinoic acid receptors[15] and β_2-adrenergic receptors[16] suggest an important role for post-translational palmitoylation of the conserved cysteine residues in the functional coupling of the receptors to their effector systems. All G protein-linked receptors cloned to date contain this conserved sequence, supporting a role for palmitoylation in receptor regulation.

Cloning of Important Monoamine G Protein-Linked Receptors

The high degree of homology among the G protein-coupled receptors has enabled many of the genes encoding these receptors to be cloned in a relatively short time. The number of receptor genes cloned has revealed that the diversity of receptor subtypes is much greater than suggested by pharmacological binding studies. For example, homology to the β_2-adrenergic receptor permitted cloning of the genes for serotonin 5-HT_{1A}, dopamine D_2, and adrenergic α_{2B} receptors. The D_2 receptor sequence was used to identify a novel highly related D_3 receptor which was not previously revealed by ligand-binding studies. The D_3 receptor has been localized to limbic areas of the brain (see Receptor Localization, earlier) and absent in basal ganglia. This unique receptor distribution in conjunction with its binding profile suggest that it might be an important target for new neuroleptic drugs.[5]

The dopamine D_1 receptor was cloned via D_2-receptor homology and independently by a polymerase chain reaction (PCR) approach using oligonucleotide primers for conserved transmembrane regions of catecholamine receptor genes. Similarly, the D_4 and D_5 receptors, which have high homology to the D_2 and D_3 receptors, have recently been cloned.[17,18] Clozapine, an atypical neuroleptic with a low probability of inducing tardive dyskinesia, has an order-of-magnitude-higher affinity for the D_4 receptor in transfected cells, suggesting that clozapine interacts with the D_4 receptor. The D_5 receptor shows a binding profile similar to the D_1 receptor, but exhibits a tenfold higher affinity for dopamine, the endogenous receptor agonist.

Th serotonin 5-HT_{1C} receptor was cloned by functional expression.[19] The resulting sequence was then used as a probe to identify the closely related 5-HT_2 receptor.[20,21] 5-HT_{1C} and 5-HT_2 are G_p-linked receptors which are coupled to the phosphoinositol hydrolysis second-messenger system.

The Ligand-Gated Receptor Family

Another superfamily of signal transduction proteins are receptors which couple the binding of a neurotransmitter or ligand directly to an intrinsic membrane ion channel. These ligand-gated ion channels mediate rapid (millisecond) postsynaptic effects initiated by the ligand-gated conductance of ions through the channel. Acetylcholine, glutamate, and aspartate are neurotransmitters which gate channels selective for cations (Na^+, K^+, and Ca^{++}). Receptor activation leads to ion conductance through the channel, which depolarizes the postsynaptic cell. Gamma-aminobutyric acid and glycine are inhibitory transmitters which gate chloride (Cl^-) channels. Opening of these channels tends to hyperpolarize the postsynaptic cell membrane potential, which increases its depolarization threshold.

The subunit structure of the GABA$_A$ receptor ($\alpha_2\beta_2$) was originally determined following its purification from bovine cerebral cortex by benzodiazepine-affinity chromatography.[22] Cloning of cDNAs encoding α and β subunits was achieved using peptide sequences derived from the purified receptor. Reconstitution studies with the cloned α and β subunits failed to yield receptors that mimicked the in vivo GABA$_A$ pharmacology. More recent DNA homology cloning has revealed additional receptor subunits (γ and δ) and subtypes of subunits, $\alpha1$-$\alpha6$, $\beta1$-$\beta3$, $\gamma1$-$\gamma2$, and $\delta1$.[23,24] The subtypes are encoded by distinct, but highly related DNAs. Coexpression of the α, β and γ_2 subunits results in a functional receptor with the predicted benzodiazepine binding and modulation.[23] All three subunits (α, β, and γ) appear to be required for the expression of functional benzodiazepine receptors.[23,24] The benzodiazepine response varies with the α subunit expressed, a finding consistent with the hypothesis that the α subunit is involved in benzodiazepine binding.

Cloning with cDNA has led to predicted protein sequences for other ligand-gated ion channel receptors, including the nicotinic cholinergic, glycine, and kainate (a glutamate receptor subtype) receptors. The receptor-ion channel complexes are multimeric proteins of two or more subunits encoded by separate homologous genes. Several subunit stoichiometries have been observed: ($\alpha_2\beta_2$), ($\alpha_2\beta_3$), and ($\alpha_2\beta\gamma\delta$). The ligand-gated receptor gene superfamily members share a common structural architecture: (1) four hydrophobic transmembrane sequences, M_1-M_4, are present in each subunit at roughly homologous positions following a large NH$_2$-terminal extracellular domain; (2) a structural loop formed by conserved cysteine residues and other invariant or conserved amino acids in a domain of the N-terminal region; (3) an invariant proline in a conserved protein environment in M_1 which is believed to introduce a bend in the α helix which may keep the ion channel closed in the absence of neurotransmitter; (4) an abundance of serine and threonine residues in M_2, which probably contribute to the hydrophilic lining of the channel. See Figure 2–3 for a diagrammatic representation of a single subunit.

Cloned receptor genes can be functionally expressed in heterologous cell systems such as nonneuronal cells in culture via DNA-mediated gene transfer or in *Xenopus laevis* oocytes following microinjection of synthetic mRNA.[25] The expressed re-

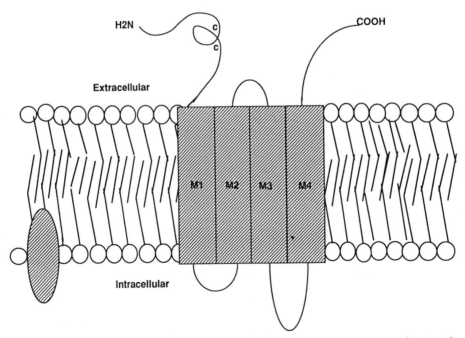

Figure 2–3. Schematic diagram of a typical single subunit of a ligand-gated receptor showing the four membrane-spanning domains (M_1–M_4), extracellular aminoterminal end containing a disulfide bridge between two cysteines forming an extracellular loop, an extracellular carboxyterminal end, and a large intracellular loop between the third and fourth transmembrane domains.

ceptors display pharmacological binding profiles similar to those of the native receptor in neuronal tissues. Furthermore, they can interact with G proteins in the heterologous system to couple to second-messenger signaling pathways. The functional effector expression can be sufficiently robust to permit the expression cloning of full-length receptor cDNA clones from cDNA libraries. In the case of single polypeptide receptors, functional expression of the unknown cloned gene has aided in the identification of the gene by characterizing it pharmacologically and functionally. Reconstitution studies with cloned subunits of multisubunit receptors can be done to determine the configuration of the native receptor.

TRANSDUCTION

Transduction of a signal occurs by a variety of mechanisms after binding of a ligand to a cellular receptor. The G protein-coupled superfamily of receptors acts through several different pathways. Presumably, the specificity of the coupling resides in the type of G protein to which the receptor is coupled. The best-studied system is the adenylyl cyclase activation cascade. Binding of a compound such as NE to a β-adrenergic receptor stimulates the formation of cAMP via adenylyl cyclase after activation of G_s. Formation of cAMP produces an increase in the activity of a cAMP-dependent protein kinase (pro-

tein kinase A), which phosphorylates a variety of proteins important in regulating cellular functioning[26] (Fig. 2–4). A number of other receptors activate adenylyl cyclase as well. Another well-studied system is the adenylyl cyclase inhibitory pathway. For example, binding of NE to an α_2-adrenergic receptor inhibits cAMP formation by activation of G_i. Thus, depending on the receptor type that NE binds to, α_2-adrenergic or β-adrenergic, and the G protein to which the receptor is linked, there is either an inhibition or activation of the cAMP system.

The Phosphoinositide Cascade

The phosphoinositide system (PI) represents a different second-messenger pathway. Activation of phospholipase C via activation of a receptor linked to G_p cleaves phosphatidyl-inositol-bisphosphate (PIP_2) into inositol-trisphosphate (IP_3) and diacylglycerol (DAG), both of which act as second messengers. Inositol-trisphosphate binds to a specific receptor on the endoplasmic reticulum, triggering the release of calcium into the cytoplasm (Fig. 2–5). Diacylglycerol stimulates protein kinase C, which then phosphorylates a variety of substrates.[27] Norepinephrine binding to an α_1-adrenergic receptor stimulates phospholipase C and the PI system. The cAMP and PI systems interact, in that phosphorylation of the IP_3 receptor by a cAMP-dependent protein kinase decreases the ability of IP_3 to release calcium.

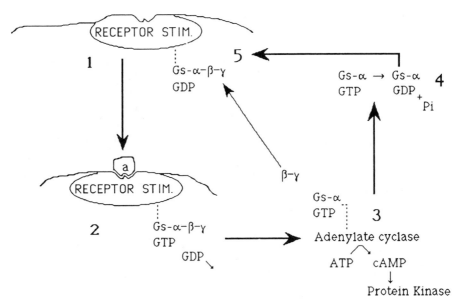

Figure 2–4. G_s protein activity: (1) Unoccupied receptor is associated with G_s (G stimulatory) protein with α, β, and γ subunits and GDP. Upon binding of agonist (2), GTP displaces GDP and the β and γ subunits dissociate from the α subunit (3). The G_s-α-GTP complex activates adenylyl cyclase, which catalyzes the formation of cAMP from ATP. Protein kinase A is then activated by cAMP, which is later degraded by phosphodiesterase. Cleavage of the bound GTP by GTPase (4) dissociates the complex from adenylyl cyclase, and the β and γ subunits reassociate (5), thus preparing the complex for another round. G-inhibitory (G_i) has a similar structure, but with a different α subunit and inhibits adenylyl cyclase activity.

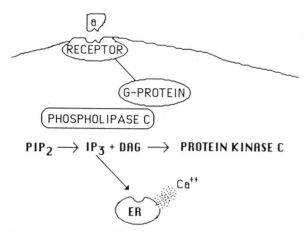

Figure 2–5. Phosphotidyl-inositol pathway: Binding of an agonist (a) to receptor activates phospholipase C (PL-C) via a G protein. PL-C cleaves phosphatidyl-inositol-bisphosphate (PIP$_2$) into inositol-trisphosphate (IP$_3$) and diacylglycerol (DAG). IP$_3$ binds to a specific receptor on the endoplasmic reticulum (ER) and triggers the release of calcium into the cytoplasm. DAG activates protein kinase C, which in turn phosphorylates a variety of cellular substrates.

Ion Channel Activation

A second class of cellular responses to receptor activation is the opening or closing of ion channels. Gamma-aminobutyric acid receptors, which are subdivided into GABA$_A$ and GABA$_B$ subtypes, act directly via chloride channels (GABA$_A$) or by calcium and potassium channels (GABA$_B$) linked to G proteins. The effects of drugs on GABA receptors include modulation of many diverse behavioral states such as anxiety, sleep, muscle tension, seizure susceptibility, learning, and memory. In the CNS, benzodiazepine binding sites are found in close association with the GABA$_A$ receptor–Cl–channel complex. A number of different drugs have been shown to exert their effects through interaction with this GABA$_A$–Cl–ionophore complex. Binding of benzodiazepines to benzodiazepine binding sites associated with GABA$_A$ receptors increases GABA-stimulated chloride channel opening, which hyperpolarizes the membrane and inhibits cell firing. Benzodiazepines and barbiturates bind to different sites on the GABA$_A$ receptor–Cl–channel complex and mediate their behavioral effects by potentiating the inhibitory activity of GABA.[28] Electrophysiological measurement of GABA-evoked membrane conductance changes in *Xenopus* oocytes microinjected with GABA$_A$-receptor RNA shows that benzodiazepines achieve their potentiation by increasing the frequency of channel opening, while barbiturates prolong the duration of channel opening.[21]

Clinical Importance of Second-Messenger Systems

A recently explored area of therapeutic intervention has been at the level of the second-messenger effector enzymes. Initially there was a conceptual bias against the development of drugs acting at this level because it was believed that anything acting after the receptor would lack the selectivity required. However, there now appears to be great diversity, and hence potential selectivity, in the structure of the effector enzymes. Molecular cloning has shown the existence of five isoforms of phospholipase C,[29] seven isozymes of protein kinase C,[30] and five families of cyclic nucleotide phosphodiesterases[31] with unique tissue distributions. Rolipram, a selective cAMP phosphodiesterase type IV antagonist,[31] effectively blocks reserpine-induced hypothermia in rats, a test frequently used to predict antidepressant activity. Inhibitors of other phosphodiesterase isoforms are inactive and preliminary clinical trials confirm rolipram's predicted antidepressant activity. Thus, drugs acting at the level of the second-messenger generating enzymes show promise as a new class of pharmacological agents with selectivity achieved by targeting specific enzyme isoforms.

REGULATION

In the presence of an agonist, the β-adrenergic receptor shows a compensatory decrease in both ligand binding and adenylyl cyclase stimulation. This is a well-known biochemical effect induced by chronic exposure to most clinically effective antidepressives. What cellular mechanisms might account for this phenomenon? There are a number of points along the signal transduction pathway where alterations might occur (Figs. 2–4 and 2–5). The affinity of the receptor or the total number of receptors (B$_{max}$) might be decreased. Alternatively, the receptor could be uncoupled from the effector system through disruption of its linkage to the appropriate G protein. The cAMP or protein kinase products or inositolphosphate pathway products could also feed back and inhibit earlier interactions or modify proteins involved in the signal transduction pathway.

Receptor Desensitization (Down-Regulation)

Investigators using several different model systems have shown that preincubation of β-adrenergic receptors with their agonists results in a decrease in receptor number (B$_{max}$). This phenomenon has been termed desensitization. Agonist-induced β-receptor desensitization is associated with internalization or phosphorylation of the receptor.[32–34] The time course and extent of phosphorylation and desensitization parallel each other. A number of serine and threonine residues, potential phosphorylation sites, were identified in the third cytoplasmic loop (important in G protein interactions) and the COOH-terminal sequence of the receptor (see Structure, earlier). Protein kinase C and cAMP-dependent kinase are both capable of phosphorylating some of these sites. It appears that receptor phosphorylation occurs through the same mechanism of cAMP-mediated activation of protein kinase, thus providing a negative feedback mechanism for the signal transduction system.

Agonist-induced phosphorylation and desensitization were also observed in mutant cells lacking G_s and the adenylyl cyclase-kinase system.[35] This finding suggested the existence of a kinase selective for the agonist-occupied β-receptor independent of G protein activation. Such a novel selective kinase was found, β-adrenergic receptor kinase (βARK). Phosphorylation of the β-receptor by βARK causes an 80 per cent reduction in the activation of G_s.[36] Many other adenylyl cyclase-coupled systems undergo agonist-induced desensitization, and it is reasonable to think that other receptor-specific kinases will be found. β-Adrenergic receptor kinase is capable of phosphorylating the α_2-adrenergic receptor (G_i-linked) but not the α_1-adrenergic receptor (G_p-linked). These findings suggest that adenylyl cyclase-coupled receptors may utilize common regulatory mechanisms that are distinct from those utilized by the PI-linked receptors.

Potential phosphorylation sites on G_s have also been identified, and phosphorylated G_s appears to inhibit interaction with agonist-activated receptors. Protein kinase C is capable of phosphorylating these sites. G Protein phosphorylation might be a mechanism for heterologous desensitization: the desensitization of heterogeneous receptors mediated through the same G protein [e.g., exposing cells to prostaglandin (PGE_1) induces desensitization of both PGE_1 and β-adrenergic receptors]. The role of G protein phosphorylation in the regulation of signal transduction requires further investigation.

Receptor Sensitization

Current data suggest that postsynaptic receptors chronically deprived of synaptic input, through denervation or exposure to receptor antagonists, increase in number (B_{max}), thus becoming "supersensitive." This supersensitivity is also referred to as "up-regulation." Most of the model systems used to study sensitization and desensitization have been adenylyl cyclase-linked systems. Investigations of 5-HT_2 and the 5-HT_{1C}-receptor regulation, both linked to the PI second-messenger system, suggest that generalizations derived from one effector system may not hold for the PI-linked receptors. The expected up-regulation following denervation of 5-HT_2 receptors [chemical lesion such as 5,7-dihydroxytryptamine (5,7-DHT)] is not observed.[37] In addition, there is no apparent effect on receptor-mediated PI hydrolysis. In contrast, the 5-HT_{1C}-receptor–mediated PI hydrolysis in rat choroid plexus is supersensitive following 5,7-DHT lesions, but no increase in receptor density is detected. Treatment with antagonists does not produce the expected supersensitivity and up-regulation of the 5-HT_2 and 5-HT_{1C} receptors, but, paradoxically, induces a down-regulation, a de-

crease in receptor density, and desensitization of PI hydrolysis. These results are controversial due to the possibility of irreversible binding of drugs or their metabolites. Studies of the mechanisms underlying these effects are ongoing.[38]

Autoreceptors

Presynaptic autoreceptors have been described in virtually all the classical neurotransmitter systems: adrenergic, cholinergic, dopaminergic, GABAergic, and serotonergic. These receptors respond to neurotransmitters in the cleft by inhibiting further transmitter release from the cell in which they are found. Thus, autoreceptors represent a mechanism whereby individual neurons can self-regulate the amplitude of their chemical signal through a feedback mechanism. In general, agonists/antagonists acting at the presynaptic autoreceptor exert an effect opposite that at a postsynaptic receptor (i.e., α-adrenergic presynaptic receptor antagonists increase release of norepinephrine from a NE neuron).

Clinical Role for Autoreceptors

Presynaptic autoreceptor subsensitivity has been proposed as a mechanism of action for many antidepressant drugs, but most of the evidence comes from ex vivo studies in experimental animals. Clinical evidence in humans is either lacking or fails to support the development of autoreceptor subsensitivity; however, this is still controversial. It is possible that CSF and plasma metabolite levels typically used in clinical studies may not provide a rigorous enough test of the hypothesis. Furthermore, some of the in vitro studies may not have differentiated between presynaptic and postsynaptic receptor effects.

There are at least three distinct mechanisms whereby autoreceptors might regulate neuronal activity: (1) regulation of neurotransmitter synthesis; (2) regulation of neurotransmitter release; (3) and regulation of impulse activity. Dopamine autoreceptors in different regions of the CNS have been found to differ with respect to these mechanisms.[39] Stimulation of autoreceptors to inhibit DA activity in distinct regions of the CNS without affecting other regions or postsynaptic D_2 or D_1 receptors would be highly desirable and might eliminate undesirable side effects common with antipsychotic drugs (extrapyramidal reactions). Intensive effort is currently being devoted to finding agents selective for DA autoreceptors and to more clearly define the DA-autoreceptor situation.

There is evidence suggesting that lithium induces a 5-HT autoreceptor subsensitivity, but these effects develop rapidly while the clinical effects require weeks to months to appear. Therefore, it seems unlikely that lithium's effects on 5-HT release play a significant role in lithium's mechanism of action. Lithium's ability to potentiate the effect of other antidepressant drugs in depressed nonresponders may involve this effect on 5-HT release.

Serotonin reuptake inhibitors, such as fluoxetine, sertraline, fluvoxamine, and clomipramine, are the drugs of choice for the treatment of obsessive-compulsive disorder (OCD).[40] While their primary mechanism of action is to inhibit 5-HT reuptake and thereby increase the concentration of 5-HT at the synapse, the therapeutic effect is thought to result from a progressive desensitization of the presynaptic 5-HT$_{1A}$ receptors, enhancing 5-HT release and inducing a down-regulation of 5-HT$_2$ receptors. The delay in onset of the therapeutic effect is consistent with this mechanism. The newer generation 5-HT–selective reuptake inhibitors, such as fluoxetine and fluvoxamine, are generally devoid of the troublesome side effects frequently associated with tricyclic antidepressants like the anticholinergic, antihistaminergic, and adverse adrenergic cardiovascular effects. These agents are also effective in the treatment of major depression and, probably, panic disorder.

CONCLUSION

An implicit goal in biological psychiatry has been to understand the neural mechanisms underlying clinical psychiatric syndromes. The recent "receptor revolution" of the late 1970s and 1980s led to a dramatic increase in the number of known receptors, a clearer understanding of many drug actions, and the discovery of a few more selective drugs, but fell short of expectations that it would bring new insights into the pathophysiology of psychiatric diseases. For example, there is a better understanding about the mechanism of action of a variety of antianxiety drugs such as benzodiazepines, barbiturates, and alcohol acting to potentiate the effect of GABA at the GABA$_A$ receptor-chloride channel, but this has not led to the hoped-for understanding of the causes of neural substrates mediating anxiety.

The application of molecular biological techniques made possible the discovery of the G protein-linked receptor gene superfamily, the G protein gene superfamily, and the ligand-gated receptor gene superfamily. The rapid progress in receptor research is exemplified by the recent cloning of three new dopamine receptors, D$_3$, D$_4$, and D$_5$.[5,16,17] The cloning of these receptors and others that will follow provide new molecular tools to gain further insight into the role receptors play in psychiatric diseases. This information will lead to the development of more effective psychotropic medication by achieving higher specificity for target receptors and identifying novel receptor targets.

Our present knowledge regarding receptors and neuronal activity in normal and disease states derives primarily from animal research, postmortem studies, and peripheral metabolite studies in humans. Each of these approaches has limitations, but probably the greatest is the lack of animal models for the cognitive, emotional, and communicative functions of the human brain. Only the human brain has highly developed frontal lobes and has evolved elaborate verbal and written communication systems as well as the capacity for abstract and imaginative thought. It is these uniquely human characteristics that appear to go awry in many psychiatric diseases. For these reasons, the in vivo study of both normal and diseased human brains before and during drug treatment using imaging techniques such as positron emission tomography (PET) scanning or magnetic resonance imaging (MRI) should help us learn more about receptor function in normal and diseased states in the human brain.

While much has been learned about the structure of receptor subtypes using molecular biological approaches, a new era is beginning in which these strategies are being used to unravel the complexities of receptor regulation. The goal is to learn how receptors are controlled at all levels, from gene transcription, coupling, and uncoupling to G proteins or ion channels, effector enzymes responsible for second-messenger synthesis, and positive or negative feedback mechanisms regulating their response to changes in the synaptic milieu. Results of these ongoing studies will undoubtedly reveal new targets for selective drug intervention, representing many, if not all, the steps in the signal transduction cascade. The next generation of psychotropic medications is likely to be more effective, with fewer side effects if they can effectively target a particular receptor subtype or enzyme with a restricted tissue distribution. This more comprehensive knowledge of receptor regulation is likely to yield insight into the neural mechanisms underlying psychiatric disorders.

Clearly, there will always be patients who are not helped by a particular drug no matter how good a drug might be. For a number of reasons, often quite complex, they fail to respond or they experience intolerable side effects. Advances in psychiatric therapy for these individuals does not measure how far we have come, but how far we have to go. At the very least, new strategies in drug development will result in an increase in both the number and the diversity of drugs available. In addition, more selective and specific medication with fewer side effects should become available, making pharmacological management more efficacious in the therapeutic approach to patients.

ACKNOWLEDGMENTS

The authors gratefully acknowledge the support of the National Institute of Mental Health (MH 39437), the Spunk Fund, The John Merck Fund, and the endowment fund of the Nancy Pritzker Laboratory. JEK is the recipient of a research fellowship from the Dana Foundation. RDC is the recipient of a Research Scientist Award from the NIMH (MH 00219). The authors thank Dr. Bryan Roth for his critical reading of the manuscript.

REFERENCES

1. Creese I, Burt D, Snyder SH: Biochemical actions of neuroleptic drugs: Focus on dopamine receptor. *In* Iversen LL, Iversen SD, Snyder SH, eds. Handbook of Psychopharmacology. Vol 10. New York: Plenum Press, 37–89, 1978.
2. Kuhn R: The treatment of depressive states with G22355 (imipramine hydrochloride) Am J Psych 115:459–464, 1958.
3. Mansour A, Meador-Woodruff JH, Bunzow JR, et al: Localization of dopamine D2 receptor mRNA and D1 and D2 receptor binding in rat brain and pituitary: An In situ hybridization-receptor autoradiographic analysis. J Neuroscience 10(8):2587–2600, 1990.
4. Young WS, Kuhar MJ: A new method for receptor autoradiography: [³H]-Opioid receptors in rat brain. Brain Res 179:255–270, 1979.
5. Sokoloff P, Giros B, Martres MP, et al: Molecular cloning and characterization of a novel receptor (D3) as a target for neuroleptics. Nature 347:146–151, 1990.
6. Snyder SH, Yamamura H: Antidepressants and the muscarinic cholinergic receptor. Arch Gen Psychiatry 34:236–239, 1977.
7. U'Prichard DC, Greenberg DA, Sheehan PP, Snyder SH: Tricyclic antidepressants: Therapeutic properties and affinity for α-noradrenergic receptor binding sites in the brain. Science 199:197–198, 1978.
8. Richelson E: Tricyclic antidepressants and the H1 receptors. Mayo Clinic Proc 54:669–674, 1979.
9. Blue ME, Yagaloff KA, Mamounas LA, et al: Correspondence between 5-HT2 receptors and serotonergic axons in rat neocortex. Brain Res 453:315–328, 1988.
10. Seggal MR, Yousif MY, Lyon RA et al: A structure-affinity study of the binding of 4 substituted analogues of 1-(2,5-dimethoxyphenyl)-2-aminopropane at 5-HT2 serotonin receptors. J Medicinal Chem 33:1032–1036, 1990.
11. Weiss ER, Kelleher DJ, Woon CW et al: Receptor activation of G proteins. FASEB J 2841–2848, 1988.
12. Ross EM: Signal sorting and amplification through G protein-coupled receptors. Neuron 3:141–152, 1989.
13. Strader CD, Sigal IS, Dixon RAF: Genetic approaches to the determination of structure-function relationships of G protein-coupled receptors. Trends Pharm Sci (suppl):26–30, 1989.
14. Lefkowitz JR, Caron MG: Adrenergic receptor. Models for the study of receptors coupled to guanine nucleotide regulatory proteins. J Biol Chem 263:4993–4996, 1988.
15. Ovchinnikov YA, Abdulaev NG, Bogachuk AS: FEBS Lett 230:1–5, 1988.
16. O'Dowd BF, Hnatowich M, Caron MG, et al: Palmitoylation of the human β₂-adrenergic receptor. J Biol Chem 264(13):7564–7569, 1988.
17. Van Tol HHM, Bunzow JR, Guan HC, et al: Cloning of the gene for a human dopamine D4 receptor with high affinity for the antipsychotic clozapine. Nature 350:610–614, 1991.
18. Sunahara RK, Guan HC, O'Dowd BF, et al: Cloning of a gene for a human dopamine D5 receptor with higher affinity for dopamine than D1. Nature 350:614–619, 1991.
19. Julius D, MacDermott AB, Axel R, Jessel M: Molecular characterization of a functional cDNA encoding the serotonin 1C receptor. Science 241:558–564, 1988.
20. Pritchett DB, Bach AWJ, Wozny M, et al: Structure and functional expression of cloned rat serotonin 5-HT₂ receptor. EMBO J 7:4135–4140, 1988.
21. Julius D: Molecular biology of serotonin receptors. Ann Rev Neurosci 14:335–360, 1990.
22. Schofield, PR, Darlison MG, Fujita N, et al: Sequence and functional expression of GABAA receptor shows a ligand-gated receptor super-family. Nature 328:221–227, 1987.
23. Schofield PR: The GABAA receptor: Molecular biology reveals a complex picture. Trends Pharm Sci 10:476–478, 1989.
24. Luddens H, Wisden W: Function and pharmacology of multiple GABAA receptor subunits. Trends Pharm Sci 12:49–51, 1991.
25. Lester HA: Heterologous expression of excitability proteins: Route to more specific drugs? Science 241:1057–1063, 1988.
26. Kammer GM: The adenylate cyclase-cAMP-protein kinase A pathway and the regulation of the immune response. Imunol Today 9(7–8):222–229, 1988.
27. Hokin LE: Receptors and phosphoinositide-generated second messengers. Ann Rev Biochem 54:205–235, 1985.
28. Olsen RW, Yang J, King RG et al: Barbiturate and benzodiazepine modulation of GABA receptor binding and function. Life Sci 39:1969–1976, 1986.
29. Rhee SG, Suh PG, Ryu SH, Lee SY: Studies of inositol phospholipid-specific phospholipase C. Science 244:546, 1989.
30. Shearman MS, Sekiguchi K, Nishizuka Y: Modulation of ion channel activity: A key function of the protein kinase C enzyme family. Pharmacol Rev 41(2):211, 1989.
31. Breavo JA, Reifsnyder DH: Trends Pharm Sci 11:150–155, 1990.
32. Chuang DM, Costa E: Evidence for internalization of the recognition site of β-adrenergic receptors during receptor subsensitivity induced by (-)isoproterenol. Proc Natl Acad Sci USA 76:3024–3028, 1979.
33. Chuang DM, Kinnier WJ, Farbe L, Costa E: A biochemical study of receptor internalization during β-adrenergic receptor desensitization in frog erythrocytes. Mol Pharmacol 18:348–355, 1980.
34. Sibley D, Strasser RH, Caron MGG, Lefkowitz RJ: A novel catecholamine activated adenosine cyclic 3′,5′-phosphate independent pathway for β-adrenergic receptor phosphorylation in wild type and mutant S49 lymphoma cells: Mechanism of homologous desensitization of adenylyl cyclase. Biochemistry 25:137–1377, 1986.
35. Strasser RH, Caron MGG, Lefkowitz RJ: Homologous desensitization of adenylyl cyclase is associated with phosphorylation of the β-adrenergic receptor. J Biol Chem 260:3883–3886, 1985.
36. Benovic JB, Bouvier M, Caron MG, Lefkowitz RJ: Regulation of adenylyl cyclase-coupled β-adrenergic receptors. Ann Rev Cell Biol 4:405–428, 1988.
37. Sanders-Bush E: Adaptive regulation of central serotonin receptors linked to phosphoinositide hydrolysis. Neuropsychopharmacology 3(5–6):411–416, 1990.
38. Roth BL, Hamblin M, Ciaranello RD: Regulation of 5-HT₂ and 5-HT₁C serotonin receptor levels: Methodology and mechanisms. Neuropsychopharmacology 3(5–6):427–433, 1990.
39. Meltzer HY: Presynaptic receptors: Relevance to psychotropic drug action in man. Presynaptic receptors and the question of autoregulation of neurotransmitter release. Ann NY Acad Sci 604:353–371, 1990.
40. Levine RJS, Hoffman ED, Knepple ED, Kenin M: Long-term fluoxetine treatment of a large number of obsessive-compulsive patients. J Clin Psychopharmacol 9:281–283, 1989.

3

ELECTROENCEPHALOGRAMS AND EVENT-RELATED POTENTIALS IN CLINICAL PSYCHIATRY

GEORGE FEIN, Ph.D. and ENOCH CALLAWAY, M.D.

Windows on the Mind

Brain electrical activity recorded from the scalp is a source of information about underlying brain structure and function which carries with it minimal risk for the subject. In addition, brain electrical activity can resolve events that take place over the course of a few milliseconds. These two useful properties are shared both by records of ongoing electrical activity, known as the electroencephalograph (EEG); and by EEG phenomena time-locked to specific events, known as event-related potentials (ERP). This chapter will review contributions made by studies of EEGs and ERPs to the understanding of mental processes, to the development of psychopharmacological agents, and to the diagnosis and treatment of psychiatric conditions. This order of presentation is used, since a critical appreciation of clinical applications requires some background understanding of the basic psychophysiological and psychopharmacological studies.

Brain electrical activity involves current flow in the brain, which results in an electric and magnetic field. The electric field can be measured via electrical potential differences between points on the scalp, while the magnetic fields can be measured using supercooled magnetometers [the magnetoencephalogram (MEG)]. Magnetoencephalogram recording equipment is more than an order of magnitude more expensive than that required for EEG or ERP recording. The major theoretical advantage of the MEG was that it could more accurately localize intercranial sources, since the magnetic field is not affected by the low conductivity of the skull. However, the excitement about the potential of MEG has been tempered by Cohen and colleagues' recent demonstration that good localization accuracy (on the order of 1 cm, which is very close to that of MEG) can be achieved from scalp recorded electrical activity.[1]

Besides being noninvasive and relatively easy to record, EEGs and ERPs have, from the start, shown remarkable sensitivity to psychological variables. All this has generated a perennial hope that EEGs and ERPs might someday provide electrical "windows on the mind." For those interested in the human mind, this has had an enormous appeal, and the majority of the pioneers in the field have been psychiatrists, psychologists, and psychophysiologists. It is ironic that practical applications have been easier to achieve in branches of medicine that are less interested in the mind.

History of Technical Advances

Although electrical activity of nervous tissue had been studied in the eighteenth century by pioneer physiologists such as Galvani, the human EEG was first described by Berger, a German psychiatrist, in 1924. Berger also described the EEG's relationship to states of consciousness, its sensitivity to psychopharmacological agents, and its relationship to epileptic activity.

After Berger, there were technical improvements, particularly in the design of amplifiers and recorders, and naturally there were many clinical developments, particularly in the study of epilepsy. However, the next major developments came with the advent of relatively low-cost digital computers in the 1960s. Digital computers facilitated major advances in time-series analysis of the ongoing EEG, and made possible the study of ERPs, where the response to multiple stimuli must be summed to yield an adequate signal-to-noise ratio to detect and measure the ERP. Both of these methodologies had been available via electromechanical procedures, but the floodgate of studies by the ordinary investigator came with the development of the digital computer and of efficient algorithms for spectral analysis (the Fast-Fourier Transform). A more recent major advance was the demonstration in 1972 by Jewett and colleagues[2] that averaging (over 1000) potentials recorded at the scalp could disclose the minute potentials generated in brainstem structures. These potentials were said to be recorded in the far field; before their work, only cortical (near-field) evoked potentials had been thought to be accessible in humans.

Finally, some mention must be made of recent developments[3] that may at first glance seem of interest only to the practicing electrophysiologist. Examples include recent work on dipole source localization, on the effects of the recording reference, on methods for measuring changes in the evoked potential response to repeated stimuli, on reference-free recording methods such as the current source density, and on application of on-line pattern recognition to the study of communication between brain structures.

For the clinician, these somewhat formidable topics are of interest both because of the new frontiers and clinical applications they portend and because obsolete and misleading techniques, such as linked-ear reference EEG recordings, are still being used in some commercially available brain mapping systems. These new developments reflect two important and interrelated trends in ERP and EEG research. The first is an acknowledgment that brain biophysics must be taken into account if the field is to progress significantly. The second is the willingness of investigators to make an investment in increased computational capabilities and more complicated statistical and biophysical models of the EEG and ERP. The microcomputer revolution has made these developments possible, as tremendously powerful yet inexpensive computers are now available. Investigators at the forefront of EEG and ERP research can develop new methods that are computationally beyond the scope of clinical application in the secure knowledge that microcomputer technology will facilitate the clinical application of their methods in a few short years.

CONTRIBUTIONS TO UNDERSTANDING THE HUMAN MIND

The Physiological Substrate of Dreams

In two seminal studies Aserinsky and Kleitman[4] and Dement and Kleitman[5] described the psychophysiology of several stages of sleep. In particular, they described a stage of sleep called rapid eye movement (REM) sleep, which was characterized by rapid, conjugate eye movements, a low-voltage fast EEG resembling arousal (thus also known as paradoxical sleep), and loss of muscle tone. When awakened from REM sleep, subjects almost always recalled dreams of the sort that had long been the fuel for many psychoanalytic theories.

Instead of relying on memories that could be retrieved on awakening (or even worse, on the couch days later), the student of dreaming could collect dreams "fresh off the press." This made possible studies of the relationship between daytime and presleep events and subsequent dream content and between dream content and body and eye movements during the dream event. Although many a hunter has seen his dog go through coordinated hunting movements during a dream, now, via experimental awakenings, the relationship between such dream content

and eye movements during the dream were open to investigation.

Electroencephalogram-assisted psychological investigation of dreaming continues, and constitutes a field in its own right. For this review, suffice it to say that the new technology put to rest Freud's theory that dreams are "guardians of sleep," fulfilling wishes that would otherwise awaken the sleeper. In fact, not all dreams are wish-fulfilling and many of them actually awaken the sleeper.

Dissection of Information Processing

The sensitivity of the human ERP to cognitive processes was apparent in the earliest studies. For example, while stimulus intensity was obviously reflected both in ERP amplitude and latency, very weak stimuli were found to evoke large responses if they were significant for the subject.

The Contingent Negative Variation

Intensive and psychologically sophisticated work on the relationships between ERPs and attention was stimulated by Grey Walter's discovery of the contingent negative variation (CNV) in 1964.[6] When there is warning stimulus that is followed by a second stimulus that commands the subject to make a response, then, between the warning and response, a frontal negativity develops, which is "reset" when the response is executed. This CNV has been extensively studied and dissected into an earlier, somewhat more frontal orienting response, and a later, more central, readiness response which, in turn, overlaps a premotor potential that contains a component arising from the motor cortex.

The P300

The best studied ERP event sensitive to cognitive operations is the so-called P300, discovered by Sutton et al. in 1967.[7] This is a vertex/midline-parietal positive component occurring about 300 msec after a stimulus. Much of our knowledge about the P300 is due to the extensive work of Donchin and his colleagues. For example, the degree to which a stimulus is surprising is related to P300 amplitude. P300 latency has been shown to be sensitive to a variety of stimulus parameters (e.g., intensity, complexity) but is relatively insensitive to parameters which influence the response required by the stimulus. This property allows the P300 to be used in serial information processing experiments as a tool for distinguishing experimental manipulations which affect stimulus processing from those that affect response processing.

The association of P300 latency with stimulus evaluation rather than response selection and initiation was established in a classic experiment in which McCarthy and Donchin[8] used a display which contained either the word "LEFT" or "RIGHT." Uppercase words required a response with one hand, while lowercase words required a response with the other hand. Obviously, responding with the side contrary to the displayed word (i.e., with the right hand to LEFT) involved a response conflict, and slowed the response. The words LEFT and RIGHT could be degraded by appearing in a matrix of Xs or of letters, and the more distracting letters also slowed responding. Degraded stimuli slowed both P300 and reaction time, while response conflict slowed reaction time without slowing P300 latency.

More recently, it has become evident that the P300 is not a unitary phenomena, but rather is made up of a number of subprocesses. One of the most useful partitioning of P300 was Corschesne's distinction between P3A and P3B.[9] P3A is a more anterior component, which acts like an orienting response to stimulus novelty; while P3B is more posterior component and reflects aspects of active stimulus evaluation, as described above. Electrophysiological paradigms for measurement of P3A amplitude and latency effects are among the first to give the investigator access to frontal cortex mechanisms.

The Question of How Early Attention Begins to Operate

Does attention represent only conscious selection and editing, or are filtering and selection operations accomplished by central nervous system operations that are so early and peripheral as to be inaccessible to consciousness? The phenomenological speculations on this topic are beyond the scope of this review. The flavor of a more physiological argument is reflected in the classic studies by Hernandez-Peon and Jouvet,[10] who recorded ERPs from the cochlear nucleus of a cat in response to click stimuli and found that the ERPs were suppressed when the cat was shown a rat held under a bell jar. This was taken as evidence for attentive processes filtering auditory input at this very early level. Worden and Marsh later demonstrated that this effect of the rat on the cat's click ERP was abolished when head position, ear position, and intra-auricular muscle activity were controlled.[11] Since then, there has been a continuing attempt to determine when effects of attention can influence ERPs and what particular attentional mechanisms are involved at each level.

Very early attention-sensitive components of the ERP have been described by a variety of workers (e.g., Hillyard and colleagues[12]; Naatanen[13]). For example, studies of these "mismatch negativity" components which occur at about 100 msec after a stimulus, indicate sensitivity to changes in pitch, location in space, and sense modality. There appears to be a combination of early slow waves and discrete components that sum to produce the early ERP negativity. Factors such as a requirement for rapid sensory processing and the complexity of the changing feature affect the latency of the mismatch attentional component.

The search for evidence of attention-related changes at the level of the brainstem continues. The existence of corticofugal tracts going to the retina and cochlea provide a neuroanatomical basis for expecting such early sensory gating; but so far, convincing evidence for that has not been seen in far-field evoked potentials. In fact, since they are so insensitive to attention, far-field evoked potentials can be used to assess sensory functions without the necessity of the subject cooperating and paying attention (or even being conscious).

Human Information Processing

Event-related potential components provide a sequence of timing markers for information processing events from stimulus onset to response. Thus, latencies of the various ERP components provide tools for exploring models of human information processing. Changes in the latency of a particular component in response to an experimental manipulation provides evidence about when (in the temporal sequence of information processing between stimulus and response) the experimental manipulation produced its effect.

A useful example is found in Duncan-Johnson and Kopel's use of the sensitivity of P300 latency to speed of stimulus processing (see The P300, earlier) to settle a controversy regarding the nature of the Stroop effect.[14]

The Stroop effect refers to the slowing of response that occurs when one tries to name the color of ink used to print the name of another color. For example, with the word "RED" printed in green ink, the subject is supposed to say "Green." It takes longer to name a color used to print a conflicting color-word than to name the color of a spot. There had been a longstanding controversy as to whether that slowing is due to response conflict or stimulus interference. In the response conflict theory, the automatic tendency to read print sets up motor patterns that must be cleared before the proper response can be made. In the stimulus interference theory, the automatic processing of the word interferes with the less practiced evaluation of the color.

As noted above, P300 latency is affected by manipulations of stimulus evaluation and not by manipulations of response selection and initiation. Duncan-Johnson and Kopel recorded P300s to determine whether the Stroop effect involved alterations of stimulus or response processes or both. They found that P300 latency was unaffected by the color-name conflict, while reaction times were strongly affected. Thus, they showed that response conflict was the operative factor. Their experiment illustrates the use of ERPs as a tool for examining the information processing operations affected by specific tasks or experimental manipulations.

Localization of Cognitive Functions in the Cortex

A major focus of EEG and ERP research during the past two decades has been the delineation of functional differences between the two cerebral hemispheres. Electroencephalograph experiments use local diminution of alpha cavity (8 to 12 Hz) as indicating that a specific cortical region is active during a task. Evoked-response potential experiments use visual hemifield or dichotic listening paradigms, where stimuli are input preferentially to one or the other hemisphere and the resulting ERP component latencies are compared. If ERP latencies are earlier with input to one hemisphere, that hemisphere is inferred to be more efficient in processing the stimulus inputs. The major findings of this body of work is that the left hemisphere is "specialized" for verbal, sequential, analytic processes, while the right hemisphere is specialized for visual-spatial, synthetic processes. Exactly what is meant by specialized is much more complicated. Galin[15] has discussed the implications of these findings for psychiatrists. For example, it is important to distinguish among the concepts of capability, efficiency, and competence.

Davidson and his colleagues,[16] using the ongoing EEG, have generated an intriguing body of results pertaining to the role of the left and right prefrontal cortices in affective function. They have shown that the left anterior region is specialized for approach and the right anterior region is specialized for withdrawal, and have consistently found diminished left-sided anterior activation in depressed subjects, which is interpreted as indicating an approach-system deficit. This finding has been recently corroborated in positron emission tomographic (PET) studies, and is consistent with work suggesting that depressed individuals are characterized primarily by decreased positive affect. Their model suggests that individuals who display this frontal asymmetry in the resting state, when subject to environmental stress, are more vulnerable to withdrawal, a negative affective state, and depressive disorders.

Exciting and provocative extensions of these paradigms have been made in the study of infant temperament. A number of investigators have described a temperamental category observed early in life called behavioral inhibition, which involves heightened wariness and fear in unfamiliar and novel situations. Behaviorally inhibited children are at risk for affective and anxiety disorders, and their parents have a higher incidence of such disorders compared to parents of uninhibited children. On baseline EEG, inhibited 10-month-old infants demonstrate decreased left-sided anterior activation, and this pattern predicts persistent behavioral tendencies in these children. These studies provide compelling evidence that persistent behavioral tendencies have a biological (most likely genetic) basis, and that ongoing brain electrical activity is a sensitive marker of the underlying biological phenomena.

PRACTICAL APPLICATIONS

Nonpsychiatric Applications

The most clearly established clinical applications of ERPs and EEGs have more relevance to neurology, audiology, and surgical monitoring than to psychiatry and psychology. While these applications will not be discussed in detail, it seems useful to list some of them briefly.

Triage

Triage is one important service that EEGs and ERPs currently render. They do this by virtue of the fact that they reflect gross brain damage and brain death. Selection of patients (e.g., trauma victims, neonates) for limited treatment resources, and the decision to terminate life support are examples where electrophysiological measures contribute to decision making.

Sensory Testing

Brainstem auditory evoked potentials and somatosensory evoked potentials are used to measure the integrity of primary sensory systems in infants who cannot respond verbally to sensory stimulation. Since these ERPs are present even under anesthesia, they are also regularly used in the operating room to monitor the integrity of sensory pathways (e.g., optic nerve, auditory nerve, spinal cord) during surgical procedures. More recently, the ongoing EEG has been used as an indirect measure of the integrity of blood supply to the CNS during cardiac and cerebrovascular surgery.

Epilepsy

Epilepsy is the original domain of the clinical electroencephalographer. A good neurologist never treats an abnormal EEG, nor fails to treat seizures even though the EEG may be normal. Nevertheless, the EEG can be a source of welcome reassurance when it supports a clinical decision. In the operating room, the EEG plays a more critical role in decision making by locating seizure foci for excision.

EEGs and ERPs in Psychopharmacology

The intimate relationships between brain electrical activity and CNS function finds a natural application in pharmacodynamic studies.[17] With the possible exception of nootropics (e.g., piracetam), centrally acting drugs alter brain electrical activity, often in a characteristic manner for specific classes of drugs. If one wants to determine when and for how long a drug acts on the CNS, one cannot rely on blood levels, since the blood-brain barrier is not a passive membrane. Among the several methods for directly examining drug action in the brain are: (1)

measures of behavior; (2) single-photon computed tomography (SPECT) or positron emission tomography (PET) imaging; (3) magnetic resonance spectroscopy; and (4) EEGs or ERPs or both. Of these alternatives, EEG/ERP measures are often easier, cheaper, and more reliable. One hitch is that the time course of a drug's effect on the EEG and on a particular behavior need not be highly correlated, so one cannot predict the time course of CNS behavioral effects from the time course of EEG effects. If one's primary interest is in the behavioral effects of a drug, then the behavior of interest should be the primary variable examined.

In addition to data on pharmacodynamics, the EEG signature of a drug can predict its psychopharmacological profile with some accuracy. Neuroleptics slow fundamental EEG frequencies, while benzodiazepines cause a characteristic increase in high-voltage beta (20 Hz) activity. Stimulants produce arousal and speed early ERP components (but not P300), while anticholinergics cause a low-voltage EEG (paradoxical arousal), but slow ERP components. More elaborate classifications of drugs have been developed empirically, so that properties of a new drug can be assessed while dose/response and time/response relationships are being determined. As one would expect when a practical application exists, there are commercial laboratories that perform such pharmaco-EEG analyses for the drug industry.

One might hope that EEG and ERP measures could be used clinically to monitor medication levels. At present, however, they offer no competition to the measurement of drug blood levels. Leaving aside issues of sensitivity and reliability, it is easier to draw blood than to hook a patient up for EEG recording.

Finally, ERP measures can help in pinpointing the specific information processing operations affected by a drug. Because of this, the use of pharmacological agents together with ERPs provides powerful paradigms both for studying the effects of drugs on human information processing and also for determining the neurochemical substrate of various aspects of human information processing.[18] For example, aminergic stimulants (e.g., amphetamine) speed reaction time without having much effect on P300. Hence, they are speeding it principally by acting on response processing, after stimulus processing is completed. In contrast, noradrenergic agents can act on components that occur earlier than 200 msec, with clonidine slowing the yohimbine speeding latencies.

Diagnosis of Sleep Disorders

Polysomnography is a general term referring to the simultaneous recording of several different physiological variables during sleep. At present, the major use of the EEG in the clinical sleep laboratory is for sleep staging and for the recording of nocturnal seizures. For the most part, the EEG is an ancillary measure that helps to pinpoint the sleep stage during which other primary disturbances occur. Examples include respiratory function (e.g., sleep apnea), muscle activity (e.g., nocturnal myoclonus), and penile tumescence (e.g., the differential diagnosis of psychogenic versus somatic impotence).

Psychiatric Diagnosis

The uses of the EEG and ERP in psychiatric diagnosis can be roughly divided into two classes, depending on whether the electrophysiological measures are seen as reflections either of underlying physiological abnormalities or else of psychological dysfunction. Thus, if one believes that psychiatric illness represents a physiological derangement of the brain, one can use the EEG or ERP to search for manifestations of this derangement. On the other hand, if one is concerned with the psychological aspects of mental illness, then the EEG and ERP promise a more objective way of studying changes in sensory and cognitive operations.

It seems logical that if evoked potentials are sensitive to psychological and physiological processes, they should be powerful tools for psychiatric diagnoses. Unfortunately, this has not been demonstrated to be the case. However, there are a variety of commercial devices using EEGs and ERPs as psychiatric diagnostic aids, and there is ample commercial advertising presenting the position that EEGs and ERPs provide valuable psychiatric diagnostic and prognostic information.[19] This review can serve its purposes best by trying to present a balanced but largely contrary argument.

It is indeed the case that EEGs and ERPs are altered in psychiatric disease. The major problem has to do with the specificity of abnormalities. Psychiatric patients are likely to blink more and move more than normals. They often attend less well and may be generally more poorly motivated than a normal control population. They are often on drugs that alter both the EEG and the electrical properties of the skin. All these can be a source of differences between patient and control populations and even among patient groups. Even when impressive differences between clinical groups are reported, it is risky to predict clinical applications, for the level of patient motivation and artifact control achieved by a highly motivated research team may be hard to duplicate in a routine clinical situation. Clever computer algorithms can never really clean up dirty data—garbage in; garbage out.

Physiological Approach

Recovery Cycles

An important physiological paradigm is the study of recovery cycles, where one compares the response evoked by a stimulus on its first presentation with the response evoked by that stimulus when it quickly follows another stimulus. Recovery cycles are important because they test the sensory systems under conditions of stress, which are more likely to bring out subtle abnormalities.

Roemer and his coworkers have done an enormous body of work studying the relationship between evoked potential recovery cycles (and other measurements) and psychiatric diagnoses.[20] Their work has been marked by meticulous laboratory techniques and advanced multivariate statistical analyses. They and others have repeatedly demonstrated the ability to statistically distinguish between the EEG and ERPs of a wide variety of psychiatric disorders. That these ERP measures would tell the clinician something he didn't already know about a particular patient remains to be shown in a convincing way.

One particularly promising recent finding concerns the auditory P50 recovery cycle.[21] Schizophrenics' and their relatives' P50 responses appear to recover to a greater degree from an initial stimulus than do normal controls. Manics show a similar abnormality, which normalizes when they improve, while the deficit tends to be unrelated to clinical state in the schizophrenic. If this finding holds up, it may prove to be a useful tool in the diagnosis of schizophrenia, in the early detection of people at risk for schizophrenia, and perhaps in genetic studies. These promises, however, remain to be fulfilled.

Cortical Localization

There are certain cognitive operations and certain emotional reactions that can be more or less localized in the cerebral cortex. Some of the evidence for that assertion comes from the observation that the EEG and ERP reflections of local cortical changes can be associated with specific cognitive operations and emotional states (see Localization of the Cognitive Function in the Cortex, earlier). If psychiatric diagnostic entities are related to cortical dysfunctions, then it should follow that EEG and ERP topographic mapping could be applied to psychiatric diagnosis.

It is well known that left-hemisphere strokes are more often associated with depression, and so one might expect right-hemisphere activity to do better than left-hemisphere activity in depression. The work of Davidson's group (see Localization of the Cognitive Functions in the Cortex, earlier) has extended this notion of lateralized affect to the association of approach with left (and avoidance with right) prefrontal cortical activity. Thus there is reason to expect a relationship between right prefrontal dominance and vulnerability to depression.

Neuropsychological deficits in psychosis (the distinction between mania and schizophrenia being less clear than some would have us believe) have suggested frontal lobe dysfunction, while temporal lobe epilepsy and psychosis have been associated. Thus abnormal frontotemporal activity might be expected in psychosis. Finally, there is evidence to

suggest that left temporal lobe abnormalities are more common than right in psychotic patients.[22]

There is no shortage of reports on correlations between EEG and ERP cortical localizations and pathology in psychiatric patients, but few have stood the test of replication. Perhaps the most replicated findings deal with schizophrenic hypofrontality. In support of the EEG and ERP studies, there are now data from PET scan studies in which schizophrenics show reduced frontal activation during tasks that call on frontal cortical operations. Unfortunately, nothing has been reported that suggests ultimate clinical utility. That, however, is less than surprising in view of the fact that schizophrenia is the name for a syndrome, and is not a diagnosis in the traditional medical model.

It seems more likely that some basic information processing or behavioral concept (like Davidson's avoidant personality) would correlate with aspects of EEG activity, and both would require the consideration of biopsychosocial mediating variables before being related to psychopathology.

Reduced P300 Amplitude as a Possible Genetic Marker For Alcoholism

Begleiter and colleagues[23] have amassed compelling evidence that reduced P300 amplitude in alcoholics is a physiological marker of a genetic predisposition to alcoholism and to other addictive behaviors. The primary findings are: (1) the P300 amplitude is reduced in chronic or abstinent alcoholics in large sample studies; (2) that this reduction is carried primarily by the subset of alcoholics who have a positive family history for alcoholism; (3) after controlling for a positive family history for alcoholism, decreased P300 is not associated with extent of alcohol use; and (4) decreased P300 is present in the adolescent offspring of alcoholics who have a strong genetic loading for alcoholism, even though these offspring never drank alcohol themselves. These findings have been consistently replicated by other investigators and are being used in a large, multicenter study of the genetics of alcoholism.

Brute Force

Another branch of the physiological school has followed the premise that if enough data are gathered, the patterns which discriminate subtle CNS abnormalities can be revealed through complicated statistical and computer analyses. The clearest example of this approach is reflected in the work of John and his associates.[24] Gathering EEG and ERP data from multiple electrode locations, under a variety of recording conditions, in very large samples of various normal and abnormal populations, they used sophisticated multivariate statistics to identify EEG and ERP patterns specific to certain abnormalities. The ability of this approach, which they called neurometrics, to discriminate reliably between psychiatric diagnoses and to predicted drug response remains to be demonstrated. For example, early studies claimed that neurometrics could distinguish dyslexic children from normal readers, which would have been of major benefit for the clinician. Unfortunately, subsequent work has not supported this claim.

Independent replication of results is essential! No amount of statistical sophistication can make up for the absence of someone else getting the same results in another setting. The problem of independent evaluation and replication of some commercial qualitative EEG systems is further compounded by their use of proprietary databases. John's group has generally been willing to share their databases, but some other groups keep theirs secret. Large databases are expensive to accumulate, so the desire for secrecy is understandable, but it does set up yet another barrier to independent evaluation.

Psychophysiological Approach

VARIABILITY

The second approach to the use of evoked potentials in psychiatric diagnosis might be called the psychophysiological approach. Instead of looking for physiological signs, psychological questions are asked using EEGs and ERPs. Again, there is no lack of statistically significant findings.

The most ubiquitous abnormality in the ERPs of psychiatric patients is increased variability. This may include variability in amplitude and variability in component latencies. If, because of psychopathology, psychological processes are not going smoothly and attention waxes and wanes, then there will be greater than normal ERP variability. In addition, there are often other information processing malfunctions in psychiatric patients. Anything that reduces reliability of information processing will increase variability.

One effect of latency variability is to reduce amplitude in average ERPs. When a particular ERP component occurs at the same time in each individual sample, then it will produce a larger event in the average than will a component that occurs at varying times from trial to trial. Indeed, the effectiveness of averaging depends on the assumption that the event to be recovered from the embedding noise is time-locked to stimulus onset. Thus, some reports of reduced amplitudes of ERP components in psychiatric disease actually reflect increased variability.

Careful and expert attention to the motivation of patients, the selection of controls, and single-trial ERP analysis can remove or identify variability. Work in laboratories that exercise such careful controls suggests that there are ERP amplitude changes in psychiatric illness that are independent of poor motivation and increased variability.

SPEED OF INFORMATION PROCESSING

Attention affects the amplitude of the evoked potential more than its latency. By contrast, age and dementing illness prolong latency. This has lead to the hope that one might distinguish between pseudodementia (depression) and true dementia on the basis of P300 latency.

Again, there are statistically significant data supporting this contention, although their utility in practice is questionable. One finds undemented depressed people with long latency P300s and demented people without depression with P300 latencies that are not abnormal for their age. Furthermore, most clinicians would choose to treat an apathetic and withdrawn patient for depression even if they suspected they were dealing with dementia. The risk of missing a treatable depression is in general much worse than the risks of administering an antidepressant to a purely demented patient.

NEURAL EFFICIENCY

No review would be complete without some mention of the use of ERP latencies to measure intelligence. Some years ago, the idea of assessing "neural efficiency" with ERPs was advanced, and there were dreams of developing truly culture-free IQ tests based on ERP measures. There is a residual from that period of enthusiasm in current military studies of ERP measures as tools to use in selecting personnel for special tasks. There is little in the open literature from which to evaluate that work. In general, however, the story seems to be the familiar one. There are correlations between ERP measures and intelligence (with "r" around .4) but they are not large enough to be of practical value.

Psychiatric Treatment

Biofeedback

There are many correlations between brain physiology, scalp EEG, and mental processes. While ordinarily one thinks of both EEG and mind as arising from brain, the limitations of such a Newtonian view are quickly apparent. Obviously, mental processes can have effects on brain physiology, and through biofeedback, the EEG can also be elevated to the starting point of the causal sequence. This has been illustrated in the use of brain-wave feedback to help in achieving meditation-like states, and in achieving brain states where epileptic seizures are less likely.[25]

Voluntary control of the EEG is an old trick. Anyone with strong alpha (10 Hz occipital) activity and a vivid visual imagination can turn on alpha by closing their eyes, and turn it off by conjuring up a vivid visual image. The relaxed, immobile, but alert state favored by meditators is associated with alpha and with organized theta (8 Hz parietal) activity, and so it follows that feedback of brain-wave activity could help one achieve such a state, just as EMG feedback can help one learn to relax muscles, and temperature feedback can help one learn to dilate skin blood vessels.

The use of EEG biofeedback to obtain "alpha states" reached its peak popularity along with psychodelic drugs and various exotic meditative practices during the 1960s. There is no doubt that some control of the EEG can be learned, and reason to believe that biofeedback can be of use in such an endeavor. There have been reports of benefits ranging from psychoanalytic insights to maha samadi, but nothing convincing enough to stem the dwindling of interest in the procedure.

One of the more intriguing chapters in that story had to do with the effect of EEG biofeedback training on seizure frequency. Those studies were carefully controlled, but the time and effort required has not apparently sustained clinical interest.

Seizure Monitoring in Electroconvulsive Therapy

There is ample evidence that subconvulsive doses of current through the brain are not effective in treating depression, and may cause more post-treatment confusion that convulsive doses. On the other hand, it stands to reason that the smaller the current passed through the brain, the better, since large currents can produce brain damage. Without muscle paralysis, the dose of current can be titrated to produce a clear tonic-clonic seizure. However, with anesthesia and neuromuscular blockade, the peripheral evidence of a seizure may be obscured. Thus, some experts advise monitoring EEG activity during ECT so that an effective seizure can be guaranteed at the same time as current dose is being minimized.

CONCLUSIONS

The hope that developed in the 1960s and 1970s that electrophysiology would provide an electrical window on the mind for the diagnosis and elucidation of neuropsychiatric disorders has not been realized. However, one must keep in mind that much the same can be said about all other methodologies of biological psychiatry. The disappointment and disenchantment with the psychiatric yield of various methodologies (including electrophysiology) reflects the unrealized hope that simple solutions would be forthcoming for very complicated problems. One of the major problems is that psychiatric diagnosis, even in its most improved modern incarnation (e.g., DSM-III-R), is at a very early stage in its scientific development and deals with categories of patient's symptoms and signs, rather than with dysfunctional biological or physiological systems. In retrospect, since electrophysiological measures reflect the functioning of physiological systems and specific psychological operations, it was an unreasonable expectation that specific and sensitive electrophysiological abnormalities would differentiate phenomenological categories of abnormal functioning.

In recent years, as more sophisticated analysis methods and research paradigms have come to the fore, the excitement and high expectations for electrophysiological investigation have been rekindled. If the expectations are to be met, it is crucial that future research has strong foundations both in brain biophysics and physiology, and in the psychological constructs that underlie the behaviors being studied via electrophysiological methods.

REFERENCES

1. Cohen D, Cuffin BN, Yunokuchi K, et al: MEG versus EEG localization tests using implanted sources in the human brain. Ann Neurol 28:811–817, 1990.
2. Jewett D, Romano HW, Williston JS: Human auditory evoked responses: Possible brain stem components detected on the scalp. Science 167:1517–1518, 1970.
3. Gevins A, Remond A: Handbook of Electroencephalography and Clinical Neurophysiology. Vol 1. Methods of Analysis of Brain Electrical and Magnetic Signals. Amsterdam: Elsevier, 1987.
4. Aserinsky E, Kleitman N: Regularly occurring periods in eye motility and incomitant phenomena during sleep. Science 118:273–274, 1953.
5. Klelitman N: Sleep and Wakefulness. 2nd ed. Chicago: University of Chicago Press, 1963.
6. Walter WG, Cooper R, Aldridge VJ, et al: Contingent negative variation: An electrical sign of sensori-motor association and expectancy on the human brain. Nature 203:380–384, 1964.
7. Sutton S, Tueting P, Zubin J, John ER: Information delivery and the sensory evoked potential. Science 155:1436–1439, 1967.
8. McCarthy G, Donchin E: A metric for thought: A comparison of P3 latency and reaction time. Science 211:77–80, 1981.
9. Corschesne E, Hillyard SA, Galambos R: Stimulus relevance, task relevance and the visual evoked potential in man. Electroencephalogr Clini Neurophysiol 39:131–143, 1975.
10. Hernandez-Peon R, Scherrer H, Jouvet M: Modifications of electrical activity in cochlear nucleus during "attention" in unanesthesized cats. Science 123:331–332, 1956.
11. Worden FG: Attention and auditory electrophysiology. In Stellar E, Sprague JM, eds. Progress in Physiological Psychology. Vol. 1. New York: Academic Press, 1966.
12. Hillyard, Coles MGH, Donchin E, et al: Psychophysiology: Systems, Process and Applications. New York: Guilford Press, 1986.
13. Naatanen R: The role of attention in auditory information processing as revealed by event related potentials and other brain measures of cognitive functioning. Behav. Brain Sci 13:201–288, 1990.
14. Duncan-Johnson CC, Kopel BS: The Stroop effects: Brain potentials localize the source of interference. Science 214:938–940, 1981.
15. Galin DW: Implications for psychiatry of left and right cerebral specialization. Arch Gen Psychiatry 31:572–583, 1974.
16. Henriques JB, Davidson RJ: Regional brain electrical asymmetries discriminate between previously depressed and healthy control subjects. J Abnormal Psychol 99:22–31, 1990.
17. Itil TM, Itil KZ: The significance of pharmacodynamic measurements in the assessment of bioavailability and bioequivalence of psychotropic drugs using CEEG and dynamic brain mapping. J Clin Psychiatry 47(suppl):30–27, 1986.
18. Naylor H, Halliday R, Callaway E: Biochemical correlates of human information processing. In Vernon AP, ed. Biology of Intelligence. New Jersey: Ablex Publishing Corporation, (in press).

19. Luchins DJ, McCarley RW, Morihisa JM, et al: Quantitative electroencephalography: A report on the present state of computerized EEG techniques. APA Task Force Report on Computerized EEG. New York: American Psychiatric Association, 1990.
20. Roemer RA, Shagass C: Replication of an evoked potential study of lateralized hemispheric dysfunction in schizophrenics. Biol Psychiatry 28:275–291, 1990.
21. Adler LE, Gerhardt GA, Franks R, et al: Sensory physiology and catecholamines in schizophrenia and mania. Psychiatry Res 31:297–309, 1990.
22. Roberts GW, Done DJ, Bruton C, Crow TJ: A "mock up" of schizophrenia: Temporal lobe epilepsy and schizophrenia-like psychosis. Biol Psychiatry 28:127–143, 1990.
23. Begleiter H, Porjesz B, Bilhari B, et al: Event related brain potentials in boys at risk for alcoholism. Science 225:1493–1496, 1984.
24. John ER: Neurometrics: Clinical Applications of Quantitative Electrophysiology. Hillsdale NJ: Lawrence Erlbaum, 1977.
25. Orne MT, Weiss T, Callaway E, Strobel CF: Biofeedback: Report of the task force on biofeedback of the American Psychiatric Association. New York: American Psychiatric Association, 1979.

4

NEURO IMAGING: Uses in Psychiatry

LEWIS R. BAXTER, M.D., BARRY H. GUZE, M.D., and
CHARLES A. REYNOLDS, Pharm. D.

As medicine evolves from a practice to a science, accurate, specific diagnosis becomes essential for the proper selection and management of available therapies. One reason psychiatry has lagged behind other medical disciplines is that, until recently, there have been no techniques available to monitor the biochemistry and physiology of the living human brain. With the rapid development and expanding availability of computerized brain imaging techniques, this is now changing. We will review briefly the use of these technologies in modern psychiatric diagnosis and their potential use in the selection of appropriate treatment in the future. The review will be limited; those interested in a more detailed introductory description of imaging methods are referred elsewhere.[1]

Presently, the clinical use of brain imaging techniques is largely confined to structural imaging with x-ray computed tomography (CT) and conventional magnetic resonance imaging (MRI). These are used to separate psychiatric disorders from traditional neurological entities where brain structure is physically altered. We will focus on these techniques.

Newer "functional brain imaging" technologies such as positron emission tomography (PET), single-photon emission computed tomography (SPECT), and magnetic resonance spectroscopy (MRS), which can measure ongoing physiological and biochemical processes in the living brain, are beginning to demonstrate potential clinical utility. Although functional brain imaging will be reviewed only briefly here, clinical applications of these techniques are near. Clinicians are advised to be alert for developments.

STRUCTURAL BRAIN IMAGING

The most commonly used structural brain imaging techniques today are x-ray computed tomography and magnetic resonance imaging. The pneumoencephalogram and skull film are largely obsolete for psychiatry. It is well known that neurological illnesses with definable structural lesions may masquerade as psychoses, depression, and personality change (Table 4–1). This might seem to suggest that a structural brain scan should be performed on every psychiatric patient. However, with CT scanning, radiation exposure is not inconsequential; and with both CT and MRI, expense and, in some cases, patient tolerability may be prohibitive.

There is general agreement that any patient with focal neurological symptoms including a movement disorder, or with an unexplained new-onset delirium or dementia, warrants a structural brain scan. Although there is no universal agreement beyond these symptoms, we agree with Weinberger[2] that a structural brain scan is indicated for first-onset psychosis of unknown etiology, prolonged catatonia (especially if there is anything atypical in the clinical picture), and anorexia nervosa. Major depression or personality change with onset after age 50 should,

TABLE 4-1. STRUCTURAL BRAIN DISEASES ASSOCIATED WITH PSYCHIATRIC SYMPTOMS[a]

Brain Disease Associated with Psychosis and Personality Change or Both	Brain Disease Associated with Depression	Brain Disease Associated with Movement Disorder	Brain Disease Associated with Dementia
Huntington's disease	Subdural hematoma	Huntington's disease	Alzheimer's disease
Encephalitis	Tumor, granuloma, abscess	Idiopathic cerebral ferrocalcinosis (Fahr's disease)	Pick's disease
Lupus erythematosus	Normal pressure hydrocephalus	Wilson's disease	Multi-infarct dementia
Tumor, granuloma, abscess	Lupus erythematosus	Basal ganglia infarct	Normal pressure hydrocephalus
Trauma	Cerebral infarction	Olivopontocerebellar atrophy	Abscess
Metachromatic leukodystrophy	Trauma	Carbon monoxide, manganese poisoning	Tumor
Wilson's disease	Multiple sclerosis	Hallovorden-Spatz disease	Spongiform encephalopathology (Creutzfeldt-Jacob disease)
Kuf's disease	Arnold-Chiari mal-formation	Tumor, granuloma	Lupus erythematosus
Idiopathic cerebral ferrocalcinosis (Fahr's disease)	Huntington's disease	Lupus erythematosus	Metachromatic leukodystrophy
	Binswanger's disease	Multiple sclerosis	Kuf's disease
			Binswanger's disease
			Arnold-Chiari malformation
			Subdural hematoma

[a] Adapted with permission from Weinberger DR: Am J Psychiatry 141:12, 1984.

likewise, indicate a need for a structural brain scan, especially when there is not a clear family history of a similar disorder.

In fact, any disorder thought to be psychiatric that does not fit the typical presentation or, even when typical, does not respond to conventional therapy, should alert the clinician to the advisability of a structural brain scan. A conventional electroencephalogram (EEG) should be considered at the same time, since the EEG is highly sensitive not only to seizure phenomenon but also to gliomas, although with poor specificity.

CHOOSING BETWEEN X-RAY COMPUTED TOMOGRAPHY AND MAGNETIC RESONANCE IMAGING FOR STRUCTURAL BRAIN STUDIES

Magnetic resonance imaging is more costly than CT scanning—in most centers about twice so. Magnetic resonance imaging does offer superior tissue contrast and, of course, is without x-ray exposure (2 to 3 rads for most CT head studies). In fact, there are few known medical risks to a simple MRI study (e.g., pacemakers, metallic implants). Contrast media used with either CT or MRI can be a medical risk and should not be used routinely. Contrast should be used only in subsequent studies if an initial noncontrast study has identified a lesion or if clinical data suggest it is clearly warranted (e.g., high suspicion of an infiltrating brain tumor).

For the anxious or agitated patient in whom sedation may not be used, CT may be preferable to MRI. A complete MRI survey of the brain now takes approximately 45 minutes, whereas an adequate CT study can be completed in approximately 15 minutes.

Some large patients may not be able to fit in many present MRI devices, whereas they can be accommodated in a CT. Further, claustrophobic patients may find MRI much more difficult to tolerate than CT, in which only the top of the head is within the scanner.

Beyond these financial and physical considerations, the choice between MRI and CT is largely determined by the suspected lesion (Table 4-2). Magnetic resonance imaging gives superior tissue contrast for most brain lesions. Further, there are certain regions of the brain, such as the inferior temporal lobes, cerebellum, and brainstem, where overlying bony structures result in high degrees of x-ray attenuation and artifacts that lead to poor visualization with CT. Suspected lesions in these regions generally warrant an MRI examination. Many pathological processes, particularly gliomas in children, have a predilection for these regions.

There are also certain brain tissues which are not well differentiated from others by CT. Diseases that involve these tissues are consequently not well evaluated with CT. White matter diseases, such as multiple sclerosis and multi-infarct dementia, are common examples. Vascular malformations and infiltrating gliomas are other examples. Some degenerative illnesses such as Huntington's disease can be identified earlier in their course with MRI due to its superior sensitivity to small degrees of structural change, compared to the lower resolution CT. Magnetic resonance imaging is also superior in visualizing midline structures and identifying atrophic changes.

Still, CT does have its place outside of cost containment. Magnetic resonance imaging scanning

TABLE 4–2.   RECOMMENDATIONS FOR PSYCHIATRIC USE OF MAGNETIC RESONANCE IMAGING (MRI) IN RELATION TO COMPUTED TOMOGRAPHY (CT)[a]

MRI Instead of CT	CT Instead of MRI	MRI After CT

Anatomical regions suspected
  Temporal lobes
  Cerebellum
  Subcortical structures
  Brainstem
  Spinal cord
Particular diseases suspected
  White matter or demyelinating disorders
  Seizure focus
  Dementia
  Infarction
  Neoplasm (other than meningeal)
  Vascular malformations (including angiographically occult)
  Huntington's disease (and other degenerative diseases)
Children (posterior fossa, temporal lobe, midline)
CT contraindicated to avoid
  Radiation
  Iodine-based contrast material
  Intravenous procedure
	No localizing abnormalities present
	No specific disease suspected that would be better evaluated with MRI
	Suspected pathology well studied with CT
	  Meningeal tumor (primary or metastatic)
	  Pituitary lesions
	  Calcified lesions
	  Acute subarachnoid or parenchymal hemorrhage
	  Acute parenchymal infarction
	MRI contraindicated
	  Pacemaker
	  Aneurysm clip
	  Ferromagnetic foreign body
	  Pregnancy
		CT abnormal but not diagnostic
		Equivocal or normal CT but high index of suspicion for disease likely to be seen better with MRI
		Normal CT but atypical symptoms or course
		Normal CT but strong clinical or emotional need for reassurance with MRI

[a] Adapted with permission from Garber HJ, et al: Am J Psychiatry 145:2, 1988.

does not identify calcified lesions or acute bleeding well. Acute hemorrhaging and basal ganglia calcification (Fahr's disease) are also best identified on CT. Since MRI does not define the boundary between the brain and the skull well, CT has been a superior technique for meningeal tumors (primary or metastatic) and subdural hematomas. Computed tomography is, of course, also indicated when the patient contains significant amounts of magnetic material, such as an implanted pacemaker.

The need for careful medical monitoring during the imaging procedure may make it impossible to insert the patient along with his monitoring equipment into an MRI scanner. Likewise, pregnancy may make it impossible to fit in an MRI scanner; and although there is no convincing evidence of any damage to the fetus from exposure to high magnetic fields, most centers are reluctant to scan pregnant women.

Table 4–2, adapted from Garber et al.,[3] summarizes considerations in choosing between MRI and CT. Magnetic resonance imaging should be used instead of CT when the suspected neuropathology would be better visualized by MRI. Furthermore, MRI may be indicated after CT when atypical psychiatric symptoms or clinical presentations have not been adequately evaluated by CT alone. This last condition is, in all probability, not common. There is a high concordance between MRI and CT findings when these tools are used as screening examinations in psychotic patients.[4]

SEDATION FOR BRAIN IMAGING STUDIES IN PSYCHIATRY[5–8]

The use of sedation for brain imaging of the agitated psychiatric patient deserves consideration. We will confine our remarks to sedation for structural imaging, since the drugs used may in and of themselves alter the processes studied with functional imaging.

The first consideration is, "Is sedation necessary?" Even grossly psychotic patients will often respond with adequate cooperation if the clinician gives a careful explanation of the need for the study and how it is done. Further, if the patient can be accompanied by a familiar person with whom he or she has a good alliance, management is almost always easier.

Table 4–3 gives average doses of appropriate, commonly used agents for sedation in adults. However, there is no "one-dose-fits-all" schedule for any psychoactive drug. You should always titrate for optimal effect. In addition, one must consider interactions with other drugs and medical conditions with any particular agent chosen.

Droperidol is a particularly good agent in the psychotic patient; it is more sedating, yet with a significantly shorter half-life than haloperidol. Lorazepam is a good choice for nonpsychotic patients. If used intravenously, it is best to start with 0.5 to 1.0 mg and titrate up with additional doses every 3 to 5 minutes until the desired effect is obtained. Final dosage commonly ranges from 1 to 8 mg by this

TABLE 4–3. ADULT MEDICATION DOSAGES

Drug	Dosage[a]	Onset (minutes)	Comments
Chloral hydrate	500–2 gm p.o.	30–60	May experience some GI distress
Secobarbital	100 mg p.o.	15–30	
Droperidol	2.5–10 mg IM or IV	3–10	EPS rare, postural hypotension possible
			More sedating than haloperidol
Lorazepam	2–4 mg p.o., IM, or IV	15–30	Less respiratory suppression than diazepam
			OK IM
Diazepam	2–10 mg p.o.	15–30	Do not give IM-poor absorption, sterile abscesses
	2–10 mg IV	1–5	
Amobarbital	100–200 mg p.o. or IM	45–60	Do not give faster than 50 mg/min IV
	100–20 mg IV	<2–5	Laryngeal spasm a risk
			Usual IM maximum = 500 mg
			Need muscle mass for IM use

[a] p.o.; orally; IM, intramuscularly; IV, intravenously; GI, gastrointestinal; EPS, extrapyramidal symptoms.

route. Both droperidol and lorazepam are handled well in the patient with liver dysfunction. We do not recommend midazolam; there is a significant risk of respiratory arrest, and it does not last long enough for any clinical imaging procedures.

Sedation of children requires special care. There is a significant risk of "paradoxical reactions," wherein the patient becomes more agitated with low to moderate doses of sedatives. This same problem is also not rare in the elderly or in adults with gross structural or metabolic brain pathology. Although similar agents can be used in children as in adults, there are too many individual considerations for us to feel confident about responsible use of extensive dosage tables for children. For general use, however, chloral hydrate is probably the best choice, although it can be irritating if aspirated, and there have been some concerns expressed recently about the carcinogenic potential (in animals) of its metabolites. Usual, safe doses are 50 mg/kg (to a maximum of 2 gm) p.o. or p.r.n. ½ hour before the procedure. The use of other, more risky agents, such as thiopental, should be relegated to those quite familiar with their use and risks in radiological procedures.

FUNCTIONAL BRAIN IMAGING TECHNIQUES

Presently available functional brain imaging techniques are PET, SPECT, and MRS.

Magnetic resonance spectroscopy relies on a separation of the magnetic resonance signal of a given element into different chemical forms. The most commonly used MRS approach is proton MRS. In this method, the proton signals from water are suppressed and the spectra from less-abundant forms of hydrogen are examined. Spectroscopy can also be performed for other chemical nuclei, such as ^{31}P. This permits the examination of adenosine triphosphate (ATP), inorganic phosphate, phosphomonoesters, and phosphodiesters.

Localization of this biochemical information currently is difficult with MRS and requires large brain areas to be examined which do not conform to specific neuroanatomic structures. Also, acquisition times can be long and may be difficult for many psychiatric patients to tolerate. Furthermore, only certain elements where the isotopes are paramagnetic may be studied. Magnetic resonance spectroscopy requires a high magnetic field strength of great homogeneity, precluding use of all but the top-of-the-line MR scanners currently available. Absolute quantification also presents significant difficulties.

Positron emission tomography and SPECT have certain similarities. In each technique, a tracer substance is injected into the subject. This tracer chemical is attached to a radiation-emitting isotope. The radiation signal is picked up by an array of detectors located around the subject. These detectors convert the signal from the radiation into a digital electrical signal. This signal is in proportion to the distribution and concentration of the tracer. It is reconstructed as a brain map of the rate of the biochemical reaction being studied.

In PET, the compound to be traced is labeled with a positron-emitting isotope. A positron is the antimatter equivalent of the electron, and decays by colliding with an electron to produce two high-energy gamma rays which are emitted at 180 degrees from each other. This dual, simultaneous, signal is what gives PET a higher resolution than SPECT, which uses the signal from a single x-ray photon emitted from a traditional nuclear medicine isotope such as ^{123}I or ^{99m}Tc.

For both SPECT and PET, information from these radioactivity events is picked up by sensors and processed by the computer in a tomographic fashion similar to CT. The concentrations of the tracer substances used are so small that they do not perturb the underlying physiological processes being studied, and thus allow PET and SPECT to make accurate measurements of these processes.

Presently, the major limitations of PET are the need for a cyclotron to produce the very short lived positron-emitting isotopes, and the need for synthesis equipment to make the tracer compound of interest rapidly and at high purity and sterility. Although small medical cyclotrons and automated chemical synthetic equipment are beginning to make PET available at larger medical centers for clinical use, it is SPECT that presently has by far the wider availability.

Single-photon emission computed tomography is done with conventional nuclear medicine cameras. The compounds used in SPECT have substantially longer half-lives than the positron emitters used in PET. They are also available commercially.

To date, SPECT has mainly been used to image blood flow. Positron emission tomography has been used mostly to study glucose metabolism and blood flow. However, both techniques have the potential to measure many brain biochemical processes, such as neurotransmitter turnover rates, the densities of neuroreceptors, etc. Most of this latter work has been done with PET, where positron-emitting isotopes of naturally occurring atoms (e.g., carbon, nitrogen, oxygen, fluorine) can be substituted for stable atoms in organic substances. These isotopes do not alter the activity of the compound of interest. The large atoms typically used for SPECT isotopes, such as iodine and technetium, do not occur commonly in biological systems and have proved more difficult to attach effectively to tracers of interest to psychiatrists.

Magnetic resonance spectroscopy also provides quantitative regional measurements of biochemical and physiological processes in vivo.[9] It is noninvasive and does not expose patients to ionizing radiation. Furthermore, it has no known side effects, and because of that appears ideally suited for longitudinal studies of patients. Its major weakness is that it is presently insensitive compared to PET and SPECT.

POTENTIAL CLINICAL APPLICATIONS OF FUNCTIONAL IMAGING

Functional imaging has its clearest potential clinical application in two areas: temporal-lobe-origin epilepsies and Alzheimer's-type dementia. Many PET studies of glucose metabolism have demonstrated that, in the interictal state, seizure foci in temporal lobe epilepsy are usually profoundly hypometabolic. This, combined with EEG data, gives very accurate localization of many temporal lobe seizure foci.

In Alzheimer's-type dementia, a score of studies demonstrate that early in the clinical course of this illness there is profound, biparietal glucose hypometabolism.[10] Since glucose metabolism and blood flow are, under almost all circumstances, highly correlated in the human brain, it is not surprising that SPECT studies of Alzheimer's disease looking at blood flow indices have also tended to indicate a biparietal abnormality.

The differentiation of early Alzheimer's-type dementia from traditional psychiatric illnesses, particularly severe depression with cognitive impairment in the elderly, is often a difficult differential diagnosis problem. Positron emission tomographic studies of major depression, albeit in young to late middle-age adults, have demonstrated lateral prefrontal hypometabolism, but not the parietal deficits seen in Alzheimer's disease.[10,11] Similar lateral prefrontal cortex findings have been seen in schizophrenia. Thus, there is the *potential* of using PET and SPECT to identify Alzheimer's disease in patients who might otherwise be considered purely psychiatric. However, it must be pointed out that patients with Alzheimer's disease can have other illnesses concomitantly, particularly secondary depression. Identifying an Alzheimer's disease pattern on PET or SPECT scanning would not necessarily be a reason for foregoing an empirical, clinical trail of an antidepressant in an individual with any depressive signs and symptoms.

Another indication for PET would be in the rare case of an individual whose family history is not known and who presents with psychiatric symptoms, prior neuroleptic exposure, and bilateral chorea. Huntington's disease exhibits profound caudate nucleus glucose hypometabolism long before there are structural changes demonstrable by MRS or CT,[12] whereas such metabolic loss is not seen in tardive dyskinesia.

Early work with receptor ligands for PET and SPECT hold the greatest promise for the future. There is some indication that schizophrenia may show a lower density of dopamine receptors than seen in normals, though this is still controversial.[13,14] Brain imaging techniques that can visualize specific neurotransmitter system may be critical in the diagnosis of specific psychiatric illnesses in the future.

Equally impressive, and technologically closer at hand, functional imaging techniques have clearly demonstrated the potential ability to measure the effectiveness of a drug at blocking neuronal receptors and also assessing brain drug levels.[15] Magnetic resonance spectroscopy has shown potential to measure lithium and fluorinated psychotropic drug concentrations and pharmacokinetics in brain. One day, such tests may prove useful in deciding which drugs, and at what dosages, will be best for specific patients. This has the potential of obviating the empirical clinical trials—requiring weeks and exposing patients to significant side effects—now necessary before either best dosage or even efficacy can be known.

ACKNOWLEDGMENT

Supported in part by a NIMH Research Scientist Development Award (MH00752-03) (LRB).

REFERENCES

1. Andreasen NC, ed: Brain Imaging: Applications in Psychiatry. Washington, DC: American Psychiatric Press, Inc., 1989.
2. Weinberger DR: Brain disease and psychiatric illness: When should a psychiatrist order a CAT scan? Am J Psychiatry 141:1521–1527, 1984.
3. Garber HJ, Weilburg JB, Buonanno FS, et al: Use of magnetic resonance imaging in psychiatry. Am J Psychiatry 145:1084–1088, 1988.
4. Cohen BM, Buonanno F, Keck PE, et al: Comparison of MRI and CT scans in a group of psychiatric patients. Am J Psychiatry 145:1084–1088, 1988.
5. Lofstrom JB: Risk evaluation and patient assessment in sedation. Acta Anaesthesiol Scand 32(suppl 88):17–20, 1987.
6. Lundgren S: Sedation as an alternative to general anesthesia. Acta Anaesthesiol Scand 32(suppl 88):21–23, 1987.
7. Mindus P: Anxiety, pain and sedation: Some psychiatric aspects. Acta Anaesthesiol Scand 32(suppl 88):7–12, 1987.
8. Nakata MC: Sedation in pediatric patients undergoing diagnostic procedures. Drug Intell Clin Pharm 22, 711–715, 1988.
9. Guze BH: Magnetic resonance spectroscopy: A technique for functional brain imaging. Arch Gen Psychiatry 48:572–574, 1991.
10. Guze BH, Hoffman JM, Baxter LR, et al: Functional brain imaging and Alzheimer's type dementia. Alzheimer Dis Assoc Disorders, 3:103–109, 1991.
11. Baxter LR: PET studies of cerebral function in major depression and obsessive-compulsive disorder: The emerging prefrontal cortex consensus. Ann Clin Psychiatry, 3:103–109, 1991.
12. Mazziotta JC, Phelps ME, Pahl JJ, et al: Reduced cerebral glucose metabolism in asymptomatic subjects at risk for Huntington's disease. N Engl J Med 316:357–362, 1987.
13. Wong DF, Wagner HN, Tune LE, et al: Positron emission tomography reveals elevated D_2 dopamine receptors in drug-naive schizophrenics. Science 234:1558, 1986.
14. Farde L, Wiesel FA, Halldin C, Sedvall G: Central D_2 dopamine receptor occupancy in schizophrenic patients treated with antipsychotic drugs. Arch Gen Psychiatry 45:71–76, 1988.
15. Sedval G, Farde L, Porsson A, Wiesel FA: Imaging of neurotransmitters in the living human brain. Arch Gen Psychiatry 43:995–1005, 1986.

5

HORMONAL REGULATION OF BEHAVIOR

CHARLES B. NEMEROFF, M.D., Ph.D. and K. RANGA R. KRISHNAN, M.D.

In this chapter, we discuss each of the endocrine axes and their alterations in the major psychiatric disorders. Space constraints preclude an encyclopedic review of this area, and the interested reader may refer to Copolov and Rubin.[1]

GROWTH HORMONE

The secretion of growth hormone (GH) is regulated by both neural and endocrine influences, both stimulatory and inhibitory. This control is achieved by at least two hypothalamic hormones, growth hormone-releasing hormone (GRF) and somatostatin. These hormones are synthesized and released from neurons in the hypothalamus. In addition, there is evidence that catecholamines and indoleamines, primarily dopamine, norepinephrine, and serotonin, act to modulate the release of these hypothalamic hormones. In view of the role of catecholamines and indoleamines in regulating GH secretion, and their putative role in the pathophysiology of affective disorders and schizophrenia, GH regulation in patients with these psychiatric disorders have been conducted.[2]

Affective Disorders

Growth hormone is secreted in pulses that are highest in the first few hours of the night. Age is an important determinant of GH secretion; GH secretion decreases with increasing age. Mendlewicz et al.[3] studied the 24-hour secretion of plasma GH in 16 patients with major depression (eight unipolar and eight bipolar) compared with eight age- and sex-matched controls. Both unipolar and bipolar depressed patients secreted more GH than normal subjects, and this hypersecretion occurred during waking hours rather than during sleep. In this study, a relationship between nocturnal GH secretion and depression was not found. Schilkrut et al.[4] reported that GH secretion was disturbed during the night in depressed patients, and that depressed patients had a diminished nocturnal GH release. They suggested that GH abnormalities in depressed patients were secondary to disrupted sleep architecture, and also reported a diminished association between nocturnal GH spikes and slow-wave sleep. Mendlewicz et al.[3] also found a diminished association between nocturnal GH spikes and slow-wave sleep stages, and suggested that this finding may be related to the inhibitory effect of diurnal hypersecretion of GH.

Several reports suggest that the dopaminergic regulation of GH secretion is not altered in depression.[2] Clonidine, an α_2-adrenergic agonist, stimulates GH release. An attenuated GH response to clonidine has been observed in depressed patients by several investigators.[5] Indeed, the blunted GH response to clonidine is considered by many to be the most reproducible and specific finding in the biology of affective disorders.

Recently, Dinan and Barry reported that the GH response to orally administered desmethylimipramine (DMI) is blunted in depressed patients, both endogenous and nonendogenous subtypes, when compared to controls. Their studies suggest diminished α_2-adrenergic responsiveness in depression.[6] With the availability of synthetic GRF, the GH response to GRF in patients with depression could be studied. The results from these studies have been discordant.

Alzheimer's Disease

Growth hormone regulation has also been studied in Alzheimer's disease, primarily because patients with Alzheimer's disease have a significant reduction in central nervous system concentration of somatostatin.[7] If patients with Alzheimer's disease have a longstanding reduction in the availability of hypothalamic somatostatin, then alterations in pituitary GH secretion may result. We did not, however, find a difference between Alzheimer's patients and control subjects in the GH response to GRF.[8] It would appear that the GH response to GRF may be altered primarily in individuals with the early-onset form of the disease, and its use as a diagnostic adjunct for Alzheimer's disease, if any, would be limited to those subjects.

Schizophrenia

Plasma GH concentrations are of interest in schizophrenia research because GH secretion is, to some extent, under the influence of dopamine, the catecholamine neurotransmitter thought to play a preeminent role in the pathophysiology of schizophrenia. Although there is considerable evidence for a pathophysiological role for the mesocorticolimbic dopamine system in schizophrenia, there is little evidence for a role of the tuberoinfundibular dopaminergic system in this disorder. The major methodological problem in studies of GH and schiz-

ophrenia is the effect of neuroleptic treatment, and possible confounds related to nonspecific factors such as weight, weight change, etc. Well-designed studies controlling for all these factors and involving a large number of subjects need to be undertaken to clarify the issue of whether the tuberoinfundibular dopaminergic system and its control of GH secretion is pathologically involved in schizophrenia.

Anorexia Nervosa

Basal plasma GH concentrations are elevated in greater than 50 per cent of patients with anorexia nervosa.[9,10] Growth hormone concentrations in these patients are related to body weight and weight loss and return to normal after the patients start eating a normal-calorie diet.[10,11] Growth hormone changes are probably related to the low-calorie diet and are similar to those seen in individuals with malnutrition.[12] The GH response to insulin is blunted in anorexia nervosa.[10] A blunted GH response to L-dopa and apomorphine has also been reported in these patients.[11,13] These abnormalities are also corrected by refeeding. Growth hormone alterations in anorexia nervosa are probably related to changes in food intake and thus may be secondary to the illness rather than being primarily involved in the etiopathogenesis of the disorder.

HYPOTHALAMIC-PITUITARY-ADRENAL AXIS

Because the hypothalamic-pituitary-adrenal (HPA) axis plays an integral role in the pathophysiology of stress, and stress has long been thought to precipitate episodes of affective disorder in genetically vulnerable individuals, it has been the best studied of all the endocrine axes in psychiatric disorders. An understanding of the physiological regulation of the HPA axis is necessary to evaluate HPA axis disturbances reported in certain psychiatric disorders.

For several years, adrenocorticotrophic hormone (ACTH) was considered as the sole agent regulating cortisol release from the adrenal cortex. Recent evidence suggests that this view may be too simplistic.[14] At the anterior pituitary corticotroph, a number of factors regulate the secretion of ACTH. These include corticotropin-releasing factor (CRF), vasopressin, somatostatin, vasoactive-intestinal polypeptide, catecholamines (both α- and β-adrenergic mechanisms), angiotensin, and glucocorticoids. Corticotropin-releasing factor is the major modulator of the ACTH response to stress, with vasopressin playing an adjunctive role. In contrast, the stress response to hemodynamic (hemorrhage) stimuli seems to be primarily mediated by vasopressin. Norepinephrine, via a central α_1-adrenergic mechanism, plays an important role in regulating HPA-axis activity in humans. Dopamine has little effect on HPA-axis activity, serotonin exerts a stimulatory influence, whereas gamma-aminobutyric acid (GABA) and opioid peptides inhibit HPA-axis activity.

Affective Disorders

The HPA axis has been most intensively studied in patients with affective disorders.[15] Patients with affective disorders during the depressed phase exhibit increased secretion of cortisol as measured by 24-hour urinary free cortisol. Moreover, depressed patients show elevated plasma corticosteroid concentrations which are highest in the most severely depressed subjects. Plasma glucocorticoid levels return to normal following successful electroconvulsive therapy (ECT) or antidepressant treatment. Sachar et al.[16] investigated the cortisol production rate in depressed subjects by measuring isotopically labeled cortisol metabolites in urine before treatment and after recovery. The cortisol production rate was elevated during the illness and returned to normal in most subjects after recovery. Several studies suggest that the degree and extent of ACTH rise does not parallel that observed with cortisol. These findings suggest that there is an increase in the sensitivity of the adrenal cortex to ACTH in depressed subjects. Further studies suggest that the enhanced cortisol response observed after high doses of ACTH may reflect adrenocortical hypertrophy, rather than an increased sensitivity to the ACTH receptors.[17]

The blunted ACTH response to CRF in depression is not merely due to the hypercortisolemia and resultant negative feedback. The corticotroph may be sensitized to CRF, possibly by increased secretion of vasopressin. It is possible that there is an increase in pituitary gland size in depression. Indeed, utilizing magnetic resonance imaging, we have recently shown in a study of 19 depressed patients and 19 age- and sex-matched controls, that the pituitary gland is enlarged in depressed patients.[18]

Dexamethasone Suppression Test

The dexamethasone suppression test (DST) is undoubtedly the most intensively studied single test of HPA-axis activity in patients with depression. In a landmark publication, Carroll et al.[19] reported that DST nonsuppression had a 67 per cent sensitivity and a 96 per cent specificity for the diagnosis of melancholia in psychiatric patients hospitalized on a research unit. Since the publication of this report, numerous investigators studied this phenomenon with both concordant and discordant results. Summarizing a vast literature, the DST is unlikely to be useful as a screening test for melancholia or major depression. However, the DST does appear to be useful in distinguishing between subjects with melancholia from those with schizophrenia, and patients with psychotic depression from patients with schizophrenia.

The Role of Corticotropin-Releasing Factor in the Pathogenesis of Depression

Because CRF is the major physiological regulator of the HPA axis, by virtue of its potent action on ACTH secretion, it was plausible to posit CRF hypersecretion as a major contributor to the hypercortisolemia observed in patients with major depression. In addition, direct central administration of CRF produces behavioral effects remarkably similar to the cardinal signs and symptoms of major depression including decreased libido, decreased appetite, psychomotor alterations, and disturbed sleep. These findings led to the measurement of CRF in cerebrospinal fluid (CSF) of drug-free patients with major depression, and patients with other psychiatric diagnoses. Several studies support the hypothesis that CRF is hypersecreted in depressed patients, resulting in both behavioral signs and symptoms, and increased HPA-axis activity.[20]

Schizophrenia

The DST nonsuppression rate in schizophrenia varies from 0 to 70 per cent, with a mean rate of approximately 20 per cent. The range appears to reflect the type of patients, activity of the patients, presence of associated symptoms of depression, and the effects of hospitalization.[21] The CRF stimulation test has also been conducted in patients with schizophrenia. Cortisol and ACTH responses to CRF in patients with schizophrenia appear to be normal.[22] In most studies in which CSF CRF concentrations have been measured, schizophrenic patients exhibit normal values.

Alzheimer's Disease

Occurrence of DST abnormalities in patients with Alzheimer's disease has been attributed to hippocampal pathology. Sapolsky et al.,[23] in a series of elegant studies, have demonstrated that the hippocampus is of major importance in regulating HPA axis activity. Glucocorticoid feedback at the level of the hippocampus is responsible for turning off the HPA-axis response to stress. Thus, in Alzheimer's disease, destruction of hippocampal neurons and loss of the feedback system may account for increased rates of DST nonsuppression.

THE HYPOTHALAMIC-PITUITARY-THYROID AXIS

Although patients with primary hypothyroidism exhibit many of the signs and symptoms of major depression, considerable evidence has accumulated over the past decade that supports the hypothesis that a sizeable proportion of drug-free depressed patients exhibit abnormalities in the hypothalamic-pituitary-thyroid (HPT) axis, and these alterations may contribute to depressive symptoms.

The Thyrotropin Response to Thyrotropin-Releasing Hormone In Depression

Shortly after the discovery of the chemical identity of thyrotropin-releasing hormone (TRH), a TRH stimulation test was standardized. Thyrotropin-releasing hormone (500 μg) is administered intravenously over 1 minute and blood samples are collected at 30-minute intervals for 2 to 3 hours. Several investigators, beginning with the pioneering observations of Prange et al.[24] have observed that approximately 25 per cent of depressed patients, though euthyroid by any of the usual endocrinological criteria, exhibit a blunted thyroid-stimulating hormone (TSH) response to TRH. Although the best-documented cause of an attenuated TSH response to TRH is hyperthyroidism, little evidence of excessive thyroid hormone secretion in depression has been found. One putative mechanism to explain the blunted TSH response to TRH in drug-free depressed patients would be chronic hypersecretion of TRH, which theoretically could result in a reduced number of TRH receptors on the adenohypophyseal thyrotrophs, receptor "down-regulation."

The specificity of the elevated CSF concentrations of TRH in depressed patients has been evaluated in a few small studies. In drug-free patients with anorexia nervosa, CSF TRH levels are not increased,[25] nor do patients with Alzheimer's disease, anxiety disorders, or alcoholism show any alterations in CSF TRH.[26]

Symptomless Autoimmune Thyroiditis and Depression

Although the blunted TSH response to TRH in depressed patients has received considerable attention, approximately 15 per cent of depressed patients exhibit an exaggerated TSH response to TRH. This finding was studied most intensively by Gold et al.[27] and has led to the realization that a sizeable number of depressed patients with exaggerated TSH responses to TRH and normal baseline plasma TSH and thyroid hormone concentrations have, by definition, grade III hypothyroidism.

In spite of years of concerted study, it is almost remarkable how little we know of the role of the HPT axis in the pathophysiology of affective disorders. Nevertheless, considerable progress has been made in recent years. First, it is evident that a sizeable proportion of depressed patients, in particular those with bipolar illness, exhibit relatively high rates of autoimmune thyroiditis, as evidenced by the presence of antithyroid antibodies. The issue of treatment of depressed patients with symptomless autoimmune thyroiditis remains an issue of paramount importance. Is treatment with exogenous thyroid hormone alone sufficient to normalize their mood state? There are anecdotal accounts of treating such patients successfully with T_4 alone, and there is a large literature review by Prange et al.[28] demon-

strating reduced effectiveness of tricyclic antidepressants in patients with frank hypothyroidism. The high rate of autoimmune thyroiditis and subclinical hypothyroidism in bipolar patients is of interest in view of the recent studies of Bauer and Whybrow who reported therapeutic responses of rapid-cycling bipolar patients to high doses of thyroid hormones.[29]

The blunted TSH response to TRH observed in approximately 25 per cent of depressed patients, as well as in abstinent alcoholics, remains mechanistically enigmatic. Our studies would suggest that chronic TRH hypersecretion, as evidenced by increased CSF TRH concentrations, results in adenohypophysial TRH receptor down-regulation. The finding of an inverse relationship between CSF TRH concentrations and the TSH response to TRH in our pilot study of alcoholic patients supports this view.

Finally, there is a large literature on the use of thyroid hormone, usually T_3, to potentiate the therapeutic effects of tricyclic antidepressants and to convert antidepressant nonresponders to responders. This phenomenon was first observed by Prange and coworkers[30] in depressed patients, and this has recently been reviewed.[31]

CONCLUSION

We have described alterations in three of the major neuroendocrine axes in psychiatric disorders: the HPA, HPT, and GH systems. There is unequivocal evidence that each of these are altered in patients with affective disorders. It seems likely that these alterations are due to pathophysiological changes within the CNS of these patients. This neuroendocrine window strategy has been particularly fruitful in research in affective disorders and, to a lesser extent, anorexia nervosa, but not very helpful in schizophrenia or Alzheimer's disease. Moreover, alterations in secretion of the hormones of the hypothalamic-pituitary-gonadal axis and of prolactin secretion in the major psychiatric disorders have been less closely scrutinized, and the extant findings remain less robust and more discordant. As more multidisciplinary tools become available, the specific brain areas mediating these abnormal neuroendocrine responses in patients with psychiatric disorders will be elucidated. Whether these neuroendocrine changes are responsible for the behavioral signs and symptoms of these diseases remains unclear.

ACKNOWLEDGMENTS

We are grateful to Nancy Winter for preparation of this manuscript. The authors are supported by NIMH MH-42088, MH-40524, MH-40159, MH-45975, MH-46791, and MH-44716.

REFERENCES

1. Copolov DL, Rubin RT: Endocrine disturbances in affective disorders and schizophrenia. *In* Nemeroff CB, Loosen PT, eds. Handbook of Clinical Psychoneuroendocrinology. New York: Guilford Press, 1988:760–194.
2. Risch SC, Lewine RJ, Kalin NH, et al: Limbic-hypothalamic-pituitary-adrenal axis activity and ventricular-to-brain ratio studies in affective illness and schizophrenia. Neuropsychopharmacology (in press).
3. Mendelwicz J, Linkowski P, Brauman H: TSH responses to TRH in women with unipolar and bipolar depression. Lancet 2:1079–1080, 1979.
4. Schilkrut R, Chandra O, Osswald M, et al: Growth hormone during sleep and with thermal stimulation in depressed patients. Neuropsychobiology 1:70–79, 1975.
5. Charney DS, Henninger GR, Steinberg DE et al: Adrenergic receptor sensitivity in depression: Effects of clonidine in depressed patients and health controls. Arch Gen Psychiatry 39:290–294, 1982.
6. Dinan TG, Barry S: Responses of growth hormone to desipramine in endogenous and non-endogenous depression. Br J Psychiatry 156:680–684, 1990.
7. Nemeroff CB, Kizer JS, Reynolds GP, Bissette G: Neuropeptides in Alzheimer's disease: A post-mortem study. Regul Pept 25:123–130, 1989a.
8. Nemeroff CB, Krishnan KRR, Belk BM, et al: Growth hormone response to GHRF Alzheimer's disease. Neuroendocrinology 50:663–666, 1989.
9. Landen J, Howarth N, Greenwood FC: Plasma sugar free fatty acid, growth hormone response to insulin II in patients with hypothalamic or pituitary dysfunction or anorexia nervosa. J Clin Invest 45:437–449, 1966.
10. Marks V, Howarth N, Greenwood FC: Plasma growth hormone levels in chronic starvation in man. Nature 208:686–687, 1965.
11. Casper RC, Davis JM, Pandey GN: The effect of nutritional status and weight changes on hypothalamic function tests anorexia nervosa. *In* Vigensky RA, ed. Anorexia Nervosa. New York: Raven Press, 1977:137–147.
12. Garfinkel PE, Brown GH, Stancer HC, Moldofsky H: Hypothalamic pituitary function in anorexia nervosa. Arch Gen Psychiatry 32:739–744, 1975.
13. Sherman B, Halmi KA: Effect of nutritional rehabilitation on hypothalamic pituitary function in anorexia nervosa. *In* Vigensky RA, ed. Anorexia Nervosa. New York: Raven Press, 1977:211–224.
14. Krishnan KRR, Ritchie JC, Manepalli AN, et al: What is the relationship between plasma ACTH and cortisol in normal human and depressed patients. *In* Schatzberg AF, Nemeroff CB, eds. HPA Axis, Physiology, Pathophysiology and Psychiatric Implications. New York: Raven Press, 1988:115–127.
15. Stokes P, Sikes CR: The hypothalamic-pituitary-adrenocortical axis in major depression. Endocrinol Metab Clin North Am 17:1–18, 1988.
16. Sachar E, Hellman L, Fukushima D, Gallagher T: Cortisol production in depressive illness. Arch Gen Psychiatry 23:289–298, 1970.
17. Krishnan KRR, Ritchie JC, Saunders WB, et al: Adrenocortical sensitivity to low dose ACTH administration in depressed patients. Biol Psychiatry 27:930–933, 1990.
18. Krishnan KRR, Doraiswamy PM, Lurie SN, et al: Pituitary size in depression. J Clin Endocrinol Metab 72:256–259, 1991.
19. Carroll BJ, Feinberg M, Greden JF, et al: A specific laboratory test for the diagnosis of melancholia. Arch Gen Psychiatry 38:15–22, 1981.
20. Nemeroff CB: The role of corticotropin-releasing factor in the pathogenesis of major depression. Pharmacopsychiatry 21:76–82, 1988.
21. Evans DL, Golden RJ: The dexamethasone suppression test. A review. In Loosen PT, Nemeroff CB, eds. Handbook of Clinical Psychoneuroendocrinology. New York: Guilford Press, 1987:313–335.
22. Roy A, Pickar D, Doran A, et al: The corticotropin releasing hormone stimulation test in chronic schizophrenia. Am J Psychiatry 143:1393–1397, 1986.
23. Sapolsky R, Armine M, Packar MA: Stress and glucocorticoids in aging. Endocrinol Metab Clin 16:965–980, 1987.
24. Prange AJ, Wilson IC, Lara PP, et al: Effects of thyrotropin-releasing hormone in depression. Lancet 1:999–1002, 1972.
25. Lesem MD, Kaye WH, Bissette G, et al: Low CSF immunoreactive-TRH levels in anorexia. Proceedings of the American Psychiatric Association, 143rd Annual Meeting, New Research Abstracts, 240, 1990.
26. Roy A, Bissette G, Nemeroff CB, et al: Cerebrospinal fluid thyrotropin-releasing hormone concentrations in alcoholics and normal controls. Biol Psychiatry 28:767–772, 1990.
27. Gold MS, Pottash ALC, Extein I: Hypothyroidism and depression. JAMA 245:1919–1922, 1981.
28. Prange AJ, Wilson IC, Breese GR, Lipton MA: Hormonal alteration of imipramine response: A review. In Sachar EJ, ed. Hormones, Behavior and Psychopathology. New York: Raven Press, 1976:41–67.
29. Bauer MS, Whybrow PC: Rapid cycling bipolar affective disorder. II. Treatment of refractory rapid cycling with high-dose levothyroxine: A preliminary study. Arch Gen Psychiatry 47:435–440, 1990.
30. Prange AJ, Wilson IC, Rabon AM, Lipton MA: Enhancement of imipramine antidepressant activity by thyroid hormone. Am J Psychiatry 126:457–469, 1969.
31. Prange AJ, Loosen PT, Wilson I, Lipton MA: The therapeutic use of hormones of the thyroid axis in depression. *In* Post CR, Ballenger J, eds. Neurobiology of Mood Disorders. Baltimore: Williams & Wilkins, 1980:311–322.

THE LABORATORY IN PSYCHIATRY

JOHN F. GREDEN, M.D.

GENERAL HISTORY AND DEFINITIONS

It is difficult for clinicians to make consistently accurate medical decisions when judgments must be based solely on clinical history and physical examination. It always has been; it always will be. Recognizing this fact, clinicians have long sought to develop laboratory tests—standardized, technical procedures designed to improve diagnostic and treatment monitoring skills. Historically, tests focused upon "analysis" of selected body fluids, such as urine, saliva, or sputum, with clinicians assuming that consistent abnormalities in these fluids would reflect underlying disease processes. Early efforts were limited to visual characterization, weight measurements, and smell, but as technology improved, quantitative measurements and analytic techniques expanded. Access to other parts of the body, such as blood and spinal fluid, also became possible.

The objective for most laboratory tests was to identify or quantify some variable that presumably indicated or "marked" the presence of an underlying pathophysiological process, thus aiding diagnosis. Some tests also proved valuable in monitoring treatment progress. Because these technical, standardized procedures conventionally were developed and "tested" in scientific laboratories, they became known colloquially as laboratory "tests." Because they also "mark" the presence of disease and sometimes change with severity, they occasionally are referred to as laboratory "markers" or "correlates."

The laboratory has become an integral part of medical practice. It also is controversial. Most consider laboratory assessments indispensable to good clinical practice. Others suggest that reliance upon laboratory measures has become exaggerated, and that the lab interferes with the traditional doctor-patient relationship, causes decay of conventional diagnostic skills, contributes to escalating costs, and sometimes exposes patients to unnecessary risks. As with most such debates, there are elements of truth in both perspectives. The laboratory is indispensable to modern medicine, but not always well used.

THE LABORATORY IN PSYCHIATRY

The past two decades have been characterized by an explosion of interest in the role of the laboratory in psychiatry. Thousands of articles have been published. Numerous symposia have focused solely upon proposed new tests. Extramural grant funding to evaluate new laboratory measures increased dramatically during the 1980s.

Behind this flourishing growth is a substantial and intriguing history.[1] For example, Gall's attempts in the early 1800s to develop the field of phrenology by quantifying and categorizing "bumps" or prominences on the skull and then linking these with personality features represented his attempt to develop a standardized laboratory measure of personality. If this chapter were being written during Gall's era, phrenology assuredly would have been on the list of laboratory procedures available to clinicians. That it is not is primarily attributable to the fact that subsequent studies failed to confirm Gall's claims of a close linkage between skull configuration and personality.

Comparable to phrenology, many laboratory tests are introduced but then fail after an initial period of optimism, becoming victims to the unrelenting scrutiny of the scientific process. Other tests are extremely successful. Some, such as serologic tests for syphilis, have dramatically changed the course of both general medicine and psychiatry.

Most medical and psychiatric laboratory markers have not been born in actual clinical settings. Instead, their introduction is preceded by important advances in other fields of science, notably chemistry, genetics, physics, mathematics, electrophysiology, and computer sciences. To illustrate, when chemical assays gained in sophistication, it enabled psychiatric clinicians to search for substances shown to be linked to abnormal perceptions, cognitions, affect, or behaviors. Examples included measurement of porphyrins to diagnose porphyria; ceruloplasmin levels measured for patients suspected of having Wilson's disease; thyroid measures being applied for cases of mental retardation due to myxedema; or the Wasserman Test used for screening patients who might have central nervous system (CNS) syphilis (a diagnosis that accounted for perhaps 20 per cent of patients in public psychiatric hospitals in the early twentieth century). The development of radioimmunoassay technology was especially important for assessing CNS diseases, since it enabled measurement of substances present in small concentrations.

Combinations of scientific advances further expanded the horizons of the psychiatric laboratory. To illustrate, breakthroughs in physics, nuclear medicine, neurochemistry, and computer sciences were combined by clinical investigators to enable imaging of brain anatomy and function,[2–5] leading to positron emission tomography (PET), single-photon emission computed tomography (SPECT), and magnetic resonance imaging (MRI) scanning. This pattern reflects the value of collegial interactions between psychiatry and other sciences.

Few laboratory tests can be considered specifically "psychiatric" in nature. Perhaps this is one reason why some psychiatrists have questioned the value of laboratory assessments, despite their well-documented impressive impact on patient well-being.

The laboratory in psychiatry, while not having the dominant role that it does in some medical specialties, already is important. It will play a progressively greater role in the future. Thus, all clinicians treating patients with psychiatric disorders need to understand the rationale for tests, the types of tests currently available, appropriate reasons for ordering them, common sources of variance that interfere with diagnostic performance, common pitfalls in interpreting results, and their relative financial impact (when used wisely, they often result in profound reductions in cost; when used inappropriately, they accelerate costs[6]). It is the objective of this chapter to address these issues. Detailed instructions on how to use and interpret specific tests have been published elsewhere.[7–10]

RATIONALE OF PSYCHIATRIC LABORATORY TESTS

The ideal laboratory test should be closely linked to a known underlying pathophysiological process; should be present when the "disease" is present, absent when the disease is not present; should quantifiably reflect severity of the known pathophysiology; should change in close temporal relationship with changes in the pathophysiology (ideally within minutes, hours, or days); and should be safe, of acceptable cost, repeatable at frequent time intervals, and free of influence by confounding variables such as age or concomitant medications.

There are no laboratory tests in any specialty of medicine that meet all these criteria. *None*. Yet, many clinicians continue to use this rigorous litany as their standard criteria for acceptance when a new test is proposed.

Barriers to developing laboratory tests for psychiatric patients are greater than for most specialties of medicine. There are three primary reasons. First, specific etiologies or pathophysiological processes are unknown for most psychiatric diagnoses. Second, there is profound overlap in clinical features, longitudinal course, and response to treatment for many psychiatric diagnoses (e.g., depression, eating disorders, panic, generalized anxiety disorder, and obsessive compulsive disorders have many clinical features in common; so do mania, psychotic depression, and schizophrenia). Such heterogeneity may reflect common denominators in pathophysiology, making it difficult to develop specific tests for specific DSM-III-R diagnoses. A third reason is that the brain, the location of major psychiatric pathophysiologies, has been difficult to investigate. It is well-protected, encased in the skull—an enigma, a hidden frontier.

INDIRECT LABORATORY CORRELATES

The brain's inaccessibility forced investigators to seek indirect strategies that presumably "mark" abnormalities in selected brain regions believed to be linked to various syndromes. The neuroendocrine strategy, for example, was designed to test the hypothesis that the imbalance of neurotransmitters in the limbic system responsible for depression concomitantly would produce neuroendocrine dysregulation, such as excessive secretion of cortisol or failure to suppress cortisol following the dexamethasone suppression test (DST). The hypothesis was generally confirmed, in that abnormal hypothalamic-pituitary-adrenal (HPA) test results tend to be present in many patients when the disease of depression is present, presumably because of a relatively close linkage to the same underlying pathophysiology. Unfortunately, specificity for the neuroendocrine strategy for depression per se was far less than desired, but efforts continue to improve clinical performance, and the neuroendocrine strategy served as a catalyst to promote many more indirect research efforts, such as tagging a dopaminergic ligand with a radioisotope and using PET scanning data to evaluate the number and density of dopamine receptors in selected brain areas of patients with schizophrenia.

Indirect hypotheses for new laboratory tests will continue to be required as long as we lack certainty about underlying pathophysiological processes. As we gain more information about etiology of psychiatric disorders, the search for laboratory tests will become more direct and sophisticated.

TYPES OF LABORATORY TESTS IN PSYCHIATRY

Laboratory tests in psychiatry can be arbitrarily categorized into six groups and are listed in alphabetical order. (Table 6–1): (1) biochemical; (2) brain imaging; (3) electrophysiological; (4) genetic; (5) neuroendocrine; (6) neuropsychological; and (7) miscellaneous, including pharmacological challenge strategies.

TABLE 6–1.   TYPES OF LABORATORY TESTS IN PSYCHIATRY

Biochemical
Brain imaging
Electrophysiological
Genetic
Neuroendocrine
Neuropsychological
Miscellaneous (including pharmacological challenge strategies)

REASONS FOR ORDERING LABORATORY TESTS IN PSYCHIATRY

There are three primary reasons for ordering a laboratory test for a patient with a psychiatric problem: (1) to aid in diagnosis; (2) to aid in nondiagnostic treatment decisions; and (3) for forensic purposes. In the future, a fourth reason may join this list—to screen and identify normal individuals to determine if they are at high risk for subsequent development of selected psychiatric disorders. Genetic screening and measurement of metabolites in cerebrospinal fluid to assess risk of suicide may be examples of this application.

Knowing the reason for ordering a laboratory test is a crucial starting point. Thus, each of these reasons will be reviewed in greater detail.

Diagnosis

Laboratory tests often aid the clinician in ruling in or ruling out a particular diagnosis. Rarely do tests make a diagnosis on their own merit, and even more rarely in the absence of other information. Indeed, an important conceptual axiom for the beginning clinician would be that "laboratory tests do *not* make diagnoses: clinicians make diagnoses, sometimes with the aid of laboratory tests."

When striving to make an accurate diagnosis, seven critical factors should be considered for every patient: (1) onset, including age and type (e.g., gradual, precipitous); (2) premorbid personality and functioning (how was the individual feeling prior to actual onset?); (3) family or genetic history; (4) longitudinal course (e.g., gradual deterioration versus episodic and recurrent); (5) clinical signs and symptoms; (6) laboratory test results; and (7) response to prior treatment. Laboratory tests clearly represent only one element in the necessary data pool for formulating a diagnosis.

Unfortunately, clinicians and investigators often fail to obtain concomitant information about all seven of these critical factors. This increases the risk that new syndromes will be "coined" and given new names when they may have the same or similar underlying pathophysiology. This pattern is a major reason for the heterogeneity that often plagues our nosology and serves as a curse for development of diagnostic laboratory tests. Prior to concluding that any laboratory result is specific for a given diagnosis,

test results must be compared to those from other patient subgroups, and from matched nonpatient controls. Ideally, these groups should be as homogeneous as possible. In "real life," laboratory data often end up being compared from two presumably different diagnoses (e.g., major depressive episode versus dysthymia) when these disorders actually are closely related. If overlap or insignificant differences are found, the specificity of the test is criticized. In actuality, it may be the nosological system that is flawed and that the two disorders ought not to be considered as separate and distinct, but as different ranges of severity of the same disorder. When considered from this perspective, it is evident that laboratory data often—certainly not always—may be providing more valuable information than our existing nosologic system. Nosologists do not routinely incorporate this perspective, however. Ideally, laboratory validation should be required before any new diagnoses are accepted. Past experience confirms that it is dangerous to uncritically accept existing diagnostic terms as the "gold standard."

Several axioms summarize these points: (1) the value of any given laboratory test must be considered in the context of why it is ordered; (2) a single laboratory test may be superb for one purpose, such as monitoring treatment, while poor for another, such as diagnosis; (3) diagnostic heterogeneity is a potent enemy of laboratory test development; and (4) laboratory data and clinical assessment data (onset, course, signs and symptoms, response to treatment, and outcome/prognosis) should be evaluated iteratively, rather than judging the value of laboratory data solely on the basis of existing nosological categories.

Four concepts are essential for interpreting laboratory data when used to aid diagnosis[11,12]:

1. *Sensitivity* of a test refers to its ability to identify true-positives or those individuals with the disease in question, such as by detecting a substance responsible for or closely associated with a disease.

2. *Specificity* of a test refers to the goal of excluding false-positives, thus identifying the normals in a sample; a specific test would detect the substance in question, but no others.

3. *Referent levels or values* refer to the fact that a range of laboratory results is obtained from most tests and that each value reflects a different probability that pathophysiology is present. Diagnostic likelihood thus changes depending upon where in that range a lab value lies. Referent values vary with the disease in question, the population studied, and the reasons for ordering the test.

4. *Confidence level* refers to the likelihood of finding true-positive cases, or those with the disease, by use of different referent levels.

The reason that these terms are so important is that most psychiatric disorders—comparable to most disorders in medicine—encompass a range of abnormality or severity. The human body simply does not work in "on-off" fashion for most functions. Therefore, another axiom would be that clinicians would be well advised to discard the outdated and misleading concept of "normal versus abnormal," and learn to approach diagnosis using referent values, noting that with changes in the actual laboratory result, there are relative changes in sensitivity, specificity, and confidence level.

Diagnostic laboratory tests are usually evaluated for the first time in research settings—protected environments with homogeneous, severe, medication-free patients. Initial diagnostic performance often is favorable in such unique settings. Following introduction into clinical practice, for many reasons diagnostic tests characteristically become less sensitive and less specific. In traditional clinical settings, patients usually are less homogeneous and less severe (especially if testing is done in ambulatory settings), the disorder being sought is less prevalent than it tends to be in specialized units, and confounding sources of variance are more widespread, including use of drugs, alcohol, tobacco, and medications. Medications often are being changed or withdrawn in clinical settings and this may represent a greater source of physiological variance than administration of an agent. Thus, poorer diagnostic performance initially should be anticipated in clinical settings. If given a chance, however, many tests undergo gradual refinement. To illustrate, tests designed to aid neurologists in diagnosing a possible brain tumor have become more numerous and sophisticated (Table 6–2). Old tests are not always discarded, but often simply augmented by additional strategies. Tests then are used in combinations or in sequences, a pattern that may be extremely helpful if used knowledgeably, or extremely misleading if used carelessly. As illustrated in Table 6–2, tests used to diagnose psychiatric diagnoses also are undergoing advances in development. Thus, the shortcomings of a single test (e.g., the DST) should not serve as a rationale to reject an entire strategy. Patience and understanding about laboratory developments are essential if progress is to occur. If initial expectations of practicing psychiatrists are excessive—as they appear to have

TABLE 6–2. HISTORICAL PROGRESSIONS OF DIAGNOSTIC LABORATORY TESTS: EXAMPLES IN NEUROLOGY AND PSYCHIATRY

To Aid Neurologists in Diagnosing Brain Tumor or Space-Occupying Lesion	To Aid Psychiatrists in Diagnosing Limbic-HPA Dysregulation and "Depression"
Neurological exam	Psychiatric exam
EEG	17-OHCS or 17-KGS
Pneumoencephalogram	24-hr UFC
Radioisotope brain scan	Plasma cortisol
Arteriogram	DST
CT scan	CRH challenge test
MRI scan	Neuropeptides
rCBF, PET, or SPECT scan	DST/CRH test

TABLE 6–3. AXIOMS FOR USING PSYCHIATRIC DIAGNOSTIC LABORATORY TESTS

Laboratory tests do *not* make diagnoses; clinicians make diagnoses, sometimes with the aid of laboratory tests

Laboratory tests represent only one component of the data pool required for diagnosis and should never be considered in isolation

Psychiatric laboratory tests usually have higher sensitivity, specificity, and confidence levels when initially evaluated in research settings, and decreased performance when introduced into clinical practice

Diagnostic performance of a laboratory test may improve when combined with other tests, but care should be taken to insure that one testing process does not interfere with others

Low prevalence of a disease dramatically decreases diagnostic performance; prevalence can be increased by prior clinical screening

No laboratory tests have perfect sensitivity, specificity and confidence levels; clinicians need to be realistic in their expectations about tests

Laboratory tests are probability statements; clinicians should abandon concepts of "normal versus abnormal," and learn to use reference values, noting that confidence levels for a diagnosis change with the actual laboratory result

Sensitivity and specificity have inverse relationships for most laboratory tests; the clinician should decide whether to select reference values that maximize sensitivity or specificity based on treatability of the disease in question

  High specificity for diseases with no treatment and poor prognosis [e.g., human immunodeficiency virus (HIV) infection or Alzheimer's disease]

  High sensitivity for diseases with known, safe treatments and good prognosis (e.g., panic disorder, depression)

been—all test strategies will be promptly categorized as disappointing failures. This would bode poorly for our future.

Genetic principles for scientific interpretation of diagnostic laboratory data receive intriguingly little attention in medical school. Many clinicians never learned them, have forgotten them, or assume them to be unimportant. In contrast, they are vital. Some of the more important axioms are summarized in Table 6–3.

Treatment

Diagnosis tends to receive most attention, but the majority of laboratory tests in medicine probably are ordered to monitor treatment. There are three primary reasons for ordering tests during treatment: (1) monitoring progress; (2) documenting compliance or adequacy of treatment; and (3) identifying complications.

Monitoring Progress

To be valuable to clinicians in monitoring treatment, a test generally needs to be state-related (i.e., able to reflect severity of the pathophysiology and change in close temporal relationship with changes in the disease; be relatively safe, noninvasive, and inexpensive; and have prompt turnaround). Fortunately, for psychiatrists, a few tests meet these criteria. More can be expected to do so.

Several *biochemical tests* have well-established indications for serial monitoring to determine if the disease process is improving, remaining stable, or worsening. These include drug screens for pharmacological substances in plasma, blood, or urine in patients suspected of abusing drugs; and measures of toxicology (e.g., in patients diagnosed as having heavy metal intoxication).[13]

Electrophysiological measures have important applications in serial monitoring of treatment progress.[14,15] Patients with cognitive or behavioral abnormalities secondary to complex partial seizures should be monitored with periodic electroencephalograph (EEG) tests during treatment to monitor the underlying pathophysiology. Patients with narcolepsy and psychiatric manifestations similarly can be monitored with multiple sleep latency measures during treatment until stability has been achieved. Polysomnography findings of shortened rapid eye movement (REM) latency, impaired sleep efficiency, and increased REM density have been hypothesized to be of diagnostic value for depressed patients, and this is being studied in many research settings, but serial monitoring of depressed patients with sleep EEG assessments is still in the stage of research assessment, as are tests of psychomotor function.[16,17]

Several *neuroendocrine tests*—especially of the HPA axis—have been studied rather thoroughly as potential markers for monitoring treatment. Early HPA studies with the DST clearly indicated that for most depressed patients, nonsuppression was state-related.[18] While not totally specific, DST levels were generally higher during severe depression, less abnormal during mild depression, and absent during euthymia. Based on this observation, extensive work was conducted to determine if repeated use of the DST could be used to monitor progress. Early reports were promising. Subsequent studies conducted in more clinical settings predictably were less clear-cut. Nevertheless, in 1985, Arana and Baldassarani[19] conducted a meta-analysis of 145 patients from 13 studies to assess whether DST "normalization" correlated with outcome. The data showed that 81 per cent of those who normalized a previously nonsuppressive DST had good outcome, compared with only 23 per cent of those who failed to normalize. Non-normalization earlier had been hypothesized to predict a high risk of relapse.[20] The American Psychiatric Association compiled a task force to assess this issue in 1987[21] and concluded, on the basis of a meta-analysis, that "non-normalization may be a poor prognostic sign. This highly relevant potential clinical application of the DST requires further investigation." Subsequent studies unfortunately have not been forthcoming, partially because the profession at large became disappointed that the DST did not meet lofty expectations. While having been studied perhaps more than any test other than EEGs, serial neuroendocrine measures still must be considered a research tool, with many factors remaining to be assessed (e.g., serial plasma dexamethasone concentrations).[22] However, based on available data, it would appear reasonable to recommend that patients with well-documented affective pathophysiology—regardless of specific DSM-III-R diagnosis—and a nonsuppressive DST should have repeat testing completed during the course of treatment; if DST results remain nonsuppressive, medications certainly should be continued, the patient should be monitored closely, consideration should be given to assess adequacy of plasma concentrations if tricyclics are being used, treatment augmentation with additional medications might be considered, or alternative diagnoses should be assessed, such as a mild Cushing's disease secondary to a pituitary microadenoma. All these options are generated only with the aid of laboratory data.

The only other neuroendocrine test that has been studied meaningfully for serial monitoring is the thyroid releasing hormone/thyroid stimulating hormone (TRH/TSH) thyroid challenge test. Data still are sketchy, but persistent abnormalities suggest ongoing pathophysiology.

Neuropsychological testing has a long tradition of being used for serial monitoring. Examples include assessment of memory function in patients with head injuries and suspected Alzheimer's disease. Detailed reviews of these tests as well as new advances to be anticipated in this field are published elsewhere.[10]

In research settings, *brain imaging* measures sometimes have been repeated to monitor longitudinal course. It is intriguing to note how readily many clinicians accept the value of brain imaging measures as diagnostic tools for serial monitoring, despite the paucity of data. This is especially true for EEG spectral topography (brain mapping), for which we have witnessed a proliferation of equipment and an increase in the number of studies in clinical settings, despite the absence of well-established diagnostic sensitivity, specificity, or documented change during treatment. It should be remembered that pictures of brain anatomy and function are mathematical constructs derived from measures of brain flow, glucose metabolism, distribution of a radioisotope, receptor binding, or electrical activity, and not photographs per se. Clinical use of brain imaging tests is still in the research stage of development, except for the possible exception of using PET imaging to aid neurosurgeons in the localization of a seizure focus prior to surgical intervention.

One serial application of brain measures that has been relatively well studied involves abnormal ventricular brain ratios (VBR), found in some patients with schizophrenia.[23] Specifically, patients with negative symptoms (e.g., anhedonia, alogia, amotivational syndrome, apathy) are more prone to have enlarged lateral ventricles, as measured by VBR. This finding is among the better established in psychiatry, and since it may have long-range treatment and prognostic implications, it appears reasonable to suggest that schizophrenics with evidence of enlarged ventricles or abnormal ventricular:brain ratios should have repeat CT or MRI scans—perhaps annually or every several years until stability is demonstrated—to determine if the abnormality is progressive. With this exception, there are no well-established uses for repeat brain imaging with computed tomography (CT), MRI, rCBF, PET, or SPECT scans for patients with psychiatric diagnoses. Such applications predictably will emerge, but only after there are better-identified linkages between brain imaging findings and underlying pathophysiology.

There are no well-established applications to date for *serial* monitoring of *genetic tests* for specific psychiatric disorders.

Rating scales represent perhaps the simplest examples of standardized instruments to monitor progress. Scales such as the Hamilton Depression Rating Scale, the Yale-Brown Obsessive Compulsive Inventory, and The State-Trait Anxiety Index conventionally are not considered laboratory tests, but perhaps should be. All good rating scales have undergone a rigorous process of development comparable to that of lab tests, including comparisons among patients with the disease in question, those with other types of disease, and normal controls. They also have been refined to the point where there is good inter-rater reliability and concurrent and construct validity. Rating scales are among the most valuable, easy, and inexpensive tools for monitoring progress during treatment. Many are designed to be self-rated, completed by patients before they see the clinician, scored in a minute or so, and readily incorporated into the medicolegal record. Busy clinicians may find it helpful to send a rating battery by mail to patients prior to their first appointment, so that data are available at the time of assessment. Rating scales generally save time, since most can be distributed, completed, and collected by trained technicians, nurses, or secretaries. Sadly, rating scales are not used widely by most practicing clinicians. They should be.

Documenting Compliance or Treatment Adequacy

COMPLIANCE

Patients do not always comply with their psychiatrist's recommendations. More disturbing, they sometimes disguise or even lie about this lack of compliance, even when asked directly. Lack of compliance can prevent improvement, increase the risk of relapse, or produce inappropriate uncertainty about diagnosis.

Laboratory tests sometimes help psychiatrists to determine if patients are complying with pharmacological treatment, since many medications can be measured in plasma or blood.[24] These include most antidepressants, neuroleptics, benzodiazepines, or anticonvulsants. Laboratory confirmation of compliance should be considered for patients who are refractory, have multiple relapses, or who convey other signs suggesting that noncompliance might be occurring. This simple process might enable beneficial alterations in treatment strategy (e.g., the use of a depot neuroleptic for noncompliant patients with schizophrenia). The small cost often proves to be a worthwhile investment considering the dramatic reductions associated with prevention of even a single repeat hospitalization.

TREATMENT ADEQUACY

Prescription of a treatment does not always produce favorable outcome, even when that treatment is known to be efficacious. For favorable outcome to occur, most treatments need to be adequate in both dosage and duration. Laboratory tests have long been available to quantify adequacy of treatment.[25] These are especially valuable for patients with affective disorders. While some controversy remains, current clinical indications would endorse periodic assessments of treatment adequacy for patients receiving tricyclic antidepressants, lithium, or carbamazepine. Adequate data have been compiled for only three heterocyclic agents—imipramine, desipramine, and nortriptyline. For any of these, if plasma concentrations are inadequate (or below the therapeutic window for nortriptyline), dosage should be increased. For imipramine, the clinician is striving to achieve levels about 200 ng/ml, combining both imipramine and desipramine (DMI) levels. For DMI, levels should be higher than 125 ng/ml. For nortriptyline, the projected range is 50 to 150 ng/ml. If levels are found to be in the toxic range or above the therapeutic window for nortriptyline, dosage should be decreased. Perhaps a majority of treatment failures in patients with major unipolar depressive episodes may be attributable to inadequate medication levels. This problem is easily identified and usually easily remedied. Again, the results clearly are worth the small fee for a plasma level, since adequacy of treatment may prevent weeks, months, or even years of a refractory course. A related application occurs when some patients switch pharmaceutical brands of tricyclics or switch to a generic product. An unknown percentage subsequently experience changes in plasma levels and a return of symptoms, probably because of different pharmacokinetics. Again, a simple laboratory test might provide valuable information to the clinician. Most affective disorders have a lifetime course. Thus, many—perhaps most—may require long-term or lifetime maintenance,[26] a phenomenon that is just being discovered by many clinicians. During that maintenance, whenever there are major fluctuations in clinical status, plasma levels should be compiled to assess adequacy. Finally, a small number of patients fail to metabolize heterocyclic antidepressants adequately, and quickly achieve toxic levels. If undiagnosed and unchecked, severe consequences may result (cardiac risks especially increase), or patients will not comply and treatment will fail. For those complaining of untoward symptoms, especially anticholinergic in nature, testing of plasma levels is indicated to rule out toxicity.

In all situations, the blood sample should be obtained approximately 10 to 14 hours following the last dose, usually in the morning. Proper collection techniques are essential and should be well known by all established laboratories. The same laboratory should be used consistently for each patient, since labs will vary in their results.

Considering all available evidence, it seems unreasonable to not utilize tricyclic plasma levels to greater extent in clinical practice. Despite this, most physicians do not do so, especially those in primary care settings.[24] It should be noted that effective or adequate plasma levels have *not* been determined for a number of medications, including some widely prescribed antidepressants such as fluoxetine. For these treatments, plasma levels would not be indicated.

The monitoring of treatment adequacy for patients receiving lithium has a well-established history.[27,28] Insufficient lithium levels are associated with a higher risk of relapses in bipolar patients. Intriguingly, the need to monitor lithium levels was accepted without debate by clinicians, probably because of concerns about toxicity.

Carbamazepine levels initially were shown to have relevance during the treatment of patients with temporal lobe epilepsy or partial complex seizures. When carbamazepine was introduced as a treatment for refractory bipolar patients, monitoring of levels similarly was recommended, striving to reach a therapeutic window between 4 and 12 mg/ml. In reality, this level is based on an assumption that there might be similarities between bipolar patients and those with epilepsy, and minimal data have been compiled to support this window in psychiatric patients. However, carbamazepine promotes its own metabolism; thus, it seems prudent for psychiatrists to check levels 5 days after full dosage has been achieved, and then once again 3 to 4 weeks later to insure that levels have not dropped. After that, testing of carbamazepine levels would only be indicated if there were a deterioration in clinical course.

To date, effective therapeutic plasma levels have not been identified for neuroleptics. There are no current clinical indications for monitoring neuroleptic levels, other than to confirm compliance.

Identifying Complications

Some treatments have inherent risks. When it is determined that a patient needs a treatment despite known risks, serial monitoring may identify known complications at an early stage, while possibly still reversible. Two important examples are with patients receiving carbamazepine (Tegretol) and clozapine (Clozaril), both known to occasionally produce hematological complications, specifically agranulocytosis or aplastic anemia or both, and hepatic toxicity. While hematological side effects probably occur in fewer than 5 per cent of patients treated with either agent, they can be serious and life threatening. Thus, serial monitoring of hematological and hepatic measures is essential for those being treated. For carbamazepine, this should occur before treatment and at least every 2 weeks for the first 2 months of treatment. Then, if values are stable, testing can be conducted once every 2 to 3 months. For clozapine, hematological testing should be conducted weekly. Traditionally, primary clinicians have been responsible for monitoring the risk of complications. This tradition recently was challenged when a pharmaceutical firm linked availability of clozapine to mandatory laboratory screening conducted by a dedicated agency, for a substantial fee. This policy presumably emerged because of fear that clinicians would fail to monitor adequately. A stirring debate reversed the mandatory nature of this policy. The primary clinician retains responsibility. It is a weighty responsibility. Policies and monitoring schedules need to be clear-cut, with effective time-cue mechanisms so that periodic checks are not forgotten.

Forensic

Laboratory data have long been used as evidence in judicial settings. Sometimes, tests are specifically ordered for legal purposes, usually to determine the presence, absence, or severity of some pathophysiological process so that this information can be used as evidence in court proceedings. Other times, they are ordered for defensive purposes. Regardless of stated rationale, the procedures for using a test for forensic reasons should be stringent and the same as those employed in good clinical practice.

Screening or Risk Assessment

As test sophistication improves, it may be possible to use tests to screen patients to determine if they are at risk for selected psychiatric disorders. For example, once Huntington's disease became localized on chromosome 4, genetic screening for this disorder became possible. Other genetic screens (cystic fibrosis, neurofibromatosis) already are available. Heterogeneity (e.g., the fact that schizophrenia may be of multiple subtypes and may have different etiologies) may make it difficult to identify genetic screens for some psychiatric disorders, but with the astonishing breakthroughs in molecular genetics and ongoing efforts to map the genome, it is reasonable to predict that trait screens will be available for selected psychiatric disorders within a decade.

State-related biochemical or neuroendocrine screening is more precarious and susceptible to sources of variance, but the potential value to clinicians is profound. For example, many clinicians struggle to assess and quantify risk for suicide. Recent research, while still in developmental stages, would suggest that patients with low levels of serotonin metabolite [5-hydroxyindoleacetic acid(5-HIAA)] in cerebrospinal fluid (CSF),[28] high levels of plasma or CSF methoxyhydroxyphenylglycol (MHPG), and elevated glucocorticoid levels might be at especially high risk.

TYPES OF PSYCHIATRIC LABORATORY TESTS IN CURRENT PRACTICE

It is striking to note how few tests are widely employed in current psychiatric practice. These are listed in Table 6–4.

General Guidelines for Commonly Used Tests

Lithium

Plasma samples for lithium levels should be obtained at approximately the same time of day at each sampling, ideally 11 to 13 hours after the last dose was ingested. Assessment of thyroid function (T_3, T_4, TSH, and antithyroid antibodies) should be conducted before treatment and repeated annually, paying special attention to TSH changes. Renal function (creatinine, creatinine clearance, and 24-hour urine volume) also should be evaluated annually for all patients receiving long-term maintenance lithium. Pregnancy testing should occur before starting women of childbearing age on lithium, since the fetus is especially susceptible to lithium-induced thyroid changes.

Antidepressants

With tricyclic antidepressants, dosage should be increased as rapidly as safely tolerated, and plasma levels tested 4 or 5 days after the last dosage adjustment, when the patient can be assumed to be at steady state, ideally after about 2 weeks of treatment. Psychiatrists should request laboratory personnel to include active metabolites in their assessment, since these are relevant when considering treatment adequacy. It should be noted that plasma levels for tricyclics have been reported to be of value for children as well as adults.[24] Psychiatrists might also wish to advise mothers receiving antidepressants to avoid breastfeeding their babies, since most antidepressants appear to be secreted in breast milk.

TABLE 6–4. PATTERNS OF UTILIZATION OF PSYCHIATRIC LABORATORY TESTS

In Current Practice
  Medication levels
    Lithium
    Selected antidepressants
    Carbamazepine/anticonvulsants
  Medication "screens" (blood, urine, exhaled breath)
    Substances of abuse
    Alcohol
  Medical/neurological "screens"
    Electroencephalography (EEG)
    Computed tomography (CT) or magnetic resonance imaging (MRI)

Should be Considered for More Widespread Use
  Panic disorder
    Challenge tests (e.g., lactate challenge)
  "Depressive" symptoms (depression, anorexia, schizoaffective disorder, panic disorder)
    Hypothalamic-pituitary-adrenal screening and monitoring (e.g., DST, CRH test)
    Thyroid challenge tests (TRH/TSH) and thyroid screening (T_3, T_4, TSH, and autoantibody screens)
    Polysomnography (sleep EEG) for refractory cases
  Schizophrenia
    CT or MRI brain imaging
  Anxiety
    Drug screen for caffeine, ephedrine, phenylpropanolamine (PPA), amphetamines, or cocaine

Possible or Likely in the Future
  Genetic screening
  Brain imaging using PET and SPECT
  Dim-Light Melatonin Onset (DLMO) for chronobiological and seasonal disorders
  Multiple Sleep Latency Test, genetic typing and polysomnography for patients suspected of narcolepsy
  CSF 5-HIAA for assessment of suicidal risk
  Pharmacological challenges for diagnosis of schizophrenia (amphetamine or methylphenidate challenge test)
  Combinations

Research Tests With an Uncertain Future
  Psychomotor measures (e.g., facial electromyography, pupillometry, limb motility)
  Psychoimmunology measures (e.g., natural killer cell, mitogen stimulation or lymphocytes)
  Biochemical and receptor studies (e.g., α_2-adrenergic, ^{3}[H]imipramine, plasma HVA, dopamine β-hydroxylase)
  Neuroendocrine tests (e.g., melatonin, melanocyte stimulating hormone, growth hormone)

Medication Screening

When medication screens are conducted on blood, urine, or exhaled breath, it is important to note that the routine drug screens often used in many hospital laboratories lack the sensitivity that psychiatrists often desire.[13] In many settings, drug screens are conducted by thin-layer chromatography (TLC). Performance would be improved by using enzymatic assays, antibody-based tests (which often have 100-fold greater sensitivity), or gas chromatography–mass spectroscopy (GC-MS), which may have a 1000-fold increase in performance. Urine samples should ideally be the first voiding of the morning, and supervised. These guidelines should be part of routine orders when drug screens are ordered in hospital settings. For interpretive purposes, a negative screen does not mean the absence of substance abuse, especially if TLC is used. To illustrate, TLC detects cocaine use only up to 12 to 24 hours after last use, compared to 2 to 3 days after last use for radioimmunoassay (RIA) or enzyme immunoassay, and 7 to 10 days after last use for GC-MS. Conversely, if a positive result is obtained using TLC, a second testing with a more specific approach should be ordered to confirm a positive result before using laboratory data to support a diagnosis of substance abuse. This may be problematic in some circumstances, because days or weeks may pass before a second test is ordered, and during this interval, the individual may be able to refrain from prior drug use. If temporal circumstances dictate, and the laboratory offers GC-MS, it should be ordered specifically.

Table 6–4 (under "Should be Considered for More Widespread Use") lists tests that the author believes would benefit clinical practice if used more commonly. This listing will be considered provocative by some, premature by others. Each of the tests on this list are safe, relatively well-established, and has the potential to focus diagnosis and treatment efforts, thus helping to avoid inappropriate or prolonged treatments, refractoriness, or wrong treatment. If a lactate challenge test helped confirm an uncertain diagnosis of panic disorder, for example, and patients were treated early with imipramine, phenelzine, or alprazolam, morbidity could be limited, in some cases secondary agoraphobia could be prevented, and patterns of dependency on alcohol or benzodiazepines might be prevented.

A separate comment is warranted with regard to greater use of the DST for patients with affective features. During the past several decades, psychiatrists were relatively preoccupied with searching for specific tests for individual psychiatric conditions, and the DST was the focus of this effort. The effort may have been unwise and misguided. As described in other sections of this chapter, our nosology may be too heterogeneous to enable us to develop specific tests for many psychiatric conditions. The newest perspective is to use test results to inform us about commonalities of pathophysiology. It is intriguing to note that while the DST clearly lacks specificity for depression per se, DST nonsuppression is predominantly found in a range of conditions that are responsive to heterocyclic or monoamine oxidase inhibitor (MAOI) treatments. These include delusional depression, nondelusional depression, schizoaffective disorder (depressed type), anorexia nervosa, panic disorder, and dysthymia. Abnormal HPA results in this case may be indicating a common pathophysiological underpinning for all these disorders, with differences in clinical features dependent upon differences in age, gender, severity, chronicity, or involvement of other neurotransmitters (e.g., dopamine). Thus, the DST, while not making a specific diagnosis of depression, might be conveying important information to the clinician that the patient is likely to be responsive to an agent such as imipramine. Such a prospect warrants further systematic investigation.

MAJOR SOURCES OF VARIANCE IN CLINICAL UTILIZATION OF THE LABORATORY

Laboratory tests in all fields of medicine are subject to error.[1,6,11,12] Table 6–5 lists generic sources of variance common to many tests. It is essential to note that each test has unique factors that may produce variability. Some are modified by age, others are not. Some test results differ tremendously between men and women; others show no meaningful differences. Some assays have excellent repeatability and reproducibility; others are extremely labile, and subject to assay drift. Even tests that are assumed to be well established and accurate often are subject to assay error. To illustrate, split samples from the same specimen were sent to different commercial laboratories to measure tricyclic plasma concentrations, and values ranged from 50 to 150 per cent of the actual value. Laboratories are not perfect. Results from one laboratory cannot be uncritically extrapolated to another. Laboratory personnel often seem to understand that better than clinicians.

One factor that alters the performance of all diagnostic tests is the prevalence of the disease in question. If a disease is scarce in the population being tested, even if a test has a desired low false-positive

TABLE 6–5. MAJOR SOURCES OF VARIANCE IN CLINICAL UTILIZATION OF THE LABORATORY

Assay variance
Age
Severity
Prevalence of the disease in the clinical setting
Concomitant medications, drugs, alcohol, tobacco, caffeine, or medication washout
Failure to use referent levels

rate, the number of false-positive results may equal or exceed the number of true-positives. Diagnostic performance might thus be considered poor, because of low specificity. In actuality, the test might be excellent, if only this concept were understood. The phenylketonuria (PKU) screening test is an example of a test that has excellent sensitivity, excellent specificity, but is poor in "making" a diagnosis because of the low prevalence of PKU in the population. In the past, a number of studies seeking to assess the impact of newly proposed psychiatric tests failed to even consider the role of prevalence, and yet concluded that the test was inadequate in performance. Hopefully we have learned from prior errors.

PHILOSOPHICAL PERSPECTIVES: WHAT CAN THE LABORATORY TEACH US?

Most clinicians evaluate the value of a laboratory test on the basis of its day-to-day impact on clinical decision making. The laboratory is capable of doing more. It has been and continues to be important in teaching psychiatrists many long-term philosophical lessons about the diseases that burden our patients.

For example, laboratory data played a major role in forcing modern societies to rethink mystical concepts about etiology of psychiatric disease; this battle is not yet won. Psychoimmunology, electrophysiology, and brain imaging data, by demonstrating covert and overt linkages between internal and external events and bodily functions, have challenged antiquated concepts of a mind-body dichotimization. Laboratory results repeatedly remind us how commonly psychopathology is linked to medical disease, how important it is for psychiatrists to retain medical skills and orientation, and how mental health treatments that fail to incorporate a thorough medical assessment will usually be doomed to failure. Lab data even prompt us to rethink poorly conceptualized treatment delivery models. For example, current data reveal that many patients with depression, schizophrenia, or other diagnoses have concomitant use of pharmacological substances that may cause or at least contribute to their symptoms. Considering that comorbidity between drug abuse, alcoholism, and other psychopathologies is the norm in many clinical settings rather than the exception, it makes little sense to perpetuate separate treatment networks, to have different regulatory policies for psychiatric and substance abuse disorders, or different third-party funding guidelines. Yet, this still remains the case.

Intelligent use of the laboratory requires understanding and skill. Considering the major role played by the laboratory, and the assuredly greater role it will play in the psychiatry of the future, perhaps all physicians ought to spend a segment of their training in a laboratory. To know the lab is to love it.

REFERENCES

1. Greden JF: Laboratory tests in psychiatry. In Kaplan HI, Sadock BJ, eds. Comprehensive Textbook of Psychiatry. IV. Baltimore: Williams and Wilkins, 1985:2028–2033.
2. Sokoloff L: Relationships among local functional activity, energy metabolism and blood flow in the central nervous system. Fed Proc 40:2311–2316, 1981.
3. Kety SS, Woodford RB, Harmel MH, et al: Cerebral blood flow and metabolism in schizophrenia. Am J Psychiatry 104:765–770, 1948.
4. Ingvar DH, Franzen G: Distribution of cerebral activity in chronic schizophrenia. Lancet 2:1484–1486, 1974.
5. Sokoloff I: The radioactive deoxyglucose method. In Agranoff BW, Aprison MH, eds. Advances in Neurochemistry. New York: Plenum Publishing Corporation, 1982:1–81.
6. Griner PF, Glaser RJ: Misuse of laboratory tests and diagnostic procedures. N Engl J Med 307:1336, 1982.
7. Gold MS, Pottash ALC: Diagnostic and Laboratory Testing in Psychiatry. New York: Plenum Medical Book Company, 1986.
8. Widmann FK: Clinical Interpretation of Laboratory Tests. 9th ed. Philadelphia: FA Davis Company, 1983.
9. Hall RCW, Beresford TP: Handbook of Psychiatric Diagnostic Procedures. Vol. II. Medical & Scientific Books, Spectrum Publications, Inc., 1985.
10. Zappulla RA, LeFever FF, Jaeger J, Bilder R: Windows on the Brain: Neuropsychology's Technological Frontiers. Ann NY Acad Sci 620:1991.
11. Galen RS: Application of the predictive value model in the analysis of test effectiveness. Clin Lab Med 4:685, 1982.
12. Galen RS, Gambino SR: Beyond Normality: The Predictive Value and Efficiency of Medical Diagnoses. New York: John Wiley & Sons, 1975.
13. Vereby K, Martin D, Gold MS: Drug abuse: Interpretation of laboratory tests. In Gold MS, Pottash ALC, eds. Diagnostic and Laboratory Testing in Psychiatry. New York: Plenum Medical Book Company, 1986:155–167.
14. Struve FA: Clinical electroencephalography as an assessment method in psychiatric practice. In Hall RCW, Beresford TP, eds. Handbook of Psychiatric Diagnostic Procedures. Vol. II. Medical & Scientific Books, Spectrum Publications, Inc., 1985:49–73.
15. Karacan I, Williams RL: Sleep electroencephalography. In Hall RCW, Beresford TP, eds. Handbook of Psychiatric Diagnostic Procedures. Vol. II. Medical & Scientific Books, Spectrum Publications, Inc., 1985.
16. Greden JF, Carroll BJ: Psychomotor function in affective disorders: An overview of new monitoring techniques. Am J Psychiatry 138:1441–1448, 1981.
17. Greden JF: Tests of psychomotor function. In Hall RCW, Beresford, TP, eds. Handbook of Psychiatric Diagnostic Procedures. Vol. I and II. Medical & Scientific Books, Spectrum Publications, Inc., 1985.
18. Greden JF, Gardner R, King LD, et al: Dexamethasone suppression tests in antidepressant treatment of melancholia: The process of normalization and test-retest reproducibility. Arch Gen Psychiatry 40:493, 1983.
19. Arana GW, Baldessarani RJ, Orsteen M: The dexamethasone suppression test for diagnosis and prognosis in psychiatry. Arch Gen Psychiatry 42:1193–1204, 1985.
20. Greden JF, Albala AA, Haskett RF, et al: Normalization of dexamethasone suppression test: A laboratory index of recovery from endogenous depression. Biol Psychiatry 15:449–458, 1980.
21. APA Task Force Report on Laboratory Tests in Psychiatry: The dexamethasone suppression test: An overview of its current status in psychiatry. Am J Psychiatry 144:1253–1262, 1987.
22. Devanand DP, Sackeim HA, Lo E, et al: Serial dexamethasone suppression tests and plasma dexamethasone levels. Arch Gen Psychiatry 48:525–533, 1991.
23. Olson SC, Nasrallah HA, Coffman JA, Schwarzkopf SB: CT

and MRI abnormalities in schizophrenia: Relationship
with negative symptoms. *In* Greden JF, Tandon R, eds.
Negative Schizophrenia Symptoms: Pathophysiology and
Clinical Implications. Washington DC: American Psychiatric Press, Inc., 1991:145–160.

24. Preskorn SH, Gold MS, Extein I: Therapeutic drug level monitoring in psychiatry. *In* Gold MS, Pottach ALC, eds. Diagnostic and Laboratory Testing in Psychiatry. New York:
Plenum Medical Book Company, 1986:131–154.

25. Task Force on the Use of Laboratory Tests in Psychiatry:
Tricyclic antidepressants—blood level measurements and
clinical outcome: An APA task force report. Am J Psychiatry 142:155, 1985.

26. Frank E, Kupfer DJ, Perel JM, et al: Three-year outcomes for
maintenance therapies in recurrent depression. Arch Gen
Psychiatry 47:1093–1099, 1990.

27. Coombs HI, Coombs RR, Mee UG: Methods of serum lithium
estimation. *In* Johnson FN, ed. Lithium Research and
Therapy. New York: Academic Press, 1975:165–179.

28. Cooper TB, Carroll BJ: Monitoring lithium dose levels: Estimation of lithium in blood and other body fluids. J Clin
Psychopharmacol 1:53–61, 1981.

29. Roy A, De Jong J, Linnoila M: Cerebrospinal fluid monoamine metabolites and suicidal behavior in depressed patients. Arch Gen Psychiatry, 46:609–612, 1989.

7

GENETICS OF PSYCHIATRIC DIAGNOSIS AND TREATMENT

ELIZABETH S. BOWMAN, M.D. and JOHN I. NURNBERGER, JR., M.D., PH.D.

Major psychiatric disorders, like many other medical conditions, appear to result in part from inherited predisposition. The primary evidence for this is
from genetic epidemiological studies. Twin, adoption, and family studies are helpful in determining if
illnesses are inherited, the mode of inheritance, how
much risk relatives have for developing the illness,
and what other kinds of illnesses (spectrum conditions) may result from different expressions of the
same gene(s).

Twin studies provide a general estimate of heritability by enabling comparison of rates of illness concordance in monozygotic (MZ) and dizygotic (DZ)
twins. If an illness is under genetic control, the concordance in MZ twins should be greater than that of
DZ twins. If the concordance in MZ twins is less
than 100 per cent, environmental influences are presumed to be present. Comparing biological parameters in MZ twins who are illness-discordant may assist in identifying those environmental influences.

Adoption studies attempt to separate genetic and
environmental influences on illness prevalence. In
one method, illness rates are compared in the biological and adoptive families of adopted persons with
and without the illness. Genetic transmission is im-
plied if the prevalence of the illness is greater in the
biological relatives of the ill adoptees than among
the biological relatives of well adoptees. In another
method, the adopted-away children of ill and well

parents are studied. If adopted-away offspring of ill
parents have an increased incidence of the illness,
genetic transmission is supported.

Family studies, conducted by direct examination
of all available family members, provide more reliable information on illness rates than are found by a
family history provided by a few informants. Family
studies may provide information about the mode of
genetic transmission and the relatives' risk of manifesting the illness (morbid risk). Family studies are
consistent with a genetic contribution if the relatives
of ill persons have higher rates of the illness than the
relatives of well persons. Putative spectrum conditions should also aggregate in families of ill persons.

In high-risk studies, the offspring of patients with
an illness are studied before they pass through the
age of risk. Biological markers and rates of spectrum
conditions in offspring of patients and controls may
be compared. Follow-up studies may compare the
traits of offspring who later become ill and those
who do not. By studying offspring in both the premorbid and ill states, biological markers that are illness state-dependent can be separated from those
which are disease trait markers.

Pathophysiological traits may be distinguished
from genetic linkage markers. A trait that is associated with illness within a family may represent a
specific genetic susceptibility factor and may help
clinicians identify relatives at risk. The study of link-

age of an illness to a genetic marker of known location can help identify the chromosomal location of the gene for the illness. During the past decade, the possibilities for such studies have been vastly expanded by the availability of deoxyribonucleic acid (DNA) markers and efficient methods of DNA assessment.

Use of the above strategies has greatly improved our knowledge of the genetic contribution to the occurrence of psychiatric illnesses. A summary of current genetic findings for major heritable disorders is listed below.

AFFECTIVE DISORDERS

Over the past 50 years, twin studies of major [unipolar (UP) and bipolar (BP)] affective disorders have consistently shown evidence for heritability. The concordance in MZ twins (65 per cent in pooled data) has consistently been higher than that for DZ twins (14 per cent). Heritability estimates by various methods ranges from 60 to 70 per cent, comparable to the heritability of coronary heart disease and hypertension. Bertelsen et al.[1] found that concordance in MZ twins increased as the severity of the proband's illness increased: concordances ranged from 33 per cent in UP probands with less than three episodes, to 80 per cent in bipolar BP I probands (the proband is the initially ascertained patient in a genetic study). Concordance in BP II was 78 per cent and was 59 per cent in unipolars with three or more episodes.

Adoption studies support a genetic hypothesis for affective disorder, but genetic factors are more prominent in families with BP disorder than in those without. The largest study of adopted BP probands found a 31 per cent risk for affective disorder in biological relatives compared to 2 per cent in relatives of controls. The risk in families of adopted BP probands was similar to that for nonadopted bipolars

(26 per cent). Adoption studies that include a broader class of affective disorders in probands show evidence for both genetic and environmental influences: adoptive relatives of affective probands had rates of affective illness that were in excess of the rates found in adopted relatives of controls. However, there is a 15-fold increase in suicide in biological relatives of depressed adoptees, compared to families of control adoptees. Suicide itself may be heritable independent of psychiatric diagnosis.

Family studies have consistently shown that affective illness aggregates in families. Pooled data from 14 studies of 5280 relatives of BP probands show a 7.9 per cent risk of BP disorder and an 11.7 per cent risk for UP depression in relatives. Pooled results from nine studies of 3797 relatives of UP probands show a 2.7 per cent risk for BP illness and a 15.6 per cent risk for UP illness. For comparison, three studies of 1177 relatives of controls found a 0.8 per cent risk for BP and a 3.7 per cent risk for UP illness in relatives.[2]

Studies of various forms of affective illness show that they appear to be related in a hierarchical manner (Fig. 7–1).[3] In a large two-center study, relatives of schizoaffective probands were more likely than controls to have schizoaffective, BP, and UP illness (40 per cent risk for affective disorder), while relatives of BP probands had less overall risk (25 per cent) for affective disorder and were likely to have BP or UP illness. Relatives of UP probands had a 20 per cent overall risk for affective disorders (mostly UP). Multifactorial models that include genetic and environmental factors are consistent with this and several other data sets. The relatives of probands with early onset of illness generally appear to have a higher risk than relatives of later-onset probands.

Linkage studies in BP illness have not yet yielded reproducible results. A study of the Old Order Amish showed BP illness linked to chromosome 11, but the linkage was not supported with extension of this pedigree or in studies of other BP families. Link-

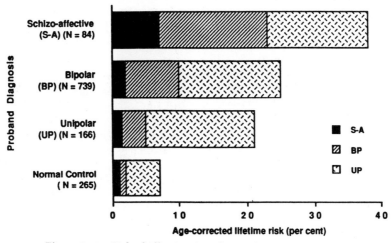

Figure 7–1. Risk of affective disorders in first-degree relatives.

age to markers in the Xq27-Xq28 chromosome has been reported by several groups, but this has not been replicated by others studying sizeable series of pedigrees.

No definitive biological marker for heritability of mood disorders has been discovered, but several candidates exist. Sensitivity to rapid eye movement (REM) sleep induction by cholinergic agonists associates with affective illness in pedigrees and has been found in well-state BP patients and some UP patients. Twin studies have suggested that this marker is heritable. Melatonin suppression by light has been found to be supersensitive in BP patients and some of their offspring.

Affective-spectrum illness studies indicate that some UP illnesses are genetically related to BP, but some are not. Bipolar II illness appears partially genetically related to BP I and to UP. There is no evidence that genetic vulnerability to rapid-cycling BP illness differs from BP vulnerability in general. Several studies show that cyclothymia is probably genetically related to BP disorder.

Studies of schizoaffective patients have generally found that their relatives have an increased incidence of both affective disorders and schizophrenia. It may be possible to distinguish between an episodic type of schizoaffective illness and a chronic form, but this is controversial. Studies of schizophrenic and bipolar patients have typically found that the families of each have no increased risk for the other illness; however, some families of schizophrenics have an increased incidence of depression.

ALCOHOLISM

While genetic factors clearly contribute to the development of alcoholism in some patients, the mechanism is heterogeneous and shows interaction with environmental factors. Twin studies of both sexes have consistently placed the heritability of the amount of alcohol consumption at 30 to 40 per cent, but males have shown higher heritability (37 per cent than have females (25 per cent).[4] Monozygotic twins show higher rates of concordance for alcoholism than DZ twins in most studies.

Family studies have found that the rate of alcoholism among relatives of alcoholic probands is 25 to 35 per cent in male relatives and 5 to 10 per cent in female relatives, compared to 5 to 10 per cent in male and 1 to 3 per cent in female control relatives. Adoption studies show both male and female offspring of alcoholics to have an increased risk for alcoholism compared to controls, with most of the excess risk restricted to male adoptees.

Large Swedish adoption studies and family studies have divided alcoholism into two types. Type 1 is "milieu-limited," has onset after age 25, accounts for female alcoholics, is uncomplicated by antisocial behaviors, and requires both genetic and environmental factors for alcoholism to develop. Its heritability is approximately 20 per cent. Type 2 alcoholic families show male-to-male alcoholism transmission with early onset in men, and low-frequency somatization but little alcoholism in women. Type 2 alcoholism is highly heritable (about 90 per cent) and may be under the control of a single genetic locus. Sons of type 2 alcoholics have a ninefold increase in risk, regardless of adoptive environment. Bohman et al.'s 1987 large adoption study found type I and II transmission and a third pattern in which the common vulnerability is expressed as alcoholism and antisocial behavior in men and high-frequency somatization in women.

A number of biological markers have been associated with alcoholism and are relatively independent of alcohol intake. Male alcoholics and their sons show decreased slow-wave activity on electroencephalogram (EEG) and have smaller amplitude P300 and N430 components in evoked-potential studies. Platelet monoamine oxidase (MAO) activity and adenylate cyclase activity are both lower in alcoholics compared to controls, and platelet MAO is lower in type 2 than in type 1 alcoholism. Sons of alcoholics have also been found to have reduced behavioral and endocrine responses to alcohol as compared to controls. The activity of the alcohol-metabolizing enzyme aldehyde dehydrogenase (ALDH) is under genetic control. Inheritance of various isoenzymes may influence risk for alcoholism. For example, an inherited ALDH I deficiency, found in 25 to 53 per cent of Asians, is associated with a flushing response to alcohol, and those with this deficiency appear to have a lower rate of alcoholism than other Asian subjects. Linkage studies have not yet linked alcoholism to any particular chromosome; an association with the A1 allele of the D_2 dopamine receptor gene in the q22-q23 region of chromosome 11 has been reported, but this finding awaits successful replication.

ALZHEIMER'S DISEASE

A genetic basis for Alzheimer's disease (AD) is now firmly established for early-onset families and is suspected in late-onset families. Three patterns have been seen:

1. Recent work has focused on the long arm of chromosome 21 where studies of numerous early-onset families (age less than 60 years) have found linkage to several loci (D21S13-16 and D21S1/S11)) close to the centromere. These early onset families have an autosomal dominant pattern of transmission with nearly complete penetrance.

2. Most late-onset families and some highly inbred Volga German families have demonstrated no linkage to chromosome 21.

3. Some AD may be nonfamilial in pattern.

Goate et al.[5] concluded that there is no evidence of genetic heterogeneity for AD within early-onset families and that differences between early- and late-onset families may be due to nongenetic forms of late-onset AD. Farrar et al.[6] studied 70 families and concluded that early-onset AD has an autosomal dominant pattern (a conclusion supported by other studies), but late-onset AD has at least two etiologies—autosomal dominant in some families, and other genetic or shared environmental factors in others. In this study, the risk of AD for offspring was 53 per cent with early-onset parents and 86 per cent with late-onset parents. The excess risk in late-onset families occurs after age 78 and reaches 86 per cent by age 87. The risk for men and women in early-onset families is equal, but data are inconclusive for later-onset families.

Much attention has been given to the fact that the Alzheimer's locus is near the gene for beta-amyloid precursor protein (APP) on chromosome 21. The APP cleavage product, amyloid, is found in abnormally high amounts in the brains of AD patients. Recently, Goate et al.[5] demonstrated a mutation on the APP gene in two unrelated early-onset AD families, suggesting that some cases of AD could be related to this mutation.

ANTISOCIAL PERSONALITY DISORDER

Several twin studies provide evidence of a genetic diathesis for antisocial personality disorder (ASP). Concordance for criminality in Danish studies is 51 per cent and 26 per cent for male MZ and DZ twins, respectively, and 35 per cent and 14 per cent for female MZ and DZ twins.[7]

Adoption studies have pointed to both genetic and environmental factors in the development of sociopathy, with the combination of both factors being more than additive in conferring risk. If both adoptive and biological parents are antisocial, the risk for ASP in offspring is nine times that of the general population. The adopted-away offspring of criminal mothers as well as those of criminal fathers have been found to have an excess of criminality compared to controls. Adoption studies support the observation that women require relatively more genetic predisposition before manifesting ASP. Adoption studies indicate that while alcoholism and ASP are found in the same families, they are transmitted at least partially independently. Some authors have hypothesized a predisposition to illness that may be expressed as sociopathy in men and somatization in women: the prevalence of Briquet's syndrome is increased in female relatives of sociopathic probands and sociopathy is increased in male relatives of Briquet's probands.

An XYY karyotype has been identified as a possible biological marker for criminality. In a large Danish study, 41 per cent of XYY but only 9.3 per cent of XY males had criminal convictions. Decreased IQ and increased height may be mediating variables associated with risk for criminality in XYY males.

PANIC DISORDER, PHOBIAS, AND OTHER ANXIETY DISORDERS

There is increasing evidence for a genetic contribution to anxiety disorders and to a relationship with depression. Family studies of panic disorder probands show a 22 to 25 per cent incidence of panic in first-degree relatives compared to 2 per cent in controls, and show familial incidence in 61 to 67 per cent of families. Relatives of agoraphobics have an excess of all types of anxiety disorders and have twice the rates of agoraphobia found in control families. Studies of anxiety neurosis have found an excess of that disorder and of panic disorder in relatives, but replication using modern diagnostic criteria is needed to interpret these results.

There is overlap within the anxiety disorders and between the anxiety disorders and depression.[8] A person with an anxiety disorder has an increased lifetime risk of having another anxiety disorder or having depression. Several studies have found no increase in major depression in relatives of panic and other anxiety probands, but others find that the risk of depression in panic proband families is identical to that in depression proband families, and both groups have higher rates than controls. Families of probands who have both panic and depression are at increased risk for depression, anxiety disorders, and alcoholism.

ATTENTION DEFICIT DISORDER

Most studies have concluded that there are important family-genetic risk factors in attention deficit disorder (ADD), and that ADD is associated with a spectrum of other psychiatric illnesses, most notably anxiety, depression, and conduct disorders. One twin study found that genetic effects accounted for around half the variance in hyperactivity. An adoption study found an association between hyperactivity in adopted offspring and attentional difficulties in biological parents.

A link between ADD or learning disorders and Tourette's syndrome (TS) has been proposed, but a systematic family study found that TS and ADD segregated independently. McClellan et al. found that rates of ADD were significantly greater (29 per cent) in offspring of parents with depressive and panic disorders than in offspring of controls (13 per cent). Biederman et al.[9] found that relatives of ADD probands had a significantly greater risk for ADD (25 per cent), antisocial disorders (25 per cent), and mood disorders (27 per cent) than did relatives of psychiatric and normal controls. The risk for antisocial disorder may be related to ADD: ADD relatives of ADD probands had significantly higher risk for antisocial disorder (61 per cent) than did relatives who did not have ADD (19 per cent). Attention deficit disorder has also been linked with minor physical anomalies in families. Some evidence supports the division of

ADD into that associated with conduct disorder (related to adult antisocial personality) and that associated with cognitive problems only.

AUTISM

Recent studies of infantile autism point to genetic factors in its incidence. Family studies show a 2.7 per cent recurrence risk for siblings, a rate 50 times higher than in the general population. In Jorde et al.'s[10] study, the familial aggregation of autism does not extend beyond sib pairs; this may be related to reduced fertility among autistic subjects or to the existence of spectrum forms of the disorder. Twin studies have found 36 per cent of MZ twins but 0 per cent of DZ twins to be concordant for autism, and around 90 per cent of MZ and 10 per cent of DZ twins to be concordant for a broader range of social and cognitive impairments. While numerous single-gene disorders have been found in autistics, fragile X has been best studied. Fragile X has been reported in 8.0 per cent of 363 autistic males and 12.1 per cent of 33 autistic females, compared with an estimated population prevalence of about 0.1 to 0.2 per cent.

EATING DISORDERS

Studies of anorexia nervosa and bulimia point to the heritability of eating disorders and to a link with depression. A twin study of anorexia found a higher concordance rate in MZ (56 per cent) than in DZ twins (5 per cent).[11] An increase in eating disorders in the relatives of bulimics compared to controls has not been found consistently.

Studies of the risk of depression in families of eating disorder probands are contradictory. Studies have found an increased risk of depression in relatives of: (1) anorexics versus controls; and (2) bulimics versus anorexics. One study found the risk for depression in both anorexic and bulimic families to be as great as the risk in depressive proband families. Most but not all studies of families of bulimics have found higher rates of UP illness than in control relatives. It is not clear whether this is dependent on the presence of affective illness in the proband. Some studies found no difference in the incidence of affective disorders in families of eating disorder probands with and without depression, but another study found a higher incidence of affective disorder in first-degree relatives of depressed bulimics than in relatives of nondepressed bulimics. Recent studies have not confirmed earlier associations between HLA types and bulimia or anorexia.

SCHIZOPHRENIA

Evidence from genetic research indicates that schizophrenia is likely caused by the interaction of genetic predisposition and environmental influences. A pooling of all twin studies shows that MZ concordance is 33 per cent (range: 14 to 59 per cent), compared to 8 per cent (range: 0 to 10 per cent) in same-sex DZ twins when a strict definition of schizophrenia is used. Heritability is 49 per cent (MZ concordance) and 9 per cent (DZ concordance) when broader definitions are used.

Heston, in 1966, found more schizophrenia (16 per cent) in adopted-away offspring of schizophrenic mothers than in controls (0 per cent). Studying biological relatives of schizophrenic and control adoptees, Kety et al. found that significantly more (8.7 per cent) relatives of schizophrenic-spectrum adoptees than of control relatives (1.9 per cent) suffered from some schizophrenic disorder. Rates of schizophrenia in the adoptive families did not differ between the two groups. More recently, application of DSM-III criteria to personally interviewed subjects has confirmed the essential results of earlier studies: adopted-away biological relatives of schizophrenics have significantly higher rates of schizophrenia than do biological relatives of controls.

Pooled data from a number of family studies show that the risk for schizophrenia is 8 to 10 per cent for siblings of schizophrenics (versus 1.2 per cent for controls), 3 to 5 per cent for parents, 12 per cent for children of one schizophrenic parent, and 46 per cent for children of two schizophrenic parents. Second-degree relatives have a 2 to 4 per cent risk. Family study data from American studies show that the first-degree relatives of schizophrenics have 8 to 18 times more risk of schizophrenia than first-degree relatives of controls.

The consistent finding of higher heritability estimates in twin studies when using a broader definition of schizophrenia suggests the existence of a spectrum of disorders genetically related to schizophrenia. An excess risk for schizotypal personality has been found in some family studies of schizophrenic probands. Gershon et al.[12] found that relatives of schizophrenics had a 6 per cent risk for all psychoses, and relatives of schizoaffective probands had an 11 per cent risk of psychoses.

In 1988, a chromosomal translocation involving the glucocorticoid receptor region of chromosome 5 was reported in a family with schizophrenia. Subsequently, a linkage study reported segregation of schizophrenia and schizophrenia-spectrum disorders with the long arm of chromosome 5 in seven British and Icelandic families. Four other studies, however, did not replicate this finding.[13] Studies in larger samples of schizophrenic families are underway and may shed further light on this controversial area.

Studies of biological markers have found an association between HLA-A9 and paranoid schizophrenia, but linkage studies to the HLA locus have yielded both positive and negative findings. Smooth pursuit eye movement deficits, found in both schizophrenics and their well relatives, represent the most promising marker and may be an alternate manifestation of a single illness gene with a dominant inheritance pattern. Ongoing high-risk offspring studies have identified attentional deficits as possible predictors of schizophrenia.

SOMATIZATION DISORDERS

Some evidence points to a genetic contribution to somatization disorders (SD), but studies are not conclusive. One twin study of SD showed a nonsignificantly higher rate of concordance in MZ twins (29 per cent) than in DZ twins (10 per cent); environmental factors (e.g., somatization as a learned response) were felt to influence the concordance rates. Several studies have found significant increases in somatoform disorder among female relatives of Briquet's probands and an increased risk of ASP and alcoholism among male relatives, leading to the speculation that a common vulnerability may be expressed as somatization in women and ASP in men. The relative contribution of genetics and environmental learning in the production of SD awaits further studies.

TOURETTE'S SYNDROME AND OBSESSIVE-COMPULSIVE DISORDER

Recent studies strongly point to the heritability of TS and to genetic connections with obsessive-compulsive disorder (OCD) and chronic multiple tics (CMT), both of which may be variant phenotypes of the TS gene. Several studies have found increased rates of OCD in TS patients compared to controls and increased rates of OCD in the relatives of TS probands. Rates of OCD do not differ between families of TS probands with and without OCD. Two studies concluded the mode of inheritance of TS is autosomal dominant. Heterozygosity for the gene is proposed to account for less severe tic symptoms. Using the assumption that a single major locus accounts for TS symptoms, ongoing studies using DNA probes have excluded linkage for more than 50 per cent of the autosomal genome.[14]

GENETIC CONTRIBUTIONS TO TREATMENT RESPONSE

Research on the genetic contributions to response to psychotropic medications is sparse in comparison to the numerous studies on the heritability of psychiatric illnesses. Most studies have focused on the effect of a family history of illness on responses to antidepressants, lithium, and neuroleptics. Studies on the familial concordance of treatment response itself are rare. The key question for clinicians is whether a family history is helpful when choosing medication for the individual patient.

Antidepressants

Regulation of the rate of metabolism may be one mechanism by which genetic endowment affects response to tricyclics. The rate of oxidative metabolism is the primary determinant of serum levels of a set dose of these drugs. Twin and family studies have shown that the rate of hydroxylation of secondary amine tricyclics is controlled mainly by genetic factors and is strongly associated with a person's debrisoquine hydroxylation phenotype, a phenotype which can be determined by a simple laboratory test and used to predict the rate of metabolism of desipramine and nortriptyline.[15] Persons who are slow hydroxylators are at risk of developing excessive blood levels of secondary amine tricyclics, either when formed from the tertiary amines or when given per se.

It is not clear if there are differences in antidepressant response between individuals on a genetic basis, independent of pharmacokinetic considerations. Retrospective surveys of depressed patients whose relatives had also been treated with antidepressants showed that 20 of 22 pairs of relatives had similar responses when treated with antidepressive agents of the same class (tricyclics or MAOIs), but only 7 of 18 pairs had similar responses when treated with agents of a different class. This suggests a familial similarity in response to antidepressants, but does not clarify if such a response is due to pharmacokinetic factors, receptor effects, or familial environmental effects.

One study of endogenously depressed tricyclic responders and nonresponders showed that independent of illness state, age, and illness severity, responders had significantly less excretion of tyramine-O-sulphate after a dose of tyramine than did nonresponders. Diminished excretion also existed in some never-depressed first-degree relatives. It may be that tyramine excretion can be used as a marker of tricyclic-responsive depression.

Racial differences in response to psychotropic medications indicate possible genetic effects on drug response, but cultural factors cannot be ruled out.[16] Asians have shown higher antidepressant levels on a fixed dose of desipramine than have caucasians. The genetically based differences in metabolism of desipramine in Chinese apparently affects other pathways in addition to hydroxylation and leaves 30 per cent of Asians at risk for toxicity from routine doses of tricyclics. Some evidence suggests that Asians also require lower plasma antidepressant levels, suggesting that racial differences in response may not simply be due to differences in metabolism. Hispanics require lower doses of antidepressant medication and report more side effects at dosages half the caucasian therapeutic dose. African-American depressed patients have been reported to have significantly higher fixed-dose blood levels and to experience more improvement than caucasians with similar doses of antidepressants. The difference may possibly be due to the significantly higher blood levels for a given dose in African-American patients. These findings suggest clinicians should initially employ lower doses of antidepressants in black, Hispanic, and Asian patients, and should consider monitoring blood levels to ensure adequate treatment without toxic effects.

Lithium

A number of studies have addressed the question of whether a family history of affective illness predicts response to lithium, but results have not been consistent. One study showed that a BP family history predicted a lithium antidepressant response, but two studies failed to find this.[17]

Studying first-degree relatives of patients with mood-incongruent psychosis, Sautter et al.[18] found that relatives of lithium responders had a significantly greater risk of having schizophrenia or schizoaffective disorder as compared with relatives of nonresponders. Lithium-responsive probands also showed a remitting course in their illness rather than a deteriorating course. The relatives of lithium responders and nonresponders did not differ in risk of schizophreniform disorder, UP depression, or BP disorder.

Kendler's 1991 review of mood-incongruent psychotic affective illness found that compared with mood-congruent psychotic and nonpsychotic UP depressed patients, patients with mood-incongruent psychosis have lower response rates to lithium, higher familial rates of schizophrenia, and lower familial rates of affective illness. Kendler's study implies that a family history of schizophrenia may lead to a poorer response to lithium by contributing to the occurrence of mood-incongruent psychotic symptoms in affective disorders (as opposed to merely having an affective disorder without psychosis or having mood-congruent psychosis). Sautter's findings, however, show that *within* the group of patients with mood-incongruent psychosis, a higher family risk of schizophrenia is associated with a better response to lithium. At the present time, more research is needed to better define the relationship between family history of psychiatric illnesses and lithium responsiveness in psychotic affective disorders.

Asians have been reported to require lower oral dosages and blood levels of lithium than caucasians, but there are no reported differences among African-Americans, caucasians, and Asians in clinical response to lithium or in lithium blood levels in response to a single dose of lithium. Blacks, however, do show a significantly longer plasma lithium half-life than caucasians or Asians.

Twin studies of lithium RBC:plasma ratio have shown that the body's handling of lithium at the cellular level is genetically determined, but the implications of treatment response are not clear. At the present time, a family history of affective disorder is more helpful in predicting lithium nonresponse with mood-incongruent affective psychoses than in predicting the response of patients with other types of affective disorders.

Neuroleptics

A relationship between genetic factors and neuroleptic response in schizophrenia has not been demonstrated in controlled studies. Family history studies have been contradictory and true family studies have not yet been performed. The studies which have been done are inconclusive in demonstrating a relationship between a family history of schizophrenia spectrum disorders and neuroleptic response. A small cerebellar vermis : brain ratio has been associated with good therapeutic response to neuroleptics in schizophrenics in one study.

There are several family history studies that provide preliminary data on the likelihood of experiencing side effects from neuroleptics. A family history of Parkinson's disease may predispose to parkinsonian side effects from neuroleptics. A family history of affective disorder may predispose to parkinsonian-like side effects or to tardive dyskinesia. This work needs confirmation by family study methods.

Some racial differences in neuroleptic levels and side effects have been found. Asians exhibit extrapyramidal side effects at lower dosages than do blacks or whites. In one study, Chinese were found to have a 52 per cent higher plasma haloperidol concentration (on a fixed dose) compared to weight- and sex-matched non-Asians.

More research is needed to clarify the effect of genetic endowment on response to psychotropic medications. The kinds of studies that are most informative are often the most methodologically difficult and the most time consuming to conduct. Prospective studies of the response of at-risk relatives to particular medications are needed to clarify the relationship of family history to treatment response. Such studies would take years to conduct and are ethically difficult, since the choice of medication for ill persons may be restricted by study designs. Studies that employ systematic direct evaluation of relatives, utilizing standardized diagnostic methods, are needed. Treatment-blind family studies are needed, as are double-blinded studies of biological markers and treatment response. In addition, studies which rigorously control for medication blood levels and dosages based on body weight are needed.

REFERENCES

1. Bertelsen A, Harvald B, Hauge M: A danish twin study of manic-depressive disorders. Br J Psychiatry 130:330, 1977.
2. Nurnberger JI Jr, Gershon ES: Genetics of affective disorders. *In* Paykel, ed. Handbook of Affective Disorders. 2nd ed. (in press), 1992.
3. Gershon ES, Hamovit J, Guroff JJ, et al: A family study of schizoaffective, bipolar I, bipolar II, unipolar, and normal control probands. Arch Gen Psychiatry 39:1157, 1982.

4. Devor EJ, Cloninger CR: Genetics of alcoholism. Ann Rev Genet 23:19, 1989.
5. Goate A, Chartier-Harlin M-C, Mullan M, et al: Segregation of a missense mutation in the amyloid precursor protein gene with familial Alzheimer's disease. Nature 349:704, 1991.
6. Farrar LA, Myers RH, Cupples LA, et al: Transmission and age-at-onset patterns in familial Alzheimer's disease: Evidence for heterogeneity. Neurology 40:395, 1990.
7. Cloninger CR, Christiansen KD, Reich T, et al: Implications of sex differences in the prevalences of antisocial personality, alcoholism, and criminality for familial transmission. Arch Gen Psychiatry 35:941, 1978.
8. Weissman MM: The epidemiology of anxiety disorders: Rates, risks, and familial patterns. J Psychiatr Res 23(suppl 1):99, 1988.
9. Biederman J, Faraone SV, Keenan K, et al: Family-genetic and psychosocial risk factors in DSM-III attention deficit disorder. J Am Acad Child Adolesc Psychiatry 29(4):526, 1990.
10. Jorde LB, Mason-Brothers A, Waldmann R, et al: The UCLA-University of Utah epidemiologic survey of autism: Genealogical analysis of familial aggregation. Am J Med Genet 36:85, 1990.
11. Holland AJ, Sicotte N, Treasure J: Anorexia nervosa: Evidence for a genetic basis. J Psychosom Res 32:561, 1988.
12. Gershon ES, DeLisi LE, Hamovit J, et al: A controlled family study of chronic psychoses. Arch Gen Psychiatry 45:328, 1988.
13. Crowe RR, Black DW, Wesner R, et al: Lack of linkage to chromosome 5q11-q13 markers in six schizophrenia pedigrees. Arch Gen Psychiatry 48:357, 1991.
14. Pakstis AJ, Heutink P, Pauls DS, et al: Progress in the search for genetic linkage with Tourette syndrome: An exclusion map covering more than 50% of the autosomal genome. Am J Hum Genet 48:281, 1991.
15. Spina E, Steiner E, Ericsson O, et al: Hydroxylation of desmethylimipramine: Dependence on the debrisoquin hydroxylation phenotype. Clin Pharmacol Ther 41:314, 1987.
16. Lawson WB: Racial and ethnic factors in psychiatric research. Hosp Community Psychiatry 37:50, 1986.
17. Nurnberger JI Jr: Pharmacogenetic approaches to the study of brain function. In Vogel F, Sperling K, eds. Human Genetics. Berlin-Heidelberg: Springer Verlag, 1987:484.
18. Sautter FJ, McDermott BE, Garver DL: A family study of lithium-responsive psychosis. J Affective Disord 20:63, 1990.

PART II

CLINICAL DISORDERS

Section A

ORGANIC DISORDERS

8

DSM-IV:
Organic Disorders

GARY J. TUCKER, M.D.

The proposed changes for DSM-IV of the Organic section of DSM-III-R consist of two major structural changes, refinement of the criteria for delirium and dementia, and the proposed addition of a postconcussive syndrome and the addition of specific subtypes of personality disorders secondary to lesions of the central nervous system. These changes primarily affect diagnostic precision, but there should be little effect on traditional treatment of these disorders.

MAJOR RECOMMENDED CHANGES
FROM DSM-III-R

A core group was complemented by a large group of national and international experts, all primarily interested in organic conditions. This group included psychiatrists, neurologists, and neuropsychologists. Perhaps of most concern to the Work Group and consultants was the implication of the category name itself, "Organic Disorders." With the advances in the scientific understanding of behavioral disorders, it seemed rather arbitrary to divide the nomenclature into "organic conditions" and "nonorganic conditions," thus implying that a certain number of behavioral conditions were not organic. While this suggestion has stirred controversy in the literature,[1] most of the field is supportive of eliminating this distinction.[2] Even the argument that the organic conditions are related to a known etiology and the other conditions have as yet not had a specific etiology delineated is difficult in that

whether the etiology is known or not yet known, it is still important to recognize that behavioral disorders are due to changes in the central nervous system.

Two major proposals and options were made to eliminate this false dichotomy: (1) that the name be changed completely, and (2) that the categories of dementia, delirium, and amnestic disorders were large and encompassing enough to stand on their own as freestanding categories in the nomenclature,[3] much as do affective disorders, psychotic disorders, etc.[4] Most seemed in favor of changing the name entirely, and for nosological "neatness," it was felt that an overarching category was necessary. Consequently, the term that was felt to be most defining of the current categories listed under the Organic Disorders was that they all manifested themselves primarily by changes in *cognition*. Therefore, the use of the term "Cognitive Impairment Disorders" as the overarching category was felt most appropriate. This recognizes the fact that there are also cognitive changes in schizophrenia, depression, obsessive-compulsive neurosis, and other conditions but, for the organic disorders, cognitive dysfunction is the major defining characteristic. However, there will be two options for the field to consider. The first is the use of a completely new term, such as "Cognitive Impairment Disorders," or letting the conditions stand alone in the nomenclature as "Delirium," "Dementia," or "Amnestic Disorders."

The second major change, in part, was necessitated by removal of the term "organic," but in reality, was driven by a desire to make the nomenclature more compatible with the way clinicians think. When most clinicians are confronted with someone with an anxiety disorder or an affective disorder, they immediately begin to think in terms of differential diagnosis. Part of this differential diagnosis must consider all the biological and psychological causes for this condition. Consequently, it was decided that a more appropriate term for "Organic Anxiety Disorder" or "Organic Affective Disorder," and so on, would be "Second Anxiety Disorder due to ——— Axis III Condition" or "Secondary Affective Disorder due to ——— Axis III Condition." A more appropriate place for them in the diagnostic schema would be in the major home-base such as the section on anxiety disorders or the section on affective disorders. Consequently, the section on anxiety disorders would then have a primary list of anxiety disorders and two types of secondary anxiety disorders, those related to an Axis III condition and those related to a substance-induced condition.

Several issues related to this change have yet to be resolved including: How do you attribute the strength of the etiological relationship between the Axis III condition and the supposed behavioral change? In the literature review, the strength of such associations was found to be mostly on the case report level rather than through systematic studies. The second problem was related to how similar the criteria for a secondary anxiety disorder must be in order to be labeled a secondary disorder. Did it have to meet the criteria for the primary disorder exactly, or did it have to meet more of a "sounds like" criteria? As these secondary conditions are often confounded by medical conditions, it was felt that it would be better to have criteria that are less stringent than the home-based diagnostic criteria.

SPECIFIC RECOMMENDED CHANGES IN DIAGNOSTIC CRITERIA

The major change suggested for delirium is an attempt to increase compatibility with ICD-10. For that reason, the "A" criterion returned to an impairment of consciousness with a reduced ability to focus or sustain or shift attention rather than attention alone. There was a feeling that the change to "attention" in DSM-III-R from DSM-III overly narrowed the category. Another change recommended was precipitated by the difficulty in diagnosing delirium in demented patients. Consequently, the "B" criterion is proposed to be changed to, "changes in cognition which are not better accounted for by a preexisting, established, or evolving dementia." As dementia is one of the predisposing factors toward delirium, it was felt important to suggest such a change. It was also felt that it would be useful to have a mixed type of delirium, as it is clear that one can have delirium both from an Axis III condition and from a substance-induced situation (Table 8–1).

Changes in the dementia section were intended to

TABLE 8–1. PROPOSED ORGANIZATION FOR COGNITIVE IMPAIRMENT DISORDERS, DELIRIA, DEMENTIA, AND AMNESTIC DISORDERS

Deliria
  Delirium due to an axis III condition
  Substance-induced (intoxication/withdrawal) delirium (specific substance)
  Delirium due to multiple etiologies
  Delirium due to unknown etiology
  Delirium not otherwise specified
Dementia
  Dementia due to an axis III conditions
  Dementia of the Alzheimer's type
  Vascular dementia
  Dementia due to other axis III conditions
  Substance-induced (intoxication/withdrawal/residual) dementia
  Dementia due to multiple etiologies
  Dementia due to unknown etiology
  Dementia not otherwise specified
Amnestic disorders
  Amnestic disorder due to an axis III condition
  Substance-induced (intoxication/withdrawal/residual) amnestic disorder
  Amnestic disorder not otherwise specified
Cognitive impairment disorders
  Cognitive impairment disorder not otherwise specified due to an axis III condition
  Substance-induced cognitive impairment disorder not otherwise specified
  Cognitive impairment disorder not otherwise specified

make DSM-IV more compatible with the National Institute of Neurologic and Communicative Disorders and Stroke (NINCDS) criteria and the Alzheimer's Disease and Related Disorders Association (ADRDA) criteria. This was accomplished by changing the "A" criterion to "multiple cognitive deficits, as manifested by memory impairment and impairment of language, apraxia, agnosia, and disturbances in executive functioning," leaving out the personality change criteria. Specific criteria for dementia due to Axis III conditions, dementia of the Alzheimer's type, vascular dementia, and mixed etiology dementia were also included. It was also recognized that one of the most common causes for psychiatric and behavioral management of patients with dementia is related to the behavioral symptoms associated with them. Consequently, it is proposed that the ability to diagnose specific behavioral states such as depressed mood, delusions, hallucinations, behavioral disturbances, communication disturbances, motor skill disturbances, etc., be included in the diagnostic schema.

The amnestic disorders were little changed and the course can now be stipulated in terms of being either transient or persistent.

RECOMMENDATIONS FOR NEW CATEGORIES FOR DSM-IV

From the literature reviews, it became apparent that many of the commonly used terms such as "frontal lobe syndrome," and "temporal lobe syndrome," had little support for diagnostic specificity within the literature. The literature consisted primarily of case reports, while many of the systematic studies that investigated these syndromes showed that lesions in other parts of the brain could cause similar symptomatology. Thus, these historical syndromes had little specificity with regard to anatomical location of the injury. However, there are specific behavioral changes related to insults of the central nervous system. These conditions include a disinhibited state, an emotional labile state, an aggressive state, an apathetic state, or a mixture of the above. The work group felt that it would be more precise to use these terms as descriptive modifiers of the secondary personality disorders (formerly "Organic Personality Disorders").

Another diagnostic category that is present in ICD-10 and for which we have no current stipulation in DSM-III-R is postconcussive disorder. The literature review in this area showed that there is a consistent syndrome after head trauma, and we are in the process of recommending that this be included in the options.

Other descriptive terms which will probably be included are tardive dyskinesias and the various drug-induced movement disorders.

REFERENCES

1. Lipowski ZJ: Is organic obsolete? Psychosomatics 31:342–344, 1990.
2. Spitzer RL, First M, Tucker GJ: Organic mental disorders and DSM-IV. Am J Psychiatry 148:3, 1991.
3. Spitzer RL, Williams JBW, First M, et al: A proposal for DSM-IV: Solving the "organic/nonorganic" problem. J Neuropsych Clin Neurosci 1:126–127, 1989.
4. Popkin MK, Tucker GJ, Caine E, et al: The fate of organic mental disorders in DSM-IV: A progress report. Psychosomatics 30:438–441, 1989.

9

ALZHEIMER'S DISEASE

J. PIERRE LOEBEL, M.D., STEPHEN R. DAGER, M.D., and
MARGARET A. KITCHELL, M.D.

CLINICAL PRESENTATION AND COURSE

In 1906, Alois Alzheimer, a psychiatrist, described the case of a 51-year-old woman who presented with suspiciousness followed by progressive memory impairment and other cognitive and behavioral disturbances until her death 4½ years later.[1] The clinical features which he described remain the classic clinical description of this disorder. New information is poorly assimilated, so that a typical early manifestation is to forget recent events or mislay objects. Interests begin to narrow and work and the activities of daily living become more slipshod. There is decline in the ability to exercise proper judgment, together with personality deterioration. Dysphasia, dyspraxia, and agnosia become evident, as well as problems in maintaining the stream of thought and speech, and disorientation in time and space. Behavior can adopt disorganized, disinhibited, and sometimes violent forms. Psychotic phenomena may occur. Later stages proceed inexorably to cachexia, motoric disturbances which may include seizures and loss of sphincter control, and death.

While the presentation as described is the most common, there have been attempts to delineate alternative or unusual patterns of decline, possibly related to subtypes. The distinction between early- and later-onset types has been revived, with some[2] claiming that this distinguishes etiology (greater genetic load in the former), neuropathology (predominance of plaques over tangles in the latter), neurochemistry (a greater decrease of choline acetyltransferase and other neurotransmitters in the former), clinical presentation (more severe symptoms in the former with earlier onset of myoclonus and seizures), and natural history (more rapid progression in the former). The genetic contribution is currently under intensive investigation, with indications of autosomal dominant transmission in several large family pedigrees and multifactorial, age-dependent expression estimated at 65 per cent or more in the remaining cases.[3] These considerations remain controversial, and management is not fundamentally influenced by them.

PREVALENCE AND IMPACT

In the 65- to 74-year-old population of the United States, prevalence has been estimated as 3 per cent, increasing to 47.2 per cent in those over 85 years. Females predominate. On postmortem examination, approximately 50 per cent of all cases of clinically diagnosed dementia are due to Alzheimer's disease, signifying that between 1 and 5 million persons are affected to some degree by this condition at the present time in the United States.[4]

DIAGNOSTIC PROCESS

To make the diagnosis of Primary Degenerative Dementia of the Alzheimer type (DAT) in accordance with the criteria set out by DSM-III-R, the history is taken, a physical examination performed, the mental status assessed, with special reference to cognitive functions, and efforts made to exclude other forms of dementia (Table 9–1). The latter is important in view of the high incidence of both misdiagnoses and concurrent other illnesses.[5] The laboratory screening tests which have been recommended for assistance in making the differential diagnosis are listed in Table 9–2; selection among them should be guided by the clinical considerations pertaining to each case. Neither the cerebral atrophy seen on computed tomography (CT) nor the hypoactivity revealed by positron emission tomography (PET) are currently of sufficient sensitivity and specificity to be definitive for diagnosis. If anticipated improvements in techniques, reduction in costs, and the establishment of norms for comparison occur, brain imaging techniques will become more clinically relevant.

Neuropsychological testing has a place in establishing the diagnosis of DAT, delineating the cerebral localization of the disorder, and measuring severity.[6] Reevaluation over time is often helpful. Using these approaches, autopsy-validated diagnostic accuracy is now approximately 90 per cent.

TABLE 9–1.   DIFFERENTIAL DIAGNOSIS OF DEMENTIA[a]

Primary dementias
  Alzheimer's disease
  Pick's disease
  Creutzfeldt-Jakob disease
Dementias secondary to other illness
  Psychiatric
    Depressive disorders
    Schizophrenia
    Factitious/conversion disorder
  Somatic
    Major organ-system impairment
    Endocrine
    Infections
    Tumor (primary CNS and paraneoplastic)
    Neurologic
      Nutritional (B_{12}, folic acid, and alcohol-related)
      Huntington's disease (chorea)
      Parkinson's disease
      Progressive supranuclear palsy
      Hydrocephalus
      Subdural hematoma
    Vascular (multi-infarct dementia)
Toxicity (iatrogenic, industrial, and heavy metal)

[a] Adapted with permission from Read S: The dementias. In Sadavoy J, Lazarus LW, Jarvik LF, eds. Comprehensive Review of Geriatric Psychiatry. Washington DC: American Psychiatric Press, Inc., 1991:290.

TABLE 9–2.   RECOMMENDED LABORATORY SCREENING IN THE DIAGNOSIS OF DEMENTIA

Blood studies
  Complete blood cell count
  Hematocrit
  Hemoglobin level
  Sedimentation rate
  Serum urea nitrogen and creatinine
  Serum glucose
  Sodium, potassium, chloride, carbonate
  Calcium, phosphorus
  Vitamin B_{12}, folic acid
  Liver function tests, including bilirubin, albumin
  Thyroid function tests
  Serological tests for syphilis
  Toxicology screen
Urinalysis
Electrocardiogram
Chest x-ray
Computed tomographic (CT) brain scan
Electrocardiogram
Stool examination for occult blood

TREATMENT

Investigations into the etiology, pathogenesis and neuropathophysiology of DAT are being vigorously pursued, but no conclusions which enable specific treatment of the primary lesion(s) have been reached.

Principles of Management

Reduction of "Excess" Disabilities

As with other chronic illnesses, in the absence of established etiology management necessitates approaches along many fronts, with the primary objective being to reduce "excess" disabilities (i.e., those secondary to the impact of the primary condition). Since the disease is protean in its manifestations and progressive, different clinical challenges will be posed during the course of the illness. This is best responded to by a team approach, allowing for a flexible response with whatever special service or expertise is most appropriate. The team should include or be able as needed to draw upon the services of all medical specialties, social work, nursing, home health and related care providers (including respite care), as well as experts on legal and financial matters.

Support for Caregivers

Since the duration of the illness, although variable, is often lengthy and most patients are cared for at home for considerable periods of time, a vital aspect of management is the provision of support for the caregivers, who are frequently under considerable stress.[7] This is especially important to stave off institutionalization for as long as feasible.

Maintenance of Everyday Routines

Routines of everyday living need to be maintained as consistently as possible. While there have been few systematic studies, clinical observation indicates (and families confirm), that emphasis should be on familiarity of routine and environment; adjustments of the pace, clarity, and content of communication to the patient's ability to absorb; and repeated reassurance by explanation and comportment.

Ensuring the Optimal Functioning of All Sensory Modalities

Together with treatment of coincident somatic illness, the mental state will benefit from ensuring the optimal functioning of all sensory modalities, such as by refraction and other ophthalmic care, adequate illumination, hearing aids (especially important in the case of suspicious, paranoid patients), and proper dentures. Attention needs to be paid to nutrition, and vitamin supplementation may be helpful.[8]

Role of the Caregiver in the Morale of the Patient

The patient with DAT should be approached in a hopeful manner tempered with due caution, in order to maintain the sense of autonomy and self-esteem of the patients and the morale of the caregivers. Symptomatic treatment of the patient in an individualized manner and meaningful support of the family is always feasible and often effective. This includes the need to be available at all times in an advocacy capacity. One patient's spouse wrote "Alzheimer's patients cannot speak for themselves and desperately need advocates. When I find my husband in less than good shape, I become angry and sad—and vocal!" The professional caregiver should do no less.

Treatment of Cognitive Impairments

Pharmacological Approaches

Although a variety of medications have been used as cognitive enhancing agents for the treatment of DAT, results have been inconsistent and mostly disappointing. In part, this may be due to the heterogeneous nature of the illness or a lack of specificity in the clinical diagnosis. Prospective studies are difficult to evaluate owing to a variable onset and course of illness. Clinical trials seeking to improve diagnostic reliability generally enroll patients with moderate to severe clinical manifestations of the disease, which probably corresponds to a similar degree of neuropathological damage.[9] However, preexisting structural damage is unlikely to be reversible.

A number of treatment strategies for DAT, based on different theories regarding its etiology, have been advanced. In the belief that DAT is related to reduced cerebral blood flow, a putative cerebral vasodilator, the ergoloid mesylate preparation Hydergine, has been the most extensively studied agent used for the treatment of DAT. It remains the only Food and Drug Administration (FDA)–approved medication for DAT in this country. Early clinical trials found overall evidence of behavioral and psychological improvement which was, however, inconsistent among individual patients.[10] Subsequent clinical trials of Hydergine have been mostly unable to demonstrate therapeutic efficacy. In part, inconsistent findings may reflect underdosing of the medication. However, at current recommended doses (3 mg/day), Hydergine appears to be generally ineffective for the treatment of DAT.[11]

Irrespective of whether the ergoloid mesylates increase cerebral blood flow, it has become clear that this is not the pathological basis for DAT. As there is also evidence to suggest that the ergoloid mesylates exhibit metabolic enhancement and α-adrenergic antagonism as well as having serotonin and dopamine agonist properties, it is difficult to postulate a specific mechanism of action in individual cases of improvement.

Among the "nootropic" or metabolic enhancing agents whose possible value in the treatment of DAT has been of interest for over three decades, piracetam has been one of the more extensively evaluated. Piracetam, a cyclic derivative of gamma-aminobutyric acid (GABA), has been reported to increase phosphorylation of adenosine diphosphate (ADP) to adenosine triphosphate (ATP) and thus accelerate the release of acetylcholine. Although studies have reported improvement in attention span and decreased agitation, enhancement of cognitive functioning was not sustained.[12]

Piracetam has not been released in the United States. However, several homologues are in the process of being developed in this country. One such agent, oxiracetam, has been extensively evaluated for the treatment of both DAT and multi-infarct dementia, with unimpressive clinical results overall, although individual patients have substantially improved. For example, in a single-blind study conducted at our center, there was an overall lack of improvement during a 16-week trial of oxiracetam (1600 mg/dy) among six mild to moderately severe

DAT patients. An exception was a patient who experienced substantial clinical improvement, both behaviorally and on neurocognitive testing, which was sustained during the 16-week treatment trial. When oxiracetam was discontinued, the patient experienced progressive clinical deterioration over 5 months, which remitted when the medication was re-started. The patient remained on oxiracetam at a dosage of 1600 mg/day for approximately 5 years, with continued moderate improvement up until the time of his demise due to unrelated causes. In the face of postmortem findings of well-advanced neuropathological changes consistent with severe Alzheimer's disease, the patient was able to regain and retain his ability to socialize and maintain functions of daily living while on the medication.[12]

Instead of nonspecific metabolic enhancement, a number of neuropharmacological strategies for treating DAT have focused on specific neurotransmitter systems. The well-established observation that a loss of cholinergic neurons is involved in the pathophysiology of DAT has been the impetus for efforts to manipulate the cholinergic mechanism of neurotransmission in a variety of ways. Attempts to increase acetylcholine synthesis through the administration of precursors such as choline and lecithin have been mostly disappointing.[13]

An alternative approach to dietary supplementation of cholinergic precursors has been to inhibit synaptic degradation of choline through the administration of acetylcholinesterase inhibitors. In a review of 12 studies in which physostigmine was administered to patients with dementia, ten demonstrated at least some evidence of temporary improvement, which could not be wholly explained by enhancement of attention.[14] However, treatment with physostigmine is impractical clinically due to problems with short half-life, unacceptable peripheral side effects, and an inconsistent pattern of response. These promising results, however, have led to the development of centrally acting acetylcholinesterase inhibitors with longer half-lives.

Among centrally acting acetylcholinesterase inhibitors, particular interest has focused on tetrahydroaminoacridine (THA). The Food and Drug Administration (FDA) is currently appraising the results of studies, with special reference to undesirable side effects primarily involving hepatic toxicity.[15] Recent multicenter crossover studies of combination THA and lecithin have failed to demonstrate substantial improvement with THA in comparison to placebo, although the small number of DAT patients studied limits definitive conclusions.[16]

An approach which does not entail a presynaptically produced substrate has been to administer cholinergic agonists having direct postsynaptic effects. Intravenous infusions of arecholine did appear to improve cognition in one small group of DAT patients studied.[17] However, subsequent attempts with arecholine administration have been less encouraging.[18]

A number of problems occur with the peripheral administration of cholinergic agents including both peripheral side-effects and variable penetrance into the central nervous system. Due to these concerns, bethanacol has been administered directly into the central nervous system via a neurosurgically placed intrathecal pump. Although initial open study results were encouraging, further double-blind trials have failed to demonstrate consistent improvement using this approach.[19]

Investigations are still at an early stage of the neurotrophic protein nerve growth factor.[20] This may reverse cholinergic cell body atrophy, which in DAT has been hypothesized to be caused by a reversible disturbance of the trophic functions of these cells.

Although cholinergic mechanisms have been a particular focus of attention, other neurotransmitters also are affected in DAT.[21] Pharmaceutical interventions targeting the biogenic amines, such as norepinephrine and dopamine and their metabolites, or the indolamines, such as serotonin, have had some beneficial effects on disturbed behavior. It is less clear whether cognitive functions may be enhanced.

A variety of neuropeptides have been administered to DAT patients in an attempt to correct associated deficiencies, based on postmortem findings. Vasopressin is a neuropeptide that has generated interest due to its effects on enhancing memory in normal controls and learning in animals. However, administration of vasopressin to DAT patients, in controlled trials, does not produce clinically significant improvement.[22] It does have stimulatory effects that might nonspecifically improve memory performance. This may be the basis also for reports of opiate antagonist (naloxone)–induced improvements in memory, although these have been disputed.[23]

Current treatment strategies for DAT appear to be moving toward a more integrated approach combining metabolic enhancement plus augmentation of various impaired neurotransmitter and neuropeptide systems, although this treatment approach is still investigational.

Psychological Approaches

Despite earlier interest in "reality orientation" and "memory retraining," there have not been any recent advances employing psychological interventions. A different treatment approach, adapted from its application in schizophrenia, has sought to modify the "emotional expressivity" of the caregivers, this being essentially a reflection of their anger regarding the illness and of emotional overinvolvement with the patient.[24] To date, the approach appears encouraging in improving the coping abilities and decreasing stress levels of both patients and care providers.

Treatment of Noncognitive Disturbances

While cognitive disturbances are considered to be those most characteristic of and directly related to the pathophysiology of DAT, several other types of disturbance may also be present and more amenable to treatment.

Psychotic Features

The prevalence in DAT of auditory and visual hallucinations and delusions has been estimated at 10, 13, and 16 per cent, respectively. The forms taken by these phenomena are not characteristic of the illness; delusions being predominantly paranoid in nature and misidentifications of the Capgras syndrome type not infrequent.[25]

Treatment of psychotic symptoms is generally with neuroleptic agents. Some demented patients have been reported to respond well to very low doses (e.g., 0.125 mg) of haloperidol; otherwise, the use of neuroleptics in the DAT patient follows traditional geriatric psychopharmacological lines.[26] As in younger patients, no specific neuroleptic has been shown to be particularly efficacious. Special precautions are, however, needed to reduce the age-related increase in the potential for adverse side effects, although there are no reports specifically investigating the prevalence of these side effects in elderly DAT patients. In particular, anticholinergic side effects may produce confusion, oversedation, exacerbation of glaucoma, constipation, urinary retention, provocation of delirium, and orthostatic hypotension, with its attendant risks of falls and fractures. In order to reduce anticholinergic side effects, the low-sedation high-potency agents are generally preferred. A second major area of concern is the propensity of the neuroleptics to cause extrapyramidal symptoms, including tardive dyskinesia, to which the elderly appear to be especially prone.

Mood Disorders

The precipitants of depressed mood in the elderly demented patient may include all the neurochemical and psychosocial perturbations to which the elderly are prone. In addition, the individual (especially in the early stages of the illness) may experience the failing memory and functional impairments that accompany this as a threat to the integrity of the self. Depression in dementia is common, with a prevalence variously estimated at between 10 and 40 per cent depending on the degree of severity.[27] The pharmacological treatment of mood disorders occurring in patients with DAT does not differ in essence from the treatment of other elderly patients with these conditions. It is advisable to use caution in interpreting results of clinical trials of antidepressants in DAT. A study which compared efficacy of imipramine with placebo in moderately depressed DAT patients demonstrated an equivalent improvement in both conditions.[28]

Mania and hypomania occurring in DAT have been found to be responsive to lithium carbonate treatment, albeit in some cases in doses producing plasma levels lower than those recommended for therapeutic response in younger patients.

Psychotherapy with mood-disordered DAT patients poses special problems. In our experience, in both interpretative and supportive modes, psychotherapy can be of value as, for instance, in cases when with the failure of customary defenses, core conflicts emerge or when a patient with failing cognitive functions is enabled to use the therapist as an accessory ego.

Behavioral Problems

Of all aspects of care of the patient with DAT, perhaps the most troubling is the wide array of disturbed and disturbing behaviors that may become manifest during the course of the illness.[29] They are also a common source of management difficulties within long-term care facilities, although DAT is not exceptional in this respect.[30]

The associations between various behaviors and other features of the illness (e.g., severity of cognitive impairment) are beginning to be clarified, but there is as yet no widely accepted etiological underpinning or systematic approach to management.[31] With the exception of the forms of agitation described below, none of these behaviors have been found to respond specifically to any one pharmacological agent. Management therefore relies largely upon psychological interventions, including distraction, environmental manipulation with occasional need for restraints to ensure safety, and positive and negative reinforcement of the behaviors. Although it may be difficult to identify precipitating and maintaining contingencies, the effort to do so will in many cases be successful, permitting specific interventions. One of the special functions of units dedicated to the care of patients suffering from DAT is to provide behavioral modification: there are indications that these specialized DAT units may be effective in stabilizing the functional capacity of DAT patients.[32]

Especially prominent behavioral difficulties are agitation and aggression. An assessment of the contributing contingencies is the first advisable step with manipulation of these as necessary. When pharmacotherapy is resorted to, this has traditionally taken the form of neuroleptic agents, since the benzodiazepines are more prone to causing confusion, disorientation, disinhibition, oversedation, anterograde amnesia, and tolerance or dependence.[33] There continues to be a dearth of clear-cut findings upon which to base treatment decisions. However, the best-supported guidelines for intervention with neuroleptics suggest that: (1) agitated, belligerent, and psychotic manifestations respond best, albeit in a nonspecific manner; (2) withdrawn, anergic, and uncooperative behaviors respond poorly; (3) doses should be as low as possible to achieve relief in target symptoms, the medication used for as short a time as possible and with appropriate attention to possible drug side effects, especially when used with others that may also have anticholinergic properties; and (4) that, overall, these agents confer only modest benefits and also have substantial placebo effects.[34] In all cases, adverse concomitant effects that should be avoided are more important grounds on which to choose among agents than efficacy.

In addition to the neuroleptics, attempts have also been made to use benzodiazepines, antidepressants, lithium carbonate, carbamazepine, and β-blocking agents, the choice among these agents being dictated by the associated presence of, predominantly and respectively, anxiety, dysphoria, hyperactivity, irritability, and agitation.[35]

APPROACHES TO CAREGIVERS

Caregiver stress and its alleviation continues to receive considerable research attention. Conceptual frameworks for analyzing stress of the caregivers have been put forward and provide a basis for interventions.[36] There is a high prevalence of depression in this population, with the potential for "burn-out" to precipitate institutionalization of the DAT patient.[37] Factual information continues to be one of the main pillars of effective support of the caregivers—and is frequently lacking or inadequate for their experienced needs.[38,39]

In overview, a combination of information provision regarding the disease process and the resources available, instruction on the handling of specific behaviors, and supportive counseling addressed to the caregivers' own emotions have been found of benefit in reducing stress and its concomitants. National and local organizations now exist to provide these interventions, and physicians should encourage contact with these.

REFERENCES

1. Alzheimer A: Uber eine Eigenartige Erkrankrung der Hirnrinde. Allegemeine Zeitschrift fur Psychiatrie und Psychisch-Gerichtlich Medicin, 1907.
2. Rossor MN, Iversen LL, Reynolds GP, et al: Neurochemical characteristics of early and late onset types of Alzheimer's disease. Br Med J 288:961, 1984.
3. Kay DWK: Genetics, Alzheimer's disease and senile dementia. Br J Psychiatry 154:311, 1989.
4. Read S: The dementias. In Sadavoy J, Lazarus LW, Jarvik LF, eds. Comprehensive Review of Geriatric Psychiatry. Washington, DC: American Psychiatric Press, Inc., 1991:287.
5. Larson EB, Reifler BV, Sumi SM, et al: Diagnostic evaluation of 200 elderly outpatients with suspected dementia. J Gerontol 40:536, 1985.
6. Albert MS: Neuropsychological testing. In Sadavoy J, Lazarus LW, Jarvik LF, eds. Comprehensive Review of Geriatric Psychiatry. Washington, DC: American Psychiatric Press, Inc., 1991:230.
7. Cohen D, Eisdorfer C: Depression in family members caring for a relative with Alzheimer's disease. J Am Geriatri Soc 36:885, 1988.
8. Burns A, Marsh A, Bender DA: A trial of vitamin supplementation in senile dementia. Int J Geriatr Psychiatry 4:333, 1989.

9. Blessed G, Tomlinson BE, Roth M: The association between quantitative measures of dementia and of senile change in the cerebral gray matter of elderly subjects. Br J Psychiatry 114:797, 1968.
10. Yesavage JA, Tinklenberg JR, Hollister LE, et al: Vasodilators in senile dementias. Arch Gen Psychiatry. 36:220, 1979.
11. Thompson TL, Filley CM, Mitchell WD, et al: Lack of efficacy of hydergine in patients with Alzheimer's disease. N Engl J Med 323:445, 1990.
12. Dager SR, Loebel JP, Claypool K, et al: (submitted for publication).
13. Hollander E, Mohs RC, Davis KL: Cholinergic approaches to the treatment of Alzheimer's disease. Br Med Bull 42:97, 1986.
14. Whalley LJ: Drug treatments of dementia. Br J Psychiatry 155:595, 1989.
15. Marx JL: FDA queries Alzheimer's trial results. Science 240:969, 1988.
16. Gauthier S, Bouchard R, Lamontagne A, et al: Tetrahydroaminoacridine-lecithin combination treatment in patients with intermediate-stage Alzheimer's disease: Results of a Canadian double-blind crossover, multicenter study. N Engl J Med 322:1272, 1990.
17. Christie JE, Shering PA, Ferguson J, et al: Physostigmine and arecoline: Effects of intravenous infusions in Alzheimer presenile dementia. Br J Psychiatry 138:46, 1981.
18. Tarot PN, Cohen RM, Welkowitz, et al: Multiple-dose arecoline infusions in Alzheimer's disease. Arch Gen Psychiatry 45:901, 1988.
19. Harbaugh RE, Reeder TM, Senter HJ, et al: Intracerebroventricular bethanechol chloride infusion in Alzheimer's disease. Results of a collaborative double-blind study. J Neurosurg 71:481, 1989.
20. Fischer W, Wictorin K, Bjorkland A, et al: Amelioration of cholinergic neuron atrophy and spatial memory impairment in aged rats with nerve growth factor. Nature 329:65, 1987.
21. Raskind MA: Organic mental disorders. In Busse EW, Blazer DG, eds. Geriatric Psychiatry. Washington DC: American Psychiatric Press, Inc., 1989:342.
22. Peabody CA, Thiemann S, Pigache R, et al: Desglycinamide-9-arginine-8-vasopressin (DGAVP, Organon 5667) in patients with dementia. Neurobiol Aging 6:95, 1985.
23. Tariot PN, Sunderland T, Weingartner H, et al: Naloxone and Alzheimer's disease. Arch Gen Psychiatry 43:727, 1986.
24. Bledin KD, MacCarthy B, Kuipers L, et al: Daughters of people with dementia. Expressed emotion, strain and coping. Br J Psychiatry 157:221, 1990.
25. Burns A, Jacoby R, Levy R: Psychiatric phenomena in Alzheimer's disease. II. Disorders of perception. Br J Psychiatry 157:76, 1990.
26. Jenike MA: Handbook of Geriatric Psychopharmacology. Littleton, MA: PSG Publishing Company, Inc., 1985:17.
27. Wragg RE, Jeste DV: Overview of depression and psychosis in Alzheimer's disease. Am J Psychiatry 146:577, 1989.
28. Reifler BV, Teri L, Raskind M, et al: Double-blind trial of imipramine in Alzheimer's disease patients with and without depression. Am J Psychiatry 146:45, 1989.
29. Teri L, Larson EB, Reifler BV: Behavioral disturbance in dementia of the Alzheimer's type. J Am Geriatr Soc 36:1, 1988.
30. Loebel JP, Borson S, Hyde T, et al: Relationships between requests for psychiatric consultations and psychiatric diagnoses in long-term care facilities. Am J Psychiatry 148:898, 1991.
31. Maletta GJ: Management of behavior problems in elderly patients with Alzheimer's disease and other dementias. Clin Geriatr Med 4:719, 1988.
32. Rovner BW, Lucas-Blaustein J, Folstein MF, et al: Stability over one year in patients admitted to a nursing home dementia unit. Int J Geriatr Psychiatry 5:77, 1990.
33. Bernstein JG: Handbook of Drug Therapy in Psychiatry. Boston, MA: PSG Publishing Company, Inc., 1984:172.

34. Barnes R, Veith R, Okimoto J, et al: Efficacy of antipsychotic medications in behaviorally disturbed dementia patients. Am J Psychiatry 139:1170, 1982.
35. Leibovici A, Tariot PN: Agitation associated with dementia: A systematic approach to treatment. Psychopharmacol Bull 24:49, 1988.
36. Pearlin LI, Mullan JT, Semple SJ, et al: Caregiving and the stress process: An overview of concepts and their measures. Gerontologist 30:583, 1990.
37. Zarit SH, Todd PA, Zarit JM: Subjective burden of husbands and wives as caregivers: A longitudinal study. Gerontologist 26:260, 1986.
38. Fortinsky RH, Hathaway TJ: Information and service needs among active and former family caregivers of persons with Alzheimer's disease. Gerontologist 30:604, 1990.
39. Chiverton P, Caine ED: Education to assist spouses in coping with Alzheimer's disease: A controlled trial. J Am Geriatr Soc 37:593, 1989.

10

DELIRIUM

IRA R. KATZ, M.D., PH.D.

Discussions of psychiatric therapy for delirium must consider the importance of recognizing delirium as a critical indicator of the need for medical treatment and identifying cases in which specific treatments may be indicated as well as more general approaches to the support of the patient and the management of symptoms causing danger and distress. The most important aspect of treatment must be the recognition of delirium and the evaluation of precipitating causes to allow the timely initiation of medical interventions. Therefore, the initial focus in this discussion must be on clarification of both the basic concept and the criteria for diagnosis.

It is impossible to discuss delirium without referring to historical problems in nomenclature and the definition of the term. It has at times been considered as a syndrome, defined in terms of symptomatology, and at times as a disorder, for which the diagnosis includes consideration of etiology (organic) and course (acute or subacute and reversible) as well as symptoms. Understanding the literature is complicated as a result of the use of numerous different approaches to terminology. Overlapping if not synonymous terms include acute confusional state, acute organic brain syndrome, reversible dementia, acute brain failure, and toxic or metabolic encephalopathies. The DSM-III[1] and DSM-III-R[2] definitions are similar, but not identical. Although the DSM-III-R definition is now "official," the DSM-III definition is, at this time, better validated, and it therefore remains useful. The DSM-III required evidence of "a specific organic factor judged to be etiologically related to the disturbance," while DSM-III-R is less definitive, allowing the diagnosis in the absence of such evidence if the disturbance "cannot be accounted for by any non-organic mental disorder." The latter criterion addresses the clinical reality that precipitating organic causes are, at times, not readily apparent, even after extensive diagnostic evaluations.

DELIRIUM AND DEMENTIA

Both delirium and dementia are acquired disorders in which there are diffuse disturbances in cognitive performance. In general, they differ in both clinical course and symptomatology. Delirium in DSM-III and DSM-III-R is defined as a disorder in which clinical features "develop over a short period of time (usually hours to days) and tend to fluctuate over the course of a day." In contrast, no clinical course is specified for dementia. Alzheimer's disease, of course, is a disorder characterized by an insidious onset; but cerebrovascular disease (multi-infarct dementia), head trauma, and carbon monoxide poisoning can all cause dementias of acute onset. Thus, acute onset of cognitive impairment does not necessarily indicate a diagnosis of delirium. However, as these examples suggest, it does indicate the urgent need for medical evaluation; this principle should be extended to include any acute changes in mental status.

The cardinal symptom of delirium as defined in DSM-III is "clouding of consciousness (reduced clarity of awareness of the environment), with reduced capacity to shift, focus, and sustain attention to environmental stimuli;" in DSM-III-R it is "reduced ability to maintain attention to external stimuli (e.g., questions must be repeated because attention wanders) and to appropriately shift attention to external stimuli (e.g., perseverates answer to a previous question).'' In dementia, according to DSM-III, the "state of consciousness (is) not clouded," and, in an alternative expression of the same point, the DSM-III-R definition of dementia states that deficits do not occur "exclusively during the course of delirium." The critical place of "consciousness" and "attention" in the diagnostic criteria for delirium, and the refinement of these criteria with revision of the *Diagnostic and Statistical Manual of Mental Disorders* demonstrate both the importance of deficits in attention as a central feature of delirium, and a concern that the level of consciousness and the ability to maintain attention may be difficult to assess on clinical grounds. In spite of these concerns, it has become clear that these functions can be defined in operational terms and can be reliably assessed in clinical evaluations.

Noting that problems in maintaining attention can follow from either a reduced level of consciousness (e.g., drowsiness or a difficulty in maintaining wakefulness), or from hyperarousal and distractibility, Anthony et al.[3] have developed methods for evaluating a patient's "global accessibility" and have found that it can be reliably assessed. They state:

> Accessibility was rated on a scale from 0.0–10.0 after a minimum of 2 minutes' interaction or attempted interaction (e.g., if the patient was stuporous). Usually the rating was made immediately after completion of the Minimental State Examination (MMSE), a test that often requires about 5 minutes. The basis for rating this aspect of consciousness was how well the patient kept his mind on interaction with the observer as judged by the observer. If the observer could readily engage the patient in ordinary conversation, and could keep the patient engaged throughout the interview, a high rating of 9.0–10.0 was made. If the patient could not be roused from stupor or was so agitated that no conversation was possible, a low rating of 0.0–1.0 was made. If the observer could engage the patient in conversation, but had to modify the interview to cope with drowsiness, wandering attention, or other variation in consciousness (including heightened awareness as in drug-induced deliria) a midrange rating was made unless there was an extenuating circumstance. For example, one interview was interrupted by a minor crisis on the ward that distracted the patient's attention.

Johnson et al.[4] provide explicit guidelines for assessment of attention:

> Ability to shift, focus, and sustain attention was determined by observing the patient's general attentiveness during the clinical interview and by asking the patient to perform specific tasks: (a) spell "world" forward and backward, (b) state the days of the week forward and backward, and (c) attend to, and engage in, a brief standard comprehension task. . . . A patient who had difficulty attending to a comprehension task and made one or more errors in spelling "world" backward or stating the days of

the week backward was rated as having a mild deficit. A severely impaired patient could only make brief contact or was stuporous or unresponsive.

In general, the DSM-III criteria for diagnosis of delirium have been demonstrated to have adequate inter-rater reliability in medical inpatients. The validity was established by demonstrating an association with both increased mortality and increased length of hospitalization.[5,6]

CLINICAL PERSPECTIVES

From the clinician's perspective, the importance of diagnosing delirium follows from the fact that it indicates a state of impairment that has a rather high probability of being reversible, but one where, in the absence of effective treatment, there is a high degree of vulnerability to further deterioration. The presence of the signs and symptoms of delirium suggests both an opportunity for the amelioration of cognitive deficits and a need for urgent medical intervention to prevent irreversible deterioration or death. Although this may be stated as a rule, there are a number of exceptions.

First, the symptoms of delirium do not always indicate that cerebral activity is affected by reversible toxic or metabolic brain disease. They may occur as a result of structural brain disease; specifically, cerebrovascular disease involving cerebral structures that mediate the process of attention. Symptoms of delirium have been reported primarily from infarcts in the region of the right middle cerebral artery,[7] right thalamus,[8] and the posterior circulation.[9] Although patients with irreversible dementia can experience superimposed reversible toxic or metabolic brain disease, symptoms of delirium can also arise in such patients as a result of psychosocial stress. In patients with preexisting cognitive impairment from dementia, anxiety, agitation, depression, or fatigue can affect attention, while sensory deprivation can induce perceptual distortions, or hallucinations, and lead to the diagnosis of delirium. However, clinicians should not attribute symptoms to such causes unless acute organic factors have been ruled out by medical evaluation. The term "pseudodelirium"[10,11] has been proposed to describe disorders with symptoms similar to those of delirium that occur without demonstrable organic causes, and are presumably due to the effects of stress or functional psychiatric disorders. It is not a diagnosis but, rather, a reminder that depression, anxiety, mania, schizophrenia, and other psychoses can, at times, mimic delirium, especially when they occur in elderly patients with some degree of dementia. Although it has been suggested that psychosocial stress by itself can cause delirium, there is no clear evidence that this can occur in patients without preexisting cerebral disease.

Second, there are cases in which reversible cognitive deterioration occurs in patients who do not meet diagnostic criteria for delirium. Although differences between disciplines and between individual investigators make it difficult to interpret the literature on reversible cases of dementia,[12] it is clear that a reasonable number of patients meeting diagnostic criteria for dementia have treatable causes for at least a component of their cognitive deficits.

The conclusion must be that the diagnosis of delirium is associated with a high probability that a medical illness is affecting the brain and that cerebral dysfunction can be reversible. It is, however, important to state that this cluster of symptoms does not necessarily imply reversibility and that reversible cognitive impairment can also occur in the absence of symptoms of delirium.

One of the recurring themes in the recent literature is that delirium is, as a rule, underrecognized in clinical practice. The problem is both quantitative (i.e., severe cases are more readily recognized) and qualitative (i.e., cases manifest by anxiety, psychotic symptoms, and agitation are more likely to be diagnosed than those manifest by mild to moderate depression, withdrawal, and lethargy). The magnitude of the problem is illustrated by Levkoff and coworkers,[13] who found a prevalence of delirium in acutely hospitalized elderly patients of 0.7 per cent in a review of medical records and note that systematic assessment of similar patient populations regularly demonstrates a prevalence approximately 20-fold higher or more.

CASE IDENTIFICATION

Several distinct approaches to case identification have been used in research and may be applicable to clinical practice. Folstein and coworkers have utilized cognitive screening instruments such as the MMSE as a method for case identification.[14,15] With this approach, the diagnosis of delirium involves a two-stage process in which the screening evaluation is used to identify cases of cognitive impairment that need further evaluation, and the specific diagnosis is established by clinical assessment. For research, the fact that it identifies patients with dementia as well as those with delirium may be a problem, but for clinical purposes, it is important to recognize both syndromes. Although the sensitivity of this approach to clinical diagnosis in the acute-care hospital is, in general, adequate, there are cases in which a delirious patient's performance may be within the normal range either as a result of limitations in the sensitivity of the instrument or to problems related to the fluctuating clinical course of the syndrome.

Other approaches have used the global accessibility rating,[3] checklists or structured assessments based upon the diagnostic symptoms[4] or symptoms judged to best discriminate between patients with delirium and normals or those with dementia,[16] and as a component of comprehensive assessive instruments[17] and rating scales that include items assessing both diagnostic symptoms and less-specific associated symptoms.[18-20] The findings from these approaches converge.[21-23]

In general it has been estimated that the prevalence of delirium on acute medical and surgical units is high, with reports generally ranging from 10 to 15 per cent. The prevalence in elderly patients is severalfold higher, with prevalence rates from studies of geriatric patients on medical wards in the range of 10 to 50 per cent or higher. On medical units, most cases are apparent at admission. In contrast, in surgical patients, most cases develop during the course of hospitalization. It has been estimated that 10 to 50 per cent of patients experience delirium after general surgery. The incidence varies as a function of both the nature of the patient population and the procedure. The incidence after surgical repair of hip fracture is 50 per cent or higher, probably as a result of the age and the prevalence of dementia in the patient population as well as the extent of tissue damage. A recent review of the literature has estimated that, overall, 37 per cent of elderly patients experience changes in mental status after surgery.[24] Although teaching in this area generally states that delirium is most common at the extremes of life, in the very young and very old, there has been little systematic research conducted in pediatric populations. Other groups at high risk include terminal cancer patients[25,26] and those with acquired immunodeficiency syndrome (AIDS).[27,28]

As demonstrated in the classic studies of Roth[29] and of Engel and Romano,[30] delirium can occur in several distinct contexts. In his investigations of the natural history of mental disorders of late life, Roth studied illnesses that led to psychiatric hospitalization and validated the distinction between delirium (acute confusion), dementia (senile and arteriosclerotic psychosis) and the functional psychiatric disorders of late life (affective psychosis and late paraphrenia). He characterized the clinical course of delirium by observing that acute confusion was generally characterized by a high mortality at or around the time of the index admission, with full recovery and a return to independent living in those who survived. In contrast, Engel and Romano studied delirium as a complication of medical illnesses in the acute-care hospital. They first called attention to the fact that delirium is a common complication of serious medical disorders, but that only the most severe of cases were recognized by clinicians. They also established the utility of the electroencephalogram (EEG) for establishing the diagnosis.

A more recent development in this field has been the recognition that delirium and related cognitive disorders are not limited to dramatic events requiring hospitalization or to complications of severe medical illnesses and that, instead, they can occur as part of the psychopathology of everyday life in apparently stable patients with chronic disease. The evidence comes from a number of sources. There are, for example, associations in chronic schizophrenic patients between cognitive impairment and plasma levels of anticholinergic medications.[31,32] The fact that cognitive deficits could be related to medications in patients in ongoing treatment suggests that persistent toxic encephalopathies can occur without physicians being aware that their patients are suffering from iatrogenic disease. The finding that approximately 10 per cent of patients going to a specialized clinic in a tertiary care hospital for evaluation of cognitive impairment have drug-related deficits as a component of their cognitive deterioration suggests that this phenomenon is widespread.[33-35]

Cognitive deficits can result from physiological abnormalities associated with chronic disease. The best documented example may be the association between deficits and hypoxemia in patients with chronic obstructive pulmonary disease.[36] At this time, these chronic and mild states present problems in diagnosis. Although they are toxic or metabolic encephalopathies, it is not clear whether they are best considered states of delirium, of dementia, or placed in some other category. In clinical practice, the major problems, however, are not difficulties in nomenclature, but in recognizing cases and targeting treatment. In principle, it should be possible to improve the sensitivity for case identification through longitudinal monitoring of cognitive performance in chronically ill patients. Current practice, however, ignores this possibility. No physician would treat vulnerable elderly patients or those with chronic disease without monitoring the functioning of vital systems (e.g., through repeated electrocardiograms or blood tests of renal or liver functions). In contrast, clinical practice virtually ignores the need for ongoing monitoring of the patient's cognitive and cerebral state. The most straightforward way to introduce this would be to incorporate the use of standardized mental status examinations or brief batteries of specific psychological tests into practice; this is an area in which significant advances in patient care could result from the use of low-technology, low-cost procedures. Early detection of delirium and the prevention of disability would be facilitated by proactive monitoring of elderly patients using repeated measures of cognitive status whenever medications that can affect cerebral functioning are prescribed or whenever patients have chronic illnesses that can cause physiological abnormalities affecting brain activity.

Special problems exist in the care of patients with disabling chronic diseases and those living in a supportive environment. The diagnosis of dementia explicitly, and that of delirium implicitly, requires cognitive impairment of a degree that interferes with vocational or social functioning or with activities of daily living. For individuals living independently, especially those working or sharing in the management of a home, day-to-day performance may be the most sensitive test of mental status, so that even minor deficits will result in seeking help. This may not be the case for patients with disabling illnesses and those who live in settings that are designed to compensate for deficits in self-care. In fact, systematic surveys of psychiatric symptoms in nursing homes have demonstrated that the prevalence of delirium is approximately 6 per cent.[37,38] Finding delirium with this frequency in research surveys suggests that it is often not recognized by those clinicians who are actually treating the patient. For patients who live in an environment that makes minimal demands on their intellectual capacity, significant deterioration in cognitive ability and cerebral activity can occur without apparent decrements in functioning. For such patients, early detection of deficits and the prevention of escalating disability requires ongoing monitoring of mental status.

Use of the EEG for the diagnosis of delirium may be the best established example of the use of a laboratory test for the diagnosis of any psychiatric disorder. To illustrate its value, the differential diagnosis of a withdrawn, apathetic, and uncooperative patient hospitalized for acute illness must include both delirium and depression. There may be times when the patient's responses and direct behavioral observations do not allow the distinction between them. In such cases, results from an EEG can allow the decisions about treatment to be made: a normal EEG would suggest the diagnosis of a functional disorder and the need for treatment of depression, while abnormal findings would suggest the diagnosis of delirium and the need to reevaluate the patient's medical status. Electroencephalographic changes associated with delirium can be demonstrated on both the routine clinical and computer-analyzed EEG. They include background slowing (increased delta and theta activities), low-voltage fast activity (beta), and progressive disorganization of the EEG as the patient deteriorates. Other patterns have been identified, including triphasic spike and wave complexes in certain metabolic encephalopathies and epileptiform patterns during withdrawal from alcohol, barbiturates, or benzodiazepines. As discussed below, the nature of the EEG abnormalities may be useful in identifying treatment of relevant subtypes of delirium. Since the pioneering work of Engel and Romano, the value of the EEG has been confirmed in most, but not all studies.[39-43] The apparent exceptions may be related to heterogeneity of the EEG under premorbid conditions. As with measures of cognitive status, the sensitivity of EEG measures for the detection of delirium could probably be enhanced by use of repeated longitudinal measures in vulnerable patients.

Subtypes

Lipowski has called attention to several subtypes of delirium that can be distinguished on the basis of associated psychomotor symptoms as hyperactive-hyperalert, hypoactive-hypoalert, or mixed variants.[21] The more important distinction, however, is not based on symptomatology but on physiology.

One model that can be used to define physiologically relevant subtypes is based on the observation that global accessibility can be lost in two distinct states: coma and status epilepticus. The former is manifest by a decrease and the latter by an increase in cerebral electrical activity. Delirium can be conceptualized as lying on a continuum between normal consciousness and either of these states. Delirium associated with decreased cerebral perfusion, fever, hypoxemia, hypoglycemia, and most drugs, as a rule, lies along the continuum between normal wakefulness and coma and is associated with slowing of the EEG, while that associated with withdrawal from alcohol, barbiturates, of benzodiazepines lies between normal and status epilepticus and is associated with increased low-voltage fast activity on the EEG (often in addition to slow activity). In general, clinical experience suggests that while delirium associated with states of withdrawal occurs with increased fast activity and is almost invariably associated with psychomotor changes in the direction of hyperactivity, delirium associated with other disorders and increased slow-wave activity is more variable in its behavior manifestations.

Predisposing Factors

The evaluation of patients with delirium should search for both precipitating and predisposing factors.[21] The precipitants are the acute and proximate causes of delirium. They commonly include toxic effects of medications and other substances; states of withdrawal from alcohol, barbiturates, and benzodiazepines; infections; conditions affecting cerebral perfusion, oxygen supply, and energy metabolism; other metabolic disturbances including electrolyte imbalances and the complex abnormalities associated with severe hepatic or renal disease; ictal and postictal states; and structural brain disease, including infarcts, tumors, and head trauma. In evaluating patients for precipitants it is important to consider the possibility that episodes of delirium may result from the additive or interactive effects of several abnormalities that may, by themselves appear minor and of doubtful clinical significance. Diagnostic evaluations should also consider the presence of predisposing factors, more chronic disorders, or conditions that can increase the severity of the precipitant or the sensitivity of the brain to its effects.

Conceptually, the predisposing factors can be divided into those affecting the patient's physiological and cerebral reserve. Decreased physiological reserve can result from chronic cardiac, pulmonary, or renal disease; endocrine abnormalities; or changes in drug metabolism that follow from both aging and physical illness. Patients with, for example, stable, minor degrees of heart failure will be less able to compensate for episodes of pneumonia, fever, or dehydration, and these illnesses will therefore have greater effects on cerebral perfusion and metabolism. Decreased cerebral reserve occurs when the brain is more sensitive to a physiological or pharmacological stressor. It occurs in patients with Alzheimer's disease, in patients with cerebrovascular disease, and in other conditions. In a review of medical records, Levkoff et al.[13] identified four independent risk factors associated with cases of delirium among hospitalized older patients: urinary tract infection, low serum albumin at hospital admission, elevated white cell count at admission, and proteinuria at admission; these findings represent markers for both precipitating and predisposing factors. Although this study did not identify preexisting dementia as a predictor of delirium, there is abundant evidence that it is a risk factor; in one series of 100 general hospital patients with delirium, 44 per cent had the delirium superimposed on a chronic dementia.[44] The initial treatment of patients presenting with delirium must be directed toward precipitants, but evaluations should not be considered complete until the presence of disorders affecting physiological and cerebral reserve have been considered. Treatment should be directed toward both the current episode and improving the management of chronic conditions to reduce the patient's vulnerability for future episodes.

As stressed above, the most critical aspects of the treatment of delirium consist of diagnosis, the identification of precipitants and predisposing conditions, and the prompt initiation of medical treatment. Other key components of treatment include the recognition of those cases of delirium that require specific treatment, the acute management of affective and behavioral states that represent sources of danger or distress, and the general physiological and psychosocial support of the patient.

TREATMENT APPROACHES

Specific treatment is needed for delirium accompanying withdrawal from alcohol, barbiturates, and benzodiazepines.[21] This type of delirium frequently occurs when use of these agents is discontinued at admission to the general hospital. Identification of patients at risk and the initiation of interventions designed to prevent withdrawal is necessary at this time. Obtaining a comprehensive history, and, where appropriate, continuing treatment with medications exhibiting cross-tolerance can prevent withdrawal and delirium. The importance of these considerations was demonstrated in one study that found that the presence of benzodiazepines in urine in elderly medical patients admitted to the hospital was a risk factor for delirium, and that most of the benzodiazepine users who did develop delirium had their medications discontinued at the time of hospital admission.[45] Once symptoms have developed, the diagnosis of a hyperactive delirium resulting from withdrawal can be established by history, by observing symptoms (hyperactivity and hyperarousal with autonomic symptoms support the diagnosis but are not pathognomonic), and by evaluating the EEG (looking for increased low-voltage fast activity). Diagnosis is important, of course, because this type of delirium requires specific treatment. Benzodiazepines are currently the treatment of choice for alcohol withdrawal. Early treatment of withdrawal symptoms can decrease the incidence of delirium and seizures. Although essentially all of the available benzodiazepines are effective, chlordiazepoxide, diazepam, oxazepam, and lorazepam are used most frequently. The differences between agents follow from their physical properties and pharmacokinetics rather than from fundamental differences in their pharmacodynamics. The basic strategy in treatment is to titrate patients with increasing doses of benzodiazepines until clinical improvement occurs; the object is to control symptoms without oversedation. Once symptoms are controlled, dosages should be gradually decreased; the need for monitoring during this period of downward titration is more critical when short-acting benzodiazepines are used. When hallucinations or delusions are present, it may be necessary to use neuroleptics (e.g., haloperidol) in addition to benzodiazepines. Other components of management include treatment of associated abnormalities (e.g., hypomagnesemia, dehydration, thiamine deficiency), and provision of both physiological and psychosocial support.

The treatment for barbiturate withdrawal generally involves use of barbiturates themselves. Phenobarbital is a reasonable agent because it has useful anticonvulsant properties and because its long half-life facilitates tapering. Benzodiazepine withdrawal can be treated by administration of a long-acting benzodiazepine, giving a drug such as diazepam on a frequent basis, as much as hourly, until symptoms are controlled, and then tapering gradually. If necessary, adjunctive use of a neuroleptic such as haloperidol can be used for management of psychotic symptoms.

Delirium due to the toxic effects of centrally acting anticholinergic (muscarinic blocking) medications is another condition for which specific treatment is available. Although most cases of anticholinergic-induced delirium can be treated by discontinuing the relevant drug and managing the patient supportively until the medication is cleared and symptoms remit, this is not always possible. When there is stupor or coma, when autonomic effects are severe, and when psychotic symptoms or agitation interfere with management, use of the centrally acting cholinesterase inhibitor physostigmine can be used to achieve a rapid reduction in symptoms.[46,47] The first step in the use of physostigmine should involve administration of an initial 1- to 2-mg test dose of physostigmine salicylate subcutaneously or intramuscularly followed by cautious observation of the patient. The presence of significant tissue levels of muscarinic blocking medication is confirmed if there is little or no change in peripheral autonomic symp-

toms over a period of approximately one half hour; the diagnosis of anticholinergic toxicity is disconfirmed if the patient develops symptoms of cholinergic excess, including bradycardia, tearing, excess salivation, sweating, and pupillary constriction. When the diagnosis is established, treatment should involve administration of 1 to 2 mg of physostigmine intramuscularly or by slow intravenous infusion every 0.5 to 2.0 hours, either until there is clinical improvement or there are signs of cholinergic excess. During treatment, it is necessary to monitor patients continuously for signs and symptoms of both anticholinergic toxicity and cholinergic excess. Atropine should be kept available to treat toxicity due to excess physostigmine.

The use of physostigmine for the treatment of delirium resulting from anticholinergic medications is established, but effects of physostigmine have also been reported in other conditions. Although they must be recognized as experimental, they are of interest because they may shed light on more general aspects of the pathogenesis of delirium. Reports from clinical studies that physostigmine may reverse delirium from agents that are not themselves anticholinergic, including benzodiazepines[48] and H_2 blockers,[49,50] suggest that indirect dysregulation of cholinergic neurotransmission may occur in toxicity from diverse medications, but further research in this area is clearly necessary.[51] The additional finding from studies in experimental animals that physostigmine can reverse some of the effects of hypoxia[52] suggests that the disruption of cholinergic systems may be a final common path in many toxic and metabolic encephalopathies.

PSYCHOSOCIAL MANAGEMENT

Other aspects of treatment or management are less specific but can be critical to the well-being of the patient. Psychosocial and environmental treatment of delirium is frequently neglected.[53] The goals of these interventions are not directed toward reversing the basic pathological process, but rather toward stabilization and reassurance of the patient to prevent or manage agitation, anxiety, perceptual disturbances, psychoses, and related symptoms that can interfere with medical treatment and impede recovery. Recognizing that both sensory deprivation and excess stimulation can lead to psychiatric symptoms and behavioral disturbances, the level of stimulation should be adjusted on an individual basis. Maintaining a reasonable amount of light at night may be essential to maintain orientation and to minimize frightening perceptual disturbances and illusions. Other interpersonal and environmental approaches to maintain orientation should include frequent, regularly occurring contact with nursing staff to provide information and reassurance. Given that symptoms of delirium wax and wane, it is necessary to use lucid periods as an opportunity for explaining what is happening to the patient. It should, in general, be reassuring for patients to hear that their symptoms are resulting from the way in which their medical illness is affecting the way the brain is working, but that they can expect to return to their normal state with treatment. Given the attention deficits characteristic of delirium, it will, in general, be necessary to repeat information a number of times to the patient. When appropriate, information should also be given to the family or others involved in the patient's care. Environmental elements that may be important include a view of the outside through a window, a large clock, and a calendar showing the day and the date. Helping the patient maintain a sense of familiarity with his surrounding can be useful. Visits from family should be encouraged, but it is necessary to explain to them that the patient is, at this time, cognitively impaired as a result of delirium and in need of support and reassurance from them. Patient management would be facilitated if hospitals made provision for "rooming in" of families of patients at high risk for delirium, especially the cognitively impaired elderly, just as they do for children. Having personal belongings such as photographs available can also be useful. The television or radio can provide both familiarity and a useful level of stimulation, but they can also be a source of annoyance or illusions. The key must be to tailor the nature of the environment to the needs of the individual patient, by trial and error where needed, and to give the patient as much control as is consistent with the level of impairment and the need for safety. Maintaining or restoring a sense of control is essential for all patient management, especially for those with delirium. Even when there is doubt about whether the patient can understand, it is important to identify and explain the use of medical equipment, medications, and procedures, preferably in brief, simple statements. Physiological support should be directed toward maintaining nutrition, adequate hydration, and electrolyte balance. Even when a presumed precipitant of the delirium is recognized, it is important to recognize that there may be multiple causes and that what appear to be minor abnormalities can make significant contributions to physiological instability. In addition, plans for management should recognize the likelihood that patients with delirium and those who have recently recovered may have difficulty in swallowing and may have impaired gag reflexes that place them at risk for choking and aspiration.

PHARMACOLOGICAL TREATMENT OF AGITATION

Although early detection, appropriate medical treatment, and attention to the importance of psychosocial management should minimize agitation, anxiety, and psychotic symptoms, psychotherapeutic medications can be necessary and effective when delirium is accompanied by psychiatric or behavioral symptoms that interfere with medical care or represent sources of danger and distress to the patient. In this context, the ideal agent for the treatment of agitation would be one that is effective for the control of symptoms but does not contribute to either cognitive impairment or physiological instability. According to these criteria, the best available agents are the high-potency neuroleptics.[21,54] Haloperidol is a useful prototype of this class of medication. When given orally, haloperidol is detectable in plasma within 60 to 90 minutes, with peak levels at 4 to 6 hours. After intramuscular injections, peak levels occur in 20 to 40 minutes. Although there has been essentially no controlled research in this area, clinical experience does allow the formulation of reasonable approaches to treatment. In adult patients with mild to moderate agitation, doses of, at most, 5 to 10 mg once or twice a day are usually sufficient. When agitation is severe, rapid tranquilization with intramuscular doses of 5 to 10 mg repeated every 30 to 60 minutes until symptoms are under control is reasonable. In elderly patients with mild to moderate agitation, starting doses for treatment would be in the range of 0.5 to 1.0 mg (i.e., a total daily dose of 0.5 to 3.0 mg). When rapid tranquilization is required, initial dose administration should be on the order of 0.5 mg each hour, increasing as needed if there is not a rapid response. While the literature has described the use of high-dose intravenous haloperidol either alone or in combination with benzodiazepines for the treatment of extreme agitation, such treatment is rarely necessary. The side effects of neuroleptics are those that should be familiar from the use of these drugs in other psychiatric disorders. When drug-induced parkinsonism occurs, the best approach is discontinuation of the drug or reduction of dosage; any pharmacological treatment for extrapyramidal symptoms can, in principle, exacerbate delirium. Akathisia presents a problem, because it may be difficult to distinguish from agitation due to delirium; when it is unclear if a patient has agitation due to delirium or akathisia due to neuroleptics (i.e., whether the patient is receiving too little medication or too much), the most prudent course is to attempt to discontinue the neuroleptic. There are times, for example when patients have significant liver disease or parkinsonism, when there is reason to avoid use of neuroleptics. When such patients have agitation without psychotic features, use of short-acting benzodiazepines may be a reasonable alternative. However, when prescribing such medications, it is important to recognize that they can cause excess sedation and exacerbate cognitive impairment.

REFERENCES

1. Diagnostic and Statistical Manual of Mental Disorders. 3rd ed. American Psychiatric Association, 1980:107.

2. Diagnostic and Statistical Manual of Mental Disorders. 3rd ed. (revised). American Psychiatric Association, 1987:103.

3. Anthony JC, LeResche LA, Von Korff MR, et al: Screening for delirium on a general medical ward: The tachistoscope and a global accessibility rating. Gen Hosp Psychiatry 7:36–42, 1985.

4. Johnson JC, Gottlieb GL, Sullivan E, et al: Using DSM-III to diagnose delirium in elderly general medical patients. J Gerontol Med Sci 45(3):M113–119, 1990.

5. Cameron DJ, Thomas RI, Mulvihill M, et al: Delirium: A test of the diagnostic and statistical manual III criteria on medical inpatients. J Am Geriatr Soc 35:1007–1010, 1987.

6. Thomas JI, Cameron DJ, Marianne FC: A prospective study of delirium and prolonged hospital stay. Arch Gen Psychiatry 45:937–940, 1988.

7. Mori E, Yamadori A: Acute confusional state and acute agitated delirium: Occurrence after infarction in the right middle cerebral artery territory. Arch Neurol 44:1139–1143, 1987.

8. Bogousslavsky J, Ferrazzini M, Regli F, et al: Manic delirium and frontal-like syndrome with paramedian infarction of the right thalamus. J Neurol Neurosurg Psychiatry 51:116–119, 1988.

9. Devinsky O, Bear D, Volpe BT: Confusional states following posterior cerebral artery infarction. Arch Neurol 45:160–163, 1988.

10. Lipowski ZJ: Transient cognitive disorders (delirium, acute confusional states) in the elderly. Am J Psychiatry 140:1426–1436, 1983.

11. Goldney R: Pseudodelirium. Med J Aust 1:630, 1979.

12. Maletta GJ: The concept of "reversible" dementia: How unreliable terminology may impair effective treatment. J Am Geriatr Soc 38:136–140, 1990.

13. Levkoff SE, Safran C, Cleary PD, et al: Identification of factors associated with diagnosis of delirium in elderly hospitalized patients. J Am Geriatr Soc 36:10999–1104, 1988.

14. Anthony JC, LeResche L, Niaz U, et al: Limits of the "Mini-Mental State" as a screening test for dementia and delirium among hospital patients. Psychol Med 12:397–408, 1982.

15. Rabins PV, Folstein MF: Delirium and dementia: Diagnostic criteria and fatality rates. Br J Psychiatry 140:149–153, 1982.

16. Inouye SK, van Dyck CH, Alessi CA, et al: Clarifying confusion: The confusion assessment methods: A new method for detection of delirium. Ann Intern Med 113:941–948, 1990.

17. Roth M, Huppert FA, Tym E, Mountjoy CQ: CAMDEX: The Cambridge Examination for Mental Disorders of the Elderly. Cambridge, MA: Cambridge University Press, 1988.

18. Trzepacz PT, Baker RW, Greenhouse J: A symptom rating scale for delirium. Psychiatry Res 23:89–97, 1988.

19. Miller PS, Richardson JS, Jyu CA: Association of low serum anticholinergic levels and cognitive impairment in elderly presurgical patients. Am J Psychiatry 256:342–345, 1988.

20. Lowy FH, Engelsmann F, Lipowski ZJ: Study of cognitive functioning in a medical population. Comp Psychiatry 14:331–338, 1973.

21. Lipowski ZJ: Delirium: Acute Confusional States. New York: Oxford University Press Inc., 1990.

22. Lindesay J, Macdonald A, Starke I: Delirium in the Elderly. New York: Oxford University Press, Inc., 1990.

23. Francis J, Kapoor WN: Delirium in hospitalized elderly. J Gen Intern Med 5:65–79, 1990.

24. Cryns AG, Gorey KM, Goldstein MZ: Effects of surgery on the mental status of older persons. A meta-analytic review. J Geriatr Psychiatry Neurol 3:184–191, 1990.

25. Adams F: Neuropsychiatric evaluation and treatment of delirium in cancer patients. Adv Psychosom Med 18:26–36, 1988.

26. Massie MJ, Holland J, Glass E: Delirium in terminally ill cancer patients. Am J Psychiatry 140:1048–1050, 1983.

27. Fernandez F, Levy JK, Mansell PWA: Management of delirium in terminally ill AIDS patients. Int J Psychiatry Med 19(2):165–172, 1989.

28. Holland JC, Tross S: The psychosocial and neuropsychiatric sequelae of the acquired immunodeficiency syndromes and related disorders. Ann Intern Med 103:760–764, 1985.

29. Roth M: The natural history of mental disorders in old age. J Ment Sci 101(423):281–301, 1955.

30. Engel GL, Romano J: Delirium, a syndrome of cerebral insufficiency. J Chron Dis 9:260–277, 1959.

31. Tune LE, Strauss ME, Lew MF, et al: Serum levels of anticholinergic drugs and impaired recent memory in chronic schizophrenic patients. Am J Psychiatry 139:1460–1462, 1982.

32. Perlick D, Stastny P, Katz I, et al: Memory deficits and anticholinergic levels in chronic schizophrenia. Am J Psychiatry 143:230–232, 1986.

33. Larson EB, Reifler BV, Summi SM: Diagnostic evaluation of 200 elderly outpatients with suspected dementia. J Gerontol 5:536–544, 1985.

34. Larson EB, Reifler BV, Sumi SM, et al: Diagnostic tests in the evaluation of dementia: A prospective study of 200 elderly outpatients. Arch Intern Med 146:1917–1922, 1986.

35. Larson EB, Kukull WA, Buchner D, Reifler BV: Adverse drug reactions associated with global cognitive impairment in elderly persons. Ann Intern Med 107:169–173, 1987.

36. Grant I, Prigatano GP, Heaton RK, et al: Progressive neuropsychologic impairment and hypoxemia: Relationship in chronic obstructive pulmonary disease. Arch Gen Psychiatry 44:999–1006, 1987.

37. Rovner BW, Kafonek S, Fillip L, et al: Prevalence of mental illness in a community nursing home. Am J Psychiatry 143:1446–1449, 1986.

38. Rovner BW, German PS, Broadhead J, et al: The prevalence and management of dementia and other psychiatric disorders in nursing homes. Int Psychogeriatr 2(1):13–24, 1990.

39. Obrecht R, Okhomina FOA, Scott DR: The value of EEG in acute confusional states. J Neurol Neurosurg Psychiatry 42:75–77, 1979.

40. Pro JD, Wells CE: The use of electroencephalogram with diagnosis of delirium. Dis the Nerv Syst 38:804–808, 1977.

41. Andreasen NJC, Harfrord CE, Knott JR, et al: EEG changes associated with burn delirium. Dis Nerv Syst 38:27–31, 1977.

42. Koponen H, Partanen J, Paakkonen A, et al: EEG spectral analysis in delirium. J Neurol Neurosurg Psychiatry 5:980–985, 1989.

43. Cadilhac J, Ribstein M: The EEG in metabolic disorders. World Neurol 2:296–308, 1961.

44. Purdie FR, Hareginan B, Rosen P: Acute organic brain syndrome: A review of 100 cases. Ann Emerg Med 10:455–461, 1981.

45. Foy A, Drinkwater V, March S, Mearrick P: Confusion after admission to hospital in elderly patients using benzodiazepines. Br Med J 293:1072, 1986.

46. Granacher RP, Baldessarini RJ: Physostigmine. Arch Gen Psychiatry 32:375–380, 1975.

47. Johnson AL, Hollister LE, Berger PA: The anticholinergic intoxication syndrome: Diagnosis and treatment. J Clin Psychiatry 42:313–317, 1981.

48. Nilsson E: Physostigmine treatment in various drug-induced intoxications. Ann Clin Res 14:165–172, 1982.

49. Goff DC, Garber HJ, Jenike MA: Partial resolution of ranitidine-associated delirium with physostigmine: Case report. J Clin Psychiatry 45:400–401, 1985.

50. Jenike MA, Levy JC: Physostigmine reversal of cimetidine-induced delirium and agitation. J Clin Psychopharmacol 3:43–44, 1983.

51. Pandit UA, Kothary SP, Samra SK: Physostigmine fails to reverse clinical, psychomotor, or EEG effects of lorazepam. Anesth Analg, 62:679–685, 1983.

52. Gibson GE, Pelmas CJ, Peterson C: Cholinergic drugs and 4 aminopyridine alter hypoxic-induced behavioral deficits. Pharmacol Biochem Behav 18:909–916, 1983.
53. Richeimer SH: Psychological intervention in delirium: An important component of management. Postgrad Med 81(5):173–180, 1987.
54. Conn DK: Delirium and other organic mental disorders. In J Sadavoy, L Lazarus, L Jarvik, eds. Comprehensive Review of Geriatric Psychiatry. American Association of Geriatric Psychiatry. Washington, DC: American Press, Inc., 1991.

SUGGESTED READINGS

Lipowski ZJ: Delirium: Acute Confusional States. New York: Oxford University Press Inc., 1990.
Lindesay J, Macdonald A, Starke I: Delirium in the Elderly. New York: Oxford University Press, Inc., 1990.
Francis J, Kapoor WN: Delirium in hospitalized elderly. J Gen Intern Med 5:65–79, 1990.
Beresin EV: Delirium in the elderly. J Geriatr Psychiatry Neurol 1:127–143, 1988.

11

ORGANIC MOOD, DELUSIONAL, AND ANXIETY DISORDERS

RICARDO JORGE, M.D. and ROBERT G. ROBINSON, M.D.

Organic mental disorders are mental or behavioral disturbances that are presumed to be etiologically related to permanent or temporary dysfunction of the brain. If there is not a presumed etiological relationship between the mental symptoms and the known brain dysfunction, the abnormality, by DSM-III-R convention, is termed an organic mental syndrome.

Even when used in the more restricted sense (i.e., presumed etiological relationship between brain dysfunction and mental disorder), organic mental disorders include an enormous range of mental disorders and brain dysfunctions. The most common mental disorders are cognitive impairments including dementia, delirium, substance intoxication, and substance withdrawal. Organic mental disorders, however, also include virtually all of the syndromes not associated with brain dysfunction such as depression, schizophreniform disorders, anxiety disorders, and others. Similarly, the brain dysfunctions may range from generalized brain disease such as progressive degeneration of the brain in Alzheimer's disease, to focal brain lesions produced by cerebral ischemia or brain neoplasms, to temporary toxic states such as drug intoxication. Thus, this chapter by necessity can only deal with a limited range of mental disorders and associated brain pathologies.

Over the past several years, we have been studying patients with brain lesions due to focal cerebral infarction or intracerebral hemorrhage. Our studies have generally focused on depression, but we have also studied mania,[1–4] anxiety disorders,[5] and schiz-ophrenia-like disorders.[6,7] In this chapter, we will review ours as well as other investigators' findings concerning the clinical manifestations, clinicopathological correlates, conditions, and the latest available treatments of these disorders.

ORGANIC MOOD DISORDERS

Depression

Prevalence

Our studies, as well as those of other investigators, have identified two types of depressive disorders associated with cerebral ischemia. One type is major depression, which we have defined by DSM-III symptom criteria for major depression (excluding duration criteria). The other types is minor depression, which we have defined by DSM-III symptom criteria for dysthymic depression (excluding duration criteria). In a consecutive series of 103 patients with acute cerebrovascular lesions, 27 per cent were found to meet symptom criteria for major depression, while 20 per cent showed symptoms of minor depression.[8] Virtually all other studies have identified a similar frequency of depression (ranging from 30 to 50 per cent of the population studied).[9–11]

Clinical Pathological Correlations

Our studies have consistently found a statistically significant relationship between lesion location and poststroke major depression.[12,13] Our initial finding of a significant relationship between lesion location and depression was based on a study of consecutive series of patients admitted to a stroke unit after the acute onset of a cerebrovascular lesion.[12] Major or minor depressive disorder was found in 14 of 22 patients who had an injury to the left hemisphere, but in only 2 of 14 patients who had a lesion of the right hemisphere ($\chi^2 = 9.4$, df = 1, $p < .01$). We also found that the location of the intrahemispheric lesion affected the frequency of depression. Of ten patients with a left anterior lesion (i.e., the anterior border of the lesion was less than 40 per cent of the AP distance), six had major depression, compared with one of eight patients with a left posterior lesion ($\chi^2 = 4.4$, df = 1, $p < .05$).[12]

We have also examined patients with stroke lesions restricted to either cortical or subcortical structures of the right or left hemisphere.[12] We found that 7 of 16 patients with left cortical lesions and 5 of 13 patients with left subcortical lesions had depressive disorder, while one of nine with a right cortical lesion and one of seven with a right subcortical lesion had depressive disorder ($\chi^2 = 4.0$, df = 1, $p < .05$). When we further divided patients into intrahemispheric lesion location, five of five patients with left cortical anterior lesions had depression compared to 2 of 11 patients with left cortical posterior lesions ($\chi^2 = 6.7$, df = 1, $p < .01$). When subcortical lesions were examined,[14] seven of eight patients with left basal ganglia lesions had major depressive disorder compared with one of seven patients with a right basal ganglia lesion and zero of six patients with a left thalamic lesion and zero of four patients with a right thalamic lesion ($\chi^2 = 17.0$, df = 3, $p < .001$). In addition to the relationship to brain structure involved in the lesion, we found a statistically significant correlation between the proximity of the lesion to the frontal pole and severity of depression.[13] Among patients with left cortical lesions, the correlation was $-.52$ while the correlation for left subcortical lesions was $-.68$.

Within the past year, there have been two studies that have examined the relationship between lesion location and depression following stroke.[10,15] These studies utilized very different populations from the low socioeconomic class, urban black patients that were examined in our original studies. Eastwood et al.[10] examined a group of 87 patients in Toronto, Canada who were generally elderly (mean age 63) and white (91 per cent), with 12 or more years of education (57 per cent). Patients were in a rehabilitation hospital and were examined approximately 12 weeks following stroke. Among patients with single lesions of the left, but not right, hemisphere, there was a strong correlation between proximity of the lesion on computed tomographic (CT) scan to the frontal pole and severity of depression ($r = .74$, $p < .01$).

Another study by Morris et al.[15] examined a consecutive series of 35 patients with single CT-verified ischemic brain lesions. Patients were elderly (mean age 68), white (100 per cent), lower socioeconomic class, Australian, and were interviewed in a rehabilitation hospital approximately 2 to 3 months following stroke. Although there was a tendency for depressed patients to have a higher frequency of left hemisphere lesions compared with nondepressed patients (64 per cent versus 52 per cent), the distance of the lesion from the frontal pole was strongly correlated with severity of depression ($r = .87$, $p < .001$) in the left but not the right hemisphere ($r = .06$, $p = NS$). These findings held true, however, only after patients with previous history of psychiatric disorder were removed ($r = .18$ if previous history was not removed). Although some investigators[16] have reported weaker (albeit statistically significant) relationships between proximity to the lesion of the frontal pole and severity of depression, these differences are likely due to methodological and population differences.[17] All investigators, however, who have examined this issue have found a statistically significant correlation suggesting that patients with more anterior lesions have a greater severity of depression than patients with more posterior lesions regardless of whether the lesion is cortical or subcortical.

Although one might expect a significant correlation between the severity of depression and severity of functional impairments produced by brain injury, virtually all empirical studies have failed to show a significant correlation between the severity of physical impairment and the severity of depression or have shown only weak correlation. The first investigators to address this issue were Folstein et al.,[18] who compared 20 consecutively admitted stroke patients with ten orthopedic patients. While the two groups proved to be comparable in terms of physical disabilities, stroke patients had a significantly higher frequency of depression (45 per cent versus 10 per cent). In our longitudinal study of patients with acute stroke,[8] we found that the correlation coefficient between Hamilton Depression Score and degree of impairment in activities of daily living was .37 ($p < .01$). The study of Morris et al.[11] reported no statistically significant difference between the activities of daily living (ADL) score in patients with and without depressive disorder. Eastwood et al.[10] studied stroke patients in a rehabilitation setting and reported a low but significant correlation between depression and functional physical impairment.

In summary, the correlation between depression and physical impairment following stroke does not appear to be strong. Thus, there is little evidence to support the idea that physical impairment is a primary cause of depression following stroke. There are several studies, however, which suggest that if depression develops, the patient's physical recovery tends to be significantly impaired.[19,20]

The relationship between severity of depression and severity of intellectual impairment has also shown a relatively weak correlation.[8] Fogel and

Sparadeo[21] reported the first case of a patient who developed a severe depression and marked cognitive impairments immediately after a stroke. The depression and cognitive impairments improved significantly, however, following treatment with a tricyclic antidepressant. In a study involving patients with restricted left hemisphere strokes, we found that both lesion size and depression correlated independently with severity of intellectual impairment.[22] Moreover, in a study in which patients with major depression were compared with 13 patients without mood disturbance matched for lesion size and location, depressed patients had significantly lower (more impaired) Mini-Mental State Examination (MMSE) scores than the nondepressed patients.[23]

In summary, the correlation between severity of depression and severity of cognitive impairment appears to be a weak, although significant, relationship. Intellectual impairments are related to both the size and the location of the ischemic injury as well as the severity of associated depression. Anecdotal reports have demonstrated a significant improvement in neuropsychological function after treatment with a tricyclic antidepressant.[21] As with physical impairments and depression, an important area for future research will be to demonstrate the impact of early treatment of depression upon recovery from both physical and cognitive deficits following stroke.

Treatment

Only two randomized double-blind treatment studies have been conducted to examine the efficacy of antidepressant treatment for depression following stroke. Our group conducted the first controlled study, in which 39 patients who met diagnostic criteria for either major or minor depressive disorder were treated with nortriptyline or placebo.[24] In the active group (N = 17), nortriptyline dosages were started at 20 mg/day for 1 week, 50 mg/day for weeks 2 and 3, 70 mg/day for week 4, and 100 mg/day for weeks 5 and 6. Mean serum nortriptyline concentrations were 63 ± 44 ng/ml at week 2, 74 ± 38 at week 4, and 116 ± 40 at week 6. All patients had achieved serum concentrations above 50 ng/ml by the end of the study. Eleven of the seventeen active-treatment patients completed the study. Of the six who did not complete the study, three experienced delirium, one had a syncopal episode of unknown etiology, one patient complained of dizziness, and one patient complained of oversedation. Of the 22 patients receiving placebo, 15 completed the study. Of the seven noncompleters, one developed mania, two refused to be interviewed because of lack of treatment efficacy, two died (one from a pulmonary embolism and one following a second stroke), and two were discharged from the hospital and lost to follow-up. Patients in the active and placebo groups were comparable in terms of their age, sex, socioeconomic class, marital status, family psychiatric history, prior medical illnesses, lesion size and location, neurolog-

ical symptoms, cognitive impairment, and activities of daily living. Repeated measure analysis of variance demonstrated that patients receiving nortriptyline showed a significantly greater improvement in depression as measured by both the Hamilton Rating Scale for Depression ($p = .006$) and the Zung Self-Rating Depression Scale ($p = .021$) than patients who received placebo. The active and placebo groups, however, did not differ significantly in their mean Hamilton Depression Scores until weeks 4 and 6 of treatment.

The other double-blind treatment study of post-stroke depression was conducted by Reding et al.[25] In this study, 27 patients participating in a stroke rehabilitation program were randomly assigned to treatment with either trazodone hydrochloride or placebo. Patients with and without evidence of depression were included. Trazodone was started at a nightly dose of 50 mg and then increased by 50 mg every 3 days until a nightly dose of 200 mg was achieved. Six patients receiving placebo and five patients receiving trazodone (four because of sedation and one secondary to eye discomfort) were dropped from the study. The major finding from this study was that patients who scored higher than 50 per cent on the Zung scale (N = 9) or who had a "clinical diagnosis of depression" (N = 8) tended (though statistically not significant) to have a greater improvement in their Barthel ADL score when treated with trazodone than when treated with placebo. When only patients with abnormal dexamethasone suppression tests (DST) were considered (N = 16), the seven patients treated with trazodone had a statistically significantly greater improvement in Barthel ADL score than the nine patients treated with placebo.

In summary, controlled treatment trials of depression following stroke have found a significant improvement in depression associated with the use of antidepressant medications. In each study, however, there were important medication side effects in the treated groups. None of these side effects, however, were irreversible and there were no deaths which were attributed to the use of antidepressant medication. There is evidence that the use of antidepressants in patients following stroke may improve both mood and a degree of impairment in activities of daily living.

Mania

Although mania occurs less frequently than depression, mania is another mood disorder that may result from brain ischemia caused by stroke. Krauthammer and Klerman[26] reported several cases of mania which they referred to as secondary mania, since they were associated with toxic, metabolic, or neurological disorders.

No systematic studies of mania following stroke have been conducted that would allow some estimates of the frequency of this disorder to be determined. In systematic studies of approximately 400 patients with acute stroke, we have only encountered two patients with mania. The other patients who have been included in our studies, which now number approximately 20, have been identified based on the existence of mania and secondarily found to have a brain lesion.

The relationship between lesion location and mania following stroke has been even more consistent than the association between depression and lesion location. Cummings and Mendez[27] reported two patients who developed mania following right thalamic strokes. Based on these cases and review of the literature, they concluded that secondary mania was a disorder related to damage to limbic areas of the right hemisphere. In our study of patients with secondary mania, there were nine patients with mania following stroke.[1] Eight of these nine patients had lesions exclusively in the right hemisphere, while one had a left hemisphere lesion. The brain areas involved were the orbital frontal and basal temporal cortex, thalamus and head of the caudate.

This study did not suggest, however, why most patients with right hemisphere strokes do not develop mania. We examined this issue by comparing 11 of our secondary manic patients who had positive CT scans with a group of patients who had the same size, location, and etiology of brain lesion but without mood disorder.[2] Patients with secondary mania were found to have a significantly higher bifrontal ratio (i.e., CT scan measure of subcortical atrophy at the level of the front lobes) and third ventricular : brain ratio (i.e., CT scan measure of atrophy in diencephalic brain areas) than lesion-matched controls. Family history of affective disorder was significantly more common among patients with poststroke mania (four of nine) than among patients with poststroke depression (3 of 31) (p < .05).[1]

In summary, mania following brain injury appears clinically identical to mania not associated with known neuropathology. Mania after brain injury, however, is strongly associated with injury to the right hemisphere, particularly limbic-connected areas.[28] Risk factors for the development of mania appear to be subcortical atrophy or a family history of affective disorder. These risk factors may explain why a relatively small number of patients with right hemisphere lesions develop this mood disorder.

Treatment

Although there are no systematic studies on the treatment of mania following brain injury, most of the cases of secondary mania reported in the literature showed a good response to treatment with the usual antimanic drugs (lithium and neuroleptics). Bakchine et al.[29] carried out a double-blind, placebo-controlled study in a single patient with mania following brain injury. Clonidine (600 mg/day), an α_2-adrenergic agonist, used in the treatment of hypertension, rapidly reversed the manic symptoms,

whereas carbamazepine (1200 mg/day) was associated with no mood change, and L-dopa (375 mg/day) produced an increase in manic symptoms. Some reports have also suggested that patients who develop secondary mania (particularly those associated with a high frequency of seizure disorders) may not be as responsive to lithium as patients with primary mania.[30] Anecdotal reports in the literature have also reported that some patients with secondary mania may respond to treatment with anticonvulsant drugs such as carbamazepine or valproate.[31,32]

BIPOLAR DISORDER

Some patients who experience episodes of mood disorder following brain injury have a bipolar (BP) disorder. Among a group of 19 patients with secondary mania, we found that BP patients had an episode of depression which preceded the manic syndrome but occurred after the brain lesion.[4] The unipolar (UP) manic group consisted of 12 patients who did not have depression prior to the onset of mania. Based on periods of follow-up ranging from 6 months to 5 years, some of these patients had recurrent mania, but no episodes of depression. Compared to the UP manic group, patients with poststroke BP disorder showed a significantly greater intellectual impairment as measured by MMSE scores.[4] There were no significant intergroup differences in demographic variables, handedness, personal or family history of psychiatric disease, or neurological findings. Six of the seven patients with BP disorder had subcortical lesions and right hemisphere lesions. The lesions involved the head of the caudate nucleus (two patients), thalamus (3 patients) and head of the caudate, dorsolateral frontal cortex, and basolateral temporal cortex (one patient). The remaining patient developed a BP disorder following surgical removal of a pituitary adenoma. Patients with UP mania also had lesions predominantly in the right hemisphere, but their lesions tended to be cortical rather than subcortical. Five of the twelve; patients had lesions involving the orbital frontal cortex, while another five had lesions of the basotemporal cortex. A hypothesis of unequal frequency of BP compared to UP manic disorder based on the presence of cortical or subcortical lesions was statistically substantiated (Fisher test, p < .005). Thus, BP disorder tends to be more frequent following the involvement of subcortical structures of the right hemisphere (i.e., basal ganglia or thalamus) and UP manic disorder following lesions of cortical structure of the right hemisphere (i.e., orbital frontal or basal temporal cortex).

Treatment

The treatment of secondary BP disorders has never been systematically investigated. There are reports in the literature of cases in which the usual treatment with lithium has not been successful.[30] Other cases, however, do appear to respond to lithium treatment.[28] In our follow-up of patients with UP mania versus BP disorder,[4] we did not control treatment, but we did evaluate the outcome of treatment efforts. There were a variety of treatment outcomes. Some patients did respond to lithium treatment, whereas others did not. Some patients did well on carbamazepine in combination with lithium or alone, but others failed to respond. Tricyclic antidepressants were usually effective in treating the depressive phases. Neuroleptics with or without lithium were similarly effective for treatment of mania at some times, but not at others.

In summary, the treatment of BP disorder (manic type) following brain injury is dependent upon the same regimen of pharmacotherapy that is used for primary mania. If lithium with or without neuroleptics or antidepressants does not work, carbamazepine, clonidine, valproate, or verapamil may be useful alternatives. Controlled therapeutic trials in secondary BP disorder, however, are desperately needed to provide an empirical basis for managing these disorders.

ORGANIC HALLUCINATORY AND DELUSIONAL SYNDROMES

Historically, the most common hallucinatory phenomenon associated with brain injury are those secondary to sensory loss. For example, auditory hallucinations associated with deafness are usually simple words or tunes, whereas visual hallucinations following blindness are often visions of animals or faces that are not associated with delusions. These kinds of hallucinations are recognized by the patient as being false perceptions.[7] The term "peduncular hallucinosis" has been used to describe some of these hallucinations that are associated with brainstem lesions. They have been reported with lesions of the midbrain, substantia nigra, subthalamic region, basal ganglia, thalamus, and limbic structures.[33-36]

Psychotic disorders as a complication of stroke lesions are a rare phenomena. Levine and Finklestein[37] reported on eight patients who developed secondary hallucinations after a cerebrovascular lesion. The most important finding was that all of them had right hemisphere lesions involving partially or completely the temporoparieto-occipital junction. The psychotic episodes (hallucinations and delusions) developed acutely and were present for days to months. The second important finding was that seven of the eight patients had seizures that followed the brain injury. Seizures preceded the onset of psychosis in five patients and followed the onset of psychosis in the remaining two cases. Thus, this study strongly suggested that seizures may play an important role in the pathogenesis of the syndrome.

We screened consecutive admissions of a stroke unit and a psychiatric inpatient unit during a 10-year period and found only five patients with a hallucinatory/delusional syndrome following a stroke lesion.[6] In this series with secondary hallucinations or delusions or both, all of the patients had right hemisphere lesions. We then compared these five patients with another group of five patients having cerebrovascular lesions that were matched for both location and volume in order to examine the importance of nonlesion factors in the production of this syndrome. We could not find significant between-group differences in any of the demographic variables, personal or family history of psychiatric disorder, or neurological examination. However, three of the five patients with secondary psychosis developed seizures after the stroke lesions, while none of the nonpsychotic lesion-matched controls did. In addition to seizures, however, we also found that patients with hallucinatory phenomena had significantly more subcortical atrophy as manifested by significantly larger areas of both the frontal horn and the third ventricle as compared to the lesion-matched controls. We suggested that the subcortical atrophy was probably a preexisting condition rather than a consequence of the stroke, because it was visible in the earliest CT scans taken after stroke and was present in the lateral ventricle on the opposite side of the brain from the lesion.

In summary, studies of relatively small groups of patients with hallucinatory or delusional disorders following stroke have identified three factors that appear to be important for the production of secondary psychosis: (1) a right hemisphere lesion involving the temporoparieto-occipital junction; (2) the presence of seizures some time after the brain lesion; and (3) subcortical atrophy in diencephalic regions that probably preceded the stroke.

Treatment

There are two basic approaches that have been used for the treatment of secondary delusional and hallucinatory syndromes. One of them is anticonvulsant therapy. This approach has its rationale in the frequent coexistence of seizure phenomena. In Levin and Finklestein's series,[37] however, secondary psychotic features did not usually respond to anticonvulsant treatment. Although they reported that one patient's mild delusional and hallucinatory symptoms cleared with phenytoin, other patients who received phenytoin (up to 1200 mg/day) and carbamazepine (up to 800 mg/day) showed little response to treatment. Price and Mesulam,[38] on the other hand, reported a patient whose repeated psychotic episodes (lasting from 1 day to 1 week) were controlled with phenobarbital.

The second approach to the treatment of hallucinations and delusions is the use of neuroleptic medications. Although some patients have been noted to be resistant to neuroleptic medication (e.g., trifluperazine up to 80 mg/day[37]) many patients with secondary psychotic disorders have improved with neuroleptics. Although the optimal dosages have not been established, the medications used have included both phenothiazines and butyrophenones.

ORGANIC ANXIETY DISORDER

Anxiety disorders associated with stroke have received remarkably little attention in the medical literature. We have, however, conducted one study of depression and anxiety disorder following stroke.[5] Anxiety disorder was defined by meeting DSM-III diagnostic criteria for generalized anxiety disorder excluding the duration criteria. We found a relatively high frequency of anxiety disorder among a consecutive series of patients (i.e., 29 of 98 patients). The great majority of patients with anxiety disorder, however, had major depression (23 of 29). We also found a rather low frequency of anxiety disorders without associated depression (6 of 98). The only clinical finding that distinguished the anxiety disorder (only) group from the depressed, depressed-anxious, or no disorder groups was an increased frequency of alcohol abuse (4 of 6 patients with anxiety alone versus 14 of 92 others, $p < .01$).

The anxious-depressed group had a significantly higher frequency of cortical lesions (16 of 19) compared with the major depression-only group (7 of 15, $p < .02$) or the no-disorder group (13 of 27, $p < .02$). On the other hand, the major depression-only group showed a significantly higher frequency of subcortical lesions (mainly involving the left basal ganglia) (8 of 15) compared with the anxious-depressed (2 of 19, $p < .01$) group. To our knowledge there are no studies that have examined patients for panic disorder following stroke.

In summary, anxiety disorders are very common following stroke, but they are frequently accompanied by major depression. Anxiety disorder in the absence of depression is relatively uncommon. These anxiety-plus-depressive disorders are associated with cortical brain lesions of the left hemisphere, while anxiety disorder alone may be associated with alcohol abuse.

Treatment

There have been no systematic studies or even anecdotal reports of treatment of anxiety disorders following stroke. The only available guidelines for treatment of these disorders are those used in treatment of anxiety disorders not associated with organic factors. The benzodiazepines are the most commonly used medications in generalized anxiety disorders. If the anxiety disorder is accompanied by depression, the secondary (more sedating) tricyclic medications (e.g., amitriptyline), used to treat the depressive disorder, may be beneficial in reducing both anxiety and depression. Buspirone may be useful in reducing anxiety without producing an addic-

tive drug state as the benzodiazepines are prone to do.

FUTURE DIRECTIONS

The investigation of mood, delusional, and anxiety disorders in patients with known neuropathological disorders is in its early stages. We have focused on ischemic brain injury in this chapter because there is the greatest amount of information available about these disorders, but there are numerous other causes of brain dysfunction which may add their own unique aspects to these mental disorders. In addition, our knowledge about the course, clinical manifestations, clinical correlates, and treatments of these disorders are only beginning to be established. There are many studies, particularly of anxiety disorders, which need to be done.

One of the great hopes of studying disorders in which there is a known neuropathology is that the investigation of the pathophysiology or biochemical consequences of these lesions will ultimately illuminate the mechanism of these disorders. That kind of discovery might eventually lead to the development of truly rational treatments for these disorders (i.e., treatments in which specific neuropathological changes could be targeted) rather than the kind of empirical studies that currently form the basis for our treatment decisions.

ACKNOWLEDGMENTS

The authors are indebted to Drs. Sergio E. Starkstein, Thomas R. Price, John R. Lipsey, Rajesh M. Parikh, J. Paul Fedoroff, Helen S. Mayberg, and Karen Bolla who participated in many of these studies. This work was supported by the following NIMH grants: Research Scientist Award MH 00163 and MH 40355.

REFERENCES

1. Robinson RG, Boston JD, Starkstein SE, et al: Comparison of mania with depression following brain injury: Causal factors. Am J Psychiatry 145:172–178, 1988.
2. Starkstein SE, Pearlson GD, Boston JD, et al: Mania after brain injury: A controlled study of causative factors. Arch Neurol 44:1069–1703, 1987.
3. Starkstein SE, Mayberg HS, Berthier ML, et al: Secondary mania: Neuroradiological and metabolic findings. Ann Neurol 27:652–659, 1990.
4. Starkstein SE, Fedoroff P, Berthier ML, et al: Manic-depressive and pure manic states after brain lesions. Biol Psychiatry 29:149–158, 1991.
5. Starkstein SE, Cohen BS, Fedoroff P, et al: Relationship between anxiety disorders and depressive disorders in patients with cerebrovascular injury. Arch Gen Psychiatry 47:246–251, 1990.
6. Rabins PV, Starkstein SE, Robinson RG: Risk factors for developing atypical (schizophreniform) psychosis following stroke. J Neuropsychiatr Clin Neurosci 3:6–9, 1991.
7. Starkstein SE, Robinson RG, Berthier ML: Post-stroke hallu-

cinatory syndromes. Neuropsychiatr Neuropsychol Behav Neurol, 1992 (in press).

8. Robinson RG, Price TR: Post-stroke depressive disorders: A follow-up study of 103 patients. Stroke 13:635–641, 1982.

9. Sinyor D, Jacques P, Kaloupek DG, et al: Post-stroke depression and lesion location: An attempted replication. Brain 109:537–546, 1986.

10. Eastwood MR, Rifat SL, Nobbs H, et al: Mood disorder following cerebrovascular accident. Br J Psychiatry154:195–200, 1989.

11. Morris PLP, Robinson RG, Raphael B: Prevalence and course of post-stroke depression in hospitalized patients. Int J Psychiatry Med 20:327–342, 1990.

12. Robinson RG, Kubos KL, Starr LB, et al: Mood disorders in stroke patients: Importance of location of lesion. Brain 109:537–546, 1986.

13. Starkstein SE, Robinson RG, Price TR: Comparison of cortical and subcortical lesions in the production of post-stroke mood disorders. Brain 110:1045–1059, 1987.

14. Starkstein SE, Robinson RG, Berthier ML, et al: Differential mood changes following basal ganglia versus thalamic lesion. Arch Neurol 45:725–730, 1988.

15. Morris PLP, Robinson RG, Raphael B: Lesion characteristics and post-stroke depression. Evidence of a specific relationship in the left hemisphere. Neuropsychiatr Neuropsychol Behav Neurol, 1992 (in press).

16. House A, Dennis M, Warlow C, et al: Mood disorders after stroke and their relation to lesion location. Brain 113:1113–1129, 1990.

17. Castillo CS, Robinson RG: Neuropsychiatric disorders and cerebrovascular disease. Curr Opin Psychiatry 4:101–105, 1991.

18. Folstein MF, Folstein SE, McHugh PR: Mood disorder as a specific complication of stroke. J Neurol Neurosurg Psychiatry 40:1018–1020, 1977.

19. Parikh RM, Lipsey JR, Robinson RG, et al: Post-stroke depression: Impact on activity of daily living over two years. Arch Neurol 47:785–790, 1990.

20. Synyor D, Amato P, Kaloupek D, et al: Post-stroke depression: Relationship to functional impairment, coping strategies, and rehabilitation outcome. Stroke 17:1102–1107, 1986.

21. Fogel BS, Sparadeo FR: Focal cognitive deficits accentuated by depression. J Nerv Ment Dis 173:120–124, 1985.

22. Robinson RG, Bolla-Wilson K, Kaplan E, et al: Depression influences intellectual impairment in stroke patients. Br J Psychiatry 148:541–547, 1986.

23. Starkstein SE, Robinson RG, Price TR: Comparison of patients with and without post-stroke major depression matched for size and location of lesion. Arch Gen Psychiatry 45:247–252, 1988.

24. Lipsey JR, Robinson RG, Pearslon GD, et al: Nortriptyline treatment for post-stroke depression: A double blind study. Lancet 1:297–300, 1984.

25. Reding MJ, Orto LA, Winter SW, et al: Antidepressant therapy after stroke: A double blind trial. Arch Neurol 43:763–765, 1986.

26. Krauthammer C, Klerman GL: Secondary mania: Manic syndromes associated with antecedent physical illness or drugs. Arch Gen Psychiatry 35:1333–1339, 1978.

27. Cummings JL, Mendez MF: Secondary mania with focal cerebrovascular lesions. Am J Psychiatry 141:1084–1087, 1984.

28. Starkstein SE, Boston JD, Robinson RG: Mechanisms of mania following brain injury: 12 case reports and review of the literature. J Nerv Ment Dis 176:87–100, 1988.

29. Bakchine S, Lacomblez L, Benoit N, et al: Manic like state after orbitofrontal and right temporoparietal injury: Efficacy of clonidine. Neurology 39:777–781, 1989.

30. Shukla S, Cook BL, Mukherjee S, et al: Mania following head trauma. Am J Psychiatry 144:93–96, 1987.

31. Forrest DV: Bipolar illness after right hemispherectomy. Arch Gen Psychiatry 39:817–819, 1982.

32. Pope HG, McElroy SL, Satlin A, et al: Head injury, bipolar disorder and response to valproate. Compr Psychiatry 29:34–38, 1988.

33. Geller TJ, Bellur SN: Peduncular hallucinosis: Magnetic resonance confirmation of mesencephalic infarction during life. Ann Neurol 21:602–604, 1987.

34. McKee AC, Levine DN, Kowal NW, et al: Peduncular hallucinosis associated with isolated infarction of the substantia nigra pars reticulata. Ann Neurol 27:500–504, 1990.

35. Feinberg WM, Rapcsak SZ: Peduncular hallucinosis following paramedian thalamic infarction. Neurology 39:1535–1536, 1989.

36. Lanska DJ, Lanska MJ, Mendez MF: Brainstem auditory hallucinosis. Neurology 37:1685, 1987.

37. Levine DN, Finklestein S: Delayed psychosis after right temporoparietal stroke or trauma: Relation to epilepsy. Neurology 32:267–273, 1982.

38. Price BH, Mesulam M: Psychiatric manifestations of right hemisphere infarctions. J Nerv Ment Dis 173:610–614, 1985.

12

AN OVERVIEW OF THE TREATMENT OF GERIATRIC DISORDERS

CARL SALZMAN, M.D. and CURTISS DuRAND, M.D.

The Uniqueness of Psychogeriatrics

Approximately 15 per cent of the 25 million Americans over age 65 have psychiatric disease. In addition, organic mental impairment rises from 4 per cent of those aged 65 to 74, to 25 per cent of those aged 75 and older. Evaluation and treatment of this substantial illness burden is complicated by the special characteristics of psychiatric disorders in the elderly, the large prevalence of concomitant medical disorders, the substantial use of medications and over-the-counter drugs by the elderly, and the pharmacodynamic and pharmacokinetic consequences of aging. These special considerations serve to distinguish elderly patients from younger adults in much the same way as pediatric patients must be distinguished from adult patients. This chapter will briefly summarize some of these considerations.

Americans over age 65 receive 22 per cent of all drug prescriptions;[1] and about one quarter of older people are dependent on prescription drugs for daily activities.[2] Psychotropic agents constitute a significant proportion of prescription drugs used by the elderly. In fact, sedatives and hypnotics constitute the third most common class of drugs taken regularly by older patients. Thirty per cent of older patients in general hospitals use psychotropic agents, and as many as 92 per cent of institutionalized elderly patients use these drugs.[3] Surveys of nursing homes show that older Americans receive an average of 5 to 12 medications every day.[4] Older patients take an average of eight drugs simultaneously in general hospitals. This extensive drug use increases the older patient's risk of serious drug toxicity and drug interactions. Varying dosage schedules may also lead to inadvertent errors in compliance with one or more medications.

Older people have greater difficulty with compliance because of forgetfulness, confusion about doses and schedules, problems with packaging, labels that are too small to be read easily, and containers that can be very difficult to open. Personal beliefs about medications may also influence compliance. For example, if the older patient believes taking medicine for depression is a sign of weakness, the drug may not be taken at all. Others take extra pills because they believe that "more is better."

Pharmacodynamic and Pharmacokinetic Considerations in the Elderly

There is evidence that aging alters the central nervous system's (CNS) sensitivity to psychotropic drugs due to alterations in synthesis, turnover, receptor binding, and synaptic neurotransmission in many parts of the brain. Evidence suggests that decreases in CNS norepinephrine, serotonin, dopamine, gamma-aminobutyric acid (GABA), and acetylcholine result in increased receptor-site sensitivity in areas of the brain associated with mood, cognition, and coordinated motor behavior. These changes can lead to significant changes in responsiveness to psychoactive drugs. For example, the anticholinergic effects of tricyclic antidepressants, which may be minor irritations for young adults, can lead to confusion, oversedation, unsteadiness, fecal impaction, and urinary retention in the elderly. As another example, benzodiazepines may significantly alter psychomotor functioning.[6] Comprehensive reviews of age-related alterations in psychotropic drug pharmacodynamics are available in Salzman[6] and Sunderland.[7]

Alterations in psychotropic drug pharmacokinetics also occur with age. The liberation (release from dosage form and entering into solution), absorption, distribution, metabolism, and elimination of drugs[8] changes significantly during the aging process (Table 12–1). For example, most psychotropic drugs bind extensively to albumin; increased sedation with some of these drugs has been observed in older people associated with reduced levels of plasma albumin. In addition, the marked increase in percentage of total body fat with aging increases the apparent volume of distribution of fat-soluble drugs and decreases the apparent volumes of distribution of water-soluble drugs.

Hepatic metabolism serves to (1) metabolically inactivate many but not all drugs (phase I metabolism), and to (2) transform nonpolar lipid-soluble compounds into polar water-soluble products which can then be excreted by the kidney (phase II metabolism). Phase I reactions include oxidation (e.g., phenytoin, diazepam, chlordiazepoxide, prazepam, imipramine, and chlorpromazine), reduction (e.g., clonazepam), and hydrolysis (e.g., carbamazepine,

80

TABLE 12–1. PHARMACOLOGICAL CHANGES AND THEIR CONSEQUENCES[a]

	*Pharmacological Change with Age	Clinical Consequence
Liberation	Decreased gastric secretion and motility; increased Ph	Delayed dissolution; change in degree of ionization
Absorption	Unchanged or slight delay; greater delay with antacids; increased gastric emptying time; decreased peristalsis, decreased mesenteric blood flow rate, mucosal atrophy	Do not prescribe psychotropics and antacids at same time; give sleep medication 1 hr before bed
Protein binding	Decrease with age, disease, and malnutrition; decreased albumin, increased gamma globulin and α_1 acid glycoprotein	Increased free fraction leads to potential toxicity
Volume of distribution	Often increased (except lithium) leading to delayed clearance; increased body fat, decreased blood flow rates	In combination with hepatic metabolism, clearance delayed and elimination half-life doubled or tripled
Hepatic metabolism	Decreased metabolism of most neuroleptics, antidepressants, hypnotics, stimulants, and long-acting benzodiazepines	See above: prolonged elimination half-life 24–75 hr for most psychotropics except short-acting benzodiazepines
Renal clearance	Reduced	Prolonged elimination half-life of lithium; more frequent and more severe lithium toxicity

[a] Adapted with permission from Saltzman C: Geriatric psychopharmacology. Ann Rev Med 36:217–228, 1985; and Ritschel WS: Gerentokinetics: Pharmacokinetics of Drugs in the Elderly. 23, 1988.

desipramine, imipramine, desmethyldiazepam, and propanolol). Some of the phase I products (e.g., desmethyldiazepam) are pharmacologically active. Phase II reactions, which yield water-soluble metabolites ready for excretion, include conjugation with either glucuronide or sulfate, or acetylation. Drugs which require only phase II conjugation include alprazolam, oxazepam, and lorazepam. Phase I oxidation reactions are generally impaired in the elderly, but phase II reactions are not significantly affected by age.[9]

Benzodiazepines provide good examples of the effect of age on these metabolic processes. As people age, phase I metabolism of long–half-life benzodiazepines slows, prolonging the elimination half-life of both the drug and its active metabolites by a factor of two to three as compared with younger adults, leading to increased toxicity.[4,10–12] Both the drug and its active metabolites accumulate, leading to increased toxicity. After treatment has been stopped, elimination of the parent compound and its active metabolites proceeds very slowly, leading to persistance of therapeutic and toxic effects in the older adult for days or even weeks. For example, the elimination half-life of diazepam increases from 20 hours at age 20 to about 90 hours at age 80. In contrast, the short–half-life benzodiazepines undergo only phase II metabolism (conjugation), which is unaffected by aging, and thus are eliminated at about the same rate as in younger adults. Thus, steady state and clinical response are reached much sooner and relatively little accumulation occurs, making these short–half-life benzodiazepines preferred for the elderly.

The metabolism of antidepressants is also affected by aging. Tricyclic antidepressant steady-state blood levels may be twice as long, and their elimination half-life may be two to three times as long as in younger adults.[13,14] Further, tricyclics are metabolized to potentially cardiotoxic[15] water-soluble hydroxy metabolites which are cleared by the kidney. Age-related decline in renal function [which is not necessarily reflected in blood urea nitrogen (BUN) or creatinine level] leads to significantly prolonged elimination half-life of these metabolites as well as for another water-soluble psychotropic drug, lithium.

TREATMENT OF SPECIFIC CONDITIONS

Agitation and Psychosis

There are five common sources of disturbances in behavior and thinking in older people: (1) chronic organic disorders such as dementia[60]; (2) delirium and acute confusional states; (3) paranoid psychosis of late life; (4) chronic schizophrenia; and (5) major affective disorders. When agitation and psychosis are not responsive to nonpharmacological interventions, neuroleptic drugs are often used. Studies of the effects of neuroleptics lead to four main conclusions[16–20]:

1. Although neuroleptic agents have consistent and reliable therapeutic effect in the control of agitation and psychosis in the elderly, their general therapeutic efficacy is only modest and some older patients may become worse.

2. Older patients are more sensitive than younger patients to neuroleptic side effects. The side effects that are especially frequent and troublesome in the elderly are sedation, orthostatic hypotension, and extrapyramidal symptoms (EPS). Sedation is usually not desired in the elderly, since the sedated patient may become confused and even more agitated. The elderly are more prone to orthostatic hypotensive

episodes, and neuroleptics increase that risk, with the resultant dangers of falls and fractures. Because of the increased risk of sedation and orthostatic hypotension, low-potency neuroleptics such as chlorpromazine and thioridazine are recommended less often than high-potency neuroleptics for this patient population. The elderly are also prone to more frequent and more severe EPS, especially by high-potency neuroleptics such as haloperidol and fluphenazine. In general, however, the high-potency neuroleptics are preferred, and EPS is minimized by using very low doses (Table 12–2).

3. Regardless of the choice of a neuroleptic, behavioral disruptions in older patients can often be controlled by using very small doses. For example, doses of fluphenazine or haloperidol as small as 0.25 mg one to four times a day or thioridazine 10 to 25 mg two to four times per day may be effective without inducing unwanted side effects. Liquid preparations can be used to titrate small doses.

4. Increasing age is associated with higher risk of tardive dyskinesia. There is no evidence, however, that very low neuroleptic doses in the treatment of agitation and psychosis are more likely to produce tardive dyskinesia or worsen this movement disorder in the elderly.

Since neuroleptics have many drawbacks, there have been efforts to identify other agents for the treatment of agitation in the elderly. For some older patients, especially those who are demented or who have developed neuroleptic toxicity, propranolol in divided doses of 10 to 100 mg is helpful.[18–21] In this dose range, side effects are unusual, but careful monitoring of pulse and blood pressure is important. Contraindications include bronchospastic disease or significant cardiac disease. Trazodone in doses of 75 to 200 mg/day has been reported as effective treatment of agitation and disruptive behavior.[22–25]. Increasing clinical experience suggests that it is safe and effective in some patients in doses of 50 to 100

mg/day. Buspirone is a nonbenzodiazepine antianxiety agent with dopamine-blocking properties that is reported to be effective in the control of severe agitation and disruptive behavior in dementia.[19,27] Very high doses (e.g., 20 to 80 mg) may be necessary. So far, reported side effects are not prominent. Other treatments are less predictably useful. Carbamazepine in doses of 50 to 200 mg/day has controlled chronic agitation and chronic disruptive behavior in some patients, especially those who are demented.[20,27] Lithium is also sometimes useful in the management of disruptive behavior.[18,20,28] The therapeutic range is from 150 to 600 mg/day, in divided doses. However, both carbamazepine and lithium may produce neurotoxicity characterized by increased agitation, confusion, and disorientation. Thus the clinician should use low doses and be ready to stop the drug if clinical deterioration occurs.

Depression

The use of psychotropic medications to treat depressed elderly people requires an appreciation of several age-related factors. These factors include variability of diagnosis and treatment response, and increased predisposition to side effects. Older people have a high prevalence of physical illness, use more prescription and nonprescription drugs, have higher rates of treatment noncompliance, and have age-related physiological changes that alter pharmacodynamic and pharmacokinetic properties of drugs (see earlier in chapter).

Differential diagnosis of depression in the elderly is complicated by variability of the clinical presentation of depressive symptoms, lack of reliable clinical or biological markers for psychiatric disease, and the impact of physical illness and concomitant treatments on emotional state. Therefore, when assessing the depressed elderly patient, an essential and even

TABLE 12–2. REPRESENTATIVE NEUROLEPTIC DRUGS FOR THE ELDERLY PATIENT[a]

Generic Name	Dose Range in Elderly (mg)	Relative Incidence of Side Effects			
		Sedation	*Hypotension*	*EPS*	*Anticholinergic*
Chlorpromazine	10–300	+++++	++++	+	++++
Thioridazine	10–300	++++	++++	+	+++++
Chlorprothixene	10–300	++++	++++	++	++++
Clozapine[b]	Not established	+++++	+++++	+	+++++
Loxapine	5–100	+++	++	++	++
Molindone	5–100	+	++	++	++
Perphenazine	4–32	+++	++	++	++
Thiothixene	4–20	++	++	+++	++
Trifluoperazine	4–20	+	++	+++	++
Fluphenazine	0.25–6	++	+	++++	++
Haloperidol	0.25–6	++	+	++++	+

[a] Adapted with permission from Salzman C: Principles of psychopharmacology. *In* Bienenfeld D, ed. Verwoerdt's Clinical Geropsychiatry. 3rd ed. Baltimore: Williams and Wilkins, 1990:239.
[b] Data on clozapine derived from Lieberman JA, Kane JM, Johns CA: Clozapine: Guidelines for clinical management. J Clin Pyschiatry 50:9, 329–338; and from package insert.

lifesaving step is to search carefully for a physical condition which presents with depressive symptoms.[60] Because of these facts, the specific pharmacological treatment of depression in the elderly should be preceded by a comprehensive history and physical examination as well as a pretreatment electrocardiogram (ECG).

The clinical picture of depression in the elderly is often one of an anxious, withdrawn, apathetic, fatigued patient who is preoccupied with somatic symptoms. Depressed patients over the age of 50 demonstrate more agitation, insomnia, and hypochondriasis.[29]

Drug Selection

In selecting an antidepressant drug for an older person, it is especially important to consider the impact of aging and physical illness on drug effect, the impact of drugs on physical illness, nonspecificity of drug effect, and compliance problems. As noted, age-related alterations in antidepressant pharmacokinetics lead to higher plasma levels and prolonged presence of heterocyclic agents and their toxic metabolites (Table 12–3). Older patients are also more sensitive to antidepressant side effects. Some antidepressants, for example, may exacerbate cardiac arrhythmias in older people, and anticholinergic side effects of others may markedly increase symptoms of prostatic hypertrophy, blurred vision, and symptoms associated with decreased gastrointestinal motility. Since symptom patterns in the elderly are less well defined than those of younger adults, and since

much of the research on the effects of psychotropic drugs was conducted in younger adults, prescribing principles used for younger adults may not provide an adequate guide to safe and effective treatment of elderly persons.

Heterocyclic Antidepressants

The heterocyclic group of antidepressants includes the tertiary amines and their metabolites, the secondary amines. There are no convincing data to suggest that one of these drugs is therapeutically superior to any other for the average older patient. Selection, therefore, is based primarily on the side-effect profile. Because tertiary heterocyclics produce the most intense and most frequent side effects,[30,31] they are not recommended as first-choice antidepressants for the elderly, although some studies have reported low toxicity at very low doses, such as 30 to 75 mg/day of doxepin[32] or amitriptyline[33] (see Table 12–3 for the contrast between dose ranges in the elderly and in younger adults).

The two secondary amines in wide clinical use are notriptyline, the demethylated metabolite of amitriptyline; and desipramine, the demethylated metabolite of imipramine. Desipramine produces little sedation and may be helpful for an apathetic, anergic older patient with psychomotor retardation. In some older patients, this so-called activating effect of desipramine may lead to insomnia or agitation. Desipramine is also useful for older patients who are sensitive to anticholinergic side effects or who are taking other drugs with anticholinergic properties. Nortriptyline is less activating and produces slightly less orthostatic hypotension than other antidepressants.[30,34] Thus it is recommended for the patient with a history of falls, dizziness, stroke, or others in whom orthostatic hypotension could be especially hazardous.

At high therapeutic plasma levels, all heterocyclic antidepressants as well as their metabolites tend to prolong electrical conduction, as reflected in a wider QRS interval on the ECG. At toxic levels (QRS exceeds 100 msec), heart block, ventricular arrhythmias, and even sudden death can result. Widening QRS is a contraindication to increasing the antidepressant dose regardless of blood levels.[35]

Monoamine Oxidase Inhibitors

Monoamine oxidase inhibitors (MAOIs) can be useful treatments for depressed elderly patients whose depression is characterized by withdrawal, lack of motivation, apathy, and anergia.[36–40] As with other antidepressants given to the elderly, increased sensitivity to side effects requires lower doses. Doses for the two common MAOIs commonly prescribed for older persons are phenelzine, 7.5 to 30 mg/day, or tranylcypromine, 10 to 40 mg/day. The most common side effect of MAOIs in the elderly is orthostatic hypotension. They can also cause agitation in the

TABLE 12–3. USUAL DOSES OF ANTIDEPRESSANT DRUGS IN YOUNGER ADULTS AND IN THE ELDERLY[a] AND SELECTED ELIMINATION HALF-LIVES[b]

Drug	Doses in (mg/day) Adult (<65)	Doses in (mg/day) Elderly (>65)	Elimination Half-Life (Hr)
Imipramine	50–300	25–150	23–26
Desipramine (from imipramine)	—	—	75–92
Desipramine	50–300	25–150	26
Amitriptyline	50–300	25–150	
Nortriptyline	25–75	10–35	37–45
Protriptyline	10–70	5–30	
Doxepin	50–200	25–150	
Amoxapine	50–300	15–150	
Maprotiline	50–300	25–150	32
Phenelzine	15–90	15–60	
Tranylcypromine	10–60	10–30	
Trazodone	300–600	100–300	11
Methylphenidate	—	10–40	
Dextroamphetamine	—	10–20	
Fluoxetine	20–80	20	48–72
Norfluoxetine (from fluoxetine)	—	—	168–216
Bupropion	300–450	150–300	

[a] Adapted with permission from Bienfeld D: Verwoerdt's Clinical Geropsychiatry. 3rd ed. Baltimore: Williams and Wilkins, 1990:116.
[b] Data on elimination half-lives derived from Salzman C: Clinical Geriatric Psychopharmacology. New York: McGraw-Hill, 1984:241.

elderly demented patient. When using these agents, it is essential to carefully prepare the patient and family for the dietary restrictions, since the combination of MAOIs with food containing high amounts of tyramine can cause hypertension and serious sequelae such as myocardial infarction or stroke. The risk of noncompliance with dietary restrictions precludes their use by most older outpatients. There is also an increased risk of interactions between MAOIs and other drugs.

Atypical Antidepressants

Fluoxetine may be particularly useful for the patient with dysthymic disorder with extreme fatigue or lack of motivation.[41,42] Its usefulness may be limited for some patients because of its long elimination half-life (Table 12–2). Side effects include agitation, insomnia, and gastrointestinal upset. Although dose ranges for the elderly have not been clearly established, elderly patients may respond to as little as 5 mg/day, and become severely agitated, dysphoric, and nauseated at higher doses. Some older patients, however, tolerate 20-mg doses on an every-other-day schedule. Still others may tolerate a full daily 20-mg dose.

Trazodone is recommended for patients who do not respond to other antidepressants. Side effects include sedation, dry mouth, and orthostatic hypotension. The dose range for older patients is only 25 to 300 mg/day.

Bupropion is an effective antidepressant for some elderly patients, but there is not yet sufficient clinical experience to identify the types of patients who are more likely to respond to this drug.[61] Although it can be associated with seizures in higher dosages, there are no data yet to suggest that older persons are more susceptible to this effect.[31] Excessive motoric stimulation is a common side effect. Dosage in the elderly is 150 to 300 mg/day.

Central nervous system (CNS) stimulants may be useful for some older persons who have become apathetic, withdrawn, and disinterested in their surroundings, but who are not clinically depressed. Other older persons with chronic illness can become so discouraged as to withdraw from life and become resigned to death. Starting doses of 2.5 to 5 mg of methylphenidate may produce a renewed interest in life, increased motivation, improved attention, and an enhanced sense of well-being. Methylphenidate, the CNS stimulant of choice, should be given in the morning to avoid insomnia. Dosage can be increased by 2.5 to 5 mg every 2 or 3 days until a total dose of 20 mg/day is reached. Some older patients may respond better to amphetamines. Psychomotor stimulants should not be given for depression, since they have poor antidepressant activity and may increase agitation. The most common side effects include tachycardia and mild hypertension, necessitating careful medical supervision. Tolerance may develop after several weeks of treatment. Like MAOIs, psychomotor stimulants can produce agitation and restlessness in those who are demented.

Long-Term Management

Fifty to eighty per cent of patients with one depressive episode can expect a recurrence, and the risk of recurrence increases with each additional episode.[43] Since late-life depression can be severely debilitating and potentially lethal, older patients who have had two or more depressive episodes should receive maintenance antidepressants in order to prevent additional episodes. For some, especially the very old, maintenance dosages may be as small as 25 to 50 mg/day of a heterocyclic agent.

Anxiety

Anxiety is a common symptom in late life. In older patients, symptoms of anxiety are not as clearly defined as in younger adults and the criteria for the diagnosis of an anxiety disorder are less specific. Furthermore, it may be difficult to distinguish pathological affective states in the elderly from age-appropriate worries and preoccupations. In older people with mild anxiety as well as those with anxiety of progressively increasing severity, symptoms of cognitive, emotional, and physical impairment usually accompany the anticipatory concerns. Decreases in concentration, attention, and memory are common, and dizziness, or feelings of impending faintness, of heart attack, or of "going crazy" occur. Difficulty falling asleep is almost always present, as well as alterations in appetite. Thus, anxiety in older patients may exacerbate already-existing age-related sleep and appetite disturbances.

Anxiety and depression almost always coexist in the elderly and it is usually difficult to determine whether the primary affective disturbance is a depressive or an anxious state. However, some differential diagnostic guidelines are helpful. Anxious older people tend to feel and look apprehensive and express a need that "something must be done," and this heightened state is accompanied by increased sweating, tachycardia, dry mouth, restlessness, inability to concentrate, and trouble falling asleep. In contrast, depressed older people usually appear listless, apathetic, and without energy. Rather than express a need for something to be done, they may repeat "nothing can be done." In depression, concentration difficulty is usually due to lack of interest rather than secondary to restlessness or distraction. Depressed older people tend to eat less, spend more time in bed, and may not suffer from signs of autonomic arousal such as sweating and tachycardia.

Just as anxiety may be a symptom of a physical disorder[60], it can also mimic actual cardiovascular, endocrine, and neurological illnesses that occur commonly in older people; or signs of anxiety may be misinterpreted by the older patient as signs of serious physical illness. For example, symptoms such as nausea, abdominal burning, belching, flatulence, constipation, or diarrhea that are common components of anxiety may be considered by older patients as signs of gastrointestinal disease such as cancer. Tightness in the chest, difficulty breathing, and tachycardia may be misinterpreted as early signs of heart attack. Poor memory, attention, and concentration may be feared by the anxious older person as rapidly developing Alzheimer's disease. Although a careful clinical interview (including a complete medical history from the patient and collateral informants and a mental status examination) should narrow the differential diagnosis, a physical examination and ECG are essential.

Pharmacological Treatment of Anxiety

Benzodiazepines

Benzodiazepines are the class of drugs that are predominantly used for the treatment of anxiety disorders as well as anxiety symptoms in older patients.[44] They are helpful for older patients who are in acute crisis (e.g., hospitalization, grief, change in living circumstances) or for patients with longstanding psychiatric or personality disorders that have been responsive to antianxiety treatment.

Although benzodiazepine pharmacokinetics have been well studied in the elderly (see discussion earlier in chapter), there are remarkably few studies of the appropriate therapeutic use of these drugs for the anxious older patient. Opinion regarding their use seems to be divided among experienced clinicians. For some, these drugs provide older patients with considerable symptom relief and relatively little toxicity with careful dosing. Others consider them to be especially toxic in the elderly and avoid their use except for brief crisis situations.

Older patients themselves are divided about the usefulness of benzodiazepines. Although many experience them as helpful,[45] some older patients, especially those who are mentally alert and active, express concern about benzodiazepines interfering with memory, attention, and mental agility in general. Special care should be taken for those patients who expect to drive an automobile.

Once the decision to prescribe an anxiolytic for an elderly patient has been made, the choice of drug depends on whether the clinician wishes to prescribe a long– or short–half-life compound. As discussed above, short–half-life compounds are usually recommended. Thus, oxazepam, lorazepam, or alprazolam are typically prescribed in multiple daily doses for a limited period (Table 12–4). Since there are no studies of benzodiazepine discontinuance in the elderly, clinicians must assume that these drugs may also cause intense discontinuance symptoms (such as anxiety) in older people as they do in younger adults. Long–half-life benzodiazepines may be effective for the younger, healthy older person who can comply with once-a-day dosing, but these compounds should be avoided for those who are older, physically ill, taking other drugs, or who have dementing illnesses.

When anxiety is chronic and long-term benzodiazepine treatment is indicated, frequent monitoring of the older patient's clinical and mental status is necessary. Chronic use may lead to progressive toxicity that may be confused with the signs of normal aging or early senescence. Physical dependence may develop when daily therapeutic doses of any benzodiazepine are taken for more than a few months.

Older patients as a group are more sensitive to the potential toxicity of anxiolytic drugs because of age, comorbidity, polypharmacy, and reduced drug-taking compliance. The four categories of side effects that commonly occur older people at doses lower than in younger adults are sedation, cerebellar toxicity, psychomotor retardation, and impaired cogni-

TABLE 12–4. BENZODIAZEPINES FOR ANXIOUS ELDERLY PATIENTS

Drug	Potency	Starting Dose (mg)	Dose Range (mg)	Mean Elimination Half-Life (hr) Young	Mean Elimination Half-Life (hr) Old
Short half-life					
Oxazepam[a]	Low	15	10–60	10	10
Lorazepam[a]	High	0.5	0.5–4	12	12
Alprazolam[a]	High	0.25	0.125–2	10	17
Long half-life					
Chlordiazepoxide[a]	Low	5–10	10–40	10	30
Diazepam[a]	Low	2	2–20	24	75
Chlorazepate[a]	Low	7.5	7.5–60	24	200
Prazepam[a]	Low	10	10–40	24	200
Clonazepam[b]	High	0.125	0.125–2	18–50	18–50
Quazepam[b]	Low	7.5	7.5–15	25–41	25–41

[a] Data derived from Saltzman C: Treatment of anxiety: In Saltzman C, ed. Clinical Geriatric Psychopharmacology. New York: McGraw-Hill, 1984:139.
[b] Data from Physicians' Desk Reference, 1991, and Doral formulary profile.

tive function.[4,16,46–48] Sedation may cause the older person to become confused, belligerent, and agitated, and this condition may be increased at night or by alcohol or other CNS sedative agents. Cerebellar toxicity is manifested by ataxia, dysarthria, incoordination, and unsteadiness. Psychomotor impairment in the older patient is characterized by slowed reaction time, diminished accuracy of motoric tasks, and impaired hand-eye coordination. Cognitive impairment, which is reversible, includes anterograde amnesia, diminished short-term recall, increased forgetfulness, and decreased attention.[10,11,26] These symptoms closely resemble both the early stages of dementia as well as normal age-related impairment in cognitive function.

OTHER DRUGS

Buspirone, β-blockers, antidepressants, antihistamines, and neuroleptics are also used to treat anxiety in older patients, although with less predictable effects. Buspirone has been reported to treat anxiety in healthy older people without sedation, dyscoordination, dependence,[49] or disability related to cognitive psychomotor side effects.[50] Research studies demonstrate therapeutic equivalence of buspirone with the benzodiazepines.[49,51,52,54] Clinical experience using buspirone in the elderly is still sparse, but suggests that buspirone is more effective as a treatment for agitation than as an antianxiety drug. For the treatment of anxiety, the therapeutic range is 5 to 20 mg/day.

β-Blockers, like buspirone, may substantially improve disruptive behavior in the elderly, but there are no clinical trials in older patients of their use for the subjective symptoms of anxiety,[53] for anxiety-associated autonomic symptoms, or to prevent performance anxiety. Contraindications include congestive heart failure (CHF), sinus bradycardia, greater than first-degree heart block, and asthma.

Given the observation that anxiety and depression commonly coexist in older patients, antidepressants may be indicated in mixed affective states. Desipramine or nortriptyline, 25 mg/day, for healthy patients over 60, or 10 mg/day for patients over 70, may be therapeutic. Trazodone in doses of 50 to 150 mg/day is helpful, especially if sedation is required.

Antihistamines such as diphenhydramine or anxiolytics with antihistamine properties such as hydroxyzine are occasionally useful for very–short-term management of acute anxiety. They are sedating, anticholinergic drugs that may also cause confusion, disorientation, and oversedation, and are not recommended for long-term use. The dose of hydroxyzine is 10 mg one to four times a day, with a range of up to 100 mg/day. The use of neuroleptics for treatment of anxiety as contrasted with agitation has never been demonstrated. Given their potential toxicity, neuroleptics should not play a major role in the treatment of anxious elderly patients.

Insomnia

As humans age they are inclined to spend more hours in bed, sleep fewer hours, take longer to fall asleep, and experience fragmented, interrupted, and often unrefreshing sleep. Furthermore, many drugs disrupt sleep, including caffeine, nicotine, alcohol, antihypertensives, nasal decongestants, steroids, hormones, and antiarrhythmia agents. Physical illness, pruritis, sleep apnea, arthritis, paroxysmal nocturnal dyspnea, and angina as well as depression may awaken the elderly sleeper, particularly later in the night during rapid eye movement (REM) sleep.

When drugs are used to assist sleep, there are several guidelines which should be followed. Benzodiazepines are useful for brief periods, and short–half-life agents are preferred; long-term use should be avoided whenever possible. Doses should be kept to a minimum, which often means using one fourth to one half the amount used with younger adults. For example, a triazolam dose for the older patient would be 0.125 mg at night; temazepam dose would be 7.5 to 15 mg at night. There is evidence that estazolam, a new triazolobenzodiazepine with a mean elimination half-life of 18.4 hours in the elderly, may be an effective hypnotic for short-term or intermittent use in the elderly at doses of 0.5 to 1 mg.[55] Duration of treatment of insomnia is controversial. Some prescribe a maximum of 20 doses per month for not more than 3 months. Others recommend that benzodiazepines be given only two or three times per week, or even one or two times weekly.[56,57]

It is important for the clinician to recognize that older patients frequently have difficulty discontinuing benzodiazepine hypnotics. It is not uncommon to encounter older patients taking these hypnotic agents for years, even though efficacy is questionable and side effects are likely. These include oversedation, decreased coordination, and cognitive impairment resembling dementia. Recent data suggest that this benzodiazepine-induced concentration and memory impairment is reversible when they are discontinued.[53]

REFERENCES

1. Salzman C: A primer on geriatric psychopharmacology. Am J Psychiatry 139:69–76, 1982.
2. Guttman D: A study of drug-taking behavior of older Americans. In Medication Management and Education of the Elderly. Amsterdam: Excerpta Medica, 1978:32.
3. Salzman C: Clinical Geriatric Psychopharmacology. New York: McGraw-Hill, 1984:241.
4. Salzman C: Key concepts in geriatric psychopharmacology: Altered pharmacokinetics and polypharmacy. Psychiatr Clin North Am 5:181–190, 1982.
5. Salzman C: Psychotropic drug use and polypharmacy in a general hospital. Gen Hosp Psychiatry 3:1–9, 1981.
6. Salzman C: Neurotransmission in the aging central nervous system. In Salzman C, ed. Clinical Geriatric Psychopharmacology. New York: McGraw-Hill, 1984:1984.

7. Sunderland J: Neurotransmission in the aging CNS. In Salzman C, ed. Clinical Geriatric Psychopharmacology. 2nd ed. Baltimore: Williams and Wilkins, 1992.
8. Ritschel WS: Gerontokinetics: Pharmacokinetics of Drugs in the Elderly. 1988:23.
9. Greenblatt DJ, Shader RI: Pharmacokinetics in Clinical Practice. Philadelphia: WB Saunders Company, 1985:Chapter 4.
10. Pomara N, Stanley B, Block R, et al: Adverse effects of single therapeutic doses of diazepam on performance in normal geriatric subjects: Relationships to plasma concentrations. Psychopharmacology 84:342–346, 1984.
11. Pomara N, Stanley B, Block R, et al: Diazepam impairs performance in normal elderly subjects. Psychopharmacol Bull 20:137–139, 1984.
12. Salzman C: Pharmacokinetics of psychotropic drugs and the aging process. In Salzman C, ed. Clinical Geriatric Psychopharmacology. New York: McGraw-Hill, 1984: 32–45.
13. Abernathy DR: Psychotropic drugs and the aging process: pharmacokinetics and pharmacodynamics. In Salzman C, ed. Clinical Geriatric Psychopharmacology. 2nd ed. Baltimore: Williams and Wilkins, 1992.
14. Greenblatt DJ: Pharmacokinetics of antianxiety drugs in the elderly. In Salzman C, Lebowitz B, eds. Anxiety in the Elderly. New York: Springer Publications, 1990.
15. Young RC, Alexopoulos GS, Shamoian CA, et al: Plasma 10-hydroxynortriptyline and ECG changes in elderly depressed patients. Am J Psychiatry 142:866–868, 1985.
16. Lovett WS, Stokes DK, Taylor LB, et al: Management of behavioral symptoms in disturbed elderly patients: Comparisons of trifluoperazine and haloperidol. J Clin Psychiatry 48:234–236, 1987.
17. Risse SC, Barnes R: Pharmacologic treatment of agitation associated with dementia: Geriatric seminar. J Geriatr Soc 34:368–376, 1986.
18. Salzman C: Treatment of agitation in the elderly. In Meltzer HY, ed. Psychopharmacology: The Third Generation of Progress. New York: Raven Press, 1987:1167–1176.
19. Salzman C: Treatment of agitation, anxiety, and depression in dementia. Psychopharmacol Bull 24:39–42, 1988.
20. Wragg RE, Jeste DV: Neuroleptics and alternative treatments: Management of behavioral symptoms and psychosis in Alzheimers disease and related conditions. Psychiatr Clin North Am 11:195–213, 1988.
21. Yudofsky S, Williams D, Gorman J: Propanolol in the treatment of rage and violent behavior in patients with chronic brain syndromes. Am J Psychiatry 138:218–220, 1981.
22. Greenwald BS, Marin DB, Silverman SM: Serotoninergic treatment of screaming and banging in dementia. Lancet 20:1464–1465, 1986.
23. Pinner E, Rich CL: Effects of trazodone on aggressive behavior in seven patients with organic mental disorders. Am J Psychiatry 145:1295–1296, 1988.
24. Simpson DM, Foster D: Improvement in organically disturbed behavior with trazodone treatment. J Clin Psychiatry 47:191–193, 1986.
25. Tingle D: Trazodone in dementia (letter). J Clin Psychiatry 47:482, 1986.
26. Colenda CC: Buspirone in treatment of agitated demented patient. Lancet 1:1169, 1988.
27. Leibovici A, Tariot N: Carbamazepine treatment of agitation associated with dementia. J Geriatr Psychiatry Neurol 1:110–112, 1988.
28. Holton A, George K: The use of lithium in severely demented patients with behavioral disturbance. Br J Psychiatry 146:99–104, 1985.
29. Brown RP, Sweeney J, Loutsch E, et al: Involutional melancholia revisited. Am J Psychiatry 141:24–28, 1984.
30. Salzman C, Van der Kolk: Treatment of depression. In Salzman C, ed. Clinical Geriatric Psychopharmacology. New York: McGraw-Hill, 1984:77–115.
31. Alexopoulos GS: Treatment of depression. In Salzman C, ed.

32. Laskshamanan EB, Mion CC, Frengley JD: Effective low dose tricyclic antidepressant treatment for depressed geriatric rehabilitation patients. J Am Geriatr Soc 34:421–426, 1986.
33. Robinson DS: Age-related factors affecting antidepressant drug metabolism and response. In Nandy K, ed. Geriatric Psychopharmacology. New York: Elsevier North Holland, 1979:17–19.
34. Glassman AH, Walsh T, Roose P, et al: Factors related to orthostatic hypotension associated with tricyclic antidepressants. J Clin Psychiatry 43:35–38, 1982
35. Salzman C: Clinical use of antidepressant blood levels and the electrocardiogram. N Engl J Med 313:512–513, 1985.
36. Georgotas A, Mann J, Friedman E: Platelet monamine oxidase inhibitors as a potential indicator of favorable response to MAOIs in geriatric depression. Biol Psychiatry 16:997–1001, 1981.
37. Georgotas A, Friedman E, McCarthy M, et al: Resistant geriatric depressions and therapeutic response to monamine oxidase inhibitors. Biol Psychiatry 18:195–205, 1983.
38. Zisook S: A clinical overview of monoamine oxidase inhibitors. Psychosomatics 26:240–246, 1985.
39. Jenike MA: Handbook of Geriatric Psychopharmacology. Littleton, MA: PSG Publishing Company, 1985:39–96.
40. Lazarus LW, Groves L, Gierl B, et al: Efficacy of phenelzine in geriatric depression. Biol Psychiatry 21:699–701, 1986.
41. Feighner JP, Cohn JB: Double-blind comparative trials of fluoxetine and doxepin in geriatric patients with major depressive disorder. J Clin Psychiatry 46:20–25, 1985.
42. Feigner JP, Boyer WF, Meredith CH: An overview of fluoxetine in geriatric depression. Br J Psychiatry 153(suppl 3):105–108, 1988.
43. Prien RF: Long-term maintenance therapy in affective disorders. In Rifkin A., ed. Schizophrenia and Affective Disorders. Boston: Wright, 1983:95–116.
44. Salzman C, Lebowitz B: Anxiety in the Elderly. New York: Springer Publications, 1989.
45. Pinsker H, Suljaga-Petchel K: Use of benzodiazepines in primary care geriatric patients. J Am Geriatr Soc 32:595–598, 1984.
46. Jenike MA: Anxiety disorders of old age. In Jenike MA, ed. Geriatric Psychopharmacology. Chicago: Yearbook Medical Publishers, 1989:248–271.
47. Lieberman JA, Kane JM, Johns CA: Clozapine: Guidelines for clinical management. J Clin Psychiatry 50:9, 329–338.
48. Nakra BRS, Grossberg GT: Management of anxiety in the elderly. Compr Ther 12:53–60, 1986.
49. Levine S, Napolillo MJ, Domanta AG: Open study of buspirone in octogenarians with anxiety. Hum Psychopharmacol 4:51–53, 1989.
50. Hart RP, Colenda CC, Hamer RM: Effects of buspirone and alprazolam on the cognitive performance of normal elderly subjects. Am J Psychiatry 148:73–77, 1991.
51. Napolieollo MJ: An interim multicentre report on 677 anxious geriatric out-patients treated with buspirone. Br J Clin Pract 40:71–73, 1986.
52. Robinson DS, Napoliello MJ: The safety and usefulness of buspirone as an anxiolytic in elderly versus young patients. Clin Ther 10:740–746, 1988.
53. Salzman C: Discontinuing benzodiazepines improves cognition in elderly nursing home residents. Internatl J Geriatr Psychiatry 2:1992.
54. Singh AN, Beer M: A dose range finding study of buspirone in geriatric patients with symptoms of anxiety. J Clin Psychopharmacol 8:67–68, 1988.
55. Pierce MW, Shu VS: Efficacy of estazolam: The United States clinical experience. Am J Med 88(suppl 3A):1990.
56. Gaillard JM: Place of benzodiazepines in the treatment of sleep disturbances. Rev Med Suisse Romande 107:717–720, 1987.
57. Reynolds CF, Kupfer DJ, Hoch CC, et al: Sleeping pills for the

elderly: Are they ever justified? J Clin Psychiatry 46:9–12, 1985.

58. Salzman C: Principles of psychopharmacology. *In* Bienenfeldt D, ed. Verwoerdt's Clinical Geropsychiatry. 3rd ed. Baltimore: Williams and Wilkins, 1990:239.

59. Salzman C: Treatment of anxiety. *In* Salzman C, ed. Clinical Geriatric Psychopharmacology. New York: McGraw-Hill, 1984:131–148.

60. Soreff SM, McNeil GN: Handbook of Psychiatric Differential Diagnosis. Littleton, MA: PSG Publishing Company, 1987.

61. Ayd FJ: Bupropion: A novel antidepressant—update 1989. Int Drug Ther Newslett 24(8):30–36, 1989.

62. Salzman C: Geriatric psychopharmacology. Ann Rev Med 36:217–228, 1985.

63. Bienenfeld D: Verwoerdt's Clinical Geropsychiatry. 3rd ed. Baltimore: Williams and Wilkins, 1990.

Section B

SUBSTANCE USE DISORDERS

KEEPING CURRENT WITH THE DSMs AND SUBSTANCE USE DISORDERS

MARC ALAN SCHUCKIT, M.D.

Usually, the first step in choosing a treatment is establishing an accurate diagnosis.[1] Therefore, changes in diagnostic schemes can have major impacts on the application of treatments. This chapter is based on the premise that keeping current with psychiatric therapies, including those applied to the substance use disorders, requires an understanding of the therapeutic guidelines that are paving the way for DSM-IV.

ABUSE AND DEPENDENCE IN DSM-IV

The overall process involved in the evolution of DSM-IV differs in many ways from its predecessors.[2–4] To enhance efficiency and communication, small groups were created to coordinate the work while relying heavily on a large cadre of advisors. The small Work Groups were guided by the premise that further change in the diagnostic manual should be based on data rather than philosophy. Thus, information from the published literature, reevaluations of existing data sets, and a field trial are forming the basis for decisions regarding revisions in diagnostic criteria. The committees have also recognized that the psychiatric field will benefit from stability in criteria, and that few changes should be made without adequate justification regarding their beneficial impact on establishing prognoses or selecting the most appropriate treatments.[2,5,6] In addition, our group

recognized that any criteria must be relevant to all substances of abuse, and that the definitions must be straightforward enough for clinical settings.

The group began with a review of the DSM-III-R process, culling from the literature available data on the implications of the changes that occurred in 1987. To bolster the process, the Work Group received monies from the John D. and Catherine T. MacArthur Foundation to carry out additional analyses on existing data sets, and obtained funding from both the National Institute of Drug Abuse and National Institute of Alcohol Abuse and Alcoholism to carry out a field trial.

The review of the criteria established for DSM-III-R and the scant available literature revealed some possible problems. As recently reviewed by Nathan,[7] the movement away from the emphasis on physical aspects of tolerance and withdrawal had some benefits but ignored the empirical data demonstrating the ability of these symptom sets to predict future course.[8,9] The shift in the diagnostic criteria away from the consideration of social consequences for abuse or dependence also moved away from well-established and potentially important predictors of outcome. An additional problem is that the concept of dependence in DSM-III-R became so broad that clinicians could be tempted to apply it to any condition of excessive behaviors including shopping and sexual activities, with a resulting panoply of potential disorders that go far beyond present data and that do not appear to all investigators to be appropriately grouped with substance use disorders.[10] Similarly, the broad concept of dependence may have increased the heterogeneity of labeled patients, a step that goes counter to the desire of many individuals in the field to identify relevant subtypes of substance abusers in an effort to develop more focused and effective treatment approaches. The changes in criteria may have also reduced the meaning of the concept of abuse to a label lacking any documented prognostic and treatment implications. Finally, a major criticism that encompasses all of the points outlined above is the reluctance that many clinicians and researchers have in accepting such a radical change between diagnostic manuals without having subjected the criteria set to empirical testing for concurrent and predictive validity. The field lacks meaningful comparisons of DSM-III and III-R criteria applied to a wide range of patients in diverse clinical settings which are required for fully informed decisions.

Thus, the members of the DSM-IV Work Group faced competing pressures. On the one hand, we wished to make the fewest changes possible, basing alterations on data. On the other hand, we recognized that the relatively short time between DSM-III and III-R did not allow for adequate testing of the 1987 criteria. The MacArthur Foundation–supported analyses and field trials were, therefore, established to compare the potential concurrent validity and predictive ability of DSM-III, III-R, and two potential modifications of the latter for DSM-IV. Recognizing the need for any diagnostic manual of the 1990s to relate to the International Classification of Diseases (ICD-10), the impact of this diagnostic set was also incorporated into evaluations.

The first possible approach for abuse and dependence in DSM-IV utilizes the nine items originally outlined in DSM-III-R, thus ensuring that key elements of the broad concept of dependence are maintained. However, this iteration of the criteria requires that at least one item related to tolerance or withdrawal is present for a diagnosis of dependence. In this approach, abuse is also more directly defined and incorporates social and psychological aspects of impairment in the absence of any evidence of tolerance or withdrawal.

The second proposed version of criteria for abuse and dependence also includes the original items from DSM-III-R, taking care to define more clearly many of the concepts and offer more explicit examples. The two major changes involved in this possible approach include encouraging clinicians to subtype dependence into those individuals with and without physiological aspects as well as the more clearly presented concept of abuse.

Data reanalyses supported by the MacArthur Foundation and field trials will contribute to the final decision of whether to keep DSM-III-R in an unaltered state or to change to either of the two potential versions of abuse and dependence. The final

decisions for DSM-IV will be a blend between the results of the data analyses and clinical and research preferences.

ADDITIONAL ISSUES RELEVANT TO DSM-IV

Several other developments are also being incorporated into the new diagnostic manual. These include decisions about the optimal way to deal with the relationship between psychiatric symptoms and substances of abuse, a reorganization of the original "organic" substance use diagnoses in order to conform with the proposed new approach for the cognitive disorders in DSM-IV, and more precise definitions of remission and severity.

The Work Group developed a lengthy document reviewing the complexities in the interactions between psychiatric symptoms and intoxication or withdrawal from psychoactive substances.[11] The co-occurrence of psychiatric symptom patterns and substance use is a frequent event for at least three reasons: (1) there is a high prevalence of substance use problems in society as well as high rates of anxiety and depressive disorders; (2) intoxication with drugs or withdrawal from substances can cause symptoms of anxiety, depression, and psychosis; and (3) several psychiatric disorders (e.g., schizophrenia, mania, and antisocial personality disorder) have high rates of secondary substance use problems.

Recognizing the complexity of the interactions as well as the data demonstrating that the majority of abusers of stimulant and depressant drugs have temporary and potentially severe psychiatric symptoms that are likely to disappear with abstinence, the committee recommends that a clearer presentation of the guidelines originally established in DSM-III and DSM-III-R are needed for the new diagnostic manual. Therefore, clinicians will be advised that psychiatric symptoms only observed in the context of intoxication with drugs (e.g., psychoses or states of anxiety during stimulant intoxication) as well as those seen only during the 6 weeks after withdrawal from drugs (e.g., severe depressions following cessation of heavy use of depressant drugs or stimulants) do not in themselves indicate the presence of a separate psychiatric syndrome (e.g., major depressive disorder). On the other hand, when psychiatric syndromes precede the onset of severe alcohol- or drug-related life problems or when they persist beyond 6 weeks of abstinence, the presence of another major psychiatric disorder must be suspected and, if appropriate, diagnosed. These guidelines, while implicit in the early diagnostic manuals, will now receive greater prominence, reflecting more impressive data accumulated in the past 5 to 10 years.

More than any other group of disorders in DSM-IV, the substance use diagnoses are affected by the decision to reorganize the organic disorders into cognitive sections.[12] Thus, the "traditional" organic affective and anxiety syndromes related to substances of abuse are now listed within the relevant diagnostic subsections (e.g., the affective disorders and anxiety sections). An additional change involves the recommendation that each of these disorders be listed as a three-part label indicating the drug, the condition (e.g., intoxication, withdrawal, or persisting problems), and the prominent symptom (e.g., anxiety or psychosis).

Finally, there is a need to define severity and remission more carefully. Guidelines for the former are being pilot tested in order to determine whether a count of the actual number of symptoms observed will lend itself to a logical form of scaling between mild, moderate, and severe.[13] Descriptions of remission being considered resemble those presented in the past, but with greater emphasis on the tenuousness of abstinence observed during the first 6 months following cessation of drug use, the appropriateness of recognizing whether any substance intake has occurred in the absence of major life problems, and a clinical option of dropping the diagnostic label after 3 consecutive years of complete abstention.

CONCLUSIONS

The DSM-IV Substance Use Work Group has been guided by the desire to make as few changes as possible while using data to correct potential deficiencies within DSM-III-R. The result has been the development of three diagnostic options for abuse and dependence for DSM-IV, including a continuation of the DSM-III-R approach, a compromise midway between III and III-R, and a modest alteration of the 1987 diagnostic criteria. The latter would allow for subtyping people who meet criteria for a broad concept of dependence into those who do and do not have elements of physiological withdrawal or tolerance and offers a clearer demarcation of the concept of abuse. All final decisions for DSM-IV will rest with a balance between the results from data reanalyses as well as an extensive field trial, and discussions with members of both the treatment and research communities.

ACKNOWLEDGMENTS

This work was supported by The Department of Veterans Affairs Research Service and NIAAA Grants 05526 and 69012004.

REFERENCES

1. Goodwin DW, Guze SB: Psychiatric Diagnoses. New York: Oxford University Press, 1989.
2. Pincus HA, Frances A, Davis WW, et al: DSM-IV and new diagnostic categories—holding the line of innovation. Am J Psychiatry 149:112–117, 1992.
3. Frances AJ, Widiger TA, Pincus HA: The development of DSM-IV. Arch Gen Psychiatry 46:373–375, 1989.
4. Schuckit MA, Helzer JE, Crowley TJ, et al: Deliberations of the substance use Work Group for DSM-IV. Hosp Community Psychiatry 42:471–473, 1991.
5. Zimmerman M: Why are we rushing to publish DSM-IV? Arch Gen Psychiatry 45:1135–1138, 1988.
6. Winokur G, Zimmerman M, Cadoret R: Cause the Bible tells me so. Arch Gen Psychiatry 45:683–684, 1988.
7. Nathan PE: Psychoactive substance dependence. In Widiger T, Frances A, Pincus H, et al, eds. The DSM-IV Source Book. Washington, DC: American Psychiatric Press, (in press).
8. Hasin DS, Endicott J, Keller MB: RDC alcoholism in patients with major affective syndromes: Two-year course. Am J Psychiatry 146:318–323, 1989.
9. Rounsaville BJ: An evaluation of the DSM-III substance-use disorders. In Tischler G, ed. Treatment and Classification in Psychiatry. New York: Cambridge University Press, 1987.
10. Miele GM, Tilly SM, First M, et al: The definition of dependence and behavioural addictions. Br J Addict 85:1421–1423, 1990.
11. Schuckit MA: The relationship between alcohol problems, substance abuse, and psychiatric syndromes. In Widiger T, Frances A, Pincus H et al, eds. The DSM-IV Source Book. Washington, DC: American Psychiatric Press (in press).
12. Crowley TJ: The organization of intoxication and withdrawal disorders in DSM-IV. In Widiger T, Frances A, Pincus H, et al., eds. The DSM-IV Source Book. Washington, DC: American Psychiatric Press (in press).
13. Woody GE, Cacciola J: Review of the remission criteria for DSM-IV. In Widiger T, Frances A, Pincus H, et al, eds. The DSM-IV Source Book. Washington, DC: American Psychiatric Press (in press).

14

ALCOHOL PROBLEMS

JOSEPH M. McCREERY, M.D. and R. DALE WALKER, M.D.

DEFINITIONS

The DSM-III-R operationally defines and distinguishes between abuse and dependence by using concepts that place greater emphasis on patterns of compulsive use and no longer require evidence of physiological dependence.[1] With this schema, alcohol-abusing and -dependent (alcoholic) persons are those who compulsively continue drinking in spite of evidence of alcohol's deleterious effects. Social drinkers (the majority of drinkers) are those who can stop drinking without difficulty and suffer no persistent negative effects. Generally, as overall alcohol consumption increases, abuse and dependence develop, and alcohol problems appear and increase in severity.[2] For clarity and consistency, we shall use the term "alcohol problems" to represent the concepts of alcohol abuse, dependence, and alcoholism.

PREVALENCE AND EPIDEMIOLOGY

Approximately 10 per cent of Americans have problems with alcohol, and 10.5 million adults are alcohol dependent. *Men* as a group drink more than women and have higher rates of alcohol problems. *Women* at high risk for alcohol-related problems tend to be those who are moderate to heavy drinkers, unemployed, single, young, and living with a chronic drinking partner.[3] Adolescent alcohol abuse is more common in males and is most prevalent between 16 and 18 years of age.[4] *Elderly* people have a group prevalence of alcohol problems of 2 per cent, and tend as a group to maintain stable patterns of alcohol use, with decreases in use being more frequent than increases. However, losses inherent in the aging process may result in late-onset heavy drinking, especially in persons of higher socioeconomic status.[3] *Homeless people* experience elevated risks of health problems due to their homeless status. In the 20 to 40 per cent of them who abuse alcohol, these risks are increased even more.[3] *African Americans* abstain more and drink less at all levels of alcohol use than do whites. *Hispanics* have high rates of abstinence, but have the highest rates of heavy drinking and of alcohol-related problems (especially in males) of all the racial and ethnic groups. *Asian Americans* have the lowest consumption levels and rate of alcohol-related problems of all the major American racial and ethnic groups. A genetic predisposition to the flushing response, due to an inherited isoenzyme of aldehyde dehydrogenase in 50 per cent of this population, may be partially protective. *American Indians and Alaska natives* are a culturally diverse population whose tribal groups and communities vary widely in alcohol consumption patterns, prevalence of alcohol problems, and beliefs about alcohol problems. Compared to the general population, rates of consumption are higher, but a higher percentage abstain.

ETIOLOGIES

There is no single known cause for alcohol problems, and it is highly probable that there are multiple causes. Genetic predisposition,[3,5] pharmacological factors,[6] and environmental conditions contribute to the development of alcohol problems, but none of them alone are exclusive causes, and the relative role of each varies in each individual.

The relationship between alcohol problems and psychiatric comorbidity has been documented.[7] Alcohol disorders have the highest lifetime prevalence of all mental disorders considered individually, with 13.5 per cent of the population having alcohol problems. Of the people with alcohol problems, 36 per cent will have a comorbid mental disorder, and 45 per cent will have comorbid mental disorder and/or other drug abuse problems. There are more people with both alcohol and mental disorder than with other drug and mental disorders. The association between alcohol and psychiatric problems is highest with antisocial personality disorder (ASP), and strong with drug abuse dependence, and mania. Depression and dysthymia are not strongly associated, but could be expected to be more strongly associated in a clinical sample.[8] Persons with primary mental health disorders (especially schizophrenia, bipolar disorder, anxiety disorders, and ASP) have a higher incidence of alcohol problems than the general public.[7]

TABLE 14–1. CAGE QUESTIONNAIRE[a,b]

C	Have you ever felt that you should cut down on your drinking?
A	Have people annoyed you by criticizing your drinking?
G	Have you ever felt bad or guilty about your drinking?
E	Have you ever taken a drink first thing in the morning to steady your nerves or get rid of a hangover (eye opener)?

[a] Adapted with permission from Mayfield DG, McCleod G, Hall P: The CAGE questionnaire: Validation of a new alcoholism screening instrument. Am J Psychiatry 131:1121–1123, 1974.
[b] One positive answer raises concern. More than one positive answer is a strong indication of alcohol problems.

SCREENING AND ASSESSMENT

Screening is used to determine if alcohol problems exist, and is an essential part of every medical and psychiatric evaluation. Reliable, brief, easily administered screening instruments are unfortunately underutilized in many settings, resulting in underdiagnosis of drug and alcohol problems. The CAGE questionnaire (Table 14–1)[9] and the Short Michigan Alcoholism Screening Test (SMAST) (Table 14–2)[10] are two examples of easily administered screening instruments.

Biochemical tests are less specific and sensitive than self reports, but can be a valuable tool for detecting hidden alcohol abuse disorders. Gammaglutamyl transferase (GGT) is probably the most sensitive indicator of alcohol-induced liver damage. Other tests include blood alcohol level (BAL), mean corpuscular volume of red blood cells (MCV), uric acid, and liver enzymes including aspartate aminotransaminase/glutamic oxaloacetic transaminase (SGOT), and alkaline phosphatase. Recent research focuses on elevated carbohydrate-deficient protein transferrin (CDT) as an indicator of current consumption of 60 or more gm of alcohol per day,[20] and on the possible role of alcohol metabolites (called acetylcholine adducts) in triggering immune responses that may play a role in immunological abnormalities accompanying alcoholic liver disease.[21]

Medical Consequences

These affect a wide range of organ systems with varying degrees of severity, and are listed in Table 14–3. The teratogenic effects of in utero alcohol exposure produce a spectrum of abnormalities that range from the subtle cognitive-behavioral impairment of Fetal Alcohol Effects (FAE) to the symptoms of Fetal Alcohol syndrome (FAS), a constellation of prenatal and postnatal growth retardation, craniofacial abnormalities, major organ system malformations, and central nervous system (CNS) dysfunction including mental retardation. The cognitive and intellectual impairment of FAS persist into adulthood.[23] Abstinence from alcohol during pregnancy is the only assured prevention for FAE and FAS.

WITHDRAWAL AND DETOXIFICATION

If mild to moderate alcohol problems are detected, brief intervention or brief therapy should be provided by the physician or by a community agency with appropriately trained staff. Follow-up observation of the effects are essential. Substantial or severe problems need referral for detoxification and specialized intensive treatment.

Safe withdrawal from alcohol and preparation for alcohol treatment are the goals of alcohol detoxification (detox). If detoxification is not an integral part of the treatment program, the physician may need to

TABLE 14–2. SHORT MICHIGAN ALCOHOLISM SCREENING TEST (SMAST)[a]

1	Do you feel that you are a normal drinker? (do you drink less than or as much as other people?)	(no)[b]
2	Does your wife, husband, a parent, or other near relative ever worry or complain about your drinking?	(yes)
3	Do you ever feel guilty about your drinking?	(yes)
4	Do friends or relatives think you are a normal drinker?	(no)
5	Are you able to stop drinking when you want to?	(no)
6	Have you ever attended a meeting of Alcoholics Anonymous?	(yes)
7	Has your drinking ever created problems between you and a near relative?	(yes)
8	Have you ever gotten into trouble at work because of drinking?	(yes)
9	Have you ever neglected your obligations, your family, or your work for two or more days in a row because you were drinking?	(yes)
10	Have you ever gone to anyone for help about your drinking?	(yes)
11	Have you ever been in a hospital because of drinking?	(yes)
12	Have you ever been arrested for drunken driving, driving while intoxicated, or driving under the influence of alcoholic beverages?	(yes)
13	Have you ever been arrested, even for a few hours, because of other drunken behavior?	(yes)

[a] Adapted with permission from Seltzer ML, Vinokur A, van Rooijen L: A self-administered Short Michigan Alcoholism Screening Test (SMAST). J Stud Alcohol 36(1):117–128, 1975.
[b] Responses indicative of alcohol problems in parenthesis. Scoring: Each alcohol indicative answer is given 1 point.
0–1 = no evidence of alcohol problems; 2 = possible alcohol problems; 3 or more = definite alcohol problems.

TABLE 14-3. MEDICAL CONSEQUENCES OF HEAVY PROLONGED ALCOHOL USE

Gastrointestinal	Esophageal inflammation, gastritis, exacerbation of ulcers, decreased intestinal motility and mucosal function, pancreatitis (acute and chronic)
Liver	Fatty infiltration, alcoholic hepatitis, and cirrhosis (all may exist concurrently, cirrhosis may develop de novo)
Malignancy	Risk increased, especially for oropharynx, tongue, larynx, esophagus, and liver
Cardiac	Cardiomyopathy, diminished left ventricle contractility, decreased myocardial blood flow, increased myocardial oxygen consumption, arrhythmias after heavy bouts of drinking
Vascular	Increased risk of hypertension and intracranial hemorrhage
Nutritional/metabolic	Malnutrition from inadequate intake and utilization, impaired metabolism of vitamins and minerals (especially folate, thiamine, pyridoxine, vitamin A, magnesium, and zinc)
Immune/hematopoietic	Depressed platelet production, decreased PMN production and function, depressed cell-mediated immunity (increased rates of TB), decreased T cells (especially helper cells, which could enhance risk of AIDS infection and progression)
Endocrine	Increased cortisol and catechols, abnormal testosterone metabolism in males, imbalance of sex hormone secretion in women in all phases of the menstrual cycle
Neurological	Blackouts, seizures, hallucinations, peripheral neuropathy, cortical atrophy on head CT, and cerebellar degeneration, Wernicke-Korsakoff syndrome, alcoholic dementia

facilitate the patient's transfer to the treatment program at the completion of detox.

Most people can be safely detoxed in an outpatient setting. Social detoxification (with reassurance, nursing care, personal attention, and no medications) may be effective in motivated patients with mild to moderate withdrawal and good social support. Hospitalization is necessary for those with severe medical or surgical problems, and with current or previous severe withdrawal reactions such as delirium or seizures.

Detoxification should occur in a calm and nonstimulating environment. Vital signs are monitored at a minimum of once each 8 hours. Observation should be more intense during the first 24 hours. Generous quantities of fruit juices and other fluids are encouraged.

Adequately treated alcohol withdrawal is usually uncomplicated. Tremulousness begins within a few hours of stopping or diminishing drinking after prolonged heavy use. Nausea, vomiting, headache, malaise, and/or weakness may accompany signs of autonomic hyperactivity (tachycardia, hypertension, and sweating), signs of neuronal irritation (anxiety, irritability, depressed mood, and insomnia), and perceptual distortions (transitory poorly formed hallucinations or illusions). Most symptoms resolve within 3 to 4 days.

Delirium tremens, a potentially fatal consequence of inadequate treatment of withdrawal, begins within 2 to 3 days after drinking cessation and resolves in 3 to 5 days. Delirium, marked agitation, and autonomic hyperactivity may be accompanied by physically dangerous behavior in response to delusions and hallucinations. Delirium's onset should prompt medical consultation and a search for underlying medical disease (e.g., pneumonia, pancreatitis, hepatic failure).

Generalized convulsions occur rarely during withdrawal, usually within the first 2 to 3 days, and are not usually associated with underlying epilepsy. Multiple or focal seizures should prompt neurologi-cal consultation to rule out idiopathic or post-traumatic epilepsy. Because the side effects of anti-seizure medications are potentiated by alcohol, the most effective prophylaxis is probably avoidance of alcohol.

Alcohol hallucinosis is a rare disorder in which vivid auditory or visual hallucinations or both develop within 48 hours of ceasing or reducing heavy drinking. They may persist for weeks or permanently, may not intrude into normal functioning, or may result in secondary delusions with ideas of reference and a clinical picture similar to schizophrenia.

Medications

On admission, 100 mg of thiamine is given parenterally and followed by 100 mg orally daily for the next 3 days. Multivitamins with minerals and folate (1 mg) are given daily.

Benzodiazepines are the agents of choice for treatment of withdrawal. They control symptoms of autonomic hyperactivity and neuronal irritation, and protect against progression to delirium and seizures, with a wide margin of safety. Those with long half-lives and active metabolites (chlordiazepoxide and diazepam) allow less frequent dosing and possibly less reinforcement of drug-seeking behavior, but pose a greater risk of oversedation in patients with compromised hepatic function. Intermediate–half-life agents with no active metabolites (lorazepam and oxazepam) accumulate less and are less sedating. Lorazepam has the added advantage of reliable absorption with parenteral administration.

Patients' medication requirements are variable, but rarely exceed 400 mg/day of chlordiazepoxide or 10 mg/day of lorazepam. Treating objective signs of withdrawal on an as-needed (p.r.n.) basis every 2 hours may avoid undertreatment during the first day. Twenty-five to fifty milligrams of chlordiazepoxide, or 1 to 2 mg of lorazepam, may be given orally every 2 hours with dosage adjustment as needed. On the second day, the first day's total dose may be given in four divided doses with p.r.n. doses. Subsequent daily dose reduction by 25 per cent per day is usually tolerated. An alternative oral regimen uses loading doses of 10 mg of diazepam every 1 to 2 hours at the onset of withdrawal symptoms, with discontinuation when symptoms subside.[13] The possibility of accumulation and sedation in patients with hepatic compromise must be kept in mind with this regimen.

Neuroleptics are not indicated in uncomplicated withdrawal because they lower the seizure threshold and carry the risk of tardive dyskinesia. They may be used adjunctively with benzodiazepines for severe hallucinations and preexisting psychotic disorders.

Additional pharmacological agents are being investigated for use in withdrawal. The β-adrenergic blockage of atenolol is effective against tachycardia and hypertension, but offers no protection against seizures and delirium. When administered with oxazepam, it has improved recovery time.[14] The centrally acting α_2-adrenergic agonist clonidine reduces autonomic hyperactivity, but there is disagreement about other protective effects.[15] Carbamazepine has shown indications of having equal efficacy with benzodiazepines in several small studies, and may have advantages in a small population that cannot tolerate benzodiazepines.[16] Calcium channel blockers are also being investigated.[17]

TREATMENT OPTIONS

Treatment options include brief intervention, brief therapy, outpatient therapy, and intensive treatment in an outpatient or inpatient setting. Brief intervention is probably the least expensive option, and inpatient aversion therapy, residential milieu, and insight-oriented psychotherapy are probably the most costly.

Brief intervention is extremely important in the early phases of alcohol problems, and is a critical area for physicians in interrupting the drinking cycle. If more physicians would provide this in an effective and predictable way before alcohol problems have progressed to marked severity, much individual and social morbidity could probably be prevented. The physician utilizes whatever manner of effective communication works with a patient to educate the patient to the adverse effects of alcohol use, and to inform the patient that their intake is excessive. This may be done by inviting the patient to explore and discuss the ways in which they can see alcohol having a deleterious effect on their well-being. The physician then empathetically supports this information with clinical evidence pertaining to the patient and with education about alcohol's toxic effects. Within the context of a shared mutual concern for the patient's well-being, reduction of alcohol abuse is recommended. An ongoing interactive process between physician and patient is initiated, with the physician repeatedly addressing the issue and

supporting the goal of reduced alcohol use. Subjective observations are elicited from the patient, record keeping of consumption or periodic laboratory evaluation may be introduced, and obstacles to drinking reduction are explored. Referral for more intensive treatment occurs if the situation does not improve.

Brief therapy is intermediate between brief intervention and intensive treatment, and is usually provided by trained staff at a community alcohol center. In about six outpatient sessions, patients learn specific behavioral methods for stopping or reducing drinking. These include goal setting, self-monitoring, identification of situations with high risk of drinking, and methods to avoid drinking or overdrinking.[2]

Specialized intensive treatment programs may be outpatient or inpatient based. Outpatient treatment provides the patient the opportunity to work on alcohol problems in their regular environment. Inpatient treatment usually lasts 17 to 28 days, is more expensive, and offers a safe and structured environment where the unstable patient may receive more support before returning to an environment where alcohol is readily available. Inpatient treatment is probably indicated when patients are poorly motivated, suicidal, depressed or psychotic, and when there are medical problems or disrupted social support systems.

Although studies have found no significant differences in outcome between inpatient or outpatient treatment settings, and no differences based on length of treatment,[18] the wide range of patient characteristics and treatment program structures makes an overall assessment of efficacy difficult. Many studies have focused on middle class populations where most patients were married and had jobs (a good-prognosis group). Flexible use of inpatient residential treatment programs with no fixed length of stay may be beneficial for a severely impaired population with little or no social stability or support. Ambulatory treatment options and brief intervention should be encouraged, but attempts to limit treatment options on the basis of cost only should await the results of current multicenter trials to determine which form of treatment is best for each subpopulation of patients.

COMPONENTS OF TREATMENT

Treatment components are used in various combinations in different programs, and emphasis may vary. Group psychotherapy is an essential component of most treatment programs, and when well utilized, provides a supportive environment, empathetic counselors, a confrontational (but not hostile) focus, and cognitive reinforcement of positive self-image.

Social skills training improves communication skills, assertiveness, the ability to resist peer pressure, and reduces alcohol use more than supportive therapy alone.

Alcoholics Anonymous (AA) is a self help group that many people find beneficial for maintaining sobriety or reducing drinking. Alcoholics Anonymous views alcoholism as an incurable disease for which continual abstinence is the only treatment. Participants attend a highly structured self-help group with very clear precepts. Group participation and the use of personal sponsors provides support for the individual, and Alanon and Alateen programs provide support for family members. The 12-step program involves an acceptance of being powerless over alcohol and a surrender of will to a personally defined higher power. An important theme of the AA approach is the acceptance of responsibility for one's behavior. A large percentage of first-time attenders do not return, but in heavily dependent drinkers, attendance and activity have been shown to correlate with abstinence and improved health. Although AA's claims to be the most efficacious treatment are not scientifically validated, self-help programs such as AA can be a valuable component in a comprehensive treatment program that includes other modalities of treatment.

Family therapy or partner involvement in therapy may facilitate better outcomes, and should always be a consideration when treating alcohol problems in children and adolescents. Families and children of alcoholics have a higher rate of developmental difficulties, social adjustment problems, learning difficulties, and drug and alcohol dependence later in life. Family patterns may also help initiate and maintain alcohol problems. Unmotivated people with alcohol problems may be assisted to reduce drinking or accept treatment by counseling their family members in ways of reinforcing those desired behaviors.

Aversion therapy attempts to reduce or extinguish the desire to drink by repeatedly pairing alcohol with noxious stimuli such as nausea and emesis produced by an emetic. Covert sensitization is a type of aversion therapy that uses verbal suggestion to pair imagined drinking with unpleasant experiences such as nausea or unpleasant visualizations. Success rates claimed by programs using aversion therapy have been criticized for the absence of controlled studies and because their subjects have comprised a largely homogeneous and good-prognosis group. Covert sensitization may prove to be a useful addition to broader treatment strategies for a select population of problem drinkers.

Relapse prevention attempts to maintain behavioral changes over time by increasing self-efficacy. High-risk drinking situations are identified and ranked by degree of risk. Individual strengths and resources are identified, and self-efficacy–enhancing cognitive and behavioral responses are explored. The patient explores progressively risky drinking situations in his or her environment. New coping responses and behaviors are practiced, and improved competency is noted. Periodic review explores alternatives in areas of persistent poor self-confidence. For appropriately selected participants, reductions in alcohol consumption and improvement in ratings of self-efficacy maybe facilitated.

MEDICATIONS THAT ASSIST IN MAINTAINING ABSTINENCE

Disulfiram (Antabuse) permanently inhibits the enzyme aldehyde dehydrogenase (ALDH) and causes accumulation of acetaldehyde and a toxic reaction after alcohol use. It should be used as one component in a broad-based treatment approach. Its usefulness in preventing alcohol use is probably based on a desire to avoid the symptoms of its toxic reaction with alcohol. Five to ten minutes after the use of alcohol, the toxic reaction begins with flushing, and progresses to throbbing headache, dyspnea, nausea, vomiting, chest pain vertigo, blurred vision, possible hypotension, confusion, and in severe cases, vascular collapse. The symptoms last from 30 minutes to several hours and leave the patient exhausted. Supportive therapy is usually sufficient unless severe symptoms develop, at which point medical consultation should be sought. Disulfiram is taken daily on a maintenance basis under medical supervision, and is contraindicated in pregnancy. A minimum of 12 hours must have elapsed since the last use of alcohol before the first dose is given. Sensitivity to alcohol may persist from 6 to 14 days after stopping disulfiram until new functional enzyme is secreted. The patient must be informed that alcohol use will cause illness and may possibly be fatal, and must be advised to avoid all forms of alcohol, including disguised forms in foods, medications, and cosmetics. Rare but potential side effects of disulfiram alone include mild gastrointestinal distress, decreased potency, anxiety, lethargy, dermatitis, hepatotoxicity, and peripheral neuropathy (which may be minimized by not exceeding 125 to 250 mg/day).[19] Compliance may be improved by periodic breathalizer and laboratory monitoring.

Other agents are currently being investigated. Calcium carbimide (Temposil) inhibits ALDH for 24 hours and has less side effects than disulfiram, but is not available in the United States. The opiate antagonist naltrexone may have a potential role in relapse prevention in humans. Research to date indicates that serotonin reuptake inhibitors may have a beneficial effect on reducing alcohol use in some nondepressed people with alcohol problems. Fluoxetine has been shown to alter alcohol intake in problem drinkers. Its advantages include lack of cross-reactivity with alcohol and minimal side effects. Buspirone, a nonbenzodiazepine anxiolytic with low abuse potential and no sedation, reduced anxiety and desire to drink in a group of alcoholics when given after detoxification. A recent study by Fawcett et al. reported that lithium levels of 0.4 mEq or greater were associated with a higher rate of abstinence, and that this effect did not seem to be mediated by antidepressant effects.[20] A subsequent large cooperative Veterans Administration study found lithium carbonate to be no more effective than placebo in reducing problematic alcohol consumption.[21] At this time, lithium has no role in relapse prevention other than the treatment of mood disorders responsive to lithium that are not caused by alcohol. Neuroleptics have no role in relapse prevention other than for treatment of psychosis.

TREATMENT OF PSYCHIATRIC SYMPTOMS

Anxiety, panic, depression, brief hallucinations, and mild cognitive impairment are usually transitory expressions of withdrawal symptoms, and resolve spontaneously within 1 to 2 weeks. Anxiety symptoms may remit more slowly over a few months of abstinence and usually do not represent an underlying anxiety disorder. Reassurance and adequate use of benzodiazepines during withdrawal as described above is usually sufficient treatment. The physician must be alert to the possibility of comorbid psychiatric disorders. These may be discovered by a careful history of symptoms predating alcohol problems and by persistence of severe symptoms for 2 to 4 weeks after alcohol withdrawal. A minimum of 2 to 4 weeks after withdrawal should be allowed to elapse before initiating antidepressant medication to allow adequate time for the depressive effects of excessive alcohol use to resolve.[22] If an antidepressant is indicated, fluoxetine may have advantages over tricyclic agents because of its lack of cross-reactivity with alcohol and its wider margin of safety.

The severity of pretreatment psychiatric problems is a reliable predictor of alcohol treatment response. Patients with severe underlying psychiatric disorders do poorly regardless of the type of therapy they receive, but referral to a dual-diagnosis program may provide more of the intensive treatment and support that they need for improvement to occur.

AFTERCARE

Three to six months of weekly (or more frequent) encounters are needed to support the use of new abstinence skills and facilitate early detection of and intervention for relapse. Self reports have limited reliability in aftercare and should be supplemented with collateral reports and biological tests (breathalizer, GGTP, and urine toxicology screens) as necessary. Post-treatment drinking is related to poor outcome in all levels of functioning, but evaluation of outcome should consider other aspects such as work adjustment, interpersonal relations, other substance abuse, and subjective well-being. More research is needed to define and optimally match aftercare programs to appropriate subpopulations.

REFERENCES

1. American Psychiatric Association: Diagnostic and Statistical Manual of Mental Disorders. 3rd ed. Revised. Washington, DC: American Psychiatric Association, 1987.
2. Broadening the base of treatment for alcohol problems: Report of a study by a committee of the Institute of Medicine Division of Mental Health and Behavioral Medicine. Washington, DC: National Academy Press, 1990.
3. U.S. Department of Health and Human Services: Seventh Annual Report to the U.S. Congress on Alcohol and Health From the Secretary of Health and Human Services. Rockville, MD: NIAAA, 1990.
4. Kandel D, Logan J: Patterns of drug use from adolescence to young adulthood: I. Period of risk for initiation, continued use, and discontinuation. Am J Public Health 74:660–667, 1984.
5. Cloninger CR, Bohman M, Sigvardsson S: Inheritance of alcohol abuse. Arch Gen Psychiatry 38:861–868, 1981.
6. Donovan DM, Marlatt GA: Assessment of expectancies and behaviors associated with alcohol consumption: A cognitive-behavioral approach. J Stud Alcohol 41:1153–1185, 1980.
7. Regier DA, Farmer ME, Rae DS, et al: Comorbidity of mental disorders with alcohol and drug abuse: Results from the epidemiological catchment area (ECA) study. JAMA 264(19):2511–2518, 1990.
8. Helzer JE, Pryzbeck TR: The co-occurrence of alcoholism with other psychiatric disorders in the general population and its impact on treatment. J Stud Alcohol 49(3):219–224, 1988.
9. Mayfield DG, McCleod G, Hall P: The CAGE questionnaire: Validation of a new alcoholism screening instrument. Am J Psychiatry 131:1121–1123, 1974.
10. Selzer ML, Vinokur A, van Rooijen L: A self-administered Short Michigan Alcoholism Screening Test (SMAST). J Stud Alcohol 36(1):117–128, 1975.
11. Stibler H, Hultcrantz R: Carbohydrate-deficient transferrin in serum in patients with liver diseases. Alcoholism (NY) 11:468–473, 1987.
12. Israel Y, Orrego H, Niemela O: Immune responses to alcohol metabolites: Pathogenic and diagnostic implications. Semin Liver Dis 8(1):81–90, 1988.
13. Sellers EM, Naranjo CA, Harrison J, et al: Diazepam loading: Simplified treatment of alcohol withdrawal. Clin Pharmacol Ther 34(6):822–826, 1983.
14. Kraus ML, Gottleib LD, Horowitz RI, et al: Randomized clinical trial of atenolol in patients with alcohol withdrawal. N Engl J Med 313:905–909, 1985.
15. Liskow BI, Goodwin DW: Pharmacological treatment of alcohol intoxication, withdrawal and dependence: A critical review. J Stud Alcohol 48:356–370, 1987.
16. Malcolm R, Ballenger JC, Sturgis ET, et al: Double-blind controlled trial comparing carbamazepine to oxazepam treatment of alcohol withdrawal. Am J Psychiatry 146:617–621, 1989.
17. Koppi S, Eberhardt G, Haller G, et al: Calcium-channel-blocking agent in the treatment of acute alcohol withdrawal—caroverine plus meprobamate in a randomized double-blind study. Neuropsychobiology 17:49–52, 1987.
18. USDHHS: Sixth special report to the U.S. Congress on alcohol and health from the Secretary of Health and Human Services. Rockville, MD: NIAAA, 1987.
19. Palliyath SK, Schwartz BD, Gant L: Peripheral nerve functions in chronic alcoholic patients on disulfiram: A six month follow up. J Neurol Neurosurg Psychiatry 53(3):227–230, 1990.

20. Fawcett J, Clark DC, Aagesen CA, et al: A double-blind, placebo-controlled trial of lithium carbonate therapy for alcoholism. Arch Gen Psychiatry 44:248–256, 1987.
21. Dorus W, Ostrow DG, Anton R, et al: Lithium treatment of depressed and nondepressed alcoholics. JAMA 262:1646–1652, 1989.
22. Brown SA, Schuckitt MA: Changes in depression among abstinent alcoholics. J Stud Alcohol 49(5):412–417, 1988.
23. Streissguth AP, Aase JM, Clarren SK, et al: Fetal alcohol syndrome in adolescents and adults. JAMA 265(15):1961–1967, 1991.

15

STIMULANT ABUSE:
Cocaine and Amphetamine

ROY M. STEIN, M.D. and EVERETT H. ELLINWOOD, M.D.

The current stimulant epidemic began with a surge of cocaine use in the 1970s that was apparent among the affluent and educated, due to cocaine's high price and image as a safe drug of the elite. In the 1980s, the U.S. cocaine supply and its purity increased dramatically, resulting in a much cheaper, more potent product that became accessible to a larger, poor, inner-city population. By the mid-1980s, as information about the dangers of cocaine became widespread, overall middle-class casual use of the drug began to decline, with a simultaneous escalation of dependence and sequelae among lower socioeconomic groups, especially in urban areas. Between 1985 and 1988, based on a national household survey, the number of persons in the United States who had used any cocaine in the preceding 12 months had decreased from 12 million to 8 million, but the number of frequent users did not change, resulting in an increase in the proportion of frequent users from 5 per cent to over 10 per cent of the total group who had used.[1] Between 1985 and 1988, the number of cocaine-related emergency room visits increased by over 300 per cent. By late 1989, these numbers had begun to decline slightly, but there was no accompanying decline in cocaine-related deaths.[1] Annual surveys of drug use by high school seniors indicate that cocaine use peaked in 1985 (lagging behind overall illicit drug use, which peaked in 1979) and has been decreasing since then, with 3.4 per cent reporting having used cocaine in the past month in 1988.[1]

The increase in frequent use by a subset of users has been fueled by the marketing of cocaine base, or crack, an alkalinized form that has a low melting point and is thus able to be smoked. Smoked cocaine base reaches the brain even more rapidly than the injected hydrochloride form, and without the perceived hazards associated with using needles. Effects are intense and of short duration, resulting in frequent readministration and an unprecedented liability for severe addiction. Whereas cocaine replaced amphetamines as the stimulant of choice in the late 1970s, local "miniepidemics" of methamphetamine, "ecstasy" (MDMA), and MDA rise and fall based on local marketing systems and laboratory synthesis capabilities. Recently, a smokable form of amphetamine, known as "ice," has been synthesized and marketed, possibly in response to governmental efforts to interrupt the importation of cocaine. This drug is described as having marked aggressive effects and a duration of action much longer than that of crack. If the cocaine supply does in fact diminish as a result of government interdiction efforts, the use of ice and other amphetamines will likely increase.[1]

PHARMACOLOGY

Central nervous system (CNS) stimulants enhance the central activity of norepinephrine and dopamine. Cocaine acts primarily by inhibiting the reuptake of these neurotransmitters from the synapse[2] and may also act as a direct agonist at some dopamine receptors. It also has significant local anesthetic effects, which are the bases for its medical uses.[2]

Amphetamine use results in enhanced central activity of norepinephrine and dopamine, primarily through enhancing release, as well as blocking reuptake in synaptic terminals.[3] At high doses, amphetamine also induces release of 5-hydroxytryptamine (5-HT, serotonin) and may have some direct agonist effects on 5-HT receptors.[3]

Acute stimulant toxicity most commonly results from overdose, typically following intravenous injection or smoking. Symptoms may include severe anxiety, paranoia, confusion, disorientation, hallucinations, severe hypertension and tachycardia, ventricular irritability, heart failure, respiratory depression, intracranial hemorrhage, seizures, rhabdomyolysis, and sudden death.[3]

PSYCHIATRIC AND BEHAVIORAL MANIFESTATIONS

The DSM-III-R identifies the following stimulant-induced organic mental disorders: intoxication, delirium, withdrawal, and delusional disorder.[4] Acute cocaine and amphetamine intoxication can produce perceptual disturbances, hallucinations, delirium, paranoid delusions, panic, agitation, impulsive aggressivity, and impaired judgment. Acute stimulant intoxication may be virtually indistinguishable from manic psychosis, schizophreniform disorders, or panic disorder. In a sample of patients with cocaine use disorders undergoing inpatient rehabilitation, 68 per cent had experienced distressing paranoid ideation while under the influence of the drug, with a significant proportion acting in response to these ideas by arming themselves or through violent behavior. Within individual patients, paranoia developed earlier within successive binges as use continued, consistent with a process of sensitization.[15] Chronic dependence results in generalized personality deterioration, to which adolescents are especially vulnerable because personality development can be distorted by the direct and indirect effects of stimulant use.

CLINICAL APPROACH TO STIMULANT ABUSE

In the clinical setting, the physician considers the following questions:

1. Is this patient a *user* or *potential user* of stimulants?
2. What is the intensity of involvement with stimulants?
3. Are there any *complications* present, including acute toxicity, withdrawal, or general medical, neuropsychiatric, or psychosocial disturbances related to stimulant use?
4. What are the characteristics of the user that may predispose to drug use and/or necessitate modification of treatment? Here one considers personality structure, ego strengths and deficits, social skills, vocational and social reinforcers prior to abuse, and longest planned abstinence the individual has achieved.

5. What factors in the *social environment* are affecting the individual's use or risk of use of the drug? These include the degree of association with users, abusers, and dealers; the presence of triggering cues in the environment, and the range of areas in the person's life in which drug use is involved.
6. What environmental factors are precipitating the current treatment presentation and the patient's ability to engage in effective treatment?

An evaluation that addresses these questions results in a biopsychosocial understanding of the patient that can serve as the basis for formulating an individualized, comprehensive treatment plan.

Stimulant users, like most patients with substance abuse problems, do not spontaneously volunteer the complete facts of their drug use. In order to detect use of cocaine or amphetamine, it is first necessary to maintain a high index of suspicion and to avoid being mislead by a stereotyped image of the "street" drug user. Although many patients will deny drug use even upon inquiry, a substantial proportion who would not mention it spontaneously do acknowledge it if the physician inquires about it in a matter-of-fact, professional manner. Therefore, routine, direct inquiry of all patients about use of drugs including stimulants is essential. One must be alert to "red flags" in the history, such as job loss or frequent job changes; divorce or other interpersonal disruption; arrests; complaints of depression, anxiety, lethargy, or insomnia; and abuse of other substances. Evidence of severe financial distress (e.g., accumulation of unusually large debts or thefts by a previously responsible person) points to the large financial drain engendered by cocaine dependence. Alertness to the findings on history and physical examination related to the various medical complications discussed earlier is useful in detecting covert stimulant use, although most patients will have a normal physical examination. It is essential to obtain, with the patient's permission, history from family, friends, previous treatment facilities, legal or correctional sources, etc.

Urine drug screening is helpful in detecting stimulant use. Just informing the patient of the intention to obtain a drug screen often elicits additional history of drug use. Cocaine and its metabolites are usually only detectable in urine up to 48 hours after last use, so a negative finding is pertinent only in evaluating an acute situation.[6] The convention in interpreting urinalyses is to consider the detection of benzoylecgonine as evidence of cocaine use within the last 3 days; however, recent data indicate that the metabolite may appear in the urine of high-dose, chronic users up to 3 weeks after last use.[1] Other laboratory findings are normal in most cocaine abusers. Nevertheless, it is appropriate to employ laboratory screening for hematological, hepatic, and renal abnormalities, and human immunodeficiency virus (HIV) and hepatitis B infection in the identified stimulant user.

Diagnostic evaluation can identify individuals at high risk for initiating use and for developing abuse and dependence, even when use has not begun. Risk factors which predict illicit drug use in adolescents include low grade-point average, lack of religious involvement, psychopathology, deviance, sensation-seeking behavior, early alcohol use, low self-esteem, poor relationships with parents, perceived peer drug use, and perception of drug use among adults and peers.[7]

When cocaine use is revealed by history, collateral data, or laboratory findings, careful interviewing with application of DSM-III-R criteria is required in order to define the level of use, abuse, or dependence, as these issues are critical in matching appropriate treatment to the patient. It is necessary to inquire as to frequency of use, quantity (expressed as grams and expense), route of administration, typical circumstances of use, and means employed to secure and pay for the drug.

Psychiatric disorders and other substance use disorders are common in stimulant abusers. Rounsaville and colleagues studied psychiatric diagnoses in 298 inpatients and outpatients receiving treatment for cocaine abuse or dependence.[5] Of these, 56 per cent had a current psychiatric diagnosis other than substance abuse; 74 per cent had a lifetime diagnosis. The most common diagnoses were affective disorders (44 per cent current; 60 per cent lifetime), including 5 per cent current and 31 per cent lifetime diagnoses of major depression. Most of the remaining affective diagnoses consisted of various affective personalities. Anxiety disorders were found in 16 per cent of patients, antisocial personality disorder in 8 per cent, and schizophrenic disorders in 1 per cent. Thirty-five per cent received a lifetime diagnosis of attention deficit disorder, based on relatively broad criteria that did not require childhood diagnosis or treatment of the condition. Twenty-nine per cent received a current diagnosis of alcoholism; 62 per cent had a past diagnosis. Onset of the affective disorders and alcoholism tended to occur after the development of cocaine abuse or dependence, while the anxiety disorders and attention deficit disorder preceded it. Because a clinical sample was used, these figures may not accurately reflect prevalence of disorders in the overall population of cocaine users, but they are quite relevant for the assessment of patients presenting for treatment.[5]

Every patient should be specifically evaluated for evidence of affective disorders, including major depression and various chronic "minor" mood disorders; anxiety disorders, attention deficit disorder, alcohol abuse and dependence, and personality disorders. While narcissistic personality disorder is not readily quantified with research instruments, clinical experience suggests that narcissistic traits and disorders are also common in patients attracted to heavy stimulant use. Patients whose stimulant use represents an attempt at self-medication of an underlying psychiatric disorder such as depression may present for treatment with less advanced levels of use and dependence, and may be more amenable to treatment due to their psychological distress.[8]

TREATMENT

Treatment involves: (1) managing acute complications, if present, including acute toxicity, delirium and acute delusional disorder, general medical complications, and acute withdrawal symptoms; (2) presenting the diagnostic findings to the patient and significant others in a clear, direct, and comprehensible manner; (3) developing a specific treatment plan in conjunction with the patient and significant others; (4) implementing the treatment plan; and (5) providing follow-up.

Management of Acute Complications

Acute cocaine intoxication usually resolves quickly due to the drug's short duration of action; amphetamine toxicity may last several hours. These situations can usually be handled by close observation and support, for example, in an emergency observation unit. Agitation can be treated with benzodiazepines, and psychotic features may be treated with neuroleptics if necessary. Specific medical complications are managed by appropriate specialists. β-Adrenergic blockers may aggravate cocaine-induced coronary ischemia by allowing greater unopposed α-adrenergic stimulation, and thus should be avoided in cases of angina or infarction in which cocaine toxicity is suspected.[9] Presentation of acute stimulant toxicity with hyperpyrexia and impending seizures is an acute medical emergency with high risk of fatality, and requires aggressive hypothermic measures, antiseizure medications, and cardiovascular monitoring and support. Acute hospitalization may be necessary for management of specific medical complications, as well as for sustained agitation, paranoia, and suicidal or homicidal ideation. Subsequent decisions in managing the patient who presents with acute complications must be based on an overall assessment of the level of drug involvement, as discussed below. The presentation of the stimulant user with acute complications provides an opportunity for evaluation and initiation of treatment of the underlying drug problem, as it often creates a brief window of increased receptivity and motivation on the part of the patient.

Presenting the Diagnosis

In presenting the diagnostic findings it is important to review the specific evidence, if present, that stimulant use is causing problems in the individual's life and that he is not able to control it on his own. If use is occurring at an experimental or "casual" level, a realistic discussion of the risks of continuing use, including medical complications, is necessary. In all cases, an unequivocal recommendation of abstinence from cocaine and other stimulants should be conveyed.

Developing a Treatment Plan

No single treatment modality has been convincingly demonstrated to induce and maintain long-term abstinence in cocaine-dependent patients. Most individuals receive a combination of treatment modalities, the selection of which is still based on clinical judgment and experience rather than on definitive clinical research findings. Treatment of the cocaine user needs to be based on a biopsychosocial understanding of the individual patient, paying particular attention to the presence of concurrent psychiatric disorders; relevant environmental and social factors; and to the severity of the stimulant use, abuse, or dependence. The physician should provide clear, specific recommendations about level and intensity of treatment, but the views and concerns of the patient and significant others should be actively incorporated into the plan. Given the problems in maintaining motivation and compliance in treatment, it is crucial to foster the patient's sense of collaboration and responsibility in treatment from the outset, rather than a feeling that treatment is being imposed upon him. In a substantial portion of cases, treatment is in fact being externally imposed by legal mandate or threatened loss of employment; here the clinician can help the patient acknowledge that outer boundary as a consequence of drug use while working to establish a positive alliance within treatment.

For the high-risk individual who is not yet using, major components of intervention include preventive education and risk-factor reduction. Many programs such as Drug Abuse Resistance Education (DARE) provide education about the effects and risks of illicit drug use and, importantly, teach decision-making and coping skills aimed at enabling young persons at risk to make responsible decisions and to handle pressures to use drugs. Peer-counseling programs take advantage of the fact that many young people more readily accept information from peers than from adult authority figures. Local schools and state and local substance abuse agencies can provide the practitioner with information about currently available prevention programs. Risk-factor reduction includes diagnosis and treatment of predisposing psychiatric disorders such as depression and attention deficit disorder, family counseling or formal therapy addressing family conflicts, and efforts to connect the individual at risk with sources of positive social support and acceptance. Treatment should actively address concurrent substance use disorders such as alcoholism, even when the primary or preferred substance is cocaine or amphetamine.

For the experimental or casual user, a clear recommendation of abstinence should be coupled with education and attention to risk factors for dependence, as discussed above in the preventive situation. Periodic follow-up visits are advisable; random urinalyses are useful in confirming abstinence. If use continues despite these steps, the diagnosis of abuse is warranted, and formal substance abuse treatment is recommended.

Experimental use of cocaine or other stimulants in the adolescent requires a thoughtful and measured approach. It is critical to assess the child's academic, extracurricular, and social adjustment; emotional and developmental status; and family relationships. The clinician needs to develop rapport and a degree of trust with the adolescent (no small task) in order to have any real impact on the young person's drug use in the context of an ongoing treatment relationship. The focus with the adolescent is on realistic drug education, discussion of decision-making and coping skills, and identifying and addressing matters of concern to the patient, as well as identifying any specific psychopathology. An unequivocal communication that the drug use must stop is coupled with an awareness of the hazards of overemphasizing experimental drug use and allowing it to become the focal point for preexisting family conflicts. In this circumstance, drug use may actually be reinforced if it serves the child's purposes in asserting his or her autonomy in a conflict with the parents over issues unrelated to substance use. Premature referral of a young person into formal drug treatment when only limited use has occurred carries the risk of polarizing the child against the physician and family and exposing the child to persons who are in fact more seriously involved with drugs. The importance of maintaining therapeutic alliance and trust and of providing regular, thorough follow-up cannot be overemphasized.

When the diagnosis is stimulant abuse or dependence, formal substance abuse treatment is necessary. It is inadvisable for the individual physician to undertake treatment of abuse or dependence on a solo outpatient basis without involving other treatment resources. Key issues in treatment planning include selection of treatment setting, types of psychosocial therapy to be employed, the role of self-help groups in treatment, and decisions regarding pharmacotherapy. Treatment settings include traditional outpatient programs, intensive outpatient day treatment programs, inpatient rehabilitation programs with lengths of stay from 3 to 6 weeks, long-term residential treatment, and halfway houses. Most individuals with stimulant abuse or milder degrees of dependence can enter therapy at the outpatient level directly, or after a brief inpatient detoxification. Intensive outpatient treatment with frequent therapeutic contacts may be especially important early in treatment. Inpatient rehabilitation is generally reserved for situations of outpatient treatment failure, severe dependence, presence of significant psychiatric comorbidity, or when the individual lives in an environment rich in drug availability and drug-related cues and personal contacts. Long-term residential treatment is appropriate for severely dependent patients who have had multiple relapses, and should be followed by gradual return to independent living through a stay in a halfway house. Maintenance of continuity of care as the patient moves along the spectrum of treatment intensity is essential.

BEHAVIORAL-PSYCHOSOCIAL THERAPIES

Psychosocial therapies for stimulant abuse are directed at: (1) helping the patient overcome his denial and recognize the significance of his drug abuse or dependence; (2) developing a commitment to abstinence and long-term recovery; and (3) developing specific behavioral skills that will allow him to maintain abstinence and develop non–drug-related sources of reward and pleasure. In most respects, these treatment approaches derive from treatments for alcohol dependence. The major modification is the increased attention directed to the dysphoria and anhedonia experienced during the withdrawal phase and to the powerful reinforcing effects of cocaine which result in intense craving upon exposure to reminders of stimulant use.

It is often necessary to remove the individual from the physical and social environment associated with stimulant use during the initial stages of treatment due to the overwhelming effect of conditioned craving.[8] An important first step in treatment is to "minesweep" the environment for conditioned stimuli, as well as mood-setting events which set the stage for increased potency of these stimuli (e.g., domestic quarrels). Upon return to outpatient treatment in their original community, patients may have to avoid particular individuals, parts of town or particular streets, and specific activities and objects.[10] If abstinence is maintained, the patient can be gradually reexposed to these conditioned cues in an attempt to foster extinction of the craving response. The overall goal is the development of self-awareness and self-mastery of these formerly subconscious autonomic events.

Relapse prevention therapy, originally developed for treatment of alcoholism, has been modified by Carroll and colleagues for use in treatment of cocaine dependence.[11] This approach combines behavioral, cognitive, educational, and self-control techniques. The patient and therapist identify high-risk situations in which relapse is likely and develop specific coping strategies for handling these situations. Treatment addresses conditioning factors and early warning signals of impending relapse. While attempting to prevent recurrences of drug use, the therapist and patient acknowledge the possibility that slips will occur, and develop cognitive and behavioral strategies for limiting the duration and intensity of any relapse episodes. Relapse prevention fosters stress reduction and the development of a healthier overall lifestyle.

Interpersonal psychotherapy, which was developed as a treatment for depression, has also been adapted for use in treatment of cocaine dependence.[12] This approach emphasizes a medical model of addiction and focuses on identification of the legitimate interpersonal needs that the individual was seeking to fulfill through the use of stimulants. Therapy promotes development of healthier ways of meeting these needs.[12]

Both the interpersonal and relapse prevention approaches can be applied in individual and group settings. Group therapy is important for most patients in that it provides a combination of support, acceptance, and confrontation that is hard for any individual therapist to provide consistently. Individual therapy is important for some individuals in that they can more readily develop trust and reveal personal concerns in this setting.

Involvement of significant others in treatment is often useful, affording treatment staff a view of the important relationships in the person's life and enhancing accurate monitoring of drug-use and drug-related behaviors. Family involvement may enhance the sense of support for both the identified patient and the family members, and, as treatment progresses, can facilitate development of strategies for changing maladaptive family interactions which contribute to continuing substance use.

Outcome studies of psychosocial treatments are beginning to appear. Kang et al. reported on 168 patients requesting outpatient treatment for cocaine abuse or dependence who were entered in an outcome study comparing weekly individual, group, and family therapy.[13] Follow-up at 6 to 12 months was obtained on 122, and of these, less than 20 per cent had achieved sustained abstinence.[13] The authors were unable to conclude that the cases of abstinence were attributable to the treatment, and suggested that a more intensive outpatient model involving daily visits, urine monitoring, and possibly the use of adjunctive medication might result in better outcomes. As additional treatment outcome studies appear, close attention must be paid to sample characteristics such as dependence severity, route of administration, associated psychopathology, and social variables.

SELF-HELP GROUPS

Enrollment in 12-step self-help groups is routinely incorporated into the treatment plan. Cocaine Anonymous (CA) is available in some areas; otherwise Narcotics Anonymous (NA) or Alcoholics Anonymous (AA) can be quite helpful. The clinician needs to monitor the patient's attendance at these meetings and addresses the patient's responses and level of involvement. The fact that the clinician attends to these issues on an ongoing basis serves to reinforce to the patient the significance of these groups. The clinician must be ready to deal with concerns the patient may raise regarding perceived conflicts between the 12-step philosophy and a medically based treatment model. For example, relapse prevention therapy fosters development of strategies to keep relapses from progressing, thus implying that such control is possible, whereas AA and NA suggest that full relapse is inevitable after a slip. While cognitive-behavioral strategies emphasize personal ability to gain control of one's behavior and substance use, the 12-step programs emphasize the individual's powerlessness over addiction. The clinician needs to address these concerns seriously, but also be aware that they may represent a form of resistance to full engagement in treatment. The complementary relationship of the two approaches is to be stressed.

Referral of family members to self-help groups like Al-Anon and Nar-Anon should be routinely considered.

PHARMACOTHERAPY

Pharmacological treatments are potentially useful in three aspects of stimulant dependence: (1) treatment of behavioral toxicity; (2) treatment of concurrent psychiatric vulnerabilities which contribute to stimulant use; and (3) treatment of "neuroadaptation" [i.e., evidence of CNS alterations in high-dose (typically intravenous or crack) users who manifest stimulant withdrawal, characterized by anhedonia, anergia, and intense craving].[8]

Acute behavioral toxicity related to cocaine intoxication may require brief treatment with benzodiazepines in order to control agitation, or neuroleptics for management of paranoia and other psychotic manifestations. Continuing antipsychotic medication may also be necessary for prolonged behavioral toxicity such as persistent stimulant psychosis, whose occurrence implies the presence of an underlying prepsychotic or borderline condition.[14] Neuroleptics must be used with particular caution, and at the lowest possible doses, since anhedonia resulting from dopamine receptor blockade may increase stimulant craving. Neuroleptics should be avoided when stimulant toxicity presents with hyperthermia, due to the risk of neuroleptic malignant syndrome.[8] Neuroleptic-induced lowering of seizure threshold should be considered, due to the risk of seizures in acute stimulant intoxication.

In treating stimulant abusers with psychiatric vulnerability, medication may alleviate symptoms and minimize the tendency of the user to attempt "self-medication." The most common comorbid diagnoses are affective disorders, alcoholism, and, possibly, attention deficit disorder.[5] Antidepressant medications may be used in patients with depressive disorders. Agents with noradrenergic and dopaminergic effects, such as desipramine, may be preferable. Caveats include the possibility that in some patients antidepressants will have stimulating effects which serve as conditioned cues for stimulant craving, and

possible synergism between antidepressants and cocaine in producing cardiotoxicity, in the event that the patient relapses into drug use while on medication.

The pharmacological treatment of adult attention deficit disorder (ADD) in the stimulant abuser must be approached with great caution. The drugs used to treat this condition, methylphenidate and dextroamphetamine, are stimulants with their own abuse potential, and, as in the case of antidepressants, stimulation produced by the prescribed drug may trigger further stimulant craving. In the setting of stimulant dependence, it is prudent to apply strict criteria for diagnosis, requiring the ADD to have been diagnosed and effectively treated with stimulants in childhood as a condition for treating the adult stimulant abuser with stimulant medication. If pharmacotherapy is used in these cases, very close monitoring of treatment compliance and of urine drug screens is necessary.

For the alcohol-dependent stimulant user, most aspects of the psychosocial treatment of the alcohol and stimulant abuse are similar. Disulfiram (Antabuse), especially when administered under supervision, may be a useful adjunct.

The third indication for pharmacotherapy is neuroadaptation,[8] which refers to the development of changes in the CNS as an adaptive response to chronic, high-dose stimulant exposure. Neuroadaptation is reflected clinically by the appearance of stimulant withdrawal syndrome in chronic, high-dose users. Medications may have distinct roles in four clinical phases that follow cessation of high-dose use: (1) withdrawal (1 to 4 days); (2) immediate postwithdrawal period (4 days to 3 weeks); (3) a waxing-waning phase lasting 1 to 6 months; and (4) long-term residual phase with latent potential for abuse. The latter two phases correspond roughly to the "extinction" phase described by some authors. The phased treatment of the patient with severe dependence is summarized in Table 15–1. During the initial phase of withdrawal, or acute "crash," benzodiazepines may relieve agitation and help induce much-desired sleep. Dopaminergic agonists such as bromocriptine and amantadine have been reported to alleviate acute craving, which may occur during the crash phase.[15]

In the withdrawal and immediate postwithdrawal phases, target symptoms for pharmacological intervention include depressed mood, anxiety, anhedonia, and spontaneous craving for stimulants. Antidepressants may be useful both in alleviating the depressive symptoms and anhedonia and in reducing craving. Gawin et al. reported beneficial effects of desipramine in reducing cocaine use during a 6-week study period, as compared to lithium and placebo.[16] Among the desipramine-treated group, there were significantly more periods of 3 to 4 weeks of continuous abstinence. Subjective craving was reduced in the desipramine group, but this reduction lagged temporally behind the decrease in cocaine

TABLE 15–1. TREATMENT PHASES OF PATIENT WITH SEVERE STIMULANT DEPENDENCE

Withdrawal, 1 to 4 days
  Is hospitalization because of psychosis or other dangers or extraction from environment necessary?
  Provide for sleep, rest, secure environment
  Set stage for treatment objectives with patient and support persons
Immediate postwithdrawal, 4 days to 3 weeks
  Is a dopamine agonist required or helpful in introducing patient to treatment?
  Plan treatment 2 to 3 weeks based on assessment
  Decide on antidepressant pharmacotherapy as adjunct to treatment initiation and maintenance
Waxing and waning phase lasting 1 to 6 months
  Establish psychosocial-behavioral programs based on assessment
  Continue pharmacotherapy based on degree of anergia, psychoasthemia, and anhedonia and response to treatment
  Establish means for handling long-term residual phase and means for crisis management if any initial recidivism
Long-term residual latent potential for abuse
  Cue sensitive urges and cravings extensively brought into consciousness and establish strategies for mastery
  Establish concrete and rehearsed plans for avoiding "greased slide" fall into intense abuse pattern rapidly after reinitialization of use

use. Gawin et al. hypothesize that desipramine's therapeutic effects are based on reversal of cocaine-induced loss of sensitivity in dopaminergic brain reward pathways, which may be responsible for the anhedonia experienced in cocaine withdrawal.[16]

In the waxing-waning phase, which may last many months or even years, merging into the long-term residual phase, spontaneous craving has largely resolved, but the addict continues to experience craving triggered by conditioned cues in the environment as well as internal cues such as mood states. This cue-induced craving gradually diminishes in intensity if not reinforced by further stimulant use. Ideally, a medication to be used in treatment at this stage would dampen cue-induced craving, hastening the extinction process. If specific mood states such as depression or anxiety are serving as cues, amelioration of these may also enhance recovery. Although results of longer duration trials of medications are not yet available, preliminary evidence suggests that desipramine reduces stimulus-induced craving (specifically, craving induced by cocaine administration), and may have a role in treatment extending beyond withdrawal into the extinction phase.

A concern regarding any pharmacotherapy during extinction is the possibility that medication effects will serve as cues for craving, as discussed above. Thus, drugs like amantadine and bromocriptine with immediate dopaminergic effects, which are useful during the acute crash in the relief of acute craving, may be counterproductive if administered during the later extinction phase.

Carbamazepine has been examined as another pharmacological adjunct,[17] but effectiveness in stimulant dependence has not been established in controlled trials. Flupenthixol, a neuroleptic agent, has been reported to have anticraving properties in crack users when administered as an intramuscular decanoate injection.[18] Unfortunately, studies of drug treatment for stimulant dependence are plagued by high drop-out rates; thus, the overall efficacy of the drugs in a general clinical population is likely to be lower than that reported for patients completing such studies.

The partial opioid agonist buprenorphine has been reported to markedly suppress cocaine self-administration in rhesus monkeys.[19] Use of this drug will likely be limited to opiate-dependent cocaine users due to its ability to induce opioid dependence, but it may prove an effective alternative to methadone in the mixed-dependence population.[19]

Pharmacological therapies can serve as useful adjuncts in the comprehensive behavioral and psychosocial rehabilitation of the stimulant abuser. The physician has the opportunity to utilize his or her medical authority to reinforce strongly the importance of involvement in a program of recovery. Regular urine drug monitoring and routine contacts with family and significant others are important aspects of follow-up. When the physician has referred the patient to a separate drug treatment program, ongoing communication and collaboration between the physician and program treatment staff is essential.

REFERENCES

1. U.S. Department of Health and Human Services: Drug Abuse and Drug Abuse Research: The Third Triennial Report to Congress from the Secretary, Department of Health and Human Services. Rockville, MD, U.S. Department of HHS, 1991.
2. Ritchie JM, Greene NM: Local anesthetics. In Gilman AG, Goodman LS, Rall TW, Murad F, eds. Goodman and Gilman's The Pharmacological Basis of Therapeutics. 8th ed. New York: Macmillan, 1990:311.
3. Hoffman BB, Lefkowitz RJ: Catecholamines and sympathomimetic drugs. In Gilman AG, Goodman LS, Rall TW, Murad F, eds. Goodman and Gilman's The Pharmacological Basis of Therapeutics. 8th ed. New York: Macmillan, 1990:187.
4. American Psychiatric Association: Diagnostic and Statistical Manual of Mental Disorders. 3rd ed., Revised. Washington, DC: American Psychiatric Association, 1987.
5. Rounsaville BJ, Anton SF, Carroll K, et al: Psychiatric diagnoses of treatment-seeking cocaine abusers. Arch Gen Psychiatry 48:43, 1991.
6. Jaffe JH: Drug addiction and drug abuse. In Gilman AG, Goodman LS, Rall TW, Murad F, eds. Goodman and Gilman's The Pharmacological Basis of Therapeutics. 8th ed. New York: Macmillan, 1990:522.
7. Climent CE, de Aragon LV, Plutchik R: Prediction of risk for drug abuse in high school students. Bull Pan Am Health Organ 24:77, 1990.
8. Kosten TR: Pharmacotherapeutic interventions for cocaine abuse: Matching patients to treatments. J Nerv Ment Dis 177:379, 1989.
9. Lange RA, Cigarroa RG, Flores ED: Potentiation of cocaine-induced coronary vasoconstriction by beta-adrenergic blockade. Ann Intern Med 112:897, 1990.

10. Gawin FH, Ellinwood EH: Cocaine and other stimulants. N Engl J Med 318:1173, 1988.
11. Carroll KM, Rounsaville BJ, Keller DS: Relapse prevention strategies for the treatment of cocaine abuse. Am J Drug Alcohol Abuse (in press).
12. Rounsaville BJ, Gawin F, Kleber H: Interpersonal psychotherapy adapted for ambulatory cocaine abusers. Am J Drug Alcohol Abuse 11:171, 1985.
13. Kang S-Y, Kleinman PH, Woody GE et al: Outcomes for cocaine abusers after once-a-week psychosocial therapy. Am J Psychiatry 148:630, 1991.
14. Ellinwood EH: Amphetamine psychosis. I. Description of the individuals and process. J Nerv Ment Dis 144:273, 1967.
15. Giannini AJ, Folts DJ, Feather JN, Sullivan BS: Bromocriptine and amantadine in cocaine detoxification. Psychiatry Res 29:11, 1989.
16. Gawin FH, Kleber HD, Byck R, et al: Desipramine facilitation of initial cocaine abstinence. Arch Gen Psychiatry 46:117, 1989.
17. Kuhn KL, Halikas JA, Kemp KD: Carbamazepine treatment of cocaine dependence in methadone maintenance patients with dual opiate-cocaine addiction. NIDA Res Monogr 95:316, 1989.
18. Gawin FH, Allen D, Humblestone B: Outpatient treatment of 'crack' cocaine smoking with flupenthixol decanoate: A preliminary report. Arch Gen Psychiatry 46:322, 1989.
19. Mello NK, Mendelson JH, Bree MP, Lukas SE: Buprenorphine suppresses cocaine self-administration by rhesus monkeys. Science 245:859, 1989.

16

CANNABIS DEPENDENCE

ROGER A. ROFFMAN, D.S.W. and ROBERT S. STEPHENS, PH.D.

Three men, so the story goes, arrived one night at the closed gates of a Persian city. One was intoxicated by alcohol, another was under the spell of opium, and the third was steeped in marihuana (hashish, as it was then called.)

The first blustered: "Let's break the gates down."

"Nay," yawned the opium eater, "let us rest until morning, when we may enter through the wide-flung portals."

"Do as you like," was the announcement of the marihuana addict. "But I shall stroll in through the keyhole!"

E. A. Rowell and R. Rowell[a]

When specialized therapeutic support is publicized and perceived by the potential client as sensitive to and appropriate for his or her experiences in struggling with marijuana dependence, a substantial number of individuals are likely to request assistance in quitting use of this drug. The focus of this chapter is threefold: describing the phenomenon of marijuana dependence, identifying important elements in the assessment process, and offering guidelines concerning the delivery of a brief individual intervention targeted at helping the client achieve durable abstinence.

---

[a] On the Trail of Marihuana: The Weed of Madness. Mountain View, CA: Pacific Press Publishing Association, 1939.

The authors have been funded by the National Institute on Drug Abuse continuously since 1986 for the purpose of evaluating alternative therapeutic modalities with adult chronic marijuana smokers. Much of this chapter will be based on our empirical work.[1–3] A case history will assist in highlighting aspects of the phenomenon and set the context for discussing assessment and intervention.

THE CLIENT

Tom, a 34-year-old married father of two, is employed as a machinist in a large industrial firm in the Pacific Northwest. He sought assistance in stopping marijuana use after having tried unsuccessfully on his own for several years to stop or cut back. He first smoked marijuana at the age of 15, and has been a daily smoker for 12 years. Prior efforts at stopping led to his experiencing considerable irritability, craving for the drug, and an eventual rationalization that occasional use wouldn't do harm. Inevitably, his efforts to remain moderate fairly quickly eroded to daily use.

At the time of his initial assessment, he indicated that there were several reasons why he desired to become abstinent: (1) he perceived himself as out of control with marijuana, reporting that he often smoked when he had resolved to abstain; (2) his wife complained that he spent far too much time being stoned—a state that she felt precluded their having satisfactory communication with one another; (3) both of them were worried about his being a poor role model for their children; and (4) he was aware that he had fallen into a pattern of making plans, often procrastinating in following through, and feeling self-critical as a consequence. Two additional concerns, although of a lower priority, were the possibility of being required to submit to random urine screening at his place of employment and some fear that his marijuana use might eventually threaten his health.

Tom reported no adverse consequences ensuing from his typical consumption of one or two beers twice a week. He indicated that he had casually experimented with cocaine and hallucinogens when in his early twenties, but had discontinued their use a decade earlier. Tom generally smoked marijuana each evening in his basement workshop after the children were asleep, and he also routinely got stoned on Saturday afternoons with three male high school friends with whom he played basketball.

Tom expressed ambivalence about stopping use. While he acknowledged that the stress within the marriage and his feeling out of control were major incentives for discontinuing use, he perceived one potential costly consequence being the breaking up of his close friendships with his buddies. Despite his ambivalence, Tom wanted to talk with the clinician about stopping use.

EPIDEMIOLOGY OF MARIJUANA USE AND DEPENDENCE

According to the National Institute on Drug Abuse (NIDA)-funded 1990 National Household Survey, 66.5 million Americans (age 12 and above) had ever used marijuana, 20.5 million had used it at least once in the past year, 10.2 million were considered as current users (had used it in the month preceding the survey), and 5.5 million were smoking the drug at least once each week. Current users included 5.2 per cent of those in the 12 to 17 age group, 12.7 per cent of those between 18 and 25, and 3.6 per cent of those age 26 and above.[4]

The usage of marijuana has continued to decline since 1979, when 16.7 per cent of 12- to 17-year-olds, 35.4 per cent of 18- to 25-year-olds, and 6.0 per cent of those age 26 and older were current users. Nonetheless, this drug remains the most popular illicit drug in the United States. The U.S. Department of State estimates that 105 million pounds of marijuana were available for use (after law enforcement seizures had been accounted for) in the United States in 1989.[5]

At the present time, there are no empirical data concerning the prevalence of marijuana dependence. A rough estimate can be obtained, however, by extrapolating from longitudinal research with users. One such study followed 97 marijuana smokers who had been using the drug for about a 10-year period.[6] A somewhat greater number of this sample were monthly (38 per cent) rather than daily (26 per cent) users. Using diagnostic criteria adapted from the field of alcoholism research, the authors estimated that 9 per cent of these ongoing users had become marijuana dependent (e.g., reported problems in at least three of four domains: physiological effects, control problems, personal-social problems, and adverse opinions from others). If this study's findings were used for the purpose of estimation, 9 per cent of 5.5 million users (those who used once per week or more often in 1990) would suggest that our client Tom is one of nearly a half-million individuals who are dependent on marijuana.

ASSESSING MARIJUANA DEPENDENCE

Perhaps more so than with reference to other illicit drugs, achieving precision in the assessment of marijuana dependence is an elusive task.[7] While the illegality of the drug offers the possibility of defining any use as abuse per se, this criterion is not likely to be clinically meaningful. Measures of chronicity, quantity consumed, or frequency of use, particularly in the extreme, may predict the likelihood of dependence, but not with sufficient certainty to be used as conclusive diagnostic indicators. Chronic use, even at a daily level, appears to occur without adverse social consequences in some users. To further complicate matters, defining a standard "dose" of marijuana is difficult because of the variable potency of street samples as well as the variable amounts of the drug that are absorbed as a consequence of differences in methods of inhalation and ingestion.

The absence of objective verifiable physical consequences associated with excessive marijuana use further limits assessment efforts. The user who appears in the emergency room—often a marijuana novice—is likely to be experiencing a transient panic reaction without concurrent physiological damage. Memory impairment and difficulties with concentration are likely to be reversible effects of acute intoxication. Impaired lung functioning might be found in the chronic user,[8] although this indicator is confounded in the individual who concurrently smokes tobacco. At present, there are few conclusive studies supporting the efficacy of medical examination in isolating indicators of excessive use of this drug.

As can occur with other forms of substance abuse and dependence, the individual's subjective appraisal of the consequences of his or her use may substantially distort descriptions of the drug's effects and attributions concerning causation. Some individuals will minimize the relationship between marijuana smoking and problems in their lives. Others will erroneously perceive marijuana smoking as the cause of social, occupational, or intrapersonal difficulties unrelated to its use.

Ultimately, marijuana dependence is characterized by continued use of this drug despite the experience of serious adverse consequences. The clinician's assessment must largely rely on self-report data, perhaps augmented by information acquired from others in the client's network, pertaining to impairment in various domains of functioning: interpersonal (effects on relationships), intrapersonal (effects on self-esteem, concerns about memory or concentration difficulties, feelings of being out of control), vocational (effects on work performance or general level of ambition in terms of one's career), scholastic (effects on studying, academic aspirations), health (actual or feared adverse health consequences), economic (excessive expenditure of money to acquire marijuana with a consequent inability to attend to other financial needs), legal (actual or potential arrests for possession, growing, selling), or spiritual (effects on one's sense of integrity, congruence with personal values).

Returning once again to Tom, recognizing that he is struggling with ambivalence suggests that the clinician may best assist him by encouraging Tom to identify and evaluate the negative consequences involved with use, providing information to him concerning marijuana effects[b] and the degree to which ambivalence and apprehension are common at the beginning of this effort, and being responsive to his feelings of dependence by describing the steps through which new learning gradually leads to enhanced self-confidence. Motivational interviewing[9] offers an approach to assisting the ambivalent client to achieve both clarity concerning the need to change and commitment to its accomplishment.

In the section that follows, we review recent clinical and nonclinical studies of marijuana users for the purpose of understanding users' personal appraisals of the manner in which their use of marijuana has had impact on their lives.

RECENT STUDIES OF MARIJUANA USERS

A nonclinical New York City study conducted in the mid-1980s focused on 150 daily marijuana users.[10,11] While most respondents reported that the benefits of use outweighed the negative effects, one half indicated that they wanted to cut back or stop entirely. Impaired memory was reported by two thirds of these individuals, and nearly one half disclosed that they were having difficulty concentrating, were finding that their motivation was low, or were concerned about possible health risks.

Another nonclinical study conducted at about the same time reported findings from 99 persons who were recruited for interviews through local media publicity seeking "heavy" marijuana users.[12] Nearly

half of these daily or near-daily users indicated that they experienced reduced levels of energy or motivation, difficulties with concentration or memory, or financial problems. Twenty-eight per cent had thought of seeking help in stopping use.

A Seattle study conducted in 1984 used local publicity to invite adults who were concerned about their marijuana use to phone for an anonymous interview.[13] Unlike the above two studies, this one specifically targeted concerned smokers. Of the 225 individuals who were interviewed over a 2-week period, more than 90 per cent were interested in obtaining help to stopping use. These respondents reported an average of 4.5 problems related to their marijuana smoking. Only 20 per cent appeared to be concurrently abusing alcohol or other drugs.

Finally, in 1987 and 1988, the authors enrolled 212 adult chronic marijuana smokers in a NIDA-funded marijuana cessation treatment study that compared two forms of group counseling.[1] The participants had been using the drug for an average of 15 years, and reported smoking it on an average of 79 of the 90 days preceding enrollment. Adverse consequences listed by at least 50 per cent of these individuals included feeling bad about using (87 per cent), procrastinating (85 per cent), lowered self-esteem (76 per cent), memory impairment (66 per cent), and withdrawal symptoms (50 per cent).

THERAPEUTIC MODELS

In this final section of the chapter, we will discuss a brief individual intervention for working with the adult chronic marijuana smoker. This approach follows from empirical work with minimal interventions (i.e., directed advice delivered by a clinician) which have shown promise with problem drinking[14–16] cigarette cessation,[17] and weight control.[18] The approach also draws on two theoretical models of behavior: a consideration of the clinical implications associated with differing stages of change, and a cognitive-behavioral model of relapse prevention.

Prochaska and DiClemente, based on their work in cigarette cessation, identified five stages of change through which individuals progress in overcoming addictive disorders.[19] Clinical interventions, in this perspective, need to be selected based on an appraisal of the stage in which any particular client is involved. During the *precontemplation stage*, the client is not as yet considering the possibility of modifying the behavior, although adverse consequences may be occurring. The *contemplation stage* is characterized by the client weighing the potential benefits and losses associated with continuing or ceasing the target behavior. *Decision-making* is the stage in which the client resolves to accomplish a behavior-change goal. Becoming skillful in initially achieving that goal is the work of the *action stage*. Finally, dealing with challenges to durability of the

---

[b] The Hazelden Foundation's 1989 Booklet, Marijuana: Current Facts, Figures, and Information, is helpful for this purpose.

behavior change is the primary focus of the *maintenance stage*.

The cognitive-behavioral model of relapse articulated by Marlatt and Gordon presumes that individuals who seek to overcome an addictive behavior will vary in the kinds of situations that present them with high risk for triggering slips.[20] For example, the client we have been discussing would likely be at high risk when playing basketball with his high school friends or when working alone in his workshop. The model suggests that counseling needs to assist the client in identifying his or her particular high-risk triggers (e.g., specific moods, thoughts, places, certain people, times of day, events), and to use behavioral rehearsal in developing or strengthening (or both) the client's ability to cope with these cues or triggers. Cognitive restructuring is emphasized in countering negative attributions in the event that a slip takes place; for example, "I'm a failure because I slipped after being abstinent for 6 days" is replaced by "I've been succeeding for 6 days, and something happened that I wasn't prepared for. I'll need to learn from this situation." Theoretically, the client who becomes skillful in effectively coping with relapse triggers will achieve a heightened sense of self-efficacy[21] and will subsequently be at reduced risk for relapse.

Were Tom to experience a brief individual intervention based on these models and targeted at assisting him with marijuana cessation, the following elements would be implemented:

Assessment

The clinician would inquire about Tom's pattern of marijuana use (e.g., frequency, amount, number of times per day of use, individuals with whom he gets stoned), the negative effects he has experienced, and his reasons for wanting to make a change in his use of this drug. As is often the case with many heavy users in their thirties and forties, Tom is likely to be conflicted about the substantial social changes that have taken place in recent decades. Having initiated marijuana use 15 to 25 years earlier, at a time when considerable tolerance for marijuana smoking existed in this country, these individuals are now confronted with the drug war's zero-tolerance attitudes and policies, they have fewer friends who still get high, they face the risk of urine screening at work or when applying for a new position, and they occupy family roles that they and their spouses may perceive as inconsistent with recreational drug use. In consideration of these factors, the clinician needs to be prepared to listen empathically to the client's feelings about changed attitudes and social policies. In essence, the inquiries being made in this assessment process focus on contemplation stage needs (i.e., assisting the client to inventory and evaluate reasons for quitting and those for continuing in preparation for committing to cessation).

Setting Goals

When setting goals, the client is likely to consider complete abstinence versus attempting to become a moderate smoker. If the clinician and client decide to give moderation a try, setting specific objectives within a specific time frame will facilitate evaluation of its outcome. Contracting with the client that he or she will work toward becoming abstinent in the event that moderation is not attainable provides a back-up plan. There are no empirical outcome studies that predict the level of success with a moderation goal.

Developing Coping Strategies

Helping the client prepare to stop might include the following instructions: look into support groups such as Marijuana Anonymous, set a quit date, get rid of all marijuana and associated paraphernalia, disclose to people with whom the client smokes that he or she is quitting and seeks their support, consider certain people and places that should be avoided because they present too great a risk, plan ahead for how free time will be spent in the first week of abstinence, and keep a daily log of situations in which strong urges to use occur.

Formalizing the decision to quit through the preparation of a "quit contract" can serve to reinforce the client's motivation. It can also remind him or her of the coping strategies that need to be practiced while learning to be a nonuser of marijuana.

A key component of the intervention includes anticipating and planning for future high-risk situations, and debriefing those that have recently been experienced. Returning to the case of Tom, the clinician would want to discuss alternatives to smoking late at night in his shop as well as on Saturdays following basketball games.

All of these strategies are based on the premise that the client is essentially entering a "training" period in which he or she is learning how to live without marijuana. Overcoming dependence involves facing vulnerable situations, practicing responding to them with alternative strategies, and gradually becoming competent and confident in this new lifestyle.

Maintenance

Periodic "check-ups" with the clinician are likely to enhance the client's sense of support as he or she continues to face relapse vulnerabilities. They provide an opportunity for reinforcing successes, debriefing particularly difficult situations, and brainstorming future coping strategies. They also facilitate broader consideration of factors in the client's lifestyle that may influence the durability of this behavior change.

SUMMARY AND CONCLUSIONS

Marijuana dependence may affect as many as one-half million individuals, many of whom have been using the drug for more than 10 years. Chronic users who find themselves needing support in stopping are likely to be motivated by a combination of factors including feeling badly about being unable to control the amount or frequency of use, procrastination, experiencing negative feedback from a spouse or partner, fearing being an inappropriate role model for children, and concerns about the potential for urine screening on the job. Many users, however, are also likely to express resentment with drug-war policies and changed public attitudes concerning use of this drug.

The relapse prevention theme discussed in this chapter can provide the framework for a brief therapeutic intervention that emphasizes assisting the client in setting goals, identifying likely sources of vulnerability to relapse, developing cognitive and behavioral coping strategies to deal with those vulnerabilities, harnessing social support, and making lifestyle modifications that will facilitate durable maintenance of the behavior change.

REFERENCES

1. Roffman RA, Stephens RS, Simpson ES, Whitaker DL: Treatment of marijuana dependence: Preliminary results. J Psychoactive Drugs 20:129–137, 1988.
2. Roffman RA, Stephens RS, Simpson ES: Relapse prevention with adult chronic marijuana smokers. J Chem Dependencies Treat 2:241–257, 1989.
3. Roffman RA, Stephens RS, Simpson ES: Relapse prevention and the treatment of marijuana dependence: Long-term outcomes. Paper presented at the annual meeting of the Association for Advancement of Behavior Therapy, San Francisco, 1990.
4. National Institute On Drug Abuse: The National Household Survey on Drug Abuse: Population Estimates 1990. (ADM publication no. 91-1732.) Washington, DC: U.S. Government Printing Office, 1991.
5. National Narcotics Intelligence Consumers Committee: The NNICC Report. Marijuana Digest 3:3, 1990.
6. Weller RA, Halikas JA: Objective criteria for the diagnosis of marijuana abuse. Nerv Ment Dis 168:98–103, 1980.
7. Roffman RA, George WH: *In* Donovan DM, Marlatt GA, eds. Assessment of Addictive Behaviors. New York: Guilford Press, 1988:325–363.
8. Tashkin DP, Coulson AH, Clark VA, et al: Respiratory symptoms and lung function in habitual heavy smokers of marijuana alone, smokers of marijuana and tobacco, smokers of tobacco alone, and nonsmokers. Am Rev Resp Dis 135:209–216, 1987.
9. Miller WR: Motivational interviewing with problem drinkers. Behav Psychother 11:147–172, 1983.
10. Hendin H, Haas AP, Singer MD et al: Living High: Daily Marijuana Use Among Adults. New York: Human Sciences Press, 1987.
11. Haas AP, Hendin H: The meaning of chronic marijuana use among adults: A psychosocial perspective. J Drug Issues 17:333–348, 1987.
12. Rainone GA, Deren S, Kleinman PH, Wish ED: Heavy marijuana users not in treatment: The continuing search for the "pure" marijuana user. J Psychoactive Drugs 19:353–359, 1987.
13. Roffman RA, Barnhart R: Assessing need for marijuana dependence treatment through an anonymous telephone interview. Int J Addict 22:639–651, 1987.
14. Edwards G, Orford J, Egert S, et al: Alcoholism: A controlled trial of "treatment" and "advice." J Stud Alcohol 38:1004–1031, 1977.
15. Chickheck J, Lloyd G, Crombie E: Outcome one year after a brief intervention among newly identified problem drinkers with social supports admitted to a general hospital: Preliminary results of a controlled study. Nat Inst Alcohol Abuse Alcohol Ser 17:348–354, 1985.
16. Zweben A, Pearlman S, Li S: A comparison of brief advice and conjoint therapy in the treatment of alcohol abuse: The results of the marital systems study. Br J Addict 83:899–916, 1988.
17. Schwartz JL: Review and Evaluation of Smoking Cessation Methods: The United States and Canada, 1978–1985. NIH publication no. 87-2940. Washington, DC: U.S. Government Printing Office, 1987.
18. Black DR, Coe WC, Friesen JG, Wurzmann AG: Minimal interventions for weight control: A cost-effective alternative. Addict Behav 9:279–285, 1984.
19. Prochaska JO, DiClemente CC: Stages and processes of self-change of smoking: Toward an integrative model of change. J Consult Clin Psychol 51:390–395, 1983.
20. Marlatt GA, Gordon JR: Relapse Prevention: Maintenance Strategies in the Treatment of Addictive Behaviors. New York: Guilford Press, 1985.
21. Bandura A: Self-efficacy: Toward a unifying theory of behavior change. Psychol Rev 84:191–215, 1977.

TREATMENT OF PSYCHEDELIC DRUG-INDUCED PSYCHOSES

EDWARD F. DOMINO, M.D.

HALLUCINOGEN-INDUCED PSYCHOSES

There are many mind-altering, or "psychedelic," drugs, some of which produce rather vivid illusions and hallucinations, primarily visual. Even though such compounds have different chemical structures, most have actions similar to lysergic acid diethylamide (LSD-25). Lysergic acid diethylamide-25 (commonly called LSD) and related substances are either complex or simple substituted indole alkylamines including tryptamine, dimethyltryptamine (DMT), and 5-methoxy-dimethyltryptamine. In addition, dimethyl-4-hydroxytryptamine (psilocin), dimethyl-4-phosphoryltryptamine (psilocybin), and dimethyl-5-hydroxytryptamine (bufotenine) also have hallucinogenic properties. Bufotenine is a rather poor hallucinogen, but is abused in Australia, where it is commonly obtained from the skin glands of the cane toad. Cohen's[1] classification of various psychedelic agents is still very useful. Substituted indole alkylamines and substituted phenylalkylamines including mescaline and 2,5-dimethoxy-4-methylamphetamine (DOM) are the principal substances in this class. Marijuana and various other forms of delta-9-tetrahydrocannabinol, phencyclidine (PCP) and its derivatives, various muscarinic cholinergic antagonists, and some miscellaneous substances like myristicin are also classified as psychedelic drugs but do not produce prominent hallucinations unless very large doses are taken. Hence, some would disagree that they should be classified as hallucinogens, at least not in the sense of substances such as LSD.

The most potent hallucinogen is LSD. Inasmuch as LSD is more likely to be abused, emphasis is placed on its clinical description of intoxication and treatment as the prototype for the entire group. There are several excellent detailed descriptions of these and other substances of abuse in various texts.[2–5]

Clinical Description

The usual adult oral dose of LSD is about 100 μg. Generally, mental effects occur within 1 hour and last for approximately 12 hours, with a peak effect of about 4 hours. Variation in the onset, peak, and dura-

tion of effects depends upon dosage and other factors related to, for example, absorption. Lysergic acid diethylamide produces mood changes, perceptual disturbances, and visual hallucinations. The drug produces sensory illusions and, especially, visual hallucinations with the eyes closed. A darkened environment with flickering light helps to produce marked visual imagery. In addition, there is distortion of body image. If taken at night, the patient has insomnia and is agitated. On the other hand, on the subsequent night there is a significant rebound of rapid-eye-movement (REM) sleep that is greater than expected from the previous night of sleep deprivation. Intense hallucinations in which sounds may precipitate visual sensations and brilliant changes in the intensity and vividness of various colors are characteristic of LSD ingestion. There may be euphoria as well as depersonalization. As expected, large doses of LSD produce more intense effects. The subject's psychological set and the environmental setting are very important in determining the psychological effects obtained.

Complications associated with the psychotic syndrome induced by LSD include seizures, anxiety, depression, acute panic, and paranoid states as well as flashbacks weeks later when the drug is no longer present in the body. There are significant physical signs and symptoms, which are predominantly sympathomimetic. They include mydriasis, an increase in heart rate, piloerection, hyperglycemia, and leucocytosis. Sometimes there is a marked elevation in body temperature. Deep tendon reflexes are hyperactive. In addition, salivation, lacrimation, tremor, nausea, and vomiting can occur.

Lysergic acid diethylamide has both serotonergic (5-HT$_2$) agonist/antagonist and dopaminergic agonist activity. Central nervous system (CNS) and autonomic signs and symptoms, along with a history of taking LSD, helps in the diagnosis of LSD or related hallucinogen intoxication. However, one must be cautious in relying on the history that LSD specifically was taken, since the user may not really know exactly what was ingested.

Other hallucinogens with similar properties vary in their intensity and duration of action. Some derivatives of mescaline, especially DOM and trimethoxyamphetamine, are far more potent than mescaline itself and may, in the case of DOM, be more likely to produce seizures. A phenethylamine derivative called MDMA, also known as ''ecstasy,'' is especially abused on college campuses. It has a mixture of amphetamine- and mescaline-like effects in large doses. However, in small doses it is said to increase rapport.

Laboratory Studies

Most hallucinogens usually are taken orally; although some, such as DMT, are usually smoked. Hallucinogen users also may use other substances including alcohol, marijuana, amphetamine, and phencyclidine. Sometimes, the drug experience induced by hallucinogens changes a person's way of living for a long time and he or she may become part of a subculture of drug users. Intoxicated patients may present with a variety of clinical pictures including prominent psychotomimetic effects, acute panic attacks, and other psychotic states including mania or depression.

Besides history and clinical signs and symptoms, laboratory analyses of the substance taken or of the patient's plasma and urine are important to unequivocally establish a diagnosis of hallucinogen intoxication. The doses of LSD ingested are usually so small that plasma levels of LSD are in the low ng/ml range. Analytic methods for determining LSD involve radioimmunoassay as well as high-performance liquid chromatography (HPLC) with fluorescence detection. The most specific assays involve gas chromatography–mass spectrometry (GC-MS) techniques. The latter are usually not readily available to most clinicians and require the samples to be sent to suitable analytical laboratories where it may take 1 or more days to establish the diagnosis by chemical means. Therefore, history and clinical picture of signs and symptoms usually establish the presumptive diagnosis and treatment.

Differential Diagnosis

Hallucinogen intoxication can be diagnosed on the basis of history, psychological symptoms, and the marked physiological changes that occur. As emphasized above, one must be careful not to depend upon the history too much, since frequently the user may not know exactly what was taken. A clinical picture of psychosis in which colored visual hallucinations predominate is almost pathognomonic. Hallucinogen ingestion is usually not difficult to differentiate from an acute schizophrenic or manic episode, although the acute psychotic reaction can be misdiagnosed. Most clinicians can readily distinguish, on the basis of clinical symptomatology alone, subjects who have taken hallucinogens compared to drug-free schizophrenic or manic patients, although the latter may also have taken a hallucinogen, in which case the diagnosis may be very difficult.

Treatment Approaches

Patients who abuse hallucinogens rarely have life-threatening medical problems. Instead, their problems are primarily psychological and psychiatric. Sometimes, the latter can lead to suicide or other dangerous and inappropriate behavior. Reassurance, reduction of sensory input, and supportive care are the major methods of treating hallucinogen-induced acute psychotic or panic reactions. A quiet, safe environment, preferably with persons who are familiar with the patient, are most appropriate to "talk the patient down." Neuroleptics generally are not indicated and may be contraindicated. If pharmacotherapy is needed, the administration of a benzodiazepine such as diazepam should be used. Chlorpromazine was given years ago but, especially in the case of DOM intoxication, cardiovascular collapse and seizures have occurred. If antipsychotic drugs are necessary for clinical management, the administration of haloperidol or a similar high-potency neuroleptic is preferred, although this is seldom needed. Since the latter are selective D_2 antagonists, there is a need to study selective $5-HT_2$ antagonists in humans as possible antidotes. There are data in animals that such compounds antagonize the effects of LSD but, as yet, no human data are available.

PHENCYCLIDINE-INDUCED INTOXICATION

Clinical Description

Depending upon the dose ingested, a patient intoxicated with PCP or related compounds—like the thienyl analog of PCP (TCP) and the ethyl analog (PCE)—shows widely different neurological and psychiatric signs and symptoms.[6,7] These can be subdivided into three major clinical pictures including (1) confusion, delirium, and psychosis; (2) semicoma/coma; and (3) coma with seizures. Inasmuch as PCP is an obsolete dissociative anesthetic, one may observe patients becoming progressively more obtunded and eventually comatose, or the reverse when the patient is emerging from coma and showing emerging delirium. Burns and Lerner[8] provided one of the best descriptions of the various clinical correlates of PCP signs and symptoms with blood levels as listed in Table 17–1. Milhorn[4] subdivided the above three clinical pictures into three stages. Most PCP abusers do not grossly overdose themselves to the point of semicoma and coma. Hence, the majority of patients intoxicated with PCP show a clinical picture of confusion, delirium, and psychosis, or stage I. Stage II represents stupor to mild coma, and Milhorn's stage III is a patient in deep coma.

Phencyclidine is abused primarily in the United States, mostly in large metropolitan areas of which Los Angeles, San Francisco, and Washington, DC are especially prominent. Because PCP is relatively easy to synthesize, it is abused as a relatively cheap sub-

TABLE 17–1. CLINICAL SPECTRUM OF ACUTE PHENCYCLIDINE INTOXICATION[a]

Psychosis, Confusion, or Delirium	Coma	Coma Plus Seizure
Dose (mg) 5–10	20+	70+
Plasma level 25–50 ng/ml	100–200 ng/ml	200–500 mg/ml
Behavioral state		
Confusion, blank stare	Unresponsive, immobile	Prolonged coma
Vertical or horizontal nystagmus	Spontaneous vertical or horizontal nystagmus	
Increased blood pressure	Increased blood pressure	Sustained increase in blood pressure
Gait ataxia	Increased deep-tendon muscle rigidity	Muscle rigidity
		Seizure activity
Excited, aggressive, or bizarre behavior	EEG *theta* slowing	EEG *theta* and *delta* slowing periodic slow-wave complexes
		Hypoventilation, apnea
Body temperature		
Elevated if excited	Slightly lower	Decreased

[a] Adapted with permission from Burns RS, Lerner SE: The effects of phencyclidine in man: A review. *In* Domino EF, ed. PCP (Phencyclidine): Historical and Current Perspectives. Ann Arbor, MI: NPP Books, 1981:449–469.

stitute for many street drugs. The patient may not realize that he or she has had PCP. The patient may have been told it was LSD, amphetamine, or synthetic marijuana. Phencyclidine used to be widely abused by college students in the 1970s; but in the 1990s, it has lost its appeal in favor of marijuana and alcoholic beverages. Phencyclidine users are usually young adults of either sex. As is true of many drug abusers, they may have other more serious psychiatric illnesses of which drug taking is only a symptom. This is important to remember because treatment of the acute phase of PCP intoxication is really only the first step to its proper long-term management. The same is true of other drugs of abuse, including the hallucinogens.

Disease, Environment, and Genetic Factors

When PCP was first developed as a general anesthetic, early clinical trials indicated that approximately one third of the patients showed an emergence delirium. Why only 33 per cent rather than 100 per cent of patients showed a delirium or psychosis is still unexplained, and suggests important environmental or genetic factors.

Schizophrenic patients appear to be much more susceptible to a prolonged psychotic episode due to PCP than other individuals. In addition, there are environmental and genetic factors influencing phencyclidine biotransformation in animals and humans,[9,10] but such research studies are still too preliminary to be clinically applicable at this time.

Laboratory Studies

Although a preliminary diagnosis of PCP intoxication can be made on the basis of history and clinical signs and symptoms, only a positive drug, blood, or urine specimen will unequivocally establish it. A large variety of different chemical assays are available, but the best is still GS-MS. The brain wave changes induced by PCP and its derivatives are un-

usual, and thus an electroencephalogram (EEG) may be helpful if the patient is cooperative or comatose. Serum creatinine phosphokinase (CPK) levels may be increased and the urine may contain myoglobin due to rhabdomyolysis.

Differential Diagnosis

The first step in the differential diagnosis of PCP intoxication must be on the basis of whether the patient is in coma with or without seizures, emerging from coma, descending into coma, or in a psychotic state. Obviously, the patient in coma with or without seizures has a differential diagnosis that excludes all other causes of coma and seizures. Again, history and laboratory analysis are crucial. Psychotic manifestations of PCP can be confused with catatonic schizophrenia, an acute toxic psychosis induced with hallucinogens, and various acute brain syndromes. The psychiatric manifestations of PCP may be confused with true schizophrenia or other causes of lethargy and bizarre, violent, agitated, or euphoric behavior. Phencyclidine intoxication readily induces nystagmus and cardiovascular and renal complications that are seldom seen in other psychiatric syndromes. Body-image loss (especially numbness of the entire body), feelings of being in outer space, and relatively rare hallucinations suggest PCP abuse (as opposed to hallucinogen use with LSD or related agents).

Treatment Approaches

Immediate Therapy

There are no specific antidotes for the intoxication induced by PCP and related substances. Hence, treatment is symptomatic. Comatose patients should be closely observed for the "a, b, c's"—airway, breathing, and cardiovascular status—and treated accordingly. All catatonic or comatose patients should have an intravenous line for receiving appropriate fluids.

Naloxone and glucose do not antagonize PCP-induced depression, but may be useful to rule out opioid overdose or insulin coma. Seizures are best treated with benzodiazepines, but dosage should be reasonably small so as not to deepen CNS depression. Urinary acidification does eliminate basic compounds such as PCP,[11-13] but the amount excreted usually is not very large compared to the amount ingested. Ammonium chloride, 1 to 2 gm every 6 hours to reduce urine pH close to 5.0, and forced diuresis with furosemide may be used. A systemic acidosis enhances urinary myoglobin excretion and thus causes kidney damage so that the issue of skeletal muscle injury and its hazards must be taken into account. Activated charcoal, in a dose of 1 gm/kg every 2 to 4 hours given shortly after oral PCP, reduces its absorption.

Psychological symptoms are best treated by appropriate psychological techniques without any pharmacotherapy. Neuroleptics are contraindicated until PCP is out of the body. There are reports that PCP may persist in some tissues such as fat or cerebrospinal fluid for weeks. Benzodiazepines may be helpful in managing extremely anxious or disturbed patients. Restraints are contraindicated in view of possible enhanced rhabdomyolysis unless such patients are a great danger to themselves or others.

Long-Term Therapy

Phencyclidine-intoxicated patients may have long-term residual psychological and psychiatric symptoms that require extensive psychological, psychiatric, and, possibly, pharmacological therapy. Such patients may continue to show symptoms of psychosis or depression and should be treated accordingly. High-potency antipsychotics or antidepressants may then be indicated.

REFERENCES

1. Cohen S: Psychotomimetic agents. Annu Rev Pharmacol 7:301–318, 1967.
2. Ellinghorn MJ, Barceloux DG, eds: Medical Toxicology—Diagnosis and Treatment of Human Poisoning. New York: Elsevier, 1988.
3. Goldfrank LR, Flomenbaum NE, Lewin NA, et al, eds: Goldfrank's Toxicologic Emergencies. 4th ed. Norwalk, CT: Appleton and Lange, 1990.
4. Milhorn HT Jr, ed: Chemical Dependence: Diagnosis, Treatment and Prevention. New York: Springer-Verlag, 1990:232–241.
5. Ciraulo DA, Shader RI, eds: Clinical Manual of Chemical Dependence. Washington, DC: American Psychiatric Press, 1991:1–420.
6. Aniline O, Pitts FN Jr: Phencyclidine (PCP): A review and perspectives. CRC Crit Rev Toxicol 10:145–177, 1981.
7. Domino EF: Phencyclidine. In Ciraulo DA, Shader R, eds. Clinical Manual of Chemical Dependence. Washington, DC: American Psychiatric Press, 1991:279–293.
8. Burns RS, Lerner SE: The effects of phencyclidine in man: A review. In Domino EF, ed. PCP (Phencyclidine): Historical and Current Perspectives. Ann Arbor, MI: NPP Books, 1981:449–469.
9. Pohorecki R, Rayburn W, Coon WW, et al: Some factors affecting phencyclidine biotransformation by human liver and placenta. Drug Metab Dispos 17:271–274, 1989.
10. Holsztynska EJ, Weber WW, Domino EF: Genetic polymorphism of cytochrome P450-dependent phencyclidine hydroxylation in mice: Comparison to phencyclidine hydroxylation in man. Drug Metab Dispos 19:48–53, 1991.
11. Domino EF, Wilson AE: Effects of urine acidification on plasma and urine phencyclidine levels in overdosage. Clin Pharmacol Ther 22:421–424, 1977.
12. Aronow R, Done AK: Phencyclidine overdose: An emerging concept of management. J Am Coll Emerg Phys 7:56–59, 1978.
13. Aronow R, Miceli JN, Done AK: Clinical observations during phencyclidine intoxication and treatment based on ion trapping. Natl Inst Drug Abuse Res Monogr 21:218–228, 1978.

18

NICOTINE USE

GREGORY W. DALACK, M.D., ALEXANDER H. GLASSMAN, M.D., and
LIRIO S. COVEY, Ph.D.

In the United States, addiction to nicotine occurs mainly in the form of cigarette smoking. Pipe and cigar smoking or chewing smokeless tobacco are less prevalent methods of obtaining nicotine, although they can also lead to nicotine addiction. In this chapter we review the clinical characteristics of cigarette smoking and nicotine addiction, and address the special issue of nicotine addiction and psychiatric comorbidity. We then outline treatment approaches and common pitfalls in dealing with this common and potentially lethal addiction.

It is, by now, a well-accepted fact that tobacco is addicting and that nicotine is the substance in tobacco that causes the addiction. In general, the clinical syndrome of drug addiction or dependence is well defined and involves compulsive use, despite harmful effects, of a psychoactive substance with reinforcing properties (i.e., pleasant effects) to which one develops tolerance and experiences withdrawal symptoms upon abstinence. Abundant research data confirm that nicotine meets the criteria of a dependence-causing substance, and diagnostic criteria for nicotine dependence are clearly defined in the psychiatric nomenclature.[1]

The pharmacodynamics and pharmacokinetics of nicotine are also well understood,[2] and cigarette smoking provides a unique drug delivery system, which facilitates the addiction to nicotine. During smoking, nicotine rapidly enters the bloodstream via the pulmonary vascular bed and reaches the brain faster than it would if administered intravenously. This rapid delivery, coupled with salutary effects on mood and level of arousal, is reinforcing, particularly after tolerance has developed to the unpleasant side effects of the drug. Smokers then intermittently dose themselves over the course of a day, reaching steady-state plasma nicotine levels of 10 to 50 ng/ml. It may be that over the course of the day, as tolerance to the stimulant activity of nicotine increases, smoking continues in order to ward off symptoms of withdrawal.[2]

The degree of individual addiction to nicotine can be measured; a widely used scale is the Fagerstrom Tolerance Questionnaire.[3] However, a very good estimate of an individual's level of addiction can be obtained by combining the number of cigarettes smoked per day with how early in the day the smoker begins to smoke.[4] Smoking shortly after arising marks a smoker as very unlikely to succeed in efforts to stop.

The risk of becoming addicted to nicotine is influenced by a number of issues, many of which are still poorly understood. It is clear that children of parents who are smokers are more likely to become smokers themselves, and one might postulate that environmental as well as genetic factors account for this. Hughes[5] has reviewed the available data regarding the effect of heredity on smoking and concluded that genetic factors have a small but definite effect on the likelihood of becoming nicotine dependent.

It has also become increasingly clear that there is significant comorbidity between cigarette smoking and psychiatric illness, specifically schizophrenia, alcoholism and affective disorder.[6–8]

Other evidence more specifically addresses the relationship between depression and cigarette smoking. In 1986, Kandel and Davies[8] reported follow-up data on 1004 young adults first examined nearly a decade earlier. They found that symptoms of depression at the original examination during adolescence were associated with cigarette smoking at follow-up. In 1988, we reported that a history of major depression was more common among cigarette smokers coming to a smoking cessation clinic than in the general population, and, more significantly, that such a history predicted less success in quitting.[9] Since then, two large epidemiological studies have replicated these original observations.[10,11]

It is clear that depression makes one more likely to be a smoker, and that, once addicted, a history of depression makes it harder for one to quit. Definitive data clarifying the relationships between alcoholism and smoking and between schizophrenia and smoking are lacking. It is obviously intriguing to speculate about the role of nicotine in these disorders, and further study is needed.

TREATMENT

Overview

It is important to remember that most smokers who successfully stop do so on their own. Generally, the percentage of men succeeding in cessation efforts regularly exceeds the rates seen in women. In addition, older individuals also have higher success rates than younger people.

While it has been said that stopping on one's own is the most effective treatment, such a statement is naive. Certainly, all smokers should first try to quit on their own, but the smoker who lights up before getting out of bed quickly understands that quitting will not be easy.[4] In general, smokers who are less addicted, and presumably less vulnerable to nicotine, are more successful at quitting. As a result, those smokers that remain are not a randomly selected group. Increasingly in this country, those who come to smoking cessation clinics represent a "hard core" group of heavily addicted, refractory smokers. Indeed, if a smoker trying to quit fails repeatedly on his own, he should seek treatment.

In addition to individual differences in vulnerability to nicotine addiction, motivation is a powerful determinant of success at smoking cessation. Within the same individual, motivation varies at different times of life. Hence, it is not surprising that some of the highest success rates have been seen among smokers after a myocardial infarction.

There is always a propensity to ask which treatment works best; however, in smoking cessation we believe there is a hierarchy of treatments differentially suited to various types of smokers. We start our discussion with pharmacological treatments and then come back to discuss psychological approaches. We chose to do this because the more scientifically rigorous data are available for drug treatments. This is so because drug treatments fall under the purview of governmental regulatory agencies which require systematic testing, while psychological approaches do not.

Pharmacotherapies

The best tested pharmacological approach to smoking cessation is nicotine replacement via nicotine gum. Multiple studies in both Europe and the United States have demonstrated the efficacy of the gum.[12] One often is asked, "What is the success rate with nicotine gum?" The question is not easily answered because the success rate depends heavily on the characteristics of the population of smokers participating in the study. What has been consistent is the existence of a drug-placebo difference. Lam et al.,[13] combining the results of nine studies in which more than 700 smokers received some type of psychological therapy plus either nicotine gum or placebo, found that about 23 per cent of those in the nicotine gum groups were not smoking 1 year after treatment began. In contrast, only about 13 per cent of the placebo-treated smokers were not smoking a year later.

Several interesting patterns have shown up during the testing of nicotine gum. Using the Fagerstrom Tolerance Questionnaire[3] to segregate smokers into those who are more addicted versus those who are less addicted, one finds that it is only among the more addicted that a drug-placebo difference consistently exists.[14] This suggests that nicotine gum works because it reduces withdrawal symptoms, and withdrawal symptoms are most significant among the more addicted smokers. It is also interesting to note that the administration of nicotine gum, without some sort of individual or group counseling or psychological support, produces rates of cessation no different than those seen with placebo gum under similar circumstances.[15]

It may be that the therapists using the gum are proficient in its use and, without their guidance, the gum is improperly used. Certainly, it is true that both patients and doctors are frequently not familiar with the proper use of a resin gum to deliver a medication. As a result, there is little question that physicians frequently write prescriptions for nicotine gum without appropriate instruction or without adequate follow-up to ensure that the proper instructions are being followed.

Nicotine is absorbed by the buccal mucosa at a moderate rate and only in an alkaline environment. The gum must first be chewed sufficiently so that it is broken up and begins to release nicotine. This is fairly easy for the smoker to recognize because of nicotine's characteristic taste. At that point, chewing must slow down to allow sufficient time for the nicotine released from the gum to be absorbed by the mucosa. This will generally mean 1 to 3 chews per minute over a period of approximately 20 minutes. If the gum is chewed more rapidly, the amount of nicotine released will exceed the capacity of the mucosa to absorb it, and the excess is likely to be swallowed. Once swallowed, nicotine is very irritating to the stomach and frequently results in nausea and various forms of gastrointestinal distress.[16]

Another problem that has only recently been described in the literature is the ability of acidic beverages to influence the mucosal absorption of nicotine. Many smokers, in their efforts to abstain from cigarettes, increase their use of coffee. They are seldom informed that the acidity of coffee, cola, or tea can almost completely block the absorption of nicotine from their gum.[17]

There has been a certain degree of concern that by using the gum, smokers are merely changing the route, but not the lethality, of their addiction. This perception is inaccurate. A smoker's risk for cancer and emphysema come largely from the process of smoking tobacco, not from exposure to nicotine. If, in fact, smokers merely changed their route of nicotine administration, and eliminated the tobacco vehicle, these risks would greatly diminish.

The degree to which cardiovascular risks come directly from nicotine is not entirely clear, but even if the former smoker consumed the same amount of nicotine from gum as he had in the past from cigarettes, the risks would fall. In fact, humans are unable or unwilling to extract the same quantity of nicotine from gum as they do from cigarettes. Serum levels of nicotine and its metabolites are about one half of those usually seen with cigarettes.[18] Although no long-term studies are available, any potential cardiovascular risk with chronic gum use must be considerably less than that associated with smoking. Anywhere from 13 to 38 per cent of abstinent smokers who quit smoking by using nicotine gum are still using the gum at 1 year.[19] The few people among them who might become addicted to the gum are still remarkably better off than if they were still smoking cigarettes.

The nicotine gum available in the United States contains 2 mg of nicotine, compared to a cigarette, which contains 4 to 5 mg. A 4-mg gum is available in Europe and should be on the market in this country in the near future. This stronger preparation has been shown to be a more effective aid to smoking cessation among heavily addicted smokers. The higher dose will most likely carry a higher risk for chronic use and more potential for adverse cardiovascular effects. For these reasons, it would seem prudent to restrict its use to smokers who have failed a trial of 2-mg gum. Smokers can, at present, try to increase their dose of nicotine by using two pieces of the polacrilex gum at the same time. However, the gum is very viscous and many smokers find large quantities of gum hard to chew.

Some companies are now testing nicotine patches, which avoid some of the adverse effects of the gum. The problem so far with the patch has been a high rate of skin rash or irritation.

The only other drug used as an aid in smoking cessation, for which multiple placebo-controlled trials are available, is clonidine.[20] We have conducted a meta-analysis of the nine published studies, consisting of four peer-reviewed articles and five abstracts, which leaves little doubt that clonidine increases the short-term chances that a smoker can successfully abstain from smoking cigarettes.[21] By combining results for 813 subjects across the nine trials, we found that clonidine, compared to placebo, increased the short-term abstinence rate by more than two fold. What remain to be clarified are the conditions that govern the efficacy of clonidine, and the long-term abstinence rate after treatment with clonidine. Like most treatments for smoking cessation, clonidine is clearly useful, but it is far from a panacea.

In many ways, the clinical utility of clonidine resembles that of nicotine gum. Its effect is modest, it seems to work better when given in conjunction with a behavioral counseling program,[21] and it also seems to work best for the more addicted smoker. Both drugs seem to work primarily by reducing withdrawal symptoms. However, the two drugs are not identical in terms of which symptoms they most effectively suppress. Clonidine has been shown to reduce the psychological craving for or preoccupation with cigarettes. By comparison, it has been difficult to demonstrate this characteristic with nicotine gum. On the other hand, nicotine gum does reduce the difficulties in mental concentration associated with nicotine withdrawal, while clonidine's sedative action may actually aggravate this aspect of the withdrawal syndrome. Thus, it would seem likely that some smokers will prefer one drug over the other. Clonidine has been administered both by tablet and by transdermal patch. Both routes of administration are effective.[21]

Initially, there was a concern about the effects of an antihypertensive drug on blood pressure in an essentially normotensive population. In our clinical experience with over 500 smoking cessation patients, we have not found clonidine-induced hypotension to be a problem. The most common side effects with clonidine, by far, have been sedation and dry mouth. However, the number of subjects who discontinue the medication due to either of these has been exceedingly small (unpublished data). Other side effects have been less frequent, and include skin rash, sexual difficulties, and constipation.

The technique for administering clonidine versus nicotine gum differs. When taken in tablet form, clonidine is started at a low dose and is gradually built up over several days before "quit day" to allow accommodation to side effects, especially sedation. Nicotine gum, on the other hand, is begun immediately on quit day. It is important to remember that neither pharmacological intervention is useful if the subject does not stop smoking. While both pharmacotherapies diminish withdrawal symptoms, neither will cause the subject to want to abstain.

Buspirone has recently been examined as a potential pharmacotherapy for smoking cessation. One open trial of buspirone[22] concluded that the medication diminished several withdrawal symptoms including craving, and facilitated a reduction in the number of cigarettes smoked per day. A more recent double-blind trial found that smokers seeking treatment in a cessation clinic and taking buspirone at low dose were more likely to abstain from smoking over the course of the study than the subjects on placebo. Despite the implication that buspirone facilitated cessation, a diminution in withdrawal symptoms was not demonstrated.[23] Hence, clarification of the efficacy and utility of buspirone in smoking cessation treatment requires further study.

Nonpharmacological Approaches

Whether a smoker decides to try to quit because of personal motivations or because of encouragement from a relative, friend, or physician, nonpharmacological approaches are the most common and reasonable first step to attempt smoking cessation. These include smoking withdrawal group clinics like those run by the American Cancer Society and the American Lung Association, aversive conditioning, self-help manuals, acupuncture, hypnosis, and such commercially available programs as "SmokEnders."

The distribution of self-help manuals for smoking cessation to a general population sample results in a significant increase in the 1-year abstinence rate over that of a control group; however, the overall cessation rates are small: 5 and 2 per cent, respectively.[24] Smoking withdrawal clinics vary in the specifics of the treatment, but all offer group counseling and support from group members regarding initiation and maintenance of abstinence. Self-reported quit rates with such treatments have ranged from 5 to 71 per cent success at 1-year follow-up. Despite the potential inaccuracies of self-report data, rates of success at this level of intervention are greater than with self-help manuals alone.

The few well-controlled studies examining the efficacy of acupuncture and hypnosis in smoking cessation show these approaches to be of little or no benefit. The published data on SmokEnders treatment outcome have not been rigorously collected. Hence, the often impressive cessation rates that are reported are very difficult to interpret.[25]

A physician's advice to stop smoking is a rather obvious, yet potent, approach to facilitating cessation. Definitive, direct advice from a physician, especially when given while the patient is suffering a cigarette-related illness, can increase quit rates substantially. Indeed, a well-timed, nonjudgmental admonition about the merits of smoking cessation can often synergize with a patient's enhanced motivation during pregnancy or illness.

Treatments that include aversive behavioral conditioning via rapid smoking have been shown to be the most effective treatment for smoking cessation. With appropriate medical supervision, the technique is generally safe even in smokers with cardiopulmonary disease. Along with the aversive conditioning, subjects are taught more adaptive coping skills to replace the use of cigarettes. Long-term cessation rates up to 50 per cent have been reported.[25,26]

Behavioral skills training is a more systematized approach to motivate smokers during the attempt to quit and to teach them relaxation techniques, as well as more adaptive ways to cope without cigarettes. Such training has been shown to be more effective than a control condition in which smokers share smoking experiences and receive only general information about the hazards of smoking.[27,28] However, the efficacy of behavioral skills training is most evident in the less addicted smoker.[27]

Combined Treatment

For many smokers, pharmacological treatment without other intervention, or nonpharmacological intervention alone is not effective.[28] For the more addicted smoker who is motivated to quit but who has failed smoking cessation attempts on his own or with minimal-intervention approaches, a combined approach holds the greatest promise of success. Such an approach will most often include a pharmacotherapy component, as described above, plus behavioral skills training. Kottke et al.,[29] in their review of successful treatments for smoking cessation, found

that success was correlated with the degree of face-to-face contact with the identified health care professional, the number and duration of contacts, and the number of treatment approaches applied.

At the same time, it is clear that no single treatment, however multidimensional, works for all smokers. The method for any individual smoker to achieve the goal of smoking cessation is to continue to try a variety of approaches, guided by past experience with other treatments, until cessation is achieved.

CONCLUSION

Much remains to be understood about nicotine addiction. The factors that determine individual susceptibility are complex, and may in part intersect with determinants of other psychopathology. The potentially lethal consequences of smoking are clearer than ever and will continue to propel efforts to refine our understanding of the nature and treatment of this serious condition.

REFERENCES

1. American Psychiatric Association: Diagnostic and Statistical Manual of Mental Disorders. 3rd ed. Revised. Washington, D.C.: American Psychiatric Association, 1987:167.
2. Benowitz NL: Pharmacodynamics of nicotine: Implications for rational treatment of nicotine addiction. Br J Addict 86:495–499, 1991.
3. Fagerstrom KO: Measuring degree of physical dependence to tobacco smoking with reference to individualization of treatment. Addict Behav 3:235–241, 1978.
4. Lichtenstein E, Mermelstein RJ: Some methodological cautions in the use of the tolerance questionnaire. Addict Behav 11:439–442, 1986.
5. Hughes JR: Genetics of smoking: A brief review. Behav Ther 17:335–345, 1986.
6. Hughes JR, Hatsukami DK, Mitchel JE, et al: Prevalence of smoking among psychiatric outpatients. Am J Psychiatry 143:993–997, 1986.
7. Burling TA, Ziff DC: Tobacco smoking: A comparison between alcohol and drug abuse patients. Addict Behav 13:185–190, 1988.
8. Kandel DB, Davies M: Adult sequelae of adolescent depressive symptoms. Arch Gen Psychiatry 43:255–262, 1986.
9. Glassman AH, Stetner F, Walsh BT, et al: Heavy smokers, smoking cessation, and clonidine: Results of a double-blind randomized trial. JAMA 259:2862–2866, 1988.
10. Glassman AH, Helzer JE, Covey LC, et al: Smoking, smoking cessation and major depression. JAMA 264:1546–1549, 1990.
11. Anda RF, Williamson DF, Escobedo LG, et al: Depression and the dynamics of smoking. JAMA 264:1541–1545, 1990.
12. Fagerstrom KO: Efficacy of nicotine chewing gum: A review. In Pomerleau OF, Pomerleau CS, eds. Nicotine Replacement: A Critical Evaluation. Progress in Clinical and Biological Research. Vol 261. New York: Alan R Liss, 1988:109–128.
13. Lam WC, Sacks HS, Sze PC, et al: Meta-analysis of randomised controlled trials of nicotine chewing-gum. Lancet 2:27–30, 1987.
14. Fagerstrom KO, Schneider NG: Measuring nicotine dependence: A review of the Fagerstrom tolerance questionnaire. J Behav Med 12(2):159–182, 1989.

15. Schneider NG, Jarvik ME, Forsythe AB, et al: Nicotine gum in smoking cessation: A placebo-controlled, double-blind trial. Addict Behav 8:253–261, 1983.

16. Henningfield JE, Jasinski DR: Pharmacologic basis for nicotine replacement. *In* Pomerleau OF, Pomerleau CS, eds. Nicotine Replacement: A Critical Evaluation. Progress in Clinical and Biological Research. Vol 261. New York: Alan R Liss, 1988:35–61.

17. Henningfield JE, Radzius A, Cooper TM, et al: Drinking coffee and carbonated beverages blocks absorption of nicotine from nicotine polacrilex gum. JAMA 264:1560–1564, 1990.

18. Benowitz NL: Pharmacologic aspects of cigarette smoking and nicotine addiction. N Engl J Med 319:1318–1330, 1988.

19. Hughes JR: Dependence potential and abuse liability of nicotine replacement therapies. Biomed Pharmacother 43:11–17, 1989.

20. Glassman AH, Covey LS: Future trends in the pharmacological treatment of smoking cessation. Drugs 40(1):1–5, 1990.

21. Covey LS, Glassman AH: A meta-analysis of double-blind placebo-controlled trials of clonidine for smoking cessation. Br J Addict 86:991–998, 1991.

22. Gawin F, Compton M, Byck R: Potential use of buspirone as treatment for smoking cessation: A preliminary trial. Fam Pract Recert 11(suppl 9):74–78, 1989.

23. West R, Hajek P, McNeill A: Effect of buspirone on cigarette withdrawal symptoms and short-term abstinence rates in a smokers clinic. Psychopharmacology 104:91–96, 1991.

24. Davis AL, Faust R, Ordentlich M: Self-help smoking cessation and maintenance programs: A comparative study with 12-month follow up by the American Lung Association. Am J Public Health 74:1212–1217, 1984.

25. Sachs DPL: Cigarette smoking: Health effects and cessation strategies. Clin Geriatr Med 2(2):337–362, 1986.

26. Hall RG, Sachs DPL, Hall SM, et al: Two-year efficacy and safety of rapid smoking therapy in patients with cardiac and pulmonary disease. J Consult Clin Psychol 52:574–581, 1984.

27. Hall SM, Rugg D, Tunstall C, et al: Preventing relapse to cigarette smoking by behavioral skill training. J Consult Clin Psychol 52:372–382, 1984.

28. Goldstein MG, Niaura R, Follick MJ, et al: Effects of behavioral skills training and schedule of nicotine gum administration on smoking cessation. Am J Psychiatry 146:56–60, 1989.

29. Kottke TE, Battista RN, DeFriese GH, et al: Attributes of successful smoking cessation interventions in medical practice: A meta-analysis of 39 controlled trials. JAMA 259:2882–2889, 1988.

19

OPIOID DEPENDENCE

JAMES A. HALIKAS, M.D. and KENNETH KUHN, M.D.

Some of the most exciting work in the past 20 years in neuroscience has involved the discovery of opioid receptors in the mammalian brain, and the subsequent isolation and identification of endogenous neuropeptide substances that have their primary site of action at these opioid receptor locations.[1] The original conceptualization of a system of endogenous opioids focused primarily on their natural responsiveness to pain perception and pain blockade. At the present time, there are already three different identified families of endogenous opioids, all with separate genetic regulation systems. There are at least five opioid receptor subgroups, with applications to research in schizophrenia, experimental acute psychoses, affective disorders, as well as in neuroendocrine dysregulation, with effects on satiety, appetite control, and the neurophysiology of sleep, to mention a few.[2]

EPIDEMIOLOGY

There are approximately 500,000 heroin addicts in the United States at the present time, almost half of them located in New York City.[3] Interestingly, the number of chronic heroin addicts estimated to exist in 1990 is approximately the same figure estimated in 1970. Thus, although there have been intercurrent epidemics of other drugs during the past two decades, the size of the heroin-using population has remained relatively stable.[2]

The course of the illness varies, based on a number of factors: socioeconomic issues, use patterns, situational factors, route and frequency of use, and use of other drugs. Initiation of use of narcotics generally occurs in mid to late adolescence after experimentation with multiple other drugs, beginning first with cigarettes and alcohol. For many narcotic addicts, use progresses over a 6- to 8-year period until recognition of loss of control and dependence, or interruption due to legal, medical, or social consequences bring the addict into treatment.[4] Because of intercurrent life events (particularly, criminal activities) and medical complications of illicit drug use, it is speculated that there may be up to a 2 per cent annual mortality rate among heroin addicts.[2] While there is no indication that opiate dependence is a genetically mediated disease in the same way that alcohol dependence appears to be, there does seem to be a familial association, possibly related to common socioeconomic and environmental issues present.

CONCURRENT USE OF OTHER DRUGS

In our society, narcotic use virtually never begins de novo. That is, heroin addiction proceeds from a long history of use of other drugs and alcohol. Also, the heroin user is often concurrently an abuser of alcohol, marijuana, cocaine, and benzodiazepines. As heroin addicts grow older, fully one third develop clear-cut alcohol addiction. Polydrug use, and therefore, multiple drug abuse diagnoses, is the normative condition in this population. Polydrug use complicates the clinical course, causes medical complications, and diminishes treatment responsiveness. Indeed, unless the treatment approach recognizes the polysubstance abuse, it will be inadequate to the treatment challenge.[5]

MEDICAL ASPECTS OF OPIOID DEPENDENCE

Most medical morbidity associated with opioid dependence is a consequence of the illegal nature of the addiction. Injection equipment is illegally obtained or gerryrigged, sold, shared, and repeatedly used. Consequently, increased rates of serum hepatitis, endocarditis and, more recently, human immunodeficiency virus (HIV) infection, can all be ascribed to the heroin delivery system.

Besides the risk of blood-borne infection, there is the acute problem of potential overdose. Heroin, as a narcotic, is a respiratory depressant. In susceptible individuals, it can cause a sudden pulmonary edema that is irreversible, and which may be an immunologically based response. Polysubstance abuse often causes potentiation of the respiratory depressant effects of heroin. Other medical complications that are usually not life threatening, but which serve as medical markers, include the following: multiple abscesses on the extremities, many of which leave permanent scars, secondary to the practice of subcutaneous narcotic injection, or "skin popping"; edema of the hands as a result of the sclerosing of the deep veins of the upper extremities; and the presence of "tracks," darkened, scarred, and hardened superficial veins, the most obvious mark of chronic intravenous opioid use, which are usually extensive on the backs of the forearms and in the antecubital fossae.[6]

PHARMACOLOGY OF OPIOIDS

The current definition of an opioid is any substance that interacts with the stereospecific opioid receptors located throughout the brain.[7] There are five subclasses of opioid receptors, but for the discussion regarding opioid dependence, we will focus primarily on the mu receptors, which are known to be the site of action of mu receptor agonists, such as morphine and heroin.

There are two groups of opioid analgesics considered to be dependence producing: naturally occurring opium-derived substances including heroin, codeine, morphine, and codeine derivative byproducts; and the synthetic opioids, including meperidine and methadone. An agonist is defined as any opioid substance that stimulates the stereospecific opioid receptor; an antagonist, on the contrary, does not stimulate the opioid receptor, but obstructs the receptor, so that it cannot be stimulated by an agonist.[7] Clinically, the most important opioid antagonists are naltrexone and naloxone. Naloxone is a short-acting antagonist that is given intravenously to reverse the effects of mu agonists such as morphine or heroin in the treatment of opioid overdose. A longer acting *orally* administered opioid antagonist is naltrexone, which has a 12- to 24-hour action and has an extremely high affinity for mu receptors. It can be used only after mu receptors have been completely cleared of opioid agonists with the displacement from the receptor by naloxone. Naltrexone, therefore, has a clinical utility as a long-term opioid antagonist or blockade drug to stabilize opioid-dependent patients in the postwithdrawal recovery period.[8]

The pharmacological effects of mu opioid agonists are well known: these include pupil constriction, mood elevation, respiratory depression, decrease in pain perception, drowsiness, indifference to stress, alterations in neuroendocrine function, and decrease in gastrointestinal peristalsis. Many first-time opioid abusers experience nausea and vomiting, which is, however, overridden by the mood-enhancing effects of the drug.[7]

The pharmacokinetic profile of the various mu opioid agonists is quite varied. Heroin (diacetylmorphine) is more lipid soluble and more quickly crosses the blood-brain barrier than its precursor, morphine.[7] The rapid onset of action is followed by rapid metabolism 4 to 6 hours later, which results in a rebound withdrawal and craving. Methadone has complex pharmacokinetics with storage in plasma proteins and a reduced "first-pass" liver effect.[9] The plasma "reservoir" prevents the sharp peak and rapid decline in serum levels, and results in a much longer craving blockade effect. The half-life of methadone is 18 to 36 hours, depending on metabolic rate variability. Metabolism of methadone may be slowed or enhanced by the concomitant use of other medications that affect the cytochrome P-450 microsomal hepatic enzyme system.[10]

OPIOID WITHDRAWAL SYNDROME

Rapid cessation of use of an opioid substance after 2 or more weeks of regular use will result in the following symptoms: craving for the opioid drug; nausea/vomiting; generalized myalgias; lacrimation; and rhinorrhea.[6] The patient may also have yawning, diarrhea, dilatation of the pupils, and sweating or piloerection (goose bumps) of the skin. Short-acting opioids such as morphine or heroin produce an intense withdrawal syndrome within 24 hours, with peak intensity at 48 hours. Longer acting opioids, such as methadone, present a long withdrawal syndrome, with more subjective discomfort, insomnia, restlessness, severe aching, and myalgias (complaints of deep "bone pain").[6] The physical symptoms associated with opioid withdrawal are often compared factually but disparagingly to a generalized viral syndrome, which is never life threatening and which has a time-limited course. This analogy misses the extreme severity of discomfort seen with this syndrome. Further, the psychological craving that follows in the protracted withdrawal period becomes increasingly intense and is easily triggered by cues in the environment or by memories associated with prior narcotic use. Consequently, the relapse rate for chronic heroin users is over 90 per cent in the first few weeks following the detoxification period. Patients who maintained opioid abstinence in the Lexington, KY Federal Drug Treatment Facility for over a year relapsed at astoundingly high rates within the first weeks following discharge, when they returned to their original drug-using environment. Detoxification alone for opiate dependence is therefore now considered an inadequate treatment modality.

PSYCHIATRIC COMORBIDITY IN THE OPIOID-DEPENDENT POPULATION

It has recently been recognized that opioid-dependent individuals have a high lifetime prevalence of coexistence psychiatric disorders. In a carefully done study among patients in addiction treatment, nearly 50 per cent of the men and 70 per cent of the women fulfilled diagnostic criteria for an affective disorder.[11] In that same study, one third of the men also fulfilled diagnostic criteria for alcohol dependence, and nearly 25 per cent of the women had an anxiety disorder diagnosis. Overall, 80 per cent of the opioid-dependent population had at least one other psychiatric disorder, and over 50 per cent had at least two additional diagnoses.[11] Opioid-dependent patients, with psychiatric comorbidity, have more frequent hospitalizations and a more turbulent clinical course in general. Consequently, treatment programs are now focusing on comprehensive psychiatric diagnostic screening and individualized treatment planning. The suicide rate is estimated to be three to four times greater within the opioid-dependent population than in normal control groups.[2]

TREATMENT APPROACHES

This section will focus on treatment approaches for the opioid-dependent person, with emphasis on a multimodality approach. Initial assessment must include careful psychiatric diagnosis for comorbid conditions, thorough alcohol and drug use history for concurrent substance abuse disorders, and thorough medical assessment for concurrent, possibly occult, medical disorders, before instituting therapy.

The ideal therapy should be individualized to the patient's needs. This will include an extensive psychosocial rehabilitation program that addresses educational deficiencies, vocational limitations, personal social support system, and personal motivation for abstinence. Concurrent appropriate pharmacotherapies and psychological counseling will be needed.[12] Many opioid dependent individuals eventually are placed in a narcotic substitution (methadone) program for long-term stabilization and maintenance. First treatment, however, should involve an attempt at drug-free abstinence prior to initiating any drug substitution therapy.

OPIOID DETOXIFICATION

Opioid detoxification can proceed rapidly or slowly, depending on what opiates the patient is currently addicted to, what concurrent drugs the patient is also using, the level of cooperation of the patient, and the resources available. For example, 48- to 72-hour detoxification protocols for heroin addicts include combinations of an intravenous drip of naloxone; a sedating neuroleptic medication; anticonvulsants such as carbamazepine; clonidine; and short-acting benzodiazepines. Such protocols also require round-the-clock monitoring by a nurse or physician.[13] When medical or psychiatric factors mandate inpatient treatment, a longer, 10- to 14-day, detoxification protocol can be followed. The initial methadone dose should be titrated upward with the goal of eliminating opioid withdrawal signs and symptoms without sedation. This usually requires 15 to 25 mg of methadone given every 12 hours. After a period of 2 to 3 days of stabilization, a gradual taper of 5 mg daily or every other day can proceed to a daily total dose of 20 mg. Thereafter the taper should proceed more slowly, with 2.5-mg daily decreases. Clonidine can be initiated for sedation and comfort when the patient starts having insomnia, usually at or below 10 mg/day of methadone. Clonidine requires careful orthostatic monitoring of blood pressure. Doses can be adjusted beginning at 0.1 to 0.2 mg given up to 3 to 4 times daily.[14]

After completion of the methadone taper, a period of 7 to 10 days of documented narcotic abstinence is necessary before instituting any possible use of naltrexone, the long-acting narcotic antagonist medication. After 7 to 10 days of abstinence, confirmed by a negative urine for opioids, a naltrexone challenge test of 5 mg is given orally, followed by close nursing observation for a period of up to 4 hours. The patient may then be started on 50 mg naltrexone daily to assist in opiate abstinence maintenance by creating a narcotic blockade. An alternative to waiting the several days required before beginning naltrexone maintenance therapy is to do a naloxone challenge test.[12] Naloxone is a short-acting opioid antagonist that can be given 48 hours after methadone taper. An intravenous dose of 0.4 mg (1 ml) is given and the patient is closely monitored for skin, pupil, and blood pressure changes and any subjective symptoms of discomfort suggestive of the opioid withdrawal syndrome. When the naloxone challenge is negative, it is then safe to try a low test dose of naltrexone, usually 5 mg. If naltrexone is given before opioid withdrawal is complete, there can be an intense aversive reaction, difficult to reverse because of the receptor affinity of the drug and its long duration of action.[12] This detoxification should occur in the midst of an extensive psychosocial rehabilitation program, which should include individual and group therapy, peer support groups of recovering addicts, psychoeducational programming regarding all drugs of abuse, and the development of coping skills in order to maintain a drug-free lifestyle.

MANAGEMENT OF OPIOID DEPENDENCE DURING PREGNANCY

All but very slow opioid detoxification is generally contraindicated any time during the gestation period because of risk of spontaneous abortion associated with opioid withdrawal. Finnegan has documented the clear advantages of methadone maintenance during pregnancy. Pregnant opioid addicts should be maintained on a dose of methadone that eliminates craving, since the risk of exposure to blood-borne infections and toxic contaminants associated with illicit opiates far outweighs the management problems encountered with moderate-dose (20 to 40 mg/day) methadone.[15] The goal of methadone maintenance during pregnancy is to prevent exposure of the mother and baby to any street drug products; therefore, if an outpatient maintenance dose of 80 mg is necessary, dealing with an apneic baby at birth and slow detoxification of the baby after birth is more practically managed than dealing with the complications of street drug abuse.[16]

METHADONE MAINTENANCE TREATMENT

Initial evaluation of a heroin addict involves a thorough physical examination and complete psychiatric and drug use history. If it is well documented that the patient is over 18 years of age, has had unsuccessful trials of other treatment modalities, and has a history of at least 1 year of heroin dependence, a methadone maintenance program may be offered.

The initial dose of methadone is usually between 20 and 30 mg, with the patient observed in the clinic for response to the medication. An intravenous narcotic antagonist, naloxone, should be available in case the dose of methadone results in respiratory depression and unconsciousness. Gradual titration of the dose over a period of 1 to 2 weeks to a maintenance dose of between 60 and 80 mg then occurs.[17] This maintenance dose is usually required to eliminate opiate hunger or craving and to block the effects of illicit opioids. During the first several days of this titration upward, the patient will continue to have early morning opioid withdrawal symptoms. It takes at least 3 to 5 days to establish a methadone steady-state level. It should be noted that there are several medications that will shorten the half-life of methadone by enhancing its metabolism. These medications induce the hepatic cytochrome P-450 microsomal enzyme system, and include the benzodiazepines, carbamazepine, dilantin, rifampin, and erythromycin, to mention a few.[10]

Ideally, the use of methadone blood levels drawn in the morning before the morning dose of methadone (the "trough level") is useful in determining an adequate maintenance dose, since patients will notoriously claim the need for increasing doses. A trough serum level of over 100 μg/ml of methadone usually indicates an adequate opiate blockade and elimination of opiate hunger. Clinical studies have not confirmed a clear correlation between opioid craving and stable serum trough levels. However, variation and rate of decline in serum levels does correlate with craving symptoms. After stabilization of methadone, the patient is assigned to a primary care coordinator, who will then be the primary contact for that patient at the clinic. Outcome studies have shown that several factors can improve overall outcome, including staff continuity, with one primary counselor assigned to a patient for a lengthy period of time.[18] Cultural and ethnic concordance of patients and therapists has been found to be extremely important in improving outcome. Group therapy with peers, in addition to individual counseling, improves therapy. Treatment of intercurrent comorbid psychiatric diagnoses, particularly affective episodes using antidepressants, reduces relapse and improves outcome.[19] A long-term psychosocial rehabilitation program, which allows the patient time to address educational and vocational deficits and to repair family relationships, is needed. Such a narcotic substitution therapy program requires 2 to 4 years. Thus, methadone maintenance is not to be considered a brief or transitory modality of treatment.[17]

MANAGEMENT OF CONCURRENT DRUG USE

A depressing phenomenon of the past 5 years has been the relapse into cocaine use by methadone maintenance patients.[20] Often, because of their past history of injection drug use, these patients have relapsed into intravenous cocaine use, with all of the attendant human immunodeficiency virus (HIV)-related dangers. Maintenance with methadone appears to have the side effect of reducing the aversive effects of cocaine, in imitation of the previously described "speedball." It has been found that another narcotic, buprenorphine, now available orally in the United States only in experimental protocols, may be an effective narcotic substitution therapy that does not encourage cocaine use.[21] An additional potential advantage of buprenorphine maintenance, rather than methadone maintenance, is the apparent ease with which patients can be detoxified from buprenorphine.[22]

Concurrent alcohol abuse among methadone patients is also a problem.[23] At first, this was thought to be a direct consequence of the methadone itself. It is now apparent that this is part of the aging process for these addicts, and probably reflects as yet unelucidated biological factors. As these addicts age, alcohol addiction becomes their final common pathway. Thus, vigorous psychosocial treatment and consideration of the use of disulfiram are both appropriate. Use of antidepressant medications for occult depressive episodes is also seen as a possible treatment alternative, which may prevent alcohol self-medication.

The narcotic antagonist, naltrexone, is currently the only marketed medication for narcotic abstinence maintenance. This medication, taken at a dose of 50 mg/day each morning, will block the effects of any narcotic dose taken. It does nothing to reduce or eliminate narcotic craving or hunger that prompts the narcotic use. Medications are being tested in Europe that may attenuate this narcotic hunger. In this country, the selective serotonin reuptake inhibitors such as fluoxetine and paroxetine are being tested for similar effects. Meanwhile, the clinician, when faced with the opioid-dependent individual, should be aware of the need for psychosocial rehabilitation in addition to any pharmacotherapy maintenance that is contemplated. Further, the clinician should be alert to other psychiatric conditions or drug use that may complicate the patient's condition. Finally, the clinician should be aware of treatment facilities in his or her locale that specialize in managing these patients over a long-term basis.

THERAPEUTIC COMMUNITY IN THE TREATMENT OF OPIOID DEPENDENCE

The philosophy of therapeutic communities (TC) in opioid dependence is based on the notion that the individual addict can only begin a process of recovery if he or she lives in the context of other recovering individuals. This allows the opioid-dependent person to be supported by the community, but at the same time confronted on all levels regarding the behavioral aspects and the thinking patterns associated with addiction. The community consists of an expanded group of peers, who are all in various stages of the recovery process and who work together in providing support to each other and to those individuals who are in the beginning stage of entering the recovery program. It is, therefore, a collaborative effort, with responsibility of recovery placed both on the peer community as well as the individual patient, and with an interdependence that requires mutual trust and steadfast honesty.[24]

Primary staff are degreeless professionals, who have moved up through the ranks in the hierarchy of the TC. Methods employed in the treatment process include large "encounter" or confrontational groups, group education, and assignment of tasks and expanded responsibility as individuals progress in the program. Therapeutic communities have evolved with experience, including the hiring of professionals to participate within the community itself and provide additional therapeutic intervention skills. The underlying philosophy that connects all of the variety of therapeutic communities is that fundamental change of addictive behaviors requires a full-time commitment and cannot be accomplished through time-limited isolated exposure to therapeutic modalities, such as psychotherapy. Therapeutic communities' usefulness has been well documented with hard-core patients who have failed traditional outpatient programs. The goal of the therapeutic community is to bring about a dramatic transformation in basic lifestyle and values, so when the patient does leave the community, he or she will be able to sustain the positive effects over time. There is an emphasis placed on vocational training, making up educational deficits, and learning personal integrity and self-respect. This multidisciplinary approach is felt to be necessary to modify complex human behavior that is tied in with drug seeking and addiction.[24]

Because of the time commitment, with an average stay in TC of 1 to 2 years, the treatment is considered to be an option for those patients who have failed more traditional short-term day hospital and traditional chemical dependency programs. Probably the single most successful group consists of those patients who have been intercepted by the criminal justice system and have been compelled to participate in these programs. Repeated outcome studies show a significant decrease in criminal activity following residential therapeutic confinement for this subgroup of opiate addicts.[24]

As research continues in this exciting area, diverse applications unfold and new questions are raised. While this chapter has discussed opioid dependence, its diagnosis, and clinical management, it is important to keep in mind that much of what we know in this area of clinical utility has been contributed by basic animal neuropharmacological research.

REFERENCES

1. Snyder SH: The opiate receptor and morphine-like peptides in the brain. Am J Psychiatry 135:645–652, 1978.
2. Jaffe J: In Kaplan HI, Sadock BJ, eds. Comprehensive Textbook of Psychiatry V. Vol 1. Baltimore: Williams and Wilkins, 1989.
3. Wartenberg A: In Herrington RE, Jacobson GR, Benzer DG, eds. Alcohol and Drug Abuse Handbook. St Louis: Warren H Green, Inc, 1987.
4. Halikas JA, Darvish HS, Rimmer JD: The black addict: I. Methodology, chronology of addiction, and overview of the population. Am J Drug Alcohol Abuse 3(4):529–543, 1976.
5. Benveovuto J, Bourne P: The federal polydrug abuse project initial report. J Psychedelic Drugs 7:115–120, 1975.
6. Ling W, Wesson DR: Drugs of abuse—opiates. West J Med 152:565–572 (special issue on addiction medicine), 1990.
7. Jaffe JH, Martin WR: Opioid analgesics and antagonists. In Gilman AG, Goodman LS, Rall TW, Murad F, eds. The Pharmacological Basis of Therapeutics. 7th ed. New York: Macmillan, 1985:491–604.
8. Martin WR, Jasinski DR, Mansley PA: Naltrexone, an antagonist for the treatment of heroin dependence. Arch Gen Psychiatry 28:784–791, 1973.
9. Olsen GD: Methadone binding to human plasma albumin. Science 176:525–526, 1982.
10. Kreek MJ, Garfield JW, Gutjahr CL, et al: Rifampin-induced methadone withdrawal. N Engl J Med 294:1104–1106, 1976.
11. Rounsaville BJ, Wressman MM, Kleber HD, Wilber C: Heterogeneity of psychiatric diagnosis in treated opiate addicts. Arch Gen Psychiatry 39:161, 1982.
12. Kleber HD, Topazian M, Gaspari J, et al: Clonidine and naltrexone in the outpatient treatment of heroin withdrawal. Am J Drug Alcohol Abuse 13(1, 2):1–17, 1987.
13. Bromley J: Clonidine-naltrexone detoxification of opiate addicts. Presentation at: Addiction Medicine: State of the Art Review. American Society of Addiction Medicine, San Diego, CA. Nov 11–19, 1989.
14. Gold MS, Redwovel DE Jr, Kleber HD: Clonidine in opiate withdrawal. Lancet I:929–930, 1965.
15. Finnegan LP: Clinical prenatal and developmental effects of methadone. In Cooper JR, Altman F, Brown B, Czechowicz D, eds. Research on the Treatment of Narcotic Addiction: State of the Art. Washington, DC: U.S. Government Printing Office, 1980.
16. Finnegan LP: Neonatal abstinence syndrome: Assessment and pharmacotherapy. In Rubaltelli FF, Granati B, eds. Neonatal Therapy: An Update. New York: Elsevier Press, 1986.
17. Zweben JE, Payte JT: Methadone maintenance in the treatment of opioid dependence: A current perspective. Addiction Medicine (special issue). West J Med 152(5):588–599, 1990.
18. Ball JC: A schema for evaluating methadone maintenance programs. NIDA Res Monogr Ser 95:74–77, 1989.
19. Woody GE, O'Brien CP, Rickels K: Depression and anxiety in heroin addicts: A placebo-controlled study of doxepin in combination with methadone. Am J Psychiatry 132:4, 447–450, 1975.
20. Kuhn KL, Halikas JA, Kemp KD: Carbamazepine treatment of cocaine dependence in methadone patients with dual-opiate-cocaine addiction. NIDA Res Monogr Ser 95:316–317, 1989.
21. Kosten TR, Morgan CJ, Kleber HD: Buprenorphine treatment of cocaine abuse. NIDA Res Monogr Ser 95:46, 1989.
22. Kosten TR, Kleber HD: Buprenorphine detoxification from opioid dependence, a pilot study. Life Sci 42:635–641, 1988.
23. Kreek MJ: Opiate-ethanol interactions: Implications for the biological basis and treatment of combined addictive diseases. In Harris LS, ed. Problems of Drug Dependence. NIDA Research Monograph 81. Rockville, MD: NIDA, 1987.
24. DeLeon G, Rosenthal MS: Therapeutic communities. In Dupont RL, Goldstein A, O'donnell J, eds. Handbook on Drug Abuse. Rockville, MD: NIDA, 1979:39–45.

SEDATIVE-HYPNOTIC ABUSE

MARIE LOURDES FILS-AIME, M.D.

HISTORY

Sedative-hypnotic medications belong to several chemical classes. The largest of these are the barbiturates and the benzodiazepines. The first sedative agents were introduced to clinical use in the 1840s. At the beginning of the twentieth century, the barbiturates came into widespread use. The benzodiazepine chlordiazepoxide (Librium) was introduced in 1957.[1] Because the benzodiazepines have proven to be safer than barbiturates and equally effective, they have largely replaced the older drugs. More than 2500 benzodiazepines have been synthesized today, with the hope to develop one that is safe and has a low likelihood of producing dependency. Only about 50 benzodiazepines have been used clinically.

EPIDEMIOLOGY

In 1975 there were 100 million prescriptions filled for sedative-hypnotics. Sixty million of them were for benzodiazepines. In 1985 there was a slight decrease in the total number of prescriptions for sedative-hypnotics in the United States. A vast majority, 81 million, were written for benzodiazepines.[2]

The popularity of the benzodiazepines is not restricted to the United States. In 1970, the National Institute of Mental Health (NIMH) organized an epidemiological study on benzodiazepine use in ten different countries. A total of 9.6 to 16.8 per cent of the interviewees had used these drugs in the preceding year (15 per cent in the United States). In terms of continued use for 1 month or more, the range was 3.4 to 8.6 per cent (6 per cent in the United States). A similar survey done in 1979 showed that regular daily use of benzodiazepines for 1 year or longer was by 15 per cent of the users, which constitutes about 1.6 per cent of the adult population in the United States. As can be seen from the last survey done by the National Institute on Drug Abuse[3] (NIDA) (Tables 20–1 and 20–2), a relatively low percentage of the population reports a lifetime nonmedical use of sedatives or tranquilizers.

PREDISPOSING FACTORS

There is increased probability to use a sedative-hypnotic in multisubstance abusers, alcoholics, middle-aged (over 50) or elderly women, educated persons, and those from an above average economic background, with a chronic medical illness, or with a sedentary lifestyle.[4] Interestingly, family structure, economic status, individual social function, or stressful life events were not correlated with drug use in Beijing.[5,6] It was also found that the extreme users were women, and iatrogeny was the main cause of drug abuse.[7]

MECHANISM OF ACTION

The action of the benzodiazepines is to increase the affinity of gamma-aminobutyric acid (GABA) to the GABA A–receptor. Thus, the benzodiazepines act in the brain as neuromodulators by enhancing the action of GABA, to increase the permeability of the ion channel to chloride. The fact that benzodiazepine action on the chloride channel is to increase the probability of channel openings rather than their duration could explain their relative safety in overdose.[8] Alcohol affects the GABA receptor–associated chloride flux as well, but uses a mechanism different from the benzodiazepines, which may explain their synergistic effect when used together.

PHARMACOKINETICS

The benzodiazepines are relatively lipophilic, are largely protein bound in blood plasma, but equilibrate with the brain rapidly. The different pathways in the metabolism of the benzodiazepines include reduction, oxidation, glucuronidation, and dealkylation.[9] Lorazepam and oxazepam are not extensively metabolized and are the drugs of choice for elderly patients or for patients with liver disease. Midazolam and lorazepam are water soluble enough that

124

TABLE 20–1. PERCENTAGE REPORTING NONMEDICAL USE OF ANY PRESCRIPTION-TYPE SEDATIVES IN LIFETIME BY AGE GROUP AND DEMOGRAPHIC CHARACTERISTICS: 1988.[a]

Demographic Characteristics	Age Group (Years)				
	12–17	18–25	26–34	>35	Total
Total	2.3	5.5	7.9	1.7	3.5
Sex					
Male	2.4	6.6	10.2	2.3	4.5
Female	2.3	4.5	5.7	1.1	2.6
Race/ethnicity[b]					
White	2.9	6.2	9.4	1.6	3.8
Black	0.9	2.4	2.5	2.5	2.3
Hispanic	0.9	3.3	3.5	2.0	2.5
Population density					
Large metro	2.3	4.6	10.4	2.6	4.4
Small metro	2.8	7.0	7.7	1.0	3.5
Nonmetro	f	4.9	3.8	f	2.0
Region					
Northeast	2.0	4.7	10.3	f	3.0
North central	3.2	6.6	7.1	1.2	3.3
South	2.2	5.9	6.4	1.3	3.1
West	1.6	4.3	9.7	4.1	5.0
Adult education[c]					
Less than high school	N/A[g]	8.6	10.0	1.7	3.7
High school graduate	N/A	5.5	8.1	0.7	3.5
Some college	N/A	3.8	6.9	3.2	4.1
College graduate	N/A	f	7.2	1.7	3.3
Current employment[d]					
Full-time	N/A	5.5	8.2	1.9	4.3
Part-time	N/A	5.0	8.6	5.2	5.9
Unemployed	N/A	f	10.6	f	6.0
Other[e]	N/A	6.6	5.2	f	1.5

[a] Adapted with permission from National Institute on Drug Abuse: National Household Survey on Drug Abuse, 1988. Rockville, MD: NIDA, ADAMHA, PAS, USDHHS, 1990.

[b] The category "other" for race/ethnicity is not included.

[c] Data on adult education are not applicable for 12 to 17 year olds and are missing for ten persons 18 to 25 years old, six persons 26 to 34 years old, and 13 persons 35 or older. Total refers to those 18 and older (unweighted N = 5690).

[d] Data on current employment are not applicable for 12 to 17 year olds and are missing for six persons 18 to 25 years, three persons 26 to 34 years old, and five persons 35 or older. Total refers to those 18 and older (unweighted N = 5705).

[e] Retired, disabled, homemaker, student, or "other."

[f] Low precision; no estimate reported.

[g] N/A, Not applicable.

they can be administered intramuscularly or intravenously. Diazepam and chlordiazepoxide have a long half-life and share the long-acting metabolite, N-desmethyldiazepam.[10] Their absorption is erratic after intramuscular administration. When given orally, the majority of people prefer diazepam over chlordiazepoxide,[8–10] perhaps because it equilibrates with the brain faster. This preference probably makes them less inclined to take chlordiazepoxide for nonmedical purposes.

INDICATIONS FOR SEDATIVE-HYPNOTIC USE

Physical Examination and Differential Diagnosis

Patients receiving prescriptions for sedative-hypnotics may come to physicians at times with vague complaints, such as nervousness, or with relatively specific ones, such as insomnia. The patient may request sleeping pills or the physician may feel compelled to do something because of his or her perceptions of the patient's expectations.

The presenting symptoms leading to prescribing sedative-hypnotics may be caused by many medical, mental, or neurological illnesses (Table 20–3).

A good history followed by a thorough physical examination is always necessary prior to prescribing sedative-hypnotics. Urine should be collected for drug screening to rule out substance abuse that the patient did not reveal to the physician. No medication should be prescribed without a clear diagnosis. After starting the treatment, if there is no improvement, the diagnosis should be evaluated, and the treatment changed as needed.

TABLE 20–2. PERCENTAGE REPORTING NONMEDICAL USE OF ANY PRESCRIPTION-TYPE TRANQUILIZERS IN LIFETIME BY AGE GROUP AND DEMOGRAPHIC CHARACTERISTICS: 1988.[a]

Demographic Characteristics	Age Group (Years)				
	12–17	18–25	26–34	>35	Total
Total	2.0	7.8	9.3	2.9	4.8
Sex					
Male	1.5	9.0	10.7	2.8	5.2
Female	2.7	6.6	8.0	2.9	4.4
Race/ethnicity[b]					
White	2.5	9.4	10.9	2.8	5.2
Black	0.6	f	4.8	3.9	3.1
Hispanic	1.2	4.4	3.4	3.4	3.3
Population density					
Large metro	1.9	8.2	10.4	3.5	5.4
Small metro	2.9	8.3	9.1	2.2	4.6
Nonmetro	1.2	6.4	7.9	2.6	3.9
Region					
Northeast	2.0	5.6	9.5	2.8	4.3
North central	1.8	10.9	9.9	3.2	5.4
South	2.5	8.4	8.3	2.2	4.4
West	1.4	5.3	10.5	3.8	5.2
Adult education[c]					
Less than high school	N/A[g]	12.3	14.1	1.7	4.8
High school graduate	N/A	7.0	9.2	2.4	5.0
Some college	N/A	6.9	8.0	5.0	6.0
College graduate	N/A	4.3	7.8	3.6	4.9
Current employment[d]					
Full-time	N/A	6.9	9.5	3.3	5.7
Part-time	N/A	9.5	9.6	6.6	7.9
Unemployed	N/A	8.9	14.1	f	8.9
Other[e]	N/A	8.6	7.0	1.3	2.6

[a] Adapted with permission from National Institute on Drug Abuse: National Household Survey on Drug Abuse, 1988. Rockville, MD: NIDA, ADAMHA, PAS, USDHHS, 1990.

[b] The category "other" for race/ethnicity is not included.

[c] Data on adult education are not applicable for 12 to 17 year olds and are missing for ten persons 18 to 25 years old, six persons 26 to 34 years old, and 13 persons 35 or older. Total refers to those 18 and older (unweighted N = 5,690).

[d] Data on current employment are not applicable for 12 to 17 year olds and are missing for six persons 18 to 25 years, three persons 26 to 34 years old, and five persons 35 or older. Total refers to those 18 and older (unweighted N = 5,705).

[e] Retired, disabled, homemaker, student, or "other."

[f] Low precision; no estimate reported.

[g] N/A, Not applicable.

TABLE 20-3. DISEASES THAT MAY BE ASSOCIATED WITH ANXIETY OR INSOMNIA OR BOTH

Psychiatric	Medical	Neurological
Dementia	Hyperthyroidism	Seizures
Schizophrenia	Sleep apnea	Tremors
Bipolar disorder	Excessive caffeine use	Encephalitis
Major depression	Periodic movements in sleep	Intracranial lesions
Dysthymia		
Cyclothymia	Congestive heart failure	

Sedative-Hypnotics and Alternatives in the Treatment of Insomnia

The DSM-III-R[11] categorizes sleep disorders into first-degree dyssomnias (insomnia, hypersomnia, and disorders of the sleep-wake cycle), and second-degree parasomnias (nightmares, sleep terrors, and sleep walking). To fulfill criteria for the diagnosis of insomnia, the patient must be unable to fall asleep or maintain sleep a few times a week, and the duration of the disorder must be at least 1 month. If the condition has lasted more than 3 months, it is considered chronic and benzodiazepines or other sedative-hypnotics have not been shown to be helpful. According to Mellinger et al.,[12] 85 per cent of people suffering from severe insomnia were untreated by any type of medication. Prolonged use of sedative-hypnotics by chronic insomniacs may result in rebound insomnia and poor quality of sleep, with nightmares and frequent awakenings.

Before prescribing sedative-hypnotics for insomnia, it is useful to entertain the possibility that the problem could be treated without medication. Some patients sleep or take naps during the day, thus they cannot sleep at night. Staying awake throughout the day may solve this problem. Some patients consume coffee, caffeinated soft drinks, chocolate, or tea before bedtime. Stopping the use of the stimulants close to bedtime may alleviate this problem. Elderly patients often complain of not sleeping enough. Reassurance by explaining that most adults do not need 8 to 10 hours of sleep is often helpful. If the patient feels rested, maybe fewer hours are enough.

Patients who are going through a stressful period in their lives may have difficulty falling asleep or maintaining sleep. First, the physician will have to help them understand that this loss of sleep is common and probably will be temporary. If the insomnia is caused by major depression, the depression should be treated. Even though we know that some benzodiazepines, such as alprazolam (Xanax), have some antidepressant activity,[13] they are not the drugs of choice in the treatment of depression. When the patient's mood improves, he or she will usually be able to sleep better.

Manic patients often deny having a sleeping problem, but the people living with the patient may complain that he or she does not sleep at night. Schizo-

phrenics can show a very disturbed pattern of sleep, particularly in the context of acute exacerbation of their illness. Alcoholics and substance abusers will also have problems sleeping, which could continue long after the patient stops drinking or abusing drugs.

Myoclonic movements during sleep, also called periodic movements in sleep (PMS) or nocturnal myoclonus, consist of abnormal movements, primarily of the patient's lower extremities. They could be mild or severe and disturb the patient's sleep without awakening him. Sleep apnea is an additional cause of insomnia in which respiration ceases totally. Its prevalence increases with age, and it affects men more often than women.[9] Cessation of breathing can cause frequent awakening during the night. This represents a limited list of common medical causes of insomnia that have to be considered as part of the differential diagnosis of insomnia.

In cases of insomnia not secondary to drug abuse or significant medical, neurological, or mental illnesses, a nonpharmacological approach, such as behavioral change to improve sleep hygiene with supportive therapy, should be tried first. If this approach fails, a sedative-hypnotic should be given for a short period of time.

Sedative-Hypnotic Effects on Sleep

If the physician decides to use a sedative-hypnotic, a drug with an intermediate half-life should be prescribed, rather than a very short, short- or a long-acting one, because of possible dependence or addiction, and hangover effects. The optimal sedative-hypnotic would produce drowsiness and facilitate the onset and maintenance of a state of sleep that resembles natural sleep in its electroencephalographic (EEG) characteristics and from which the recipient could be easily aroused. During wakefulness after long-acting sedative-hypnotics such as flurazepam, there is a decrease in alpha activity and an increase in fast low-voltage activity, especially beta activity. This shift to beta activity appears to correlate with the antianxiety effects of these medications. There is usually a decrease in stage 1 sleep, an increase in stage 2 sleep, and shortening of stage 4 and rapid-eye-movement (REM) sleep caused by most sedative-hypnotics.[10] In spite of these changes in sleep architecture, most patients responding to the treatment report feeling rested in the morning. During chronic use, the effects on the different stages of sleep become less pronounced.[10] The number of dreams may also increase. The efficacy to promote sleep is also usually lost during chronic administration of a sedative-hypnotic.

Sedative-Hypnotics as Muscle Relaxants and Anticonvulsants

Diazepam has been known to relieve muscle spasm associated with disseminated sclerosis, tetanus, cerebral palsy, and stroke. Some of the benzodiazepines may produce hypotonia without interfering with normal locomotion. Tolerance develops over time to the muscle relaxant effects of benzodiazepines. The benzodiazepines diazepam and lorazepam are among the drugs of choice in status epilepticus. Diazepam has been known to cause respiratory depression; this is why a close monitoring of vital signs is necessary when this drug is administered intravenously. Some benzodiazepines, such as clonazepam, may be more selective than diazepam in their anticonvulsive efficacy. The benzodiazepines do not act at the seizure focus but prevent spreading of the seizure to the subcortical area. Tolerance to the anticonvulsant effect may develop with prolonged use.

Use in Anesthesia

The benzodiazepines produce sedation that progresses to hypnosis and stupor. To be effective as an anesthetic, some of the benzodiazepines used to be combined with other central nervous system (CNS) depressants. The benzodiazepines are superior to the barbiturates as a preoperative medication. Like most sedative-hypnotics, a preanesthetic dose of a benzodiazepine will produce impairment of recent memory and will also cause retrograde amnesia for events that occur during an operation.[9]

The benzodiazepines alone can be used before minor surgical procedures. Midazolam maleate has been used to induce general anesthesia for eye surgery. It produces changes in the acid-base balance equilibrium conducive to a decrease in the intraocular pressure. The changes in hemodynamic parameters are relatively minor, which makes midazolam a good anesthetic for eye surgery, particularly in the elderly.

Treatment of Severe Agitation

In patients with severe agitation, such as bipolar patients in a manic episode and phencyclidine (PCP) intoxication, benzodiazepines combined with an antipsychotic can be very helpful in the emergency room. Lorazepam 2 mg intramuscularly every hour for three to four doses has been commonly used. The sedative-hypnotic will decrease the physical restlessness and moderate mental excitement, but alone will not clear the psychosis.

Treatment of Anxiety Disorders

Many patients will come to the physician complaining of feeling worried for no specific reason. The symptoms often are not severe enough to impair successful completion of daily activities. Benzodiazepines have in the past been found to be effective in such patients. At the present time, buspirone is the drug of choice, particularly if the patient is at risk for benzodiazepine abuse, and if the patient has not been previously treated with benzodiazepines. If in the past the patient was successfully treated with a benzodiazepine, and was withdrawn from the medication without difficulty, the same benzodiazepine can probably be administered again without difficulty.

The symptoms of panic disorder according to DSM-III-R are: (1) shortness of breath; (2) dizziness or faintness; (3) tachycardia or palpitations; (4) trembling; (5) choking; (6) nausea or abdominal distress; (7) depersonalization or derealization; (8) numbness or tingling sensations; (9) flushes or chills; (10) chest pain or discomfort; and (11) a fear of dying or going crazy. Four or more symptoms constitute a panic attack; three or less are called a limited attack. Panic disorder usually responds to treatment with tricyclic antidepressants, particularly imipramine (Tofranil), and also the monoamine oxidase inhibitor (MAOI) phenelzine (Nardil). Alprazolam (Xanax), a triazolobenzodiazepine with antianxiety as well as antidepressant properties, has been used with some success in the treatment of panic disorder, but withdrawing the medication can be problematic.

Treatment of Alcohol or Sedative-Hypnotic Withdrawal

The majority of patients who have been abusing a substance such as alcohol or a sedative-hypnotic are at risk of experiencing withdrawal upon discontinuation or upon reducing the dose. Alcohol withdrawal can be treated successfully with benzodiazepines. There is increased activity of the sympathoadrenal and hypothalamic-pituitary-adrenal (HPA) axes during withdrawal and the severity of symptoms is correlated with their activities.[8] Usually, patients with mild withdrawal are not administered benzodiazepines, but receive multivitamins, thiamine, hydration, and are provided with a quiet environment, and usually do well. According to the method of Sellers et al.,[14] using the Clinical Institute Withdrawal Assessment of Alcohol (CIWA-A), moderate (CIWA-A 20 to 25) and severe (CIWA-A above 25) withdrawal have been treated at the NIAAA with diazepam 10 mg every hour or 20 mg every 2 hours until the symptoms are controlled or the patient is sedated, with close monitoring of the vital signs. Diazepam should be given with caution to patients exhibiting withdrawal symptoms at a high blood alcohol level, because of the additive effect of these two drugs.

Repeatedly untreated or inadequately treated ethanol withdrawals may produce sensitization over time. To avoid such a development, it may be useful to treat even mild withdrawal symptoms with a benzodiazepine to prevent any progressive worsening of successive withdrawals.[8]

SEDATIVE-HYPNOTIC USE IN SPECIAL POPULATIONS

Pregnancy

During pregnancy, drugs should be withheld whenever possible, or used with caution if absolutely necessary. Benzodiazepines have been associated with the floppy infant syndrome. In the first trimester, their use has been associated with cleft lip and cleft palate. Other uncontrolled studies report intrauterine growth retardation, withdrawal syndrome, hyperbilirubinemia, and cardiac arrhythmias in the newborn. Animal studies have produced conflicting data concerning neurochemical changes in adult animals treated with sedative-hypnotics in utero.

Geriatric Populations

In the population older than 65, 15 per cent are chronic anxiolytic drug users, and this rate of regular use is five times higher than in the general population.[15] The elderly in general have nonspecific complaints. At this age, many of the elderly seen by physicians are already taking two or three medications, and the addition of a sedative-hypnotic may only increase the adverse effects.

The adverse reactions associated with cognitive impairment increase as the number of prescription drugs increases. The hepatic microsomal oxidation may decrease with age and drug elimination may be prolonged. Chronic use of a sedative-hypnotic may result in disabling CNS side effects. Fainting, dizziness, loss of balance, and bone fractures are more frequent in women using long–half-life benzodiazepines than in age- and sex-matched controls.[16] Benzodiazepines may contribute to falls in the elderly by decreasing body balance, and concomitant reduction of peripheral neurosensation in the lower extremities could aggravate the problem. Fall rates increase with age in elderly people and are greater in women than in men; however, the death rate from falls is greater for men than women.[16] The long-acting sedative-hypnotics have been associated with an increased risk of falling during the daytime. For this reason, the short-acting sedative-hypnotics should be used in the elderly. Even then, if the patient has to wake up after 2 or 3 hours after taking the medication, the risk of falling is very high.

ADVERSE EFFECTS OF THE SEDATIVE-HYPNOTICS

Sedative-hypnotics can cause physical and psychological dependence in patients on a therapeutic dose[17] and following physician's advice. Therefore, the physician should explain to the patient in advance that the medication is for a limited period of time, and that the medication could cause tolerance and abrupt discontinuation or reducing the dose could cause unpleasant withdrawal. Concomitant use of benzodiazepines undergoing oxidative metabolism with cimetidine or disulfiram (Antabuse) could increase their side effects by increasing their blood level via decreasing their hepatic clearance.

The most common side effects are drowsiness, ataxia, psychomotor impairment, marked sedation, respiratory depression, hypersensitivity reactions, exacerbation of porphyria, fatigue, anterograde amnesia, disorientation and sleeplessness, nausea, and headaches.[2,9,10] These reactions could be much more severe in the elderly patient. Rare reports describe agranulocytosis and jaundice.

Abuse and Dependence

It is well known at this time that use of sedative-hypnotics even in therapeutic doses can cause abuse or dependence. First, let us clarify these definitions according to the DSM-III-R. For the diagnosis of dependence, the patient must exhibit three of the following symptoms: (1) the substance is often taken in larger amounts or over a longer period than the person intended; (2) a persistent desire or attempts to cut down or control the substance use; (3) frequent intoxication or withdrawal symptoms interfering with social occupations; (4) limitation of occupational or recreational activities because of substance use; (5) continued substance use despite knowledge of medical problems; (6) marked tolerance; (7) withdrawal; (8) the substance is taken to relieve or avoid withdrawal symptoms; (9) the symptoms persist for at least 1 month or over a longer period of time.

The DSM-III-R definition of substance abuse includes these symptoms: (1) maladaptive pattern of psychoactive substance use indicated by either continued use despite knowledge of a persistent or recurrent problem caused (or exacerbated) by use of the psychoactive substance, or recurrent use in situations in which use is physically hazardous; (2) symptoms of the disturbance have persisted for at least 1 month or have occurred repeatedly over a longer period of time.

A review showed that after 1 to 4 weeks of detoxification in an inpatient setting, 84 per cent of previous sedative-hypnotic abusers were still abusing sedative-hypnotics after discharge. A 5-year follow-up showed that 50 per cent were abusing drugs or alcohol with significant social deterioration, and 8 per cent had committed suicide. Intellectual impairment was still as high as during admission in slightly more than half of the original group.[18]

Overdose and Suicide

Barbiturate overdose is associated with a high incidence of death. The risk of death from overdose has been reduced considerably since the shift from barbiturates to benzodiazepines. The number of suicides by drug overdose in the United States increased between 1953 and 1963 from 735 to 2666, and the barbiturates remained responsible for 75 per cent of drug suicides.[7]

A survey was conducted in the United States and Canada in the latter part of 1976. The combined population was 79.2 million. Diazepam was found to be present in 1239 cases of death. Drugs alone caused death in 914 cases. The remaining 375 fatalities were due to other causes. Only two persons died after having taken only diazepam.[19] Sedative-hypnotic drugs are the chemical agents most commonly used for committing suicide.[9] Physicians could reduce the availability of the drugs by prescribing small amounts during frequent visits.

Treatment of Sedative-Hypnotic Overdose

Overdose of short-acting barbiturates has the highest mortality rate. The treatment is both symptomatic and supportive. Special attention should be given to the airway because of the possibility of barbiturates to cause respiratory depression. Blood pressure should be maintained in the beginning with intravenous fluids. Overdose of benzodiazepines may cause respiratory depression, nystagmus, confusion, and slurred speech.[10] As with the barbiturates, the respiration and vital signs should be monitored closely, and intravenous fluids and artificial respiration given as needed.

Withdrawal

Abrupt discontinuation of a sedative-hypnotic can produce a severe withdrawal syndrome.[20] The symptoms may include delirium and grand mal seizures. Withdrawal can also develop on low therapeutic doses. It is usually less severe, but can nevertheless be distressful.

The short-acting drugs, like alprazolam (Xanax) and lorazepam (Ativan), because of their rapid elimination from the body, may produce a more severe withdrawal syndrome, with earlier onset, than the long-acting drugs. The following symptoms are often encountered: anxiety, agitation, psychosis, perceptual disturbances, gastrointestinal disturbances, hyperthermia, neuromuscular irritability, grand mal seizures, and delirium. The sedative-hypnotic delirium resembles the alcoholic delirium tremens. Mild withdrawal symptoms include anxiety that may be worse than the condition for which the drug was originally prescribed, as well as rebound insomnia, dizziness, headache, anorexia, weight loss, vertigo, tinnitus, and blurred vision. The withdrawal can start 1 to 10 days after cessation of the drug and its duration may last from a few days to several weeks. Gradual reduction of the dose usually prevents the development of a severe withdrawal syndrome. Hollister and Csernansky[9] first noted withdrawal symptoms in 50 per cent and seizures in 8 per cent of subjects receiving diazepam 120 mg/day for 21 consecutive days. With diazepam, because of its slow

rate of elimination, symptoms may appear 4 days after the last tablet or, in some cases, 1 to 2 weeks after cessation of the drug intake.

Treatment can be started by inquiring about the patient's daily use of sedative-hypnotics. Most of the time the patients overestimate their daily intake, while a few may underestimate their drug use. In the detoxification process, phenobarbital is preferable to pentobarbital because of its longer half-life and greater antiseizure activity. If the selected drug is diazepam, 20 mg p.o. should be given every 2 hours until the patient shows sedation or intoxication. If the patient appears intoxicated after two doses, he is considered nontolerant and no further medication is given.

When using phenobarbital, 30 mg is considered equivalent to 100 mg of pentobarbital. After receiving a maximum dose in the first day, medication should be tapered daily by 30 mg for phenobarbital and 10 mg for diazepam.[21] The drugs should be given four times a day and careful monitoring should be done between doses. According to the patient status, modifications can be done whenever it is necessary, which means increasing the dosage if there are signs of withdrawal, or withholding it if there is sedation. Detoxification can be accomplished over a period of 7 to 10 days.

For alprazolam (Xanax) it is recommended to taper the medication no faster than 0.5 mg every third day. The usual regular daily dose for meprobamate is 800 mg in four divided doses. It should be tapered slowly by no more than 10 per cent every other day to avoid convulsions. Alkalization of the urine may accelerate the process. Rickels et al.[22] reported that people with certain personality traits, neuroticism, lower education, and more severe depressive and anxious symptoms are at high risk for relapse after completing withdrawal. The severity of withdrawal was associated more with the baseline personality, high Eysenck neuroticism score, female sex, and mild to moderate alcohol use, than with the benzodiazepine half-life or daily dosage. Clonazepam has been used with some success to treat high-dose alprazolam dependency.[23] Propranolol has also been used to treat sedative-hypnotic withdrawal. It appears to decrease the severity of the withdrawal syndrome and may accelerate the detoxification process.

BUSPIRONE HYDROCHLORIDE

To solve the problem of physiological and psychological dependence to therapeutic doses of anxiolytics, buspirone hydrochloride (Buspar) appears to be the safest alternative. It is the first of a new class of anxiolytic agents, the azaspirodecanediones. Buspirone is not related to the benzodiazepines chemically or pharmacologically. It has proven efficacy and safety in the treatment of generalized anxiety disorder, is well tolerated without causing drowsiness, and has shown no potential for abuse. Buspirone does not impair psychomotor performance, nor does it produce anterograde amnesia. There is no synergistic effect between alcohol, the sedative-hypnotics, and buspirone.[24] Abrupt discontinuation of buspirone does not produce a withdrawal syndrome. The major drawback is that buspirone takes 1 week or more before the manifestation of its anxiolytic effect.

BENZODIAZEPINES AND THE NEW YORK STATE REQUIREMENT FOR TRIPLICATE PRESCRIPTIONS

A letter in a recent issue of *The Lancet*[25] deplores the new trend evident in New York State, which consists of an increase of 17 per cent in prescriptions for meprobamate, a much more dangerous drug in overdose than the benzodiazepines. Prescriptions for chloral hydrate rose by 158 per cent compared to a 4 per cent increase in the rest of the country, and barbiturate prescriptions went up by 41 per cent compared to an 11 per cent decline in the rest of the country.

James Egnot, from the New York State Department, Division of Public Health Protection, provided the following figures on recent drug use in New York State. There was a 95 per cent decrease in benzodiazepine use since January 1, 1989, in a group of patients numbering 3400 suspected of diverting drugs. This group includes any patient who has been using more than $500 in pharmacy services in at least 1 month, between September and November of 1988. There has been a 76 per cent reduction in prescriptions dispensed by some pharmacies suspected of being "pill mills." There is a 31 per cent decrease in drug overdose involving the benzodiazepines, and street prices of the drugs have increased two to five times. Alcohol consumption did not increase with the decrease in benzodiazepine use. We received figures concerning alcohol use in New York State from Mr. Steven Zych of the New York State Taxation and Finance Department. There was a steady decrease in alcohol use from 453,000,448 gallons in 1988 to 445,773,881 gallons in 1989, and 436,346,866 gallons in 1990. Tax collections have been higher because of tax increases on alcoholic beverages.

The practice of requiring triplicate prescriptions was devised to prevent the abuse of benzodiazepines, and it may be succeeding. However, turning back the clock to the use of barbiturates will probably increase the total of deaths by overdose and increase drug dependence. Thus, the ultimate result of this change in practice is currently unknown.

CONCLUSIONS

In spite of the large number of prescriptions written for sedative-hypnotics, their abuse is relatively limited.[25,26] Surveys show that many patients who receive the medicines from their physicians actually take lower doses than prescribed. Most patients who have been prescribed sedative-hypnotics for a short period of time have been able to stop the medications without difficulties. However, these medications can produce dependence in vulnerable patients, even when taken in therapeutic doses.

The minority of patients who end up abusing sedative-hypnotics often use them concomitantly with other substances such as alcohol, cocaine, or heroin,[2] and most of the time the sedative-hypnotic is not their primary substance of abuse.

To minimize the risk of sedative-hypnotic abuse, after elimination of medical, neurological, mental, and environmental causes of the presenting complaint of anxiety or insomnia, a nonpharmacological approach should be first considered. If this approach fails, a low-dose sedative-hypnotic should be tried with caution and for a limited period of time. The participation of the patient in the decision making is recommended, and this cooperation will facilitate treatment. Appropriate psychotherapy, exercise, and abstinence from alcohol are often necessary ingredients of the treatment plan. If buspirone or antidepressants fail to give the desired effect, the sedative-hypnotics could be used. Many patients are suffering from chronic anxiety or chronic insomnia. Even though benzodiazepines have not been demonstrated to work on chronic insomnia, on rare occasions the decision to prescribe a sedative-hypnotic for a long term may be in the best interest of the patient and could improve the patient's quality of life. Such a decision always requires a close follow-up.

ACKNOWLEDGMENT

The author would like to acknowledge the many helpful suggestions and comments provided by Dr. Markku Linnoila. Without his help and encouragement, this chapter could not have been written.

REFERENCES

1. Salomon C: Brief review of the history of hypnotics. Nouv Press Med 8:2511, 1979.
2. Miller NS: Benzodiazepine use in clinical practice: Suggestions for prevention. Am J Prev Psychiatry 2:16, 1990.
3. National Institute on Drug Abuse: National Household Survey on Drug Abuse, 1988. Rockville, MD: NIDA, ADAMHA, PHS, USDHHS, 1990.
4. Bergman H: Alcohol and drugs in the treatment of alcoholism: A comparison of men and women. Br J Addict 547:553, 8491.
5. Fleischhacker WW, Barnas C, Hackenberg B: Epidemiology of benzodiazepine dependence. Acta Psychiatr Scand 74:80, 1986.
6. Jiang Z: Drug abuse among residents of Beijing: An epidemiologic survey of 1,822 households. Chung Hua Shen Ching Ching Shen Ko Tsa Chih 23:66, 1990.
7. Allgulander C: History and current status of sedative-hypnotic drug use and abuse. Acta Psychiatr Scand 73:465, 1986.

8. Nutt D, Adinoff B, Linnoila M: Benzodiazepines in the treatment of alcoholism. In Galanter M, ed. Recent Developments in Alcoholism. Vol 7. Treatment Research. Washington, DC: American Medical Society on Alcoholism, 1988:283.

9. Hollister LE, Csernansky JG: Clinical Pharmacology of Psychotherapeutic Drugs. 3rd ed. New York: Churchill Livingstone, 1990.

10. Goodman LS: Goodman and Gilman's The Pharmacological Basis of Therapeutics. 7th ed. New York: Macmillan, 1985.

11. American Psychiatric Association: Diagnostic and Statistical Manual of Mental Disorders. 3rd ed. Revised. Washington, DC: American Psychiatric Association, 1987.

12. Mellinger GD, Bolter MD, Uhlentuth EH: Prevalence and correlates of the long term use anxiolytics. Arch Gen Psychiatry 251:375, 1984.

13. Garvey J, Tollefson GD: Prevalence of misuse of prescribed benzodiazepines in patients with primary anxiety disorder or major depression. Am J Psychiatry 143:1601, 1986.

14. Sellers EM, Naranjo CA, Harrison M, et al: Diazepam loading: Simplified treatment of alcohol withdrawal. Clin Pharmacol Ther 34:822, 1983.

15. Sussman N: Diagnosis and drug treatment of anxiety in the elderly. Geritr Med Today 10:1, 1988.

16. Sorock GS: Falls among the elderly: Epidemiology and prevention. Am J Prev Med 24:282, 1988.

17. Woods JH, Katz JL, Winger G: Use and abuse of benzodiazepines. Issues relevant to prescribing. JAMA 260:3476, 1988.

18. Ross HE: Dependence on sedative-hypnotics: Neuropsychological impairment yields dependence and clinical course in a 5 year follow-up study. Alcohol Clin Exp Res 13:810, 1989.

19. Finkle BD, McCloskey KL, Goodman LS: Diazepam and drug associated deaths in the United States and Canada survey. JAMA 242:429, 1980.

20. Schweizer E, Rickels K, Case WG, et al: Long-term use of benzodiazepines: Effects of gradual tapering. Arch Gen Psychiatry 47:908, 1990.

21. Perry PJ, Alexander B: Sedative-hypnotic dependence: Patient stabilization, tolerance testing, and withdrawal. Drug Intell Clin Pharm 20:532, 1986.

22. Rickels K, Schweizer E, Case WG, et al: Long-term therapeutic use of benzodiazepines: Effects of abrupt discontinuation. Arch Gen Psychiatry 47:899, 1990.

23. Albeck JH: Withdrawal and detoxification from benzodiazepine dependence: A potential role for clonozepam. J Clin Psychiatry 48:43, 1987.

24. Goa KL, Ward A: Buspirone. A preliminary review of its pharmacological properties and therapeutic efficacy as an anxiolytic. Drugs 32:114, 1986.

25. Woods JH, Katz JL, Winger GD: Restricting benzodiazepine prescribing. Lancet 337:295, 1991.

26. Pies R: Benzodiazepine abuse: How real, how serious. Psychiatr Times 8:13, 1991.

21

DUAL DIAGNOSIS:
Concept, Diagnosis, and Treatment

RICHARD K. RIES, M.D. and NORMAN S. MILLER, M.D.

The co-occurrence of an alcohol/drug (substance) disorder with another psychiatric disorder is defined as a "dual diagnosis." Unfortunately, the term dual diagnosis is so vague that it has acquired multiple connotations in its popular usage. The term most often implies that the two independent conditions occur together.[1] However, it may also refer to psychiatric syndromes that either are induced by substance use or that lead to substance use and self-medication. Most prevalence studies of comorbidity do not provide etiological relationships between the psychiatric syndromes and the alcohol/drug use.[2] Similarity of drug-induced versus non–drug-related symptoms may create significant false-positive diagnoses, as several authors have pointed out.[3] This practice makes it difficult to ascertain correct diagnoses, and consequently, true prevalence rates for comorbid disorders. For discussion purposes, we define substance disorder as drug and/or alcohol abuse/dependence.

The temporal assignment of one disorder (primary) preceding another (secondary) longitudinally does not necessarily denote causality. The two disorders may arise independently in time and have no causal relationship.[1] The "primary/secondary" distinction has also been used to denote that one disorder is underlying or central to the other disorder, implying a direct causal role for the primary disorder. Although one disorder may cause another, the interaction between psychiatric and substance disorders is frequently assumed and not demonstrated longitudinally in studies that examine comorbidity in psychiatric populations.

Prevalence in General Populations

The findings of the Epidemiologic Catchment Area (ECA) study for the prevalence rates of DSM-III disorders indicate that psychiatric disorders associated with alcohol/drug dependence are common. While one third of the total population in the ECA sample met lifetime criteria for a psychiatric diagnosis, among those with the DSM-III diagnosis of alcoholism, almost half (47 per cent) had an additional psychiatric diagnosis,[2] though these rates may include false-positive "drug-induced" disorder, as pointed out above.

The ECA data revealed that alcohol dependence was the most common diagnosis at 13.7 per cent of the general population. Phobia was the second most common psychiatric diagnosis at 12.8 per cent, followed by drug abuse and dependence at 6.9 per cent, depression at 5.1 per cent, antisocial personality disorder at 2.5 per cent, obsessive-compulsive disorder at 2.5 per cent, dysthymia at 1.5 per cent, panic disorder at 1.5 per cent, cognitive dysfunction at 1.1 per cent, and anorexia at 0.1 per cent. Thus, alcoholism is the most common disorder in comparison to other psychiatric disorders.

In alcoholic women, phobias and depression, followed by antisocial personality, panic, schizophrenia, and mania were the psychiatric disorders cited in descending prevalence. Interestingly, the *relative risk* for a psychiatric diagnosis for women with alcoholism in relation to the general population is greatest for antisocial personality and least for depression and phobias, owing to the high rates of these latter disorders among nonalcoholic women in the general population. Furthermore, the prevalence of *relative risks* for psychiatric disorders is the same for women alcoholics as for men alcoholics, suggesting a common contribution from the alcoholism.[2]

Prevalence in Patient Populations

Studies of patient populations have assessed the co-occurrence of psychiatric disorders and alcohol/drug disorders. These studies are biased toward a more severely affected patient population, and they report a high association of alcohol dependence with drug dependence and with other psychiatric disorders. It is possible that psychiatric symptoms motivate the alcoholic or drug-dependent patient with psychiatric comorbidity to seek treatment. Studies suggest that the comorbid patient may have a more severe course; greater psychopathology; and more medical, psychological, and social consequences.

The co-occurrence of alcohol dependence with other drug dependence is common, especially in younger populations.[4] Over 80 per cent of alcoholics under the age of 30 are dependent on another drug, most often marijuana, followed by cocaine, sedative-hypnotics (benzodiazepines/barbiturates), and opiates. Studies of drug-dependent patient populations have found a rate of alcohol dependence of 80 to 90

per cent in cocaine addicts, 50 to 60 per cent in marijuana abuser, 50 to 75 per cent in opiate addicts, and 25 to 50 per cent in benzodiazepine addicts.[5]

Other studies indicate that dual-diagnosis patients have a poorer prognosis. Dual-diagnosis patients tend to be younger, more often male, and have poorer medication compliance. In addition, they are nearly twice as likely to be rehospitalized during 1-year follow-up.

Underdiagnosis and Misdiagnosis

Despite the high prevalence of drug and alcohol dependence in psychiatric populations, there is substantial evidence that these disorders are underdiagnosed and misdiagnosed. Inpatient psychiatric program directors estimated the underdiagnosis or misdiagnosis or both of alcoholism as occurring 60 per cent of the time. Drug use and dependence is also underdiagnosed. The most commonly used drugs in addition to alcohol are cannabis, cocaine, sedative-hypnotics, and opiates. Some studies have correlated psychiatric syndromes with type of drug use. Stimulant drug users are frequently misdiagnosed as schizophrenics, depressant drug users as depressives, and multiple drug users as personality disorders—often antisocial and borderline types.[1] Few studies have followed these patients longitudinally to determine how much (or many) of the psychiatric syndromes were drug induced, and if so, to what degree the symptoms resolved.

Other Diagnostic Considerations

Psychoactive drugs and alcohol produce psychiatric syndromes through several pharmacological mechanisms:

1. Acute and chronic intoxication with stimulants and withdrawal from depressants causes central nervous system (CNS) hyperexcitability that can mimic anxiety disorders such as phobic disorder, obsessive-compulsive disorder, panic disorder, and generalized anxiety disorder.

2. Acute and chronic intoxication with depressants and withdrawal from stimulants can mimic major depression.

3. The depressive syndrome diminishes rapidly over days in the majority of alcoholics and drug addicts, but persists in a minority.

4. Psychotic symptoms can be produced during intoxication with stimulants and hallucinogens, and during both withdrawal and intoxication from depressants.

5. Although less well documented, alcohol and drug dependence can produce disturbances in personality such as antisocial, narcissistic, and hysterical behaviors.

Cognitive deficits, and to a lesser extent depression, are correlated with advancing age and sex. Some studies demonstrate greater cerebral atrophy in older alcoholics. Women alcoholics tend to show greater prevalence of affective symptoms and other psychiatric disorders than their male counterparts. Women who are dependent on drugs also show a significant rate of depression.

The course of patients having both substance dependence and a psychiatric disorder linked temporally to substance use more closely follows that of the alcohol/drug disorder. Although drug-induced psychiatric syndromes have similar symptoms as major depressive, psychotic/personality disorders, the sociodemography, family histories, and early life courses more closely resemble those observed for alcoholics than for those with other psychiatric disorders.

A CLINICAL MODEL FOR TREATMENT OF DUALLY DIAGNOSED PATIENTS

There is a paucity of research on specific treatment interventions for drug and alcohol dependence in psychiatric patient populations. Most of the studies to date have been anecdotal, nonrandom, and have used eclectic forms of treatment that are likely hard to reproduce. Although increased psychiatric severity as measured by the Addiction Severity Index (ASI) has been shown to predict poor response to addictive treatment in drug/alcohol populations, the ASI has not been carefully studied in psychiatric populations. Only recently have positive reports of the use of "dual focus" treatment programs been introduced,[6-11] although they have not as yet been assessed by well-designed and controlled studies. Given this "state of the art," we can, however, describe components of dual diagnosis treatment that have been clinically described as useful and which are currently used in our own programs.

Some Definitions

We can view the psychiatric treatment system as composed of acute, subacute, and longer term treatment settings. Acute treatment includes that supplied in emergency rooms and acute care inpatient units. Subacute treatment includes either inpatient stabilization following acute treatment (usually a few days to up to a few weeks of inpatient treatment), or initial outpatient visits at which the patient may be relatively unstable, but not in an acute condition. The "longer term" phase refers to outpatient treatment, or for a distinct minority, may refer to chronic long-term inpatient care. For discussion purposes we will separate the disorders into (1) substance (drug/alcohol) disorder and (2) psychiatric—meaning any other nonsubstance psychiatric disorder. Sections on acute and subacute treatment will be functionally divided into psychiatric diagnosis, behavioral management, and medication management; and correspondingly, substance diagnosis, behavioral management, and medications.

Acute Phase

Acute Psychiatric Diagnosis

Acute psychiatric settings include patients with the most severe forms of psychopathology and behavioral dyscontrol. This psychiatric severity may be caused or complicated by (1) medical/neurological conditions; and (2) drug intoxication/withdrawal. Thus, psychiatric diagnosis of the most acute dual diagnosis conditions should first attempt to rule out potentially lethal medical and toxic conditions that can mimic or complicate "functional" psychiatric conditions. This requires good medical personnel and facilities. The behavioral presentation of an agitated, incoherent, uncooperative, and psychotic individual with alcohol on breath may be identical whether observed in a decompensated schizophrenic who drank only on the day of admission or in an alcohol- and cocaine-dependent person with a toxic paranoid psychosis, who may also have head trauma. Thus the diagnostician should ask: (1) Does the patient have a potentially lethal medical disorder, head trauma, or other CNS disease? (2) Is the patient toxic or intoxicated? and (3) Is the patient in withdrawal?

Differentiation between drug-induced and "functional" psychoses is often difficult because of (1) little or unreliable information from the acute patient, (2) other sources of information may not yet be located, and (3) acute psychotic states often mimic each other. The rapid recognition of drug- or medically induced disorders is usually more important at this stage than subdiagnosis within the functional psychotic disorders, since acute and specific medical interventions may be needed to prevent seizures, respiratory impairment, and other conditions. Once drug- or medically induced disorders have been controlled or ruled out, the acute management of most psychotic psychiatric disorders can proceed.

Acute Psychiatric Behavioral Management

Psychiatric behavioral management focuses on acute symptom clusters rather than DSM-III-R diagnosis. Primary concerns are management of danger to self or others, violence, and agitation. Behavioral techniques include stimulus reduction, reassurance, limit setting, and physical restraint. At this stage, most patients are unable to participate in groups, and group involvement may in fact worsen behavior by providing too much stimulation.

Acute Psychiatric Medication Management

Medication for acute psychotic management is more symptomatic than diagnostically determined. Once medical, CNS, intoxication, or withdrawal symptoms are worked-up and clarified, most treatment will be focused on agitation, manic symptoms, and/or psychosis. In addition, certain patients with previous documented psychiatric diagnosis and known medication response may be started on longer term but less acutely helpful medications such as lithium. However, the most potent acute medication alternatives are either benzodiazepines or neuroleptics. We have been increasingly using high-dose benzodiazepines for treatment of acute agitation, mania, psychosis, and sleep disorder.[12] Benzodiazepines have replaced about 80 per cent of our previous neuroleptics use. This is because (1) benzodiazepines are less toxic, causing no dystonia or tardive dyskinesia; (2) benzodiazepines have a more predictable and safe sedative response; (3) benzodiazepines are not listed as "antipsychotics" and thus do not need court approval in involuntary patients (as occurs in some states); (4) benzodiazepines also treat sleep disturbance and sedative/alcohol withdrawal symptoms—one or both of which are usually present in acute dual-diagnosis patients. The main concern with benzodiazepines is that they are significantly addictive in patients with addictive histories and potentially dependence inducing in others.[13,14] Therefore, in dual-diagnosis patients, benzodiazepines should be tapered and discontinued as the acute phase resolves. We suggest using benzodiazepines like steroids (i.e., if you use them, use enough to do the job, starting with high-dose and building in a taper). "As needed" (p.r.n.) benzodiazepines will often cause drug-seeking behavior in dual-diagnosis patients. Neuroleptics will still be needed in most schizophrenic and some manic psychotic individuals; however, benzodiazepines may be all that is needed in drug-induced psychoses, mania, or reactive psychoses.[12]

Acute Substance Diagnosis

The focus here is differentiating intoxication or withdrawal or both from psychiatric or medical conditions. The details and extent of addictive behavior and lifestyle will come later. History, auxiliary information, toxicology screens, vital signs, and physical exam will help to determine types of drugs and the presence of withdrawal or intoxication. Evaluating the amount of denial is important because much historical information may be distorted, minimized, and rationalized by the patient in the active stages of drug and alcohol dependence.

Acute Substance Behavioral Management

Behavioral interventions in acute intoxication or withdrawal syndromes can be extremely helpful. Decreasing stimulation and "talking down" those intoxicated on stimulants or hallucinogens to decrease paranoia and agitation is well known. Relaxation and breathing exercises may also decrease withdrawal symptoms from alcohol/sedatives. Beginning intervention in addictive disease by linking the substance use and current symptoms should begin, but gets more focus in the subacute phase when the patient has better memory and concentration.

Acute Substance Medication Management

Medication for the acute phase will be for managing (1) intoxication, (2) withdrawal, or (3) medical complications. Intoxication should be managed symptomatically, with most cases needing only time and observation. More invasive techniques such as the use of nalorphine should be restricted to emergency room staff familiar with their use. Short-acting stimulant intoxication (cocaine) will usually resolve with little or no treatment, but in severe cases or with longer acting stimulants, the use of benzodiazepines in the range of 4 to 8 mg of lorazepam (or equivalent per day) is recommended. Acute withdrawal symptoms are of most concern with alcohol/sedatives or opiates or both. Protocols for management of drug-specific withdrawal syndromes are available, and new rapid withdrawal treatments for benzodiazepines, alcohol, opiates, and cocaine have been developed.[15–20]

Subacute Phase

Subacute Psychiatric Diagnosis

The patient's acute behavioral, toxic, or withdrawal syndromes should be resolving. More definitive diagnosis becomes possible as clinical course is observed. More history can be obtained from the patient, other sources, previous records, and other treatment providers. The major focus of psychiatric diagnosis is differential diagnosis between resolving (1) acute but temporarily induced conditions from (2) more enduring psychiatric conditions such as bipolar illness or schizophrenia. Major non−substance-related psychiatric disorders need differentiation in order to begin disorder-specific medication treatments.

Subacute Psychiatric Behavioral Management

Psychiatric and behavioral interventions will involve focusing on the stabilization of the patient, including psychotic, depressive, and manic features. Anxiety that was obscured by psychosis may become more prominent. Limit setting, beginning socialization, and symptom- or diagnosis-specific therapy will be started. Group therapy on problem definition and discharge planning should be initiated. Important questions here include: Are the content and form of psychiatric interventions consistent with chemical dependency interventions or are they conflicting? How can psychiatric and chemical dependency interventions best compliment each other and serve the treatment objective of the patient?

Subacute Psychiatric Medications

Psychiatric medications should change from symptomatic treatment (such as the use of benzodiazepines for sedation), to more diagnostically determined (such as the use of lithium or carbamazepine for bipolar manic features). Symptomatic medications such as benzodiazepines or other sedatives may continue through this period; however, unless the patient is documented as not responding to other types of medications, potentially addictive medications should be tapered and stopped during this phase of treatment. Because medication compliance may have been problematic in the past, the appropriate use of medications from both psychiatric and chemical dependency perspectives must be carefully discussed.

Substance Subacute Diagnosis

As patients become more coherent and additional history is developed, differential diagnosis of drug/alcohol dependence can be assessed in conjunction with the psychiatric diagnosis. The course of any withdrawal symptoms and results of toxicological screen can also be used as supportive data in diagnosis. Differential "dual-diagnostic" questions should include: Is there substance dependence or abuse? What drugs? What is the interaction between substance use and type with the development of the admitting psychiatric syndrome? Was use increasing or decreasing? Were psychiatric symptoms induced are exacerbated by the substance intoxication or withdrawal or exacerbated? How much denial or admission of drug use is present? Has the patient ever been to drug/alcohol treatment or any of the Anonymous programs. Are there "beneficial" effects from drugs that the patient expresses (e.g., socialization, self-medication of symptoms, self-medication of psychiatric medication side effects, relief from akinesia and anhedonia)? What have been negative consequences (e.g., suicide attempts, medical problems, psychiatric admission, loss of money, legal)? What is the HIV status and risk? The answers to these questions will guide drug- and alcohol-dependence intervention and treatment both through the course of subacute inpatient psychiatric treatment and afterward, for referral to specific outpatient programs.

Subacute Substance Behavioral Management

As the patient becomes more coherent, relating the patients' admitting symptoms and life problems with their drug dependence is necessary. This can be done in one-to-one sessions, groups, or both. If the focus remains only on decreasing psychiatric symptoms, the addiction denial system rapidly takes over and is often hard to penetrate in the future. Thus, while most psychiatric staff are trained to help decrease the intensity of stress and symptoms in "typical" psychiatric patients, the dual-diagnosis patient must be continually reminded of drug and alcohol problems and behaviors (i.e., staff needs to increase stress) in order to prevent denial from sealing over their ability to deal with their addiction. A balance between comfort and confrontation needs to be found. Psychiatric staff must spend as much time

focusing on addiction-related issues as with medication side effects or other psychiatric therapies with which they are more familiar. A trained chemical dependency therapist should be available to psychiatric units to work with patients, families, and staff. In addition to one-to-one interventions, other useful modalities include a drug and alcohol discussion group, availability of Alcoholics Anonymous (AA) or other 12-step meetings, and drug- and alcohol-intervention—related pamphlets or other literature.[6–8,11] There are numerous well-made drug and alcohol videos that focus on topics ranging from brain chemistry, to denial and family dysfunction. We have found these quite helpful in stimulating patient discussion as well as educating staff.

Resocialization, communication, and time management functions of inpatient psychiatric groups can be as easily met in a therapy group focused on drug and alcohol problems as with any other more typical "psychiatric" focus, such as assertiveness. Including family or other important people in the persons' life into the treatment setting to focus on both psychiatric and drug/alcohol intervention should be done at this point.

Medications

Most medications for drug and alcohol management will be tapered and stopped at this point, since they will usually be related to time-limited withdrawal conditions. However, some medications for addiction will need to be maintained, and fall generally into three areas: (1) health maintenance (e.g., vitamins, minerals, and prescribed symptomatic medications to be given to chronic alcohol users or others who have had poor nutrition; medical care)[15]; (2) antidrug use or antiwithdrawal or both (e.g., Antabuse for alcoholism, or the use of methadone for heroin dependence)[15]; (3) anticraving (potential but controversial therapies included here would be tricyclic antidepressants or carbamazepine to reduce cocaine craving and relapse).[17–20] The ongoing use of medications such as Antabuse, antidepressants, carbamazepine, and methadone will demand that patients be available and capable of outpatient follow-up with regular and careful medical supervision. This will usually demand a case manager.

Subacute Stage Discharge or Transition Planning

Discharge from most acute care psychiatric inpatient units will usually occur between 1 and 3 weeks after admission. During the "subacute" phase, psychiatric diagnosis should be better clarified, psychiatric behavioral and medication management plans should be consolidated, drug/alcohol history and diagnosis should be clarified, and intoxication and withdrawal states should be mostly resolved. For most patients, the 1 to 3 weeks of hospitalization will have focused more on acute symptom management and "intervention" rather than diagnostically determined "treatment" of core conditions. Treatment will hopefully have been started sometime toward the middle or end of hospitalization; however, the bulk of ongoing treatment will occur after discharge. For subacute outpatients, the more severe should have been referred to inpatient treatment, and the less severe should be undergoing what we have described directly above. Following acute and subacute phases, planning for longer term treatment begins. Treatment planners at this stage face these key issues:

1. Are there ongoing psychiatric diagnoses or treatment needs?

2. Does the psychiatric condition qualify for public/private mental health center services?

3. Are there ongoing substance diagnoses or treatment needs?

4. Does the drug/alcohol condition qualify for public/private substance abuse services?

5. Are there dual-diagnosis services available, and if so, who should or does qualify for services?

The discharge needs of a patient admitted as an intoxicated psychotic (described in the Acute Psychiatric section) will vary greatly. Of the two etiological examples given, most cocaine/alcohol-dependent patients with a drug-induced (and temporary) psychosis will have little or no major psychiatric sequelae by discharge. The focus after acute stabilization should be primary chemical dependency treatment. Continued involvement with "mental health" may even reinforce denial by giving psychological rationales. On the other hand, the schizophrenic who drank only on the day of admission will need primary psychiatric treatment with a basic amount of substance abuse intervention and education provided on site at the mental health center. He would not qualify for chemical dependency services. The schizophrenic who is chronically psychotic and also dependent on substances will need concurrent treatment for both psychiatric and substance abuse (i.e., "integrated dual-diagnosis treatment."[6-11]

Longer Term Issues With Special Focus on Chronically Mentally III

Patient Treatment Matching and Dual-Diagnosis Typology

Patient/treatment matching paradigms need to define schemes of patient typology and treatment typology. Because the focus of this section is on the chronically mentally ill patient, we will assume that the bulk of outpatient psychiatric diagnosis and care will be provided through the public mental health system. A model for use with private care or less severely mentally ill patients is given elsewhere. Given funding and limitations, most mental health centers only accept patients who have major, chronic psychiatric disorders with resulting significant psychosocial and economic dysfunction. Diagnosis at the end of subacute hospitalization or the beginning of outpatient treatment with a new patient should attempt to classify both psychiatric and chemical dependency diagnoses according to elements of nosology as well as treatment systems qualifications (usually severity). We developed the following diagnostic groupings and have found them useful.

DUAL-DIAGNOSIS TYPOLOGY

Type I. High-severity psychiatric–high-severity substance

Type II. High-severity psychiatric–low-severity substance

Type III. Low-severity psychiatric–high-severity substance

Type IV. Low-severity psychiatric–low-severity substance

High-severity psychiatric means that the patient suffers from a chronic psychiatric disorder that causes major dysfunction in psychological, cognitive, social, economic, and job functions. Most of these patients fall into diagnostic groups which include schizophrenia, bipolar disorders, recurrent severe depressive disorders, paranoid disorders, and some of the more dysfunctional personality disorders such as schizoid, schizotypal, and borderline. Low-severity psychiatric includes most major depressions, dysthymic and anxiety disorders (which resolve relatively rapidly with treatment), most personality disorders, and temporary drug-induced psychiatric disorders. Patients in the low-severity psychiatric grouping will have relatively little or no psychosocial and less economic impairment related to their psychiatric syndrome when it is adequately treated or resolved. High-severity drug/alcohol disorder includes patients who qualify for a DSM-III-R diagnosis of psychoactive substance dependence. Low-severity drug/alcohol disorder includes those who qualify for a DSM-III-R diagnosis of psychoactive substance abuse or those with drug or alcohol use that has a measurable but minor impact on their psychosocial function.

Treatment Typology

One of the rationales for defining the four typologies above is related to the structure of our care systems. Most acute treatment of dual diagnosis occurs through the psychiatric system due to the severity of psychopathology and behavioral dyscontrol. As patients move from acute to subacute state and the diagnostic process is developed, longer term outpatient requirements can be determined. The outpatient systems of care, however, are usually in parallel and are primarily based in either the mental health or chemical dependency systems. For discussion purposes we will define the following conditions:

1. Sequential treatment is defined as treatment occurring within one system (either the psychiatric system or the chemical dependency system) followed by treatment in the other system.

2. Parallel treatment is concurrent but separate treatment.

3. Integrated treatment is the co-occurrence of psychiatric treatment and chemical dependency treatment within a single agency. Staff are cross-trained and many should be cocertified in both chemical dependency and mental health.

As discussed above, most acute psychiatric conditions (especially types I and II) will need acute stabilization on a highly staffed psychiatric unit due to the degree of psychopathology and behavioral dyscontrol. Chemical dependency units are not usually staffed or architecturally designed to deal with such patients. However, as acute symptoms resolve, subacute and longer term treatment needs become more apparent. Our experience suggests that most type I patients need integrated dual-diagnosis treatment, especially in the subacute and longer term stages. Type II patients can be referred to either an integrated program or a mental health center program with a less intensive amount of chemical dependency intervention (parallel treatment). Once psychiatrically stable, type III patients should be referred to the outpatient or inpatient chemical dependency system with either psychiatric consultation (parallel or integrated service) in the case of ongoing less severe psychiatric disorder or no further psychiatric consultation if the patient had only a drug-induced psychiatric state that was resolved. Type IV patients will probably not present to inpatient units of either type, but are more likely encountered in outpatient clinics. A dual approach for the psychiatric clinician has been described elsewhere for type IV patients.[3]

Integrated Outpatient Dual-Diagnosis Program Issues

A significant number of chronic psychiatric patients with or without dual diagnoses may be non-motivated or unable to take part in either traditional psychiatric or substance treatment programs. Case management has been a response to (1) assist patients' movement into a recovery track, or (2) acknowledge that certain patients are unable or noncompliant to readily improve. The case manager keeps the patient as functional as possible and decreases costs and morbidity associated with the patients' condition. Case management can also be applied to dual-diagnosis patients, both in recovery and maintenance. The maintenance track, by our definition, means that patients have problems with compliance, motivation, or have such severe conditions that improvement is not imminent. The focus of case management is to decrease morbidity and costs associated with the patients' condition. The

case manager should always encourage movement of the patient from the maintenance condition into the recovery track. Most therapy will involve one-to-one interaction between the patient and the case manager in monitoring needed medications, providing needed support while confronting drug/alcohol dependence, and attempting to decrease overall morbidity. The case manager will usually be a protective payee and will manage most financial affairs. Chemical dependency intervention will involve one-to-one educational sessions with a case manager, a minimal amount of group videos or discussion or both, and potential reading material. Using the AA model, the case manager should enlist patients in the recovery track to act as co-interventionists for certain other patients who are in the maintenance track. Since patients with both major mental and major drug/alcohol disorders have usually lost housing, family ties, and the ability to work, motivation toward improvement must be through positive enticements rather than negative incentives or limits. Most have nothing left to lose.

The recovery track will involve patients who express a willingness to improve in both their psychiatric and addiction conditions. Motivation and the patient's own expectations seem to be key factors in identifying short-term reported abstinence and compliance with therapy.[9] These factors likely also apply to long-term outcome. The recovery track should not only involve more intense therapeutic interventions, but should also include positive rewards (e.g., better housing, better food, better activities, tickets to local sports events, movies) as part of the therapeutic context. These advantages must be known by both maintenance and recovery track individuals such that all patients see that compliance and motivation pay off. Likewise, in taking away drugs from patients, there needs to be something else to "fill in the gap." Since many chronic psychiatric patients say that drug/alcohol use temporarily provides excitement or helps them to feel "normal," activities that provide these experiences must be designed and available to those in the recovery track. Drug-free housing that supports recovery and involves on-site recovery groups is important. Dual-diagnosis or "persuasion" groups[6,7] that focus not only on intervention, but on recovery issues, should be occurring numerous times per week. These groups may focus on relapse prevention or other techniques, but need to be consistent with AA (i.e., 12-step recovery program) as outlined by several authors.[6–8,21–23] As patients become more coherent and socially appropriate, involvement with AA groups that include other dual-diagnosis patients should occur. Most urban centers across the country have a growing number of AA groups that involve dual-diagnosis patients. For patients who are unable or unwilling to use 12-step groups, facilitator-led recovery groups using relapse prevention models are useful.[21–23] The recovery track should involve vocational training as patients' abilities to earn new monies improve, thus providing even more rewards for those in the recovery track. Drug- and alcohol-related videos should be included in the dual-diagnosis program discussion groups. Since many of these patients will have come from dysfunctional families, getting patients involved with the adult-children-of-alcoholics literature, videos, and at times, therapy groups, will provide further recovery, though this requires more stability of both substance and psychiatric disorder. As patients become more involved with recovery programs, the issue of medication use needs continued focus. Patients may experience well-meaning 12-step program members, especially Narcotics Anonymous (NA), who are against all drug and medication use. Patients need to be educated that they may well interact with such individuals, and need to practice how to cope with antimedication messages or discussions. However, most AA and many NA members are supportive of proper use of psychiatric medications, and AA has produced a pamphlet in support of the use of most psychiatric medications (but not medications that induce tolerance and dependence). Understanding the relationship and potential conflicts between substance recovery and use of psychiatric medications is complex, but can be rewarding both for clinicians and patients. Added training in the area of addictions is available through several professional societies that involve psychiatrists as well as other physicians. These include: American Academy of Psychiatrists on Alcohol and Addictions (AAPAA); American Society of Addiction Medicine (ASAM), Association for Medical Education and Research on Substance Abuse (AMERSA), and the Alliance for Mentally Ill Chemical Abusers (AMICA).

CONCLUSIONS

Dual-diagnosis conditions have important clinical, research, and training implications for the practice of psychiatry in the coming years. Currently, a minority of psychiatrists have had adequate supervised training in addictive disorders, but training programs are improving in this area. This chapter was developed to help the psychiatric clinician who encounters dually diagnosed patients within the context of clinical care. Outcome studies are in progress; however, much remains to be learned about what actually works with these often difficult patients.

ACKNOWLEDGMENTS

This work was partially supported by Health and Human Services Research Grant #5 RO1 DA 04864-03.

REFERENCES

1. Lehman AF, Myers CP, Corty E: Assessment and classification of patients with psychiatric and substance abuse syndromes. Hosp Community Psychiatry 40(10):1019–1025, 1989.
2. Reiger DA, Farmer ME, Rae DS, et al: Comorbidity of mental disorders with alcohol and other drug abuse. JAMA 264(19):3511–2518, 1990.
3. Ries RK: In Roy-Byrne PP, ed. Alcoholism and anxiety: new findings for the clinician. Washington DC: American Psychological Association Press 6:123–149, 1989.
4. DeMilio L: Psychiatric syndromes in adolescent substance abusers. Am J Psychiatry 146(9):1212–1214, 1989.
5. Miller NS, Mirin SM: Multiple drug use in alcoholics: Practical and theoretical implications. Psychiatr Ann 19(5):248–255, 1989.
6. Minkoff K: An integrated treatment model for dual diagnosis of psychosis and addiction. Hosp Community Psychiatry 40(10):1031–1036, 1989.
7. Osher FC, Kofoed LL: Treatment of patients with psychiatric and psychoactive substance abuse disorders. Hosp Community Psychiatry 40(10):1025–1030, 1989.
8. Ries RK: Substance abuse intervention on inpatient psychiatry. Subst Abuse 10:28–32, 1989.
9. Ries RK, Ellingson T: Dual diagnosis—a data based inpatient pilot study. Hosp Community Psychiatry 41(11):1230–1233, 1990.
10. Thacker W, Tremaine L: Systems in serving the mentally ill substance abuser: Virginia's experience. Hosp Community Psychiatry 40(10):1046–1049, 1989.
11. Wallen M, Weiner H: The dually diagnosed patient in an inpatient chemical dependency treatment program. Alcohol Treat Q 5(1/2):197–218, 1988.
12. Easton MS, Janicak PG: The use of benzodiazepines in psychotic disorders: A review of the literature. Psychiatr Ann 20(9):535–544, 1990.
13. Ciraulo DA, Sands BF, Shader RI: Critical review of liability for benzodiazepine abuse among alcoholics. Am J Psychiatry 145(12):1501–1506, 1988.
14. Griffiths RR, Wolf B: Relative abuse liability of different benzodiazepines in drug abusers. J Clin Psychopharmacol 10(4):237–243, 1990.
15. Schuckit MA: In Drug and Alcohol Abuse—a Guide to Diagnosis and Treatment. 3rd ed. New York: Plenum Press, 1989.
16. Ries RK, Cullison S, Horn R, Ward N: Benzodiazepine withdrawal: Clinician's ratings of carbamazepine treatment versus traditional taper methods. J Psychoactive Drugs 23(1):73–76, 1991.
17. Malcolm R, Ballenger JC, Sturgis ET, Anton R: Double-blind controlled trial comparing carbamazepine to oxazepam treatment of alcohol withdrawal. Am J Psychiatry 146:617–621, 1989.
18. Vaughan DA: Frontiers in pharmacologic treatment of alcohol, cocaine, and nicotine dependence. Psychiatr Ann 20(12):695–710, 1990.
19. Gawin FH, Fleber HD, Byck R, et al: Desipramine facilitation of initial cocaine abstinence. Arch Gen Psychiatry 46:117–121, 1989.
20. Halikas J, Kemp K, Kuhn K, et al: Carbamazepine for cocaine addiction? Lancet 1(8638):623–624, 1989.
21. Evans K, Sullivan JM: In Dual Diagnosis: Counseling the Mentally Ill Substance Abuser. New York: The Guilford Press, 1990.
22. O'Connell DF, ed. In Managing the Dually Diagnosed Patient: Current Issues and Clinical Approaches. New York: The Haworth Press, 1990.
23. Daley DC, Moss H, Campbell F: In Dual Disorders: Counseling Clients with Chemical Dependency and Mental Illness. Center City, MN: Hazelden Foundation Press, 1987.

Section C

SCHIZOPHRENIA

22

THE IMPLICATION OF CRITERIA CHANGES FOR DSM-IV SCHIZOPHRENIA

SAMUEL J. KEITH, M.D. and SUSAN M. MATTHEWS, B.A.

We have seen a dramatic evolution of the psychiatric diagnosis of schizophrenia in the United States. A wide range of influential figures and scientific forces have taken us from a narrow conceptual framework for the illness, to a considerably broader one, to the more recent emphasis on a narrow approach as defined in DSM-III-R. Foremost in the evolution has been the requirement of specific psychotic symptomatology (the "A" criterion of schizophrenia) for a diagnosis of schizophrenia to be made. It is these specific criteria that not only *separate* the current diagnosis from the past, but also provide the opportunity to move in a direction of increased reliability of the diagnosis and its symptomatology.

Operationally, the past 15 years have seen a continuing move toward the scientific necessity of developing reliable criteria.[1] Drawing heavily on the German phenomenologists like Kurt Schneider and work by the St. Louis (Feighner et al.) and New York (Spitzer) groups, the two principles involved have been that symptoms should be *specific to one illness and not occur in others;* and that they be *readily observed and agreed upon by observers.* Thus, specific and quantifiable symptoms or periods of time have been selected to make the criteria for schizophrenia.

As currently defined in the United States by DSM-III-R, schizophrenia is a mental illness with core features: psychotic symptoms—hallucinations and delusions; the chronicity of the illness requires a 6-month period of illness; deterioration in functioning; and an exclusion of affective or mood components or established organic etiology. The treatment implications of such a primarily symptom-based diagnosis is toward the reduction and elimination of symptoms. Psychopharmacology, with its intrinsic capacity to reduce symptomatology, has become the standard not only for schizophrenia, but for other disorders—depression and anxiety—as well. Of particular importance to note is the role of positive symptoms in the definition and treatment implications of schizophrenia. Hallucinations and delusions, of both specific and general nature, have become the hallmark of the illness, and their elimination the hallmark of successful treatment. The emphasis on their fleeting presence ("1 week or less if successfully treated") has emphasized their definitional importance, but also created the possibility of a large class of false-positives for those people who may have an acute psychotic illness of transient nature. Further, because the remaining requirement of 6 months of illness may be composed of prodromal and residual symptoms, the reliability and validity of this rather extensive and cumbersome list of symptoms assumes considerable importance. Additionally, it has been noted that the DSM-III-R criteria has placed somewhat less emphasis on the negative symptoms of the illness—and our treatments have generally been ineffective in treating them.

The current revision of DSM will be addressing each of the following areas:

1. Psychotic features and their duration.
2. The role of negative symptoms.
3. The utility of prodrome and residual symptoms.

PSYCHOTIC FEATURES AND THEIR DURATION

Psychotic Features

The overall awkwardness of the A criterion in DSM-III-R has led to the suggestion that for teaching, and even clinical purposes, a division into positive and negative symptoms would be useful. Further, the question of whether the division of positive symptoms on the basis of generalized hallucinations and delusions versus specific schneiderian symptoms and bizarre delusions merits continuation will be examined in the field trials. Although historically accepted as being pathognomonic for schizophrenia, the specificity of schneiderian symptoms has been challenged by many over the past decade. The reliability of deciding whether a delusion is bizarre (impossible, implausible, or unusual), makes this an area under consideration for revision. The issue of negative symptoms will be considered in a separate section.

Duration

The current DSM-III-R criteria requires a 6-month duration of *illness* for the diagnosis of schizophrenia. However, in terms of psychotic symptoms (A criterion), it requires only 1 week, and even that has a proviso. The exact criteria requires 1 week *"or less if successfully treated"* of psychotic symptoms; the remaining 5 months, 3 weeks may be composed of either prodrome or residual symptoms.

The significance of duration becomes quite apparent, particularly with initial-onset patients. The DSM-III-R criteria implies that characteristic psychotic symptoms *may* be "successfully treated" in less than 1 *week,* or in any event, that 1 week of psychotic symptoms is sufficient to meet the diagnosis of schizophrenia. If this is correct, then many patients who would be classified as schizophrenic under DSM-III-R criteria would fall into the International Classification of Diseases (ICD-10) category of acute schizophrenia-like psychotic disorder. For the well-established case of schizophrenia (long course of psychotic symptoms with progressive deterioration), meeting criteria for the diagnosis is not difficult. The major group of concern would be those who respond to treatment within a 1- to 4-week period. It appears likely, however, that very few psychotic episodes leading to schizophrenia last less than 1 month, and because the DSM-III-R allows those with brief psychotic experiences to qualify for a diagnosis of schizophrenia or at least schizophreniform illness, we know almost nothing about those patients whose psychosis is short-lived.

At the present time, closure on duration of psychotic symptoms is difficult to make and no solution will be universally satisfactory. The impact of having an idiosyncratic national diagnostic system (as ICD-10 moves toward the 1-month duration) may ultimately tip the balance. At this point it may, however, be the best option to adopt the 1-month duration of psychotic symptoms as a base requirement for entering the schizophrenia spectrum. Whether to then extend a category from 1 month to 6 months called schizophreniform, and beyond 6 months, schizophrenia, will require a judgment on whether there is data to support this dichotomization. At least in doing it this way, there will be a nesting of schizophreniform/schizophrenia within what the ICD-10 will be identifying as schizophrenia.

NEGATIVE SYMPTOMS

There is perhaps no other area in schizophrenia phenomenology research that has grown as rapidly as that on negative symptoms. From the conceptual work of Huglings-Jackson,[2] to the seminal work of Strauss et al.,[3] to the clinical research applications of Crow,[4] to the codifying and classifying work of Nancy Andreasen,[1] this field has moved into prominence in the diagnosis and treatment of schizophrenia. As noted above, negative symptoms have proven to be quite treatment resistant despite their critical importance in accounting for outcome variance. The sole negative symptom in the DSM-III-R A criterion is flat affect. Other negative symptoms are captured in the residual symptoms and the deterioration in functioning requirement. The DSM-IV will be giving acute consideration to expanding the A criterion to include such negative symptoms as avolition, alogia, and anhedonia—constructs difficult to define, but important in our overall understanding of schizophrenia.

THE UTILITY OF PRODROMAL AND RESIDUAL SYMPTOMS

There has been considerable discussion in the literature over what constitutes a prodromal symptom. Currently, it is reasonably accurate to say that prodrome has become a heterogeneous group of behaviors related in a temporal manner to the onset of psychosis. The concept of schizophrenia or schizophreniform illness having a gradual onset of insidious course is one that has historically been a critical component of the illnesses. What has conflicted contemporary psychiatry are issues of how best to capture and characterize these clinically accepted phenomenon. With residual symptoms, there has been relatively less debate, because for the most part these symptoms are collected prospectively following psychotic symptomatology—a phenomenon that will color many aspects of the patient's future life, including the confidence with which we assess residual symptoms. With prodrome, however, we are usually in the position of having to assess potentially "low-grade" symptoms retrospectively—inescapable for reasons of efficiency and acceptable because of the place of retrospective data in the history of psychiatry and medicine in general. Critical, then, becomes the characterization of the components of prodrome in terms of their reliability and duration.

The role of prodromal and residual phases of schizophrenia and schizophreniform illnesses will also characterize a significant difference between ICD-10 and DSM-III-R. The ICD-10 recognizes that the prodrome exists, but has chosen not to include its characterization or duration into the diagnostic criteria. In practical terms, this difference between the two diagnostic systems is highlighted with the first-episode patient. For DSM, the characteristic psychotic symptoms may assume somewhat less significance in terms of *duration*, with the only requirement being that they be present for 1 week (or less if successfully treated) at some point. The remainder of the criteria for diagnosis for the first-episode patient is dependent on the accurate assessment of the presence of *prodrome*. If the symptoms that brought the patient to psychiatric attention are of relatively recent onset, a diagnosis of schizophreniform (provisional) is made, with a 6-month time clock started. After the 6-month time period has elapsed, if either psychotic or residual symptoms persist, a diagnosis of schizophrenia is made.

If there has been an insidious onset, and the presence of characteristic symptoms is established, then the diagnosis hinges on an accurate, retrospective dating of prodromal symptoms for up to 6 months in the past. Further, if the highest degree of difficulty in diagnosis lies with the first-episode patient, then the focus of a discussion of "6 months" becomes in actuality the utility, reliability, and implication of prodrome as defined in DSM, because *after* 6 months of manifest *illness* (either active psychotic symptoms or residual symptoms as assessed prospectively), the diagnosis becomes considerably easier regardless of the system used.

While it becomes clear that the symptoms of prodrome can be reasonably assessed in terms of presence or absence, there are two substantial problems. First is the conceptual problem created by combining "prepsychotic" symptoms (e.g., markedly peculiar behavior, odd beliefs, unusual perceptual experiences) with "negative-like symptoms" (e.g., marked social isolation, blunted or inappropriate affect, marked lack of initiative). It seems logical that these may be from entirely different domains of psychopathology. The clinical implications of the onset of psychosis are different for those who have had

longstanding negative or negative-like symptoms as compared to a group without or whose psychosis began relatively recently (e.g., 2 months) with prepsychotic symptoms only. Second, possibly leading from the above, is that the prepsychotic symptoms, while easier to date for onset, occur relatively closer to the beginning of frank psychotic symptoms than 6 months; and the negative-like symptoms, which are longer in duration, are quite difficult to date in terms of onset.

Whether to incorporate prodromal and residual symptoms into the diagnostic criteria will be the first decision point. Our recommendation takes into consideration that ICD-10 will not be using them in their diagnostic criteria. For DSM to include them as part of the diagnostic classification will leave us with a conflicting nosology. We would prefer, therefore, to recommend their use as a means of characterizing, not classifying.

One further possibility is that the two types of prodromal symptoms (and possibly three, if role functioning is considered as a separate domain) be disentangled, with prepsychotic and frank psychotic symptoms being used for onset dating, therefore reducing the amount of time required to meet criteria; and negative-like symptoms or frank negative symptoms being used as a characterizing or subtyping variable in a presence-or-absence manner either preceding or following the onset of the characteristic A criterion symptoms.

SUMMARY

There are a number of changes that may well take place in the revision of the current DSM-III-R criteria. The prevailing Zeitgeist of conservatism in regard to change, except where there is empirical evidence to support the change, will no doubt dominate the ultimate decisions. That is an acceptable standard, because allowing opinion *only* to dominate would leave nosology in a tenuous state. The changes proposed and under serious consideration in the ongoing field trials are important. We have seen how the role of diagnosis shapes the treatment response, and with the increasing emphasis on negative symptoms, treatments will need to address this area. Further, data have been sorely lacking in the area of acute psychotic (nonschizophrenic) illnesses, in no small part because they had been defined almost out of existence by the DSM-III-R criteria for schizophrenia. With the extension of positive symptoms requirement from 1 week (or less if successfully treated) to 1 month, there is an inherent encouragement to carefully assess the early presentation of psychotic illness without assigning the stigmatizing and negative treatment implications of the immediate diagnosis of schizophrenia. The additional emphasis on negative symptoms should also lead to a better therapeutic armamentaria than currently exists for this constellation of symptoms. Both of these changes will make welcome contributions to the field and should be seen as substantial challenges and opportunities for the field.

REFERENCES

1. Andreasen N: The American concept of schizophrenia. Schizophr Bull 15:519–531, 1989.

2. Huglings-Jackson J: In Taylor J, ed. Selected Writings. London: Hodder & Stroughton, Ltd., 1931.

3. Strauss J, Carpenter WT, Bartko J: The diagnosis and understanding of schizophrenia. Part III. Speculations on the processes that underly schizophrenia symptoms and signs. Schizophr Bull 1:61–69, 1974.

4. Crow TJ: Molecular pathology of schizophrenia: More than one disease process? Br Med J 280:66–68, 1980.

23

SCHIZOPHRENIA:
An Overview of Pharmacological Treatment

STEVEN G. POTKIN, M.D., LAWRENCE J. ALBERS, M.D., and
GLENN RICHMOND, M.D.

Schizophrenia is a brain illness of unknown etiology. Schizophrenia is primarily a disorder of thinking, although some dysfunction of mood can also be present. It frequently begins insidiously, with prodromal symptoms such as the development of peer and family problems and difficulties in school. The onset of psychotic symptoms usually occurs in the late teens or early twenties. Both sexes are affected in equal numbers despite a mean later onset of 6 years and frequently milder course in women. Schizophrenia is most likely not a single entity, but rather a syndrome in which different etiological factors act singly or in combination to produce the disorder. This disorder of thinking frequently manifests itself by "positive" (active psychotic) symptoms such as prominent hallucinations and fixed false beliefs, known as delusions. The delusions are often of a persecutory nature or bizarre in content. They may embrace impossible, improbable, or contradictory ideas. Many schizophrenic patients also have "negative symptoms," such as a loss of feeling for others, lack of goal-directed behavior and drive, decreased interest in pleasurable activities, and reduced emotional range referred to as blunted affect. Typically, schizophrenic patients are oriented to time, place, and person. Less commonly, patients may show "deficit" syndromes characterized by left-right confusion and abnormalities in stereognosis and graphesthesia.[1] Schizophrenic persons often have motoric abnormalities consisting of unusual mannerisms or stereotyped movements. These movements make the ill individual stand out in a crowd.

Some schizophrenic patients have positive, negative, and deficit symptoms during the initial stages of illness, while others develop their negative and deficit symptoms with progression of their illness. Most schizophrenic patients do not return to baseline functioning and have a chronic downward course, although symptom fluctuations are typical, while in others, the course of illness over time is one of slow gradual improvement with a progressive loss of positive symptoms and an increased ability to function. Few individuals with schizophrenia, however, will demonstrate a complete recovery.

With antipsychotic treatment, an increasing number of patients have been able to leave the hospital and function in the community. Approximately 70 per cent of schizophrenic patients benefit from neuroleptic treatment, but less than 5 per cent show a full restitution to a premorbid state. Approximately 15 per cent fail to respond satisfactorily to standard treatments. Treatment-refractory schizophrenics are refractory only to current medications and are not incapable of responding. Clinically relevant responses, at times dramatic, are observed in one third of such refractory patients placed on clozapine, an atypical antipsychotic.[2]

Occasionally, schizophrenic patients have brief periods of relative symptom remission, which serves to remind us that the schizophrenic nervous system has the potential to function normally.

Lifetime prevalence of schizophrenia is approximately 1 per cent worldwide. The National Institute of Mental Health (NIMH)-sponsored Epidemiological Catchment Area (ECA) study gives a lifetime US prevalence of 0.6 to 1.9 per cent for the four cities surveyed. The life expectancy of a schizophrenic person is slightly decreased, and there is a very high incidence of suicide associated with this illness. The suicide rate for schizophrenia is at least ten times that for normals and approximates that for persons with depressive illness.[3]

ETIOLOGY

Although the etiology of schizophrenia is unknown, there is a genetic predisposition to developing schizophrenia. A 17-fold increased risk in developing schizophrenia occurs when a member of one's nuclear family is schizophrenic. Family, adoption, and twin studies are consistent with a genetic predisposition as well as a role for nongenetic factors. Offspring of monozygotic twins who are discordant for schizophrenia inherit equally an increased tendency to develop schizophrenia. In spite of the healthy twin having no overt symptoms, he still passes the same genetic predisposition to his offspring.[4] There are no definitive tests to diagnose schizophrenia. Structural brain abnormalities have been observed in groups of schizophrenics. These abnormalities include enlargement of the cerebral ventricles, cortical atrophy, and reduction of the temporal lobes. Cellular abnormalities in medial temporal lobe structures are also observed. These brain abnormalities, however, are not pathognomonic for a diagnosis of schizophrenia and can be observed in other illnesses.

Schizophrenia can be differentiated from schizophreniform and brief reactive psychotic disorders by its duration of illness being greater than 6 months, and from bipolar mood disorders or schizoaffective disorder by its course and persistence of psychotic symptoms relative to the mood disturbance. The severity and character of symptoms distinguishes schizophrenia from the eccentric cluster of schizoid, schizotypal, or paranoid personality types. Malingering or factitious illness may relate to secondary gain and should be considered in the differential diagnosis.

Ruling out a treatable/reversible etiology of a psychotic presentation is of primary importance. Some of the medical illnesses that may mimic a schizophrenic disorder are listed in Table 23–1.

Routine laboratory work-up, a careful physical and neurological examination, a comprehensive family and social history, and medical history including currently used prescription and over-the-counter medications and drugs of abuse will aid in appropriate diagnosis. The laboratory workup should include complete blood count (CBC), thyroid, liver and renal function tests, B_{12} and folate, screening for syphilis, acquired immunodeficiency syndrome (AIDS), and drugs of abuse. To further investigate selected patients, computer tomography (CT), magnetic resonance imaging (MRI), or electroencephalogram (EEG) may be helpful. It is our practice to obtain a comprehensive neurological and medical work-up including an MRI for all first-episode schizophrenic patients.

Before pharmacological treatment with neuroleptics is begun, several days of drug-free evaluation are important to adequately observe the patient, complete the laboratory work-up, and obtain full history. Confirmatory history from family members, employ-

TABLE 23–1. DIFFERENTIAL DIAGNOSIS OF SCHIZOPHRENIA AND RELEVANT LABORATORY TESTS

Disorder	Laboratory Test
Epilepsy	EEG
CNS tumor (focal neurological abnormalities)	MRI
CNS infection	CBC, LP, RPR, HIV
CNS degenerative diseases	MRI, neuropsychological testing
B_{12} deficiency and anemias	Serum B_{12}, folate, CBC
Endocrine/metabolic	Blood and urine (ceruloplasmin, prophyrins, etc.)
Heavy metal poisoning	Blood, urine, x-ray
Occupational exposure	Blood, urine
Systemic lupus erythematosus (LE)	LE prep, ANA, anti-DNA
Drugs	Toxicology screen
Alcohol (especially paranoia, hallucinosis, or deficit states)	
Anticholinergic (disorientation), bromides	
Hallucinogens (phencyclidine)	
Stimulants (e.g., amphetamine)	
Psychiatric	
Mood disorders	
Other psychotic disorders (e.g., delusional disorder)	
Personality disorders	

CNS, central nervous system; EEG, electroencephalogram; MRI, magnetic resonance imaging; CBC, complete blood count; LP, lumbar puncture; RPR, rapid plasma reaction; HIV, human immunodeficiency virus; ANA, antinuclear antibody; DNA, deoxyribonucleic acid.

ers, roommates, or others is necessary because the schizophrenic person may be unable to provide essential details.

Schizophrenia, in summary, is a lifelong illness, usually beginning at the onset of early adulthood. It is a devastating illness that attacks many of our most human aspects, such as the capacity to make sense of our perceptions, to relate emotionally to others, and to think clearly. The treatment of this challenging disease requires an understanding of brain functioning, neuropsychiatry, pharmacology and psychotherapy, and a flexible approach to integrate drug treatment with supportive, educational, psychiatric, and family therapy. It is important to emphasize that treatment is given to a patient who may require continued assistance in housing, vocation, nutrition, legal, social, and diverse medical needs.

PHARMACOLOGICAL TREATMENT

Successful treatment of schizophrenia requires detailed knowledge of antipsychotic drugs. The first of these drugs, reserpine and chlorpromazine, were very sedating and produced decreased motor activity and symptoms similar to Parkinson's syndrome. Because of the marked sedative effects, these antipsy-

chotic drugs were initially called "major tranquilizers." The term major tranquilizer is misleading, because many of the subsequent antipsychotic compounds are not very sedating, and sedatives such as barbiturates and chloral hydrate have no antipsychotic efficacy. Antipsychotic drugs affect the thinking disorder and the abnormal perceptions of schizophrenia without necessarily causing sedation. Another term for these drugs is "neuroleptic" (i.e. nerve-take hold of), because the first-generation antipsychotic drugs had strong effects on motor behavior, and consequently, motor inhibition was believed to be a necessary property for antipsychotic activity. Due to the overlap of the term neuroleptic with motor side effects, novel agents such as clozapine are called atypical antipsychotics or atypical neuroleptics to distinguish their ability to be antipsychotic without producing many motor effects and/or because of their atypical pharmacology. In practice, the terms antipsychotic and neuroleptic are used interchangeably.

There are seven classes of neuroleptic drugs defined on the basis of their chemical structure (Table 23–2 and Appendix I). These drugs do not produce tolerance, addiction, or withdrawal. Within the class of phenothiazines there are three subclasses. The aliphatic or alkylamino (e.g., chlorpromazine) are the least potent and are usually prescribed in doses

TABLE 23–2. CLASS OF NEUROLEPTIC DRUGS

Class	Example	Common Brands	Available Doses
Phenothiazine			
Aliphatic	Chlorpromazine	Thorazine	Tablets: 10 mg, 25 mg, 50 mg, 100 mg, 200 mg Oral concentrate: 30 mg/ml, 100 mg/ml IM injection: 25 mg/ml
Piperidine	Thioridazine	Mellaril	Tablets: 10 mg, 15 mg, 25 mg, 50 mg, 100 mg, 200 mg Oral concentrate: 30 mg/ml, 100 mg/ml
Piperazine	Fluphenazine	Prolixin Permital	Tablets: 1 mg, 2.5 mg, 5 mg, 10 mg Oral concentrate: 5 mg/ml IM injection: 2.5 mg/ml Enanthate depot injection: 25 mg/ml Decanoate depot injection: 25 mg/ml
	Perphenazine	Trilafon	Tablets: 2 mg, 4 mg, 8 mg, 16 mg Oral concentrate: 16 mg/5 ml Injection: 5 mg/ml
	Trifluoperazine	Stelazine	Tablets: 1 mg, 2 mg, 5 mg, 10 mg Oral concentrate: 10 mg/ml Injection: 2 mg/ml
Thioxanthenes	Thiothixene	Navane	Capsules: 1 mg, 10 mg, 20 mg Oral concentrate: 5 mg/ml Injection: 2 mg/ml, 5 mg/ml
Butyrophenones	Haloperidol	Haldol	Tablets: 0.5 mg, 1 mg, 2 mg, 5 mg, 10 mg, 20 mg Oral concentrate: 2 mg/ml Injection: 5 mg/ml Decanoate depot injection: 50 mg/ml, 100 mg/ml
	Pimozide	Orap	Tablet: 2 mg
Benzamides	Sulpiride		Not available in the United States
	Clozapine	Clozaril	Tablets: 25 mg, 100 mg
Dibenzodiazepine	Loxapine	Loxitane	Capsules: 5 mg, 10 mg, 25 mg, 50 mg Oral concentrate: 25 mg/ml Injection: 50 mg/ml
Dihydroindolones	Molindone	Moban	Tablets: 5 mg, 10 mg, 25 mg, 50 mg, 100 mg Oral concentrate: 20 mg/ml

of several hundred milligrams. The piperazine group (e.g., fluphenazine) are much more potent and prescribed in tens of milligrams. The piperidine group (e.g., thioridazine) are moderately potent and prescribed in intermediate dosage. Potency refers to the dose required to achieve antipsychotic effects. For example, 10 mg of haloperidol is equal in antipsychotic efficacy to 500 mg of chlorpromazine (see Table 23–4). It should be noted that between classes as well as within each class, considerable variability is present in the relative potency of these agents in blocking dopaminergic, adrenergic, muscarinic, serotonergic, and histaminic receptors. This property was noted 40 years ago when chlorpromazine was marketed as Largactyl, so named because of its large number of actions in the central nervous system.

No body of evidence suggests that any single agent in Table 23–2 is more efficacious than any other in treating schizophrenia. The exception may be the superior efficacy of clozapine in treatment-resistant patients. Scientific literature does not provide guidance in choosing one neuroleptic over another, and prescribing relies on empirically based trial-and-error method. Statistically, groups of schizophrenic patients respond equally to these agents; however, most clinicians believe that an individual patient may respond to one antipsychotic compound better than another, but there is no guidance in choosing that agent. A patient's past history of medication response and response history in ill family members is helpful.

How does one go about choosing the right antipsychotic medication? As a general guideline, it is best to become familiar with one representative of each class of neuroleptic drug, including the three subclasses of phenothiazines. By obtaining experience with this short list of seven or eight antipsychotic agents, one can gain considerable flexibility in treating schizophrenic patients. Pimozide and sulpiride can be excluded from the list because pimozide is only approved for Tourette's syndrome in the United States although it is an effective neuroleptic, and sulpiride is not marketed in the United States.)

General Guidelines

1.   Time. It is important to wait sufficient time for the drug to achieve an antipsychotic effect. While a minority of schizophrenic patients respond in hours to several days, most hospitalized patients require 1 to 2 weeks of antipsychotic medication to show a significant response. Outpatients respond more slowly, with an average of 2 to 4 weeks. Patients with longstanding symptoms may require additional time to respond.

2.   Target symptoms. It is important to differentiate the need for sedating a patient from a need for antipsychotic medication (as described below). Neuroleptics are equivalent in antipsychotic efficacy, but are not equivalent in sedative properties.

Sedation is related to the potency of the drugs at the histaminic and muscarinic receptors.

3.   Dosage. The half-lives of neuroleptic medications are usually 12 to 36 hours. Thus, when steady state is achieved, most patients can be maintained with once-a-day dosing. The dose is often given at night to take advantage of sedation. Rarely, a patient will require divided doses because of persistent side effects.

4.   Changing medications. Despite the lack of careful studies, experienced clinicians believe that if a patient does not respond to one class of agents, there is a greater likelihood that he will respond to an agent from another class than to one from the same class.

5.   Compliance and side effects. Due to motoric side effects and sedation, many schizophrenic patients do not like the way their bodies feel on antipsychotic medications. Antipsychotic medication interference with sexual functioning is more common than usually recognized. Proper recognition and management of side effects will contribute to compliance and to having a positive experience on neuroleptic medication. When medications appear to be no longer effective, it is essential to be certain the patient is actually taking the prescribed drug. Liquid concentrate and depot (long-lasting) intramuscular formulations can be useful in these situations.

6.   Education. Many schizophrenic patients are not told that they have schizophrenia. Often the illness is often not explained to them and they are not told what to expect. It is extremely important for the clinician to ask the patient what he believes his diagnosis is and what that means. By empathetically understanding the patient's perspective, one can improve the therapeutic alliance. It is important to emphasize that schizophrenia is a serious condition for which there is no cure, but is not hopeless and will require continued long-term contact with psychiatrists and other mental health professionals.

Therapeutic and Side Effect—How to Choose An Antipsychotic

Biologically active endogenous compounds or exogenous drugs exert many of their effects by binding in a highly specific "lock-and-key" fashion to receptors. Receptors are specialized proteins located on cell surfaces and influence cellular activity. The degree of binding of neuroleptics to receptors in human brain and peripheral tissue explains many of the therapeutic effects and side effects of these drugs. The most relevant studies for comparing and understanding the therapeutic effects and side effects of neuroleptics are from human brain and peripheral tissue binding studies.[5,6]

Many side effects of neuroleptic medications can be understood by their receptor binding profiles. In Tables 23–3 and 23–4, receptor blockade and possible clinical consequences are detailed. Available

TABLE 23–3. SIDE EFFECTS RELATED TO RECEPTOR BLOCKADE

Receptor	Possible Side Effects
D_2 receptor	Extrapyramidal movement disorders (acute dystonias, pseudoparkinsonism)
	Prolactin elevations and subsequent gynecomastia and ovulatory dysfunction
Serotonin S_2 receptor	Sexual dysfunction, ejaculatory and orgasmic disturbances
	Hypotension?
Histamine H_1 receptor	Sedation and drowsiness
	Weight gain?
	Potentiation of alcohol and sedatives
Muscarinic receptor	Blurred vision and dry mouth
	Constipation and urinary retention
	Memory dysfunction
	Sinus tachycardia
	Drowsiness and fatigue
	Erectile dysfunction
α_1 Receptor	Postural hypotension, dizziness
	Reflex tachycardia
	Ejaculatory dysfunction

binding data, however, do not satisfactorily differentiate central and peripheral side effects. The tightness of binding or the affinity can be expressed by the moles of drug needed to block 50 per cent of the receptors. The greater the postsynaptic receptor occupancy by neuroleptics, the greater the blockade of function of that receptor. Table 23–4 is a modified version of Richelson's 1988[5] data such that molar affinities have been converted to the percentage of receptor occupancy expected at the average clinical dose prescribed. This table allows relative comparisons of the receptor profiles of various neuroleptics in dosages that are clinically useful. The average clinical dose is primarily based on clinical studies that have empirically compared different neurolep-

tics in groups of schizophrenic patients,[7] and not from extrapolations from binding studies. The percentage of receptor occupancy from Table 23–4 should be used as a guide in choosing one neuroleptic over another, or in switching neuroleptics to optimally choose a side effect profile that is individualized for a particular patient and his stage of illness. This table does not take into account differences in absorption, presence of active metabolites, or differences in volume of distribution. Extrapolations from in vitro binding to in vivo binding and consequent alterations in neuronal functioning are relative estimates only and do not necessarily imply a one-to-one correspondence.

D_1, D_3, D_4, and D_5 dopamine receptors, sigma, and PCP receptor affinity data have not been included in Table 23–4 because the clinical relevance of binding to these receptors is currently unknown. H_2 And α_2 binding is also excluded. H_2-Receptor blockade results in decreased gastric acid secretion, which is only of clinical significance for thiothixene and chlorpromazine. α_2-Receptor blockade interferes with the antihypertensive effects of clonidine, alpha-methyl dopa, and guanabenz, and is clinically relevant for clozapine, chlorpromazine, and thioridazine because of their strong α_2 affinities.

Antipsychotic efficacy is generally believed to be a function of D_2-receptor blockade. All antipsychotics on Table 23–4 produce greater than 94 per cent D_2-receptor occupancy except for molindone, loxapine, clozapine, and haloperidol. The failure to achieve equivalent in vitro D_2-receptor occupancy with clinically useful doses of antipsychotics suggests that antipsychotic efficacy is not solely due to D_2 blockade. In vivo position emission tomography (PET) brain imaging studies, however, demonstrate 70 to 85 per cent D_2-receptor blockade with all neuroleptics at clinical doses (except clozapine).[8] Clozapine

TABLE 23–4. PERCENTAGE OF RECEPTOR BLOCKADE FOR NEUROLEPTICS AT THE USUALLY PRESCRIBED CLINICAL DOSAGE

	Average Dose	Chlorpromazine Equivalents (mg)	Percentage of Receptor Occupancy				
			D_2	Muscarinic	H_1	α_1	S_2
Phenothiazines							
Aliphatics							
Chlorpromazine	600	100	98	93	99	100	100
Piperazines							
Perphenazine	60	10	98	5	91	89	94
Trifluoperazine	30	5	93	5	36	60	72
Fluphenazine	10–15	2	95	1	40	61	42
Piperidines							
Thioridazine	600	100	97	98	98	99	97
Mesoridazine	300	50	94	82	99	99	99
Thioxanthenes							
Thiothixene	20	3	98	1	82	71	17
Loxapine	75	12.5	57	17	95	78	98
Dibenzodiazepines							
Clozapine	360	60	78	98	100	99	100
Dihydroindolones							
Molindone	50	8–10	43	0	0	4	2
Butyrophenones							
Haloperidol	10–15	2	83	0	1	75	35

has only 40 to 50 per cent D_2 blockade. Molindone and loxapine have not been evaluated with PET. With all neuroleptics, D_2 blockade occurs within a few days, while a full antispychotic response usually requires several weeks. The lag in clinical response is not understood and raises questions regarding the causal link between receptor occupancy and therapeutic efficacy.

There are two types of acetylcholinergic receptors: nicotinic and muscarinic. Central and peripheral muscarinic blockade is relevant to commonly observed neuroleptic side effects. Inspection of Tables 23–3 and 23–4 suggests that side effects due to muscarinic blockade such as memory deficits, blurred vision, urinary hesitancy, and constipation would occur most with clozapine and thioridazine, and least with fluphenazine, thiothixene, molindone, and haloperidol. The affinities could suggest switching from thioridazine to haloperidol in a patient who develops memory disturbances or urinary hesitancy. Conversely, a patient who develops akinesia and shuffling gait with haloperidol may be switched to thioridazine.

Parkinson symptoms are observed when the balance between dopamine and acetylcholine activity in the brain is altered such that D_2 dopamine–receptor blockade is not matched by a corresponding blockade of muscarinic receptors. From Table 23–4, the parkinson symptoms could be reduced by choosing a neuroleptic with more intrinsic muscarinic blockade or a higher muscarinic to D_2 ratio such as thioridazine, or adding an anticholinergic compound such as benztropine (see Table 23–6) or decreasing the dose of haloperidol. Too low a reduction in neuroleptic could result in more psychotic symptoms. Changing to thioridazine could cause more sedation because of its potent H_1 blockade, or postural hypotension and sexual dysfunction because of its strong affinity for the α_1 receptor. Dopamine-acetylcholine balance can also be reestablished by using the dopamine releasing agent, amantadine.

Several clinical cases are provided to familiarize one with use of the Tables. New drugs can be added to Table 23–4, using the equation:

receptor occupancy = Ka
$\times$ (concentration of drug)/1 + Ka
$\times$ (concentration of drug) where Ka is the affinity
and the (concentration of drug)
is dose/molecular weight $\times$ 1/1750 liters.

Receptor profiles of new drugs will aid in anticipating side effects and integrating them into use with current antipsychotics.

Case 1

A 28-year-old Asian male with paranoid delusions is treated with 20 mg of haloperidol. He develops a twisting of his neck, similar to torticollis, which he can momentarily overcome with voluntary effort. He is placed on 4 mg of benztropine, b.i.d. The torticollis disappears, but he develops urinary retention requiring a catheter. Because of urinary retention, he stops his medication, and has difficulty walking without falling. He has lead pipe rigidity of the upper extremities, a fixed facial expression, and dry skin. The questions to be asked are: Why did the torticollis develop? What is responsible for the urinary retention and the emergence of symptoms following stopping his medications?

The diagnosis is that administration of the strong D_2 but weak muscarinic blocking drug haloperidol, caused an imbalance between acetylcholine and dopamine in the central nervous system, leading to the side effect of dystonia. This diagnosis is confirmed by the rapid response to the anticholinergic compound benztropine, which helped restore central acetylcholine dopamine balance; however, the result of benztropine was also to produce too much peripheral anticholinergic activity manifested by the urinary retention. On stopping the medications, the parkinsonian symptoms reappeared, leading to difficulty in walking, lead pipe rigidity, and masked facies. The parkinsonian symptoms appeared because the half-life of benztropine is much shorter than that of haloperidol, so the haloperidol is still exerting D_2 blocking dopamine activity while the benztropine is no longer available to reduce the cholinergic tone commensurate to the dopamine blockade.

The appropriate treatment would be to continue with benztropine, perhaps at 2 mg b.i.d., to use a lower dose of haloperidol, or to switch to medication like thioridazine, which has both dopamine blocking activity and intrinsic anticholinergic activity. It is unusual to see a difference in cholinergic sensitivity between the peripheral and central nervous systems as observed in this case. The patient may require peripheral cholinergic augmentation with a drug like bethanechol (Urecholine) for his urinary retention.

From Table 23–4, the strongest S_2 blockers would be chlorpromazine and clozapine. Ketanserin, an antihypertensive, is a very potent S_2 and alpha$_1$ blocker, and so it is not surprising that hypotension is observed with chlorpromazine. However, clinically, more hypotension is observed with clozapine than with chlorpromazine, suggesting that blockade of a single receptor in isolation without simultaneously considering other receptors effects may be too simplistic in explaining all side effects. Some new agents, Risperidone and Amperozide, are more selective for the S_2 receptor and are reported to have antipsychotic activity.

The simultaneous use of several neuroleptics does not increase efficacy and can produce confusing irrational prescribing; therefore, it cannot be recommended. A rare exception may be the use of a sedative neuroleptic such as chlorpromazine at night combined with a less sedating drug in the morning, such as haloperidol.

Plasma Neuroleptic Concentrations and Clinical Response

It is often assumed that antipsychotic medications have a wide therapeutic index. The measurement of neuroleptic blood levels has been primarily used to determine compliance; however, evidence indicates that a relatively narrow therapeutic window exists for some antipsychotics. Van Putten et al.[9] found a decrease in clinical response in patients with haloperidol levels greater than 12 ng/ml or less than 2 ng/ml. Nonresponders outside the 2- to 12-ng/ml window generally improved when these dosages were either lowered or raised to get them into therapeutic range. Several other studies have also found a curvilinear relationship between plasma haloperidol levels and clinical response with therapeutic windows approximately in the range of 3 to 22 ng/ml. While the evidence for a therapeutic window is most convincing for haloperidol, some literature suggests that this may hold true for other neuroleptics, especially butaperazine.

Alternatives to Neuroleptics

Currently, there is no effective alternative to neuroleptic treatment. Acute exacerbations of psychosis can be effectively treated with electroconvulsive treatment (ECT) especially in patients who have been ill only a few years and have some affective symptoms. Electroconvulsive therapy, however, has a very limited role in the long-term management of schizophrenia. Reserpine, a dopamine depleter, has antipsychotic efficacy, but is difficult to use and has many side effects. Numerous treatments have been suggested by case studies or open trials that have been proven to be ineffective in subsequent double-blind controlled studies. The initial enthusiasm of uncontrolled trials suggest that schizophrenic patients respond to expectations, attention, and a positive therapeutic environment. A reduction of symptoms is observed in 10 to 25 per cent of patients treated with placebo.

The following primary treatments have no greater benefit than placebo: megavitamins, hemodialysis, gluten-free diets, diets free of allergens or food colors, baclofen; antidepressants, fenfluramine, and acupuncture. Treatments that are probably not effective as the primary treatment include: high-dose propranolol, carbamazepine, lithium, alprazolam, endorphins, alpha-methylparatyrosine, methadone, and nalaxone. There are insufficient data to conclude if high-dose diazepam, cholecystokinin (CCK), and phenytoin have a beneficial role in schizophrenia.

Adjunctives to Antipsychotics

Some treatments are useful adjunctives to neuroleptic treatment. Lithium can decrease violent episodes and improve both positive and negative symptoms even in patients without affective symptoms. Carbamazepine can be effective in patients with temporal lobe abnormalities on EEG despite lack of overt seizures and has been reported to decrease aggression. Adjunctive propranolol may decrease assaultive behavior. Recent studies suggest that alprazolam as an adjunctive is not effective in schizophrenia unless the patient also experiences panic attacks. Adjunctive antidepressants can improve social withdrawal and depressive symptoms. In order to institute the appropriate treatment, it is important to distinguish concurrent affective disorder (comorbidity) from negative symptoms, neuroleptic-induced akinesia, demoralization, or an understandable situational reaction to being schizophrenic.

Discontinuing Neuroleptics

Not all patients benefit from neuroleptics. When stopping neuroleptics or when placed on placebo, some patients improve. In most of these patients the improvement is short lived and psychotic decompensation is observed within weeks to months. However, a few schizophrenics derive no positive benefit from neuroleptics and do better without them, apparently because they are free of side effects. There is no clear way to identify such persons, and frequent follow-up is necessary to detect early signs of relapse. There is some evidence, however, that interrupting neuroleptic treatment may create long-lasting difficulties. The longer a patient is psychotic without treatment, the more refractory the illness and the worse the prognosis.[10,11] There is also a suggestion from recent studies that each exacerbation of psychotic behavior becomes increasingly more difficult to treat. Repeated administration of subthreshold doses of dopamine agonists such as amphetamine or cocaine can produce a permanent cumulative effect on behavior (e.g., kindling of seizures in animals). It is possible that the dopamine excess associated with psychosis can similarly sensitize the brain toward progressively more severe psychotic episodes. For patients with two or more episodes of psychosis, continued treatment with antipsychotics is essential. In the latter stages of illness, some chronic schizophrenic patients may no longer require neuroleptic treatment.

How to Begin Treatment

The severity of psychosis and agitation, patient size and age, ethnic background, and concurrent mental illnesses are factors considered in choosing the initial dosage. For high-potency neuroleptics such as haloperidol, 5 or 10 mg can be administered on the first day, often without need for further increase. For low-potency antipsychotics and those most prone to cause sedation or hypotension, a slower titration is recommended. For the first week or two, divided doses may help alleviate side effects until tolerance to those effects develop in most individuals. Dosage to achieve antipsychotic efficacy is not correlated with the development of side effects (e.g., sedation with clozapine usually occurs at a subtherapeutic dose) and production of parkinsonian symptoms is not necessary for a therapeutic response to high-potency antipsychotics. Clozapine treatment is recommended to begin at 25 to 50 mg the first day, with a subsequent very slow titration due to the high incidence of hypotension and sedation, to which tolerance usually develops. In the authors' experience, however, many of the early side effects are paradoxically decreased by a rapid titration. For all neuroleptics, a slower titration schedule should be considered for the elderly and those of Asian ancestry because of their increased sensitivity to side effects.

Treatment of Acute Psychosis in Schizophrenia

The onset of action of antipsychotic medication is generally between 10 and 14 days. One question that arises is: How should an acutely psychotic and often agitated patient be managed during the first 2 weeks of treatment? Treatment of an acutely psychotic patient should be adjusted to prevent harm to the individual and others as well as to decrease subjective distress. The use of seclusion and restraint should be minimized or eliminated, if possible. The lowest effective dose of neuroleptic should be used to decrease the short- and long-term side effects of these medications.

Rapid neuroleptization, the use of high doses of antipsychotic medication, during the first few weeks of treatment of acute psychosis has been a common practice. The efficacy of rapid neuroleptization, however, is not supported by clinical evidence. A 10-day double-blind study of acutely ill schizophrenics failed to show any difference in clinical benefit between those receiving gradually increasing doses of haloperidol up to 100 mg/day at 5 and 10 days versus those receiving 10 mg/day for the entire 10 days.[12] In a review, Baldessarini et al.[13] concludes that doses of neuroleptic in excess of 500 to 600 mg of chlorpromazine equivalents in the first days or weeks of treatment does not add further clinical benefit regarding antipsychotic effects. Recently, Rifkin et al.[14] treated a group of 87 schizophrenics in a 6-week double-blind study using 10, 30, or 80 mg of haloperidol per day. The results revealed no significant difference in clinical outcome between groups. Thus, doses greater than 10 mg/day provided no additional benefit to treating schizophrenic exacerbations.

Although clinical research does not support the practice of rapid neuroleptization, how can an acutely psychotic agitated patient best be treated when moderate doses of neuroleptic are initially unable to manage combative behavior? There is some evidence that treatment with a benzodiazepine alone is just as effective in the first 24 hours as haloperi-

dol.[15] Perhaps early improvement in symptoms is due to sedation rather than antipsychotic effects of medications. The use of sedative medications adjunctly with neuroleptics can often prove invaluable. Sedating a patient early in the treatment process can allow time for neuroleptic medication to take effect. Sedatives should be tapered when psychotic agitation resolves. Barbituates are effective sedatives, but they induce microsomal enzymes, often leading to tolerance within a few days. Benzodiazepines are as effective and have a more benign side effect profile. A double-blind study of 24 disorganized, acutely ill schizophrenics compared a combination of haloperidol and clonazepam versus haloperidol and placebo over 4 weeks.[16] No difference was found between groups in the final clinical outcome; however, those treated with clonazepam had a significant decrease in psychotic excitement along with less extrapyramidal symptoms (EPS) and required a lower dosage of anticholinergic medications. Along with clonazepam (Klonopin), lorazepam (Ativan) is frequently used to control psychotic agitation and has the advantage of an intramuscular formulation. Recent evidence indicates that midazolam (Versed), a short-acting benzodiazepine with a rapid onset of action (approximately 15 minutes), is just as effective and might be preferred for acute emergencies in patients not yet fully evaluated, although the currently available parenteral formulations are highly concentrated and can lead to inadvertent overdosing.

As-needed (p.r.n.) doses of neuroleptic may be given to patients by clinicians who mistake akathisia for an increase in psychotic agitation. Giving more neuroleptic in the form of a p.r.n. can further exacerbate the akathisia and may lead to a cycle of increased frequency of p.r.n.'s and unnecessary increases in routine antipsychotic medication. Patients on adequate doses of routine neuroleptic should receive benzodiazepine p.r.n.'s if needed and neuroleptic p.r.n.'s should be avoided. Another possible approach to control psychotic agitation without resorting to high neuroleptic doses is to initially treat patients with sedating low-potency neuroleptics such as chlorpromazine or thioridazine. These neuroleptics combine antipsychotic properties with intrinsic sedation, probably because of their potent H_1 blockade. After the acute psychosis is controlled, patients can be switched to a neuroleptic with a different affinity profile (Table 23–4) if side effects continue to be a problem.

Side Effects

Antipsychotic medications induce a number of side effects. The most common are referred to as EPS because the effects take place in the striatum and not in the descending voluntary pyramidal or corticospinal tracts. Extrapyramidal symptoms are due to postsynaptic blockade of striatal dopamine receptors, resulting in an imbalance of dopamine and acetylcholine. High-potency antipsychotics, such as halo-peridol and fluphenazine, are more likely to cause EPS than low-potency antipsychotics such as chlorpromazine and thioridazine. This is because of the very low muscarinic receptor occupancy relative to D_2-receptor occupancy of these high-potency drugs in contrast to the greater muscarinic relative to D_2-receptor occupancy of the lower-potency antipsychotics (see Table 23–4).

Types of EPS include acute dystonic reactions, parkinsonian syndrome, and akathisia (Table 23–5). Acute dystonic reactions can be very disturbing and frightening. Dystonic reactions usually occur within the first hours to days and are especially common in young males. A dystonic reaction is a sustained contraction of the muscles of the neck, mouth, or tongue. Dystonic reactions can also manifest as spasms and distortions of the back (opisthotonos) or extraocular muscles with the eyes elevated and fixed in position (oculogyric crisis). With voluntary effort, the dystonic reactions can be briefly overcome. Dystonic reactions are frequently misdiagnosed as hysteria or tetany.

Antipsychotic drug–induced parkinsonian syndrome is clinically similar to classic idiopathic Parkinson's disease, with mask-like facies, cogwheel rigidity, motor retardation, and shuffling gait. Tremor at rest is less frequent than with idiopathic Parkinson's syndrome. A parkinsonian syndrome is usually of slower onset than an acute dystonic reaction, generally occurring after weeks of antipsychotic treatment.

Akathisia (ants-in-the-pants syndrome) presents as subjective feelings of restlessness and a need to pace. The patient has difficulty sitting still and may express feelings of anxiety and tension. It is often misdiagnosed as agitation or increased psychosis. Akathisia typically appears within the first weeks of antipsychotic treatment, but may occur anytime during the course of treatment.

Case 2

A large 32-year-old black male is placed on 30 mg of haloperidol because of paranoid ideation and hearing voices. The patient is initially withdrawn, but constantly speaks to voices. Two days later, he is aggressively pacing up and down the hall but only occasionally shouting at people. He is viewed as threatening and requested by staff to sit still. The patient refuses and is placed in seclusion and restraints. The neuroleptic dose is increased to 50 mg

of haloperidol. At 50 mg, the voices lessen but the patient looks more agitated and hostile. What is the diagnosis?

In this case the patient's akathisia, which developed after haloperidol treatment, was misdiagnosed as psychotic agitation. Because of the patient's imposing size and fear of potential violence, his need to pace was misinterpreted as psychotic agitation and the haloperidol dosage was increased. The patient was unable to voluntarily control his pacing and ended up in restraints. This diagnosis is supported by the observation that as the agitation increased, the hallucinations decreased. On a decreased dose of medication of 10 mg of haloperidol, the voices continued to abate, and the akathisia was much less severe.

The first choice for treatment of EPS is consideration of antipsychotic dose reduction. Extrapyramidal symptoms are most frequently treated with anticholinergic drugs to reestablish the dopamine acetylcholine balance. For acute dystonia, immediate relief is obtained with 2 mg of benztropine intramuscularly or other parenteral anticholinergics. Prescribed doses are listed in Table 23–6. These are usually prescribed in divided doses because of short half-lives (6 to 12 hours). Extrapyramidal symptoms usually are not troublesome when sleeping, so an h.s. dose may not be required. Amantadine, a dopamine agonist, in doses of 200 to 300 mg/day, is also effective. The concomitant neuroleptic prevents the dopamine agonism from exacerbating the psychosis. Akathisia often does not respond to anticholinergic medications. Propranolol in doses from 30 to 120 mg/day in divided doses is often effective.

As previously mentioned, low-potency antipsychotics are less likely to result in EPS because they have more intrinsic anticholinergic properties (see Table 23–4). Addition of anticholinergics to these antipsychotics should be undertaken cautiously, since cumulative adverse anticholinergic effects may occur. Adverse peripheral anticholinergic effects include dry mouth, blurred vision, constipation, and urinary hesitancy (see Table 23–3). A severe central anticholinergic reaction can develop with confusion.

TABLE 23–5. MOST FREQUENT TEMPORAL DEVELOPMENT OF NEUROLEPTIC-INDUCED MOVEMENT ABNORMALITIES

Acute dystonia—hours to days
Parkinsonism—days to weeks
Akathisia—weeks to months
Tardive dyskinesia—months to years

TABLE 23–6. MEDICATION FOR EPS IN MG/DAY USUALLY PRESCRIBED b.i.d. OR t.i.d. BECAUSE OF RELATIVELY SHORT HALF-LIVES

Medication	Proprietary Name	Dose (mg/day)
Anticholinergic		
Benztropine	Cogentin	2–6
Trihexyphenidyl	Artane[a]	4–15
Biperiden	Akineton	2–8
Diphenhydramine (also potent H_1 antagonist)	Benadryl	50–300
Dopamine releasing		
Amantadine	Symmetrel[a]	100–300

[a] Not available as parenteral formulations.

The syndrome may include dry flushed skin and confusion ("dry as a bone, red as a beet, and mad as a hatter"), tachycardia, and dilated pupils. The elderly are more susceptible to combinations that produce adverse anticholinergic effects and to α_1-mediated hypotension.

Case 3

> A 30-year-old patient stopped taking his haloperidol 10 mg/day and benztropine 2 mg/day b.i.d. yesterday and now complains of stiffness and a twisted neck. Why did he develop motor symptoms? What is the appropriate treatment?

The patient was taking haloperidol and benztropine with the net effect of decreasing both dopamine and acetylcholine transmission comparably so no movement abnormalities occurred. The half-life of haloperidol is more than 18 hours, while that of benztropine is approximately 8 hours. When the medications were stopped, benztropine disappeared from the system much quicker than haloperidol. In the new balance, the dopaminergic blocking activity of the still present haloperidol was not compensated for by the benztropine. The appropriate treatment would be to reinstitute benztropine for several days.

Case 4

> A 65-year-old female patient with a 40-year history of schizophrenia is taking 300 mg of chlorpromazine at night and 2 mg of trihexyphenidyl (Artane) b.i.d. She has taken these medications for at least 10 years and has been relatively stable living in a board and care. She is admitted because of difficulty sleeping and social withdrawal. A diagnosis of depression is made, and she is placed on doxepin 100 mg q.h.s. Doxepin was chosen because of its strong sedating effects. Two days later she becomes confused and does not know where she is. She is agitated and has a pulse of 120. What caused her deterioration in mental state?

The patient was chronically maintained on two potent anticholinergic drugs chlorpromazine and trihexyphenidyl. Following the addition of a strong anticholinergic antidepressant, she develops central anticholinergic syndrome characterized by confusion and tachycardia, dry mouth, and hot dry skin. Management should include discontinuing the trihexyphenidyl and considering using less anticholinergic neuroleptics such as fluphenazine, thiothixene, or haloperidol, and less anticholinergic antidepressants such as trazodone or bupropion. Trazodone is very sedating and lacks cholinergic activity. To confirm the diagnosis, 0.5 mg of physostigmine was given intravenously. The delirium cleared in 10 minutes but reoccurred several hours later because of physostigmine's short half-life. This situation could have been prevented if the total anticholinergic load

was considered before choosing an antidepressant or prescribing trihexyphenidyl. Loss of cholinergic receptors as a function of aging is an additional important consideration in this case.

A controversy exists over using antiparkinsonian agents prophylactically or only with the occurrence of EPS.[17] Arguments in favor of waiting include the fact that many patients never develop EPS, possible anticholinergic side effects (described above), and abuse potential (especially trihexyphenidyl). Other concerns include adding another medication and cost. Distress from EPS argues in favor of starting anticholinergics immediately for prophylaxis. Extrapyramidal symptoms can jeopardize medication compliance and doctor-patient rapport. When patients report being "allergic" to medication, they usually are referring to acute EPS. Further, some aspects of EPS are subtle and difficult to diagnose yet troublesome to the patient. Since some patients are at high risk of developing EPS, and since future compliance and therapy may be jeopardized, a case-by-case decision is appropriate. This would include determining if anticholinergics are contraindicated (e.g., enlarged prostate which already compromises urination, acute-angle glaucoma) or if a patient is at high risk for development of EPS (e.g., male under 45 years, Asian ancestry). A p.r.n. order should be included when prophylactic anticholinergic treatment is not used. A decision to taper and discontinue anticholinergic medications can be made after 4 weeks to 6 months of concomitant use of anipsychotic and anticholinergic medications. Despite evidence that continued antiparkinsonian treatment is unnecessary for most patients, once anticholinergics are started, they unfortunately are usually continued indefinitely.

Neuroleptic Malignant Syndrome

Neuroleptic malignant syndrome (NMS) is a relatively uncommon disorder associated with the use of antipsychotic medications, occurring with a frequency between 0.02 and 2.4 per cent.[18] The etiology remains an enigma. Classic manifestations include hyperthermia (38°C), severe muscle rigidity, confusion, and autonomic instability. Any of these in isolation or combination should raise a high level of suspicion in an individual taking antipsychotic medication. Laboratory tests to further assist in making a diagnosis of NMS include an elevation in creatine phosphokinase (CPK) (greater than 1,000 units/ml) and leukocytosis. The mortality rate associated with NMS has been reported as high as 10 per cent; therefore, treatment in an intensive care unit may be required. Antipsychotic medication should be immediately discontinued and supportive treatment initiated. Bromocriptine, amantadine, and dantrolene are effective treatments for NMS. Reinstitution of antipsychotic medication with a drug from a different class can be considered, if necessary, after resolution of the NMS, although NMS can reoccur.

Tardive Dyskinesia

Patients treated long term with neuroleptics can develop involuntary repetitive, rhythmic, purposeless movements. These movements most commonly include the mouth, tongue, and cheek. Chewing, puckering, grimacing, or tongue darting or twisting movements are most often observed. Involvement of other body parts including piano-playing movements of the fingers or toes, and trunk twisting can be seen. It can be difficult to distinguish these movements from schizophrenic stereotypies and mannerisms. Tardive dyskinesia (TD) symptoms are increased by anxiety or a distracting task, can be voluntarily suppressed for a short time, and are absent during sleep. The incidence is not clearly known, but well-controlled data[3] suggest 3 per cent new cases per year, although not everyone will develop TD. Most cases are mild and not noticed by the patient, family, or friends. Only 25 per cent of those with TD have symptoms that cause social or physical dysfunction. All neuroleptics appear to be equal in their capacity to cause TD, with the exception of clozapine. Clozapine rarely causes TD, if at all. The duration of treatment with neuroleptics rather than the total dose of neuroleptic is probably more important in producing TD. The only way to prevent TD is not to use neuroleptics. This must be considered and discussed with the patient and family when intending to treat a patient for more than 6 months with neuroleptics.

There is no effective treatment for TD. Most cases remit after stopping neuroleptics, but this is frequently impossible because of psychotic relapse. Fortunately, TD is not necessarily progressive, even with continued neuroleptic treatment. The best advice is to use the lowest dose of neuroleptic possible and only in cases where there is clear benefit such as schizophrenia, and very sparingly in other disorders such as affective disorder, dementia, mental retardation, and anxiety.

Prevention of Tardive Dyskinesia

Some authors suggest that periodically removing patients from neuroleptic drugs might help prevent TD similar to every-other-day use of prednisone. This suggestion is not supported by the literature. Patients with drug holidays of several months had more irreversible tardive dyskinesia than those without holidays.[19]

Other Side Effects and Considerations

Clozapine is unusual in causing sialorrhea. It has a high incidence of dose-related seizures, and weight gain. Weekly monitoring of neutrophils is required because of the approximate 1 per cent incidence of agranulocytosis associated with its use. Clozapine is currently approved only for treatment of schizophrenia when standard antipsychotic treatments have failed due to lack of efficacy or occurrence of severe side effects. Clozapine has the lowest incidence of EPS and may not cause TD. Prevailing theory is inconsistent with the co-occurrence of tardive dyskinesia and EPS; however, about 20 per cent of the time both conditions are observed simultaneously. Antipsychotic medication has also been associated with cardiovascular effects (increased heart rate and conduction delays), lowering seizure threshold (especially clozapine), hematological suppression (agranulocytosis), skin rash and pigmentary changes, ocular changes (retinitis pigmentosa with high-dose thioridazine), cholestatic jaundice (especially chlorpromazine), weight gain, reduced libido, and sexual dysfunction. D_2 blockade in the pituitary elevates prolactin and can cause amenorrhea, gynecomastia, and galactorrhea. Clozapine is unique in not elevating prolactin. Neuroleptics should be used only when indicated during pregnancy, but are relatively safe to the fetus. There are no human data indicating teratogenesis, although animal data suggest the possibility of some teratogenesis. While abrupt discontinuation of neuroleptic drugs does not produce a formal withdrawal syndrome, a few cases of nausea, vomiting, diarrhea, insomnia, or nightmares of several days duration have been reported.

Maintenance Therapy

Once a patient has recovered from a psychotic episode, it is not known how long to continue antipsychotic treatment. Even with the continuation of antipsychotic treatment, 30 to 40 per cent of patients may experience a relapse. It is sometimes difficult to determine if the patient becomes ill after stopping their medication or becomes ill and then stops medication. However, approximately 70 per cent of patients without prophylactic neuroleptics relapse over a 1-year period. The risk of developing TD must be considered in weighing the decision for prophylactic treatment.

For first-episode patients, continued antipsychotic treatment following remission should continue for a year before considering a trial off medication. For patients with more than one psychotic episode, continued maintenance treatment is indicated. Dosage reduction during maintenance has been reported to have some benefits (e.g., patients may feel better and have fewer side effects), although there is some increased risk of relapse at doses less than 300 mg/day of chlorpromazine equivalents. Some advocate use of neuroleptics only with the reoccurrence of psychotic symptoms. Recent findings of this targeted treatment dosage strategy suggest a higher incidence of relapse.[20,21]

Depot Neuroleptics

The use of long-acting injectable neuroleptics has become an integral part of maintenance treatment with many schizophrenics. Fluphenazine enanthate and decanoate and haloperidol decanoate are currently the only available preparations in the United States; however, foreign psychiatrists can choose from a larger selection. Depot neuroleptics insure greater compliance than oral preparations and avoid problems with gastric absorption. The side effects from depot neuroleptics are similar to oral preparations, but the incidence of severe akinesia can be high in patients receiving large doses. Several diverse formulae are available to convert from oral fluphenazine and haloperidol to depot; however, our approach is to begin with 12.5 to 50 mg of fluphenazine every 3 weeks or 50 to 100 mg of haloperidol every 4 weeks and carefully follow.

PSYCHOSOCIAL TREATMENT OF SCHIZOPHRENIA

The use of antipsychotic medication is clearly superior to psychotherapy in the treatment of schizophrenia. This does not mean, however, that psychotherapy or other psychosocial treatments are not valuable components of an overall treatment approach. Insight-oriented psychotherapies have been shown to be no more beneficial than supportive treatments.[22] Psychoanalytic or insight-oriented psychotherapy can be counterproductive and is inappropriate in the treatment of most persons with schizophrenia. Two psychosocial treatments that consistently improve outcome when combined with drug therapy are family therapy and social skills training.

Schizophrenic persons are not indifferent to their physical and social environment. The emotional climate of the family has been shown to play an important role in the relapse of schizophrenia. Vaughn and Leff[23] observed that schizophrenic patients who returned home to environments in which there are high levels of negative emotional attitudes (high expressed emotion), experienced a 51 per cent relapse rate after 9 months, compared to 13 per cent of those returning to low-expressed-emotion homes. High expressed emotion refers to the number of critical comments about a schizophrenic person or instances of infantilizing or emotional overinvolvement by care takers. Treating patients from high-expressed-emotion environments with family therapy along with medication produced a significant decline in relapse rate compared to those treated with medication and individual therapy.[24]

Group therapy in the form of social skills training can also significantly decrease schizophrenic relapse. Some goals of social skills training are to teach coping strategies, to improve socialization and vocational skills, and to establish a therapeutic alliance in which a patient is able to effectively communicate about important aspects of treatment such as medication side effects. A study[25] that combined social skills training with family therapy revealed an additive effect in decreasing relapse when both treatments were administered. Family therapy combined with medication, and social skills training combined with medication, both had lower incidences of relapse than medication alone. The combination of family therapy and social skills decreased relapse even further. In summary, the effectiveness of pharmacological treatment can be enhanced by psychosocial intervention and should be part of the treatment of all persons with schizophrenia.

ACKNOWLEDGMENTS

The authors wish to thank E. Richelson for his useful discussions on receptor affinities and side effects; and to M. Zona, and L. Plon for their helpful comments regarding ideas expressed in this manuscript; and C. Hsueh, C. Aurang, and A.L. Gamido for their technical assistance in preparing this manuscript.

REFERENCES

1. Buchanan RW, Kirkpatrick B, Heinrichs DW, et al: Clinical correlates of the deficit syndrome of schizophrenia. Am J Psychiatry 147(3):290–294, 1990.
2. Kane J, Honigfeld G, Singer J, et al: Clozapine for the treatment-resistant schizophrenic: A double-blind comparison with chlorpromazine. Arch Gen Psychiatry 45:789–796, 1988.
3. Caldwell CB, Gottesman II: Schizophrenics kill themselves too: A review of risk factors for suicide. Schizophr Bull 16(4):571–589, 1990.
4. Gottesman II, Bertelsen A: Confirming unexpressed genotypes for schizophrenia. Arch Gen Psychiatry 46:867–872, 1989.
5. Richelson E: Neuroleptic binding to human brain receptors: Relation to clinical effects. Ann NY Acad Sci 537:435–442, 1988.
6. Seeman P: Dopamine receptors and the dopamine hypothesis of schizophrenia. Synapse:133–152, 1987.
7. Davis JM: Comparative doses and costs of antipsychotic medication. Arch Gen Psychiatry 33:858–861, 1976.
8. Sedvall G: PET imaging of dopamine receptors in human basal ganglia: Relevance to mental illness. Trends Neurosci 13(7):302–308, 1990.
9. Van Putten T, Marder SR, Wirshing W, et al: Neuroleptic plasma levels in treatment-resistant schizophrenic patients. In Angrist B, Schultz C, eds. The Neuroleptic-Nonresponsive Patient: Characterization and Treatment. Washington, DC: American Psychiatric Press, Inc, 1990:69–85.
10. Crow TJ, McMillan JF, Johnson AL, et al: The Northwick Park Study of first episodes of schizophrenia: II. A randomized controlled trial of prophylactic neuroleptic treatment. Br J Psychiatry 148:120–127, 1986.
11. May PRA: Treatment of Schizophrenia: A Comparative Study of Five Treatment Methods. New York: Science House, 1968.
12. Donlon PT, Hopkin JT, Tupin JP, et al: Haloperidol for acute schizophrenic patients. Arch Gen Psychiatry 37:691–695, 1980.
13. Baldessarini RJ, Cohen BM, Teicher MH: Significance of neuroleptic dose and plasma level in the pharmacological treatment of psychoses. Arch Gen Psychiatry 45:79–91, 1988.
14. Rifkin A, Doddi S, Karajgi B, et al: Dosage of haloperidol for schizophrenia. Arch Gen Psychiatry 48:166–170, 1991.
15. Lerner Y, Lwow E, Levitin A, et al: Acute high-dose paren-

    teral haloperidol treatment of psychosis. Am J Psychiatry 136:1061–1064, 1979.

16. Altamura AC, Mauri MC, Mantero M, et al: Clonazepam/haloperidol combination therapy in schizophrenia: A double blind study. Acta Psychiatr Scand 76:702–706, 1987.

17. Lake RC, Casey DE, McEvoy JP, et al: The "pros" and "cons" of anticholinergic prophylaxis. Psychopharmacol Bull 22:981–984, 1986.

18. Caroff SN, Mann SC, Lazarus A, et al: Neuroleptic malignant syndrome: Diagnostic issues. Psychiatr Ann 21:130–147, 1991.

19. Jeste DV, Potkin SG, Sinha S, et al: Tardive dyskinesia: Reversible and persistent. Arch Gen Psychiatry 36:585–590, 1979.

20. Herz MI, Glazer WM, Mostert MA, et al: Intermittent vs maintenance medication in schizophrenia. Arch Gen Psychiatry 48:333–339, 1991.

21. Carpenter WT, Hanlon TE, Heinrichs DW, et al: Continuous versus targeted medication in schizophrenic outpatients: Outcome results. Am J Psychiatry 147(9):1138–1148, 1990.

22. Gunderson JG, Frank AF, Katz HM, et al: Effects of psychotherapy in schizophrenia. II. Comparative outcome of two forms of treatment. Schizophr Bull 10:564–598, 1984.

23. Vaughn CE, Leff JP: The influence of family and social factors on the course of psychiatric illness. Br J Psychiatry 129:125–137, 1976.

24. Falloon IR, Boyd JL, McGill CW, et al: Family management in the prevention of exacerbations of schizophrenia. N Engl J Med 306:1437–1440, 1982.

25. Hogarty GE, Anderson CM, Reiss DJ, et al: Family psychoeducation, social skills training, and maintenance chemotherapy in the aftercare treatment of schizophrenia. Arch Gen Psychiatry 43:633–642, 1986.

24

PARANOID DISORDER:
Clinical Features and Treatment

ALAN BREIER, M.D.

The roots of the modern concept of paranoid disorder can be traced to the early Greeks. As reviewed by Lewis,[1] the term "paranoia" was used by the Greeks in a general sense to denote craziness. Although Hippocrates referred to the delirium accompanying fevers as paranoia, the concept was not considered a technical diagnostic entity until the nineteenth century. In 1863, Kahlbaum[2] used the term paranoia for a disease that was characterized by delusions that were persistent and unchanging throughout the course of the illness. Emil Kraepelin[3] also viewed paranoia as a separate entity, differentiating it from dementia praecox, paraphrenia, and manic-depressive insanity. In Kraepelin's schema, paranoia was characterized by persistent delusions, lack of hallucinations, preservation of the personality, and a nondeteriorating course of illness. In contrast, dementia praecox was characterized by early age of onset and mental deterioration, paraphrenia by the presence of prominent hallucinations, and manic-depressive because of its primary mood component. Other twentieth century theorists disagreed with the view that paranoia was a separate disease entity. Freud,[4] Schneider,[5] and Kolle,[6] considered paranoia to be a form of schizophrenia, whereas Specht[7] believed paranoia was a subtype of affective illness.

The concept of paranoia and the separateness of paranoid disorder as a discrete psychotic illness are still somewhat controversial today. The lack of agreement about paranoid disorder has led to a range of definitions and terms including delusional disorder, simple delusional disorder, monosymptomatic psychosis, paranoid personality disorder, paranoia, and paranoid psychosis. However, recent data from descriptive, course-of-illness, and genetic studies support the view that paranoid disorder is a distinct diagnostic entity, a view which is reflected in DSM-III-R's description of delusional (paranoid) disorder.

In this chapter, the clinical features and treatment of paranoid disorder are discussed. First, the phenomenology, demography, course of illness, and genetics will be reviewed. Then, issues relevant to the differential diagnosis will be discussed. Lastly, the pharmacotherapy and psychological therapy of paranoid disorder is examined.

CLINICAL FEATURES

Phenomenology

The core phenomenological feature of DSM-III-R paranoid disorder is a persistent delusion in the absence of organic factors initiating or maintaining the disorder and other psychiatric illnesses, such as schizophrenia and mood disorder, which could be the primary cause of the delusions. The delusions must persist for a minimum of 1 month and are most commonly persistent for several years. Also, accompanying hallucinations are unusual. When hallucinations occur, they are not a prominent part of the clinical picture. The so-called negative symptoms (e.g., flat affect, poverty of speech, lack of social drive) common to subgroups of schizophrenic patients are uncommon in paranoid disorder. However, paranoid patients may exhibit social isolation secondary to suspiciousness. Generally, patients with paranoid disorder have one delusional theme as opposed to multiple delusions. According to DSM-III-R, patients with paranoid disorder are classified according to the theme of their delusion (Table 24–1). The types of delusions recognized by DSM-III-R are erotomanic, grandiose, jealous, persecutory, and somatic. The DSM-III-R stresses that the delusions in paranoid disorder must not be bizarre, which means that they involve situations that could occur in real life, such as being followed, poisoned, having a disease, and being deceived by a family member.

Demography

As noted above, the concept of paranoia has been in use for hundreds of years, but it was not until relatively recently that the basic demographic features of the illness came to light. Kendler[8] reviewed available epidemiology and sociodemographic data

TABLE 24–1.   DSM-III-R SUBTYPES OF DELUSIONAL (PARANOID) DISORDER

Erotomanic type
  Delusional disorder in which the predominant theme of the delusion(s) is that a person, usually of higher status, is in love with the subject
Grandiose type
  Delusional disorder in which the predominant theme of the delusion(s) is one of inflated worth, power, knowledge, identity, or special relationship to a deity or famous person
Jealous type
  Delusional disorder in which the predominant theme of the delusion(s) is that one's sexual partner is unfaithful
Persecutory type
  Delusional disorder in which the predominant theme of the delusion(s) is that one (or someone to whom one is close) is being malevolently treated in some way; people with this type of delusional disorder may repeatedly take their complaints of being mistreated to legal authorities
Somatic type
  Delusional disorder in which the predominant theme of the delusion(s) is that the person has some physical defect, disorder, or disease
Unspecified type
  Delusional disorder that does not fit any of the previous categories (e.g., persecutory and grandiose themes without a predominance of either), delusions of reference without malevolent content

of patients with paranoid disorder and compared this information with patients with affective illness and schizophrenia.

Paranoid disorder constitutes between 1 and 4 per cent of all psychiatric admissions, and between 2 and 7 per cent of all psychotic admissions.[8] Two psychiatric population surveys[9,10] indicate that the prevalence of paranoid disorder is 24/100,000 and 30/100,000, respectively. It appears that approximately 25 per cent of patients with paranoid disorder are in active treatment at any given point in time.[8] Although available data from clinic surveys suggest paranoid disorder is a relatively rare illness, it is possible that it is more common than previously thought. A substantial number of paranoid disorder patients may be outside of the mental health system and therefore do not appear in incidence and prevalence studies using psychiatric clinic records.

The majority of studies indicate that the peak age of first psychiatric admission is between 40 and 49 years of age.[8] This is substantially older than age of first admission for schizophrenia and, depending on the sample characteristics, is moderately older than first admissions for affective illness. It should be noted that age of first admission is not a precise reflection of age of onset. This issue may be particularly relevant to paranoid disorder because onset may be insidious and the course of illness appears to be less severe than some psychotic illnesses such as schizophrenia so that patients may delay their first psychiatric contact. Thus, it is likely that actual onset may predate first psychiatric admission by a substantial time period for many patients. With regard to gender distribution, the majority of studies indicate a greater preponderance of females with paranoid disorder, with an average ratio of 55 per cent females to 45 per cent males affected.[8] This is contrasted with a relatively even gender distribution for schizophrenia and a greater female preponderance for affective illness. An analysis of marital status from seven first-admission studies revealed that only 32 per cent of paranoid disorder patients had never married, a rate that is similar to affectively ill patients and far less than found among schizophrenic patients.[8] The relatively high marital rate may be because of the later onset of the illness.

In summary, the available demographic data demonstrates that paranoid disorder does not closely resemble either schizophrenia or affective illness. Thus, these data support the relative diagnostic separateness of this illness.

Course of Illness

Opjordsmoen[11] reported the results of a comparative long-term outcome study of 301 first-admission patients who had delusions as a prominent feature of their illnesses. The DSM-III diagnoses of the sample were paranoid disorder (N = 53), schizophrenia (N = 94), schizophreniform disorder (N = 47), schizoaffective disorder (N = 35), major affective disorder (N = 54), and other (N = 18). After a mean follow-up period of 30 years, it was clear that schizophrenic patients had the poorest outcomes and affective disorder patients had the best outcomes. Patients with paranoid disorder and the other psychotic illness had outcomes between schizophrenia and affective disorder. Eighty per cent of paranoid disorder patients had married, and 52 per cent were employed, which indicates relatively good functional levels. Fifty-five per cent of paranoid disorder patients were receiving no treatment and 27 per cent were being seen by nonpsychiatric practitioners, which supports the notion that the majority of paranoid disorder patients may be outside the mental health system. Available data indicates that paranoid disorder runs a stable, unremitting course.

Family History

There is presently a paucity of data about the familial transmission of paranoid disorder. Winokur[12] examined the prevalence of psychopathology in the families of 29 patients with simple delusional disorder (i.e., paranoid disorder with exclusionary criteria for hallucinations) and the families of 29 age- and sex-matched mixed psychiatric patient controls. He found significant differences between the groups when personality traits consisting of suspiciousness, jealousy, secretiveness, and delusions were combined with greater levels of these characteristics in the delusional disorder families.

Family studies have been used to examine the relationship between paranoid disorder and other psychiatric illness, particularly schizophrenia and affective illness. Using a rediagnosed sample of the Danish adoption study, Kendler and colleagues[13] failed to find an increased prevalence of paranoid disorder in family members of schizophrenics. In another study comparing family members of schizophrenics and paranoid disorder, Kendler and Hays[14] again failed to find increased prevalences of schizophrenia in the paranoid cohort, although there was increased prevalences of schizophrenia among the schizophrenic family members. In addition, affective illness was equally uncommon among paranoid and schizophrenic relatives. Thus, these studies provide genetic support for the diagnostic separation of paranoid disorder from schizophrenia and affective illness.

DIFFERENTIAL DIAGNOSIS

The differential diagnosis of paranoid disorder generally involves ruling out specific psychiatric, neurological, and metabolic/endocrine illnesses. The psychiatric illnesses that can mimic paranoid disorder include schizophrenia, mood disorder with psychotic features, and substance abuse syndromes. Schizophrenia is characterized by prominent hallucinations, bizarre delusions, and formal thought disorder. Paranoid disorder encompasses nonbizarre delusions, and hallucinations and formal thought disorder are not prominent. In addition, the age of onset of schizophrenia is typically in the second and third decades, whereas the age of onset for paranoid disorder tends to be in the fourth and fifth decades. Perhaps the most challenging differential involves ruling out mood disorder with psychotic features. This illness often has nonbizarre delusions without prominent hallucinations and formal thought disorder. The critical issue in differentiating mood disorder with psychosis from paranoid disorder is the prominence and temporal relationship of the mood syndrome. Depressive features may be a component of paranoid disorder but if they occur, are not prominent and occur after the onset of paranoid disorder. In contrast, in a primary mood disorder, the affective component is prominent and usually occurs prior to the onset of psychotic features. With regard to substance abuse syndromes, amphetamine, alcohol, and cocaine abuse are the most common disorders that may produce a syndrome similar to paranoid disorder.

A large number of neurological and metabolic/endocrine disorders should be considered in the differential diagnosis of paranoid disorder. For example, monosymptomatic delusions can be the initial presentation for some dementing illnesses including Huntington's, Alzheimer's, and Pick's diseases. Brain tumors can also present a clinical picture that resembles paranoid disorder. Metabolic/endocrine/autoimmune disorders to be included in the differential are thyroid disturbances, hypopituitarism, uremia, Addison's disease, and central nervous system (CNS) lupus. Additional neurological, metabolic, and endocrine disorders that have delusions as part of their clinical pictures have been reviewed.[15]

TREATMENT

There is a glaring lack of information in the scientific literature regarding the treatment of paranoid disorder. In fact, we were unable to find any published reports of double-blind, clinical trials of patients with paranoid disorder. Consequently, it has been necessary to extract principles of treatment from strategies that have proven efficacy in related disorders and apply them to paranoid disorder. However, pending the necessary double-blind studies, it is unclear if treatment experience gleaned from related illnesses are generalizable to paranoid disorder patients.

Pharmacotherapy

The mainstay of treatment for psychosis are the neuroleptic drugs. There is unequivocal evidence that neuroleptics are superior to placebo for the treatment of delusions. The majority of data about the efficacy of neuroleptic drugs comes from studies of schizophrenic patients and, as stated above, the extent of the generalizability of these data to paranoid disorder patients is unknown. There are data, however, about the use of neuroleptics in paranoid disorder from open-labeled studies and case reports.

Munro[16] reported an open treatment trial of pimozide for 26 patients with "monosymptomatic hypochondriacal psychosis," an illness comparable to DSM-III-R paranoid disorder, somatic type. Pimozide was administered in dosages that ranged from 2 to 12 mg/day. He found that 19 patients (63 per cent) had an "excellent" response with a complete or near complete remission of symptoms and a satisfactory return to full social functioning. Improvement was generally seen during the first week of treatment. An additional seven patients (23 per cent) had a "fair" response characterized by partial improvements in social functioning. The patients were followed-up 6 months to 4.5 years later and found that all but three patients still required active pimozide treatment.[16] Because pimozide has not been compared with other neuroleptics, it is unknown if pimozide has superiority for the treatment of paranoid disorder.

Other uncontrolled studies have found similar results. The treatment of paranoid patients (N = 19) and schizophrenic patients (N = 13) with prochlorperazine and methotrimeparazine revealed no significant differences between the two groups even though 89 per cent of paranoid patients and 62 per cent of schizophrenic patients received some improvement from the treatments.[17] Bilikiewicz et al.,[18] in a study of nine patients with paranoid disorder, found that chlorpromazine was clinically effective in all cases. In a 6-week comparison of sulforidazine and thioridazine in 15 paranoid disorder patients, Blanc and colleagues[19] found that both treatments were effective and that sulforidazine was more effective than thioridazine.

Our clinical experience with paranoid disorder patients reveals that patients tend to derive some benefit from neuroleptics, although complete elimination of delusions is rare. In particular, somatic and erotomanic type paranoid disorder appear less responsive to neuroleptics than persecutory type. This observation should be considered preliminary, pending assessment in controlled studies. Poor compliance with neuroleptic treatment is a serious obstacle to effective treatment and appears relatively common among patients with paranoid disorder. The lack of compliance is related to the failure of many patients to acknowledge they have an illness that requires treatment. Also, parkinsonian side effects, which appear to be common and poorly tolerated among paranoid patients' treatment, adversely affect compliance.

Following are two cases of paranoid disorder seen in our clinic:

Case 1

The patient was a 35-year-old employed, divorced male at the time he was admitted to our outpatient clinic. He had a 5-year history of a fixed persecutory delusion consisting of a belief that coworkers harassed him through a variety of methods including adding harmful chemicals to his food and spraying his apartment with harmful gases. He had no evidence of a primary affective disorder, thought disorder, hallucinations, or clouded sensorium. He had no history of drug/alcohol abuse, and organic, neurological, and metabolic/endocrine disorders were ruled out. His diagnosis was paranoid disorder, persecutory type.

He had a normal childhood with good social functioning and school performance. At age 19, he apparently became less social, although he did go on to marry at age 27. He completed 3.5 years of college and was gainfully employed throughout his twenties. There was no family history of psychiatric illness.

His treatment and course of illness was marked by trials of a variety of neuroleptics including thiothixene 5 to 10 mg/day, trifluoperazine 20 mg/day, perfenazine 28 to 32 mg/day, fluphenazine 20 mg/day and fluphenazine decanoate 1 cc every 2 weeks. It appears he derived a good response from previous neuroleptics, with the response characterized by decreased intensity of the delusional beliefs to a point where their veracity was questioned by the patient. However, there is no evidence that the delusions completely abated. The patient developed significant levels of akathisia with each neuroleptic, which led to a pattern of noncompliance followed by exacerbation of paranoid belief and symptoms of tension, anger, and mild depression. He eventually dropped out of our clinic because of a refusal to take neuroleptic agents.

Case 2

The patient was a 23-year-old unemployed single male who had a 5-year history of fixed paranoid delusions. Beginning at age 18, the patient became progressively more suspicious of strangers, leading to marked social withdrawal to a point where he would not leave his home because of fear of being harmed. He had marked ideas of reference as evidenced by approaching strangers who may be smiling or laughing, and he would accuse them of laughing at him. He was so suspicious during his evaluation with us that he would not permit more than one staff member in the room at a time because he feared being overpowered. He also exhibited anxious and depressive symptoms. He had no history of hallucinations, formal thought disorder, or impaired sensorium. Temporal lobe epilepsy, other neurological disorders, and metabolic/endocrine abnormalities were ruled out. Although depressive symptoms were present, the onset of paranoia preceded depressive symptoms and persisted during nondepressive periods. Paranoid symptoms persisted in the absence of alcohol use. Diagnosis was paranoid disorder, persecutory type.

The patient had a normal childhood with no impairments in school and social functioning. He completed high school, achieving above average marks. He was considered outgoing and popular in high school. There was a history of alcohol and marijuana use in teenage years. Family history was remarkable for alcohol abuse in the patient's father.

The course of illness and treatment was marked by no history of hospitalizations and a number of pharmacological trials. Thioridazine alone and thioridazine in conjunction with carbamazepine were initially tried, with only mild reduction in paranoid symptoms. Next, fluphenazine 5 to 10 mg/day was initiated and found not to be effective. Imipramine and fluphenazine combination were then tried, but the patient developed urinary retention and the regimen was discontinued. Lastly, alprazolam 1.5 mg/day in conjunction with thioridazine 75 mg/day neuroleptic was initiated and found to significantly reduce anxious and depressive symptoms, but paranoid symptoms persisted without diminishment.

There has been limited experience with neuroleptic-augmenting agents such as benzodiazepines, lithium, carbamazepine, and antidepressants in the treatment of patients with paranoid disorder. Future studies will be needed to determine if these agents are useful. For patients with secondary anxiety and depression, augmenting neuroleptic therapy with benzodiazepines and antidepressants, respectively, may be indicated. In addition, family history of pharmacotherapeutic response may guide the choice of augmenting agent.

There may be a role for newer atypical neuroleptics in the treatment of paranoid disorder. Kane and colleagues[20] have demonstrated that clozapine, in comparison to chlorpromazine, has superior efficacy for several symptoms of schizophrenia including delusions in severely ill "treatment-resistant" patients. It will be important to determine if clozapine's superiority generalizes to less ill patients and specifically to patients with paranoid disorder. For the past 2 years, we have been examining the efficacy of clozapine in schizophrenic outpatients in a 10-week double-blind study.[21] Our preliminary experience suggests that clozapine has limited efficacy for monosymptomatic stable delusions and appears more effective for formal thought disorder, hallucinations, hostility, and impulsive behavior. Another rationale for considering atypical neuroleptics in the treatment of paranoid disorder is that some of these agents, such as clozapine and remoxpride, have little if any parkinsonian side effects. Thus, these agents may be better tolerated and improve compliance.

Psychotherapy

Traditional psychoanalytically oriented psychotherapy has been proven to be an ineffective treatment for primary psychotic disorders.[22] May and Tuma[22] reported that traditional psychotherapy alone was not superior to standard hospital management, and psychotherapy plus neuroleptics were only marginally superior to neuroleptics alone. There is evidence that psychoeducationally oriented psychotherapy is an effective treatment for patients with primary psychotic illnesses.[23-26] Although the majority of these studies involved schizophrenic outpatients, the principles of psychoeducation may be applicable to paranoid disorder patients. Falloon and colleagues[24] compared the efficacy of the family-based psychoeducational approach and traditional individual case management. The family-based approach was designed to improve problem-solving capacity, enhance social skills, and reduce interactional stress. After 9 months, the family psychoeducational group had significantly fewer relapses, fewer hospitalizations, lower levels of psychotic symptoms, and required less neuroleptic medication to maintain stability.

Another goal of psychoeducational psychotherapy of paranoid and other psychotic illnesses is to provide the patient and family with current information about the etiology, pathophysiology, prognosis, clinical features, and treatment of the illness. Along these lines, psychotic patients in our clinic are assisted in developing insight into the fact that they have a serious psychiatric illness. This is often difficult with paranoid patients because they may strongly reject the suggestion that their delusional beliefs are not real. However, in the context of a trusting, therapeutic alliance, patients may acknowledge they have an illness without necessarily disavowing the delusional beliefs. Illness recognition facilitates compliance with medication, involvement with mental health agencies, and may improve personal judgment and decision making in social and occupational domains.

We have developed a model for self-control and coping with psychotic symptoms that may be integrated into a psychoeducational approach to the treatment of paranoid disorder.[27] The model involves three sequential phases. In the first phase, termed self-monitoring, patients develop an awareness of the existence of psychotic or prodromal symptoms. The second phase is called self-evaluation, which involves correctly recognizing the self-monitored behaviors as psychotic phenomena. The third phase, termed self-control, involves employing specific personal stratgeies to reduce symptoms. Examples of these strategies include reducing stimuli, brief periods of social isolation, and using distractors.[27]

CONCLUSION

Paranoid disorder is an illness that is associated with characteristic demography and course of illness. Genetic studies provide evidence to validate its diagnostic separateness from schizophrenia and affective illness. It is unknown if paranoid disorder is associated with unique pathophysiological processes. Many psychiatric, neurological, and metabolic/endocrine illnesses may present with delusions and therefore must be considered in the differential diagnosis of paranoid disorder. Uncontrolled studies suggest that neuroleptics are useful in the treatment of patients with paranoid disorder. These observations must be confirmed by double-blind studies. Behaviorally oriented psychotherapeutic approaches may offer a useful adjunct to the pharmacotherapy of this illness. Because of the significant levels of morbidity associated with this illness, it will be important for future research to focus on the treatment and etiology of paranoid disorder.

REFERENCES

1. Lewis A: Paranoia and paranoid: A historical perspective. Psychol Med 1:2–12, 1970.
2. Kahlbaum K: Die Gruppirung der Psychischen Krankheiten. Danzig: Kafemann, 1863.
3. Kraepelin E: Manic depressive insanity and paranoia. In Barclay RM, ed. Psychiatrie, ein Lehrbuch fur Studierende und Artze. 8th ed. Edinburgh: Livingstone, 1921.
4. Freud S: The Disposition of Obsessional Neurosis, standard ed. London: Hogarth Press, 1958: Vol 12, 318.
5. Schneider K: Clinical Psychopathology. New York: Grune & Stratton Inc., 1959:108.
6. Kolle K: Die Primare Verruckheit (Primary Paranoia). Leipzig: Thieme, 1931.
7. Specht G: Ueber den/pathologischen affect in der chronischen paranoia. Leipzig: Bohme, 1901.
8. Kendler KS: Demography of paranoid psychosis (delusional disorder). A review and comparison with schizophrenia and affective illness. Arch Gen Psychiatry 39:890–902, 1982.
9. Stromgren E, quoted by Lemkav P, Tietze C, Cooper M: A survey of statistical studies on the prevalence and incidence of mental disorders in sample populations. Public Health Rep 58:1909–1926, 1943.
10. Larsson T, Sjorgren T: A methodological, psychiatric and statistical study of a large Swedish rural population. Acta Psychiatr Scand 89(suppl):1–250, 1954.
11. Opjordsmoen S: Delusional disorders. I. Comparative long-term outcome. Acta Psychiatr Scand 80:603–612, 1989.
12. Winokur G: Familial psychopathology in delusional disorder. Compr Psychiatry 26:241–248, 1985.
13. Kendler KS, Gruenberg AM, Strauss JM: An independent analysis of the Copenhagen sample of the Danish adoption study of schizophrenia. III. The relationship between paranoid psychosis (delusional disorder) and the schizophrenia spectrum disorders. Arch Gen Psychiatry 38:985–987, 1981.
14. Kendler KS, Hays P: Paranoid psychosis (delusional disorder) and schizophrenia. Arch Gen Psychiatry 38:547–551, 1981.
15. Cummings JL: Organic delusions: Phenomenology, anatomical correlations, and review. Br J Psychiatry 146:184–197, 1985.
16. Munro A: Monosymptomatic hypochondriacal psychosis. Br J Hosp Med 24:34–38, 1980.
17. Ey H, Bohard F: Resultats d'une therapeutique medicamenteuse dans les delires chroniques. Evolution Psychiatrique 35:151–195, 1970.
18. Bilikiewicz T, Sulestrowski W, Wdowiak L: Les resultats du traitement de la paranoia et de la paraphrenie par le largactil. Annee Medico-Psychol 115:52–69, 1957.
19. Blanc M, Borenstein P, Brion S, et al: Etude comparative del l'activite de deux neuroleptiques. Encephale 59:97–161, 1970.
20. Kane J, Honigfeld G, Singer J, Meltzer H, et al: Clozapine for the treatment-resistant schizophrenic: A double-blind comparison with chlorpromazine. Arch Gen Psychiatry 45:789–796, 1988.
21. Breier A, Buchanan RW, Kirkpatrick B, et al: Clozapine treatment in schizophrenic outpatients: Preliminary results from a double-blind efficacy study. International Congress on Schizophrenia Research, April, 1991.
22. May PRA, Tuma AH: Treatment of schizophrenia: An experimental study of five treatment methods. Br J Psychiatry 111:503–510, 1965.
23. Goldstein MJ, Rodnick EH, Evans JR, et al: Drug and family therapy in the aftercare treatment of acute schizophrenia. Arch Gen Psychiatry 35(10):1169–1177, 1978.
24. Falloon IRH, Boyd JL, McGill CW, et al: Family management in the prevention of exacerbations of schizophrenia: A controlled study. N Engl J Med 306(24):1437–1440, 1982.
25. Leff J, Kuipers L, Berkowitz R, et al: A controlled trial of social intervention in the families of schizophrenic patients. Br J Psychiatry 141:121–134, 1982.
26. Hogarty GE, Anderson CM, Reiss DJ, et al: Family psychoeducation, social skills training, and maintenance chemotherapy in the aftercare treatment of schizophrenia. Arch Gen Psychiatry 43:633–642, 1986.
27. Breier A, Strauss JS: Self-control in psychotic disorders. Arch Gen Psychiatry 40:1141–1145, 1983.

25

THE TREATMENT OF SCHIZOAFFECTIVE DISORDER

SAMUEL G. SIRIS, M.D.

Schizoaffective disorder is a diagnostic concept that has represented a substantial conundrum for psychiatry over the years. Certain patients present with clinical symptomatology that appears to be a mixture of features present in narrowly defined cases of schizophrenia and affective disorder, and lack of clarity with regard to how best to classify these cases spawned the concept of "schizoaffective disorder." As late as DSM-III, schizoaffective disorder was a diagnosis of last resort, without specified criteria, to be employed only when other more explicitly diagnosed conditions could not be established. As a legacy of this approach, relatively few treatment studies have been conducted specifically on patients with schizoaffective disorder, in relationship to other psychiatric conditions of comparable severity. Nevertheless, sufficient numbers of patients continue to present with disorders appropriately diagnosable as schizoaffective that attention clearly needs to be paid to their proper diagnosis and treatment.

Today, competing concepts continue to exist with regard to the proper place of schizoaffective disorder within psychiatric nosology. Five distinct theses are advanced: (1) schizoaffective disorder is a form of affective disorder; (2) it is a form of schizophrenia; (3) it is a separate psychiatric disorder apart from any other; (4) it represents a region on a continuum which runs between affective disorder and schizophrenia; and (5) it represents a confluence of independent affective and schizophrenic diatheses. Moreover, it has been argued that schizoaffective disorder is itself heterogeneous.[1-4] Formulations for organizing the subtypes include the following distinctions: (1) mostly affective versus mostly schizophrenic; (2) manic versus depressive; (3) unipolar versus bipolar; (4) chronic versus nonchronic; and (5) remitting versus nonremitting. Not surprisingly, the way schizoaffective disorder has been diagnosed and subtyped has powerfully influenced the demographic, clinical, and family diagnostic correlates that have been found, as well as the treatment implications that have emerged. For example, schizoaffective manics have been found in several studies to have a high family history prevalence of bipolar disorder, whereas schizoaffective depressed patients have a low rate of bipolar illness in their families, but a relatively high rate of unipolar affective disorder as well as a substantial prevalence of schizophrenia.[1]

This observation has been used for validation of the unipolar/bipolar distinction in schizoaffective disorder. Other validators of this distinction are clinical, demographic, and course similarities observed between schizoaffective mania and affective psychosis, whereas schizoaffective depression seems more closely to resemble schizophrenia in terms of these parameters.[2,5] For example, whereas the long-term outcome in schizoaffective mania has often been described as resembling that of bipolar disorder, schizoaffective depression has often been described as having a less favorable long-term prognosis with a course more likely to parallel that of schizophrenia. On the basis of these findings, the present review incorporates the schizoaffective manic/schizoaffective depressive distinction.

DIFFERENTIAL DIAGNOSIS

The differential diagnosis of schizoaffective mania includes, obviously, psychotic mania. The DSM-III-R distinction for this differential is both longitudinal and cross-sectional. In addition to a disturbance that has met full criteria for the manic syndrome, this definition requires a period of at least 2 weeks of substantial psychotic symptomatology (hallucinations or delusions or both) in the absence of prominent mood symptoms. It also requires certain characteristic schizophrenia-like symptoms to occur in the context of the psychotic episode.[6] (The reader should remain mindful that many of the studies upon which the treatment recommendations in this chapter are based utilized other means of distinguishing between mania and schizoaffective mania,[7] which require only cross-sectional assessment of symptomatology.) Excited or agitated schizophrenic patients can present a number of features in common with schizoaffective mania. However, in this case, the full syndrome of mania is not present. Finally, organic mental disorders, in particular the effects of abused substances such as psychostimulants, are an important differential for schizoaffective mania.

Toxicology screens for potential substances of abuse are therefore indicated in any newly admitted patients for whom the diagnosis of schizoaffective mania is being considered.

The differential diagnosis for schizoaffective depression includes psychotic depression. Once again, specific symptoms suggestive of a schizophrenic psychosis are important to the diagnosis, as is a 2-week period of hallucinations or delusions or both in the absence of prominent mood symptoms.[6] Also, again, it is important to rule out potential medical/organic sources of symptomatology, including both those that could make a depressed patient appear psychotic, and those that could make a schizophrenic patient appear depressed.[8] The negative symptoms of schizophrenia can resemble depression-like symptomatology in several important regards,[9,10] but in these instances the full syndrome of depression is not present.

Additionally, the syndrome of secondary depression in schizophrenia (also known as postpsychotic depression) can closely resemble schizoaffective depression or can follow it.[11] In this case, the full depressive syndrome occurs when the patient is no longer flagrantly psychotic. Some cases of secondary depression in schizophrenia in fact meet the DSM-III criteria for schizoaffective disorder. However, present drafts of the tenth revision of the International Classification of Drugs (ICD-10) include secondary depression in schizophrenia as a separate diagnostic category. Therefore, this review will consider its treatment, but will do so in a separate category for clarity. A further important differential for the secondary depression syndrome in schizophrenia is the syndrome of neuroleptic-induced akinesia.[11–13] This is a motor side effect syndrome in which spontaneity is compromised on an extrapyramidal basis. It can bear great phenotypic resemblance to depression, and can be particularly difficult to recognize when it is not accompanied by such tell-tale features as stiffness or reduced accessory motor movements.

THE TREATMENT OF SCHIZOAFFECTIVE MANIA

Acute Treatment

The pharmacological agents most frequently investigated and used in the treatment of schizoaffective mania are neuroleptics, lithium, and their combination.[2,14] Interestingly, although each of these agents is apparently helpful in this condition, direct correlations between the type of symptomatology (i.e., psychotic or affective-like) and pharmacological agent (i.e., neuroleptic or lithium) have often not been found.

The few studies that have compared lithium and neuroleptics in the treatment of schizoaffective mania have revealed little difference in the efficacy of these two agents.[2,14] The one exception to this pattern, however, occurred in the largest study to be undertaken.[15] This was a cooperative Veterans Administration (VA) study that had the weakness of using DSM-II diagnostic criteria, but it was the only study to separate patients on the basis of their level of activation. Although lithium was found to have equivalent efficacy to chlorpromazine in moderately active patients, chlorpromazine was found to be more beneficial among "highly active" patients. In several studies, neuroleptics were found to be more sedating than lithium. This nonspecific neuroleptic effect can be clinically useful for many excited schizoaffective manics. However, sedation is generally prominent only with low-potency neuroleptics (i.e., chlorpromazine), and it is not clear if that specific utility would be observed with high-potency neuroleptics. The trade-off, therefore, seems to be that by making an excited psychotic schizoaffective manic sleepy with a low-potency neuroleptic, one may not only make him or her easier to manage, but may also make him or her more prone to the side effects that generally accompany low-potency neuroleptics such as constipation, dry mouth, and orthostatic hypotension.

Combined treatment with lithium plus a neuroleptic may be a more effective treatment for schizoaffective mania than a neuroleptic alone.[2,14,16] The counterbalancing consideration with regard to this approach, of course, is the increased risk of side effects involved in using two treatments. The best evidence is that these side effects are merely additive, though, and that there is no special risk involved in combining lithium with a neuroleptic as long as routine cautions are observed in monitoring lithium blood levels. One interesting feature regarding the utility of adding lithium to neuroleptic in schizoaffective manic patients is that the benefit seems to extend to the entire range of their symptomatology and is not restricted to what otherwise might be conceptualized as the affective component of their presentation.

In the studies of neuroleptics and lithium in schizoaffective manic patients, dosage ranges have been used that are typical for the treatment of schizophrenia and mania, respectively. Variances that have been observed between the treatment of mania and schizoaffective mania, however, are that the resolution of the syndrome may take place more slowly and be less complete in the case of schizoaffective mania.

In light of the above considerations, a practical approach to the acute treatment of schizoaffective mania is to begin the patient immediately on neuroleptic medication, in order to bring behavioral symptoms under control as promptly as possible, while beginning to titre an appropriate dosage of lithium. Dosages of neuroleptic should be in the same ranges that are considered for the acute treatment of schizophrenia. As is the case with schizophrenia, treatment of extrapyramidal side effects with antiparkinsonian medications constitutes an important aspect of treatment as well. Since acute dystonic reactions to neuroleptic medication may be terrifying to a patient, potentially compromising subsequent compliance, prophylactic antiparkinsonian medication is usually indicated at the start of treatment. Neuroleptic medication and lithium would be continued throughout the acute treatment course, until the patient is well stabilized. At that point, because there may be a higher risk of tardive dyskinesia in patients with an affective diathesis, an attempt can be made gradually to discontinue neuroleptic medication while maintaining the lithium. The patient should be carefully watched during this interval for the emergence of recurrent symptomatology, in which case the neuroleptic can be reinstituted. Otherwise, a course of continuation treatment with lithium would begin (see later in chapter). On the other hand, if the patient for any reason appears to be intolerant to treatment with lithium, but has an adequate response to neuroleptic alone, continuing treatment can be with the neuroleptic agent, bearing in mind that longer term treatment often does not require doses as high as acute treatment.[17]

For patients who either do not respond adequately to neuroleptic medication or lithium for their schizoaffective manias, or who cannot tolerate side effects from these agents, alternative treatments are possible. These include carbamazepine,[18] sodium valproate,[19] and electroconvulsive therapy (ECT).[20,21] In these cases, doses of carbamazepine and valproate, and their target blood levels for treatment, should be the same as is the case for the treatment of affective disorders. For ECT, the treatment approach would also be the same as with affective disorders.

While the somatic treatment of schizoaffective mania is undertaken, proper psychosocial interventions and support should be made available. Usually this will include hospitalization to provide structure and limits for the patient, and help insure the minimization of the psychosocial damage that can result from inappropriate decisions and behavior. An environment should be supplied that is consistent and not excessively stimulating. Help with concrete services, decision making, and activities of daily living should be provided, and major decisions should be postponed until the patient is better able to exercise judgment in his or her own behalf. Meeting with the patient's family is also often helpful to help them understand the nature of the disorder and its treatment, and to help them cope with stresses and crises that may have emerged. The duration of hospitalization, and exact nature of psychosocial interventions, of course, will depend on the patient's particular circumstances.

Continuation and Maintenance Treatment

Organized studies of the continuation or maintenance treatment in psychiatry are rarer than studies of acute treatment. Such studies of specifically schizoaffective mania have been confined to the examination of lithium. However a number of studies of neuroleptic continuation and maintenance treatment in schizophrenia have also included patients with a schizoaffective diagnosis, allowing certain conclusions to be surmised.

Lithium has been found to possess efficacy as a prophylactic agent in broadly defined schizoaffective disorder, especially when plasma levels are maintained at 0.60 mEq/liter or above.[22] Specifically, lithium prophylaxis was found to be most useful among those patients who showed the greatest amount of affective-like symptomatology (i.e., "mostly affective" versus "mostly schizophrenic"). Additionally, lithium prophylaxis was much more effective for those patients with schizoaffective mania than for those patients who had schizoaffective depression, and more effective for those patients with a previous bipolar course. There was also a tendency, although this failed to reach full statistical significance, for patients with a family history of affective disorder to do better with prophylactic lithium, and for patients with previous schizophrenia-like symptomatology to do less well.

When maintenance treatment with lithium is undertaken, the potential long-term renal and thyroid effects need to be monitored with plasma measures of creatinine, blood urea nitrogen (BUN), T_3, and T_4 status at least every 6 months. This is in addition to more frequent routine monitoring of plasma lithium levels. It is also important for patients, and often their families, to be counseled with regard to the importance of maintaining consistent fluid and salt intake, so that their lithium levels will remain stable. They should furthermore be made aware of the early signs of lithium toxicity (e.g., diarrhea) and the need to discontinue lithium temporarily if for any reason they become dehydrated.

When continuation and maintenance treatment with neuroleptics is undertaken in patients with schizoaffective mania, the dosing strategies parallel those developed for schizophrenia.[17] As is the case with schizophrenia, neuroleptic dosage might not need to be as high as is required during acute treatment. Advantages of lowering the dosage in this manner include improved psychosocial functioning as well as a reduction in the risk of tardive dyskinesia. Although the incidence of psychotic recurrence may be higher with the reduced neuroleptic strategy, it is more than made up for by increased medication compliance and by the fact that psychotic relapses are often "slow-rolling," so that they can readily be countered by temporary neuroleptic increases. Even with relatively low doses of neuroleptic medication, however, the patient still needs to continue to be monitored for the possible emergence of subtle neuroleptic-induced akinesia. This can present with a clinical phenocopy of negative symptoms or depression, but it is usually quite treatable with adjunctive antiparkinsonian medication (see later under Treatment of Postpsychotic Depression).

Patients who required treatment with carbamazepine or valproate in order to achieve their best response may be continued on these medications for long-term treatment. Routine plasma level monitoring of these agents is indicated to assure optimal results. In addition, patients on carbamazepine should receive periodic follow-up blood counts and be monitored for any symptoms of agranulocytosis such as fever. Patients treated with valproate should receive routine follow-up liver function tests.

THE TREATMENT OF SCHIZOAFFECTIVE DEPRESSION

Acute Treatment

The outcome of treatment for schizoaffective depression has often been found to be somewhat less favorable than for schizoaffective mania. This is consistent with the notion that schizoaffective depression is more closely related to schizophrenia, but may alternatively be a reflection of less understanding of how this syndrome is best treated or the fact that lithium seems to be less specifically efficacious in these cases.

The issue of the usefulness of tricyclic antidepressants during an acute episode of schizoaffective depression is not entirely clear. The earlier of two major studies that addressed this issue found a higher response rate for amitriptyline combined with clorpromazine than for either agent used alone.[23] In this view, the responsiveness of schizoaffective disorder to this combination was similar to the response of psychotic depressions,[2,24] a condition to which it is phenotypically similar and from which it is separated by a dividing line varying according to the diagnostic system employed. The more recent study that examined actively psychotic schizoaffective depressed patients, however, did not find the addition of a tricyclic antidepressant (amitriptyline or desipramine) to haloperidol plus benztropine to be beneficial. Indeed, there was the suggestion that the addition of the tricyclic antidepressant may have retarded recovery from psychosis.[25] In addition to using slightly different diagnostic criteria, the latter study had also made an attempt to rule out the syndrome of akinesia. Had akinetic patients inadvertently been included in the earlier study, they may have benefited from the combined medication on the basis of additive anticholinergic activity. Therefore, it is probably advisable to treat psychotic patients with schizoaffective depressions first with a neuroleptic, but without an antidepressant, working to achieve the maximum antipsychotic response while continuing to be mindful of potential akinetic symptoms which could present similarly to depression.

Lithium may show some benefit in schizoaffective depressions, but this is less likely to be dramatic than for patients with schizoaffective mania.[2,14,26] Indeed, if we may extrapolate from data for patients with psychotic depressions, those patients who are most likely to respond favorably to lithium may be those who have a history of bipolar-type mood changes.[27] One other instance where lithium may be useful is when it is added to the neuroleptic-tricyclic combination in otherwise nonresponsive schizodepressions. Electroconvulsive therapy is another modality that can often be beneficial in schizoaffective depressions,[2] an observation which is not a surprise, since ECT is known to be a very useful treatment modality in psychotic depression.[27]

Appropriate psychosocial supports are important for patients during treatment of schizoaffective depression. Of prime concern is the issue of suicide. Young males from higher socioeconomic backgrounds, with high early life performance expectations and who are experiencing hopelessness, may be especially vulnerable to suicide,[28] but all schizoaffective depressed patients require careful evaluation for suicidal potential. Hospitalization may be required in this regard. Hospitalization and family interventions may also be valuable for all the same reasons as discussed above in the context of schizoaffective mania.

Continuation and Maintenance Treatment

There are few systematic data on the continuation or maintenance treatment of schizoaffective depressions. In the absence of controlled experience for guidance, the prudent course is to continue treatment with whatever medication, or combination of medications, was most effective during the acute treatment phase. Cautions with regard to long-term treatment with these agents, as discussed in the continuation and maintenance treatment section for schizoaffective mania, should be observed.

Treatment of depressive syndromes that occur in the course of schizoaffective disorder, but which are not accompanied by flagrant psychotic symptoms, are considered in the following section.

THE TREATMENT OF POSTPSYCHOTIC DEPRESSION

The concept of postpsychotic depression in schizophrenia is applied to those patients who are diagnosed as suffering from schizophrenia when they are psychotic, but who subsequently develop a syndrome of depression when they are no longer flagrantly psychotic.[11] This concept is also referred to as secondary depression in schizophrenia. Patients satisfying this concept may also be diagnosed as having schizoaffective disorder under certain diagnostic systems, and so their treatment is properly considered in this chapter. Additionally, certain schizoaffective patients may continue to experience depressive syndromes after the resolution of flagrant psychotic symptomatology. These patients would be considered to have postpsychotic depression as well.

As indicated in the differential diagnosis discussion above, a major confound of the diagnosis of postpsychotic depression is the syndrome of neuroleptic-induced akinesia.[12,13] This extrapyramidal motor side effect can mimic all the symptoms of depression, and can occur in a form subtle enough that gross motor effects such as cogwheeling, stiffness, or reduced accessory motor movements are not apparent. The appropriate approach in the treatment of postpsychotic depression, therefore, after observing the patient for a week or two in order to ascertain that the syndrome is not a transient disappointment reaction or the prodrome of a new psychotic episode, is to lower the neuroleptic dosage if this can be done without a reexacerbation of psychotic symptomatology. If the neuroleptic dose cannot be further lowered, a vigorous trial of antiparkinsonian medication should be pursued.[11] Importantly, the therapeutic effect of antiparkinsonian medications occurs quickly in the case of akinesia, within a few days to a week, so that lengthy courses of treatment to assess effects are not required. However, if antiparkinsonian medication is effective in counteracting neuroleptic-induced akinesia, prolonged adjunctive treatment with the antiparkinsonian agent may be indicated.

When postsynaptic depression-like symptomatology is stable and does not respond to antiparkinsonian medication, the question of the use of adjunctive antidepressant medication arises. On this topic, the literature is divided.[11] Several studies have failed to find a usefulness for adjunctive antidepressants in this circumstance. But other studies have found a benefit of adding antidepressants to neuroleptics in well-defined cases of postpsychotic depression, and those studies finding a benefit have tended to be stronger methodologically. The most positive study utilized the combination of fluphenazine decanoate, benztropine (2 mg p.o. t.i.d.) and imipramine (built up gradually over 3 weeks to a dose of 200 mg p.o. h.s.).[29] A trial of 6 to 9 weeks is required to test fully the benefit of neuroleptic-antidepressant combination.[11] Proper controlled studies with monoamine oxidase inhibitor antidepressants have not yet been reported.

Only one study involving maintenance treatment with adjunctive antidepressant for postpsychotic depression, among responders, has been reported.[11,30] That one study supports the thesis that long-term maintenance treatment with a tricyclic antidepressant added to a neuroleptic may be both beneficial and safe.

SUMMARY AND CONCLUSIONS

Schizoaffective disorders represent an area of diagnostic and conceptual uncertainty within psychiatric nosology. Nevertheless, a number of therapeutic agents that have been developed for the treatment of psychosis or affective disorders have been found to have potentially useful roles in the treatment of schizoaffective patients. This chapter has utilized currently popular distinctions within the realm of schizoaffective disorder (i.e., schizoaffective mania, schizoaffective depression, and postpsychotic depression) to organize strategies of acute and maintenance therapeutic approaches.

REFERENCES

1. Clayton PJ: Schizoaffective disorders. J Nerv Ment Dis 170:646–650, 1982.
2. Levitt JJ, Tsuang MT: The heterogeneity of schizoaffective disorder: Implications for treatment. Am J Psychiatry 145:926–936, 1988.
3. Coryell W, Keller M, Lavori P, et al: Affective syndromes, psychotic features, and prognosis: I. Depression. Arch Gen Psychiatry 47:651–657, 1989.
4. Coryell W, Keller M, Lavori P, et al: Affective syndromes, psychotic features, and prognosis: II. Mania. Arch Gen Psychiatry 47:658–662, 1989.
5. Maj M, Perris C: An approach to the diagnosis and classification of schizoaffective disorders for research purposes. Acta Psychiatr Scand 72:405–413, 1985.
6. American Psychiatric Association: Diagnostic and Statistical Manual of Mental Disorders. 3rd ed. Revised. Washington, DC: American Psychiatric Press, 1987.
7. Spitzer RL, Endicott J, Robins E: Research diagnostic criteria: Rationale and reliability. Arch Gen Psychiatry 35:773–782, 1978.
8. Bartels SJ, Drake RE: Depressive symptoms in schizophrenia: Comprehensive differential diagnosis. Compr Psychiatry 29:467–483, 1988.
9. Carpenter WT Jr, Heinrichs DW, Alphs, LD: Treatment of negative symptoms. Schizophr Bull 11:440–452, 1985.
10. Siris SG, Adan F, Cohen M, et al: Post-psychotic depression and negative symptoms: An investigation of syndromal overlap. Am J Psychiatry 145:1532–1537, 1988.
11. Siris SG: Diagnosis of secondary depression in schizophrenia: Implications for DSM-IV. Schizophr Bull 17:75–98, 1991.
12. Rifkin A, Quitkin F, Klein DF: Akinesia: A poorly recognized drug-induced extrapyramidal behavioral disorder. Arch Gen Psychiatry 32:672–674, 1975.
13. Van Putten T, May PRA: 'Akinetic depression' in schizophrenia. Arch Gen Psychiatry 35:1101–1107, 1978.
14. Goodnick PJ, Meltzer HY: Treatment of schizoaffective disorders. Schizophr Bull 10:30–48, 1984.
15. Prien RF, Caffey EM, Klett CJ: A comparison of lithium carbonate and chlorpromazine in the treatment of excited schizoaffectives. Arch Gen Psychiatry 27:182–189, 1972.
16. Biederman J, Lerner Y, Belmaker RH: Combination of lithium carbonate and haloperidol in schizoaffective disorder: A controlled study. Arch Gen Psychiatry 36:327–333, 1979.
17. Kane J: Treatment programme and long-term outcome in chronic schizophrenia. Acta Psychiatr Scand 82(suppl 358):151–157, 1990.
18. Okuma T, Yamashita I, Takahashi R, et al: Clinical efficacy of carbamazepine in affective, schizoaffective, and schizophrenic disorders. Pharmacopsychiatry 22:47–53, 1989.
19. Brown R: U.S. experience with valproate in manic depressive illness: A multicenter trial. J Clin Psychiatry 50 (3, suppl):13–16, 1989.
20. Ries RK, Wilson L, Bokan JA, et al: ECT in medication resistant schizoaffective disorder. Compr Psychiatry 22:167–173, 1981.

21. Black DW, Winokur G, Nasrallah A: Treatment of mania: A naturalistic study of electroconvulsive therapy versus lithium in 438 patients. J Clin Psychiatry 48:132–139, 1987.
22. Maj M: Lithium prophylaxis of schizoaffective disorders: A prospective study. J Affective Disord 14:129–135, 1988.
23. Brockington IF, Kindell RE, Kellett JM, et al: Trials of lithium, chlorpromazine and amitriptyline in schizoaffective patients. Br J Psychiatry 133:162–168, 1978.
24. Spiker DG, Weiss JC, Dealy RS, et al: The pharmacological treatment of delusional depression. Am J Psychiatry 142:430–436, 1985.
25. Kramer MS, Vogel WH, DiJohnson C, et al: Antidepressants in 'depressed' schizophrenic inpatients: A controlled trial. Arch Gen Psychiatry 46:922–928, 1989.
26. Lerner Y, Mintzer Y, Schestatzky M: Lithium combined with haloperidol in schizophrenic patients. Br J Psychiatry 153:359–362, 1988.
27. Nelson JC, Mazure CM: Lithium augmentation in psychotic depression refractory to combined drug treatment. Am J Psychiatry 143:363–366, 1986.
28. Caldwell CB, Gottesman II: Schizophrenics kill themselves too: A review of risk factors for suicide. Schizophr Bull 16:571–589, 1990.
29. Siris SG, Morgan V, Fagerstrom R, et al: Adjunctive imipramine in the treatment of post-psychotic depression: A controlled trial. Arch Gen Psychiatry 44:533–539, 1987.
30. Siris SG, Cutler J, Owen K, et al: Adjunctive imipramine maintenance in schizophrenic patients with remitted post-psychotic depressions. Am J Psychiatry 146:1495–1497, 1989.

26

TARDIVE DYSKINESIA

DANIEL E. CASEY, M.D.

Since neuroleptics were first introduced in the 1950s, it has been well recognized that they also produce neurological side effects of motor system disturbances. These were initially limited to the acute extrapyramidal syndromes (EPS) of akathisia, dystonia, and parkinsonism. However, in the late 1950s, motor syndrome abnormalities that persisted long after the drugs were discontinued began to be recognized. Tardive dyskinesia was first described in German in 1957.[1] Subsequent descriptions in French[2] and in English by Danish investigators[3] confirmed this late-onset persisting dyskinetic syndrome. The term "tardive dyskinesia" was developed in 1964.[4] Since tardive dyskinesia may persist, it has come to be recognized as one of the major limitations to neuroleptic use. Thus the careful review of proper indications for prescribing these compounds and capable management of tardive dyskinesia is required.

CLINICAL DESCRIPTION

Tardive dyskinesia is characterized by the late onset of involuntary repetitive purposeless movements that occur in predisposed patients. The typical symptoms may include orofacial dyskinesias of chewing, vermicular tongue movements, occasional tongue protrusion, lip smacking, puckering and pursing, rotatory and side-to-side jaw motion, movements of the forehead, and irregular eye blinking rates. Other body areas may be involved, with choreoathetosis of the upper and lower limbs that can be accompanied by bizarre movements in the head, neck, or hips. Rarely, tardive dyskinesia involves irregular breathing or swallowing to cause aerophagia, belching, and grunting noises.[5]

The atypical forms of tardive dyskinesia, tardive dystonia, and tardive akathisia, have been noted for many years in case reports or small studies, but they have recently received considerably more attention. Tardive dystonia resembles the abnormal postures of acute neuroleptic drug-induced dystonia, with sustained abnormal postures of torticollis, blepharospasm, oculogyric crisis, grimacing, and truncal torsion, that can persist for months or years after neuroleptics are discontinued.[6,7] Tardive akathisia resembles the restlessness of acute akathisia, but also persists after neuroleptic drugs are discontinued.[8] There is much debate as to whether these different syndromes represent distinct pathophysiological mechanisms or are better understood as symptom clusters that represent the spectrum of the tardive dyskinesia syndrome, but involve a common pathophysiology.[9]

EPIDEMIOLOGY

Prevalence

The number of existing cases at a specified time (prevalence) varies greatly across the literature from 0.5 to 80 per cent.[9,10] This wide range is undoubtedly accounted for by the many contributions of different variables, such as age and gender of patients studied, past and present drug treatment, and criteria for diagnosis. Conservative estimates of tardive dyskinesia prevalence rates average 15 to 20 per cent, but may approach 70 per cent in high-risk groups, such as the aged. In contrast, spontaneous dyskinesias, which clinically resemble tardive dyskinesia but, by definition, occur in patients who have never had treatment with neuroleptics, occur at a prevalence of 0.5 to 5 per cent. The lower end of this estimate involves younger patients, whereas the higher prevalence rates are found in the elderly.

Incidence

The number of new tardive dyskinesia cases occurring in a specified time (incidence) is approximately 3 to 5 per cent per year.[11,12]

DIFFERENTIAL DIAGNOSIS

Idiopathic-Spontaneous Dyskinesias

The explanation of abnormal movements in psychotic patients has been controversial since the time of Kraepelin and Bleuler. Kraepelin believed that dyskinesias were an integral part of the biological basis of psychosis, whereas Bleuler explained these abnormal movements on a psychic rather than anatomical basis.[9] Stereotypes and mannerisms of psychosis as well as other abnormal movements must be considered in a differential diagnosis. Neurological disorders of focal or segmental dystonias that include orofacial dyskinesia, blepharospasm, oromandibular dystonia, laryngeal and pharyngeal dystonias, and torticollis must also be considered. Tourette's syndrome, a disorder of involuntary tics and vocalizations, starts in childhood and continues with a fluctuating course through adult life. Simple, persisting tics in isolated muscle groups as well as dental problems can also appear as idiopathic dyskinetic movements.

Neuroleptic-Induced Acute Extrapyramidal Syndromes

The acute extrapyramidal syndromes induced by neuroleptic drugs must be carefully considered, as they may coexist with tardive dyskinesia. These acute-onset syndromes occur with the initiation of neuroleptics and gradually resolve within a period of days to weeks in most patients when the drugs are discontinued. These syndromes of dystonia (briefly sustained abnormal postures), akathisia (subjective and objective signs of restlessness), and parkinsonism (tremor, rigidity, bradykinesia) must be in a differential diagnosis of drug-induced movement disorders.

Other Drug-Induced Dyskinesias

Many other drugs can produce abnormal movement disorders. These include chronic use of anticholinergics, antihistaminics, and stimulants. Several anticonvulsants, oral contraceptives, chloroquine, and other malarial drugs can also provoke reversible orofacial and limb dyskinesias.[5]

Hereditary and Systemic Illnesses

Hereditary neurodegenerative syndromes of Huntington's disease and Wilson's disease should be diagnostic considerations. Alzheimer's disease patients may also develop dyskinesias in the later stages of their illness. Endocrinopathies of hyperthyroidism, hypoparathyroidism, and hyperglycemia, as well as systemic lupus erythematosus, chorea associated with pregnancy, Sydenham's chorea, central nervous system infections, and space-occupying lesions can also be associated with hyperkinetic dyskinesias.[5]

RISK FACTORS

Patient Variables: Age, Gender, Psychiatric Diagnosis, and Other Factors

There is a strong positive correlation between increasing tardive dyskinesia prevalence and incidence with increasing age.[9,13] Females are usually at greater risk for tardive dyskinesia (approximately 1.7 : 1.0 ratio). Patients with affective disorders and nonpsychotic diagnoses appear to be at higher risk than those with schizophrenia.[14] Acute EPS has been associated with tardive dyskinesia that occurs early in neuroleptic treatment, but this association has not been well correlated with later onset tardive dyskinesia. Diabetes mellitus has also been recently shown as a possible risk factor for tardive dyskinesia.[15] Finally, concurrent central nervous system injury is inconsistently associated with increased tardive dyskinesia risk.

Treatment Variables: Neuroleptic Dose and Duration

Though many retrospective studies do not show a consistent correlation between tardive dyskinesia and total neuroleptic dose or duration of treatment, more recent prospective studies do show such an association.[9,10,12,16] The relationship between neuroleptic drug blood levels and tardive dyskinesia is more complicated, as there is no consistent relationship between these two factors.[9,17]

Neuroleptic Drug Type

Until recently, there was no consistent clinical evidence to indicate that any one neuroleptic drug was more or less liable to produce tardive dyskinesia. Advocates of any particular drug could gather limited evidence to argue in favor of their own particular perspective, but opponents could gather equally unconvincing data to argue in favor of their compound. However, the recent addition of clozapine, which is carefully restricted because of a 1 to 2 per cent risk of agranulocytosis, clearly has a much lower tardive dyskinesia risk. To date, there have been no convincingly described cases of clozapine-induced tardive dyskinesia.[18]

Other Drug Factors

Compulsory periods of neuroleptic drug discontinuation have been offered as a "drug holiday" method for decreasing tardive dyskinesia risk. However, it has not been shown that this strategy is beneficial, and it may increase the risk of tardive dyskinesia.[19] Additionally, it exposes many psychotic patients to the unacceptable risk of psychotic relapse. Anticholinergics have been associated with increased tardive dyskinesia risk in some studies, but not in others. Anticholinergic agents often increase symptoms in existing cases of tardive dyskinesia, but the data are controversial as to whether anticholinergics increase the risk of developing tardive dyskinesia.

COURSE AND OUTCOME

Though it is commonly believed that tardive dyskinesia is irreversible and will inevitably worsen with continued neuroleptic treatment, observations to the contrary have been noted since the first reports.[1,2] These beliefs have led to admonitions against using neuroleptics in psychotic patients with tardive dyskinesia. However, a review of the long-term outcome data show that these strict limitations are unwarranted. Long-term outcome rates widely vary across studies, but there is a pattern of improvement of 50 per cent or more in many patients followed for 5 years or longer. Positive factors associated with a favorable outcome are young age, lower neuroleptic drug exposure, and duration of follow-up. Yet, many patients remaining on low to moderate doses of neuroleptics have equally favorable outcomes. These findings are encouraging and indicate that neuroleptics in low to moderate doses are not contraindicated in psychotic patients with tardive dyskinesia and who benefit from neuroleptic therapy.[17]

PATHOPHYSIOLOGY

The pathophysiology mechanism(s) underlying tardive dyskinesia is unknown. The theory of dopamine receptor hypersensitivity is the most commonly cited explanation of tardive dyskinesia, though there are many inadequate features of this hypothesis.[9,17] The theory proposes that dopamine in the nigrostriatal pathway becomes functionally overactive, purportedly due to increased numbers of dopamine receptors, as a consequence of chronic neuroleptic drug-induced blockade of dopamine receptors.

Direct evidence of central nervous system abnormalities has not been found. Evaluations of structural abnormalities (neuroimaging, light microscopic) and biochemical (cerebral spinal fluid, dopamine D_1 and D_2 receptor quantification in postmortem studies) and endocrinological (prolactin and growth hormone) parameters have not reliably shown significant differences between tardive dyskinesia and nontardive dyskinesia cohorts.[9,17]

Indirect data for a role of neuroleptics in tardive dyskinesia can be used to support the dopamine receptor hypersensitivity hypothesis. Chronic neuroleptic treatment produces tardive dyskinesia, and acute neuroleptic treatment will suppress existing dyskinesias. Discontinuing neuroleptics may unmask covert tardive dyskinesia. Conversely, dopamine agonists usually increase tardive dyskinesia. Though these data are usually used to argue that dopamine has a primary role in tardive dyskinesia, it is possible that it plays only a secondary or tertiary role by having a remote modulatory effect on an as yet unknown primary pathophysiology.

TREATMENT

Preventing and managing tardive dyskinesia is a clinical challenge. Unfortunately, some patients will develop tardive dyskinesia in spite of one's best efforts. However, when neuroleptic drugs are prescribed in accordance with recommended guidelines, their benefits greatly outweigh their risks. The most appropriate indications for acute and chronic neuroleptic therapy are for those patients with schizophrenia or other psychotic symptoms that benefit from treatment. Patients with neuroses and character disorders are best treated with therapies that do not involve neuroleptics. Periodically reviewing a patient's diagnosis and the need for extended neuroleptic therapy will go a long way toward reducing the prevalence and morbidity of tardive dyskinesia.

The algorithm (Fig. 26–1) offers a strategy for both reducing the risks of developing tardive dyskinesia and for managing the syndrome once it occurs.[20] Initially, one must be aware of the possibility of tardive dyskinesia occurring in any patient on neuroleptics. A high degree of vigilance for the onset of mild ab-

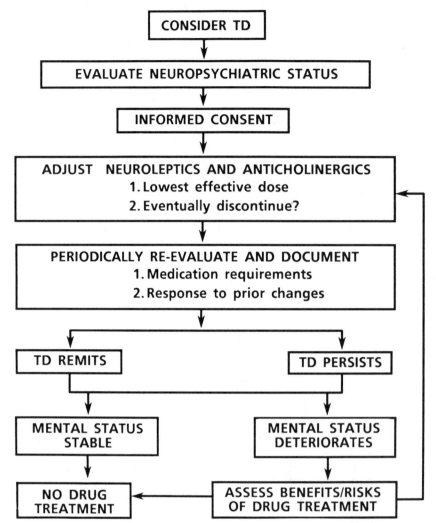

Figure 26–1. An algorithm for managing tardive dyskinesia. (Adapted with permission from Casey DE, Gerlach J: *In* Harvey C. Stancer, Paul E. Garfinkel, Vivian M. Rakoff, eds. Guidelines for the Use of Psychotropic Drugs: A Clinical Handbook. Jamaica, NY: Spectrum Publications, Inc. 1984:184.)

normal movements in patients is essential to early detection and appropriate interventions.

Thoroughly evaluating the patient provides a solid data base for managing both the neurological and psychiatric symptoms. It is always necessary to prioritize what symptoms are most important to control in the patient at this time because initiating a treatment intervention for one set of symptoms may adversely affect other symptoms. In most cases, especially those with psychoses, the mental status takes priority over tardive dyskinesia and should be the primary consideration of therapy.

After a careful evaluation of the available information, it is important to discuss with the patient the risks and benefits of treatment and no treatment. Since many psychotic patients cannot adequately appreciate issues related to treatment decisions, it is worthwhile involving a concerned family member in the consent discussions. Discussing these issues on a frequent basis with patients and their families will

increase their knowledge and engage their participation in the treatment plan.

The goal of drug therapy is to adjust neuroleptics and anticholinergics to the lowest effective dose that provides adequate control of psychotic symptoms and motor side effects. In many patients it will be possible to reduce these drug doses and maintain the therapeutic benefit. However, in some patients it may be necessary to raise drug doses to adequately control symptoms.

The effect of drug treatment interventions should be periodically reassessed and documented. By careful monitoring and documentation over extended periods, a patient's response to drug therapy can be well delineated.

Tardive dyskinesia will either remit or persist. In most cases when tardive dyskinesia improves, it does so over many months to years, though there are exceptional cases of rapid resolution.

The patient's mental status will also remain stable

or deteriorate. If the psychosis exacerbates, it is necessary to review the risks and benefits of neuroleptic treatment and reenter the algorithm at the beginning.

In some patients it may be worthwhile considering specific drug therapy to treat the tardive dyskinesia. Unfortunately, there are no uniformly safe and effective therapies. Many agents have been used to treat this disorder, but with limited and varying degrees of success.[9,10,21] Thus, it is possible to conclude that there are many treatments or no treatments for tardive dyskinesia.

Drugs affecting dopamine are the most widely studied agents in tardive dyskinesia. In rare cases where the disorder is severe or life threatening, neuroleptic drugs have been used to suppress dyskinetic symptoms so that a patient can function. However, in the majority of cases, it is not appropriate to use neuroleptics solely to suppress tardive dyskinesia. Other drugs that decrease dopamine function, such as reserpine and tetrabenazine have had variable results in suppressing tardive dyskinesia and may also carry a risk that is similar to continued neuroleptic therapy, since these compounds also reduce dopamine neurotransmission. Several patients receiving the atypical neuroleptic clozapine have had tardive dyskinesia greatly improve.[22] It is not yet known if clozapine has a specific therapeutic effect on tardive dyskinesia or whether the benefit is because the drug allows spontaneous recovery to take place.

The strategy of desensitizing the hypersensitive dopamine system by flooding it with dopamine agonists has been tried with only limited success. Thus it is not recommended and carries the risk of exacerbating psychosis.[9] In some patients with tardive dystonia, benefit has been observed with dopamine agonists, such as L-dopa or bromocriptine or the atypical antagonist clozapine.

Cholinergic compounds, such as choline and lecithin, taken as dietary supplements for precursor loading of cholinergic synthesis have not been consistently successful. Additionally, these agents, like most other compounds (with the exception of neuroleptics), have not been studied over the very long term and may carry late-onset risks of their own. Anticholinergic compounds usually aggravate existing tardive dyskinesia or may unmask covert dyskinetic symptoms. Thus they are not recommended as standard therapy for tardive dyskinesia. Yet, in a subgroup of patients with tardive dystonia, high doses of anticholinergics appear to be beneficial.[6,7]

A competing hypothesis to explain tardive dyskinesia proposes that it is due to gamma-aminobutyric acid (GABA) hypofunction. As clinical tests of this hypothesis, agents which have increased GABA either through direct agonism or inhibition of the catalytic enzymes, have only produced variable results in tardive dyskinesia.[9,23] Benzodiazepines have also been helpful in some patients with tardive dyskinesia. It is not clear whether these drugs are working through a GABA mechanism, through some other

specific effect on the underlying pathophysiology, or have only a nonspecific sedative effect.

Many other compounds affecting serotonergic, adrenergic, neuropeptide, opiate, and other neurotransmitter systems have all produced variable and inconsistent results.[9,10,21] Recent interest has developed in using high-dose vitamin E as a treatment for tardive dyskinesia,[24] but it is unknown whether this will eventually produce consistently beneficial results.

CONCLUSION

Tardive dyskinesia is a major limitation to the use of neuroleptics. However, when these drugs are prescribed appropriately to patients who respond to them, the benefits far outweigh the risks. Successful treatment strategies include a high degree of vigilance for the early onset of symptoms, careful assessment of both the psychiatric and neurological parameters, drug dosage adjustment to achieve the lowest effective doses, and periodic review and documentation of the treatment plan. Until new drugs for psychosis are developed that do not produce tardive dyskinesia, a thoughtful and considered approach is the best method for managing this troublesome syndrome.

ACKNOWLEDGMENTS

Kristina Wells prepared the typescript. This work was supported in part by funds from the Veterans Affairs Research Program and by NIMH grant no. 36657.

REFERENCES

1. Schönecker M: Ein eigentumliches syndrom im oralen bereich bei megaphenapplikation. Nervenarzt 28:35–36, 1957.
2. Sigwald J, Bouttier D, Raymondeaud C: Quatre cas de dyskinesie facio-bucco-linguo-masticatrice a l'evolution prolongee secondaire a un traitment par les neuroleptiques. Rev Neurol (Paris) 100:751–755, 1959.
3. Uhrbrand L, Faurbye A: Reversible and irreversible dyskinesia after treatment with perphenazine, chlorpromazine, reserpine, and electroconvulsive therapy. Psychopharmacologica 1:408–418, 1960.
4. Faurbye A, Rasch PJ, Bender Peterson P, et al: Neurological symptoms in the pharmacotherapy of psychoses. Acta Psychiatr Scand 40:10–26, 1964.
5. Casey DE: The differential diagnosis of tardive dyskinesia. Acta Psychiatr Scand 63(suppl 291):71–87, 1981.
6. Burke RE, Fahn S, Jankovic J, et al: Tardive dystonia: Late-onset and persistent dystonia caused by antipsychotic drugs. Neurology 32:1335–1346, 1982.
7. Gardos G, Cole JO, Salomon M, et al: Clinical forms of severe tardive dyskinesia. Am J Psychiatry 144:895–902, 1987.
8. Barnes TRE, Braude WM: Akathisia variants and tardive dyskinesia. Arch Gen Psychiatry 42:874–878, 1985.
9. Casey DE: Tardive dyskinesia. In Meltzer HY, ed. Psychopharmacology: The Third Generation of Progress. New York: Raven Press, 1987:1411–1419.

10. Baldessarini RJ, Cole JO, Davis JM, et al: Tardive dyskinesia: A task force report. Washington, DC: American Psychiatric Press, 1980.

11. Barnes TRE, Kidger T, Gore SM: Tardive dyskinesia: A 3-year follow-up study. Psychol Med 13:71–81, 1983.

12. Kane JM, Woerner M, Weinhold P, et al: Incidence of tardive dyskinesia: Five year data from a prospective study. Psychopharmacol Bull 20(1):39–40, 1984.

13. Saltz BL, Kane JM, Woerner MG, et al: Prospective study of tardive dyskinesia in the elderly. Psychopharmacol Bull 25(1):52–56, 1989.

14. Casey DE: Tardive dyskinesia and affective disorders. L'encephale 14:221–226, 1988.

15. Ganzini L, Heintz R, Hoffman WF, et al: The prevalence of tardive dyskinesia in neuroleptic-treated diabetics. Arch Gen Psychiatry 48:259–263, 1991.

16. Toenniessen LM, Casey DE, McFarland BH: Tardive dyskinesia in the aged. Arch Gen Psychiatry 42:278–284, 1985.

17. Casey DE: Tardive dyskinesia. West J Med 153:535–541, 1990.

18. Casey DE: Clozapine: Neuroleptic-induced EPS and tardive dyskinesia. Psychopharmacology 99:S47–S53, 1989.

19. Jeste DV, Potkin SG, Sinha S, et al: Tardive dyskinesia—reversible and irreversible. Arch Gen Psychiatry 36:585–590, 1979.

20. Casey DE, Gerlach J: Tardive dyskinesia: Management and new treatment. In Stancer HC, Garfinkel PE, Rakoff VM, eds. Guidelines for the Use of Psychotropic Drugs: A Clinical Handbook. New York: Spectrum Publications, Inc. 1984:183–203.

21. Jeste DV, Wyatt RJ: Therapeutic strategies against tardive dyskinesia. Arch Gen Psychiatry 39:803–816, 1982.

22. Lieberman J, Johns C, Cooper T, et al: Clozapine pharmacology and tardive dyskinesia. Psychopharmacology 99:S54–S59, 1989.

23. Nguyen JA, Thaker GK, Tamminga CA: Gamma-aminobutyric acid (GABA) pathways in tardive dyskinesia. Psychiatr Ann 19(6):302–309, 1989.

24. Elkashef AM, Ruskin PE, Bacher N, et al: Vitamin E in the treatment of tardive dyskinesia. Am J Psychiatry 147(4):505–506, 1990.

27

NEUROLEPTIC MALIGNANT SYNDROME

JOHN M. DAVIS, M.D., PHILIP G. JANICAK, M.D., and ARIFULLA KHAN, M.D.

The neuroleptic malignant syndrome (NMS) is an acute disorder of thermoregulation and neuromotor control, carrying a reported mortality rate of 21 per cent. The most frequent symptoms of NMS include: fever, often greater than 40°C (104°F); severe muscle rigidity, typically "lead pipe" or "plastic"; altered consciousness, usually with clouding of the sensorium, possibly progressing to stupor or coma; and autonomic changes most characterized by fluctuating blood pressure, tachypnea, and diaphoresis.

Neuroleptic malignant syndrome was originally described by Delay and Deniker.[1] Stanley Caroff played a particularly important role in the development of our knowledge in a seminal paper that reviewed the literature and established many of the cardinal and associated features of NMS.[2] Major clues as to pathophysiology also proceeded from clinical observations. The first was that an identical syndrome occurred in parkinsonian patients whose antiparkinsonian drugs were reduced.[3] Although relatively uncommon, the fact that an identical syndrome can occur with a rapid decrease in do-

paminergic medication is consistent with the notion that NMS is caused by neuroleptic-induced dopamine blockade.

Neuroleptic malignant syndrome can occur with a wide variety of neuroleptics, including atypical drugs such as tiapride, sulpiride, and clozapine. In addition, it occurs with dopamine-blocking agents used for other purposes, such as phenothiazine antiemetics (e.g., metoclopramide); neuroleptics as adjuncts to anesthesia (e.g., droperidol); or amoxapine, an antidepressant with a neuroleptic metabolite. The antidepressant fluoxetine has also been reported to cause NMS by an unknown mechanism, as have dopamine-depleting agents (e.g., reserpine) and combined antagonist and depleting agents (e.g., tetrabenazine). This suggests that NMS is caused by a decrease in dopaminergic tone, and supports the therapeutic benefit of a dopaminergic agonist. Conversely, if dopamine agonists have an anti-NMS effect, this provides additional evidence supporting a decreased dopamine hypothesis. In our view, the symptoms and pharmacology are the same in several situations, with an NMS-like syndrome occurring after the withdrawal of antiparkinsonian agents, such as carbidopa/L-dopa, amantadine, and bromocriptine. Given this evidence, the term neuroleptic malignant syndrome is probably a misnomer, and a better name might be the "hypodopaminergic, hyperpyrexia syndrome." Levinson and Simpson[4] have also questioned the homogeneity of this syndrome, feeling that the term "EPS with fever" may be more descriptive and less misleading, since its morbidity and mortality are primarily due to the complications of prolonged immobility and muscle contractions, rather than from a direct effect of these drugs.[4] In addition, in the majority of the cases they reviewed, there was either a clear or probable medical explanation for fever other than the neuroleptic; however, a subsequent review by Addonizio et al.[5] did not find this relationship. The evidence for a dopaminergic factor and the generally negative work-up in almost all cases suggests this is a specific disorder.

EPIDEMIOLOGY

Recently, Keck et al. reported an incidence of NMS ranging from 0.02 to 2.4 per cent in a large number of neuroleptic-treated patients and found there was a 0.67 per cent pooled mean estimate.[6] Further, a significant proportion (i.e., 40 per cent) of these patients were diagnosed as having affective disorders. The ratio of males:females who develop NMS is 3:2, and the mean reported age is about 40 years old. Other possible risk factors include the presence of an organic mental disorder; agitation; dehydration; the rate, route, and dose of antipsychotic; and the use of concurrent psychotropics, especially lithium. The most commonly implicated neuroleptic agents are the high-potency, low-dose group (e.g., haloperidol, fluphenazine). This high rate may be due to the preferential use of these drugs, the fact that they are often chosen for the medically compromised patient, and their use in high-dose rapid tranquilization regimens. Neuroleptic malignant syndrome occurs with both the oral and depot preparations, but the length of the episode seems to be more severe with the depot form.

In approximately 80 per cent of cases, NMS occurs within the first 2 weeks of treatment with a neuroleptic or after an increase in the dosage. It must be emphasized, however, that NMS can occur at any time during antipsychotic drug use. Typically, the syndrome progresses rapidly, developing fully in 24 to 48 hours, and lasts for an average of 7 to 14 days, but up to 30 days is not unusual. The duration is usually twice as long when depot agents are involved. Shalev and Munitz[7] have made several important contributions to our understanding of NMS in their review article. They noted that most cases occurred in the first few days of treatment and that many cases oc-

curred with a dose escalation of the type often used in rapid tranquilization. Their data suggest that NMS is associated with a sudden decrease in dopaminergic tone; although it is also quite true that some cases of NMS occur unexpectedly in patients who have been on the same dose for many months or years. This is important, particularly in light of the increased incidence of NMS seen upon withdrawal of dopaminergic antiparkinsonian medication.

DIAGNOSIS

Clinical Signs and Symptoms

Neuroleptic malignant syndrome includes several core symptoms, but all are not present in every case. These symptoms include fever (often greater than 40°C); severe muscle rigidity, with a lead pipe presentation as opposed to cogwheeling; an altered state of consciousness ranging from clouding of the sensorium to coma; and autonomic instability often associated with profound diaphoresis. While some patients have elevated blood pressure, others are normotensive, and still others are hypotensive. Hypotension is a poorer prognostic sign, indicating a failure of the body to sustain a normal blood pressure. Rosenbush and Stewart found that 33 per cent of patients had a labile blood pressure.[8] There are also a number of secondary symptoms, including such autonomic manifestations as respiratory distress, pallor, flushing, and incontinence; other motor disturbances (i.e., parkinsonian-like syndromes, tremor, sialorrhea, dystonic reactions, chorea, oculogyric crisis, and dyskinesia); and less frequent neurological symptoms such as dysphagia, akinetic mutism, aphonia, dysarthria, hyperreflexia, ataxia, extensor plantar responses and posturing.

Laboratory Findings

Patients with NMS almost always have elevated creatine phosphokinase (CPK) levels. Increases are usually in the 2000 to 15,000 v/Liter range and rarely above 100,000 V/liter. The absence of an elevation in CPK would speak against the diagnosis of NMS; however, it is nonspecific and can also be markedly increased with agitation, many forms of strenuous physical exercise, dystonic reactions, or intramuscular injections (high-sensitivity, low-specificity test). Often, agitated psychotic patients are given intramuscular injections, further increasing CPK levels. Serum glutamic oxaloacetic transaminase (SGOT), serum glutamic pyruvic transaminase (SGPT), and lactate dehydrogenase (LDH) are usually elevated, indicating liver involvement. White cell elevations range from 15,000 to 30,000/μL, with a shift to the left occurring in about 40 per cent of cases. The electroencephalogram (EEG) is usually normal, but may show diffuse slowing or other nonspecific abnormalities.

DIFFERENTIAL DIAGNOSIS

Malignant Hyperthermia

In malignant hyperthermia (MH), muscle rigidity and fever develop rapidly following exposure to inhalation anesthetic agents and succinylcholine. Its basis appears to be a genetic, muscle membrane defect in which the sarcoplasmic reticulum has a hypersensitive calcium release mechanism, leading to increased muscle contraction.[9] The human ryanodine receptor (the calcium release channel of the sarcoplasmic reticulum) has been cloned and the ryanodine receptor gene has been mapped to region q13.1 of the human chromosome 19. This location is close to the genetic markers for MH susceptibility (using the muscle test response to caffeine and halothane) in man or the halothane sensitivity gene in the pig model of MH. These two lines of evidence suggest that a mutation of this gene is responsible for human MH as well as the halothane sensitivity phenotype in pigs. This also implies that information from the pig is valid. It is notable that neuroleptics delay and attenuate halothane-induced MH in the pig.

There is a strong hereditary factor in malignant hyperthermia, with 80 per cent of an MH patient's family members also susceptible to this disorder. The genetic studies, however, only clearly identify autosomal dominant inheritance in less than 50 per cent of the families. In approximately 20 per cent of other families, the episode seems to be an isolated sporadic case. Some propose a polygenic multifactorial inheritance pattern, although others propose an autosomal dominant trait with low penetrance and variable expressivity. It is certainly clear that many patients with MH have had a prior history of uncomplicated anesthesia on one or more occasions. Malignant hyperthermia is triggered during anesthesia, and the onset of the hypermetabolic response occurs rapidly, with body temperature increasing at 1°C every 5 minutes. Anesthesiologists treat the disorder with 2.5 mg/kg of dantrolene, often repeated every 5 to 10 minutes to a total of 10 mg/kg. It is relevant to note that droperidol is a safe anesthetic for patients with malignant hyperthermia, though it is a neuroleptic and can cause NMS.

Hermesh et al.[10] reported a systematic study on the possible occurrence of MH and found no evidence that electroconvulsive therapy (ECT) produced it in 20 patients who had NMS or in 108 first-degree relatives. Of these, 16 index patients and 37 relatives had either surgery or ECT or both. Furthermore, there is no body of case reports suggesting that NMS and MH occur differentially in the same persons or families or both. This suggests, but does not prove, that these two syndromes are not genetically related, but given the low incidence of MH and NMS, a very large sample would be required to reject the null hypothesis. Since the temperature elevation seen in NMS is probably secondary to muscle rigidity, the use of muscle relaxants is a logical course of action.

Finally, given that MH shares its symptoms with NMS and both are successfully treated with a muscle relaxant, dantrolene, some common pathophysiology is likely.

Succinylcholine, used in ECT, is a known triggering agent for MH; therefore, psychiatrists should be aware of this complication in patients who have had a personal or family history of this disorder. We know of only one report, however, of possible MH in a patient undergoing ECT.[11] This case received concomitant neuroleptics as well as ECT and developed a temperature of 39.5°C (101.8°F) and rigidity shortly after each of the last three ECTs. The patient later had an abnormal muscle biopsy response to halothane, indicating a susceptibility to MH. Since MH only occurs during inhalation anesthesia with or without succinylcholine, the question of differential diagnosis pertains only to patients undergoing this procedure while also receiving neuroleptics. The temporal association of hyperthermia with three ECT treatments and succinylcholine suggests that this was MH and not NMS.

Lethal Catatonia

Acute lethal catatonia involves sustained agitation progressing to hyperpyrexia, withdrawal, catatonia, cardiovascular collapse, and death. A sodium amytal interview may be helpful in making the differential diagnosis. Patients with this clinical presentation who are taking neuroleptics should be assumed to have NMS and treated as such (see later in chapter).

Heat Stroke

The differential diagnosis between NMS and heat stroke is a common and practically important issue. Heat stroke is generally categorized into two variants: classical and exertional types. Classical heat stroke occurs during extreme heat waves associated with high humidity lasting for 5 or 6 days, with the elderly at particular risk. Patients suddenly develop a temperature as high as 41.6°C (107°F) or above and associated coma. It is also a common occurrence in pilgrammages to Mecca, where in a single year there were over 1000 reported cases and undoubtedly many more went unrecognized. In treating heat stroke, it is important to avoid packing the body in ice which can cause intense vasoconstriction. The aim is to cool the body core temperature, but severe vasoconstriction keeps heat in. In treating pilgrims, a net bed is used and the patient is subjected to tepid water sprays with high air movement, causing the temperature to fall at rates of 0.5°C/min.

In exertional heat stroke, even though high environmental temperature and high humidity are important, extreme exercise is the proximal cause. This type can occur in a wide variety of sporting, physical, or training activities. During a marathon, runners frequently develop temperatures of 40°C (104°F), and on occasion in marathons or marches, patients can develop temperatures in excess of 42.2°C (108°F) with associated heavy sweating.

In classical heat stroke there is a failure of the sweating mechanisms and patients often have dry skin, whereas in exertional heat stroke there is often marked perspiration. It is important to note that anticholinergics may predispose to heat stroke. For example, there is a large clinical literature from the 1930s recounting the experience of physicians in the Indian British Army Medical Corps. They reported on cases undergoing surgery who received preanesthetic anticholinergic medication and concluded that in high environmental temperatures, high doses and heavy draping must be avoided. Since anticholinergics, antiparkinsonian drugs, some antipsychotics, and some antidepressants all have high anticholinergic properties, they may predispose psychiatric patients to common or exertional heat stroke during the height of summer. In addition, an extremely psychotic patient could have exertional heat stroke because of the associated agitation. Heat stroke is not NMS, which develops in the absence of a high heat load, but there may be a possible relationship, and knowledge of the pathophysiology of heat stroke might be important in understanding the pathophysiology of NMS. Treatments for exertional heat stroke include cooling, and fluid supplements (usually intravenous).

Others

Viral encephalitis, tetanus, and other infections can be mistaken for NMS. Cerebrospinal fluid findings (increased WBC protein, decreased glucose) as well as other physical and laboratory evidence of infection should make the distinction clear. Some hypertonic states such as decorticate or decerebrate rigidity, hypocalcemic tetany, and strychnine poisoning may also mimic NMS especially if they are complicated by infection. As alluded to previously, syndromes similar to NMS may be produced by other types of drug treatment including other dopamine antagonists such as metoclopramide (Reglan); abrupt withdrawal of dopamine agonists (e.g., L-dopa); dopamine-depleting agents (e.g., reserpine); combined antagonist and depleting agents (e.g., tetrabenazine); amoxapine, as well as other antidepressants such as fluoxetine; or phenothiazine antiemetics. Neurotoxicity similar to NMS has been reported with the combination of lithium and with an antipsychotic.

TREATMENT

The most important step to effective treatment of NMS is early recognition and prompt withdrawal of the offending agent. In addition, instituting supportive measures as quickly as possible may be lifesaving. If the patient is receiving an antiparkinsonian agent, it probably should be continued; however,

data are lacking to support this approach and care must be taken to avoid a worsening of mental status and a possible temperature increase. If there is reasonable certainty that the syndrome is severe NMS, the patient should be transferred to a medical setting in which intensive observation and treatment can be provided. A variety of supportive measures can be used, including cooling blankets, ice packs, or an ice-water enema. The goal is to return the temperature to normal. In addition, one should treat complications and give supplemental oxygen with or without mechanical ventilation (the amount of oxygen and the method of delivery will depend on the patient's needs).

Because of the nature of the disorder, there are no controlled studies; however, most authors suggest a trial with dantrolene, bromocriptine, amantadine, L-dopa, or some combination of these agents. The initial dose of dantrolene should be 2 to 3 mg/kg over 10 to 15 minutes. The total dosage should not exceed 10 mg/kg/day, because of possible hepatotoxicity. The dosage range reported is 0.8 to 10 mg/kg/day. Initially, intravenous administration may be necessary until symptoms have resolved sufficiently for the patient to take oral medication. Given orally, the initial dosage range is 100 to 200 mg/day in divided doses, and up to 700 mg/day may be given in a 24-hour period. The typical oral dosage of bromocriptine is 2.5 to 10 mg three times daily; with increases up to 60 mg/day. Some have used bromocriptine in conjunction with dantrolene, with similar dosage patterns. The oral dose of amantadine is 200 to 400 mg/day in divided doses. L-Dopa plus carbidopa (Sinemet) has been infrequently used, and efficacy is not well documented. Dosage of carbidopa is 25 mg plus L-dopa 100 mg (three to eight times daily). The calcium channel blocker nifedipine has also been used to treat NMS, and further data on this drug would be important, given its beneficial effect in a single case report.[12] As to the specific effectiveness of a given drug treatment, many cases of NMS have resolved completely with conservative measures alone (i.e., withdrawing neuroleptics and instituting supportive therapy). Thus, it can be difficult to assess the benefit of any given drug when it is combined with these measures.

RETREATMENT STRATEGIES

An important issue is the retreatment strategy for patients who have developed an episode of NMS, recovered, and now require further treatment. As the NMS subsides, many patients have a reemergence of psychosis or agitation, the conditions for which the neuroleptics were first indicated. Since the disorder itself is often severe, an effective treatment is needed, but early reinstitution of neuroleptics may significantly increase a possible recurrence of the NMS episode. Electroconvulsive therapy is an effective treatment for psychotic and severe mania, depression, catatonia, schizophrenic excitement, and schizoaffective disorders.[14] However, its use for the treatment of NMS is controversial, since some patients have died or developed cardiac arrest during ECT, while others benefited when it was given during or shortly after an episode had resolved.[13] Recently, we reviewed the world literature and found a mortality rate of 10 per cent when ECT was employed during an episode of NMS.[15] This compares to a 21 per cent mortality rate in patients who received only nonspecific treatment for their episode. Further, in the three deaths with ECT, neuroleptics were continued before, during, and after ECT. Thus, the failure of the NMS to improve may have been due to the continued administration of neuroleptics. There were also other cases when neuroleptics were continued with ECT throughout the episode of NMS, and the outcomes were not favorable, though the patients survived. Again we emphasize the importance of discontinuing neuroleptics whenever the possibility of NMS is suspected. Consideration of alternative non-neuroleptic interventions should also be explored, especially in light of reports that affectively disordered patients with psychotic features may be more susceptible to tardive dyskinesia (TD) and NMS. The use of lithium or alternative treatments such as valproate for bipolar disorders, may be more appropriate after the episode of NMS has resolved. Further, in psychotic manic episodes, lower doses of neuroleptics in combination with lithium may be as effective as higher doses and perhaps diminish the possibility of an NMS recurrence.[16]

If a neuroleptic is necessary, treatment should be instituted as long as possible after an episode (i.e., at least 2 weeks). Wells and his coworkers[17] reviewed 41 cases of neuroleptic rechallenge after an episode and noted that 7 of 11 patients had a recurrence when rechallenged within 5 days or less; however, only 10 of 33 experienced a recurrence when challenged after 5 days.[17] Rosenbush et al.[18] found only 1 out of 13 cases had a recurrence when rechallenged after 2 weeks.[18] We would also suggest prophylactic concomitant bromocriptine for several weeks, with gradual tapering after that time period. Such prophylactic approaches during the retreatment phase have been attempted in a few patients, but there are no controlled studies. Nevertheless, it seems like a sensible strategy and poses little additional risk.

Since as many as 50 per cent of patients reexposed to a neuroleptic again develop the syndrome, we would suggest choosing an antipsychotic from a different family, and preferably a lower potency agent such as thioridazine. However, the recommendation to use thioridazine or a neuroleptic from a different family is based on common sense, not supportive empirical data. We would further recommend starting on a very low dose and titrating up slowly in a hospital setting to carefully monitor clinical response and temperature, as well as neurological and mental status. Using low doses will not necessarily jeopardize chances for an adequate clinical re-

sponse. For example, we have recently found evidence for a therapeutic effect with low-dose trifluoperazine.[19] One third of 37 psychotic patients showed a good response during a 2-week trial on a fixed dose of 5 mg b.i.d. On this dose, most responders fell into a medium plasma level category, and the five patients with the highest plasma levels were all nonresponders. Thus, at this relatively low dose of trifluoperazine, a large percentage of patients showed adequate response, and some may even have benefited from a reduction in dose (and plasma level), theoretically minimizing the risk of NMS. This finding is consistent with a growing body of literature indicating that "less may indeed be more" when it comes to the dose of neuroleptic. An alternate neuroleptic that has been considered is clozapine; however, three recent case reports indicate that this agent alone may also induce NMS.[20–22] We know of a fourth unpublished case and two cases with clozapine-other drug combinations. Benzodiazepines (e.g., lorazepam) have also been recommended to avoid or at least minimize the dose of antipsychotic.

COMPLICATIONS

A number of serious complications have been reported with NMS. In a review of the literature, we found an average mortality rate of 21 per cent in patients treated only with nonspecific interventions.[23] Most symptoms or historical variables failed to predict mortality from NMS; however, the highest temperature reported in an episode and the state of consciousness were highly predictive of survival versus death. The immediate cause of death was usually associated with rhabdomyolysis and myoglobinuria leading to acute renal failure in about 25 per cent of patients with a severe episode. Significant cardiac complications, such as an acute myocardial infarction with pulmonary edema and cardiac arrest have also occurred. Pulmonary complications include aspiration pneumonitis, pulmonary embolism, and hypoxia due to hypoventilation secondary to chest wall restriction. In a small number of cases, other problems such as the anterior tibial syndrome, *Escherichia coli* fascitis, hepatitis as well as hepatic failure, and disseminated intravascular coagulation (DIC) have occurred.

We also found that the specific drug treatment with dantrolene or dopaminergic agonists or both significantly reduced the mortality rate of NMS (i.e., 10 per cent versus 21 per cent), and did so uniformly in both mild, moderate, and severe cases.[23] To test the significance of this finding, we performed case-controlled analyses using as our control the mortality rate of NMS patients who had not received any specific treatment. Thus, by definition, the control group consisted of patients who had not received bromocriptine, amantadine, other dopamine agonists, dantrolene, any form of dopa, or ECT. This was not a controlled prospective study, but rather a retrospective evaluation of the clinical literature. Bromocriptine, amantadine, and dantrolene were superior to no treatment as related to clinical efficacy, recurrence of NMS, and mortality. The number of patients treated with ECT and dopa is too small to arrive at definite conclusions. And while we had a comparison group for the percentage that died, this was clearly subject to possible bias. For example, when clinicians observe a dramatic immediate benefit from a drug, they may be more likely to report it than to report a lackluster or untoward response. Likewise, severe cases leading to death are more likely to be reported. While we can speculate about these possibilities, we do not know how they may have influenced the case report literature. Our predicament is that double-blind studies cannot be done; hence, we must rely on clinical case reports.

CONCLUSIONS

In summary, NMS is an underrecognized but serious complication of drug treatment. Effective and at times lifesaving management requires early recognition and prompt intervention with supportive measures, and specific drug treatments. After an episode of NMS, retreatment strategies may include ECT, non-neuroleptic alternatives, low-potency antipsychotics, lower doses of higher potency agents, as well as clozapine, benzodiazepines or both.

REFERENCES

1. Delay J, Deniker P: Drug-induced extrapyramidal syndromes. In Vinken PJ, Bruyn GW, eds. Handbook of Clinical Neurology, Vol 6: Diseases of the Basal Ganglia. Amsterdam, Holland: North Holland, 1968:248–266.
2. Caroff SN: The neuroleptic malignant syndrome. J Clin Psychiatry 41:79–83, 1980.
3. Kuno S, Komure O, Mizuta E, et al: Neuroleptic malignant syndrome associated with withdrawal of antiparkinsonian drugs. Movement Disorders 5(suppl 1):171, 1990.
4. Levinson DF, Simpson GM: Neuroleptic-induced extra-pyramidal symptoms with fever. Arch Gen Psychiatry 43:839–848, 1986.
5. Addonizio G, Susman VL, Roth SD: Neuroleptic malignant syndrome: Review and analysis of 115 cases. Biol Psychiatry 22:1004–1020, 1987.
6. Keck PE, McElroy SL, Pope HG: Epidemiology of NMS. J Clin Psychiatry 21:148–151, 1991.
7. Shalev A, Munitz H: The neuroleptic malignant syndrome: Agent and host interaction. Acta Psychiatr Scand 73:337–347, 1986.
8. Rosenbush P, Stewart T: A prospective analysis of 24 episodes of neuroleptic malignant syndrome. Am J Psychiatry 146:717–725, 1989.
9. MacLennan DH, Duff C, Zorzato F, et al: Ryanodine receptor gene is a candidate for predisposition to malignant hyperthermia. Nature 343:559–561, 1990.
10. Hermesh H, Aizenberg D, Lapidot M, Munitz H: Risk of malignant hyperthermia among patients with neuroleptic malignant syndrome and their families. Am J Psychiatry 145:1431–1434, 1988.
11. Lazarus A, Rosenberg H: MH during ECT. (Letter to the editor). Am J Psychiatry 148:541–542, 1991.
12. Hermesh H, Molcho A, Aizenberg D, Munitz H: The calcium antagonist nifedipine in recurrent neuroleptic malignant syndrome. Clin Neuropharmacol II:552–555, 1988.
13. Addonizio G, Susman VL: ECT as a treatment alternative for patients with symptoms of neuroleptic malignant syndrome. J Clin Psychiatry 48:102–105, 1987.
14. Janicak PG, Easton MS, Comaty JE, et al: Efficacy of ECT in psychotic and nonpsychotic depression. Convulsive Therapy 5(4):314–320, 1989.
15. Davis JM, Janicak PG, Sakkas P, et al: ECT in the treatment of NMS. Convulsive Therapy 7(2):111–120, 1991.
16. Janicak PG, Bresnahan DB, Sharma RP, et al: A comparison of thiothixene with chlorpromazine in the treatment of mania. J Clin Psychopharmacol 8:33–37, 1988.
17. Wells AJ, Sommi RW, Crismon ML: Neuroleptic rechallenge after neuroleptic malignant syndrome: Case report and literature review. Drug Intell Clin Pharm 22:475–480, 1988.
18. Rosenbush P, Stewart TD, Gelenberg AJ: Twenty neuroleptic rechallenges after neuroleptic malignant syndrome in 15 patients. J Clin Psychiatry 50:295–298, 1989.
19. Janicak PG, Javaid JI, Sharma RP, et al: Trifluoperazine plasma levels and clinical response. J Clin Psychopharmacol 9:340–346, 1989.
20. Miller DD, Sharafuddin MJA, Kathol RG: A Case of clozapine-induced NMS. J Clin Psychiatry 52:99–101, 1991.
21. Anderson ES, Powers PS: NMS associated with clozapine use. J Clin Psychiatry 52:102–104, 1991.
22. DasGupta K, Young A: Clozapine-induced NMS. J Clin Psychiatry 52:105–107, 1991.
23. Sakkas P, Davis JM, Hau J, Wang Z: Pharmacotherapy of NMS. Psychiatr Ann 21:157–164, 1991.

28

TYPICAL ANTIPSYCHOTIC MEDICATION:
Clinical Practice

S. CHARLES SCHULZ, M.D. and MARTHA SAJATOVIC, M.D.

The treatment of schizophrenia was revolutionized by the discovery of the first specific antipsychotic medication, chlorpromazine, in 1949 and its subsequent introduction around the world. Chlorpromazine and other antipsychotic agents reduced the symptoms of psychosis in patients with schizophrenia and other psychotic disorders, rather than merely sedating patients. The reduction in symptoms not only relieved the suffering of schizophrenic patients but, by reduction of psychosis, patients were better able to participate in other forms of psychosocial treatment. Studies of antipsychotic medications in the following decades demonstrated them to be the mainstay of the treatment of schizophrenia around which other interventions were arranged.

Although introduced to North America in the early 1950s and utilized in the treatment of millions of patients, there have been significant advances in the last decade in the use of the typical antipsychotic medications, including refinement of dosing strategies and improved management of side effects. These advances are important in day-to-day practice, as they improve patients' comfort and compliance.

The focus of this chapter on the use of typical antipsychotic medications should not be taken as an endorsement of use of medication alone in the treatment of schizophrenia. Use of these powerful medications is maximized in the context of a therapeutic relationship so that symptoms, discomforts, side effects, and diagnostic reassessment can occur. Also, there is considerable empirical support for reduction of relapse rates with utilization of psychosocial therapies such as psychoeducationally oriented family therapy and social skills training.

What follows is an overview of the current practice of medication treatment of schizophrenia with the typical antipsychotic medications. Following a tabulation of the classes of medication, the process of selection of specific medication and dosing strategies will be described. Recognition and management of side effects, maintenance medication usage, and strategies for managing poor response precede a concluding discussion of informed consent.

In this chapter, the term "antipsychotic medica-tion" will be used throughout, although the term neuroleptic is in wide use and is synonymous with the traditional antipsychotic drugs. The antipsychotic drugs are further subclassified by chemical structure.

ANTIPSYCHOTIC DRUGS

Antipsychotic Drug Classification

The antipsychotic medications are composed of eight separate classes of drugs. These are: (1) phenothiazines, (2) thioxanthenes, (3) dibenzazepines, (4) butyrophenones, (5) diphenylbutylpiperidines, (6) indole compounds, (7) benzamides, and (8) amine-depleting agents. Table 28-1 reviews some of the most commonly prescribed antipsychotic medications.

Since the introduction of the first antipsychotic medication, chlorpromazine, in the 1950s, phenothiazines have remained one of the most utilized and well known classes of antipsychotic drugs. However, it is important to note that the term phenothiazine is not synonymous with antipsychotic, as there are numerous other classes of antipsychotic drugs with differing chemical structures. All phenothiazines have a common tricyclic structure. The subtypes of phenothiazines are aliphatic (e.g., chlorpromazine), piperazine (e.g., trifluoperazine, fluphenazine), and piperidine (e.g., thioridazine, mesoridazine).

Thioxanthenes are antipsychotics that are somewhat structurally similar to the phenothiazines. Subtypes of thioxanthenes are aliphatic (chlorprothixene) and piperazine (thiothixene).

Dibenzoxazepines also have a tricyclic nucleus. Until recently, the only dibenzoxazepine available in the United States was loxapine. Clozapine is a dibenzoxazepine that has recently become available in the United States. It is described as an atypical antipsychotic due to its minimal neurological side effects.

Structurally quite different from the phenothiazines, the butyrophenones are more potent drugs

176

TABLE 28–1. CLASSIFICATION OF ANTIPSYCHOTIC MEDICATIONS[a]

Generic	Relative Potency	Usual Daily Dose Range (mg/day)
Phenothiazines		
Chlorpromazine	100	50–10000
Thioridazine	100	50–800
Perphenazine	10	8–64
Fluphenazine	2	1–60
Thioxanthenes		
Thiothixene	5	6–120
Butyrophenones		
Haloperidol	2	1–50
Dihydroindolones		
Molindone	10	15–225
Debenzoxazepines		
Loxapine	10	10–160

[a] Tabular format adapted with permission from Kane J; Baltimore, Williams & Wilkins, 1989.

that have come into common usage. Haloperidol is a widely used butyrophenone antipsychotic. Droperidol is used primarily as an anesthetic agent or occasionally in psychiatric emergencies.

The diphenylbutylpiperidines are structurally similar to butyrophenones. Pimozide is the only currently available drug of this class in the United States. Indole compounds are another class of antipsychotics. Molindone is the only available indole in the United States.

Benzamides are in general use as antipsychotic agents only outside of the United States. Metoclopramide (Reglan) is a benzamide commonly used to treat gastroenterological problems, and though it has been associated with extrapyramidal symptoms, it does not improve psychosis.

The amine-depleting agents such as reserpine are rarely used as antipsychotic agents due to their limited efficacy compared to other antipsychotic drug classes, their strong side-effect profile, and potential to induce depression.

Mechanism of Action

The examination of the mechanism of action of the antipsychotic medications led to examination of a dopamine hypothesis of schizophrenia.[1] Studies of receptor blockade indicated antipsychotic activity appears to be due to dopamine receptor blockade. Peroutka and Snyder[2] studied 22 antipsychotic medications and their relative affinity for dopamine, serotonin, adrenergic, and histamine receptors. There was a close correlation between dopamine receptor affinity and antipsychotic potency, and no significant correlation with other receptors. However, other neurotransmitter systems may also be important in antipsychotic activity. Atypical antipsychotic effect may be related to preferential dopamine blockade in the mesolimbic system, with little or no blockade in the nigrostriatum, or there may be an

interaction between dopaminergic and serotonergic systems such that a critical dopamine/serotonin balance is achieved.[3] Though one antipsychotic may be more potent than another, it appears that in equivalent doses, all antipsychotics are equally efficacious.

The dopamine blockade properties may help explain some of the neurological, neuroendocrine, and autonomic side effects. However, these drugs also affect receptors in the noradrenergic, cholinergic, serotonergic, and histaminergic systems. This is reflected in the varying side-effect profiles of different antipsychotic drugs. Higher potency drugs, with greater relative dopamine receptor affinity, have an increased incidence of extrapyramidal and parkinsonian symptoms; whereas lower potency drugs have less of these apparently dopamine-related side effects, but are associated with more sedation and orthostatic hypotension.

IMPLEMENTATION OF ANTIPSYCHOTIC TREATMENT

Selection of Antipsychotic

Once the decision has been made to treat schizophrenic symptoms, the clinician must then decide on a specific choice of antipsychotic medication. Overall, the antipsychotics are safe medications, with a wide therapeutic index, and are nonaddictive. Although the various antipsychotic medications are equally efficacious in treating schizophrenia, there may be differences among individuals in how a person responds to the antipsychotic effects of these drugs. For the schizophrenic patient who has never been on antipsychotic medications, antipsychotic choice should be tailored to an individual patient's treatment requirements. This can be determined by an assessment of side-effect profiles. For example, elderly patients who may be more vulnerable to orthostasis would do better on low doses of a higher potency agent to reduce their risk of sedation and falls. In general, for agitated, psychotic hospitalized patients, the nonsedating/higher potency agents provide the clinician a better opportunity to observe antipsychotic effect, as there is less chance of sedation being misinterpreted as change in psychotic symptoms. However, high-potency-agent use may be limited by the presence of neurological side effects such as acute dystonias or akisthesia. Some university groups have indicated that the addition of benzodiazepines may help control anxiety symptoms in agitated schizophrenic patients rather than using high doses of sedating antipsychotic agents. In some cases, mildly agitated outpatients may benefit from the effects of a sedating (i.e., perphenazine) antipsychotic medication.

Dosing Strategies

The usual clinical practice in starting antipsychotic medication is to begin with low doses of medication (about 300 to 500 mg chlorpromazine equivalents) and increase the dose every several days if there is no improvement. While this method treats psychosis, it may lead to excessively high dosage, as antipsychotic medications generally require 5 to 7 days to reach steady state, and maximum drug effect may not occur for 4 to 6 weeks. It appears from most studies that low to moderate doses of antipsychotic (10 to 20 mg haloperidol) are as effective as high doses, although lowest effective dose of antipsychotic medication will vary among individuals. A recent study by Rifkin et al.[4] examined acute treatment of schizophrenic patients randomly assigned to 10, 30, or 80 mg/day of haloperidol. The study found no advantage to treating newly admitted schizophrenic patients with more than 10 mg/day of haloperidol and also illustrated that regardless of dose, the rate of change was similar across dose groups. Using a low but effective dose of antipsychotic medication is preferred in an attempt to diminish neurological side effects and decrease the risk of tardive dyskinesia.

For the acute treatment of schizophrenic patients, it is usually safest to give an oral dose of a high-potency agent (i.e., 5 mg haloperidol). Peak plasma concentration of most antipsychotics is reached in 2 to 4 hours after oral dose. Although antipsychotic medication has a half-life that allows once-a-day dosing, this should begin after steady state has been reached—after 7 dys of twice-daily dosing. Antipsychotic medication may also be given intramuscularly (IM) in the acute stage of treatment (2 to 5 mg haloperidol IM). Peak plasma concentration is reached in approximately 30 minutes.

If the patient is initially agitated or combative, the clinician may add a benzodiazepine such as lorazepam (1 to 2 mg) or diazepam (5 mg) to the antipsychotic regimen. The benzodiazepine may be given with the repeated dosages of antipsychotic or cautiously on a p.r.n. basis.

Rapid neuroleptization is a method of treating acute psychosis with repeated doses of IM antipsychotic medication every 30 to 60 minutes, until the desired clinical effect is achieved. This method requires close medical supervision due to risk of hypotension or laryngeal dystonia. Any apparent benefit of initial high-dose antipsychotic medication to the agitated schizophrenic patient may be due to sedation. Empirical research does not support this approach as especially more efficacious than standard doses or use of added benzodiazepines.

Patients initially begun on antipsychotic medication are usually given divided dosages, two to four times a day. This decreases acute adverse effects and helps maintain sustained bioavailability. Once plasma steady state is reached and the patient has had relative stabilization of his psychiatric symptoms, dosage may be changed to a once-a-day basis because antipsychotic elimination half-life is approximately 20 to 30 hours. Sedative effects of antipsychotic medication usually persist for approximately 3 to 4 hours after ingestion, so that once-a-day bedtime dosage is effective, well tolerated, and reduces daytime side effects.

The use of blood levels to determine appropriate antipsychotic dosage may help determine lowest effective dose and studies have suggested a medication therapeutic window. Haloperidol is the most studied and is optimally therapeutic at plasma levels of 5 to 15 ng/ml. Higher doses may be associated with suboptimal responses.[5] It is possible that basing clinical dosage on a therapeutic plasma level range for antipsychotic medication may become more common practice in the future.

Poor Response to Traditional Antipsychotics

Use of Augmenting Agents

Despite the demonstrated empirical efficacy of the traditional antipsychotic medications, as many as 30 per cent of patients with schizophrenia show a suboptimal response to treatment. In the last decade, clinicians and investigators have focused more attention on the problem of poor response, including a crisper definition of an adequate antipsychotic trial, testing of augmenting medications, and trials of atypical antipsychotic medication.

The definition of poor response to treatment has received considerable attention, with testing of clozapine as a treatment of last resort in the United States. Patients entering this trial were considered to be not responsive to antipsychotic medication if at least three medicines from at least two classes, at doses of 1000 chlorpromazine equivalents had been tried for at least 6 weeks each. Objective rating scales (BPRS) were used to assess symptoms and prospective criteria were established to separate response from nonresponse. In practice, if a patient remains significantly symptomatic despite such an effort, assessment of other causes of psychosis should be entertained. This should be followed by an examination of psychosocial treatment, including compliance and medication blood levels. The research definition of nonresponse needs to be balanced by the patients' overall needs as assessed by the clinician.

Currently, if poor response to antipsychotics is noted, the addition of other psychotropic medications is warranted and is supported by placebo-controlled empirical research. Lithium carbonate administered in doses that achieve a blood level of approximately 1.0 mEq/liter has been shown to be useful in some poorly responsive schizophrenic patients. Careful monitoring in the initiation of this treatment, especially in neuromuscular symptoms, is warranted. Benzodiazepines added to antipsychotic medication has been shown to diminish symptoms of psychosis in poor responders. For example, doses of alprazolam of 2 mg/day can be useful. Careful attention to disinhibition and slow tapering when the medication is discontinued are important. Carbamazepine has been extensively studied as an augmenting medication for persistent symptoms of schizophrenia, but does not appear to be useful for unselected nonresponders. However, it may be quite effective for schizophrenic patients with violent episodes or nonepileptic schizophrenia patients with electroencephalographic (EEG) abnormalities. Other augmenting medications such as calcium channel blockers, propranolol, and reserpine have been tested with mixed results, but are not currently used frequently.[7]

Side Effects and Management

Side effects of antipsychotic drugs can be divided into neurological effects and non-neurological effects. In general, high-potency agents are more frequently associated with neurological adverse effects, while low-potency agents are more frequently associated with non-neurological effects.

Neurological Adverse Effects

The neurological side effects may be best understood in the context of dopamine receptor blockade and the receptor's changes secondary to neuroleptic treatment.[8] Table 28–2 lists medications used to treat neurological adverse effects.

Acute dystonias are muscular spasms of the face, neck, trunk, or extremities that occur in 10 to 15 per cent of all patients on antipsychotics, usually during the early phase of treatment. Patients may experience dysphagia, facial grimacing, tongue twisting, back spasm (opisthotonus), eye deviation (oculogyric crisis), or neck spasms (torticollis). Life-threatening laryngospasm may also occur, generally at very high doses. Acute dystonias are most prevalent in young male adult and adolescent patients, and pa-

tients with previous history of acute dystonias. Often, tolerance develops to dystonic effects. Rapid intervention of acute dystonia is indicated to reduce the significant discomfort. Intramuscular diphenhydramine (50 mg IM) can bring quick symptom reduction. This should be followed by regular dosing of anticholinergic/antiparkinsonian drugs (e.g., benztropine 2 mg b.i.d. orally). Laryngospasm requires immediate intravenous treatment (e.g., diphenhydramine 25 to 50 mg IV).

Some clinicians advocate beginning patients prophylactically on anticholinergic medications when starting an antipsychotic agent. This is probably not indicated in all cases, particularly for older patients who are prone to anticholinergic toxicity. Prophylactic anticholinergic use may be indicated in adolescents, young adult male patients, those with prior history of acute dystonias, or patients so resistant to taking antipsychotic medications that development of an acute dystonia may prevent any future antipsychotic medication compliance. For patients newly begun on anticholinergic agents, it is reasonable to reassess need for continuation of the anticholinergic after 2 to 3 weeks on oral anticholinergic medications.

Antipsychotic-induced parkinsonism presents as bradykinesia, rigidity, masked facies, and drooling. Tremor may occur, but is less consistent than that associated with idiopathic parkinsonism. Symptoms usually occur within the first month of antipsychotic treatment and is dosage dependent. Approximately 10 to 15 per cent of patients on antipsychotics experience parkinsonism, with greatest prevalence in women and the elderly. Some tolerance may develop to parkinsonian effects. Rabbit syndrome is a focal, perioral tremor that may be a late-onset, drug-induced parkinsonian effect. Treatment of drug-induced parkinsonism is with antiparkinsonian agents

TABLE 28–2.   MEDICATION USED TO TREAT NEUROLOGICAL ADVERSE AFFECTS[a]

Generic Name	Trade Name	Dosage Forms (mg)[b]	Usual Daily Dose (mg)
Anticholinergic agents			
Benztropine	Cogentin, Tremin, etc. (generic)	(T) 0.5,1,2; (V) 1/ml	1–6
Biperidin	Akineton	(T) 1; (A) 5/ml	2–10
Cycrimine	Pagitane (not actively marketed)	(T) 2.5	2.5–15
Diphenhydramine	Benadryl, etc. (generic)	(C) 25,50; (L) 50/ml; (A + V) 10 or 50/ml	25–100
Ethopropacine	Parsidol	(T) 10,50	50–200
Orphenadrine	Disipal, Norlex, etc. (generic)	(T) 50,100; (L) 30/10 ml; (A) 60/2 ml	50–300
Procyclidine	Kemadrin	(T) 5	5–30
Trihexylphenidyl	Artane, Pipanol, etc. (generic)	(T) 2,5; (L) 2/5 ml	5–15
Atypical agents			
Amantadine	Symmetrel	(C) 100; (L) 50/ml	100–300
Specialized agents			
Bromocriptine	Parlodel	(T) 2.5; (C) 5	5–50
Dantrolene	Dantrium	(C) 25,50,100; (V) 20/60 ml	60–600
Propranolol	Inderal	(T) 10,20,40,60,80,90; (A) 1/ml	20–120

[a] Adapted with permission from Baldessarini R; Chemotherapy in Psychiatry, Harvard University Press, Copyright 1977 by the President and Fellows of Harvard College, 1985.
[b] Dosage forms: (T) tablets; (C) capsules; (L) syrup or other liquid for oral use; (A or V) ampules or vials for parenteral administration (diphenhydramine is also available in syringes, 50 mg/ml).

such as trihexylphenidyl 2 mg b.i.d. to t.i.d. or amantadine 100 mg t.i.d. (Table 28–2). Parkinsonian effects may be minimized or avoided by dosage reduction or changing to an alternative lower potency agent. Care must be taken in dosage reduction not to administer doses that are so low that relapse of illness occurs.

Akathisia is a subjective feeling of restlessness that is characterized by psychomotor activity, usually in the legs, seen in 20 per cent or more of patients on antipsychotics. The patient may pace endlessly, be unable to sit or stand still, and appear quite distressed. Akathisia is observed more frequently with high-potency agents and is often undiagnosed, as the patient's behavior may be mistaken for a worsening of psychosis. Akathisia occurs within days to several months of starting antipsychotic medication, and is dose related. The pathophysiology of akathisia is not known, and it is of interest that noradrenergic blocking agents can reverse symptoms. The primary management of akasthisia is to find the lowest effective dose of medication or to try a less potent medication such as perphenazine. Some patients respond to propranolol (30 to 120 mg/day). Other less-studied alternatives are benzodiazepines (clonazepam 1.0 mg p.o. b.i.d.) and benztropine (1 to 2 mg b.i.d.).

Tardive dyskinesia (TD) is a syndrome secondary to prolonged antipsychotic treatment, as 4 per cent of patients will develop TD during each year of treatment in the first 7 years of treatment. All antipsychotics except the atypical agents (e.g., clozapine) can lead to TD. Tardive dyskinesia is a syndrome of involuntary, repetitive, abnormal movements of the mouth, head, neck, trunk, or extremities. Movements may be choreiform, athetotic, or tonic contractions. The most common manifestations of TD are perioral and facial movements such as tongue darting, chewing movements, and grimacing. Tardive dyskinesia may range from barely perceptible movements to incapacitating truncal spasms. Risk of developing TD is associated with prolonged use of antipsychotics, and is increased in women, those over age 50, and those with affective illness. The etiology of TD is not clear, but may be due to a "supersensitivity" of dopamine receptors.[8] Because TD is irreversible in many cases, prevention by appropriate use and dose of antipsychotics is essential. There is no definitive treatment for TD, although preliminary observations of patients diagnosed with TD show diminished symptoms when treated with the atypical antipsychotic, clozapine. Management consists of careful use of the lowest effective dose of antipsychotic medication and continued reassessment of treatment requirements. While brief "drug holidays" do not appear to decrease potential to develop TD, if the patient's illness is such that he can be maintained off antipsychotics for long periods of time, this could diminish the potential of developing TD.

Individuals on antipsychotics should receive regular, periodic assessment for involuntary movements. Some states have mandated Abnormal Involuntary Movements Scale (AIMS) examinations every 6 months at their hospitals. When tardive dyskinesia is initially diagnosed, the clinician should consider reducing medication, if possible. Usually, sudden reduction or discontinuation will transiently increase TD movements (withdrawal dyskinesia), but some individuals may then experience slow resolution of TD symptoms, while others will have no change in movements. An increase in medication will temporarily appear to improve TD symptoms, but this is not seen as a viable treatment option. When using antipsychotics for prolonged periods, as is the case with schizophrenia, it is crucial to advise patients and families of the risks and benefits of medication treatment, particularly addressing tardive dyskinesia.

Neuroleptic malignant syndrome (NMS) is a condition of progressive worsening (24 to 72 hours) of muscle rigidity, autonomic instability (hyperpyrexia, sweating, flushing, tachycardia, blood pressure fluctuations) and obtundation and/or agitation. There is often elevation in white blood cell count (WBC), and creatine phosphokinase (CPK) elevation may lead to renal failure. Seizures and arrhythmias may occur. Although NMS can occur at any point in antipsychotic treatment, over 60 per cent occurs in the first 2 weeks of treatment. The mortality rate ranges from 4 to 22 per cent.[9] The condition is more prevalent in males. Management consists of early recognition of NMS, immediate discontinuation of antipsychotic medication, and supportive treatment of symptoms (e.g., IV fluids, antipyretics). There may be some benefit in using bromocriptine (5 mg p.o. t.i.d. to q.i.d.) or dantrolene (1 to 3 mg/kg/day IV not to exceed 10 mg/kg/day), in acute NMS.

An additional neurological adverse effect associated with antipsychotic treatment is lowering of seizure threshold. This is especially true of low-potency phenothiazines and loxapine. Molindone and some of the other high-potency agents are thought to be less epileptogenic, and could be considered in schizophrenic patients with underlying seizure disorder. Patients on antipsychotic medication who develop seizures may need to be maintained on anticonvulsant medication (carbamazepine, phenytoin) in order to continue antipsychotic treatment.

Non-neurological Side Effects

Sedation is perhaps the most common non-neurological side effect secondary to antipsychotic medication. It is most frequently associated with low-potency agents (chlorpromazine, thioridizine) and is due to histaminergic and possibly adrenergic blockade. Daytime sedation can be minimized by giving all or most of the medication at bedtime.

Anticholinergic effects of antipsychotic medication are both peripheral and centrally acting. Peripheral effects include dry mouth, constipation, blurred vision, mydriasis, and urinary retention. These symptoms may be particularly problematic in older patients. Patients with narrow-angle glaucoma may experience worsening of illness. These patients should be treated cautiously, along with close ophthalmological treatment and follow-up. Anticholinergic effects are greatest with low-potency agents. Dosage reduction, use of a higher potency agent, or the addition of amantadine may be needed to manage symptoms. Central anticholinergic toxicity may occur, although this is rare with antipsychotics used alone in therapeutic doses. The toxic syndrome is characterized by agitation and clouding of consciousness, tachycardia, urinary retention, fever, and mydraisis. Seizures and arrhythmias may occur. Treatment is with 1 to 2 mg physostigmine salicylate IM or IV repeated as needed every 30 minutes. Mild cases may be managed with immediate discontinuation of anticholinergic-associated drug and symptomatic treatment.

Orthostatic hypotension may occur with any antipsychotic, although it is most common with large doses of low-potency antipsychotics and is due to α-adrenergic blockade. Orthostasis is most severe within the first several days of treatment and tolerance usually develops. Management consists of patient education in minimizing effects of orthostasis (i.e., arising slowly from a supine position), encouraging good fluid intake, and monitoring vital signs, particularly in the first week of treatment. Orthostatic crisis may require the use of pressor agents. In these cases, an α-adrenergic pressor (metaraminol) is used.

Endocrine effects of antipsychotics are associated with dopamine blockade and elevated prolactin. This can result in gynecomastia and galactorrhea. Women may experience secondary amenorrhea and have a false-positive pregnancy test. Other adverse effects are diminished libido in both sexes, and impotence or retrograde ejaculation (with thioridazine) in men. Amantadine may be of some benefit.

Skin changes may be seen occasionally with antipsychotics. Photosensitivity reactions occur in 3 per cent of patients on chlorpromazine, and to a lesser extent with other agents. Sun screen should be used by patients exposed to bright sun, or severe burn may result. Allergic dermatitis may also occur. Prolonged use of chlorpromazine has been associated with a blue-gray discoloration of sun-exposed skin.

Ophthalmological effects may occur, particularly with long-term high-dose chlorpromazine therapy. Patients develop brownish, granular deposits in the anterior lens and posterior cornea. These may also occur with thiothixine. They do not impair vision.

Thioridazine in doses greater than 800 mg/day has been associated with a retinopathy similar to retinitis pigmentosa. This potentially progresses to blindness even after medication discontinuation. Retinopathy is unlikely with thioridazine doses less than 800 mg/day.

Cholestatic jaundice may occur in 1/10,000 patients on chlorpromazine and may occur with other phenothiazines. For unclear reasons, the incidence of antipsychotic drug-induced jaundice has decreased over the last three decades. Jaundice usually occurs in the first 5 weeks of treatment, and is preceded by a flu-like syndrome. The jaundice resolves with discontinuation of medication.

Agranulocytosis is a rare side effect of typical antipsychotic agents. It is usually seen within the first 2 months of treatment. Checking a complete blood count (CBC) is indicated if a patient develops symptoms of infection. Clozapine, an atypical antipsychotic, has a 1 to 2 per cent yearly incidence of agranulocytosis.[6] Weekly hematological monitoring is necessary. If a leukopenia occurs, medication should be discontinued immediately.

Maintenance Treatment

Maintenance antipsychotic medication effectively reduces relapse in schizophrenia. After the initial treatment of an acute episode, patients may continue on oral medication, or the psychiatrist may alternatively elect to treat with a long-acting depot antipsychotic. Only haloperidol, usually given IM every 4 weeks, and fluphenazine, usually given IM every 2 weeks, are available in depot forms. Advantages to long-acting injectable antipsychotics are potential for increased compliance, convenience, and possibly less risk of relapse.[10] Disadvantages to long-acting injectable antipsychotics include diminished flexibility in dosing adjustment and potential complication of adverse side effects (i.e., NMS). Usual initial doses are fluphenazine decanoate 12.5 to 25.0 mg IM, or haloperidol decanoate 50 mg IM. Subsequent injection doses are determined empirically based on patient tolerance of the medication and clinical determination of lowest effect antipsychotic dosage. This is usually fluphenazine decanoate 12.5 to 50 mg IM every 2 to 3 weeks, or haloperidol decanoate 50 to 100 mg IM every 4 weeks. Recent research suggests that doses of prolixin decanoate below 25 mg may be efficacious in some patients.[11]

Schizophrenic patients on maintenance antipsychotic treatment should receive the lowest effective dosage of medication. This is usually determined empirically, although recent advances in measuring blood levels may be of assistance. In many cases, patients may be maintained on lower doses than those used in acute treatment (less than 10 mg/day haloperidol p.o.). Key points in establishing lowest effective dose treatment are close communication with patients and families, frequent reassessment, and strong psychosocial support. Too rapid reduction of antipsychotic medication may result in relapse.

Consent to Treatment

It is important for schizophrenic patients and their families to participate in treatment planning. This includes being informed of and understanding benefits and potential risks of antipsychotic medications.

Patients should know potential adverse effects of medications, including risk of TD. Empirical studies have shown that explanation of the risks of TD following acute reduction of symptoms does not lead to discontinuation of treatment.

At this time, the American Psychiatric Association does not recommend written informed consent to medication treatment. However, it is necessary to document in the patient chart that the patient is understanding, and has given informed consent to treatment, particularly with regard to long-term effects of antipsychotics.

CONCLUSIONS

In summary, the introduction of the specific antipsychotic medications have had a profound effect on the treatment of schizophrenia. Symptoms are reduced in many patients, and when maintenance treatment is combined with psychosocial treatment, relapse rates are low. Careful attention to the emergence of side effects and their management can lead to greater patient comfort and compliance. As not all patients receive full benefit from antipsychotic medication treatment, the psychiatrist should be aware of the benefits of augmentation strategies or use of the newer atypical antipsychotic medications.

REFERENCES

1. Meltzer HY, Stahl SM: The dopamine hypothesis of schizophrenia: A review. Schizophr Bull 2:19–76, 1976.
2. Peroutka SJ, Snyder SH: Relationship of neuroleptic drug effects at brain dopamine, serotonin, alpha adrenergic and histamine receptors to clinical potency. Am J Psychiatry 137:1518–1523, 1980.
3. Meltzer HY, Shigehiro M, Lee J: Classification of typical and atypical antipsychotic drugs on the basis of dopamine D-1, D-2 and serotonin$_2$ pk$_i$ values. J Pharmacol Exp Ther 251(1):238–246, 1989.
4. Rifkin A, Seshagiri D, Basawaruj K, et al: Dosage of haloperidol for schizophrenia. Arch Gen Psychiatry 48:166–170, 1991.
5. Baldesserini BJ, Cohen BM, Teicher MH: Significance of neuroleptic dose and plasma level in the pharmacological treatment of psychosis. Arch Gen Psychiatry 45:79–94, 1988.
6. Kane JM, Honigfeld G, Singer J, Meltzer HY, and the Clozaril Collaborative Study Group: Clozapine for the treatment-resistant schizophrenic. Arch Gen Psychiatry 45:789–798, 1988.
7. Angrist B, Schulz SC: The neuroleptic-nonresponsive patient: An introduction. In Angrist B, Schulz SC, eds. The Neuroleptic-Nonresponsive Patient: Characterization and Treatment. Washington, DC: American Psychiatric Press, 1990:xvii–xxviii.
8. Clow A, Theodorou A, Jenner P, Marsden CD: A comparison of striatal and mesolimbic dopamine function in the rat during 6-month trifluoperazine administration. Psychopharmacology (Berlin) 69(3):227–233, 1980.
9. Addonizio G, Susman V, Roth S: Neuroleptic malignant syndrome: Review and analysis of 115 cases. Biol Psychiatry 22:1004–1020, 1987.
10. Schooler N, Levine J, Severe J, et al: Prevention of relapse in schizophrenia: An evaluation of fluphenazine decanoate. Arch Gen Psychiatry 37:16–24, 1980.
11. Marder SR, Van Putten T, Mintz J, et al: Low and conventional-dose maintenance therapy with fluphenazine decanoate. Arch Gen Psychiatry 518–521, 1987.

SUGGESTED READINGS

Angrist B, Schulz SC: The Neuroleptic-Nonresponsive Patient: Characterization and Treatment. Washington, DC: American Psychiatric Press, 1990.

Baldessarini R: Chemotherapy in Psychiatry: Antipsychotic Agents. Cambridge, MA: Harvard University Press, 1985.

Black J, Richelson E, Richardson J: Antipsychotic Agents: A Clinical Update. Mayo Clin Proc 60:777–789, 1985.

29

REVIEW OF PSYCHOSOCIAL TREATMENTS FOR SCHIZOPHRENIA

HUBERT E. ARMSTRONG, Ph.D.

Unlike disorders of mood, anxiety, or other psychotic disorders, the diagnosis of schizophrenia is based in part upon a deterioration from previous levels of functioning. This deterioration takes diverse forms and results in a myriad of residual functional disabilities and skills deficiencies needing therapeutic attention. Consequently, a substantial spectrum of treatment services is required. The purpose of this review is to describe some of the more popular or promising (they do not necessarily go together!) psychosocial treatments, attempt to briefly evaluate the research base for the claim of their prescriptiveness for schizophrenic patients, and discuss what promise they hold for the future treatment of this disorder.

Contemporary treatment of schizophrenia is heavily influenced by a diathesis-stress model that is attentive to the subtle interaction between a biological predisposition to the disease (diathesis) and those environmental events that stress the patient's adaptive capabilities and precipitate the appearance of the disorder or the relapse of symptoms. There is substantial evidence that combined biological and psychosocial approaches can be effective in the management of schizophrenia.[1] For most patients, pharmacotherapy will bring the florid positive symptoms of schizophrenia under control. Drug treatment will have little or no impact, however, upon the negative symptoms of the disease, the interpersonal relationship deficits, and the deteriorated quality of life so prominent among schizophrenics. Attention to these symptoms and titrating the environmental stressors that precipitate them are the agendas of the psychosocial treatments.

INPATIENT MILIEU TREATMENT

Early inpatient psychosocial treatment for schizophrenia (with apparently enviable results, even by current standards) was the "moral treatment" of the nineteenth century. It was not thought of as therapy, but as a teaching approach oriented toward socialization, the establishment of regular habits of self-control, and occupation of the mind through work and religious activity. As the medicalization of mental institutions occurred in the latter half of the century, this psychosocial emphasis was lost as psychiatrists became increasingly interested in the management of positive symptoms. In reviewing modern inpatient psychosocial treatments, Tucker et al.[2] conclude that there is little evidence of their effectiveness. A dramatic exception to this conclusion is the intensive behavior therapy program developed and evaluated by Paul and Lentz.

Paul and Lentz[3] implemented a milieu offering many hours of structured learning experiences in accordance with a carefully developed "token economy," a protocol of praise and token rewards made contingent upon appropriate behaviors. Inappropriate behavior was responded to with fines and time out (exclusion from the opportunity to receive reinforcers). The objective of the program was to enhance those skills required for successful community living. Thus Paul and Lentz's inpatient milieu was tailored to prepare the patient for practical community living. Eighty-four long-term schizophrenic patients were assigned to the experimental social learning milieu, a conventional milieu therapy condition, or to custodial care. Fourteen weeks of training produced dramatic improvement in overall functioning in the experimental group. Ninety-seven per cent of the social learning patients and seventy-one per cent of the milieu therapy patients were subsequently able to remain in the community over a "long term," while only 45 per cent of the custodial patients were able to remain in the community for 18 months or longer.

Shade et al.[4] report a similar inpatient milieu that they have implemented for the past 18 years at Camarillo State Hospital in California. The unit provides group and individually tailored training in personal and social skills for treatment-refractory and chronic schizophrenic patients. They report the discharge of 42 per cent of their patients to the community, with half of these patients successfully maintained in the community for periods ranging from 6 months to 5 years.

Drake and Sederer[5] concur that psychosocial treatment milieus can be effective on inpatient units. They warn, however, of potential negative effects of inpatient psychosocial care and provide guidelines for the effective use of this modality. They especially warn of the toxic effects of intensive and overstimulating psychosocial interactions. They recommend that inpatient psychosocial treatment should provide social support and nurturance, provide structure and education, include the family in the treatment, and, throughout the hospitalization, involve the outpatient staff who will be involved in aftercare.

Clearly, the inpatient psychosocial treatment of schizophrenic patients can be effective if carefully crafted and tailored to the long-term objectives of the patient and the circumstances of the environment where he or she will live.

PARTIAL HOSPITALIZATION

Partial hospitalization, or day treatment, is the intensive (several hours per day) outpatient milieu treatment of psychiatric patients. It is a flexible modality, with content and structure of the therapy often reflecting the strengths and opinions of staff more than established methods of demonstrated effectiveness. Currently, partial hospitalization milieus implement a vast array of socialization, vocational training, psychotherapeutic, and psychoeducational activities. One of the difficulties in evaluating this modality is the enormous diversity in methods and philosophies employed.

Luber[8] describes several advantages of partial hospitalization over alternative psychosocial modalities in the treatment of schizophrenia. It is less costly than inpatient hospitalization (with evidence that it is equally effective) for patients needing intensive care. Its outpatient context allows for flexible tailoring of programming to meet individual needs. It provides intensive treatment (if indicated) while allowing the patient to maintain social ties to the community. Finally, partial hospitalization carries the potential for implementation in a less stigmatizing fashion than other intensive treatments. This final point and the promise of avoiding the barrenness of human interaction so often evident in the hospital treatment of schizophrenia are compelling potential advantages of partial hospitalization for the psychosocial treatment of schizophrenia.

Linn et al.[7] studied the effects of day treatment programs on schizophrenic patients in ten Veterans Administration medical centers. Patients were randomly assigned to day treatment plus drugs or to drugs alone. Day treatment and drugs combined produced significantly more improvement than drugs alone at all centers, but certain centers were identified where reduced relapse, reduced symptomatology, and altered patient attitudes were significantly more evident than at others. Less effective centers had higher staff hours, a philosophy of high patient turnover, and provided more group therapy.

A particularly promising variation of partial hospitalization is the psychoeducational milieu described by Armstrong[8,9] and by Corrigan et al.[10] Called the Life Skills Program and First Step, respectively, these programs present partial hospitalization as life training schools implementing the idiom of competence (student, teacher, learning, education) rather than the idiom of pathology (patient, therapist, illness, treatment). These programs provide a curriculum of structured, skills-building classes 3 hours per day, 5 days per week. Both programs have based a curriculum upon the seven domains of human functioning considered by Lazarus[11] to need attention if significant and enduring behavioral change is to occur: behavior, affect, sensation, imagery, cognition, interpersonal, and drug. First Step employed a token economy to reinforce new skills and implemented training modules in community settings to facilitate the generalization of these skills to the community, while the Life Skills Program attended to the issue of transfer of training through outreach-oriented case management. Both programs offered drug therapy as a part of the treatment package.

First Step reported an 83 per cent decrease in hospitalization and a steady increase in learning performance and the generalization of skills. The Life Skills Program employed random assignment of patients to the psychoeducational milieu and a comparison milieu implementing socialization and group psychotherapeutic characteristics. While rehospitalization was significantly reduced by both milieus, attendance compliance was significantly better in the psychoeducational condition and self-esteem increased in this program, while it decreased in the comparison milieu. The experiences of the Life Skills Program and First Step are consistent with many observations of the effectiveness of social learning procedures with schizophrenic patients. They also suggest the therapeutic potential for comparatively demanding, promotive (of new skills), psychoeducational environments with schizophrenics when adequate structure and social support are provided.

An advantage of the partial hospitalization modality is its flexibility and capacity for tailoring to the needs of the patients a program that serves the community in which it exists. The variety of approaches available and the complexity of a therapy milieu makes a scientific analysis of the active ingredients difficult to conduct. The studies cited above suggest, however, that well-constructed partial hospitalization programs incorporating appropriate drug treatments can significantly contribute to the psychosocial treatment of schizophrenic patients.

PSYCHOTHERAPY

Individual Psychotherapy

McCarrick et al.[12] report that from 1980 to 1981, 66 per cent of schizophrenic patients in state and county mental hospitals and 95 per cent of schizophrenics in private psychiatric hospitals received individual psychotherapy. But the conduct of psychotherapy with schizophrenic patients, though time honored, receives mixed reviews. A review of the current literature on individual psychotherapy with schizophrenics leaves one with the clear view that individual psychotherapy does not play an important role in reducing symptoms, decreasing hospitalization, or enhancing community adjustment. Indeed, the observation that stressful psychotherapeutic experience can have a toxic effect on schizophrenics has been well documented. Even outcome studies with positive results usually describe a modest impact of treatments conducted over considerable time and often with results that cannot be replicated. One advocate of training with these modalities stresses the need to teach trainees that the likelihood of substantial change is low and that the "social support" aspect of therapy, an element as readily and perhaps more cost-effectively delivered by other modalities, is a significant part of any favorable result.[14]

The lack of convincing evidence for the usefulness of psychotherapy with schizophrenics has led to the virtual disappearance of research and theory in its application to this disorder. Coursey[14] laments this development and describes three areas of work with schizophrenics for which he considers psychotherapy to be well suited: human issues raised by having a chronic debilitating disorder, attempts to help the schizophrenic patient manage the disorder, and dealing with the normal psychological problems faced by persons struggling with this disorder. Coursey articulates several "basic elements" upon which he feels a meaningful psychotherapeutic approach to schizophrenia can be built. These include goals and methods mutually agreed upon by the patient and the therapist; teaching patients to carry out their own interventions toward a goal of patient empowerment; and a focus on problem-specific interventions including education, crisis intervention, and social support. Several other modalities discussed in this review are attentive to these issues, with some evidence of their effectiveness.

Group Psychotherapy

McCarrick et al.[12] report that 54 per cent of schizophrenic patients in state and county mental hospitals and 64 per cent of those in private psychiatric hospitals received group psychotherapy from 1980 to 1981. These figures are substantially below those reported earlier on the delivery of individual therapy to these patients. This is in spite of considerable evidence that group therapy is not only less costly, but is probably superior to individual therapy with these patients. Heinricks[15] cites several studies reporting superior results for this modality when concrete, practical, and nonintrospective methods are employed. These approaches are more attentive to the social isolation and withdrawal of the chronic schizophrenic and provide a better opportunity for reality testing than do individual methods. An important

further advantage of group therapy with these patients is the opportunity for continued social involvement without the demand to communicate during periods when the patient feels noncommunicative.

A distinct advantage of a group setting for the schizophrenic patient, according to Heinricks, is the context it provides for a psychoeducational focus on an understanding of medications, the demands of everyday living, and community adjustment. He summarizes several quasi-experimental studies showing high compliance rates, reduced rehospitalization, and improved social and vocational functioning as a result of this type of group therapy. He concludes that these treatments, when tailored to the individual needs of patients, offered at a time when the patient is no longer vulnerable to the toxic effects of overstimulation (after florid positive symptoms are under control), and combined with drug treatment, appear to offer substantial promise for the effective treatment of the negative symptoms and socialization deficits of schizophrenic patients.

FAMILY THERAPY

Family therapy for schizophrenia emerged in the 1950s in response to the view that abnormal family relationships may be causally related to this disorder. The current view of schizophrenia is very different, and modern family therapy approaches are designed less to "cure sick families" than to educate patients and their families about the patient's genetic vulnerabilities, the nature of the disease, and the role that stressful environments (including family environments) can play in the relapse of symptomology. A number of studies suggest that involvement by families enhances treatment compliance by schizophrenic patients as well as reducing recidivism and relapse.

The most promising approaches to family therapy with schizophrenics have not emerged from the family therapy movement but from research programs demonstrating that schizophrenic patients show increased risk of relapse and rehospitalization when exposed to high levels of criticism, hostility, and emotional overinvolvement. These characteristics have been termed "expressed emotion" (EE) and provide the basis for treatments designed to reduce them in the families of schizophrenic patients through supportive, educational, and skills-building procedures. Indeed, these procedures are often called psychoeducational and generally teach patients and families about schizophrenia, methods of problem solving, and methods of coping with stress.

Research into the effects of psychoeducational family therapy procedures has produced promising results. For example, Falloon et al.[17] compared psychoeducational family treatment to individual supportive management. Among the 18 patients receiving family therapy, only one experienced a major clinical relapse compared with 8 of the 18 patients in the control group. Hospital recidivism rates significantly favored the family therapy condition as well. Hogarty et al.,[17] studying 103 recently discharged schizophrenic patients, compared a protocol similar to Falloon's to social skills training focusing upon the patient's ability to avoid and handle conflict, a combined family education and patient skills training condition, and a fourth condition where patients received drug maintenance treatment alone (the control group). Each of the first three conditions included drug therapy as well. The control group (drug maintenance alone) experienced a 41 per cent relapse rate, while the family education group relapsed at 19 per cent, the social skills condition at 20 per cent, and the social skills plus family education group of patients experienced no relapse at all.

It has been noted that most chronic patients live in nonfamilial settings such as group homes. Drake and Osher[18] have applied family psychoeducational approaches in nonfamilial living settings, with good results. The results of psychoeducational family therapy with schizophrenic patients and those with whom they live is compelling. It appears that family interventions of this kind in conjunction with pharmacotherapy can significantly reduce the relapse rate among chronically ill schizophrenic patients.

SOCIAL SKILLS TRAINING

The deterioration of social functioning is a defining criterion for the diagnosis of schizophrenia and is as critical to the etiology and course of the disease as are positive symptoms. It is therefore not surprising that the emergence of social skills training in the behavioral literature has been viewed with great interest by clinicians working with these patients. These approaches generally specify an interpersonal skills deficiency (such as assertively refusing an unwanted overture); stage a specific interpersonal situation (in the treatment setting) where the behavior is rehearsed by the patient; and review the patient's performance, providing social reinforcement for correct behaviors, and feedback regarding desirable additional behaviors. The cycle is then repeated until a criterion level of performance is achieved. Videotaped review is often used, and coaching and modeling by the therapist and other patients (if in a group setting) are significant aspects of the process.

An excellent early review of the process of social skills training and experience with its use with schizophrenics was published by Wallace et al.[19] Though they felt that the approach was promising, they concluded that behavioral changes were often not clinically meaningful and rarely led to improved quality of life. Much work with the application of social skills training to schizophrenia was emerging about the time of those reports, however, and it is appropriate to revise those early conclusions.

Benton and Schroeder[20] conducted a meta-analysis of 27 studies appearing between 1972 and 1988 evaluating social skills training with schizophrenic or "mostly schizophrenic" subjects. For interventions to be defined as social skills training and the research be included in the meta-analysis, use of at least three of the following techniques were required: instruction or coaching, modeling (live or taped), behavioral rehearsal, role-playing, verbal feedback, video feedback, and interpersonal reinforcement or homework assignments or both. These authors found that "significant improvements" in behavioral measures occurred as a result of social skills training and that schizophrenics' perceptions of themselves as less anxious and more assertive changed accordingly. The authors found evidence of generalization to natural settings and that the differences between trained and untrained subjects increase over time. They also found some evidence for "generalized beliefs" over time in the form of superior discharge rates and lower relapse rates for patients who had received training. These authors conclude that social skills training with schizophrenics has been demonstrated to produce clinically meaningful changes in interpersonal behaviors and to do so ". . . even with simple training programs providing relatively small amounts of training."[20] They concluded that results with social skills training with schizophrenics over the period covered by their analysis provide ample evidence that this modality should be viewed as an essential component of treatment programs for schizophrenic patients.

CASE MANAGEMENT

Case management, or as it is often more descriptively called, assertive community treatment (ACT), is based upon the pioneering work of Stein and Test,[21] and provides individualized case management services to patients in the community. These services generally occur outside the office or mental health center; teach patients basic living skills; and closely monitor and accept responsibility for food, clothing, shelter, finances, vocational activities, medical care, and other basic needs. Case managers become involved with all aspects of their patients' lives. They encourage work, recreational, and community involvement, and assist the patient in locating and participating in these activities. The treatment is "assertive" in that patients are closely monitored and engaged, at the case manager's initiative, in appropriate treatments when signs of relapse occur. An interdisciplinary team supports case managers, who are generally available 24 hours a day, 7 days a week, to help stabilize the patient when crises occur.

Proponents of ACT feel that most seriously and chronically mentally ill patients, including schizophrenics, can often best be served by such programs. Others disagree and believe that ACT and similar case management approaches, though promising, cannot be as readily generalized as some have thought and that their performance does not yet warrant the replacement of other established treatments.

Olfson[22] summarizes the results from 11 studies examining ACT programs. None of these studies involved exclusively schizophrenic patients (Stein and Test's original study had 50 per cent schizophrenic subjects), though three of them reported a substantial proportion of schizophrenic patients, and it can be presumed that was the case for most of the studies, though diagnoses were generally not reported. The most replicable finding was ACT's capacity to reduce hospitalization. Olfson reports, however, that the Stein and Test finding that compensatory living cost increases were slight, was not supported by those studies investigating the issue, and that in fact there were substantial increases in living costs for these patients. While early work with ACT found no substantial shift of burden from institutions to families, subsequent researchers have not explored that issue.

Several studies have reported that ACT patients are significantly more pleased with their care than are control patients, but the Stein and Test finding that ACT patients felt more satisfied with their lives than control subjects has not been replicated. Most importantly, recent research reports have failed to replicate the early finding that ACT is superior to alternative treatments in controlling symptoms, improving social functioning, or promoting occupational functioning. But ACT programs have proven replicable and are clearly making community-based treatment for schizophrenics a reality in many communities by reducing rehospitalization.

CONCLUSIONS

Space does not allow for a discussion of a substantial number of additional developments in the psychosocial treatment of schizophrenia. Psychosocial rehabilitation centers, clubhouses, vocational rehabilitation programs, supported employment programs, and psychiatric rehabilitation techniques are all innovative approaches promising significant contributions to the psychosocial treatment of schizophrenia. These treatments, and those described in this review, are rarely "pure forms," but blends of techniques and conceptualizations that other approaches often employ and which frequently originated in the (sometimes distant) past. What is new is the methodological rigor that is now being applied to the evaluation of explicitly defined and therefore replicable protocols for treatment.

A little over a decade ago, Mosher and Kieth[23] summarized the literature to that date on psychosocial treatments of schizophrenia this way: "We know more about their effectiveness than is generally acknowledged." Thirteen years later that statement seems unnecessary. Many know much about the effectiveness of a considerable spectrum of psychoso-

cial treatment services for schizophrenic patients. Together with drug therapy to control the positive symptoms of schizophrenia, these treatments provide an array of alternatives providing a reasonable prospect for most communities in the effort to provide both hospital- and community-based treatment for the negative symptoms and social deficits of this disease.

REFERENCES

1. Liberman RP, Falloon IRH, Wallace CJ: Drug-psychosocial interactions in the treatment of schizophrenia. In Mirabi M, ed. The Chronically Mentally Ill: Research and Services. New York: Spectrum Publishing, Inc., 1984.
2. Tucker GJ, Ferrell RB, Price TRP: The hospital treatment of schizophrenia. In Bellack AS, ed. Schizophrenia: Treatment, Management, and Rehabilitation. New York: Grune & Stratton, 1984:175–191.
3. Paul GL, Lentz RJ: Psychosocial Treatment of Chronic Mental Patients: Milieu Versus Social Learning Programs. Cambridge, MA: Harvard University Press, 1977.
4. Schade ML, Corrigan PW, Liberman RP: Prescriptive rehabilitation for severely disabled psychiatric patients. In Meyerson AT, Solomon P, eds. New Developments in Psychiatric Rehabilitation. San Francisco: Jossey-Bass Inc., 1990:3–17.
5. Drake RE, Sederer LI: Inpatient psychosocial treatment of chronic schizophrenia: Negative effects and current guidelines. Hosp Community Psychiatry 37:897–901, 1986.
6. Luber RF: Partial hospitalization. In Bellack AS, ed. Schizophrenia: Treatment, Management, and Rehabilitation. New York: Grune & Stratton, 1984:219–246.
7. Linn M, Caffey E, Klett J, et al: Day treatment and psychotropic drugs in the aftercare of schizophrenic patients: A Veteran's Administration cooperative study. Arch Gen Psychiatry 36:1055–1066, 1979.
8. Armstrong HE: An educational approach to psychiatric day care. In Upper D, Ross SM, eds. Behavioral Group Therapy: An Annual Review. Champagne, IL: Research Press, 1980:125–146.
9. Armstrong HE, Cox GB, Short BA, et al: A comparative evaluation of two day treatment programs. Psycosoc Rehab J 14:53–67, 1991.
10. Corrigan PW, Davies-Farmer RM, Lome HB: A curriculum-based, psychoeducational program for the mentally ill. Psychosoc Rehab J 12:71–73, 1988.
11. Lazarus AA: Multimodal Behavior Therapy. New York: Springer, 1976.
12. McCarrick AK, Rosenstein MJ, Melazzo-Sayre LJ, et al: National trends in use of psychotherapy in psychiatric inpatient settings. Hosp Community Psychiatry 39:835–841, 1988.
13. Beck JC, Golden S, Arnold F: An empirical investigation of psychotherapy with schizophrenic patients. Schizophr Bull 7:241–257, 1981.
14. Coursey RD: Psychotherapy with persons suffering from schizophrenia: The need for a new agenda. Schizophr Bull 7:349–353, 1989.
15. Heinrichs DW: Recent developments in the psychosocial treatment of chronic psychotic illnesses. In Bellack AS, ed. Schizophrenia: Treatment, Management, and Rehabilitation. New York: Grune & Stratton, 1984:307–335.
16. Falloon IRH, Boyd JL, McGill CW, et al: Family management in the prevention of morbidity of schizophrenia. Arch Gen Psychiatry 42:887–896, 1985.
17. Hogarty GE, Anderson CM, Reiss DJ, et al: Family psychoeducation, social skills training, and maintenance chemotherapy in the aftercare treatment of schizophrenia. I: One year effects of a controlled study on relapse and expressed emotion. Arch Gen Psychiatry 43:633–642, 1986.

18. Drake RE, Osher FC: Using family psychoeducation when there is no family. Hosp Community Psychiatry 38:274–277, 1987.
19. Wallace CJ, Nelson CJ, Liberman RP, et al: A review and critique of social skills training with schizophrenic patients. Schizophr Bull 6:42–63, 1980.
20. Benton MD, Schroeder HE: Social skills training with schizophrenics: A meta-analytic evaluation. J Consult Clin Psychol 58:741–747, 1990.
21. Stein LI, Test MA: The evolution of the training in community living model. New Dir Ment Health Serv 26:7–16, 1985.
22. Olfson M: Assertive community treatment: An evaluation of the experimental evidence. Hosp Community Psychiatry 41:634–641, 1990.
23. Mosher LR, Keith SJ: Research on the psychosocial treatment of schizophrenia: A summary report. Am J Psychiatry 136:623–631, 1979.

Section D

MOOD DISORDERS

MOOD DISORDERS IN DSM-IV

A. JOHN RUSH, M.D.

There are several options under consideration for the mood disorders section of the fourth edition of the *Diagnostic and Statistical Manual of Mental Disorders* (DSM-IV).[1] These options have been based on available scientific data whenever possible. Which options are finally adopted will depend upon (1) results of data reanalysis and ongoing field trials, and (2) responses of the field to the options presented.

OVERVIEW OF MOOD DISORDERS

Categorical Revisions

The major categories within the mood disorders section will be retained in DSM-IV. These include bipolar disorder; cyclothymic disorder; bipolar disorder, not otherwise specified (NOS); major depressive disorder; dysthymic disorder; and depression, NOS. The group of organic mood disorders will be retained, though likely renamed secondary mood disorders. This group will be moved into the mood disorders section to facilitate clinical use when considering the differential diagnoses of mood symptoms. Finally, mood disorder syndromes induced by either somatic treatments or substances of abuse will be identified as substance-induced mood disorders and will be listed within the mood disorders section.

Bipolar disorder may be further divided into bipolar I (recurrent episodes of mania, with or without hypomania, and major depression), bipolar II (recurrent hypomanic and major depressive episodes but without manic episodes), and bipolar disorder, NOS. Bipolar II disorder may be included under major de-

pression, recurrent instead of being classified as a bipolar variant.

Major depressive disorder (or major depression) will still come in single or recurrent forms. Dysthymic disorder may be narrowed so that if clear-cut major depressive episodes occur in the course of a chronic "dysthymic level" of symptoms, then major depressive disorder with antecedent dysthymic disorder could be diagnosed. Alternatively, dysthymic disorder may be modified to specify with and without major depressive episodes. Depression, NOS may be expanded, either by text examples or by additional categories to include minor depression, recurrent brief depression, or mixed anxiety/depression (see later in chapter).

Course Modifiers

Both DSM-IV and the *International Classification of Diseases,* tenth revision (ICD-10)[2] will likely further emphasize the prior course of illness for various diagnoses, including the mood disorders, because prior course of illness assists in (1) prognostification for individual patients; (2) deciding on longer term maintenance treatments; (3) selection of acute treatment (e.g., phototherapy for a seasonal pattern; anticonvulsants for rapid cycling bipolar disorder); (4) prediction of the course of a disorder in a patient over time (e.g., postpartum onset of mania or severe (psychotic) depression may herald a bipolar disorder); or (5) distinguishing etiologically distinct disorders from each other (e.g., probands with highly recurrent major depressive episodes are more likely found in pedigrees with either recurrent major depressive disorder or bipolar disorder).[3]

Symptom Feature Modifiers

Both DSM-III[4] and DSM-III-R[5] attempt to specify selected symptom features (e.g., psychotic, melancholic) present at the nadir of the episode to assist in treatment selection. The DSM-IV will likely continue both the "psychotic symptom features" and "melancholic symptom features" modifiers. It may also adopt a third modifier, "atypical symptom features," to designate the weight-gaining, overeating, oversleeping depressed patients who may also demonstrate interpersonal rejection sensitivity, and a feeling of leadened weight or paralysis in their limbs, but who continue to demonstrate a mood that is reactive—indeed, often overreactive—to negative as well as positive events.[6–8] These patients are unlike those with melancholic features in which the mood is unreactive and the capacity for pleasure is lost. Atypical symptom features may apply to depressive episodes of bipolar, major depressive, and dysthymic disorder.

Let us now turn to specific mood disorders and detail the options under consideration for inclusion in DSM-IV for each condition.

BIPOLAR DISORDERS

For *bipolar I disorder*, the current DSM-III-R criteria will be used. The only revision might be to require a minimal time period to establish the diagnosis of a manic episode (e.g., 7 days), except when the patient's state is so severe as to require intervention/treatment before the required time period has elapsed.

The description of *bipolar I disorder, mixed phase* may require revision if the "rapid cycling" course modifier (see later in chapter) is adopted. Presently, the term "mixed phase" has at least two related but potentially different clinical referents. Mixed phase refers to patients who switch or alternate quickly between short, severe depressive and manic phases with no euthymic intervals or it can also refer to an affective episode during which (even within the same 24-hour period) symptoms meet criteria for *both* manic and major depressive episodes simultaneously without obvious, clear-cut polarity shifts. If both the rapid cycling course modifier and the minimal duration criteria for a manic episode are adopted, then mixed phase would by definition refer only to cases of *simultaneous* presentation of both manic and major depressive symptoms. Situations in which there is a rapid alternation between poles would be designated as either rapid cycling bipolar I disorder (in which the requirement of 7 days for mania and 14 days for depressive episodes is retained) or as rapid cycling bipolar II disorder or bipolar disorder, NOS.

Bipolar II disorder is characterized by recurrent major depressive episodes accompanied by recurrent episodes of hypomania.[9,10] In DSM-III-R, this condition is categorized under bipolar disorder, NOS. If one or more manic episodes occurs, the diagnosis is changed to bipolar I disorder.

Bipolar II disorder is an option as a specific category in DSM-IV because (1) it has prognostic relevance[11–14]; (2) family studies suggest that first-degree relatives of probands with bipolar II disorder have a higher incidence of bipolar II disorder than do first-degree relatives of unipolar or bipolar I probands[15–19]; (3) it may signal a cautionary note in the use of antidepressant medication (although whether rapid cycling is induced by tricyclics in bipolar II disorder is not well established) (Bauer MS, Whybrow PC, unpublished findings); (4) it may raise the notion of lithium maintenance more strongly than for recurrent unipolar depression by some reports[20,21]; but not others[22]; and (5) in about 11 per cent of bipolar II disorder patients, a diagnosis of bipolar I disorder may be expected over 5 years[23] compared to only 4 per cent for unipolar patients.

However, to ensure that recurrent major depressive disorder is not artificially converted into a bipolar disorder variant, duration criteria (e.g., 3 to 7 days) for a hypomanic episode would likely be added. Further, hypomanic episodes must be distinctly different from the patient's usual state to prevent "a few good days" from being mistakenly labeled as a hypomanic episode, thereby creating many false-positive diagnoses of bipolar II disorder. Finally, more than one clear-cut hypomanic episode might also be required to reduce false-positive diagnoses. Recall that bipolar II disorder might be subsumed under major depression, recurrent, as is planned for ICD-10.

If bipolar II disorder is adopted, *bipolar disorder, NOS* would consist of various bipolar conditions that are insufficiently clear-cut in their clinical presentations to be definitively considered either bipolar I or bipolar II disorders. Examples of bipolar, NOS entities include single or recurrent hypomanic episodes without interepisode subsyndromal depressive symptoms (which if continuous, would be diagnosed as cyclothymic disorder) and without major depressive episodes (which if present, would call for a diagnosis of bipolar II disorder). Alternatively, a patient with bipolar disorder, NOS might meet the severity but not the duration criteria for all previous and current major depressive or manic episodes.

Distinguishing labile, bipolar-like symptomatology found in bipolar disorder, NOS from the affective lability found in borderline personality disorder, intermittent cocaine or other substance abuse, or other conditions associated with bipolarity and lability of mood symptoms will continue to be a clinical diagnostic exercise and a challenge for further research.

Course modifiers available for bipolar disorder include "seasonal pattern," "rapid cycling," "descriptors of interepisode symptomatology," and "with postpartum onset" (which applies to the most recent episode). A seasonal pattern (fall onset, spring offset) has been reported for major depressive episodes in both bipolar I and II disorders. While phototherapy efficacy studies have not focused *exclusively* on the depressive episodes of either bipolar I or II disorders, both conditions are often included within the seasonal affective disorder (SAD) group (as is recurrent major depressive disorder with a seasonal pattern) (see Terman et al.[24] for a review). The DSM-III-R allows and DSM-IV will likely continue the seasonal pattern modifier for both bipolar I and II disorders, but not for the residual bipolar disorder, NOS group, as these patients have not been studied with phototherapy.

The rapid-cycling course modifier could apply to bipolar I, bipolar II, and bipolar, NOS disorders. For the first two conditions, it requires that at least four affective (manic, hypomanic, or major depressive) episodes occur within the year immediately preceding the diagnosis. For bipolar disorder, NOS, a rapid cycling pattern could describe cases with four or more manic or major depressive episodes based on symptom severity, but that do not meet the duration requirement for these episodes within the preceding year.

The rationale for the rapid cycling modifier rests on several findings: (1) compared to nonrapid cyclers, rapid cycling bipolar disorders have a disproportionate incidence (up to 90 per cent) of females in most[25–28] but not all studies[29]; (2) treatment with lithium alone appears *less* effective[25,27,30]; (3) anticonvulsants may be particularly effective either alone or in combination with lithium[31–34]; (4) prognosis is poorer[25,27,35]; (5) high-dose thyroid may be effective[36–38]; (6) thyroid axis disorders may cause a rapid cycling pattern in some patients[27,28,39]; and (7) antidepressants contribute to a rapid cycling pattern in 33 to 50 per cent of such patients.[27,40–42] While rapid cycling *may* be a phase of certain bipolar disorders (i.e., at times patients display rapid cycling patterns, whereas at other times they do not[23]), such a designator may still have relevance to treatment selection, prognosis, and indeed, may influence the type of initial medical and psychiatric evaluation conducted on those patients.

Regarding symptom feature modifiers, "psychotic symptom features," "melancholic symptom features" or "atypical symptom features" modifiers can be specified for major depressive episodes seen in the course of either bipolar I or II disorder. Only sparse data are available, however, to suggest that treatment selection is particularly affected by some of these symptom feature modifiers for depressive episodes in the course of bipolar disorder (Himmelhoch J, et al., unpublished findings).

Classically, bipolar disorders have interepisode periods that are largely free of mood and other symptoms. The initial onset of the disorder is typically precipitous (i.e., without antecedent psychopathol-ogy). Sometimes, however, the initial episode of mania or depression is heralded by subsyndromal symptomatology (e.g., cyclothymic disorder, subsyndromal depressive symptoms).[3]

Course modifiers are being considered to specify mood-related psychopathology (1) antecedent to the initial onset of bipolar disorder (i.e., before the first episode of mania, hypomania, or major depression) and/or (2) between full-blown mood episodes in the course of bipolar disorder. The antecedent mood symptomatology may have value in predicting the subsequent degree of interepisode recovery (at least in the untreated state). The level of residual interepisode symptomatology may have prognostic value, and it obviously forms a baseline against which to judge the overall efficacy of treatment for specific patients. For example, in patients who have not previously exhibited interepisode symptomatology while not on antidepressant medication, but who develop such symptoms on lithium plus an antidepressant, the latter may need to be discontinued or changed.

A body of literature suggests that either (1) postpartum psychotic manic or depressive episodes are either the first clue to an ultimate bipolar (usually type I) disorder[43,46] or (2) that the early postpartum period in particular is a high-risk period for the precipitation of manic, mixed, or depressive episodes in the course of an already established, preexisting bipolar disorder.[47–50] In addition, it appears that a postpartum mood episode is very likely to repeat itself in subsequent postpartum periods.[44,51–52] Thus, the modifier "with postpartum onset" would apply to major depressive or manic episodes in bipolar I or II disorders, as it has implications for both prognosis and prophylactic treatment.

Cyclothymic Disorder, as in DSM-III-R, will require at least 2 years of mood symptoms with both "poles" observable and with few, if any, euthymic periods. Those with cyclothymic disorder often have multiple hypomanic episodes, but by definition, they do not enter full major depressive episodes. However, if such episodes should evolve in those previously meeting criteria for cyclothymic disorder, then bipolar II disorder with antecedent cyclothymic disorder is diagnosed (rather than two different bipolar diagnoses). The treatment implications for cyclothymic disorder continue to remain unclear.

DEPRESSIVE DISORDERS

There are no symptom or duration criteria changes planned for the DSM-IV category of *major depressive disorder*. However, this entity will continue to be classified as single or recurrent. There is an ongoing field trial to evaluate the reliability of the differential diagnosis of dysthmyic and major depressive disorders. Results from this field trial could lead to a higher symptom number threshold (e.g., six or seven of the nine DSM-III-R criterion symptoms to diagnose a major depressive episode) compared to the current (DSM-III-R) requirement of five of the nine criterion symptoms. Alternatively, adding a requirement of significant functional impairment, as in the research diagnostic criteria (RDC)[53] to help differentiate a troubled time period (e.g., situational adjustment reaction or grief) from a major depressive episode is being considered, although empirical data to support this change are currently lacking.

With regard to *dysthymic disorder*, the ongoing field trial to optimally differentiate it from major depressive disorder (e.g., are there more cognitive and less vegetative symptoms?) could lead to revised criteria for this category.

No criteria changes will be specified for *depression, NOS* in DSM-IV, as this category's greatest clinical utility is its use in identifying unclear cases. Case examples will be provided in the text or indeed may be considered as additional categories in and of themselves. The following three categories are under discussion.

Minor depression, as initially defined by the RDC, consists of some of the symptoms of major depression and other symptoms—not criterion symptoms for major depression—that come and go over time, but which are present for at least 2 weeks at a time. That is, this condition is like major depression by duration and possibly course, but not by severity. It may or may not have the chronic multiyear pattern seen in dysthymic disorder. Based on the Epidemiological Catchment Area (ECA) study data, substantial short-term morbidity is associated with minor (subsyndromal) depressive symptoms. Treatment responses, familial aggregation, and biological findings remain to be clarified, however.

Recurrent, brief depression is characterized by recurrent (six to ten times/year), brief (usually 3 to 7 days) episodes that meet severity but not duration criteria for a major depressive episode. It occurs more often in females, it is not related to the menstrual cycle, and is associated with a familial history of mood disorders and substantial morbidity.[54] The treatment implications for this category are yet to be clarified.

Mixed anxiety/depression is being considered for both DSM-IV and ICD-10. By definition, it would consist of some depressive and anxiety symptoms (probably of the type found in major depressive disorder or generalized anxiety disorder). However, these symptoms would not meet or have previously met criteria for any other formal mood or anxiety disorder (e.g., major depression, panic disorder, generalized anxiety disorder). Some practitioners feel that such patients are commonly encountered in primary care settings. Whether this is a *distinct* entity based on familial, treatment response, prognostic, or biological measures is unknown.

Turning to course modifiers, the seasonal pattern course modifier for recurrent major depressive disorder will be retained in DSM-IV because it (1) has implications for selecting phototherapy,[24] and (2) has prognostic significance (i.e., it repeats more often than not from year to year). Whether such a seasonal pattern is familial, is associated with a unique biology, predicts a good or poor response to specific antidepressant medications, or ultimately evolves into a nonseasonal or more chronic pattern remain unanswered questions, however.

Major depressive episodes may end completely or only partially. If the latter occurs, (1) the likelihood of a subsequent episode is higher, (2) the need for additional treatment may be indicated, and (3) the prognosis following subsequent episodes is for continuing incomplete interepisode recovery. Thus, an option for DSM-IV is to specify "with partial or complete interepisode recovery" for major depressive disorder.

Regarding antecedent symptomatology (prior to onset of the first episode of major depression), the option to specify "with or without antecedent dysthymic disorder" is being considered, as clinical impression currently suggests that (1) this pattern is predictive of poorer interepisode recovery, (2) it may suggest additional or differential acute treatment interventions (e.g., combination of medication and psychotherapy), and (3) it may suggest a longer continuation treatment phase to attain and maintain a more thorough, longer lasting euthymic state prior to discontinuation in order to improve the ultimate prognosis.

Turning to symptom feature modifiers, "with psychotic symptoms" (i.e., with hallucinations or delusions) is specified as part of the severity descriptors for a major depressive episode in DSM-III-R for both bipolar and major depressive disorders. The DSM-IV will retain the option to specify these. The treatment implications of psychotic features include a low placebo response rate[55–57] and a better response to a neuroleptic plus a tricyclic than to the latter alone.[56,58–60] In addition, psychotic features can be presently (DSM-III-R) and will continue to be (DSM-IV) divisible into those that are mood congruent or mood incongruent, as the latter appears associated with a poorer prognosis and likely, therefore, associated with the need for extended neuroleptic treatment.

Melancholic symptom features were broadened from DSM-III to DSM-III-R.[61] Melancholic symptom features will likely be retained in DSM-IV, but simplification of the criteria is under consideration by either (1) returning to the DSM-III list, but requiring either pervasive anhedonia or unreactive mood, or (2) noting the key symptoms in the text. The rationale for retaining this modifier is that it predicts a positive response to electroconvulsive therapy (ECT)[62–66] and to tricyclic medication in some[67–70] but not all studies.[71–73] When defined narrowly, these features are associated with a positive family history[74–76]; when defined more broadly, they are not.[77,78]

Atypical symptom features vary in definition

among the groups studying them.[79–88] They include overeating, oversleeping, weight gain, reactive mood, interpersonal rejection sensitivity, leaden paralysis, marked anxiety, sleep onset insomnia, phobic symptoms, etc. Two types, "A" (anxious) and "V" (vegetative) have been proposed.[89]

The rationale to consider atypical symptom features for DSM-IV is based on the potential clinical utility in identifying those patients for whom tricyclic antidepressants are not particularly effective compared to monoamine oxidase inhibitors (MAOIs). This finding has been reported by some[7,8,88,90,91] (Rabkin JG, et al., unpublished findings), but not all.[83,86] Results of a soon-to-be-published crossover study[92] suggests that 68 per cent of patients who fail on tricyclics subsequently respond to an MAOI, while 39 per cent of those who fail on an MAOI respond to imipramine. The argument for the atypical modifier is that tricyclics are not particularly effective, whereas MAOIs are. Atypical features are associated with a younger age at onset.[93,94] Whether these symptoms run in families, repeat across episodes, or are associated with an identifiable or unique biology is not known, although rapid eye movement (REM) latency is not characteristically reduced in this type of mood disorder.[95] The relationship between atypical and melancholic symptom features during an episode and over the course of the illness remains to be clarified. Some preliminary follow-up data[96] suggests that atypical symptoms may be more likely earlier in the course of major depressive disorder, whereas melancholic features more likely appear later.

OTHER MOOD SYNDROMES

Mood disorder syndromes can be caused by various systemic disorders (e.g., Huntington's disease, multiple sclerosis). The DSM-IV may identify them as *secondary mood disorders* (i.e., secondary to Axis III diagnoses) with the etiology specified. Mood disorder syndromes can also be caused by intoxication or withdrawal from substances of abuse, such that a specific time period free of these substances is required to render the diagnosis of an independent mood disorder. In addition, selected somatic treatments (e.g., reserpine, ECT) can induce mood disorder syndromes (e.g., a major depression, hypomania). These conditions would be identified as *substance-induced mood disorders* with the presumed cause(s) specified and listed within the mood disorders section.

The DSM-III-R reduced the number of diagnostic hierarchies that were included in DSM-III, which will likely continue in DSM-IV. For example, by DSM-III, patients who met criteria for both panic disorder and major depressive disorder, the major depression but not the panic disorder was diagnosed, while both conditions are diagnosed in DSM-III-R. While this trend provides completeness for re-

searchers, it still leaves the practitioner with the difficulty of sorting out the primary diagnosis (i.e., which diagnosis merits treatment first?). The case with alcoholism and depression may illustrate one of the several clinical methods to sort out this dilemma. Evidence suggests that up to 70 per cent of individuals with alcoholism meet criteria for major depression upon admission to a hospital, but less than 15 per cent still meet this criteria 1 month later (after being alcohol and drug free without specific pharmacological intervention for the depression) (Schukit MA, unpublished findings). In this case, the diagnosis of depression may be precluded until a 1-month alcohol-free period has passed to avoid false-positive diagnoses of depression. In other cases, the prior history of illness (e.g., which came first in time, panic disorder or major depression?) may help the clinician select treatment, although research has not yet addressed this issue.

The DSM-IV mood disorders section will undoubtedly not close the book on the nomenclature for these conditions. Hopefully, it will strike a balance between what is known at this time with reasonable certainty, what experienced clinicians find practical and useful, and what researchers need to launch future investigations.

ACKNOWLEDGMENTS

The author would like to express his appreciation to David Savage for secretarial assistance and to Kenneth Z. Altshuler, M.D., Stanton Sharp Professor and Chairman for his administrative support. Special thanks are expressed to the members of the DSM-IV Mood Disorders Work Group, David Dunner, M.D., Ellen Frank, Ph.D., Martin Keller, M.D., Donald Klein, M.D., to those who conducted literature reviews, Michael Thase, M.D., Mark Bauer, M.D., Alan Schatzberg, M.D., Peter Whybrow, M.D., Alan Rothschild, M.D. and Jan Weissenburger, M.A., as well as to the many correspondents. A particular indebtedness is owed to Alan Frances, M.D. and Michael First, M.D. for their thoughtfulness, diligence, and support throughout the entire process. Much of this chapter draws upon the thoughtful reviews conducted by the DSM-IV Work Group on Mood Disorders which will be published in the DSM-IV Source Book in 1992.

Preparation of this report was supported in part by a Mental Health Clinical Research Center Grant (MH-41115) from NIMH to the Department of Psychiatry, University of Texas Southwestern Medical Center at Dallas.

The views expressed herein are those of the author and do not represent the official position of the DSM-IV Task Force or the American Psychiatric Association.

REFERENCES

1. American Psychiatric Association: Diagnostic and Statistical Manual of Mental Disorders. 4th ed (DSM-IV). Washing-

ton, DC: American Psychiatric Association (in preparation).

2. World Health Organization: International Classification of Diseases. 10th revision (ICD-10). Geneva, Switzerland: World Health Organization (in preparation).

3. Goodwin FK, Jamison KR: Manic-Depressive Illness. New York: Oxford University Press, 1990.

4. American Psychiatric Association: Diagnostic and Statistical Manual of Mental Disorders. 3rd ed (DSM-III). Washington, DC: American Psychiatric Association, 1980.

5. American Psychiatric Association: Diagnostic and Statistical Manual of Mental Disorder. 3rd ed. Revised (DSM-III-R). Washington, DC: American Psychiatric Association, 1987.

6. Liebowitz M, Quitkin F, Stewart J, et al: Phenelzine v. imipramine in atypical depression. Arch Gen Psychiatry 41:669, 1984.

7. Liebowitz M, Quitkin F, Stewart J, et al: Antidepressant specificity in atypical depression. Arch Gen Psychiatry 45:129, 1988.

8. Quitkin F, McGrath P, Stewart J, et al: Phenelzine and imipramine in mood reactive depressives: Further delineation of the syndrome of atypical depression. Arch Gen Psychiatry 45:787, 1989.

9. Dunner DL, Gershon ES, Goodwin FK: Heritable factors in the severity of affective illness. Am J Psychiatry 123:187, 1970.

10. Dunner DL, Gershon ES, Goodwin FK: Heritable factors in the severity of affective illness. Biol Psychiatry 11:31, 1976.

11. Dunner DL: Subtypes of bipolar affective disorder with particular regard to bipolar II. Psychiatr Dev 1:75, 1983.

12. Dunner DL: Stability of bipolar II affective disorder as a diagnostic entity. Psychiatr Ann 17:18, 1987.

13. Dunner DL, Fleiss DL, Fieve RR: The course of development of mania in patients with recurrent depression. Am J Psychiatry 133:905, 1976.

14. Coryell W, Keller M, Endicott J, et al: Bipolar II illness: Course and outcome over a five-year period. Psychol Med 19:129, 1989.

15. Gershon ES, Hamovit J, Guroff JJ, et al: A family study of schizoaffective, bipolar I, bipolar II, unipolar and normal control probands. Arch Gen Psychiatry 39:1157, 1982.

16. Coryell W, Endicott J, Reich T: A family study of bipolar II disorder. Br J Psychiatry 145:49, 1984.

17. Fieve RR, Go R, Dunner DL, et al: Search for biological/genetic markers in a long-term epidemiological and morbid risk study of affective disorders. J Psychiatr Res 18:425,1984.

18. Endicott J, Nee J, Andreasen N, et al: Bipolar II: Combine or keep separate? J Affective Disord 8:17, 1985.

19. Andreasen NC, Rice J, Endicott J, et al: Familial rates of affective disorder. Arch Gen Psychiatry 44:461, 1987.

20. Fieve RR, Kumbaraci T, Dunne DL: Lithium prophylaxis of depression in bipolar I, bipolar II and unipolar patients. Am J Psychiatry 133:925, 1976.

21. Dunner DL, Stallone F, Fieve RR: Prophylaxis with lithium carbonate: An update (letter to the editor). Arch Gen Psychiatry 39:1344, 1982.

22. Kane JM, Quitkin FM, Rifkin A, et al: Lithium carbonate and imipramine in the prophylaxis of unipolar and bipolar II illness. Arch Gen Psychiatry 39:1065, 1982.

23. Coryell W, Keller M, Endicott J, et al: Bipolar II illness: Course and outcome over a five-year period. Psychol Med 19:129, 1989.

24. Terman M, Terman JS, Quitkin FM, et al: Light therapy for seasonal affective disorder: A review of the efficacy. Neuropsychopharmacology 2:1, 1989.

25. Dunner DD, Fieve R: Clinical factors in lithium carbonate prophylaxis failure. Arch Gen Psychiatry 30:229, 1974.

26. Tondo L, Laddomada P, Serra G: Rapid cyclers and antidepressants. Int Pharmacopsychiatr 16:119, 1981.

27. Wehr T, Sack D, Rosenthal N, et al: Rapid cycling affective disorder: Contributing factors and treatment response on 51 patients. Am J Psychiatry 145:179, 1988.

28. Bauer M, Whybrow P, Winokur A: Rapid cycling bipolar affective disorder. I: Association with grade I hypothyroidism. Arch Gen Psychiatry 47:427, 1990.

29. Joffe R, Kutcher S, MacDonald C: Thyroid function and bipolar affective disorder. Psychiatry Res 25:117, 1987.

30. Prien R, Kupfer DJ, Mansky P, et al: Drug therapy in the prevention of recurrences in unipolar and bipolar affective disorders: Report of the NIMH collaborative study group comparing lithium carbonate, imipramine, and lithium carbonate-imipramine combination. Arch Gen Psychiatry 41:1096, 1984.

31. Okuma T, Inanaga K, Otsuki S, et al: A preliminary double-blind study of the efficacy of carbamazepine in prophylaxis of manic-depressive illness. Psychopharmacology 73:95, 1981.

32. Kishimoto A, Ogura C, Hazama H, et al: Long-term prophylactic effects of carbamazepine in affective disorders. Br J Psychiatry 43:327, 1983.

33. Post R: Approaches to treatment-resistant bipolar affectively ill patients. Clin Neuropharmacol 11:93, 1988.

34. Post R, Rubinow D, Uhde T, et al: Dysphoric mania. Clinical and biological correlates. Arch Gen Psychiatry 46:353, 1989.

35. Roy-Byrne P, Post R, Uhde T, et al: The longitudinal course of recurrent affective illness: Life chart data from research patients at the NIMH. Acta Psychiatr Scand 71(suppl 317):3, 1985.

36. Gjessing R: Rhythm and periodicity. In Gjessing L, Jenner A, eds. Contribution to the Somatology of Periodic Catatonia. Oxford: Pergamon Press, 1976:209.

37. Stancer H, Persad E: Treatment of intractable rapid-cycling manic-depressive disorder with levothyroxine: Clinical observations. Arch Gen Psychiatry 39:311, 1982.

38. Bauer M, Whybrow P: Rapid cycling bipolar affective disorder. II: Treatment of refractory rapid cycling with high dose thyroxine, a preliminary study. Arch Gen Psychiatry 47:435, 1990.

39. Cowdry R, Wehr T, Zis A, et al: Thyroid abnormalities associated with rapid cycling bipolar illness. Arch Gen Psychiatry 40:414, 1983.

40. Wehr T, Goodwin FK: Rapid cycling between mania and depression caused by maintenance tricyclics. Psychopharmacol Bull 15:17, 1979.

41. Wehr T, Goodwin FK: Tricyclics modulate frequency of mood cycles. Chronobiologia 6:377, 1979.

42. Wehr T, Goodwin FK: Rapid cycling in manic-depressives induced by tricyclic antidepressants. Arch Gen Psychiatry 36:555, 1979.

43. Dean C, Kendell RE: The symptomatology of postpartum illness. Br J Psychiatry 139:128, 1981.

44. Davidson J, Robertson E: A follow-up study of postpartum illness. Acta Psychiatr Scand 71:451, 1985.

45. Meltzer ES, Kumar R: Puerperal mental illness, clinical features and classification: A study of 142 mother-and-baby admissions. Br J Psychiatry 147:647, 1985.

46. Platz C, Kendell RE: A matched control follow-up and family study of "puerperal psychoses." Br J Psychiatry 153:90, 1988.

47. Pugh TF, Jerath BK, Schmidt WM, et al: Rates of mental disease related to childbearing. N Engl J Med 268:1224, 1963.

48. Paffenbarger RS: Epidemiological aspects of parapartum mental illness. Br J Prev Soc Med 18:189, 1964.

49. Kendell RE, Wainwright S, Hailey A, et al: The influence of childbirth on psychiatric morbidity. Psychol Med 6:297, 1976.

50. Nott PN: Psychiatric illness following childbirth in Southampton: A case register study. Psychol Med 12:557, 1982.

51. Paffenbarger RS, Steinmetz CH, Pooler BG, et al: The picture puzzle of the postpartum psychoses. J Chronic Dis 13:161, 1961.

52. Protheroe C: Puerperal psychosis: A long term study, 1927–1961. Br J Psychiatry 115:9, 1969.

53. Spitzer RL, Endicott J, Robins E: Research diagnostic criteria:

Rationale and reliability. Arch Gen Psychiatry 35:773, 1978.

54. Angst J, Merikangas K, Scheidegger P, et al: Recurrent brief depression: A new subtype of affective disorder. J Affective Disord 19:87, 1990.

55. Glassman AH, Roose SP: Delusional depression: A distinct clinical entity? Arch Gen Psychiatry 38:424, 1981.

56. Chan CH, Janicak PG, Davis JM, et al: Response of psychotic and nonpsychotic depressed patients to tricyclic antidepressants. J Clin Psychiatry 48:197, 1987.

57. Anton RF, Burch EA: A comparison study of amoxapine versus amitriptyline plus perphenazine in the treatment of psychotic depression. Am J Psychiatry 147:1203, 1990.

58. Glassman AH, Kantor SJ, Shostak M: Depression, delusions and drug response. Am J Psychiatry 132:716, 1975.

59. Frances A, Brown RP, Kocsis JH, et al: Psychotic depression: A separate entity? Am J Psychiatry 138:831, 1981.

60. Kocsis JH, Croughan JL, Katz MM, et al: Response to treatment with antidepressants of patients with severe or moderate nonpsychotic depression and of patients with psychotic depression. Am J Psychiatry 147:621, 1990.

61. Zimmerman M, Spitzer RL: Melancholia: from DSM-III to DSM-III-R. Am J Psychiatry 146:20, 1989.

62. Mendels J, Cochran C: The nosology of depression: The endogenous-reactive concept. Am J Psychiatry 124:1, 1968.

63. Rao VAR, Coppen A: Classification of depression and response to amitriptyline therapy. Psychol Med 9:321, 1979.

64. Gibbons RD, Clark DC, Davis JM: A statistical model for the classification of imipramine response in depressed inpatients. Psychopharmacology 78:185, 1982.

65. Abou-Saleh MT, Coppen A: Classification of depression and response to antidepressive therapies. Br J Psychiatry 143:601, 1983.

66. Crow TJ, Deakin JFW, Johnstone EC, et al: The Northwick Park ECT trial. Predictors of response to real and simulated ECT. Br J Psychiatry 144:227, 1984.

67. Bielski RJ, Fiedel RO: Subtypes of depression—diagnosis and medical management. West J Med 126:347, 1977.

68. Prusoff BA, Paykel ES: Typological prediction of response to amitriptyline: A replication study. Int Pharmacopsychiatr 12:153, 1977.

69. Prusoff BA, Weissman MM, Klerman GL, et al: Research diagnostic criteria subtypes of depression. Arch Gen Psychiatry 37:796, 1980.

70. Simpson GM, Pi EH, Gross L, et al: Plasma levels and therapeutic response with trimipramine treatment in endogenous depression. J Clin Psychiatry 49:113, 1988.

71. Coryell W, Turner R: Outcome with desipramine therapy in subtypes of nonpsychotic major depression. J Affective Disord 9:149, 1985.

72. Georgotas A, McCue RE, Cooper T, et al: Clinical predictors of response to antidepressants in elderly patients. Biol Psychiatry 22:733, 1987.

73. Paykel ES, Hollyman JA, Freeling P, et al: Predictor of therapeutic benefit from amitriptyline in mild depression: A general practice placebo-controlled trial. J Affective Disord 14:83, 1988.

74. Leckmann JF, Weissman MM, Prusoff BA, et al: Subtypes of depression: Family study perspective. Arch Gen Psychiatry 41:833, 1984.

75. McGuffin P, Katz R, Bebbington P: Hazard, heredity and depression. A family study. J Psychiatr Res 21:365, 1987.

76. von Knorring L: Morbidity risk for psychiatric disorders in relatives of patients with neurotic-reactive depression. In Racagni G, Smeraldi E, eds. Anxious Depression: Assessment and Treatment. New York: Raven Press, 1987:63.

77. Zimmerman M, Coryell W, Stangl D: Iowa discriminant index for endogenous depression: Family history correlates. Psychiatry Res 16:45, 1985.

78. Andreasen NC, Scheftner W, Reich T, et al: The validation of the concept of endogenous depression: A family study approach. Arch Gen Psychiatry 43:246, 1986.

79. West ED, Dally PJ: Effects of iproniazid in depressive syndromes. Br Med J 1:1491, 1959.

80. Sargant W: Some newer drugs in the treatment of depression and their relation to other somatic treatments. Psychosomatics 1:14, 1960.

81. Robison D, Nies A, Ravaris C, et al: The monoamine oxidase inhibitor, phenelzine, in the treatment of depressive-anxiety states. Arch Gen Psychiatry 29:407, 1973.

82. Ravaris C, Nies A, Robinson D, et al: A multiple-dose, controlled study of phenelzine in depression-anxiety states. Arch Gen Psychiatry 33:347, 1976.

83. Ravaris C, Robinson D, Ives J, et al: Phenelzine and amitriptyline in the treatment of depression. Arch Gen Psychiatry 37:1075, 1980.

84. Rowan P, Paykel E, Parker R, et al: Tricyclic anti-depressant and MAO inhibitor: Are there differential effects? In Youdim M, Paykel E, eds. Monoamine Oxidase Inhibitors: The State of the Art. New York: John Wiley and Sons, 1981:125.

85. Rowan P, Paykel E, Parker R: Phenelzine and amitriptyline: Effects on symptoms of neurotic depression. Br J Psychiatry 14:475, 1982.

86. Paykel ES, Rowan PR, Rao B, et al: Atypical depression: Nosology and response to antidepressants. In Clayton P, Barrett J, eds. Treatment of Depression: Old Controversies and New Approaches. New York: Raven Press, 1983:237.

87. Davidson J, Giller E, Zisook S, et al: An efficacy study of isocarboxazid and placebo in depression, and its relationship to depressive nosology. Arch Gen Psychiatry 45:120, 1988.

88. Quitkin F, Stewart J, McGrath P, et al: Phenelzine versus imipramine in the treatment of probable atypical depression: Defining syndrome boundaries of selective MAOI responders. Am J Psychiatry 145:306, 1988.

89. Davidson J, Miller R, Turnbull C, et al: Atypical depression. Arch Gen Psychiatry 39:527, 1982.

90. Quitkin FM, McGrath PJ, Stewart JW, et al: Atypical depression, panic attacks, and response to imipramine and phenelzine. Arch Gen Psychiatry 47:935, 1990.

91. Klein DF: The pharmacological validation of psychiatric diagnosis. In Robins L, Barrett J, ets. Validity of Psychiatric Diagnosis. New York: Raven Press, 1989.

92. Quitkin FM, Harrison W, Stewart JW, et al: Response to phenelzine and imipramine in placebo nonresponders with atypical depression: A new application of the crossover design. Arch Gen Psychiatry 48:319, 1991.

93. Pollitt J, Young J: Anxiety state or masked depression? A study based on the action of monoamine oxidase inhibitors. Br J Psychiatry 119:143, 1971.

94. Sovner R: The clinical characteristics and treatment of atypical depression. J Clin Psychiatry 42:285, 1981.

95. Quitkin F, Rabkin J, Stewart J, et al: Sleep of atypical depressives. J Affective Disord 8:61, 1985.

96. Akiskal HS, Bitar A, Puzantian V, et al: The nosological status of neurotic depression. Arch Gen Psychiatry 35:756, 1978.

31

MAJOR DEPRESSION

GARY D. TOLLEFSON, M.D., Ph.D.

WHAT IS IT?

The core symptoms of major depression (MD), from DSM-III-R,[1] include a disturbance in appetite or change in weight, insomnia or hypersomnia, a reduction in normal interests or pleasures, low energy or fatigue, low self-esteem, poor concentration or difficulty making decisions, psychomotor agitation or retardation, and feelings of hopelessness/suicidal ideation. These should have occurred for a minimum of 2 weeks and in the presence of some impairment in daily function. Evidence suggests that MD is associated with a neurochemical dysequilibrium analogous to other brain disorders. Studies in correlative neuroanatomy have drawn associations between the signs and symptoms of MD and regional brain foci. This and other data support the existence of biological factors in MD, but fail to conclusively address whether their role is etiological.

DIFFERENTIAL DIAGNOSIS

The physician should first exclude other primary organic etiologies or drugs that mimic MD. Table 31–1 summarizes some commonly cited examples of the organic mood syndromes. The physician should not be lulled into assuming that the incidence of such syndromes is rare.

DEPRESSION IN THE MEDICALLY ILL PATIENT

Wells et al. reported that the prevalence of psychopathology in the medically ill patient significantly exceeded that of a matched-control population.[2] As a general guideline, psychiatric complications are most commonly encountered among diseases or drugs impacting central nervous system (CNS) function. It is noteworthy to underscore the lack of specificity of individual MD signs or symptoms, especially in the medically ill patient. A greater reliance should be placed on the cognitive features of depression when interviewing the medically ill patient.

In the presence of dementia (e.g., Alzheimer's or infarct), DSM-III-R suggests that if the dementia symptoms predominate over mood features, then the diagnosis is dementia with depression. Conversely,

if MD features are at least as prominent as those of dementia, MD can be diagnosed. Across nondementiform medical/drug scenarios, mood impairment not directly caused by the physical illness can be diagnosed MD. However, the sensitivity, specificity, and reliability of an MD diagnosis in a medically ill population is not well established. As a general guideline, where MD is suspect in the medically ill patient:

1. Optimally manage the medical problem.
2. Where possible, substitute a less centrally active agent or lower the dosage(s) of the concurrent medical therapeutic(s) capable of altering mood.
3. Intervene where drug/alcohol abuse is suspected.
4. Introduce supportive/insight-oriented therapies in good prognosis medical disorders with mild depression.
5. Strongly consider adding aggressive pharmacotherapy in poor or chronic prognoses with moderate to severe depressive disorder.

PREVALENCE

Major depression can affect any age group; however, recent surveys suggest the peak prevalence occurs between ages 20 to 45 years[3] and then declines. Episodes beginning later in life may have a more precipitous onset and a greater degree of symptom severity. Data drawn from the National Institute of Mental Health (NIMH)-sponsored Epidemiologic Catchment Area (ECA) survey also revealed that 3 per cent of a general population survey had MD in a 6-month period.[3] Major depression appears more common amongst females than males (2 : 1). However, in the ECA data, no significant differences were seen regarding ethnicity, race, or socioeconomic status. Age-specific features such as behavioral (adolescent) or cognitive (the elderly) disturbance may also characterize MD.

ANXIETY

A differential diagnosis of anxiety and depression is rendered more difficult because of their significant overlap of symptoms. From a phenomenological per-

TABLE 31–1. EXAMPLES OF MEDICAL CONDITIONS PRESENTING WITH DEPRESSION

Malignancies producing paraendocrine products[a]
  Bronchogenic (ACTH)
  Lymphoma (PTH)
  Hepatoma (insulin)
  Lung (IADH)
CNS impairment
  Tumor
  Uremia
  Demyelination
  Hepatic encephalopathy
  Hypoxia
Drugs that can induce depression
  Steroids
  Narcotics
  Anticonvulsants
  Antineoplastics
  Dopamine agonists
  Hormonal agents
  Histamine blockers
  Sedative hypnotics
  Prostaglandin inhibitors
  Centrally active antihypertensives
Infections
  Intracranial
  Viral pneumonia (postacute phase)
  Hepatitis
  Viral mononucleosis
Others
  Collagen vascular disease (e.g., lupus cerebritis)
  Wilson's disease
Deficiencies
  Niacin
  Pyridoxine
  Electrolyte
  B_{12} and/or folic acid
Endocrine
  Pituitary insufficiency
  Hypothyroidism
  Diabetes mellitus
  Hyperparathyroidism
  Hypoglycemia
  Adrenal excess or insufficiency

[a] ACTH, adrenocorticotropic hormone; PTH, parathyroid hormone; IADH, inappropriate antidiuretic hormone.

spective, anxiety symptoms commonly manifest during MD; in contrast, symptoms of dysphoria frequently occur independent of symptom severity in primary anxiety disordered patients. Primary anxiety features may also exist alone for years before being complicated by depression. Recent studies indicate that patients experiencing comorbid anxiety and depression may have a more guarded prognosis, atypical response patterns to somatic therapies, and an increased risk of suicidal ideation/activity.[4,5] Treatment may increasingly be driven by the symptom complex presenting to the clinician at a given time. With improved longitudinal data and better clinical criteria, it will be easier in the future to differentiate these two disorders.

Another exclusion is uncomplicated bereavement. While considerable symptom overlap also exists here, MD is more likely to include self-depreciation, suicidality, and/or marked functional impairment

and/or an extended time duration in contrast to bereavement.

The differential diagnosis of MD also includes a number of commonly encountered "other" psychiatric maladies. For example, depressive features occurring in a schizophrenic patient should be classified as a depressive disorder, not otherwise specified (NOS); or an adjustment disorder with depressed mood. The coprevalence of alcohol and other drug abuse disorders with depression is high.

PREDISPOSING FACTORS

A history of chronic physical disease increases the risk of depression. A family history of MD also increases proband risk; while more robust amongst bipolars, unipolar MD is also more common among first-degree relatives than in the general population. As noted above, alcohol-dependent individuals or a proband with a positive family history have an increased likelihood of MD. Abuse of other drugs, including cocaine, also represent risk factors. Major depression also develops after psychosocial disruption (i.e., stress may induce physiological changes implicated in MD).[6,7]

COURSE

The onset of MD is variable. Some patients experience a sudden onset, whereas others have a protracted prodrome lasting months. Episode duration is unpredictable; however, a common dictum is that the mean duration of an untreated episode is approximately 9 months. While complete recovery from an MD episode is often achieved, a substantial minority of MD patients continue to manifest residual depressive features. Concurrent psychosocial stress is another variable associated with a suboptimal outcome.

An association between MD and neuroendocrine dysregulation, as demonstrated through the exogenous administration of hormonal probes, has been extensively reported.[8,9] Investigations of serial neuroendocrine testing suggest their possible utility as biological outcome predictors.[10]

COMPLICATIONS

The literature suggests one third of mood disordered patients develop a psychoactive substance abuse or dependency problem or both. Major depression is also complicated by the risk of suicide. In the absence of effective treatment, a conservative estimate is that approximately one in six MD patients will make a suicide attempt. Avery and Winokur argued that the aggressive application of pharmacotherapy with adequate therapeutic dosing are inversely related to the risk of suicidal behaviors.

BIOLOGICAL THEORIES OF MAJOR DEPRESSION

A detailed discussion of the numerous advances in this area are beyond the scope of this chapter. The interested reader is referred to Gold and colleagues.[6,7]

The original catecholamine hypothesis posited a relative norepinephrine (NE) deficiency within the synaptic cleft during MD. Early supporting studies demonstrated decreased 3-methoxy-4-hydroxyphenyloglycol (MHPG). At present low pretreatment MHPG may only predict bipolar depressed responders. In unipolar patients, more recent direct assays have suggested an activation of NE systems. Clearly a "monoaminergic" approach is overly simplistic. Evidence for the role of serotonin (5-HT) in MD is substantial and includes metabolite studies, plasma tryptophan, platelet or neuronal 5-HT uptake and imipramine binding, postmortem 5-HT receptor analysis, neuroendocrine challenge studies, acute tryptophan depletion, and the robust track record of a number of novel selective 5-HT agents. Additional literature suggests involvement of dopaminergic, cholinergic, gamma-amino butyric acid, peptids, second messengers, etc. It is quite plausible that subtypes of MD exist.

LABORATORY MANIFESTATIONS IN MAJOR DEPRESSION

Contemporary psychiatric research is dominated by articles on the neurobiology of MD.[6,7] Putative tests have been based on neuroendocrine dysfunction [Dexamethasone Suppression Test (DST)], and hypothalamic-pituitary-thyroid axis [thyrotropin-releasing hormone (TRH) stimulation test], and sleep architecture [shortened rapid eye movement (REM) latency]. Despite this extensive effort, to date we are without a definitive biological marker that is both sensitive and specific enough to be clinically useful.

PHARMACOTHERAPY

Tricyclic Antidepressants

The tricyclic antidepressants (TCA) have been part of our antidepressant armamentarium for over 30 years. While efficacious in 65 to 75 per cent of MD patients, the TCAs are relatively nonspecific. They demonstrate both 5-HT or NE activity or both but are also competitive antagonists at histamine, cholinergic, and peripheral α-NE receptors. None of these latter interactions appear directly related to their therapeutic profile. Rather they mediate their side-effect profile (Table 31–2).

The various TCAs appear equipotent. All are char-

TABLE 31–2. POTENTIAL CLINICAL CONSEQUENCES OF RECEPTOR BLOCKADE

	Antidepressant Receptor Affinity		
	Tricyclics	*Heterocyclics*	*Fluoxetine*
Cholinergic (dry mouth, constipation, blurred vision)	High	Low	Low
Histaminergic (sedation, drowsiness, weight gain)	High	Variable	Low
α_1-Adrenergic (postural hypotension, dizziness)	High	High	Low
Cardiac	High	Low to medium	Low

acterized by a wide interindividual range in their hepatic or "first-pass" metabolism. Thus, each has an approximate dosage range. However, given their relatively narrow therapeutic index, it is advisable to begin with a conservative dosage. Tricyclic antidepressant pharmacokinetic variability means that it is frequently necessary to titrate dosage upward to achieve a therapeutic plasma concentration. Adverse myocardial effects, often in proportion to plasma level, represent a major concern. Some of the TCAs, in a quinidine-like manner, alter cardiac conduction distal to the bundle of His. Cardiac complications are usually related to toxicity or a preexisting disorder. Additional cardiovascular side effects can include fluid retention or edema with exacerbation of concomitant congestive heart failure. Miscellaneous TCA side effects are numerous and include allergic dermatological reactions, elevated liver function tests, tremor, agitation, seizure, pseudoparkinsonian features, and, rarely, agranulocytosis.

Newer "Heterocyclic" Antidepressants

The newer second-generation agents are structurally unique molecules (i.e., nontricyclic).[11] These agents apparently do not work any faster, and are of comparable efficacy with the conventional TCAs. However, their safety profile is often more favorable. This is attributable to their neurotransmitter specificity, which minimizes concomitant adverse risks and contributes to favorable therapeutic index in overdosage.

Fluoxetine Hydrochloride

Fluoxetine (Prozac) is a second-generation antidepressant chemically unrelated to the TCAs or other available agents. It is a propylamine derivative and the first marketed from a group of highly selective 5-HT reuptake blockers. Fluoxetine is extensively metabolized in the liver, with an elimination half-life of 2 to 3 days (its active metabolite norfluoxetine, 7 to 9 days). Ease of administration is one of the advantages of this agent. Fluoxetine is usually initiated at 20 mg once daily. The majority of patients respond to this starting dose; however, occasional higher titration may be necessary. The relationship of therapeutic effect and plasma levels of fluoxetine or its metabolites is poorly defined at this time.

In contrast to the conventional TCAs, fluoxetine has minimal binding activity at cholinergic, histaminic, or α-adrenergic receptors. Thus, the side effects commonly associated with TCA are infrequently seen with fluoxetine. In clinical trials fluoxetine appears to be better tolerated than conventional TCAs. When not well tolerated, anxiety, restlessness, insomnia, rash, or gastric distress predominate. A further advantage of fluoxetine has been the lack of associated weight gain or frank weight loss with extended therapy.

Bupropion Hydrochloride

Bupropion (Wellbutrin) is structurally similar to phenylethylamine. In contrast to classical TCAs, it is a weak blocker of acetylcholine, serotonin, and norepinephrine. The mechanism of action of bupropion is unknown, but has been speculated as dopaminergic. The relationship of therapeutic effect to plasma levels of bupropion or its metabolites is also unknown.

Bupropion is rapidly absorbed and hepatically metabolized. Half-life of the initial phase is 1 to 2 hours; half-life of the second phase is 14 hours. Bupropion manifests four basic metabolites: morpholinol, threo-amino alcohol, erythro-amino alcohol, and erythro-amino diol. These metabolites have been reported to be approximately one half as potent as the parent drug. Like other antidepressants, it manifests a 2- to 3-week lag to onset. Bupropion is routinely started at 75 mg, three times daily. It may be titrated to a single maximum dose of 150 mg three times daily or a total of 450 mg/24 hours. Bupropion appears to have comparative efficacy with reference TCAs (e.g., amitriptyline).

Bupropion was voluntarily withdrawn in 1986 from a postmarketing surveillance study of seizure incidence. Study outcome revealed an approximate incidence of 0.4 per cent (4/1000). Controlled prospective studies of general antidepressant-induced seizure rates are lacking but estimated to be 1 to 2/1000.

The most frequently encountered adverse events with bupropion include agitation, dry mouth, insomnia, headache, nausea and vomiting, constipation, or tremor. As with fluoxetine, bupropion manifests lower anticholinergic, antihistaminic, and hypotensive cardiac risks. Similar to fluoxetine, a number of bupropion patients reportedly lose weight during treatment. The drug's therapeutic index is favorable, with the exception of convulsion.

Monoamine Oxidase Inhibitors

At least two monoamine oxidase (MAO) subtypes have been distinguished by their respective substrate and inhibitor specificities. Type A MAO preferentially deaminates NE and 5-HT and is selectively inhibited by clorgyline. Type B MAO (phenylethylamine degrading) is sensitive to deprenyl or pargyline. Human platelet contains only MAOB. There appears to be no significant correlation between MAOB in cerebral cortex and platelet. Most conventional MAO inhibitors (MAOI) are nonselective (i.e., exert effects upon both type A and type B. While the catecholamine hypotheses of MD suggests a significant role for type A in the treatment of depression, clinical trials have been less conclusive.

Clinical indications for the MAOIs include TCA-refractory MD, panic disorder, and "atypical" depression. The latter has been characterized by mood reactivity with at least two of the following: hyperphagia, hypersomnia, extreme fatigue, or lifelong rejection sensitivity. In atypical forms of depression, MAOI response appears superior to either TCA or placebo. Four MAOIs with neuropsychiatric indications are currently available in the United States and include isocarboxazide, phenelzine, tranylcypromine, and deprenyl.

Possible MAOI side effects include weight gain; postural hypotension; insomnia/drowsiness; and mild anticholinergic complaints such as tremor, sensory disturbance, excessive sweating, or rash. Standard drug and dietary restrictions are strongly indicated with this class of drug to minimize a sympathomimetic crisis. This hyperadrenergic state is often characterized by severe headache, diaphoresis, mydriasis, hypertension, neuromuscular excitation, and potential cardiac dysrhythmia.

Other cardiovascular effects are also infrequent and rarely dictate drug discontinuation. The MAOIs do lower supine blood pressure. However, they appear to have little effect on heart rate or cardiac conduction in contrast to the conventional TCAs.

Overdosage with a MAOI can be fatal. Clinical symptoms may sometimes demonstrate a latency up to 12 hours. Toxicity often includes neuromuscular agitation, mental confusion, autonomic arousal, hyperthermia, involuntary movements, convulsions, and altered consciousness complicated by circulatory collapse.

Trazodone

Trazodone (Desyrel) is a triazolopyridine derivative with antidepressant activity. Trazodone exhibits its apparent antidepressant activity at postsynaptic 5-HT receptors. The drug is extensively metabolized, with its main route of elimination via the kidneys. The elimination half-lives for the parent and metabolites are approximately 6 and 13 hours, respectively. In clinical studies, trazodone appears of similar efficacy to the conventional TCAs. In head-to-head comparison, trazodone may require approximately twice the milligram dosing associated with imipramine or equivalent TCAs.

Trazodone is minimally interactive at non–5-HT receptors. Thus, in clinical studies, it has been practically devoid of anticholinergic and antihistaminic side effects. However, its principle metabolite does possess moderate presynaptic α_2-NE receptor blockade, thus carrying moderate risk of postural hypotension. Trazodone (perhaps through its 5-HT mechanism) has soporific properties. This has been both advantageous (for the induction of sleep) and disadvantageous (subjective feelings of tiredness, fatigue, or lethargy that are dose dependent). The experience with trazodone to date suggests that it is less likely than TCAs to induce cardiovascular complications. There has been one reported case of heart block. Trazodone may cause ventricular ectopic beats in some patients. While not limited to trazodone only, there have been several hundred cases reported of priapism. Male patients with a history of erectile dysfunction should be considered suboptimal candidates for the initiation of trazodone. Where abnormal or persistent erectile function develops concurrent with trazodone, the drug should be discontinued. Priapism may represent a medical emergency. Common side effects experienced with trazodone include sedation, behavioral changes, hostility, agitation, and "forgetfulness." Incidence of seizures appears to be low. Trazodone has proven to have a relatively wide therapeutic index, rendering it among the safest agents. There is inadequate data to establish a meaningful association between plasma trazodone levels and clinical outcome at this time.

In overdosage ranging up to 5 gm, the predominant symptom has been drowsiness. Coma is rare. Lethality is most likely to be associated when trazodone was consumed with other drugs.

Lithium

The therapeutic potential of lithium was not recognized until the late 1940s when Cade reported lithium's antimanic effect. Lithium demonstrates a number of unique chemical properties. It bears a CNS profile similar to several monovalent and divalent cations. However, its precise mechanism of action is unknown. At present the only approved indications for lithium are the treatment of acute mania or the maintenance therapy of bipolar affective disorder. Studies in both situations have demonstrated that lithium is clearly superior to placebo. Lithium also appears to offer an adjunctive benefit to conventional antidepressants among incomplete responders. A thorough medical and psychiatric history should be completed prior to the initiation of lithium therapy including baseline renal and thyroid function testing. In the absence of renal compromise, initial dosages of lithium for augmentation are approximately 600 to 900 mg/day. Lithium is rapidly and completely absorbed from the gastrointestinal tract. Depending on the formulation, it reaches a peak serum level within 1 to 5 hours. Unlike other agents used in the treatment of depressive disorders, lithium has no metabolites, is not protein bound, and is renally excreted.

Because lithium has a half-life of approximately 24 hours, 5 days may be necessary to reach a steady-state blood concentration. Thus, serum lithium levels are generally not obtained in less than 5 to 7 days after a dose change was made unless toxicity is suspected. In the medically ill or older patient, the half-life of lithium may increase. The narrow therapeutic index of lithium (e.g., two to three times the therapeutic concentration) means the physician should be vigilant for toxicity. Adverse drug interactions are one pathway. The thiazide diuretics reduce the net clearance of lithium (relative to other monovalent cations) and may cause a substantial increase in serum lithium concentrations. Other diuretics, not active in the proximal convoluted tubule, may be safer. Recent evidence also suggests that the nonsteroidal anti-inflammatory drugs decrease lithium clearance. In contrast, those agents which enhance filtration/clearance (e.g., aminophylline, caffeine) have the reverse effect (i.e., lower lithium concentrations). Additionally, the amount of dietary sodium and fluid intake should be held relatively constant during pharmacotherapy.

Like all psychotropic medications, lithium has a profile of side effects and toxicity. The common side effects include sedation, thirst, weight gain, tremor, diarrhea, and fluid retention. Less common but noteworthy reactions include hair loss, euthyroid goiter or hypothyroidism, sinus node dysfunction/ectopy, anorexia, polyuria/polydipsia (diabetes insipidus), and aggravation of preexisting dermatological conditions such as acne or psoriasis.

Electroconvulsive Therapy

Electroconvulsive therapy (ECT) is clearly effective in both bipolar and unipolar patients. Electroconvulsive therapy is particularly effective where these diagnoses are complicated by psychotic features. However, controlled studies of ECT as a prophylactic treatment are lacking. Electroconvulsive therapy techniques have become considerably refined in electrode placement and stimulus waveform, among other aspects. Increased intracranial pressure/mass effect continues to be the principle contraindication. Additionally, any patient considered a poor risk for general anesthesia may not be appropriate for ECT. While mechanisms are yet unknown, the receptor/neurotransmitter profiles of ECT closely resemble those of the tricyclic antidepressants, especially in postsynaptic β-noradrenergic down-regulation.

Nonresponse or Tolerance

The nonresponding patient should trigger questions around drug selection, compliance, adequate dose and duration of treatment, and consideration of comorbid physical/psychosocial issues. Based on a 1982 NIMH collaborative program on the psychobiology of depression,[12] over half of depressed patients received anxiolytics instead of an antidepressant. Only about one third had received antidepressants; and then, only one in ten received an adequate dosage. Among those who received tertiary care consultation, only three fourths received an antidepressant. However, 30 per cent of inpatients received less than 100 mg TCA dosage or equivalent. If an adequate dose of one antidepressant has not been effective or well tolerated, an alternative category should be considered. Data would support use of one secondary amine TCA (e.g., nortriptyline or desipramine) or fluoxetine as first-line categories. The atypical antidepressant bupropion (Wellbutrin) can be considered as a second-line intervention when one or both of the above agents have been unsuccessful. If the patient has failed trials of these distinctly different antidepressants, augmentation therapy with lithium for at least 2 to 3 weeks should be considered. Augmentation lithium levels should be in the 0.5- to 0.9-mEq/liter range. Alternatively, the combination of a TCA or trazodone (postsynaptic site of action) and fluoxetine (presynaptic) can be considered. Remember to conservatively dose the former in light of increased TCA plasma levels associated with fluoxetine's concomitant administration. Another possible adjunct awaiting controlled evaluations is the serotonin 1A partial agonist, buspirone. Thereafter, if clinical response has not been seen, consideration of MAOI, ECT, or newer investigational compounds may be necessary. However, selective 5-HT reuptake blockers and MAOIs may be a superior early choice to the TCAs in the treatment of atypical depressive disorders. Comparative trials of an MAOI versus fluoxetine suggest comparable efficacy, the latter associated with fewer adverse events. Studies of bupropion in atypical depression are lacking. An alternative strategy is to select among the available antidepressants based on certain unique symptomatic factors (Table 31–3).

Mechanisms of Action

The original theories of antidepressant activity were based upon the assumption that these drugs blocked the reuptake of one or more amines. While this is achieved within several days of administration in vitro, clinical response typically requires 2 to 4 weeks. Advances in the ability to assess drug/receptor interactions led to an alternative explanation. Clinical efficacy exhibits a temporal relationship to receptor sensitivity or density modifications or both consequent to drug administration. Four hypotheses have been proposed: (1) β-adrenergic receptor down-regulation; (2) α_2-adrenergic receptor down-regulation; (3) α_1-noradrenergic up-regulation; and/or (4) the net enhancement of central serotonin neurotransmission (e.g., via 5-HT$_2$ receptor affinity reduction).

Of these four hypotheses, a great deal of interest

TABLE 31–3. PREDICTION OF RESPONSE[a]

Target Symptoms	Agent(s)[b]
Agitation	BDZ + AD/buspirone + AD
Psychotic	NL + AD/amoxapine/ECT
Obsessive	Fluoxetine/clomipramine
Retarded	Bupropion
Bipolar (rapid cycler)	Carbamazepine/valproate/verapamil
"Atypical"	Phenelzine/fluoxetine
Insomnia	BDZ + AD; trazodone + other AD
Bipolar (depressed)	Lithium + AD
Obesity	Bupropion/fluoxetine
Peptic ulcer	Doxepin/imipramine

[a] Treatment selection based upon a subclassification of mood disorders
[b] AD, antidepressant; NL, neuroleptic; ECT, electroconvulsive therapy; BDZ, benzodiazepine.

centers around the enhancement of synaptic 5-HT. A wide spectrum of antidepressant treatments are associated with an increase in 5-HT activity. Preclinical data suggest that conventional TCAs act at postsynaptic 5-HT receptors, whereas the newer selective 5-HT reuptake blockers [e.g., fluoxetine (Prozac), the MAOIs, and possibly the partial 1A agonist buspirone (Buspar)] alter presynaptic autoreceptor sensitivity.

Unfortunately, none of the above theories totally explain activity of the full spectrum of antidepressants currently available. Other systems implicated include: (1) selective enhancement at the gamma-aminobutyric acid-B site, (2) dopamine receptor alteration, and (3) postsynaptic enhancement of the second messenger adenosine 3,5-monophosphate.

Patient Education

Initiation of an antidepressant should include patient education regarding the biological aspects of the disease, awareness of the 2- to 4-week response latency, knowledge that antidepressants are not addictive and in most cases need not be taken lifelong, and an informed discussion of alternatives and the risks of no treatment.

Therapeutic Drug Monitoring

Therapeutic drug monitoring (TDM) can enhance both the safety and efficacy of pharmacotherapy. Many of the therapeutic and adverse reactions associated with psychotropic drugs are concentration dependent. Conversely, one of the major reasons for nonresponse to pharmacotherapy is inadequate dosing. Response disparity can be explained in part by wide interindividual differences in "first-pass metabolism" (i.e., differing hepatic degradation rates prior to the drug's systemic availability).

Through the use of TDM, the physician has available (at least for the conventional antidepressant drugs) a technique to assist in dosage adjustment, maximize therapeutic efficacy, and minimize potential toxic effects. The percentage of responders to conventional TCA therapy without the advantage of TDM has been reported in the range of 40 to 60 per cent. By using concurrent plasma level monitoring, TCA response rates reportedly may be increased to 70 to 80 per cent. Clinical studies in TCA recipients suggest that 1 in 50 physically healthy individuals receiving 100 mg (of a reference TCA) may generate a supratherapeutic concentration and potential toxicity. Tricyclic antidepressants represent one of the leading causes of death from drug overdosage. Thus, the narrow therapeutic index of TCA underscores the value of TDM in select cases.

Therapeutic drug monitoring has its limitations. It may not reflect "real" pharmacodynamic (receptor site) activity, nor does it always account for multiple active metabolites. Psychotropic drugs with useful concentration/response relationships include amitriptyline, imipramine, nortriptyline, desipramine, and lithium. The utility in maximizing treatment outcome amongst several of the so-called second-generation agents is limited by sparse data at this time.

PSYCHOTHERAPY

The spectrum of nonpharmacological treatments for depression clearly contributes to our total treatment armamentarium for MD. In the past 25 years, several new variations, many of them short term, have been introduced (e.g., cognitive therapy, interpersonal therapy). In concert, more traditional analytically oriented treatments have undergone an adaptive process. Karasu wrote an excellent review on several contemporary psychotherapeutic models.[13] Relative to dynamic psychotherapy, cognitive therapy is more standardized and time limited. It is based on discreet and directed learning experiences. The therapeutic relationship is highly collaborative and empirical. Therapeutic interventions strive to alter/improve adverse cognitive assumptions/attributes. Successful participation should facilitate the individual's ability to self-monitor their negative cognitions, analyze the related situation supporting that belief, understand how it mediates mood and behavior, and substitute more "healthy" or reality-oriented conclusions for a dysfunctional belief system. Evidence suggests cognitive therapy may be useful in the prophylaxis of recurrent depression (the premise being that enhanced self-control and mastery "rehearses" the individual to recognize and restructure cognitions).

A third approach for the mood disorders is interpersonal psychotherapy. Interpersonal therapy is not linked to any single cause or theoretical explanation for the mood disorder. Rather, a disturbance in mood is enmeshed within the individual's social milieu. If the individual is experiencing a disturbance in his or her current social role with suboptimal interpersonal experience (in childhood or adult life), it may assume a role in depression and its recurrence. The

origins of the interpersonal model derive from the contributions of Adolph Meyer and Harry Sullivan. Interpersonal psychotherapy operates with a high priority on gratifying and intimate relationships rather than personality dynamics. The qualitative aspects of a relationship are held superior to the quantitative number. Most recently, Klerman and colleagues have embellished the techniques of interpersonal psychotherapy. Four major interpersonal areas or problems can be commonly associated with MD, including: (1) complicated bereavement, (2) interpersonal role disputes or conflict, (3) problematic transitions of role (e.g., difficulty transcending developmental landmarks or life events), and (4) the presence of interpersonal deficits (e.g., inadequate social skills, isolation, frequent disruption of relationships). In interpersonal therapy, the therapist functions as an advocate for the patient. There is a significant element of support. The therapist is directive in providing advice and reassurance. The therapeutic relationship may be very active and is not based on transference, but rather is oriented toward "realistic problem solving" and the maintenance/promotion of individual independence and autonomy. Successful interpersonal therapy enhances interpersonal skills and flexibility in response to an everchanging social milieu. The therapeutic process may include reconstruction of current conflicted relationships or, where possible, previous ones. One essential net gain is a reduction in dependency through a better understanding of the symptomatic nature of their illness.

While the comparative advantages and disadvantages of these different forms of psychotherapy is beyond the scope of discussion here, several assumptions can be made. The psychodynamic approach clearly requires a verbal, psychologically minded patient. It is capable of achieving significant individual depth in a search for inward solutions. Cognitive therapy may have a broader patient application, although optimal outcomes would be with individuals capable of logical thinking and motivated to comply with tasks. However, in comparison to an analytic focus, some patients may find cognitive psychotherapy to be more superficial or not detailed. Interpersonal psychotherapy offers particular advantages for the depressed patient currently in the midst of relationship distress, regardless of whether that distress was etiologic. Critically, however, it may overemphasize the role/importance of significant relationships and may not be globally applicable to all patients.

Common features of symptom-reducing psychotherapies include: (1) careful differential diagnosis; (2) educational information regarding the diagnosis, prognosis, and treatment plan; (3) requires the capacity on the part of the patient to form a therapeutic alliance; (4) provide structure, explanation and plan, measures symptomatic outcome; and (5) can rediagnose and consider alternative or concurrent therapies if the initial approach has not been successful. According to Rush, psychotherapy as a sole treatment intervention is indicated for individuals with: a shorter duration of their current episode (e.g., less than 1 year); evidence or anticipated good interepisode recovery; no major concomitant personality problems; depression of mild to moderate severity and nonpsychotic, nonbipolar in character (A. John Rush, M.D., personal communication).

COMBINED SOMATIC-NONSOMATIC TREATMENT

At present there are over 20 studies that have examined the efficacy of psychotherapy in comparison or in combination with the pharmacotherapy of MD.[14] Most studies have employed cognitive or interpersonal psychotherapies over a relatively short treatment duration. Based on these data, psychotherapy and pharmacotherapy appear approximately equivalent in mild nonbipolar depressions. Further evidence suggests a possible synergistic effect for the combination. At worst case, there is no evidence for a poorer or more negative outcome from combined somatic and psychotherapeutic treatments.

The NIMH collaborative study of the treatment of depression studied over 250 outpatients who were randomly assigned one of four treatment conditions: cognitive therapy, interpersonal psychotherapy, imipramine, or a placebo clinical management. Patients were treated for 16 weeks. Sixty-eight per cent completed at least 15 weeks consisting of 12 sessions of treatment. In general, all active treatments were superior to placebo. Over two thirds of the patients on active treatment were symptom free by conclusion of the protocol. More patients in the placebo-clinical management cell dropped out or were withdrawn than with other treatment modalities. At the end of 12 weeks, both psychotherapies and imipramine were equivalent in their reduction of depressive symptoms. However, imipramine may have had a more rapid initial onset of action. Among the less severely depressed group there were no differences among the treatments. In contrast, in those with a Hamilton Rating Scale for Depression score of 20 or greater, imipramine and interpersonal psychotherapy were associated with significantly better outcomes.

Recently, Frank et al. completed a randomized 3-year trial in 128 recurrent MD patients.[14] All patients were initially treated with a combination of interpersonal psychotherapy and imipramine and then randomized. Five cells were employed and included imipramine and medication clinic, imipramine plus interpersonal psychotherapy, placebo plus medication clinic, interpersonal psychotherapy alone, and interpersonal psychotherapy plus placebo. A survival analysis demonstrated a highly significant and prophylactic effect for imipramine when maintained in an average dosage of 200 mg. A modest prophylactic effect was also observed for monthly interper-sonal psycotherapy. Interpersonal psychotherapy alone or with placebo was superior to medication clinic plus placebo. Both groups receiving active imipramine had significantly superior survival times (approximately 130 weeks versus 45 weeks for placebo recipients) with a slightly better performance achieved by the group receiving combined psychotherapy.

SUMMARY

The complex nature of the depressive syndrome is evident in terms of its multiple causes, clinical manifestations, and differential response to treatment. No single therapeutic modality has been uniformly successful in all patients with a depressive disorder. Psychotherapy or somatic treatments for MD can be effective alone or in combination. Future research will better characterize and refine depressive subtyping so as to develop a reliable scheme for the predetermination of optimal treatment.

ACKNOWLEDGMENT

Special thanks to Ms. Joan Mudge for her assistance in the preparation of this chapter.

REFERENCES

1. American Psychiatric Association: Diagnostic and Statistical Manual Mental Disorders. 3rd ed. Revised. Washington, DC: American Psychiatric Association, 1987.
2. Wells KB, Golding JM, Burnam MA: Psychiatric disorder in a sample of the general population with and without chronic medical conditions. Am J Psychiatry 145:976–981, 1988.
3. Robbins LN, Helzer JE, Weissman MM, et al: Lifetime prevalence of specific psychiatric disorders in three sites. Arch Gen Psychiatry 41:949–958, 1984.
4. Cloninger CR: Comorbidity of anxiety and depression. J Clin Psychopharmacol 10:43S–43S, 1990.
5. Grunhaus L: Clinical and psychobiological characteristics of simultaneous panic disorder in major depression. Am J Psychiatry145:1214–1221, 1988.
6. Gold PW, Goodwin FK, Chrousos GP: Clinical and biochemical manifestations of depression in relation to the neurobiology of stress: I. N Engl J Med 319:347–353, 1988.
7. Gold PW, Goodwin FK, Chrousos GP: Clinical and biochemical manifestations of depression in relation to the neurobiology of stress: II. N Engl J Med 319:413–420, 1988.
8. Kathol RG, Jaeckle RS, Lopez JF, Meller WH: Pathophysiology of the HPA axis abnormalities in patients with major depression: An update. Am J Psychiatry 146:311–317, 1989.
9. Nemeroff CB: Clinical significance of cycle neuroendocrinology in psychiatry: Focus on the thyroid and adrenal. J Clin Psychiatry 50 (suppl 5):13–20, 1989.
10. Targum SD: Persistent neuroendocrine dysregulation in major depressive disorder: A marker for early relapse. Biol Psychiatry 19:305–318, 1984.
11. Rudorfer MV, Potter WZ: Pharmacokinetics of antidepressants. In Meltzer HY, ed. Psychopharmacology: The Third Generation of Progress. New York: Raven Press, 1987:1353–1361.

12. Weissman MM, Jarrett RB, Rush JA: Psychotherapy and its relevance to the pharmacotherapy of major depression: A decade later (1976–1985). *In* Meltzer HY, ed. Psychopharmacology Third Generation Progress. New York: Raven Press, 1987:1059–1068.

13. Karasu TB: Toward a clinical model of psychotherapy for depression: I. Systematic comparison of three psychotherapies. Am J Psychiatry 147:133–147, 1990.

14. Frank E, Kupfer DJ, Perel JM, et al: Three year outcomes from maintenance therapies in recurrent depression. Arch Gen Psychiatry 47:1093–1099, 1990.

32

MOOD DISORDERS: Acute Mania

ROBERT M. POST, M.D.

Bipolar illness is a common major psychiatric illness, with approximately 0.9 per cent of the U.S. population meeting modern diagnostic criteria. In contrast to unipolar affective illness, where females predominate, the ratio of male : female subjects is approximately equal in bipolar disorders. In bipolar I disorder, either the current or previous manic episode has required hospitalization. This contrasts with bipolar II disorder, where there is a current or previous hypomania or less severe mania not requiring hospitalization. In bipolar I individuals, females compared with males may show greater rapidity of cycling, a preponderance of depressive episodes, and more hospitalizations for depression.

Given an initial history of mania, the illness almost universally tends to be recurrent. Thus, the focus on acute treatment in this chapter needs to be considered in the context of overall pharmacoprophylaxis of the disorder. This is all the more the case in light of recent data showing that adolescent manics are at extremely high risk for relapse (92 per cent relapse within the first 18 months after lithium discontinuation), and still incur substantial risk (37 per cent will have a recurrent episode within 18 months) even if they are maintained on their lithium.[1]

Increased psychomotor activity is the hallmark of the syndrome. In bipolar illness, mood may be euphoric, dysphoric, or irritable, and accompanied or not by psychotic features, including the occurrence of Sneiderian-positive symptoms (such as thought insertion and thought control), which have previously been thought to be found exclusively in schizophrenia. The diagnosis of bipolar II disorder may be more difficult to make based on a more subtle set of symptoms. Due to the positive subjective aspects of hypomania—namely, mood elevation, sociability, increased energy, and decreased need for sleep—a patient may deny the pathological aspects of the syndrome. These latter might include social intrusiveness, poor judgment, sexual and financial indiscretions, argumentativeness, boundless energy, sense of entitlement and grandiosity bordering on delusional, spending sprees, and a variety of other signs and symptoms that may be noticed more by family members than by the patients themselves. Consequently, family participation in the intake interview may be useful. Denial of illness can itself be a hallmark of hypomania and mania.

Elicitation of a positive family history of the disorder, if present, is helpful not only in elucidating possible genetic mechanisms, but also in possibly predicting pharmacological response. Substantial literature supports the view that a family history of affective illness in a first-degree relative is associated with a higher incidence of lithium response than in patients without such a family history,[2] although these latter patients may respond well to carbamazepine or some other treatment. It is of interest that a considerable number of studies document that important psychosocial stressors and other negative life events may be related to initial manic episodes, but are less likely to be associated with later occurrences.[3] These data are consistent with a sensitization model in which initial episodes may often be precipitated or triggered by environmental psychosocial factors, whereas later episodes, after successive recurrences, may occur more autonomously.

There are no definitive laboratory markers of the acute manic syndrome; the diagnosis is made based on the presentation of the patient. Since a wide variety of causes of secondary mania have been elucidated, these warrant consideration in the differential diagnosis.[4] Many drugs, including psychomotor stimulants, can be associated with the induction of mania. Medical illnesses such as hyperthyroidism and right frontal or diencephalic strokes have also been associated with mania. Subtle neurological signs and symptoms should additionally be sought in the history and physical exam, since multiple sclerosis can often present with unrealistic euphoria and outright rapid cycling bipolar illness in a minority of instances. Bipolar illness is rarely associated with complex partial seizures, although the presentation can be classical when it does occur. There is considerable evidence as well as debate regarding the reliability and specificity of findings in bipolar illness of ventricular dilation, temporal lobe structural abnormalities, and possible lesions identified in computed tomographic (CT) scan or magnetic resonance imaging (MRI) studies. These findings, like a burgeoning set of related findings in the schizophrenias, suggest the possibility of neurobiological alterations underlying manic syndromes, either as a vulnerability or more primary factor involved in its pathophysiology. While cerebrospinal fluid elevations in norepinephrine itself or its metabolites have been described in manic and dysphoric syndromes, these too remain controversial and are in need of further systematic investigation both in their own right and as possible predictors of subsequent pharmacological response.[5]

Some aspects of the phenomenological presentation or subtype of mania are, however, useful in projecting the proportion of pharmacological responders. While those presenting with traditional euphoric mania show a high degree of response to lithium (60 to 80 per cent response), those presenting with dysphoric mania show an extremely poor rate of lithium response (20 to 40 per cent). Rapid cycling (i.e., presenting with a history of four or more episodes in the prior year) is also associated with less lithium responsiveness.[6,7] Moreover, the pattern of manic and depressive episodes is highly associated with lithium response. Those beginning with a manic episode that switches into a depression and then is followed by a well interval (MDI) tend to be highly responsive to lithium, while the converse is true in those beginning with a depression, switching into a mania and then into a well interval (DMI).[8] Comorbid alcohol and substance abuse is also associated with a poor response to lithium, as are schizoaffective illness and some types of secondary mania.

Thus, while lithium carbonate remains the mainstay for the acute and long-term treatment of the disorder, there is increasing recognition that it is not infallible and that there is need for alternative or adjunctive treatments, as discussed in this chapter. It is important to note from the outset, however, that there are no good predictors for pharmacological responsivity among these alternative treatments. Indeed, it is clear that response to one anticonvulsant, such as carbamazepine, does not predict response to another, such as valproic acid, or vice versa. Thus,

systematic sequential clinical trials in each individual are often required in order to assess adequate responsivity among the acute antimanic treatments used alone or in combination.

While neuroleptics remain the only other, Food and Drug Administration (FDA)-approved treatment besides lithium for acute manic psychosis, there are important reasons to consider alternative agents such as carbamazepine and valproate before neuroleptics are tried. Given the likely proposition that pharmacological responsivity in the acute manic syndrome may help predict longer term prophylaxis, adequate delineation of acute response to alternative treatments becomes of paramount importance. There is also an increasing recognition of the acute and long-term side effects of neuroleptics when used alone or in conjunction with lithium carbonate.

LITHIUM CARBONATE

As indicated above, lithium is the mainstay treatment of acute mania. Blood levels to be targeted are in the range of 0.8 to 1.5 mEq/liter. Even when these levels are achieved rapidly, there is often a considerable lag in onset of maximal antimanic efficacy, requiring some 2 to 3 weeks or longer before complete effect is noted. Thus, it is often necessary to adjunctively treat the full-blown aggressive or psychotic manic patients with other drugs. These adjuncts have traditionally been the neuroleptics, although there is increasing recognition of the utility of attempting adjunctive treatment with carbamazepine or valproate instead. Neuroleptics are associated with acute extrapyramidal side effects in many instances, and a wide range of rare but serious toxicities have been recognized, including neuroleptic malignant syndrome, irreversible neurological syndromes (particularly when haloperidol is used in conjunction with lithium carbonate), and sudden death. With longer term or even intermittent administration, neuroleptics (with the exception of clozapine) are associated with tardive dyskinesia to which bipolar patients appear uniquely predisposed. Neuroleptics may also lengthen or exacerbate the next depressive phase of the illness. Thus, particularly in the case of an episode breaking through lithium prophylaxis, there is considerable merit in attempting to initially assess the acute benefit of carbamazepine or valproate rather than a neuroleptic.[9,10]

Common lithium side effects include tremor, gastrointestinal distress, diabetes insipidus, and, more rarely, hypothyroidism, psoriasis, and impaired glomerular filtration. While obtaining baseline thyroid and renal indices is desirable, the urgency of initiating treatment takes precedence; these indices can be obtained concurrently with the initiation of treatment. While some reports suggest the efficacy of lithium at higher blood levels (over 1.5 mEq/liter), these observations have not been documented systematically and higher doses and blood levels are more likely to be associated with more frequent and substantial side effects.[11] Thus, if inadequate response is achieved with moderate doses and blood levels of lithium, adjunctive strategies, which have more rapid onsets of action, may be more useful than pushing initial therapies to toxicity.

Many authorities suggest the use of high-potency oral or parenteral anticonvulsant benzodiazepines, such as clonazepam or lorazepam, for augmentation. In contrast to carbamazepine and valproate, the acute antimanic efficacy of these drugs alone has not been documented in the literature, although the sedative properties of clonazepam may usefully target initial sleep disturbance emerging as an early sign of impending mania. In this fashion, sleep may be improved acutely, perhaps helping to break the vicious cycle of relative sleep deprivation and associated induction of mania suggested by Wehr.[12] Clonazepam (0.5 to 1.5 mg h.s.) may be adequate for this purpose, although some authorities have used total doses of 2 to 4 mg or more on a daily basis.[13] Lorazepam may similarly be utilized in the range of 2 to 4 mg for h.s. dosing. The use of extremely high doses of these compounds is unlikely to be of productive therapeutic benefit in the absence of the initial positive effects of lower doses, and are likely to be associated with side effects including sedation, ataxia, and dysarthria. Similarly, there is increasing recognition that extremely high or digitalizing doses of neuroleptics have not proved more efficacious in treating acute psychosis than low or moderate doses, and may be more productive of side effects. These data, which are well documented in the treatment of acute schizophrenic psychoses, have now received parallel replication in the treatment of acute mania.

The acute and long-term benefits of clozapine in mania and schizoaffective syndromes appear promising. This drug (when its hematological side effects are adequately monitored) may prove of unique benefit in the long-term management of refractory bipolar patients, as it does not appear to cause tardive dyskinesia.

CARBAMAZEPINE

This anticonvulsant is among the best-studied treatments of acute mania. As of 1991, 19 double-blind studies have compared carbamazepine with placebo, neuroleptics, lithium, or used the ABA design.[8,14,15] These studies indicate that carbamazepine has acute antimanic efficacy in approximately two thirds of patients, with onset and rapidity of action equaling that of the neuroleptics. This is often achieved with a more benign side-effects profile than the neuroleptics and a more positive reception by patients who are not saddled with neuroleptic-induced parkinsonian side effects, akathisia, or dysphoria. In contrast to treatment of acute depression, where slow dose increases are often required, the treatment of manic patients may be initiated more aggressively, with initial doses of 400 to 600 mg/day and increasing by 200 mg daily or every third day, depending on tolerability and side effects. Dizziness, ataxia, sedation, and diplopia are often early signs of high doses of carbamazepine; these signs will disappear with either holding the dose constant (if side effects are mild) or reducing it. Moreover, since carbamazepine induces its own hepatic metabolism after 2 or 3 weeks of therapy, doses that were not initially tolerated will be readily accepted at a later time. Drug half-life will decrease from 20 to 30 hours to 10 to 20 hours with chronic administration.

While the traditional 6- to 12 µg/ml blood-level window has been touted as appropriate for the treatment of seizure disorders, there is a poor relationship of blood level and degree of clinical response, either in epilepsy or acute mania. In the face of this situation, it appears more appropriate in individual patients to titrate dose against early side effects rather than resort to a hypothetical optimal range for dose or blood level. While some patients eventually may not tolerate more than 400 to 600 mg/day, others may tolerate as much as 1800 to 2000 without side effects. At higher doses and blood level ranges, however, side effects are more likely to occur. These include not only the ones previously mentioned, but also hyponatremia and, very rarely, water intoxication. Thus, in the face of a confusional element in the presentation, the clinician should obtain serum sodiums in order to rule out hyponatremia.

A pruritic rash, usually occurring in the second to fourth week of therapy, is a common (10 to 15 per cent) accompaniment of carbamazepine treatment and usually requires discontinuation because of the concern that a very small minority of these rashes could progress to severe dermatological complications including exfoliative dermatitis and Stevens-Johnson syndrome. Some patients not responsive to other treatment modalities have been able to be continued or restarted on carbamazepine under the cover of prednisone (40 mg/day) treatment, but this should be reserved for patients who show no other evidence of systemic allergy.

As illustrated in Table 32–1, the side-effects profile for carbamazepine is considerably different from that of lithium and valproate, which appear to share many signs and symptoms in common. In contrast to lithium, carbamazepine tends to decrease total white count in a high proportion of patients. This benign white count suppression is distinguishable from the rarer idiosyncratic occurrence of agranulocytosis and aplastic anemia, estimated to occur in 1/125,000 patients.[16] Benign white count suppression from carbamazepine is thought to occur on the basis of inhibition of colony stimulating factors (CSF) in the bone marrow, and is reversed in vitro and clinically by treatment with lithium carbonate.[17] However, it is unlikely that lithium would reverse the idiosyncratic bone marrow suppression. Hyponatremia with carbamazepine may be prevented or reversed by con-

TABLE 32–1. COMPARATIVE CLINICAL AND SIDE-EFFECTS PROFILES OF LITHIUM, CARBAMAZEPINE, AND VALPROATE
(Preliminary Clinical Impressions)

	Valproate (50–120 μg/ml)	Lithium (0.5–1.5 mEq/liter)	Carbamazepine (4–12 μg/ml)
Clinical profile[a]			
Mania	++	++	++
Dysphoric	++	(+)	(++)
Rapid or continuous cycling	++	+	++
Family history negative	?	+	++
Depression	(+)	(+)	(+)
Prophylaxis			
Mania	++	++	++
Depression	+	++	++
Seizures			
Generalized, CPS	++	0	++
Absence	++	0	0
Paroxysmal pain syndromes	0	0	++
Side effects[b]			
White blood count	—	↑	↓
Diabetes insipidus	—	↑	↓
Thyroid hormones T_3, T_4	↓	↓	↓
TSH	?	↑	—
Serum calcium	?	↑	↓
Weight gain	↑	↑	(-)
Tremor	↑	↑	—
Memory disturbances	(↑)	(↑)	(↑)
Diarrhea, GI distress	(↑)	(↑)	—
Teratogenesis	↑	(↑)	(↑)
Psoriasis	—	(↑)	—
Pruritic rash (allergy)	—	—	↑
Agranulocytosis, aplastic anemia	—	—	(↑)
Thrombocytopenia	(↑)	—	(↑)
Hepatitis	(↑)	—	(↑)
Hyponatremia, water intoxication	—	—*	↑
Dizziness, ataxia, diplopia	—	—	↑
Hypercortisolism, escape from dexamethasone suppression	?	—	↑

[a] Clinical efficacy: 0, none; +, effective; ++, very effective; ( ), equivocal.

[b] Side effects: increase; decrease; ( ), inconsistent or rare; —, absent; ?, unknown; *, effect of lithium predominates over that of carbamazepine.

current treatment with demeclocycline or possibly lithium. When carbamazepine and lithium are used in conjunction, there appears to be a greater degree of suppression of T_4 and T_3, but no greater increase in thyroid stimulating hormone (TSH) levels than observed with lithium alone.[17] The decrements in thyroid indices usually do not require thyroid replacement, as hypothyroidism is extremely rare during carbamazepine treatment. This stands in contrast to the more typical need for thyroid supplementation to prevent lithium-induced goiter, marked increases in TSH, and, in rare instances, overt hypothyroidism. Other infrequent side effects of carbamazepine include induction of arteriovenous (A-V) block, hypersensitivity with lymphadenopathy, and hepatotoxicity. It appears relatively safe in overdose, especially in comparison with traditional tricyclics. Use during pregnancy, which was originally reported as safe, is no longer recommended because syndromes of developmental delay, minor craniofacial abnormalities and spina bifida have been observed.

Pharmacokinetic interactions with other drugs are common with carbamazepine. Patients should be warned that erythromycin (and its antibiotic analogues), verapamil, diltiazem, isoniazid, and propoxyphene (Darvon) substantially increase levels and produce marked toxicity. Conversely, carbamazepine may markedly decrease levels and associated efficacy of haloperidol, several antidepressants, and, most notably, birth control pills. Patients should therefore be placed on higher dosage forms of oral contraceptives while being treated with carbamazepine.

VALPROATE

Several recent double-blind controlled trials document the efficacy of valproate, supporting an earlier literature in uncontrolled trials.[18,19] Valproate appears to be particularly effective in dysphoric mania although, with this exception, valproate appears to show a rather similar profile of clinical efficacy to lithium carbonate (Table 32–1). However, valproate is effective in some patients who do not respond to either lithium or carbamazepine.[8,20,21]

Traditional blood levels of valproate associated

with acute antimanic response range from 50 to 120 μg/ml. Tremor appears to be dose related. Gastrointestinal (GI) distress is frequent with Depakene and less frequent with Depakote, which is enteric coated. If GI distress should occur, it has been successfully treated by some investigators with pepsid. Like lithium, and in contrast to carbamazepine, weight gain can be a problem with valproate. Valproate can also be associated with frequent increases in liver function indices, sometimes two to three times normal without progressing to serious hepatotoxicity of either a toxic metabolic or allergic basis. Patients should be warned to report immediately signs of right upper quadrant pain, anorexia, fever, and change in color of urine or stool so that drug can be immediately discontinued. The numerous cases of severe, potentially fatal hepatotoxicity have largely occurred in children under the age of 2 years and in those on combination therapy. This problem is extremely rare in adults and in those on anticonvulsant monotherapy. Anecdotal data suggest that selenium may help to prevent the hepatotoxicity of valproate thought to be based on the formation of free radicals. Alopecia is not an uncommon side effect of valproate treatment, but can be annoying, as previously straight hair may grow in curly. Anecdotal reports suggest that zinc may alleviate or prevent alopecia.

Valproate can be used in conjunction with lithium or neuroleptics without pharmacokinetic or dynamic interactions reported to date. Use of valproate and carbamazepine together has been reported in a small series of refractory epileptics and anecdotally in some patients with refractory manias. The combination is complicated from a pharmacokinetic perspective, such that lower doses of carbamazepine and higher doses of valproate may be required. This is because valproate increases levels of carbamazepine-10,11-epoxide and carbamazepine decreases valproate levels. As with carbamazepine, onset of action with valproate is often rapid, with substantial improvement occurring within the first week of treatment,[18] providing additional rationale for using these adjunctive treatments instead of neuroleptics in order to access acute responsivity. Valproate is associated with a low but substantial incidence of neural tube defects, including spina bifida, and thus should not be used during pregnancy.

OTHER ANTICONVULSANTS

The acute antimanic efficacy of *phenytoin* has not been documented, although the occasional responder has been reported in the literature. *Acetazolamide* (500 to 1000 mg/day) has been reported to be useful in some patients who do not respond to lithium and carbamazepine. Preliminary evidence from a single small study[22] suggests that it may be particularly effective in atypical psychoses associated with a dreamy, confusional state or those occur-

ring in puerperium or the premenstrual period. *Alprazolam* is to be relatively avoided in mania as it, like other more traditional unimodal antidepressant treatments, has been associated with the induction of mania.

CALCIUM CHANNEL BLOCKERS

These agents, particularly verapamil (240 to 480 mg/day), but also nimodipine (360 mg/day), have been reported effective in the treatment of acute mania. Double-blind studies exist only for verapamil, and are promising, although clinical practice has not yet achieved the same positive results as the initial studies in the literature. There is some suggestion that the clinical spectrum of action of calcium channel blockers is similar to lithium, implying that these agents will not play the same important role in lithium-refractory patients as the anticonvulsants. The calcium channel blockers are relatively benign in terms of their side-effects profile and they may ultimately have a role in patients who are unable to tolerate lithium side effects. Hypotension and cardiac side effects may be dose limiting with some agents. Verapamil and diltiazem, but not nifedipine, will also markedly increase carbamazepine levels if the two drugs are used concomitantly.

ELECTROCONVULSIVE THERAPY

Electroconvulsive therapy (ECT) appears to be a rapid-acting acute antimanic agent, as effective in treating mania as it is in treating acute depression. This modality may be worthy of consideration in the pharmacologically refractory acute manic patient or one with medical complications who is unable to tolerate other antimanic modalities. Treatment should be initiated with bilateral electrode placements, since evidence suggests that unilateral placements may be slower in onset, ineffective, or, in some instances, may exacerbate the manic syndrome. While all studies do not agree about the relative inefficacy of unilateral treatment, if one has to resort to the use of ECT in the face of so many available effective antimanic treatments, initial use of bilateral treatment would be the conservative approach during refractory mania.

CLONIDINE AND OTHER EXPERIMENTAL APPROACHES

Clonidine, an α_2-agonist drug that inhibits the firing of the noradrenergic locus coeruleus, is reported to be an acute antimanic treatment in some but not all studies.[23] Further work is required to delineate its spectrum of efficacy, including the possible use in some neuroleptic-refractory patients. Whether patients showing initial response to clonidine will demonstrate tachyphylaxis, as they apparently do in the treatment of anxiety syndromes, also remains to be documented. This agent may be particularly appropriate in the manic patient with associated hypertension.

It is of theoretical interest that the inhibitor of catecholamine biosynthesis, alpha-methyl-paratyrosine (AMPT), has been reported to produce acute antimanic effects. These data are consistent with the antimanic effects of the neuroleptics related to their dopamine-blocking properties, or clonidine and propranolol with their adrenergic-inhibiting and -blocking properties, respectively. While l-propranolol has been reported to be effective in acute mania, the inactive d-isomer also appears to share this property. Moreover, in light of the high doses required for both compounds, it is unlikely that the β-adrenergic blocking properties of these drugs is associated with their antimanic effects. Rather, a more nonspecific "membrane stabilizing" effect may be implicated. Physostigmine and other cholinergic agonists have also been reported to exert acute antimanic effects. These observations are of theoretical interest from the perspective that the acute mania syndrome can be rapidly ameliorated with an intravenous dose of physostigmine, even though the more traditional pharmacotherapies and ECT appear to exert their effects with a considerable time lag. In addition, these data suggest that either increasing cholinergic tone itself or changing cholinergic-adrenergic balance is capable of exerting antimanic effects. From the mechanistic perspective, these data suggest that a variety of biochemical manipulations are capable of exerting acute antimanic effects, as noted above.

SUMMARY

Thus, a wide-range variety of antimanic agents are currently available for the treatment of acute episodes. These drugs exert their putative antimanic effects through a variety of different neurotransmitter and receptor systems: lithium at neurotransmitter and second messenger systems; neuroleptics by blocking dopamine receptors; benzodiazepines at their central-type receptors; carbamazepine at peripheral-type benzodiazepine receptors; and valproate at gamma-aminobutyric acid (GABA) systems. This perspective of different mechanisms of action provides the theoretical rationale for sequential clinical trials in the treatment-refractory manic patient. We have observed that some patients respond to the anticonvulsant carbamazepine but not to valproate, and vice versa. Thus, until precise clinical and biological markers of acute antimanic response are delineated, the clinician should be aware of the range of alternative and adjunctive agents that can be employed until an individual's response is noted and documented. This may provide invalu-

able information for further treatment or long-term prophylaxis or both. Treatment of the acute manic episode is only the first step in the treatment of the bipolar patient. With the resolution of the acute episode, attention should immediately turn toward the prevention of future episodes.

Once an appropriate clinical regimen is found to be effective and side-effects profile optimized, it behooves the clinician to maintain prophylaxis in the vast majority of patients. Not only has lithium discontinuation, even after many years of effective therapy, been associated with a high incidence of relapse (80 to 90 per cent), but two additional liabilities of lithium discontinuation have recently been documented. There is some evidence of particular vulnerability to a new episode in the first 2 weeks following lithium discontinuation (perhaps a withdrawal syndrome[24]). We have also documented a series of cases in which lithium-discontinuation–induced episodes resulted in subsequent lithium refractoriness in patients who had previously shown excellent long-term prophylactic responses to lithium.

Therefore, given the potentially malignant nature of recurrent bipolar illness, with its incapacitating and destructive effects on social networks, finances, employment, and marriage, the clinician should be judiciously conservative in the long-term treatment of this illness. The manic patient, with his euphoria, grandiosity and denial of illness, is a prime candidate for noncompliance; therefore, close monitoring of patients is required. While systematic data have not been accumulated to document the adjunctive use of psychotherapy in the treatment of bipolar patients, this is highly recommended for a variety of reasons. First, it may help engender compliance, particularly if it includes systematic gathering and graphing of information describing the patient's prior course of illness. Such graphing (or "life charting") is instructive both retrospectively and prospectively, as the patient may gain increased appreciation for the recurrent nature of this illness and its potential catastrophic consequences. In addition, psychotherapy may help deal with acute psychosocial stressors, including funerals and anniversary reactions, which may be associated with the precipitation of manic episodes.[3] Moreover, since acute sleep loss and other physiological environmental alterations (e.g., jet lag phase changes) may be associated with the induction of mania, these can also be dealt with in the context of ongoing psychotherapy. With regular therapeutic sessions serving as an early warning system so that initial symptoms of breakthrough become evident, treatment can be rapidly and aggressively altered and augmented in order to suppress episode emergence. As has been demonstrated in the prevention of relapse of recurrent unipolar depression, it is also possible that adjunctive psychotherapy will, in its own right, be important in the prevention of episodes and the supplementation of pharmacotherapy, although this remains to be directly demonstrated.

REFERENCES

1. Strober MT, Morrell W, Lampert C, Burroughs J: Relapse following discontinuation of lithium maintenance therapy in adolescents with bipolar I illness: A naturalistic study. Am J Psychiatry 147:457–461, 1990.
2. Hanus H, Zapletalek M: The prophylactic lithium treatment in affective disorders and the possibilities of the outcome prediction. Sb Ved Pr Lek Fak Univ Karlovy 27:5–75, 1984.
3. Post RM, Rubinow DR, Ballenger JC: Conditioning and sensitization in the longitudinal course of affective illness. Br J Psychiatry 149:191–201, 1986.
4. Krauthammer C, Klerman GL: Secondary mania: Manic syndrome associated with antecedent illness or drugs. Arch Gen Psychiatry 35:1333–1339, 1978.
5. Post RM, Rubinow DR, Uhde TW, et al: Dysphoric mania: Clinical and biological correlates. Arch Gen Psychiatry 46:353–358, 1989.
6. Dunner DL, Fieve RR: Clinical factors in lithium prophylactic failure. Arch Gen Psychiatry 30:229–233, 1974.
7. Post RM, Kramlinger KG, Altshuler LL, Ketter T, Denikoff K: Treatment of rapid cycling bipolar illness. Psychopharmacol Bull 26:37–47, 1990.
8. Post RM: Alternatives to lithium for bipolar affective illness. In Review of Psychiatry, vol 3. Washington, DC: American Psychiatric Press 9:170–202, 1990.
9. Kramlinger KG, Post RM: Adding lithium carbonate to carbamazepine: Antimanic efficacy in treatment resistant mania. Acta Psychiatr Scand 79:378–385, 1989.
10. Post RM, Uhde TW, Roy-Byrne PP, et al: Correlates of antimanic response to carbamazepine. Psychiatry Res 21:71–83, 1987.
11. Gelenberg AJ, Kane JM, Keller MB, et al: Comparison of standard and low serum levels of lithium for maintenance treatment of bipolar disorder. N Engl J Med 321:1489–1493, 1989.
12. Wehr TA: Sleep loss: A preventable cause of mania and other excited states. J Clin Psychiatry 50:8–16, 1989.
13. Chouinard G, Young SN, Annable L: Antimanic effect of clonazepam. Biol Psychiatry 18:451–466, 1983.
14. Post RM: Non-lithium treatment for bipolar disorder. J Clin Psychiatry 51:8, 1990.
15. Post RM: Sensitization and kindling perspectives for the course of affective illness: Toward a new treatment with the anticonvulsant carbamazepine. Pharmacopsychiatry 23:3–17, 1990.
16. Pellock JM: Carbamazepine side effects in children and adults. Epilepsia 28:S64–S70, 1987.
17. Kramlinger KG, Post RM: Addition of lithium carbonate to carbamazepine: Hematological and thyroid effects. Am J Psychiatry 147:615–620, 1990.
18. Pope HG, McElroy SL, Keck PE, et al: Valproate in the treatment of acute mania. Arch Gen Psychiatry 48:62–68, 1991.
19. Emrich DM, Dose M, von Zerssen D: The use of sodium valproate, carbamazepine and oxcarbazepine in patients with affective disorders. J Affective Disord 8:243–250, 1985.
20. Calabrese JR, Delucchi GA: Phenomenology of rapid cycling manic depression and its treatment with valproate. J Clin Psychiatry 50:30–34, 1989.
21. Small JG: Anticonvulsants in affective disorders. Psychopharm Bull 26:25–36, 1990.
22. Inoue H, Hazama H, Hamazoe K, et al: Antipsychotic and prophylactic effects of acetazolamide (Diamox) on atypical psychosis. Folia Psychiatr Neurol Jpn 38:425–436, 1984.
23. Janicak PG, Sharma RP, Easton M, et al: A double blind, placebo controlled trial of clonidine in the treatment of acute mania. Psychopharmacol Bull 25:243–245, 1989.
24. Mander AJ, Loudon JB: Rapid recurrence of mania following abrupt discontinuation of lithium. Lancet 2:15–17, 1988.

33

CLASSIFICATION AND TREATMENT OF DYSTHYMIA

MARTIN B. KELLER, M.D., LORI A. BAKER, M.A., and CORDELIA WARD RUSSELL, B.A.

THE CLINICAL PICTURE

Dysthymia is currently defined in the DSM-III-R[1] as a persistently depressed mood present for at least 2 years, with at least two of the following symptoms: poor appetite or overeating, insomnia or hypersomnia, low energy or fatigue, low self-esteem, poor concentration or difficulty making decisions, and feelings of hopelessness. For a diagnosis of dysthymia, patients cannot be without these symptoms for more than 2 months at a time.

Exclusion criteria for dysthymia include the presence of a major depressive episode during the first 2 years of illness; a manic or hypomanic episode at any time in the patient's life; psychotic symptoms or the residual phase of schizophrenia; and/or the mood being sustained by a specific organic factor or substance.

Dysthymia may be diagnosed as either primary or secondary type, and as early or late onset. A primary diagnosis of dysthymia indicates that the disorder did not occur exclusively during the course of another chronic nonmood Axis I or II disorder, while a diagnosis of secondary dysthymia indicates the opposite. An early onset diagnosis indicates that the patient became ill at age 21 or younger, while late onset indicates first occurrence after age 21.

It is of considerable clinical interest to note that the symptoms of dysthymia, as they are defined in DSM-III-R, differ from those of major depression in severity and chronicity rather than in kind. In fact, dysthymia is often diagnosed in conjunction with an overlapping episode of major depression.[2-6] Concern that the diagnostic similarity of dysthymia and major depression may be creating a large number of artifactual dual diagnoses is being investigated by the DSM-IV Mood Disorder Task Force, and will be addressed in the DSM-IV.

EPIDEMIOLOGY

An epidemiological study of dysthymia in the general population conducted by Weissman and Myers[7] found a lifetime prevalence of this disorder of 4.7 per cent in a survey of 511 subjects. The National Institute of Mental Health (NIMH) Epidemiological Catchment Area Study, which reported the prevalence of DSM-III diagnostic categories based on interviews conducted in random population samples in three sites, found rates of dysthymia ranging from 2.1 to 3.8 per cent.[8] Weissman et al.[9] have estimated that the female:male ratio of dysthymia is 1.9:1. Other community studies have found rates of "chronic depression" ranging from 2.7 to 4.3 per cent.[9,10]

The age of onset of dysthymia has typically been considered to be in the early twenties; however, studies of early onset dysthymia have found evidence of dysthymia in children and adolescents, with age of onset ranging from 6 to 13 years.[6] A study conducted by Klein et al.[11] concluded that there was a close relationship between primary early onset dysthymia and major affective disorders. The age range of dysthymia is 18 to 65 in women and 18 to 45 for men.[9,12]

COURSE OF ILLNESS

A study of the duration of dysthymia by Rounsaville et al.[13] found that the illness may persist for 2 to 20 years, with a median duration of approximately 5 years.[2,13]

The course and outcome of dysthymia are characterized by chronicity. A 2-year naturalistic follow-up study of dysthymics by Barrett[14] found that 63 per cent of the subjects reported no improvement in their illness during the follow-up period; in some cases, subjects reported a worsening of their condition. The concomitant presence of major depressive episodes, a common phenomenon in this patient group, may also worsen the course of illness. The NIMH Collaborative Study of the Psychobiology of Depression, a prospective, naturalistic longitudinal study of depressive disorders, found that 61 per cent of patients suffering from "double depression" (dysthymia with superimposed major depressive episodes) had not recovered from their underlying dysthymic disorder after 2 years of follow-up.[15]

Keller et al.[15] also found, in a 1-year follow-up of 66 formerly double depressed patients who had recovered from the superimposed major depression, that these patients experienced high rates of relapse and recurrence. While 38 per cent of the subjects recovered from dysthymia during the follow-up period, 36 per cent relapsed into a Research Diagnostic Criteria (RDC) major affective disorder, and 26 per cent remained in a state of chronic depression. During the 1-year period following their recovery from major depression, patients with double depression experienced a declining chance of recovery from the chronic minor depression, coupled with a rising chance of relapse into a major affective episode.

FAMILY STUDIES OF DYSTHYMIA

Little is known regarding the specific genetic transmission of dysthymia. However, several studies have found evidence that a high incidence of chronic depression exists in the relatives of chronically depressed probands.[16] Klein et al.[11] reported that the offspring of patients with episodes of major depressive disorder that have high rates of dysthymic disorder. Blehar et al.[17] found evidence for the familial transmission of major depression, but concluded that genetic factors have negligible effect on the transmission of dysthymia.

BIOLOGICAL AND LABORATORY STUDIES

At this time, knowledge on the biological abnormalities related to dysthymia is considered speculative. The little data that do exist incorporate neuroendocrine strategies and neurophysical hypotheses. Roy et al.[18] reported an 18 per cent dexamethasone suppression test (DST) nonsuppression rate in dysthymic disorder. Neurophysiological correlates of dysthymic disorder include shortened rapid eye movement (REM) sleep and diminished electrodermal activity.[19,20] Akiskal et al.[21] and Hauri and Sateia[22] have found modest REM latency associations in dysthymic patients; however, both of these studies used very small sample sizes.

Miller et al.[23] found no significant differences in DST nonsuppression rates between patients with double depression (36 per cent) and episodic depression (47 per cent). In addition, no differences in DST nonsuppression rates were found between patients with early versus late onset double depression.

A study of sleep patterns and quality in dysthymics by Arriaga and colleagues[24] found that dysthymic patients experienced fragmented and superficial sleep, with no changes in REM, and a higher percentage of stage 1 sleep and reduction of slow-wave sleep as compared with normal controls.

THE DIFFERENTIAL DIAGNOSIS OF DYSTHYMIA

In order to diagnose dysthymia, the clinician must carefully differentiate between chronic or unremitting low-grade depression, chronic or unremitting episodes of major depression, depressive personality attributes, double depression,[21,25] and chronic anxiety.[11,26] Numerous boundary issues remain between major depression, double depression, and dysthymia. A clearer differentiation of these disorders is one of the goals of the DSM-IV Mood Disorders Task Force. At this time, the differentiation of these disorders depends on the timing, duration, number, and severity of depressive symptoms and not on a qualitative distinction in the symptom profile.[25]

TREATMENT OF DYSTHYMIA

Research on the treatment of dysthymia is still sparse, but studies have begun to indicate that antidepressant somatotherapy may have positive effects on this disorder, if such treatment is implemented. Some of the medications that have recently been studied include imipramine, amitriptyline, ritanserin, sulpride, tianeptine, phenelzine, and amineptine. The most recent studies on the use of these medications in dysthymic patients are summarized below.

Imipramine

A study by Kocsis et al.[27] of the use of the antidepressant imipramine in subjects with dysthymia suggests that this medication is an efficacious treatment for the disorder. These authors report favorable responses to imipramine in 45 per cent of a sample of 29 dysthymic patients, versus 12 per cent in a sample of 25 dysthymics receiving placebo. Overall, they report that 59 per cent of study completers taking imipramine, versus 13 per cent of those taking placebo, reported improvement. These authors also note that 6 weeks of imipramine somatotherapy also produced improved sociovocational functioning in this sample of dysthymic patients.[28]

Amitriptyline and Ritanserin

In a double-blind, 8-week study of 30 DSM-III dysthymics, Meco et al.[29] reported that amitriptyline 25

to 50 mg and ritanserin 10 to 20 mg showed comparable efficacy in reducing anxious and depressive symptoms. These authors suggest that the response of dysthymic subjects to these antidepressant medications supports the inclusion of dysthymia in the "affective disorders" category of the DSM.

A study of the physiological effects of ritanserin in animals and healthy volunteers by Pavia and colleagues[30] demonstrated that ritanserin significantly increased slow-wave sleep and affected sleep stage transitions during the night. The authors suggest that ritanserin's effect on sleep may contribute to the relief of dysthymic patients.

Sulpride

A Finnish study compared the benefits of sulpride 100 to 200 mg with placebo. Thirteen of twenty-two elderly depressives receiving sulpride and 13 of 24 taking placebo had SCID diagnoses of dysthymic disorder.[31] Sulpride was no more effective than placebo.

Tianeptine

Tianeptine was researched in a study of patients with major depression and dysthymia.[32] The results of this study indicated that the tianeptine, with its antidepressant and anxiolytic properties, would be suitable for a full range of depressive symptomatology. A study of tianeptine versus amitriptyline in depressed alcoholics suffering from either dysthymia or major depression by Loo et al.[33] found that tianeptine was more successful in relieving the somatic symptoms of these two disorders, and was associated with only few, rare anticholinergic effects. The authors concluded that tianeptine was a safer and more efficacious choice for the treatment of depressive disorders than amitriptyline. However, another study comparing these two medications found no significant differences in outcomes in dysthymic patients with clinically manifest anxiety.[34]

Phenelzine

A study by Stewart et al.[35] of nonmelancholic depressed outpatients with atypical features found that a significantly higher number of subjects responded to phenelzine than imipramine. The ratio of this difference was 71:48 per cent.

Even though positive effects have been demonstrated in the use of phenelzine, one small study of this medication's long-term effects suggested that patients treated with phenelzine relapsed into severe chronic depression that was refractory to other treatments.[36]

Amineptine

The tricyclic compound of amineptine was developed in France. A study by Kemali[37] found that use of this antidepressant on 324 patients with DSM-III diagnoses of major depression (29 per cent), dysthymia (60 per cent), and atypical depression (11 per cent) resulted in a positive outcome in 91 per cent of the dysthymics, 75 per cent of those with major depression, and 84 per cent of atypical depressions.

Duration of Somatic Treatment

Aronson and Shukla[38] investigated the duration of antidepressant treatment in a retrospective study of subjects with chronic depression. This study compared 26 patients with chronic depression who relapsed when antidepressant medication was tapered off after 6 to 12 months of successful treatment, to a sample of 15 subjects with episodic depression whose medication was successfully tapered. They found that the subjects who relapsed when medication was withdrawn had experienced a longer duration of illness prior to seeking treatment and were more likely to demonstrate comorbid anxiety disorders or anxiety symptoms, personality disorders, delusional depression, and dysthymic disorder than patients who did not relapse after tapering. They suggest that antidepressant treatment may "control" rather than cure depressive symptoms in this population of chronic patients.

Psychotherapy

Surprisingly little has been written about the clinical experience of psychotherapy and chronic depression.[39,40] Kocsis et al.[16] found that 76 per cent of dysthymic subjects entering a pharmacological trial had previously failed psychotherapy lasting at least 6 months. Kocsis also found that 61 per cent of dysthymics who had participated in psychotherapy for a substantial amount of time had little somatic relief.

While few controlled trials of the use of psychotherapy for treatment of dysthymia have been conducted, some investigators have suggested that cognitive and behavioral psychotherapies show promise in the treatment of depression.[23,41] Typically, these are short-term techniques designed to address depressive deficits as demonstrated in cognitions, behaviors, and affects.[42] The development of such therapies for use in the treatment of dysthymia may be an important area for future clinical research.

Exercise

Several authors have recently investigated exercise as an alternative to psychotherapy in the treatment of chronic minor depression. Greist et al.[43] reported that the effects of 10 weeks of regular exercise were equivalent to 10 weeks of cognitive behavioral psychotherapy in allieviating depressive symptoms in a small sample of subjects meeting RDC criteria for minor depression. Fremont and Craighead[44] found no difference in outcomes when they compared patients receiving cognitive therapy, supervised running, and a combination of both exercise and running. However, these studies used small sample sizes and acknowledged considerable methodological limitations.

DISCUSSION

While the work of the DSM-IV Mood Disorders Task Force will help to better define dysthymia and differentiate it from major depression and depressive character pathology, it is also incumbent upon psychiatrists and general practitioners to learn to recognize and treat this illness. Patients with dysthymia who develop concomitant episodes of major depression have a highly pernicious form of affective illness, and a low likelihood of returning to a normal state, even when they recover from the major depression. As the above-cited studies indicate, dysthymic patients have an excellent chance of benefitting from adequate antidepressant somatotherapy once their illness is recognized. Failure to treat these patients may result in chronic, debilitating depressive illness.

It is clear that further research is needed on the etiology, pathophysiology, course, symptoms, and treatment of dysthymia. With regard to treatment, the further development of the cognitive and behavioral therapies that have shown promising results in patients with major depression may be one important avenue of future investigation.

REFERENCES

1. American Psychiatric Association: Diagnostic and Statistical Manual of Mental Disorders. 3rd ed. Revised. Washington, DC: American Psychiatric Press, 1987.
2. Keller MB, Shapiro RW: "Double depression": Superimposition of acute depressive episodes on chronic depressive disorders: Am Psychiatry 139(4):438–442, 1982.
3. Akiskal HS, King D, Rosenthal TL: et al: Chronic depressions, part 1: Clinical and familial characteristics in 137 probands. J Affective Disord 3:297–315, 1981.
4. Perry JP: Depression in borderline personality disorder: Lifetime prevalence at interview and longitudinal course of symptoms. Am J Psychiatry 142(1):15–21, 1985.
5. Keller MB, Lavori PW: Double depression, major depression and dysthymia: Distinct entities or different phases of a single disorder? Psychopharmacol Bull 20(3):399–402, 1984.
6. Kovacs M, Feinberg TL, Crouse-Novak M, et al: Depressive disorders in childhood: I and II. Arch Gen Psychiatry 41:229–237 (I) and 643–649 (II), 1984.
7. Weissman MM, Myers JK: Affective disorders in a U.S. urban community: The use of research diagnostic criteria in an epidemiological survey. Arch Gen Psychiatry 35:1304–1311, 1978.
8. Robins LN, Helzer JE, Weissman MM, et al: Lifetime prevalence of specific psychiatric disorders in 3 sites. Arch Gen Psychiatry 41:949–958, 1984.
9. Weissman MM, Leaf PJ, Tischler GL, et al: Affective disorders in five United States communities. Psychol Med 18:141–153, 1988.
10. Karno M, Hough RL, Burnam AM, et al: Lifetime psychiatric disorders among Mexican Americans and non-hispanic

whites in Los Angeles. Arch Gen Psychiatry 44:695–701, 1987.

11. Klein DK, Taylor EB, Dickstein S, Harding K: The early-late onset distinction in DSM-III-R dysthymia. J Affective Disord 14:25–33, 1988.

12. Myers JM, Weissman MM, Tischler GL, et al: Six-month prevalence of psychiatric disorders in three communities, 1980–1982. Arch Gen Psychiatry 41:959–967, 1984.

13. Rounsaville BJ, Shokomskas D, Prusoff BA: Chronic mood disorders in depressed outpatients: Diagnosis and response to pharmacotherapy. J Affective Disord 2:72–78, 1988.

14. Barrett J: Naturalistic change over two years in neurotic depressive disorders (RDC categories). Compr Psychiatry 25(4):404–418, 1984.

15. Keller MB, Lavori PW, Endicott J, et al: "Double depression": Two-year follow-up. Am J Psychiatry 140(6):689–694, 1983.

16. Kocsis JH, Voss C, Mann JJ, Frances AJ: Chronic depression: Demographic and clinical characteristics. Psychopharmacol Bull 22(1):192–195, 1986.

17. Blehar MC, Weissman MM, Gershon ES, Hirschfeld RMA: Family and genetic studies of affective disorders. Arch Gen Psychiatry 45:289–292, 1988.

18. Roy A, Sutton M, Pickar D: Neuroendocrine and personality variables in dysthymic disorder. Am J Psychiatry 142:94–97, 1985.

19. Ward NG, Doerr OO: Is skin conductance a sensitive and specific marker for depression? Paper presented at the 40th Annual Meeting of the Society of Biological Psychiatry, Dallas, TX, 1985.

20. Thase M: Biological factors related to dysthymic disorder. Paper presented at the National Institute of Mental Health Workshop on Dysthymic Disorder, Washington, DC, 1986.

21. Akiskal HS, Rosenthal TL, Haykel RF, et al: Characterological depressions: Clinical and sleep EEG findings separating 'subaffective dysthymias' from 'character spectrum disorders.' Arch Gen Psychiatry 37:777–783, 1980.

22. Hauri P, Sateia MJ: REM sleep in dysthymic disorders (abstr). Sleep Res 13:119, 1984.

23. Miller IW, Norman WE, Keitner GI: Cognitive-behavioral treatment of depressed inpatients: Six and twelve month follow-up. Am J Psychiatry 146:1274–1279, 1989.

24. Arriaga F, Rosado P, Paiva T: The sleep of dysthymic patients: A comparison with normal controls. Biol Psychiatry 27(6):649–656, 1990.

25. Keller MB: Diagnostic and course of illness variables pertinent to refractory depression. In Tasman A, Goldfinger SM, Kaufmann A, eds. Review of Psychiatry. Washington, DC: American Psychiatric Press, 1990.

26. Alneas R, Torgersen S: DSM-II symptom disorders (Axis I) and personality disorders (Axis II) in an outpatient population. Acta Psychiatr Scand 78:348–353, 1988.

27. Kocsis JH, Frances AJ, Voss C, et al: Imipramine treatment for chronic depression. Arch Gen Psychiatry 45:253–257, 1988.

28. Kocsis JH, Frances AJ, Voss C, et al: Imipramine and social-vocational adjustment in chronic depression. Am J Psychiatry 145:997–999, 1988.

29. Meco G, Marini S, Mariana L, et al: Ritanserin in dysthymic disorders (DSM-III): A double-blind study versus amitryptyline (abstr). Psychopharmacology 282:1988.

30. Paiva T, Arriaga F, Wauquier A, et al: Effects of ritanserin on sleep disturbances of dysthymic patients. Psychopharmacology 96(3):395–399, 1988.

31. Kivella SL, Lehomaki E: Sulpride and placebo in depressed elderly outpatients: A double-blind study. Int J Geriat Psychiatry 2:255–260, 1987.

32. Defrance R, Marey C, Kamoun A: Antidepressant and anxiolytic activities of tianeptine: An overview of clinical trials. Clin Neuropharmacol 11(2):S74–S82, 1988.

33. Loo H, Malka R, Defrance R, Barrucand D, et al: Tianeptine and amitriptyline. Controlled double blind trial in depressed alcoholic patients. Neuropsychobiology 19(2):79–85, 1988.

34. Guelfi JD, Pichot P, Dreyfus JF: Efficacy of tianeptine in anxious-depressed patients: Results of a controlled multicenter trial vs. amitriptyline. Neuropsychobiology 22(1):41–48, 1989.

35. Stewart JW, McGrath PJ, Quitkin FM, et al: Relevance of DSM-III depressive subtype and chronicity of antidepressant efficacy in atypical depression: Differential response to phenelzine, imipramine and placebo. Arch Gen Psychiatry 46:1080–1087, 1989.

36. Donaldson SR: Tolerance to phenelzine and subsequent refractory depression: Three cases. J Clin Psychiatry 50(1):33–35, 1989.

37. Kemali D: A multicenter Italian study of amineptine (survector 100). Clin Neuropharmacol 12(2):S41–S50, 1989.

38. Aronson TA, Shukla S: Long-term continuation antidepressant treatment: A comparison study. J Clin Psychiatry 50(8):285–289, 1989.

39. Weissman MM, Akiskal HS: The role of psychotherapy in chronic depressions: A proposal. Compr Psychiatry 25:23–31, 1984.

40. Kocsis JH: Dysthymic disorder. In Karasu B, ed. Treatments of Psychiatric Disorders. Washington, DC: American Psychiatric Association, 1989.

41. Shea MT, Elkin I, Hirschfeld RMA: Psychotherapeutic treatment of depression. In Hales RE, Frances AJ, eds. Psychiatric Update: The American Psychiatric Association Annual Review, vol 7. Washington, DC: American Psychiatric Press, 1988.

42. Keller MB, Baker LA: The effects of major depression on dysthymia. Clin Adv Treatment Psychiatr Disord 4(2):4–7, 1990.

43. Greist JH, Klein MH, Eischens R, et al: Running as a treatment for depression. Compr Psychiatry 20(1):41–54, 1979.

44. Fremont J, Wilcoxon Craighead L: Aerobic exercise and cognitive therapy in the treatment of dysphoric moods. Cog Ther Res 11(2):241–251, 1987.

34

ATYPICAL DEPRESSION

JONATHAN W. STEWART, M.D., JUDITH G. RABKIN, Ph.D., M.P.H., FREDERIC M. QUITKIN, M.D., PATRICK J. McGRATH, M.D., and DONALD F. KLEIN, M.D.

Although not recognized by DSM-III[1] and DSM-III-R[2], various syndromes labeled atypical depression have been suggested for over 30 years to characterize patients preferentially responsive to monoamine oxidase inhibitor (MAOI) antidepressants. Prior to describing atypical depression in detail, we will review the use of the term in order to place it into its historical context. We will then present a description of the syndrome, its family history, laboratory findings, differential diagnosis, diagnostic criteria, and suggestions for treatment.

HISTORICAL CONTEXT

Early in the use of antidepressant medications, the term atypical depression was proposed to characterize depressed patients who both responded poorly to tricyclic antidepressants or electroconvulsive therapy (ECT) and benefitted from MAOIs.[3–5] While it is clear that such patients exist,[6] five separate groups have applied the term to different but probably overlapping syndromes.

English Group

West and Dally[3] and Sargant[5] described patients who were particularly responsive to treatment with the MAOI, iproniazid. Common characteristics included mood reactivity, initial insomnia, reversed diurnal variation, fatigue, somatic overreactivity, good premorbid functioning and personality, and poor response to imipramine or ECT. These patients tended not to display the classical endogenous symptoms of guilt, weight loss, or morning worsening. These investigators did not address the increased sleep and appetite reported by some subsequent groups.

Vermont Group

In the United States, Robinson and colleagues at the University of Vermont were among the first to undertake clinical trials with MAOIs, first comparing phenelzine to placebo,[7,8] then to amitriptyline.[9] These studies required that "enough depressive symptoms were present to warrant drug treatment."[9]

Post hoc, they found reactivity of mood, anxiety and the absence of terminal insomnia to characterize MAOI-responsive patients. Although there was a tendency for patients with endogenous depression to do somewhat better on imipramine, and those with nonendogenous depression to benefit more on phenelzine, these differences did not approach statistical significance.

Paykel, Rowan, and Colleagues

Paykel, Rowan, and colleagues have issued several reports from a study comparing phenelzine to amitriptyline in 131 depressed outpatients.[10–12] These investigators tested three different syndromes of atypical depression: anxiety with or without depression, reversed vegetative symptoms, and nonendogenous depression. Focusing on mildly to moderately depressed outpatients, they found only symptoms of anxiety to correlate with increased response to phenelzine relative to amitriptyline. Other definitions of typical or atypical depression did not differentiate the drugs.

Davidson and Colleagues

Davidson et al.[13] randomly assigned 81 depressed outpatients to 6 weeks' treatment with isocarboxazid or placebo. They required their patients to have significant anxiety (Covi anxiety score 8 or higher) and significant depression (baseline score of at least 20 on the 24-item version Hamilton Rating Scale for Depression) lasting at least 4 weeks.

Specific criteria for atypical depression were later identified for analysis of subgroups. These required mood reactivity and nonendogenicity by the Newcastle Scale. Patients with atypical depression were further divided into those with one or more reverse vegetative symptom (hyperphagia, weight gain, or evening worsening), referred to as "V"-type atypical depression, and those with none of these vegetative symptoms, referred to as "A"-type atypical depression. Isocarboxazid was more effective than placebo in patients with V-type atypical depression. The individual symptoms of high initial anxiety and interpersonal sensitivity also predicted isocarboxazid response.

215

Columbia Group

The group at Columbia University, including Quitkin, Klein, Liebowitz, Stewart, and McGrath, designed comparative trials to demonstrate phenelzine's superiority over tricyclic antidepressants in treating atypical depression. They developed criteria for atypical depression requiring reactivity of mood plus two or four associated features, including significant hyperphagia, hypersomnia, feelings of intense lethargy, and pathological sensitivity to interpersonal rejection.

Four reports support the validity of their definition of atypical depression, while several investigations of patients without atypical depression put the studies of atypical depression into perspective. Together, the original and replication studies plus two nonresponder studies represent four tests of the hypothesis that patients prospectively identified as having atypical depression are more likely to improve with phenelzine than imipramine. In all four studies, phenelzine was more effective than imipramine, although not always to a statistically significant degree.[6,14–17]

The composite picture from the studies of the Columbia group is that responses to imipramine in patients with atypical depression can be expected to be 48 per cent (95 per cent confidence limits 38 to 58 per cent), compared to an expected remission rate of 79 per cent (95 per cent confidence limits 59 to 92 per cent) in patients with simple mood-reactive depression, and 80 per cent (95 per cent confidence limits 68 to 92 per cent) in patients with melancholia. Because the Columbia criteria are the most clearly operationalized and best validated, together with the rest of the literature they provide a useful working description of atypical depression as identifying a depressive subgroup having decreased likelihood of response to tricyclic antidepressants.

CLINICAL DESCRIPTION OF ATYPICAL DEPRESSION

Symptomatology

The historical perspective suggests that atypical depression is characterized by mood reactivity and reversal of typical endogenous features of depression. The Columbia group has focused on hyperphagia (present in 47 per cent of Columbia's atypical patients) and hypersomnia (35 per cent), as well as intense feelings of lethargy (47 per cent), while other groups have also included initial insomnia and reversed diurnal variation. Pathological sensitivity to interpersonal rejection is frequent, being present in 71 per cent of patients with atypical depression.

Comorbid disorders frequently found with atypical depression include panic disorder, generalized social phobia, and personality disorders, particularly avoidant and dependent personalities. Because of the often chronic nature of atypical depression,

differentiation from these disorders is often difficult. For example, whether to attribute avoidance of social situations to social phobia or the rejection sensitivity often seen in atypical depression can be problematic. Similarly, chronically depressed patients often meet DSM-III-R criteria for dependent or avoidant personality disorder or both.

Longitudinal Course

Usual age of onset for atypical depression is before age 20. Patients with atypical depression tend to have a chronic, nonphasic course. Epidemiological studies have not included atypical depression as a diagnostic entity, so the true rate of atypical depression among depressives in the general population is unknown.

LABORATORY STUDIES

The Columbia group[18] found that the sleep of patients with atypical depression was largely equivalent to that of normal controls, but sharply different from the sleep of patients with melancholia who demonstrated the shortened rapid eye movement (REM) period latency and disrupted sleep generally reported in the literature. Patients with atypical depression have not shown abnormalities on tyramine excretion or dichotic listening tests.[19,20]

FAMILY HISTORY

West and Dally[3] reported a positive family history of depression in 36 per cent of their MAOI-responsive patients, but relative rate and type of disorder were not reported, and there was no comparison group, rendering interpretation problematic. Pare and Mack[21] proposed the existence of two genetically distinct types of depression: one that responds better to MAOIs, and the other with a preferential response to tricyclics. As evidence, they cited the observation that first-degree relatives often respond to the same class of antidepressant as the proband. Stewart analyzed family history data and found that patients with atypical depression have increased familial rates of chronic depression and atypical depression, while probands with melancholia or other nonatypical depression have increased rates of episodic major depression and melancholia (J.W. Stewart, unpublished data).

DIFFERENTIAL DIAGNOSIS

Major Depression and Dysthymia

The concept of atypical depression predates DSM-III and DSM-III-R, and cuts across the affective categories defined by the official nomenclature. Thus, a patient with major depression or dysthymia (or both) may or may not also have atypical depression, as defined here. Atypical depression, then, should be thought of as a modifier of a DSM-III-R category, rather than as a separate disorder.

Melancholia

Atypical depression can readily be differentiated from melancholia. Reactivity of mood and reversed vegetative symptoms such as hypersomnia and hyperphagia are hallmarks of atypical depression, while melancholia is often characterized by nonreactivity of mood and the classical endogenous symptoms of weight loss, early morning wakening, and morning worsening. Chronic interpersonal and vocational difficulties are more characteristic of atypical depression than melancholia.

Seasonal Affective Disorder

The symptomatology of seasonal affective disorder (SAD) includes the hyperphagia, hypersomnia, and feelings of intense lethargy characteristic of atypical depression.[22] However, the high likelihood of response of SAD to phototherapy may not be seen in atypical depression, suggesting these are different entities.[22,23] The pathognomonic feature of SAD is its characteristic winter worsening coupled with summer remissions year after year. Although atypical depression can present with an episodic course, this is not tied to the season.

Bipolar Disorder

Rather than differentiating bipolar disorder from atypical depression, the best integration of the available information at present appears to be to consider the presence of bipolar disorder and atypical depression separately. Independent of depressive subtype, a history of mania or hypomania suggests that lithium might be prudent prior to institution of antidepressant treatment. Conversely, presence of atypical depression symptomatology during depressions appears to confer preferential responsiveness to MAOI independent of whether a bipolar history is present.

Personality Disorders

Early onset, chronicity, and prominent interpersonal and vocational difficulties suggest that an alternative formulation for atypical depression might be as a personality disorder. Furthermore, two groups have independently reported superior response of borderline personality disorder to MAOI relative to placebo.[24,25] Clearly, the chaotic or withdrawn lives of rejection-sensitive and rejection-avoidant patients with chronic atypical depression can meet criteria for several personality disorders, including borderline and avoidant personalities. Nevertheless, personality theory probably would not have predicted improvement in personality traits with lifting of mood, as is often seen in successfully treated patients with atypical depression. Until specific pathophysiology is identified, however, differentiation of atypical depression from personality disorders depends on practical considerations. Since a diagnosis of atypical depression points the clinician toward treatment of demonstrated efficacy, we find atypical depression a more useful concept for these patients than personality disorder. Nevertheless, a practical differentiating feature is whether the personality-like pathology is present when the patient is not depressed; if present, there is probably also personality pathology present, while if absent, it is probably most expedient to assume that the difficulties in relationships or functioning are part of the depressive disorder.

Anxiety Disorders

Anxiety is prominent in patients with atypical depression, as are comorbid anxiety diagnoses. A simple rule seems to suffice: if the anxiety symptoms meet the criteria for an anxiety diagnosis, this should also be made and treated.

COLUMBIA DIAGNOSTIC CRITERIA

We present in detail the Columbia operational criteria for atypical depression. These criteria are only applied where the clinician has already determined that the patient meets criteria for a DSM-III-R depressive disorder. The time frame is the current episode or past 3 months, except for rejection sensitivity, which refers to any 2-year period since age 18. Presence of mood reactivity plus two of the four associated features are required to make the diagnosis of atypical depression.

Mood Reactivity (Required)

The essential criterion of mood reactivity is defined as the capacity to be cheered up, enjoy at least some activities, or otherwise respond pleasurably to positive events or experiences. Mood reactivity is rated as present if the patient can respond with a mood lift of at least 50 per cent toward a hypothetical 100 per cent of "normal mood." Significant lifting of the mood even once is considered evidence of retained capacity for mood reactivity.

Associated Features (Any Two Required)

Hypersomnia is defined as sleeping at least 10 hours a day at least 3 days a week for 3 months.

Hyperphagia is defined as any of: markedly excessive appetite or eating, or weight gain of at least 10 pounds in 3 months. Examples of excessive appetite or eating are binge eating at least 3 times a week, and wanting to eat nearly constantly.

Leaden Paralysis is defined as a physical feeling of heaviness, which must be present at least an hour a day for at least 3 days a week for 3 months. This is a physical feeling to be differentiated from lack of interest or motivation.

Rejection Sensitivity

Criteria require significant functional impairment to result from pathological sensitivity to interpersonal rejection. This feature is unique to the Columbia formulation of atypical depression and derives from Klein's conceptualization of hysteroid dysphoria, hypothesized to be a variant of atypical depression. The time frame for rejection sensitivity is any 2-year period of adulthood. Examples of functional impairment include stormy relationships due to feelings of rejection, frequently missing important responsibilities in direct response to rejection or criticism, and avoiding romantic relationships due to fear of rejection.

TREATMENT

Psychopharmacology

Phenelzine is clearly the best documented treatment for atypical depression, with response to imipramine more modest. Other things being equal, therefore, phenelzine should be the treatment of choice for atypical depression, reserving imipramine for intolerant or unresponsive patients. Phenelzine, however, presents frequent side effects, is poorly tolerated over long periods, and requires a special diet because of the "cheese reaction."[26,27] What about other classes of antidepressants? We are aware of only a single report addressing efficacy of medications other than tricyclic antidepressants (TCA) or MAOIs in atypical depression. Reimherr et al.[28] have reported efficacy of fluoxetine for atypical depression. We have systematically used fluoxetine to treat 85 patients with atypical depression in an open study. Forty-eight (56 per cent) remitted during 10 weeks' treatment with 20 mg/day, over half not until after 6 weeks' of treatment. Thirteen of twenty-three (57 per cent) patients who did not benefit from 20 mg/day improved over the next 4 weeks when the dose was raised to 40 to 80 mg/day suggesting an overall fluoxetine response of about 80 per cent in atypical depression. These suggestive findings require confirmation in double-blind studies, but seem convincing enough to assume fluoxetine's efficacy in atypical depression, and suggest it may be as effective as phenelzine. Despite phenelzine's proven efficacy, we prefer to start with fluoxetine because it is better tolerated than phenelzine and does not require a special diet.

Our approach is to discuss with the patient the relative likelihood of benefit versus problems of the various classes of antidepressants. We also discuss the fact that while one drug may have a better "track record" than another, treatment in reality is trial and error, and each trial must last 2 to 3 months before a decision can be made that a given medication is not working. Occasional patients prefer to ignore the potential problems of MAOIs or are frightened by the recent negative publicity surrounding fluoxetine, and we will generally comply with the patient's wishes in such cases. Usually, however, once a diagnosis of atypical depression has been made, we begin with fluoxetine, 20 mg/day.

Patients with comorbid panic disorder often become extremely anxious if they take 20 mg of fluoxetine. We therefore have them dissolve the contents of a capsule in water and take one fourth (approximately 5 mg) of it each of the first 3 days. Every 3 days, if tolerated, they increase the dose by 5 mg, until they are taking a whole capsule. Although the body gradually adjusts to this anxiety reaction, once it has occurred, it can be difficult to convince a patient to retry the offending medication. Beginning with a lower dose with gradual upward titration usually minimizes this effect, although occasional patients may require a slower titration before reaching 20 mg/day. By carefully warning the patient about this possible reaction and what can be done about it, we are usually able to convince patients to tolerate it until the body accommodates to it. Temporary low-dose benzodiazepines often help with fluoxetine-induced anxiety (e.g., lorazepam 0.5 to 1.0 mg b.i.d. or t.i.d., p.r.n.).

If there is no improvement after 6 weeks, in each successive week we raise the dose by 20 mg/day and leave the patient at 80 mg/day for 4 weeks before deciding that fluoxetine has been ineffective. Unfortunately, fluoxetine appears to take longer to work than most antidepressants; our mean time to remission on 20 mg/day is 5.5 weeks. Hence, we wait what for other antidepressants would be excessive time before raising the dose.

If fluoxetine is ineffective after this approximately 3-month trial, we would like to move on to a MAOI. One must wait 5 weeks, however, between discontinuation of fluoxetine and beginning an MAOI.[29] We utilize this time to institute a trial of a TCA or bupropion. Tricyclic antidepressants must be used more cautiously during fluoxetine withdrawal than otherwise, since the presence of fluoxetine may increase the blood levels of TCA, and fluoxetine is only eliminated from the system slowly. Therefore, if we have just discontinued fluoxetine, we will begin with imipramine 25 mg at bedtime for 3 days, increasing every 3 days by 25 mg/day if tolerated until the dose reaches 150 mg/day. If the patient is unimproved, we will then increase the dose by 50 mg/day each week until the total dose is 300 mg/day. If the patient is unchanged after a total of 6 weeks, imipramine is probably ineffective for this patient. However, if a patient has shown partial improvement, we will obtain an electrocardiogram and blood level. If the combined blood level is below 300 ng/ml, the

QRS is less than 0.10 and the patient is tolerating the drug, we will then increase the dose to 350 mg/day for 1 week, then 400 mg/day, explaining to the patient our rationale for exceeding the *Physicians' Desk Reference* (PDR) maximum recommended dose. If the patient still has not completely remitted, we will consider another antidepressant.

Our next choice is phenelzine. Again contrary to the PDR, there appears not to be the same danger in adding an MAOI to a tricyclic that there is when a tricyclic is added to an MAOI.[30] Hence, we taper imipramine over 1 week, advising the patient to taper more slowly if withdrawal symptoms appear, then immediately begin phenelzine. We carefully explain that it is dangerous to eat foods containing tyramine, or use sympathomimetic drugs and meperidine. We then start with 15 mg/day increasing every 3 days by 15 mg/day to 60 mg/day, if tolerated. If there is insufficient benefit after 2 weeks on 60 mg/day, and the patient is tolerating the drug, we then increase the dose to 75 mg/day for 1 week and then to 90 mg/day for an additional 2 weeks.

One general consideration is that we do not accept partial improvement as remission. We therefore push the dose of antidepressant medications to the maximum tolerated if full remission is not achieved, occasionally above the PDR recommended dose. A second general issue has to do with "augmenters." Particularly in patients refractory to several agents, augmentation trials with lithium or thyroid hormone might be warranted. Although the literature documents such procedures, the most convincing trials have been with severely depressed inpatients; we have not been impressed with the utility of lithium or thyroid augmentation in outpatients with atypical depression, so do not yet recommend them as a usual tool. In clearly refractory cases, we would first review the diagnosis, and perhaps obtain fresh laboratory testing, including a complete thyroid battery to be as certain as possible that another disorder had not been missed.

Psychotherapy

There is no literature on the use of psychotherapy in the treatment of atypical depression. Supportive psychotherapy seems indicated in any chronic disorder, and we find it quite useful in keeping patients in treatment until medication begins to work. What about psychotherapy as the only treatment? We have treated 46 patients with atypical depression with 16 sessions of cognitive therapy. Twenty-four remitted (52 per cent), 71 per cent of whom remained well during 1-year follow-up. While this response rate may seem modest, it is in the range of imipramine for these patients, and seems higher than the response rate we find to placebo in atypical depression (24 per cent). Psychotherapy as represented by cognitive therapy seems a reasonable first approach to the treatment of atypical depression, but because several medications are clearly often effective, psychother-

apy should be time-limited (e.g., 3 months), with the clear understanding of both patient and therapist that if *remission* has not occurred, vigorous trials of medication should be instituted at that point. While cognitive therapy appears to be helpful for occasional patients with atypical depression, we find more commonly that only once the medication has been helpful can the patient then work productively in psychotherapy. Hence, once the depression remits, we recommend a reevaluation of the patient's symptoms and behaviors and refer patients with continuing interpersonal or phobic-anxiety symptoms to a behaviorally oriented psychotherapist. Patients who are more interested in introspective understanding are referred to a psychodynamically oriented psychotherapist.

The most important point in treating patients with atypical depression is for neither the therapist nor the patient to accept the depression as necessary, but rather shift the treatment every 2 to 3 months if the first medication or psychotherapy is not working. The second point is not to accept a trial, particularly of medication as adequate, until there is clear-cut nonresponse to the maximum tolerated dose after at least a month on that dose.

REFERENCES

1. American Psychiatric Association: Diagnostic and Statistical Manual of Mental Disorders: DSM-III. Washington, DC: American Psychiatric Association Press, 1980.
2. American Psychiatric Association: Diagnostic and Statistical Manual of Mental Disorders: DSM-III-R. Washington, DC: American Psychiatric Association Press, 1987.
3. West ED, Dally PJ: Effects of iproniazid in depressive syndromes. Br Med J i:1491–1494, 1959.
4. Dally PJ, Rohde P: Comparison of antidepressant drugs in depressive illnesses. Lancet i:18–20, 1961.
5. Sargant W: Some newer drugs in the treatment of depression and their relation to other somatic treatments. Psychosomatics 1:14–17, 1960.
6. Quitkin FM, McGrath PJ, Stewart JW, et al: Atypical depression, panic attacks, and response to imipramine and phenelzine. Arch Gen Psychiatry 47:935–941, 1990.
7. Robinson DS, Nies A, Ravaris CL, et al: The monoamine oxidase inhibitor, phenelzine, in the treatment of depressive-anxiety states. Arch Gen Psychiatry 29:407–413, 1973.
8. Ravaris CL, Nies A, Robinson DS, et al: A multiple-dose, controlled study of phenelzine in depression-anxiety states. Arch Gen Psychiatry 33:347–350, 1976.
9. Ravaris CL, Robinson DS, Ives JO, et al: Phenelzine and amitriptyline in the treatment of depression. Arch Gen Psychiatry 37:1075–1080, 1980.
10. Paykel ES, Rowan PR, Rao B, et al: Atypical depression: Nosology and response to antidepressants. In Clayton P, Barrett J, eds. Treatment of Depression: Old Controversies and New Approaches. New York: Raven Press, 1983:237–251.
11. Rowan PR, Paykel ES, Parker RR: Phenelzine and amitriptyline: Effects on symptoms of neurotic depression. Br J Psychiatry 140:475–483, 1982.
12. Rowan PR, Paykel ES, Parker RR, et al: Tricyclic antidepressant and MAO inhibitor: Are there differential effects? In Youdim M, Paykel E, eds. Monoamine Oxidase Inhibitors: The State of the Art. New York: John Wiley, 1981:125–139.

13. Davidson JRT, Giller EL, Zisook S, et al: An efficacy study of isocarboxazid and placebo in depression, and its relation-ship to depressive nosology. Arch Gen Psychiatry 45:120–127, 1988.

14. Liebowitz MR, Quitkin FM, Stewart JW, et al: Antidepressant specificity in atypical depression. Arch Gen Psychiatry 45:129–137, 1988.

15. Quitkin FM, Harrison W, Stewart JW, et al: Response to phenelzine and imipramine in placebo nonresponders with atypical depression: A new application of the crossover design. Arch Gen Psychiatry 48:318–323, 1991.

16. McGrath PJ, Stewart JW, Nunes E, et al: Treatment of depression unresponsive to a tricyclic or to a monoamine oxidase inhibitor: A double-blind crossover trial. (Submitted).

17. Quitkin FM, McGrath PJ, Stewart JW et al: Phenelzine and imipramine in mood reactive depressives: Further delineation of the syndrome of atypical depression. Arch Gen Psychiatry 46:787–793, 1989.

18. Quitkin FM, Rabkin JG, Stewart JW, et al: Sleep of atypical depressives. J Affective Disord 8:61–67, 1985.

19. Harrison WM, Cooper T, Stewart J, et al: The tyramine challenge test as a trait marker for melancholia. Arch Gen Psychiatry 41:681–685, 1984.

20. Bruder GE, Quitkin FM, Stewart JW, et al: Cerebral laterality and depression: Differences in perceptual assymetry among diagnostic subtypes. J Abnorm Psychol 98:177–186, 1989.

21. Pare C, Mack J: Differentiation of two genetically specific types of depression by the response to antidepressant drugs. J Med Genet 8:306–309, 1971.

22. Rosenthal NE, Sack DA, Gillen JC, et al: Seasonal affective disorder: A description of the syndrome and preliminary findings with light therapy. Arch Gen Psychiatry 41:72–80, 1984.

23. Stewart JW, Quitkin FM, Terman M, et al: Is seasonal affective disorder a variant of atypical depression? Differential response to light therapy. Psychiatry Res 33:121–128, 1990.

24. Cowdry RW, Gardner DL: Pharmacotherapy of borderline personality disorder: Alprazolam, carbamazepine, trifluoperazine, and tranylcypromine. Arch Gen Psychiatry 45:111–119, 1988.

25. Parsons B, Quitkin FM, McGrath PJ, et al: Phenelzine, imipramine, and placebo in borderline patients meeting criteria or atypical depression. Psychopharmacol Bull 25:524–534, 1989.

26. Rabkin J, Quitkin F, Harrison W, et al: Adverse reactions to monoamine oxidase inhibitors: I. A comparative study. J Clin Psychopharmacol 4:270–278, 1984.

27. Rabkin JG, Quitkin FM, McGrath P, et al: Adverse reactions to monoamine oxidase inhibitors: II. Treatment correlates and clinical management. J Clin Psychopharmacol 5:2–9, 1985.

28. Reimherr FW, Wood DR, Byerley B, et al: Characteristics of responders to fluoxetine. Psychopharmacol Bull 20:70–72, 1984.

29. Sternbach H: Danger of MAOI therapy after fluoxetine withdrawal (letter). Lancet ii:850–851, 1988.

30. White K, Simpson GM: Combined MAOI-tricyclic antidepressant treatment: A reevaluation. J Clin Psychopharmacol 1:264–282, 1981.

35

SEASONAL MOOD DISORDERS

ALFRED J. LEWY, M.D. PH.D.

Seasonal mood disorders are episodes of depression or mania that recur annually at a specific season of the year.[1] A patient with a seasonal disorder reports a mood change that occurs at the same time of the year, essentially every year since first experienced. By far the most common and the most recognized of these disorders is winter depression. (Summer depression has been identified by at least one research group; however, it appears to be related to a different mechanism and to be much less prevalent than winter depression.) Indeed, winter depression has been referred to by some as seasonal affective disorder (SAD), as if it is the only type of seasonal mood disorder. Some researchers in this area prefer to use the terms SAD-winter type, and SAD-summer type, whereas other prefer simply to use the terms winter depression (or summer depression). The lat-ter system seems preferable because it is more descriptive.

Most seasonal mood disorders are unipolar. Episodes of mania that recur annually in an individual are not common, nor do the majority of winter depressives experience an impaired manic or hypomanic mood swing during the summer; moreover, there are no treatment studies on the summer mood of winter depressives. Although there are reports that some patients are bipolar,[2] many investigators think that most winter depressives do not experience an impairment of mood in the summer; consequently, the relative increase in energy and other summer mood changes experienced by these patients is considered to be a type of euthymia, sometimes referred to as hyperthymia.

CLINICAL CHARACTERISTICS

Although some winter depressives have most—if not all—of the signs and symptoms of depression, many patients do not. At one extreme, some patients are immobilized and are unable to go to work or even get out of bed. However, most patients report only modest decrements in their occupational and social functioning. Low self-esteem and negativism are present to some degree in all patients, but at least one study reports that these cognitive features follow, and therefore, presumably, are the result of the vegetative changes in sleep and appetite that are the hallmarks of this disorder.

Almost all winter depressives have decreased energy when depressed in the winter. In this regard, this type of depression appears to be of the retarded type, as opposed to the agitated type seen in some melancholic patients. Furthermore, most winter depressives sleep excessively and complain of difficulty getting out of bed in the morning—once again the opposite of melancholic or endogenous nonseasonal (particularly unipolar) major depressives who often report early morning awakening. Thus, the hypersomnia of winter depressives resembles the sleep patterns of atypical unipolar patients and many bipolar depressed patients. Despite the fact that many winter depressives sleep longer in the winter than in the summer, their main complaints relate to feeling fatigued.

In addition to sleep and energy, the other main features of winter depression are related to seasonal changes in appetite, weight, and food preference. Winter depressives generally have increased appetite and weight gain in the winter. Most patients return to their normal weight in the summer. However, some patients retain much of their winter weight in the summer and over the years become obese. In the winter, they have an increased preference for carbohydrate-containing food, whereas in the summer they have an increased preference for fruits and vegetables.

Although most patients manifest these "atypical features," there may be a small subgroup of winter depressives who have decreased sleep and decreased appetite when depressed in the winter. Some investigators adjust treatment depending on which set of symptoms is prominent.

PREVALENCE

Winter depression has been estimated to affect as much as 5 per cent of the North American population. If "subsyndromal" individuals are taken into account, this percentage increases fourfold. On a per capita basis, the further away from the equator, the more patients with this disorder are found. This appears to have something to do with winter day length decreasing with increasing latitude.

Women seem to be affected about four or five times more than men. At present, there is no explanation for this apparent sex different (which could possibly be an artifact due to a bias in reporting). However, many patients with winter depression complain that their late luteal phase dysphoria disorder (LLPDD) worsens in the winter and some women do not experience symptoms of premenstrual syndrome (PMS) at any other time of the year.

Although family or genetic studies have not been done, many patients report at least one family member (usually a parent or child) with a similar problem. There are two studies of children with winter depression. However, it seems that during the patient's twenties and thirties the disorder increases in severity and then plateaus for a given individual, provided that there is no change in one's geographical location. For example, some patients experience their first episode after moving to a higher latitude.

Within an episode there seems to be a typical course. In most individuals, the onset occurs well after the summer solstice. With shortening of day length, symptoms gradually worsen. The worst months for most patients are January and February. Symptoms appear to abate with the longer days of March and April. A given individual can often pin down a specific time in the fall when they can expect the onset of their depression and a specific time in the spring when it will remit.

The predictable time course of the illness has prevented some patients from seeking help for their disorder: by the time their symptoms have become sufficiently severe to motivate seeking of treatment, they are beginning to experience their spring remission. Over the years, many patients come to identify their winter mood as an expected and self-limited disorder, often shared by a close family member.

Winter depression has been confused with the "holiday blues," although it should be mentioned that winter depression also occurs in the southern hemisphere, where Christmas occurs in the summer. Although scattered reports of seasonal mood disorders have surfaced in the literature for two millennia, recognition of recurrent winter depression occurred only a decade ago following the discovery of light treatment. Exposure to light appears to be the treatment of choice for winter depression. Some details about the early history of light treatment might be instructive.

HISTORY OF LIGHT TREATMENT

The 24-hour light-dark cycle is the primary time cue for circadian rhythms. Seasonal rhythms, such as the estrus (reproductive) cycle, are primarily cued by day length as it changes throughout the year. A third type of effect of light is unique to melatonin, the hormone of the pineal gland: acute exposure to light immediately suppresses melatonin production. The effects of light are mediated via a neural pathway that extends from the retina to the suprachiasmatic nucleus (SCN) of the hypothalamus. The SCN is the site of the biological clock that times all circadian rhythms and has a role in the regulation of seasonal rhythms as well.[3]

Melatonin production undergoes both circadian and seasonal changes. Pineal production of melatonin occurs only during nighttime darkness. Levels are low during the day, and in the evening rise abruptly (the melatonin onset), falling at or before dawn. The duration and circadian phase of active production change during the year: in the winter, there is a circadian phase delay and a longer duration of melatonin production compared to the summer. These changes in melatonin production mediate seasonal rhythms in many animals. In addition, melatonin may feed-back on the SCN and participate in the regulation of circadian rhythms in some species, including humans.

Prior to 1980, scientists had concluded that humans did not have the same responses to light as did other species, including nonhuman primates. However, it turns out that humans require brighter light than ordinary room light to manifest these responses.[4] The first such evidence for these responses in humans was the demonstration of acute suppression of nighttime melatonin production by light about five times brighter than ordinary room light. Following this finding, a patient with recurrent winter depression was treated by exposure to light of this intensity in the early morning and early evening, scheduled to mimic spring day length.[5]

With the successful treatment of this first patient and a subsequent controlled study of nine patients the following year, the syndrome of winter depression or seasonal affective disorder was characterized.[2] A decade later, over a thousand patients have been studied and treated.

Light treatment continues to gain acceptance in the medical community. However, there are some areas that remain controversial at the present time. Although the following is only one viewpoint, it is shared by a large, perhaps majority, group of light therapists.

FOUR CRITICAL PARAMETERS FOR LIGHT TREATMENT

Intensity

There are four critical parameters for light treatment: intensity, wavelength, duration, and timing.

Intensity was the first parameter identified. Indeed, as discussed above, it was through the fact that bright light but not ordinary-intensity light can suppress nighttime melatonin production that light treatment was conceived. It was further demonstrated that the brighter the light, the greater the suppression of melatonin production. Light suppression of melatonin does not mean that melatonin either mediates the effects of light or is involved in the pathology of winter depression or other chronobiological disorders. However, it is assumed that light which is sufficiently intense to suppress human nighttime melatonin production will have antidepressant and other biological effects.

Intensity can be adjusted by the number and wattage of lamps in the fixture. Fixtures are also fitted with different types of reflectors that affect light output. However, perhaps the factor that most affects intensity is the distance between the subject and the light source. According to the inverse square law, intensity increases as an inverse function of the square of the distance from the light source. In other words, if a person is 3 feet from a light source and then moves 1.5 feet closer, intensity increases fourfold. Most companies that make light fixtures for light therapy calibrate them to inform the patient the distance that will provide an intensity of 2500 lux.

Although the eyes should be a certain distance from the light source and should remain open during light exposure, subjects are not instructed to stare directly at the light fixture. Two or three times a minute patients are asked to scan their eyes across the fixture for a few seconds. The fixture is positioned so that the light source is at a 45-degree angle to the patient. This can be achieved by asking patients to read if the fixture is placed straight ahead of them; thus, light is coming in from above. Alternatively, some patients watch television with the light fixture at one side.

Wavelength

Wavelength was the second parameter investigated. The peak wavelength for suppression of melatonin production is in the blue-green range, around 509 nm, which turns out to be the peak for the scotopic (nighttime) sensitivity curve. This wavelength is also where rhodopsin and rods are most sensitive (animal studies also show increased sensitivity for melatonin suppression at this wavelength). Once again it should be mentioned that melatonin suppression presumably indicates what will be biologically effective light and does not necessarily implicate melatonin or melatonin suppression pathologically or therapeutically. Although of scientific interest, the fact that 509 nm is found in all white light sources means that it is not of practical significance. However, it is theoretically possible that light of this wavelength would be effective at a lower intensity than white light.

Regarding safety, lamps that emit heat or infrared radiation, such as heat lamps, should not be used for bright-light treatment. To some extent, incandescent lamps also emit heat at high intensities and at close distances, and many practitioners discourage their use as well. There is some confusion in the field about lamps that emit ultraviolet (UV) light. Clearly, the eyes should be protected from exposure from sun-tanning lamps, and these lamps are not to be used for light treatment, which requires the eyes to be open. So-called full-spectrum lamps were used in the initial studies of light therapy. However, the modest amount of UV light in these lamps (which decreases with use and is removed by most plexiglass diffusers) does not appear to be necessary for light treatment. Most practitioners find that ordinary fluorescent light is just as effective as full-spectrum fluorescent light. The most conservative approach is to avoid the use of full-spectrum light except in a few select cases in which patients do not seem to respond to any other type of fluorescent light. Although the low amount of UV light emitted by full-spectrum sources is probably not more than encountered outdoors, since chronic UV light exposure has been linked to eventual cataract formation, the use of ordinary-fluorescent lamps (such as cool-white) is preferable. Certainly, aphakic patients should not be exposed to UV-emitting lamps, since the retina will be rendered susceptible to damage from UV light without the lens to absorb UV light.

Duration

A third critical parameter is duration. The longer the exposure duration, the greater the effect. To a degree, there is probably a linear relationship between intensity and duration, in that as one of these variables increases, the other variable can be decreased. For example, if two hours of 2500 lux is effective, 30 minutes of 10,000 lux should be equally effective. As indicated above, 10,000 lux can be achieved by halving the recommended distance from the light source calibrated for 2500 lux exposure.

As the intensity increases, one is increasingly concerned about ocular toxicity. Ophthalmological evaluations have so far not revealed any untoward retinal changes following bright light exposure of 2500 to 10,000 lux. It has been argued that outdoor light, even on a cloudy day, is brighter than 10,000 lux. However, the geometry of exposure from artificial light sources is different. Consequently, it is not recommended that patients with any history or evidence of eye disease be treated with bright light, unless approved by an ophthalmologist. Patients are also asked to report any untoward side effects while undergoing light treatment, even though these are unlikely.

Timing

The fourth parameter for light treatment is timing, or time of day of exposure. One of the first theories for the mechanism of action of light therapy was the "photon counting hypothesis for SAD." According to this theory, timing is not critical—only duration and intensity.[6] That is, light is antidepressant because of exposure to a critical number of photons.

A more recent theory, the "phase-shift hypothesis," argues that timing of light exposure is critical for its antidepressant effects in winter depression and other chronobiological disorders as well. Ac-

cording to this hypothesis, there are two types of chronobiological disorders, the phase-advance type and the phase-delay type. Most, if not all, winter depressives have been hypothesized to be of the phase-delay type.[7,8] This is suggested clinically by their morning hypersomnia. Recent studies have provided evidence for phase-delayed circadian rhythms in this group of patients compared to normal controls. Although it is not certain if a larger sample size will continue to support this difference, patients will nevertheless probably be shown to be delayed when depressed in the winter compared to when they are treated with bright light or when they are well in the summer; in this case, the phase-delay disturbance would be ipsative, if not normative.

Although the phase-shift hypothesis may not completely explain why winter depressives become depressed, it does explain why the depression occurs in the winter. Most humans cue to dawn rather than to dusk. With the later dawn in the winter, circadian rhythms delay and thus the circadian phase delay is exacerbated in winter depressives. Winter depression, therefore, may be seasonal in its annual recurrence; however, its underlying mechanism may be related to another (although related) type of biological rhythm—circadian rhythms.

The phase-shift hypothesis also explains why morning light is more antidepressant than light scheduled at other times of the day.[7-10] Bright light exposure when scheduled in the morning will most effectively produce a circadian phase advance (thus correcting a phase delay). Indeed, many patients relapse when switched to evening light sufficiently late in the evening, presumably because of the induced phase delay. Most, but not all studies, support the superiority of morning light including an analysis of pooled data across research centers. This issue is not completely resolved, however, because of the possibilities of (1) a circadian rhythm in light sensitivity that might be affected by prior light exposure, (2) order effects in the crossover studies, and (3) placebo effects in the parallel-design studies.

Nonetheless, the phase-shift hypothesis is considered the leading explanation for light's antidepressant mechanism of action in winter depression, as well as in other more clearly chronobiological disorders, such as advanced and delayed sleep syndrome, and difficulties associated with transmeridianal air travel ("jet lag") and adaptation to shift work. Indeed, there is no controversy regarding the fact that bright light scheduled in the morning advanced circadian rhythms (shifts them to an earlier time) and that bright light in the evening delays circadian rhythms (shifts them to a later time). A more recent hypothesis suggests that bright light is antidepressant because it increases an abnormally low circadian amplitude. This hypothesis is too new to be assessed at the present time and is actually not mutually exclusive with the phase-shift hypothesis.

Tests of the phase-shift hypothesis have determined the importance of the phase relationship between sleep (or the sleep-wake cycle) and the other circadian rhythms. When treating winter depression, sleep time is held constant. Thus, morning light advances the other circadian rhythms not only with respect to real time but also with respect to sleep. This difference reduces what may be an abnormally wide phase angle between sleep and the other circadian rhythms. Preliminary tests have shown that delaying sleep time is also an effective antidepressant in winter depressives.[11]

PRACTICAL GUIDELINES FOR LIGHT TREATMENT

Based on research concerning the four critical parameters for chronobiologically effective light, practical guidelines can be written for optimizing light treatment of winter depression.[12] Since most, if not all, patients seem to be of the phase-delay type, patients should be initially treated with 2 hours of 2500 lux scheduled immediately upon awakening. Normally, an antidepressant response can be observed within 3 to 4 days and is complete within 1 to 2 weeks. If, however, patients have to get up early to accommodate this light exposure schedule, the antidepressant response may take a few days longer (some practitioners begin light treatment on a weekend to minimize the initial advance in sleep time). Patients are also asked to avoid bright light exposure in the evening (from shopping malls, for example), which might counteract the effect of morning light.

Once a complete response has been achieved, patients frequently decrease the exposure duration, often to as little as 30 minutes. Sometimes, exposures every other day are sufficient. Treatment should continue throughout the winter, however, as relapse occurs within 3 to 4 days if it is discontinued. Should this occur, the antidepressant response can easily be obtained following reinstatement of light therapy.

Occasionally, following morning light exposure some patients complain of severe fatigue in the evening and early morning awakening. These patients may be becoming overly phase advanced. In this case, the duration or intensity of morning light should be reduced. If not scheduled too late so as to produce a phase delay, an additional exposure period in the evening will increase the energy of some patients. However, this is considered to be a placebo effect until proven otherwise.

A few patients appear to respond better to evening light than to morning light. For these individuals, we recommend exposure between 7 and 9 P.M. These patients should avoid bright light exposure in the morning and should not delay their sleep time.

NONCHRONOBIOLOGICAL TREATMENTS

In addition to scheduling bright light exposure and sleep time, winter depression has been treated with standard types of pharmacotherapy and psychotherapy. When successful, these treatments are considered to provide only symptomatic relief, although psychotherapy may be a useful adjunctive treatment for the low self-esteem and social losses that might accompany a history of untreated winter depression. Currently, research is underway to determine if a specific type of antidepressant (e.g., serotonergic) is as effective as light treatment.

NONAFFECTIVE CHRONOBIOLOGICAL DISORDERS

When treating nonaffective chronobiological disorders such as advanced and delayed sleep-phase syndrome, jet lag, and shift work maladaptation, sleep is allowed to shift to the desired time, after which it is held constant. The treatment of advanced and delayed sleep-phase syndromes is relatively straightforward. Advanced sleep-phase syndrome is characterized by early morning awakening and early evening fatigue. These people respond to bright light scheduled in the evening just before bedtime. Over several days, bedtime can be scheduled later and later until the desired time is achieved.

Patients with delayed sleep-phase syndrome have difficulty falling asleep at night and arising in the morning. Patients with this syndrome respond to bright light scheduled in the morning, as soon as they awaken. It is advisable to let them decide for themselves how quickly they should advance their time of awakening: arising 15 minutes earlier every other day often works well. These patients should be reassured that they will be able to fall asleep earlier—provided that they use the morning light. Although bright light helps these individuals advance their sleep-wake cycles, they must be motivated to adhere to the treatment regimen. In many cases, the delayed sleep-wake cycle is overdetermined; that is, there may be several reasons why they might prefer their delayed schedule.

In treating jet lag, appropriate exposure to bright light can be achieved by scheduling time spent outdoors, taking advantage of the fact that daylight is chronobiologically active, whereas indoor light is less so. When traveling through six or fewer time zones to the west, travelers are encouraged to be outdoors for an hour or two before dusk. When traveling through six or fewer time zones to the east, they are advised to be outdoors for an hour or two after dawn. This should be done for the first few days after arriving at the new destination. When traveling through more than six time zones, travelers should obtain outdoor light in the middle of the day and avoid it in late afternoon and early evening when traveling west or in the morning when traveling east. This is because bright light might shift the body clock in the opposite direction when exposure occurs at the "wrong" time of the day.

OUTDOOR VERSUS INDOOR LIGHT

The question sometimes arises, is indoor light chronobiologically active? Most indoor light intensities are so low relative to outdoor light that they are relatively ineffective. Occasionally, sunlight directly streaming through a window might be very bright, but people are always cautioned about looking directly at the sun, which is harmful to the eyes. Under most circumstances, windows act like point sources for the inverse square. That is, the closer to the window, the greater the light intensity (as the distance to the window is halved, the intensity increases by a factor of four). Therefore, at a distance of about 1 inch from a window, indirect sunlight may sometimes be sufficiently intense, but this is obviously an impractical method for light treatment.

Outdoor daylight is almost always sufficiently intense for light treatment. Once again, patients should be instructed never to look directly at the sun. Even the light on cloudy days is usually of adequate intensity for light treatment. Cloud cover around twilight might reduce light intensity to an ineffective level, and of course twilight is not sufficiently intense.

THE QUESTION OF NONSEASONAL DEPRESSION

Treatment of nonseasonal depression is controversial at the present time. Clearly, if there is a chronobiological component, bright light is indicated, at least as an adjunctive treatment. For example, bright light in the evening will usually ameliorate early morning awakening. Beneficial effects on other aspects of the depressive episode are variable.

THE QUESTION OF SUMMER DEPRESSION

Treatment of summer depression is not related to the light-dark cycle and therefore probably represents a very different type of seasonal mood disorder. Summer depressives appear to respond to a cool, dry environment, such as achieved with air conditioning.

THE ROLE OF MELATONIN

Until very recently, the role of melatonin has been conservatively assessed: it is a useful marker for the phase of the human biological clock. Perhaps it will be used clinically to distinguish phase-delayed patients from phase-advanced patients, although currently assessment of sleep time has by and large been able to accomplish this. The question arises, does melatonin participate in the pathology of chronobiological disorders and the response to light treatment? The role of melatonin is unknown in humans, although in animals it is involved in the regulation of many seasonal rhythms and may participate in the regulation of the circadian timing system as well.

Seasonal rhythms have not been well documented in humans. Indeed, winter depression is now thought to be related more to circadian rhythms, which are clearly very important in humans. Therefore, it would not be surprising if melatonin functioned as part of the human circadian timing system. As a matter of fact, melatonin receptors have recently been identified in the human SCN.

We have found that orally-administered melatonin can shift the human biological clock.[13] Similar to light, the time of day of melatonin administration is critical. However, melatonin acts opposite to light. That is, melatonin administration in the morning causes a phase delay, whereas melatonin administration in the afternoon causes a phase advance. These findings suggest a functional role for melatonin in the human circadian system. These findings also suggest that melatonin may be used in the future to treat chronobiological disorders.

REFERENCES

1. Blehar MC, Lewy AJ: Seasonal mood disorders: Consensus and controversy. Psychopharmacol Bull 26:465–494, 1990.
2. Rosenthal NE, Sack DA, Gillin JC, et al: Seasonal affective disorder. Arch Gen Psychiatry 41:72–80, 1984.
3. Lewy AJ: Biochemistry and regulation of mammalian melatonin production. In Relkin RM, ed. The Pineal Gland. New York: Elsevier Biomedical, 1983:77–128.
4. Lewy AJ, Wehr TA, Goodwin FK, et al: Light suppresses melatonin secretion in humans. Science 210:1267–1269, 1980.
5. Lewy AJ, Kern HE, Rosenthal NE, Wehr TA: Bright artificial light treatment of a manic-depressive patient with a seasonal mood cycle. Am J Psychiatry 139:1496–1498, 1982.
6. Lewy AJ, Sack RL: Minireview: Light therapy and psychiatry. Proc Soc Exp Biol Med 183:11–18, 1986.
7. Avery DH, Khan A, Dager SR, et al: Morning or evening bright light treatment of winter depression? The significance of hypersomnia. Biol Psychiatry 29:117–126, 1991.
8. Lewy AJ, Sack RL, Miller LS, Hoban TM: Antidepressant and circadian phase-shifting effects of light. Science 235:352–354, 1987.
9. Sack RL, Lewy AJ, White DM, et al: Morning versus evening light treatment for winter depression. Evidence that the therapeutic effects of light are mediated by circadian phase shifts. Arch Gen Psychiatry 473:343–351, 1990.
10. Terman M, Terman JS, Quitkin FM, et al: Light therapy for seasonal affective disorder. A review of efficacy. Neuropsychopharmacology 2:1–22, 1989.
11. Lewy AJ, Sach RL, Singer CM, et al: Winter depression and the phase-shift hypothesis for bright light's therapeutic effects: History, theory and experimental evidence. In Rosenthal NE, Blehar MC, eds. Seasonal Affective Disorders and Phototherapy. New York: Guilford Press, 1989:295–310.
12. Lewy AJ: Treating chronobiologic sleep and mood disorders with bright light. Psychiatr Ann 17:664–669, 1987.
13. Lewy AJ, Sack RL, Latham JM: Melatonin and the acute suppressant effect of light may help regulate circadian rhythms in humans. In Arendt J, Pevet P, eds. Advances in Pineal Research: 5. London: John Libbey & Co. Ltd, 1991:285–293.

36

RAPID CYCLING

SUSAN L. McELROY, M.D. and PAUL E. KECK, Jr., M.D.

Although the recurrent nature of mood disorder has been well recognized since Kraepelin's original description of manic-depressive insanity in the early 1900s, it was not until 1974 that the phenomenon of rapid cycling was clearly defined by Dunner and Fieve.[1–6] In an attempt to identify factors associated with the failure of lithium prophylaxis in patients with bipolar disorder, Dunner and Fieve found that poor outcome was primarily associated with an increased frequency of affective episodes prior to treatment.[1] Patients experiencing four or more affective episodes per year, in particular, were disproportionately represented in the prophylaxis-failure group. Dunner and Fieve coined the term rapid cycling to describe these patients. Of 55 bipolar patients studied, 9 of 11 (82 per cent) rapid cyclers failed lithium prophylaxis compared with 18 of 44 (41 per cent) non–rapid cyclers. Since then, rapid cycling has been defined in a variety of other ways, including as a continuous circular course of affective episodes with short cycles (hypomanic or manic episodes alternating with depressive episodes with at least two cycles per year),[7] and as "chronicization" of the illness (the presence of rapidly alternating, unremitting symptoms).[8] The most widely accepted operational definition of rapid cycling, however, remains the occurrence of four or more mood episodes per year.

Rapid cycling is an important clinical phenomenon for several reasons. First, it is associated with a high degree of morbidity and perhaps an increased risk of suicide. Fawcett and colleagues,[9] for instance, found that mood cycling within an episode was associated with suicide in patients with major mood disorders. Second, rapid cycling is very difficult to treat. Not only do afflicted patients respond poorly to lithium, but evidence suggests that other standard treatments for bipolar disorder, in particular antidepressants and antipsychotics, may actually induce or exacerbate cycling.[3,4,6,7] Third, rapid cycling presents in a variety of ways and thus may go unrecognized or misdiagnosed. Fourth, as reviewed below, the disorder may be more prevalent than is currently recognized.

CLINICAL CHARACTERISTICS

Rapid cycling is presumed to be rare, with prevalence estimates ranging from 13 to 20 per cent of bipolar patients.[1–7,9–14] Some investigators have argued that these rates probably overestimate the true prevalence of the disorder, since they are derived from tertiary referral centers, which presumably attract higher proportions of treatment-resistant patients.[15] However, it could also be argued that rapid cycling may be underdiagnosed. Patients may not report hypomanic episodes, or their rapid mood shifts may be unrecognized or misdiagnosed. Moreover, recent data suggest that the prevalence of rapid cycling may be increasing.[10]

Although reported in patients with recurrent major depression and schizoaffective disorder, rapid cycling appears to be most frequent among patients with bipolar disorder.[2,12] In a follow-up of their original study, Dunner and colleagues[2] found that 40 of 307 (13 per cent) bipolar patients but none of 84 patients with major depression were rapid cyclers. Wehr and colleagues[12] similarly found that all (100 per cent) of 51 patients with rapid cycling affective disorder had bipolar disorder. Kukopulous and colleagues[10] concluded that unipolar rapid cyclers were rare and "probably only apparently unipolar."

Most studies[1–7,10–14] report that rapid cycling is more common among females than males, with proportions of females ranging from 70[2] to 92 per cent.[12] Beyond differences in episode frequency, resistance to lithium prophylaxis, and female preponderance, rapid cyclers appear similar to non–rapid cyclers with respect to a variety of other features. These include the incidence of psychotic symptoms during mania, rates of bipolar I versus bipolar II disorder, age of onset, frequency of life events prior to illness onset, duration of illness, variability in the course of illness, and family history of mood disorder.[2,3] Rapid cyclers therefore experience manic, depressive, and mixed states similar to those occurring in patients with slower cycles.[2,4] Most studies report that approximately one half of rapid cyclers exhibit bipolar I disorder, with full manic episodes alternating with major depressive episodes, and the other half exhibit bipolar II disorder, with hypomanic episodes alternating with major depressive episodes.[2,10,11,16] However, Kukopulos and colleagues[7] reported that 71 of 87 (82 per cent) rapid-cycling bipolar patients displayed hypomanic but not manic episodes.

The onset of the first affective episode typically occurs in the late teens through the third decade of life, with reported mean ages of onset ranging from 19 to 40 years.[2,10] Unlike bipolar patients in general, the majority of rapid cyclers (79 to 98 per cent) begin their illness with a depressive episode.[7,12] Additionally, many patients display subclinical mood swings or symptoms prior to the onset of full affective episodes. Kukopulous and associates[10] found that of 118 rapid cyclers, the majority [104 (88 per cent)] displayed a cyclothymic or hyperthymic premorbid temperament. Six (5 per cent) patients had a dysthymic temperament, and only eight patients (7 per cent) were considered "normothymic."

The onset of rapid cycling relative to the onset of illness is variable. Although a substantial number of patients (23 to 37 per cent) exhibit rapid cycling at the onset of illness, the majority (63 to 77 per cent) appear to develop rapid cycling some time after the onset of their mood disorder—sometimes heralded by increased intensity of hypomanic episodes or the occurrence of postdepression hypomania.[7,12] Based on these data, Alarcon[4] has proposed classifying rapid cyclers into those with early or late onset. In the late-onset group, the appearance of rapid cycling is sometimes apparently spontaneous, and thus, presumably a reflection of the natural course of the illness and underlying pathophysiological mechanisms such as progressive limbic kindling or sensitization.[6] In other patients, the onset of rapid cycling may be associated with a variety of pharmacological and nonpharmacological factors, especially treatment with antidepressants (discussed in detail later in this chapter).[3,4,7,12]

The classic course of rapid-cycling bipolar disorder is of increasing frequency and severity of affective episodes over time. Most patients display a circular course, with manic or hypomanic periods alternating with depressions. However, a wide variety of patterns have been reported, including patients who exhibit non–rapid-cycling phases and spontaneous remissions. A wide range of episode frequencies have also been reported with some patients experiencing 20 to 50 episodes per year or episodes so frequent that they cannot be reliably counted.[13,14] In extreme forms, patients may display continuous cycling without interepisodic euthymic periods, or ultrafast rapid cycling—the experience of full manic and depressive syndromes within 48- or even 24-hour intervals.[14,16] It is currently unclear whether continual or ultrafast rapid cycling are substantially different from "classic" rapid cycling (with cycles lasting weeks to months), or whether they represent ends of a clinical spectrum. In a review comparing eight ultrafast rapid cyclers with 29 classic cyclers, Alarcon[4] noted that the ultrafast patients were more likely to be older, male, and to begin rapid cycling at the onset of their mood disorders.

The relationship of rapid cycling—particularly ultrafast rapid cycling—to mixed mood states or dysphoric mania is also currently unclear. This ambiguity is embedded, in part, in the DSM-III-R definition of a mixed episode as "the full symptomatic picture of both manic and major depressive episodes intermixed or rapidly alternating every few days." Thus, mixed states are currently defined by the simultaneous occurrence of manic and depressive syndromes as well as by rapid fluctuations in mood. It is conceivable that rapid cyclers might be more likely to experience dysphoric mania, either as a transitional state between mania or depression, as an extremely severe form of rapid cycling, or as an advanced form of the illness. Both rapid cycling and dysphoric mania share an increased prevalence among females, poorer response to lithium, possible induction by antidepressants, and better response to antiepileptics.[6,17] However, in a study comparing 22 patients with dysphoric mania with 26 patients with nondysphoric mania, Post and colleagues[17] found that dysphoric manics displayed less rapid cycling both in the year before and during the index episode. Patients with more rapid cycles showed significantly less dysphoria, psychosis, and anxiety compared to those with slower cycles. Post and colleagues therefore concluded that dysphoric mania was associated with less rather than more rapid cycling.

In short, the relationship between mixed states and rapid cycling remains unclear. For practical purposes, however, mixed states (including dysphoric mania) may occur in some rapid cyclers, and the presence of rapid cycling should be evaluated in any patient who presents with a mixed state.

ASSOCIATED CONDITIONS

Although its etiology is unknown, rapid cycling is associated with a variety of factors. These include female sex; bipolar I and II mood disorder more so than recurrent major depression; hormonal factors (especially overt or subclinical hypothyroidism); the menstrual cycle, postpartum period, and menopause in women; mental retardation, head trauma, stroke, multiple sclerosis, and other neurological insults or abnormalities; and exposure to pharmacological agents, especially antidepressants.[3,4,6,7] Several studies, for instance, found increased rates of overt hypothyroidism (ranging from 23 to 50 per cent) in rapid-cycling bipolar patients compared with unselected bipolar patients (ranging from 4 to 15 per cent), even when increased preponderance of females and treatment with lithium (a known antithyroid agent) are controlled for.[14] However, most rapid cyclers do not display serum thyroxine (T_4) deficiencies. Bauer and coworkers[14] have thus hypothesized that these patients may exhibit relative thyroid hormone deficiencies primarily within the central nervous system (CNS).

Of the pharmacological agents associated with the induction of rapid cycling, tricyclic antidepressants are most frequently reported. Most other antidepressants, however, have been implicated, including tetracyclics, monoamine oxidase inhibitors (MAOIs), mianserin, nomifensine, serotonergic agents, and lithium.[3,4,7] The authors have also observed exacerbation of rapid cycling coincident with use of fluoxetine, bupropion, and buspirone. Additionally, electroconvulsive therapy (ECT), tricyclic withdrawal, dopamine agonists (L-dopa, piribedil), cyproheptadine, and conjugated estrogens have also been reported to induce rapid cycling.[3,6] The precise frequency of antidepressant-induced rapid cycling is unknown, with rates ranging from 41 to 60 per cent of antidepressant-treated bipolar patients.[7,10,12] At present, it is impossible to predict which bipolar patients will be converted to rapid cyclers with antidepressant treatment. Indeed, some investigators are skeptical about whether or not antidepressants can truly induce rapid cycling. However, Wehr and Goodwin's prospective double-blind, placebo-controlled studies[6,12,15] demonstrating reversible induction of rapid cycling in response to antidepressant treatment in bipolar patients and the apparent historical increase in the prevalence of rapid cycling coincident with the advent of antidepressant agents further support the ability of these agents to induce rapid cycling.

A variety of psychiatric conditions have been reported to occur with increased frequency in patients with rapid cycling. These include panic disorder, alcohol and substance abuse, eating disorders, and premenstrual syndrome.[13] In some patients, these conditions appear to be "state dependent," as treatment resulting in stabilization of mood also results in amelioration of the comorbid condition.[13]

FAMILY HISTORY

Two studies have examined the family histories of rapid-cycling probands.[2,11] Although both studies found increased rates of bipolar disorder, most of the affected family members were not themselves rapid cyclers. In other words, rapid cycling did not "breed true." These studies support the hypothesis that rapid cycling is a variant or subtype of bipolar disorder rather than a separate illness.

BIOLOGICAL TESTS

Few studies of biological markers potentially associated with rapid cycling have been performed to date. Extensively reviewed by Goodwin and Jamison,[6] these studies have generally attempted to assess state-dependent changes in cerebrospinal fluid

(CSF), plasma, and urinary catecholamine and other [e.g., gamma-aminobutyric acid (GABA)] metabolites, and in hormones of the hypothalamic-pituitary-adrenal axis. These studies are limited by small sample sizes, increasing the risk of type-II error. In recent studies, Joyce and colleagues[18] studied daytime plasma cortisol fluctuations longitudinally across a variety of mood states in four rapid cycling patients. Cortisol elevations occurred during depressive episodes and peaked just prior to the emergence of each episode. Cortisol levels were lower but more variable in mania. Patients in this study were also receiving thymoleptic agents which may have exerted effects on cortisol secretion. Joyce's group[19] also studied the prolactin response to metoclopramide in 20 patients with mood disorders (including eight rapid cyclers) receiving maintenance thymoleptics. Female rapid-cycling patients exhibited a greater prolactin surge than non–rapid cyclers, which the authors interpreted as supporting a role for altered dopamine neurotransmission in the switch process. In a third study, Sack and colleagues[20] compared baseline and sleep-derived thyroid stimulating hormone (TSH) and cortisol levels in eight rapid-cycling bipolar patients and eight normal control subjects. Compared to controls, rapid cyclers exhibited an absent nocturnal rise in TSH, and sleep deprivation did not produce the expected increase in TSH levels. Investigating the possible relationship between rapid cycling and CNS electrophysiological abnormalities, Levy and coworkers[21] performed electroencephalograms (EEGs) in five rapid-cycling patients and 25 patients with non–rapid-cycling mood disorders. Three of the five rapid-cycling patients displayed bitemporal paroxysmal sharp waves, whereas none of the control patients had abnormal EEGs. The three rapid cyclers with paroxysmal EEG findings, however, did not manifest behavioral evidence of epilepsy.

In summary, although it appears that rapid-cycling bipolar patients frequently have neuroendocrine abnormalities, no consistent abnormality (except for hypothyroidism in a subgroup of rapid cyclers) has yet been found that differentiates rapid cyclers from other bipolar patients, and data bearing on the pathophysiology of rapid cycling remain sparse. This remains an important area of study because a greater understanding of the biological basis of rapid cycling might also shed light on the pathophysiology of bipolar disorder in general.

DIFFERENTIAL DIAGNOSIS

A variety of conditions may be characterized by affective lability of rapid mood shifts and, thus, may resemble rapid cycling and be included in its differential diagnosis. These include cyclothymia, personality disorder, alcohol or psychoactive substance abuse, premenstrual mood changes or late luteal phase dysphoric disorder, and temporal lobe epilepsy.

STUDIES OF SOMATIC TREATMENT OF RAPID CYCLERS

There are no double-blind, placebo-controlled treatment studies of a cohort of patients with rapid-cycling bipolar disorder. However, a small body of controlled data as well as a growing amount of open data suggest that a variety of treatments—in particular lithium, antiepileptics, thyroid augmentation, and bupropion alone or in combination—may be at least partially effective in some patients.

Although many rapid cyclers do not respond adequately to lithium prophylaxis, and individuals in whom rapid cycling appeared to be precipitated or exacerbated by lithium treatment have been reported, a substantial number of patients may show some degree of response to this agent.[2–4,7,16] However, improvement may sometimes be evident only when the patient is observed over extended periods of time or when concomitantly administered antidepressants are discontinued. Dunner and Fieve,[2] for instance, reported that of 29 rapid-cycling patients treated with lithium for at least 1 year, all displayed a greater percentage of time euthymic in their last year of lithium treatment compared with their pre-lithium baseline. The increased time well was due to a decrease in the percentage of time spent hypomanic or depressed. Kukopulos and colleagues[7] reported that 15 of 21 (72 per cent) rapid cyclers receiving lithium prophylaxis who were persuaded to avoid antidepressant treatment when depressed displayed complete mood stabilization. Thus, although many rapid cyclers may not respond to lithium, a substantial number may demonstrate some degrees of response, especially when lithium is administered alone over extended periods of time.

Growing evidence suggests that antiepileptic drugs, in particular carbamazepine and valproate, may be effective in some rapid-cycling bipolar patients, including those who have responded inadequately to lithium.[5] Indeed, rapid cycling may be associated with a favorable response to carbamazepine or valproate. In a double-blind, placebo-controlled study of carbamazepine in 19 acutely manic patients, Post and colleagues[22] found that a history of rapid cycling was associated with a favorable acute antimanic response. However, Wehr and colleagues[12] reported that only 2 of 27 (7 per cent) lithium-resistant rapid cyclers responded to open-label carbamazepine—often administered in conjunction with lithium or other drugs (e.g., tranylcypromine and thioridazine).

In a review of the efficacy of valproate in 37 acutely manic bipolar patients, all five rapid cyclers responded favorably, compared to 19 of 32 (59 per cent) slow cyclers.[23] In a follow-up study, six consecutive rapid cyclers (including the five in the original report) displayed responses to valproate over extended periods of time—ranging from 3 to 25 months. Two patients received valproate alone, one required supplemental haloperidol during hypomanic periods, two required concomitant lithium, and one required concomitant lithium and neuroleptic. Of note, five patients had failed previous treatment with carbamazepine. More recently, Calabrese and Delucchi[13] reported an open-label, prospective, 7.8-month study of the acute and prophylactic efficacy of valproate in manic, depressed, and mixed episodes in 55 patients with rapid-cycling bipolar disorder. Twenty (36 per cent) patients received valproate monotherapy and 35 (64 per cent) received valproate in combination with other agents, including lithium, antidepressants, and carbamazepine. Thirty-five (64 per cent) patients were resistant to treatment with lithium or carbamazepine. Nevertheless, valproate appeared particularly effective in the acute and long-term treatment of manic and mixed states, but was less effective in the acute and long-term treatment of depression. Specifically, 31 of 34 (91 per cent) and 48 of 51 (94 per cent) patients displayed a moderate or marked acute and prophylactic antimanic response, respectively; and 12 of 14 (86 per cent) and 13 of 14 (93 per cent) patients displayed an acute and prophylactic anti–mixed-state response, respectively. By contrast, 16 of 41 (47 per cent) and 39 of 51 (77 per cent) patients, respectively, displayed an acute and prophylactic antidepressant response.

In a recently completed double-blind, placebo-controlled 21-day trial of valproate in bipolar patients with acute mania, valproate proved superior to placebo in reducing manic symptoms and improving overall level of psychiatric function. However, when the 12 responders were compared to the five nonresponders, the presence of rapid cycling was not correlated with valproate response.[24] Thus, although accumulating evidence suggests that valproate may be effective in rapid cyclers, including those resistant to lithium or carbamazepine, it is unclear whether rapid cyclers are more likely to respond to valproate compared to non–rapid cyclers.

Finally, there are case reports describing the use of other antiepileptics, in particular clonazepam and phenytoin, in the treatment of rapid cyclers.[5] Of two patients receiving clonazepam, both displayed some degree of response. One patient receiving phenytoin under double-blind, placebo-controlled conditions, however, did not respond.

A number of case reports and open studies suggest that thyroid hormone treatment may exert mood stabilizing effects in some rapid-cycling bipolar patients—regardless of the patient's thyroid state.[25,26] Both levothyroxine (T$_4$) and triiodothyronine (T$_3$) have been used successfully, usually in conjunction with standard mood stabilizers or antidepressants (especially lithium, carbamazepine, and tricyclics.) Although doses standard for replacement therapy in hypothyroidism (e.g., 150 to 200 μg/day for T$_4$ and

25 to 50 μg/day for T_3) are sometimes reported effective, many patients responded only when supratherapeutic or hypermetabolic doses (e.g., 300 to 500 μg/day of T_4) were administered. Stancer and Persad[25] reported that five of eight (63 per cent) patients with rapid-cycling bipolar disorder displayed complete or near complete remission for periods of 1.5 to 9 years when treated with hypermetabolic doses of T_4 or T_3. Two other patients displayed partial remissions. Of the five complete responders, three required no other psychotropics, one required concomitant neuroleptic, and another received concomitant phenytoin. More recently, Bauer and Whybrow[26] reported that 10 of 11 (92 per cent) rapid cyclers refractory to standard regimens (typically combinations of lithium, carbamazepine, and replacement doses of T_4) displayed reduced depressive symptoms in response to the addition of hypermetabolic doses of open-label T_4 (150 to 400 mg/day) to their standard regimens. Five of the seven (71 per cent) patients with manic symptoms displayed an antimanic response. Treatment response was not dependent on baseline thyroid status, and in nine of the ten responders, supranormal serum concentrations of T_4 were necessary to induce response.

There are very few systematic studies of antidepressants in rapid cyclers. Indeed, as reviewed above, these agents may induce or exacerbate rapid cycling. Thus, discontinuation of antidepressants has been reported to sometimes result in cessation of rapid cycling. Wehr and colleagues[12] reported that 12 of 42 (29 per cent) patients ceased to cycle rapidly when antidepressants or neuroleptics or both were discontinued. However, rapid cyclers often require treatment of their depressions. It is therefore noteworthy that small open series of patients treated with the antidepressants clorgyline,[27] a selective MAO-A inhibitor, and bupropion,[28] a novel antidepressant with an unknown mechanism of action, suggest that these drugs may have mood stabilizing effects in rapid cyclers when administered alone or in conjunction with lithium or thyroid hormone. Haykal and Akiskal[28] described six patients with rapid-cycling bipolar II disorder resistant to treatment with various combinations of lithium, carbamazepine, thyroid supplementation, intermittent low-dose MAOIs, and treatment with or withdrawal from tricyclics, who demonstrated sustained alleviation of depression without induction of hypomania or mania when bupropion (300 to 450 mg/day) was added to regimens of lithium, T_4 (nonhypermetabolic doses), or combined lithium and T_4. We have observed that small or subtherapeutic doses of standard antidepressants or light therapy given in conjunction with mood stabilizers, sometimes only during depressed phases, may be effective in treating depression without the induction of cycling.

A variety of other somatic treatments have been reported effective in rapid cycling in case reports or small case series. These include calcium channel blockers (e.g., verapamil), estrogen replacement, electroconvulsive therapy (ECT), and sleep deprivation.[3,4,7]

To our knowledge, there are no systematic studies of psychosocial treatment of rapid cyclers. However, supportive psychotherapy, focusing on education about bipolar disorder in general and rapid cycling in particular, in conjunction with participation in self-help organizations such as the National Depressive and Manic Depressive Association, may often be useful in forming and maintaining a therapeutic alliance, enhancing compliance with often complex medication regimens, and in reducing the patient's sense of isolation.[6]

CONCLUSIONS AND CLINICAL IMPLICATIONS

The first step in the successful treatment of patients with rapid-cycling bipolar disorder is to recognize that the phenomenon is occurring. It is important to realize that rapid cycling can present in a variety of ways—for instance, with irritability, hostility, dysphoria, and depression as well as with clear-cut recurrent mood swings or discrete affective episodes. In most cases, a family member or close friend should be interviewed, as patients may have difficulty accurately reporting their symptoms—often not recognizing hypomanic episodes or misinterpreting ultrafast cycling or dysphoric mania as depression. Constructing a life chart of the patient's affective episodes along with concurrent psychopharmacological treatments, medical conditions, and psychosocial stressors is a particularly useful way of illustrating the course of symptoms over time (thereby helping to establish whether or not rapid cycling is occurring), identifying potential precipitants (e.g., development of hypothyroidism or exposure to antidepressant agents), and evaluating whether any treatments have been helpful or harmful over the long term.[6]

Once rapid cycling is established, a medical evaluation should be done, with particular attention to thyroid and neurological status and possible comorbid psychiatric conditions including alcohol or substance abuse. The goal of treatment is mood stabilization. If at all possible, antidepressants and neuroleptics should be avoided and treatment restricted to mood-stabilizing agents (e.g., lithium, carbamazepine, valproate, thyroid hormone augmentation). Thus, if the patient is receiving antidepressants, neuroleptics, or other potential cycle-inducing agents, these agents should be discontinued, and the subsequent course of illness reevaluated. If cycling persists, treatment with a mood stabilizer should be initiated, and response over time (preferably for at least 1 to 2 months or cycle lengths) carefully evaluated. Patients may display several patterns of response: unabated persistence of cycling; reduced frequency or intensity (or both) of mood swings but with some residual cycling; cessation of hypomanic and manic episodes but persistent depression; complete cessation of cycling; and more rarely, amelioration of depression but persistence of hypomania or mania. With persistent cycling, hypomanic, or manic symptoms, a second and maybe even a third mood stabilizer can be added to or substituted for the first. If manic symptoms are ameliorated but depression persists, another mood stabilizer or thyroid hormone may also be added. However, if depression continues to persist (as it often does), antidepressants may be indicated. In the authors experience, antidepressant treatment can be used successfully without reinducing or exacerbating cycling as long as manic symptoms are *completely* suppressed, and the antidepressant is administered carefully—often in low doses or in an "on-off" manner (the antidepressant is taken on depressed but not on euthymic or hypomanic days).

In sum, although rapid cycling has long been considered notoriously difficult to treat, heightened awareness of the phenomenon and an increased number of available treatment options provide patients with enhanced chances of achieving stabilization of their mood disorder.

REFERENCES

1. Dunner DL, Fieve RR: Clinical factors in lithium carbonate prophylaxis failure. Arch Gen Psychiatry 30:229–233, 1974.
2. Dunner DL, Vijayalakshmy P, Fieve RR: Rapid cycling manic depressive patients. Compr Psychiatry 18:561–566, 1977.
3. Roy-Byrne PP, Jaffe RT, Uhde TW, et al: Approaches to the evaluation and treatment of rapid-cycling affective illness. Br J Psychiatry 145:543–550, 1984.
4. Alarcon RD: Rapid cycling affective disorders: A clinical review. Compr Psychiatry 26:522–540, 1985.
5. Keck PE Jr, McElroy SL: Anticonvulsants in the treatment of rapid-cycling bipolar disorder. *In* McElroy SL, Pope HG, Jr, eds. Use of Anticonvulsants in Psychiatry: Recent Advances. Clifton, NJ: Oxford Health Care, Inc., 1988:115–125.
6. Goodwin FK, Jamison KR: Manic-Depressive Illness. New York: Oxford University Press, Inc., 1990.
7. Kukopulos A, Reginaldi D, Laddomada P, et al: Course of the manic-depressive cycle and changes caused by treatments. Pharmacopsychiatria 13:156–167, 1980.
8. Akiskal HS, Mallya G: Criteria for the "soft" bipolar spectrum: Treatment implications. Psychopharmacol Bull 23:68–73, 1987.
9. Fawcett J, Scheftner W, Clark D, et al: Clinical predictors of suicide in patients with major affective disorders: A controlled prospective study. Am J Psychiatry 144:35–40, 1987.
10. Kukopulos A, Caliari B, Tundo A, et al: Rapid cyclers, temperament, and antidepressants. Compr Psychiatry 24:249–258, 1983.
11. Nurnberger J, Guroff JJ, Hamovit J, et al: A family study of rapid-cycling bipolar illness. J Affective Disord 15:87–91, 1988.
12. Wehr TA, Sack DA, Rosenthal NE, et al: Rapid cycling affective disorder: Contributing factors and treatment responses in 51 patients. Am J Psychiatry 145:179–184, 1988.
13. Calabrese JR, Delucchi GA: Spectrum of efficacy of valproate in 55 patients with rapid-cycling bipolar disorder. Am J Psychiatry 147:431–434, 1990.
14. Bauer MS, Whybrow PC, Winokur A: Rapid cycling bipolar affective disorder. I. Association with grade I hypothyroidism. Arch Gen Psychiatry 47:427–432, 1990.
15. Wehr TA, Goodwin FK: Rapid cycling in manic depressives induced by tricyclic antidepressants. Arch Gen Psychiatry 36:555–559, 1979.
16. Paschalis C, Pavlou A, Papadimitriou A: A stepped forty-eight hour manic-depressive cycle. Br J Psychiatry 137:332–336, 1980.
17. Post RM, Rubinow DR, Uhde TW, et al: Dysphoric mania: Clinical and biological correlates. Arch Gen Psychiatry 46:353–358, 1989.
18. Joyce PR, Donald RA, Elder PA: Individual differences in plasma cortisol changes during mania and depression. J Affective Disord 12:1–5, 1987.
19. Joyce PR, Donald RA, Livesey JH, et al: The prolactin response to metoclopramide is increased in depression and in euthymic rapid cycling bipolar patients. Biol Psychiatry 22:508–512, 1987.
20. Sack DA, James SP, Rosenthal NE, et al: Deficient nocturnal surge of TSH secretion during sleep and sleep deprivation in rapid-cycling bipolar illness. Psychiatry Res 23:179–191, 1988.
21. Levy AB, Drake ME, Shy KE: EEG evidence of epileptiform paroxysms in rapid cycling bipolar patients. J Clin Psychiatry 49:232–234, 1988.
22. Post RM, Uhde TW, Roy-Byrne PP, et al: Correlates of antimanic response to carbamazepine. Psychiatry Res 21:71–83, 1987.
23. McElroy SL, Keck PE Jr, Pope HG Jr, et al: Valproate in primary psychiatric disorders: Literature review and clinical experience in a private psychiatric hospital. *In* McElroy SL, Pope HG Jr, eds. Use of Anticonvulsants in Psychiatry: Recent Advances. Clifton, NJ: Oxford Health Care, Inc., 1988:25–41.
24. McElroy SL, Keck PE Jr, Pope HG Jr, et al: Correlates of antimanic response to valproate. Psychopharmacol Bull 27:127–133, 1991.
25. Stancer HC, Persad E: Treatment of intractable rapid-cycling manic-depressive disorder with levothyroxine. Arch Gen Psychiatry 39:311–312, 1982.
26. Bauer MS, Whybrow PC: Rapid cycling bipolar affective high-dose levothyroxine: A preliminary study. Arch Gen Psychiatry 47:435–440, 1990.
27. Potter WZ, Murphy DL, Wehr TA, et al: Clorgyline. Arch Gen Psychiatry 33:505–510, 1982.
28. Haykal RF, Akiskal HS: Bupropion as a promising approach to rapid cycling bipolar II patients. J Clin Psychiatry 51:450–455, 1990.

REVIEW OF ANTIDEPRESSANTS IN THE TREATMENT OF MOOD DISORDERS

ELLIOTT RICHELSON, M.D.

This chapter presents information on the pharmacology and clinical use of antidepressants. This class of compounds was first introduced by researchers in the late 1950s to treat depression, a disorder of mood. Today, we know much about the biochemical effects of these drugs. However, their mechanism of therapeutic action remains speculative. Epidemiological studies show that depression afflicts, in the United States, about 5 per cent of the adult population. Also, about 1 to 2 per cent of the adult population has acute bipolar illness. Over a lifetime, about 30 per cent of the adult population will have suffered from depression. Also, if left untreated, 25 to 30 per cent of adult depressives will commit suicide.

Sixty-five to seventy per cent of patients respond to antidepressant drug therapy and can enjoy a complete recovery from their depression. Improvement is not immediate. It usually begins about 10 days into the therapy and is complete by about 8 weeks. Electroconvulsive therapy (ECT) works in another 10 to 15 per cent of patients. Therefore, there are about 20 per cent of depressed patients who are resistant to all known forms of therapy.

TREATMENT OF DEPRESSION

The mainstay for the treatment of depression is pharmacotherapy, usually in combination with some form of limited, supportive psychotherapy. The antidepressants available in the United States today include three drugs classified as monoamine oxidase inhibitors—isocarboxazid (Marplan), phenelzine (Nardil), and tranylcypromine (Parnate)—and 12 others (see Appendix IV). The so-called tricyclic antidepressants (e.g., nortriptyline or desipramine) have been the first-line drugs. Fluoxetine (Prozac) may be becoming the first choice for many clinicians.

TYPES OF ANTIDEPRESSANTS

Antidepressants approved for use in the United States until the 1970s could be classified into two groups: tricyclic antidepressants, and monoamine oxidase inhibitors (MAOI.) This classification mixed structural (tricyclic) and functional (inhibition of monoamine oxidase) criteria. A classification based upon either structure or activity would be better. Although not completely satisfactory, one can classify all currently available antidepressants as either inhibitors of monoamine oxidase or inhibitors of monoamine neurotransmitter uptake.

Some, in attempting to classify all antidepressants according to structure, have caused a great deal of confusion in the literature with the use of the terms bicyclic, tricyclic, and tetracyclic. These terms apply only to structures that have *fused* rings numbering two, three, and four, respectively. Thus, for example, the antidepressant trazodone contains four rings but is not a tetracyclic because all these rings are not fused together. Another term used incorrectly is "heterocyclic," used to classify antidepressants according to structure. This term describes any ringed compound that contains within one or more rings an atom different from carbon. Therefore, four of the eight tricyclic compounds (doxepin, imipramine, trimipramine, desipramine, and amoxapine) are heterocyclic antidepressants. Amitriptyline, nortriptyline, and protriptyline are not heterocyclic.

CLINICAL PHARMACOLOGY OF ANTIDEPRESSANTS

Pharmacokinetic studies indicate wide interindividual variation in the absorption, distribution, and excretion of the antidepressants.[1] In addition, drug clearance generally declines with aging. Appendix IV outlines the usual daily doses for projected optimal therapeutic plasma ranges of tricyclic and other antidepressants. It should be noted that the American Psychiatric Association Task Force on the Use of Laboratory Tests in Psychiatry[2] has concluded on the basis of available data that the plasma level measurements are clinically useful in certain situations for only three tricyclic antidepressants—imipramine, desipramine, and nortriptyline. Thus, because of insufficient data and contradictory results, the Task Force concluded that optimal therapeutic ranges for other antidepressants have yet to be established. Nonetheless, the *projected* ranges presented in Appendix IV can be used as a guide in clinical practice.

Therapeutic drug monitoring is most readily available for the tricyclic compounds. Reasons for monitoring these drugs have been enumerated.[3] These reasons include: to assess compliance, to maximize response, to avoid toxicity, to minimize cost for the patient, and to avoid medicolegal problems.

Of particular note is the substantiated 10- to 30-fold variation in individual metabolism (Appendix IV), which necessitates specific attention to individualization of drug dosage and emphasizes the need to monitor drug plasma levels to achieve an appropriate therapeutic response, particularly in the elderly patient. The concept of a therapeutic window (i.e., a blood level range below and above which the drug is ineffective) has been thoroughly evaluated only for nortriptyline.[2] Protriptyline and nortriptyline, in comparison with other tricyclic antidepressants, demonstrate increased potency (Appendix IV); therefore, a smaller mean daily dose of these drugs should be prescribed. The longer elimination half-life ($T_{1/2}$) for protriptyline may in part explain the requirement for a lower dosage.

The mean elimination half-lives of most of the tricyclic antidepressants in Appendix IV are in the 15- to 30-hour range. The half-lives of maprotiline, protriptyline, and fluoxetine, however, are much longer; consequently, use of these drugs results in not only the requirement of a longer time to achieve a steady state after initiation of treatment, but also the need for a longer period of observation of complications after ingestion of an overdose. Based upon pharmacokinetic considerations,[4] a rational dosing interval for an antidepressant drug is equal to its elimination half-life (Appendix IV). In practice, a single daily dose is appropriate for those drugs with half-lives of around 15 hours or greater. It is also reasonable to consider prescribing the very–long-half-life compounds—protriptyline, fluoxetine, and maprotiline—less frequently, especially in the elderly patient.

Other pharmacokinetic information of clinical importance is that these agents are highly lipid soluble and therefore have a high volume of distribution. They are also strongly bound to plasma proteins. Changes in body fat and plasma proteins with aging, therefore, can have effects on the clearance of a drug and its potency.

BASIC PHARMACOLOGY OF ANTIDEPRESSANTS

The site of the pharmacodynamic effects of antidepressants that appears to be especially relevant clinically is the synapse. By either blocking uptake (reuptake) of neurotransmitters, blocking certain neurotransmitter receptors, or inhibiting the mitochondrial enzyme monoamine oxidase, antidepressants alter the effects of neurotransmitters at the synapses. Neurotransmitters are the chemicals which neurons use to communicate with one another and with other cell types. These small molecules, usually amino acids or their derivatives, are released from the nerve ending to interact with specific receptors on the outside surface of cells. Receptors are highly specialized proteins, which in some cases have been cloned by molecular biologists and which are very selective in their ability to bind neurotransmitters. When the chemical messenger stimulates its receptor, the receiving neuron is changed electrically and biochemically as a result of the coupling of the complex of neurotransmitter and receptor to other components of the membrane in which the receptor resides. Neurons can also regulate their own activity by feedback mechanisms involving receptors on the nerve ending (autoreceptors). An example of an autoreceptor is the α_2-adrenergic receptor on noradrenergic nerve endings which modulate release of norepinephrine. When stimulated, this presynaptic receptor inhibits further release of norepinephrine.

For some biogenic amine neurotransmitters (e.g., norepinephrine, serotonin, and dopamine), it has been established that after release they are taken back into the nerve ending (a process called uptake or reuptake). Reuptake is a mechanism that prevents overstimulation of receptors in the synapse. Neurotransmission can be enhanced acutely by blocking this uptake with a drug. But blockade of uptake can ultimately diminish neurotransmission as the receptor undergoes a compensatory change and becomes less sensitive (desensitizes) to the neurotransmitter. Antidepressants of many types, probably acting by different mechanisms, can desensitize receptors for catecholamines. This effect is the basis for one hypothesis of their mechanism of action.[5]

By blocking the postsynaptic receptor with an antagonist, neurotransmitter effects can be selectively and acutely abolished. Very often with chronic blockade, the receptor undergoes another type of compensatory change and becomes more sensitive (supersensitive) to the neurotransmitter. Supersensitivity may be the mechanism of adaptation to some receptor-related side effects of certain drugs and related to the development of tardive dyskinesia following chronic treatment with neuroleptics which block dopamine receptors.

Antidepressants can block uptake of biogenic amine neurotransmitters and antagonize certain receptors. In addition, some antidepressants inhibit the activity of monoamine oxidase, a ubiquitous enzyme that is important in the degradation of catecholamines, serotonin, and other biogenic amines. Since this enzyme is present in mitochondria which are found in most cells and in the nerve ending, its inhibition results in an elevation in the concentration of neurotransmitter available for release at the synapse.

TABLE 37–1. ANTIDEPRESSANT POTENCIES[a] FOR BLOCKADE OF NOREPINEPHRINE UPTAKE INTO RAT BRAIN SYNAPTOSOME[b]

Drug	Potency
Desipramine	110
Protriptyline	100
Nortriptyline	25
Amoxapine	23
Maprotiline	14
Imipramine	7.7
Doxepin	5.3
Amitriptyline	4.2
Clomipramine[c]	3.6
Fluoxetine	0.36
Trimipramine	0.20
Bupropion	0.043
Trazodone	0.020
d-Amphetamine[d]	2.00
Cocaine[d]	0.65

[a] $10^{-7} \times 1/K_i$, where K_i = inhibitor constant in molarity. Data can be compared both vertically and across tables to find the most potent drug for a specific property and to find the most potent property of a specific drug.
[b] Data derived from Richelson E, Pfenning M: Blockade by antidepressants and related compounds of biogenic amine uptake into rat brain synaptosomes: Most antidepressants selectively block norepinephrine uptake. Eur J Pharmacol 104:277, 1984.[37]
[c] Not marketed in the United States as an antidepressant.
[d] Reference compound.

BLOCKADE OF NEUROTRANSMITTER UPTAKE BY ANTIDEPRESSANTS

Early research on uptake blockade by antidepressants was misinterpreted. Today we know that most antidepressants are more potent at blocking uptake of norepinephrine than serotonin (Tables 37–1 through 37–3). Newer antidepressants are generally

TABLE 37–2. ANTIDEPRESSANT POTENCIES[a] FOR BLOCKADE OF SEROTONIN UPTAKE INTO RAT BRAIN SYNAPTOSOME[b]

Drug	Potency
Clomipramine[c]	18
Fluoxetine	8.3
Imipramine	2.4
Amitriptyline	1.5
Trazodone	0.53
Nortriptyline	0.38
Doxepin	0.36
Protriptyline	0.36
Desipramine	0.29
Amoxapine	0.21
Trimipramine	0.040
Maprotiline	0.030
Bupropion	0.0064

[a] $10^{-7} \times 1/K_i$, where K_i = inhibitor constant in molarity. Data can be compared both vertically and across tables to find the most potent drug for a specific property and to find the most potent property of a specific drug.
[b] Data derived with permission from Richelson E, Pfenning M: Blockade by antidepressants and related compounds of biogenic amine uptake into rat brain synaptosomes: Most antidepressants selectively block norepinephrine uptake. Eur J Pharmacol 104:277, 1984.[37]
[c] Not marketed in the United States as an antidepressant.

TABLE 37–3. ANTIDEPRESSANT SELECTIVITY FOR BLOCKADE OF NOREPINEPHRINE OVER SEROTONIN UPTAKE INTO RAT BRAIN SYNAPTOSOME

Drug	NE/5-HT Selectivity
Maprotiline	470[a]
Desipramine	380
Protriptyline	290
Amoxapine	110
Nortriptyline	65
Doxepin	15
Bupropion	6.8
Trimipramine	4.9
Imipramine	3.2
Amitriptyline	2.8
Clomipramine[b]	0.19[c]
Fluoxetine	0.043
Trazodone	0.038

[a] Indicates that maprotiline is 450 times more potent at blocking uptake of norepinephrine over serotonin.
[b] Not marketed in the United States as an antidepressant.
[c] Indicates that clomipramine is about five times more potent at blocking uptake of serotonin over norepinephrine.

more selective than the older compounds at blocking uptake of one neurotransmitter over another. In addition, there are some antidepressants, such as bupropion and trimipramine, that very weakly block uptake of norepinephrine and serotonin. Bupropion is the only antidepressant more selective for blocking uptake of dopamine (Table 37–4) than other neurotransmitters. It is also the most potent of the

TABLE 37–4. ANTIDEPRESSANT POTENCIES[a] FOR BLOCKADE OF DOPAMINE UPTAKE INTO RAT BRAIN SYNAPTOSOME[b]

Drug	Dopamine Uptake Potency
Bupropion	0.16
Fluoxetine	0.063
Nortriptyline	0.059
Clomipramine[c]	0.057
Protriptyline	0.054
Amoxapine	0.053
Amitriptyline	0.043
Maprotiline	0.034
Trimipramine	0.029
Imipramine	0.020
Desipramine	0.019
Doxepin	0.018
Trazodone	0.0070
d-Amphetamine[d]	1.2
Cocaine[d]	0.37

[a] $10^{-7} \times 1/K_i$, where K_i = inhibitor constant in molarity. Data can be compared both vertically and across tables to find the most potent drug for a specific property and to find the most potent property of a specific drug.
[b] Data derived with permission from Richelson E, Pfenning M: Blockade by antidepressants and related compounds of biogenic amine uptake into rat brain synaptosomes: Most antidepressants selectively block norepinephrine uptake. Eur J Pharmacol 104:277, 1984.[37]
[c] Not marketed in the United States as an antidepressant.
[d] Reference compound.

antidepressants at this property, although much weaker than is d-amphetamine (Table 37–4).

Selectivity cannot be equated with potency, since selectivity is derived from a ratio of potencies. For example, although maprotiline is more selective (i.e., more specific) at blockade uptake of norepinephrine than is desipramine, it is much less potent than desipramine at this blockade (Appendix IV).

BLOCKADE OF NEUROTRANSMITTER RECEPTORS BY ANTIDEPRESSANTS

In general, the most potent interaction of antidepressants is at the histamine H_1 receptor (Table 37–5). In fact, of all the known pharmacological effects of all these antidepressants (Appendix IV, Tables 37–2, 37–4, and 37–5) in general, histamine H_1-receptor blockade is their most potent effect.

Histamine is a putative neurotransmitter in brain[6] where, like elsewhere in the body, it has at least two types of receptors, histamine H_1 and histamine H_2. Recently, a third histamine receptor (H_3) was identified in brain.[7] This new histamine receptor affects the presynaptic synthesis and release of histamine, as well as other neurotransmitters. Outside the nervous system, classically, histamine H_1 receptors are involved with allergic reactions and histamine H_2 receptors are involved with gastric acid secretion. Some antidepressants are exceedingly potent histamine H_1 antagonists (Table 37–5). As a result, clinicians are using them to treat allergic and dermatological problems.[8]

The next most potent effect of antidepressants is at the muscarinic acetylcholine receptor. These receptors are the predominant type of cholinergic receptors in brain, and in that organ they appear to be involved with memory and learning.[9] In addition, there is some evidence to suggest that these brain receptors are involved with affective illness.[10] Antidepressants have a broad range of affinities for human brain muscarinic receptors (Table 37–5). The most potent is amitriptyline.

There are several subtypes of the serotonin receptor.[11] We have studied binding of antidepressants to two of them, 5-HT$_{1a}$ and 5-HT$_2$, in human brain. Antidepressants are not very potent at blocking 5-HT$_{1a}$ receptors, but some are quite potent at blocking 5-HT$_2$ receptors compared to methysergide, a drug used to treat migraine headaches prophylactically.

Monoamine oxide inhibitors have very weak direct effects on neurotransmitter receptors and are practically devoid of clinically significant pharmacological activity on them. In addition, newer, so-called second-generation, antidepressants tend to be very weak at blocking these receptors. Such data predict a side-effect profile for these newer compounds different from the older antidepressants.

CLINICAL IMPORTANCE OF THE BASIC PHARMACOLOGY OF ANTIDEPRESSANT DRUGS

All the pharmacological effects of these drugs discussed above occur shortly after a patient has in-

TABLE 37–5. ANTIDEPRESSANT AFFINITIES FOR NEUROTRANSMITTER RECEPTORS OF HUMAN BRAIN[a]

Drug	Histamine H_1 Affinity[b]	Muscarinic Affinity	α_1-Adrenoceptor Affinity	α_2-Adrenoceptor Affinity	Dopamine D_2 Affinity	5-HT$_2$ Affinity
Amitriptyline	91	5.6	3.70	0.106	0.10	3.4
Amoxapine	4.0	0.10	2.00	0.038	0.62	170
Bupropion	0.015	0.0021	0.0217	0.0012	0.00048	0.0011
Clomipramine[c]	3.2	2.70	2.63	0.031	0.53	3.7
Desipramine	0.91	0.50	0.77	0.014	0.030	0.36
Doxepin	420	1.2	4.17	0.091	0.042	4.0
Fluoxetine	0.016	0.050	0.0169	0.0077	0.015	0.48
Imipramine	9.1	1.1	1.11	0.031	0.050	1.2
Maprotiline	50	0.18	1.11	0.011	0.29	0.83
Nortriptyline	10	0.67	1.67	0.040	0.083	2.3
Protriptyline	4.0	4.0	0.77	0.015	0.043	1.5
Trazodone	0.29	0.00031	2.78	0.204	0.026	13
Trimipramine	370	1.7	4.17	0.147	0.56	3.1
Diphenhydramine[d]	7.1					
Atropine[d]		42				
Phenotolamine[d]			6.7	2.3		
Yohimbine[d]				62		
Haloperidol[d]					26	
Methysergide[d]						15

[a] Data derived with permission from Richelson E, Nelson A: Antagonism by antidepressnts of neurotransmitter receptors of normal human brain in vitro. J. Pharmacol Exp Ther 230:94, 1984.[38]
[b] $10^{-7} \times 1/K_d$, where K_d = equilibrium dissociation constant in molarity. Data can be compared vertically, horizontally, and across tables to find the most potent drug for a specific property and to find the most potent property of a specific drug.
[c] Not marketed in the United States as an antidepressant.
[d] Reference compound.

gested a dose of the medication. Thus, most of the possible clinical effects to be discussed below occur early in the treatment of patients. However, with chronic administration of the drug, adaptive changes may occur that can result in an adjustment to certain side effects, the development of new side effects, and the onset of therapeutic effects. Table 37–6 lists the pharmacological properties and their possible clinical consequences. The clinician should keep in mind that the drugs that are most potent at the properties discussed are more likely to cause these possible effects than the drugs that are weak at these properties (Tables 37–1, 37–2, 37–4, and 37–5).

Evidence to date suggests that the efficacy of antidepressants is not related to selectivity or potency for their norepinephrine or serotonin uptake blockade. These data are from clinical studies[12] as well as basic studies that show the wide range of potencies of antidepressants at blocking this uptake (Tables 37–1, 37–2, and 37–4). On the other hand, clinical data suggest that potent uptake blockade of serotonin

is necessary for treatment of certain anxiety disorders[13] and obsessive-compulsive disorder.[14]

Uptake blockade of neurotransmitters likely relates to certain adverse effects of these drugs and to some of their drug-drug interactions (Table 37–6). For example, serotonin uptake blockade likely is the property that causes the serious results when an MAOI is combined with an antidepressant. In addition, researchers have reported adverse interactions between L-tryptophan, the precursor of serotonin, and fluoxetine.[15] An interaction between fenfluramine, which increases synaptic levels of serotonin, and antidepressants that are serotonin uptake inhibitors can be predicted.

There have been a number of anecdotal reports about rare effects of fluoxetine that include extrapyramidal side effects,[16] anorgasmia,[17] paranoid reaction,[18] and intense suicidal preoccupation.[19] The extrapyramidal side effects are not due to blockade of dopamine receptors, because fluoxetine is very weak at this binding site (Table 37–5). It can only be

TABLE 37–6.   PHARMACOLOGICAL PROPERTIES OF ANTIDEPRESSANTS AND THEIR POSSIBLE CLINICAL CONSEQUENCES

Property	Possible Clinical Consequences
Blockade of norepinephrine uptake at nerve endings	Tremors Tachycardia Erectile and ejaculatory dysfunction Blockade of the antihypertensive effects of guanethidine (Ismelin and Esimil) and guanadrel (Hylorel) Augmentation of pressor effects of sympathomimetic amines
Blockade of serotonin uptake at nerve ending	Gastrointestinal disturbances Increase or decrease in anxiety (dose-dependent) Sexual dysfunction Extrapyramidal side effects Interactions with L-tryptophan, MAOIs, and fenfluramine
Blockade of dopamine uptake at nerve ending	Psychomotor activation Antiparkinsonian effect Aggravation of psychosis
Blockade of histamine H_1 receptors	Potentiation of central depressant drugs Sedation drowsiness Weight gain Hypotension
Blockade of muscarinic receptors	Blurred vision Dry mouth Sinus tachycardia Constipation Urinary retention
Blockade of α_1-adrenergic receptors	Memory dysfunction Potentiation of the antihypertensive effect of prazosin (Minipress) and terazosin (Hytrin) Postural hypotension, dizziness Reflex tachycardia
Blockade of α_2-adrenergic receptors	Blockade of the antihypertensive effects of clonidine (Catapres), guanabenz (Wytensin), α-methyldopa (Aldomet), guanfacine (Tenex) Priapism
Blockade of dopamine D_2 receptors	Extrapyramidal movement disorders Sexual dysfunction (males)
Blockade of serotonin 5-HT_2 receptors	Ejaculatory dysfunction Hypotension Alleviation of migraine headaches

speculated that these reactions involve serotonin, since serotonin uptake blockade is the most potent property possessed by fluoxetine.

Potentiation of the effects of central depressant drugs, which cause sedation and drowsiness, is a drug-drug interaction of antidepressants related to histamine H_1-receptor antagonism. Histamine H_1 antagonism is probably responsible for the side effects of sedation and drowsiness. Sedation, however, may be a wanted effect in patients who are agitated as well as depressed. On a more speculative basis, this property may be responsible for weight gain and postural hypotension.

Trazodone frequently causes sedation and drowsiness in patients. Its low affinity for the histamine H_1 receptor (Table 37–5) suggests that this drug causes these side effects by other mechanisms. However, data[20,21] showing that in clinical practice trazodone achieves high blood levels (which relate to brain levels) are consistent with the idea that trazodone causes sedation and drowsiness by blocking the histamine H_1 receptor. Alternatively, α_1-adrenergic receptor blockade at which trazodone is relatively potent (Table 37–5) may also be involved with causing sedation.[22]

Muscarinic receptor blockade by these antidepressants can be responsible for several adverse effects (Table 37–6). α_1-Adrenergic receptor blockade by antidepressants may be responsible for orthostatic hypotension, the most serious common cardiovascular effect of these drugs.[23] This side effect can cause dizzinesss and a reflex tachycardia. In addition, this property of antidepressants will result in the potentiation of the antihypertensive drugs prazosin and terazosin, potent α_1-antagonists.

Antidepressants are weak competitive antagonists of dopamine (D_2) receptors (Table 37–5). The most potent compound, amoxapine, is a demethylated derivative of the neuroleptic, loxapine. It is very likely that this in vitro activity of amoxapine explains its extrapyramidal side effects.[24] and its ability to elevate prolactin levels in patients.[25] Because of this dopamine receptor–blocking property of amoxapine, some clinicians are using it in psychotic depressions.

5-HT_2 Receptors may be involved with blood pressure regulation,[26] and their blockade may cause hypotension. The reference compound for the 5-HT_2 receptor, methysergide (Table 37–5), is a 5-HT_2-receptor antagonist used classically to prevent migraine headaches. Since trazodone is about equally effective as this drug at blocking this receptor, a possible use for trazodone in preventing migraine is suggested. However, data imply that methysergide's effects in migraine may result from its action as an agonist at a 5-HT_1 receptor.[27] Although amoxapine is much more potent than is methysergide or trazodone at this receptor, its use here is precluded by its potential to cause extrapyramidal side effects.

GENERAL CLINICAL GUIDELINES

The clinician should consider any concomitant medical disorder, whether the patient is agitated or retarded, and antidepressant side effects for determining the appropriate choice of drug in any particular clinical situation. Certain clinical guidelines exist for drug choice, dosage, duration, maintenance, termination, and alternatives to treatment with antidepressants. Table 37–7 outlines these guidelines.

The first step is the appropriate choice of drug. In general, a more sedating drug (potent histamine H_1 antagonist) should be chosen for patients with episodes of agitated depression, and a less sedating drug (weak histamine H_1 antagonist) for those patients with retarded depressive episodes. History of a previous response of the patient or a family member to a particular antidepressant drug can sometimes be helpful in selecting a drug for a patient.

The second important guideline is the appropriate dose of medication. Most patients tolerate treatment best if the beginning dose is one fourth of the maximal, usual daily dose for adults (Appendix IV). The dose should be divided initially and increased in a stepwise fashion every 2 to 3 days until the maximal, usual daily dose (Appendix IV) has been achieved, if tolerated. For example, for desipramine the target dose is 200 mg/day (Appendix IV). A patient could be started on desipramine 25 mg b.i.d. for 2 days; then 25 mg t.i.d. for 2 days; then 50 mg b.i.d. for 2 days; then 50 mg t.i.d. for 2 days; and finally, if no very troublesome adverse effects are present, 100 mg b.i.d. After about 1 to 2 weeks at this target dosage, patients may take antidepressants with the longer

TABLE 37–7. CLINICAL GUIDELINES FOR USE OF ANTIDEPRESSANTS[a]

1. Appropriate choice: select on the basis of the profile of side effects, particularly sedative effects in agitated patients or on the basis of previous response or family history of a response to a particular antidepressant.
2. Adequate dose: check blood level if toxicity ensues or if response is inadequate.
3. Adequate duration: administer for a minimum of 4 months after recovery.
4. Adequate termination or maintenance: For first depressions, 4 to 5 months after recovery, taper dose gradually for 2 to 4 months and then discontinue therapy. For recurrent unipolar depression, maintain therapy with antidepressant.
5. Adequate therapy: for almost all types of depression, a combination of psychotherapy (usually, brief supportive) and antidepressants may be slightly more effective than antidepressants alone.
6. Adequate alternative: change drug; add lithium carbonate; add thyroid hormone; use MAOI in combination with a tricyclic antidepressant (avoiding imipramine), or use electroshock therapy.

[a] Reproduced with permission from Richelson E: Antidepressants: Pharmacology and clinical use. In Karasu TB, ed. Treatments of Psychiatric Disorders. 1st ed. Washington, DC: American Psychiatric Association Press, 1989: Vol. 3, 1773.[36]

elimination half-lives (around 15 hours or greater, Appendix IV) once a day at bedtime. Elderly patients may benefit from being continued on the divided dosage schedule, so that high blood levels (possibly leading to adverse effects) do not occur during the night when the patient may arise to eliminate.

Use of MAOIs requires special considerations. These are very efficacious drugs for treating depression, are well tolerated by the elderly, and should be used when a patient fails to respond to antidepressants of other classes of drugs. However, these drugs are not for all cases, because of the need for the patient on an MAOI to avoid certain foodstuffs, especially those containing tyramine, and certain drugs, especially over-the-counter cold remedies containing sympathomimetics. The clinician must make the patient aware of these important precautions when prescribing an MAOI. A convenient way to ensure that the patient has all the information in hand is to give him or her a copy of the American Medical Association Patient Medication Instruction Sheet (PMI), *MAO Inhibitor Antidepressants* (PMI 076). When a patient is not willing or able to comply with these precautions, then another type of antidepressant should be prescribed.

If the patient is taking a tricyclic antidepressant or another MAOI, then this drug should be discontinued for 10 days before starting a MAOI. To be underscored in the list of drugs that should be avoided in patients on MAOIs are meperidine, imipramine, and fluoxetine. However, it is possible to combine safely an MAOI with a tricyclic antidepressant other than imipramine in special circumstances as discussed further below.

Of the three different MAOIs currently in use in the United States (Appendix IV), phenelzine has probably been studied the most. From this research it is known that around 2 weeks are needed to achieve maximal inhibition of platelet monoamine oxidase when depressed patients are given phenelzine,[28] and about the same length of time is necessary to recover activity after the drug is discontinued. Patients with 80 per cent or greater inhibition of this platelet enzyme have a better antidepressant response than do those with less inhibition of their enzyme.[28] Although laboratories are making available the measurement of platelet monoamine oxidase, a clinically useful rule of thumb is to target a dosage of 1 mg/kg body weight per day for the patient[28] to achieve this desired level of inhibition.

As with other antidepressants, MAOIs may be started slowly. For example, when starting a patient on phenelzine, the clinician may prescribe 15 mg the first day; 15 mg b.i.d. the second day; 15 mg t.i.d. the third day; and so forth, until the target dosage is achieved.

A treatment period of 2 to 4 weeks is usually necessary before the onset of therapeutic effects of any type of antidepressant. At the outset, the patient may need a thorough explanation of the side effects to be expected and encouragement to persist with treatment until a clinical response ensues. If the clinical response is inadequate in 3 to 4 weeks and the adverse effects are minimal, the doses should be increased a step further. Underdosing is a common error in therapeutics with these drugs. As in the example above with desipramine, the dosage should be increased another 25 to 50 mg/day; with phenelzine, the dosage should be increased another 15 mg/day. However, if poor response persists after 2 more weeks at the higher dosage or if toxicity supervenes, then plasma levels of the drug, provided that it is not an MAOI, should be ascertained. Although therapeutic plasma concentrations have been firmly established for only imipramine, nortriptyline, and desipramine,[2] enough data are available for other antidepressants (other than MAOIs) to determine for problem patients or elderly patients, whether a dosage of a drug appears to be adequate. The projected optimal therapeutic plasma range presented in Appendix IV for the other antidepressants is to be used only as a rough guide.

Elderly patients are likely to require about half of the usual daily dose that is recommended for a younger adult and may require a slower escalation of the dosage to the maximal level because of their increased sensitivity to the adverse effects of antidepressants. However, underdosing can again be a mistake in treating elderly patients, and plasma levels should be utilized more often with this group. Achievement of a steady state in these patients may take longer as well.

Third, adequate duration of treatment is important. After a complete clinical response has been achieved, therapy should be continued for at least 4 to 5 months.[29]

The fourth important clinical guideline involves termination of antidepressant therapy or maintenance therapy for patients with recurrent illness. Four to five months after complete recovery, the drug dose should be tapered gradually over 2 to 4 months and then discontinued, because abrupt withdrawal of medication may predispose the patient to relapse of depressive symptoms or to uncomfortable symptoms—for example, dysesthesias and severe sleep disturbance. Maintenance therapy with the same antidepressant without lowering the dosage[30] should be used for those patients with recurrent unipolar depression.[31]

The fifth clinical guideline is that adequate therapy for almost all types of depression should include some form of psychotherapeutic alliance between the patient and doctor at least to ensure compliance with the pharmacotherapy. This may be achieved through brief (10 to 20 minutes) supportive visits with the primary physician or, in some cases, more extensive psychotherapy. However, a combination of antidepressants and psychotherapy may be only slightly more effective than antidepressants alone.[32]

Finally, adequate knowledge of alternative or adjunctive treatments for depression is important. This includes a change in primary antidepressant drug to an antidepressant of a different chemical class; the addition of lithium carbonate[33] in a dosage to achieve a blood level of 0.8 to 1.2 mEq/liter; the addition of thyroid hormone (L-triiodothyronine 25 to 50 μg/day); or the combination of a tricyclic antidepressant with an MAOI. If this latter approach is elected, the safest course is to withdraw the patient from the antidepressant for 10 days and begin both types of medications at low doses together. Combination of the tertiary amine tricyclic antidepressant imipramine or fluoxetine and an MAOI must be avoided. Electroconvulsive therapy is still the most effective for refractory depression and may be the treatment of choice in certain medical situations that contraindicate the use of antidepressant medication[34] in conditions of extremely high suicidal risk, or in depression with psychotic features. In this latter case, the combination of an antidepressant with a neuroleptic may be superior to either drug alone. Psychostimulants may also be useful to treat depression in certain medical and surgical patients, while their efficacy in more general cases of depression is not established.[35]

REFERENCES

1. Sjöqvist F, Alexanderson B, Åsberg M, et al: Pharmacokinetics and biological effects of nortriptyline in man. Acta Pharmacol Toxicol 3:255, 1971.
2. Task Force on the Use of Laboratory Tests in Psychiatry, American Psychiatric Association: Am J Psychiatry 142:155, 1985.
3. Preskorn SH: Tricyclic antidepressants: The whys and hows of therapeutic drug monitoring. J Clin Psychiatry 50:34, 1989.
4. Gibaldi M, Levy G: Pharmacokinetics in clinical practice. 2. Applications. JAMA 235:1987, 1976.
5. Sulser F: Mode of action of antidepressant drugs. J Clin Psychiatry 44[sec 2]:14, 1983.
6. Prell GD, Green JP: Histamine as a neuroregulator. Ann Rev Neurosci 9:209, 1986.
7. Arrang JM, Garbarg M, Lancelot JC, et al: Highly potent and selective ligands for histamine H_3-receptors. Nature 327:117, 1987.
8. Richelson E: Novel uses for tricyclic antidepressants. Mod Med 51:74, 1983.
9. Bartus RT, Dean RLI, Beer B, Lippa AS: The cholinergic hypothesis of geriatric memory dysfunction. Science 217:408, 1982.
10. Janowsky DS, El-Yousef MK, Davis JM, et al: A cholinergic-adrenergic hypothesis of mania and depression. Lancet 1:632, 1972.
11. Peroutka SJ: 5-Hydroxytryptamine receptor subtypes. Ann Rev Neurosci 11:45, 1988.
12. Nystrom C, Hallstrom T: Double-blind comparison between a serotonin and a noradrenaline reuptake blocker in the treatment of depressed outpatients. Acta Psychiatr Scand 72:6, 1985.
13. Evans L, Kenardy J, Schneider P, Hoey H: Effect of a selective serotonin uptake inhibitor in agoraphobia with panic attacks—a double-blind comparison of zimelidine, imipramine and placebo. Acta Psychiatr Scand 73:49, 1986.
14. Murphy DL, Zohar J, Benkelfat C, et al: Obsessive-compulsive disorder as a 5-HT subsystem-related behavioural disorder. Br J Psychiatry 155(suppl 8):15, 1989.
15. Steiner W, Fontaine R: Toxic reaction following the combined administration of fluoxetine and L-tryptophan: Five case reports. Biol Psychiatry 21:1067, 1986.
16. Bouchard RH, Pourcher E, Vincent P: Fluoxetine and extrapyramidal side effects. Am J Psychiatry 146:1352, 1989.
17. Kline MD: Fluoxetine and anorgasmia. Am J Psychiatry 146:804, 1989.
18. Mandalos GE, Szarek BL: Dose-related paranoid reaction associated with fluoxetine. J Nerv Ment Dis 178:57, 1990.
19. Teicher MH, Glod C, Cole O: Emergence of intense suicidal preoccupation during fluoxetine treatment. Am J Psychiatry 147:207, 1990.
20. Caccia S, Fond MH, Garattini S, et al: Plasma concentrations of trazodone and 1-(3-chlorophenyl) piperazine in man after a single oral dose of trazodone. J Pharm Pharmacol 34:605, 1982.
21. Abernethy DR, Greenblatt DJ, Shader RI: Plasma levels of trazodone: Methodology and applications. Pharmacology 28:42, 1984.
22. U'Prichard DC, Greenberg DA, Sheehan PP, et al: Tricyclic antidepressants: Therapeutic properties and affinity for α-noradrenergic receptor binding sites in the brain. Science 199:197, 1978.
23. Glassman AH, Bigger T Jr: Cardiovascular effects of therapeutic doses of tricyclic antidepressants. Arch Gen Psychiatry 38:815, 1981.
24. Steele TE: Adverse reactions suggesting amoxapine-induced dopamine blockade. Am J Psychiatry 139:1500, 1982.
25. Cooper DS, Gelenberg AJ, Wojcik JC, et al: The effect of amoxapine and imipramine on serum prolactin levels. Arch Intern Med 141:1023, 1981.
26. Vanhoutte PM: Does 5-hydroxytryptamine play a role in hypertension? Trends Pharmacol Sci 3:370, 1982.
27. Saxena PR, Ferrari MD: 5-HT_1-like receptor agonists and the pathophysiology of migraine. Trends Pharmacol Sci 10:200, 1989.
28. Robinson DS, Nies A, Ravaris L, et al: Clinical pharmacology of phenelzine. Arch Gen Psychiatry 35:629, 1978.
29. Prien RF, Kupfer DJ: Continuation drug therapy for major depressive episodes: How long should it be maintained? Am J Psychiatry 141:18, 1986.
30. Frank E, Kupfer DJ, Perel JM, et al: Three-year outcomes for maintenance therapies in recurrent depression. Arch Gen Psychiatry 47:1093, 1990.
31. Prien RF, Kupfer DJ, Mansky PA, et al: Drug therapy in the prevention of recurrences in unipolar and bipolar affective disorders. Arch Gen Psychiatry 41:1096, 1984.
32. Conte HR, Plutchik R, Wild KV, Karasu TB: Combined psychotherapy and pharmacotherapy for depression. Arch Gen Psychiatry 43:471, 1986.
33. De Montigny C, Grunberg F, Mayer A, Deschenes J-P: Lithium induces rapid relief of depression in tricyclic antidepressant drug non-responders. Br J Psychiatry 138:252, 1981.
34. American Psychiatric Association Task Force Report: Electroconvulsive Therapy. Washington, DC: American Psychiatric Association, 1978.
35. Chiarello RJ, Cole JO: The use of psychostimulants in general psychiatry. Arch Gen Psychiatry 44:286, 1987.
36. Richelson E: Antidepressants: Pharmacology and clinical use. In Karasu TB, ed. Treatments of Psychiatric Disorders, 1st ed. Washington, DC: American Psychiatric Association Press, 1989: Vol. 3, 1773.
37. Richelson E, Pfenning M: Blockade by antidepressants and related compounds of biogenic amine uptake into rat brain synaptosomes: Most antidepressants selectively block norepinephrine uptake. Eur J Pharmacol 104:277, 1984.
38. Richelson E, Nelson A: Antagonism by antidepressants of neurotransmitter receptors of normal human brain in vitro. J Pharmacol Exp Ther 230:94, 1984.

38

REVIEW OF PSYCHOSOCIAL TREATMENTS FOR MOOD DISORDERS

STEVEN D. HOLLON, PH.D

It has been known for several decades that a variety of pharmacological and somatic interventions are effective in the treatment of depression. Early trials with a number of psychosocial interventions were less encouraging. In general, those trials suggested that although the psychosocial interventions often had an impact on social adjustment, they were no more effective than pill placebos with respect to the amelioration of symptoms of depression and did little to enhance the efficacy of pharmacotherapy when provided in combination.[1]

This picture has changed markedly over the last decade. Recent trials have suggested that a number of the newer psychosocial interventions may approach the efficacy of the pharmacological interventions, at least for nonpsychotic, nonbipolar depressed outpatients (the pharmacological and somatic therapies remain the treatments of choice for the more severe inpatient depressions). Further, there are indications that at least one such approach, cognitive therapy, may reduce risk for subsequent relapse,[2] and that another, interpersonal psychotherapy, may not only match pharmacotherapy in terms of its effects on depression, but may simultaneously enhance the quality of social adjustment.[3] Finally, some of the newer family interventions, similar to those generating interest in the treatment of schizophrenia, may hold real promise in the treatment of bipolar affective disorder.

In the sections to follow, each of the major approaches to psychotherapy relevant to depression are discussed. These include dynamic psychotherapy, interpersonal psychotherapy, marital and family systems therapy, behavior therapy, and cognitive therapy. In each instance, the basic treatment modality is described, followed by a brief review of the existing evidence speaking to its clinical efficacy, and concluding with a discussion of the available clinical indications.

DYNAMIC PSYCHOTHERAPY

Dynamic theories of depression have changed over the years. Whereas early versions emphasized the role of retroflected anger and unconscious masochis-tic drives, later modifications have tended to focus more on the diminution of self-esteem following interpersonal loss in the context of unresolved conflict.[4] Interventions based on either model strive to produce personality change by means of promoting understanding of past conflicts and providing insight into unconscious motivations. Specific approaches can range from the more formal structure provided in classical psychoanalysis, which stresses the interpretation of the defenses and the generation and working through of a transfer neurosis, to more flexible psychoanalytically oriented psychotherapies such as time-limited dynamic psychotherapy[5] or supportive-expressive psychotherapy,[6] which stress the use of the therapeutic relationship as a model for the exploration of underlying conflicts.

To date, dynamic psychotherapy has been tested in only three trials, each involving nonpsychotic, nonbipolar depressed outpatients. In the first, Daneman found that the combination of imipramine pharmacotherapy plus psychoanalytically oriented psychotherapy was clearly superior to psychoanalytically oriented psychotherapy alone.[7] In the second, Covi and colleagues found dynamic psychotherapy no more effective than a pill placebo and the combination of drugs plus dynamic pharmacotherapy no more effective than imipramine alone in the treatment of outpatient depression.[8] In the third, Covi and Lipman found dynamic psychotherapy to be less effective than either combined treatment involving cognitive therapy or cognitive therapy alone.[9]

Although these findings, taken as a whole, provide little support for dynamic psychotherapy, the quality of the representation of dynamic therapy in these trials leaves much to be desired. In two of the three trials,[7,8] dynamic psychotherapy was combined with a pill placebo. There is reason to think that psychotherapy plus pill placebo combinations may underestimate the efficacy of psychotherapy alone.[10] Further, in the two Covi et al. trials, dynamic psychotherapy was provided in a group treatment format, hardly a standard way of operationalizing this particular modality.[7,8] Thus, although the performance of dynamic psychotherapy in controlled trials to date has hardly been impressive, it is not clear that any of these trials have operationalized the approach in a manner consistent with what is done by knowledgeable practitioners.

At this time, it would be premature to say that dynamic psychotherapy is not effective in the treatment of depression, but there is little existing evidence to support its use. Although the dynamic psychotherapies, particularly the more recently developed time-limited varieties,[5,6] might ultimately prove to be of use in the treatment of some types of depression, the burden of proof rests with its advocates. There is currently little empirical justification for withholding either pharmacotherapy or electroconvulsive therapy (ECT) from patients suffering from severe affective disorders in favor of providing dynamic psychotherapy alone.[11]

MARITAL AND FAMILY SYSTEMS THERAPY

Systems theory suggests that the interplay of forces within a marital or family system can produce and maintain individual psychopathology.[12] Traditional approaches to marital or family systems therapy for depression have been designed to provide insight into these processes or to restructure the existing system in the service of providing symptom relief. Implicit in this notion is the expectation that failure to deal with the problem at a systems level will result in the emergence of distress in some other family member. More recent approaches to family systems therapy have been less inclined to view the basic psychopathology as a consequence of a pathological marital or family system, but have emphasized the role of conflict in important relationships in maintaining or exacerbating the expression of symptomatology. Interventions based on this modified perspective have emphasized the role of providing training in crisis resolution and stress management for families with a severely afflicted member.

To date, marital or family systems therapies have been tested in two controlled trials. In the first, Friedman found few differences between marital therapy versus amitriptyline pharmacotherapy in the treatment of depressed outpatients, although pharmacotherapy worked more rapidly and psychotherapy produced greater change in marital functioning.[13] Both advantages were retained by the combined condition. In the second, Clarkin et al. found that both bipolar and unipolar female inpatients showed superior response when family sessions for spouses and relatives was added to standard milieu treatment (including pharmacotherapy).[14] However, these advantages were maintained at an 18-month naturalistic follow-up among only the bipolar females, who also showed gains in measures of social functioning. Further, male patients (particularly the nonbipolar patients) actually showed poorer short- and long-term outcomes (both with respect to symptom status and social role functioning) in the combined condition than in standard treatment.

Clearly, additional studies are needed before a clear picture of the efficacy of marital and family therapy will be apparent. Friedman's study is among those older studies often cited to support the contention that psychotherapy influences social adjustment, but has little effect on symptoms of depression.[13] The presence of apparent gender (or polarity) effects in the work by Clarkin and colleagues suggests that much remains to be learned about just who is likely to benefit from such an intervention.[14] It would clearly be premature to attempt to provide specific indications for their use, although the suggestion by Clarkin and colleagues that family counseling might enhance the efficacy of pharmacological management for female bipolar patients is one of the first empirical demonstrations of any beneficial role for the psychosocial interventions in this population.

INTERPERSONAL PSYCHOTHERAPY

Interpersonal psychotherapy (IPT) is predicated on the notion that disturbances in important interpersonal relationships (or a deficit in the capacity to form those relationships) can play a role in initiating or maintaining clinical depression. As formulated by Klerman and colleagues, the approach is a neo-sullivanian (but nondynamic) intervention that focuses on current life situations and interpersonal relationships for the purpose of resolving problems in those areas and reducing levels of distress.[15] Unlike interventions based on systems theory, interpersonal psychotherapy typically is conducted with only the identified patient participating.

Interpersonal psychotherapy has been extensively tested in the less than two decades since it was first articulated. In the first such trial, Klerman and colleagues found that a forerunner of IPT enhanced social functioning among depressed female outpatients.[16] Although it was reported to be no more effective than a pill placebo in terms of reducing relapse following successful pharmacotherapy,[17] there was some evidence that, if not combined with a pill placebo, interpersonal counseling approached the efficacy of either pharmacotherapy alone or combined treatment.[10]

In a subsequent trial, Weissman and colleagues found IPT comparable to amitriptyline alone (with each superior to a minimal contact control) and the combination of drugs and IPT superior to either single modality alone in the treatment of depressed outpatients.[18] Pharmacotherapy was associated with a rapid remission in vegetative symptoms, whereas IPT had a greater but somewhat delayed effect on mood and interest.[19] Endogenous patients were more likely to respond to pharmacotherapy than interpersonal psychotherapy.[20] Psychotherapy was not associated with any differential risk for relapse across a 1-year follow-up period, although patients previously treated with interpersonal psychotherapy did evidence greater gains in social functioning by the end of that follow-up period.[21]

In the recent National Institute of Mental Health (NIMH) Treatment of Depression Collaborative Research Program (TDCRP), interpersonal psychotherapy, like imipramine psychotherapy, was found to be superior to pill placebo in the treatment of severely depressed outpatients (cognitive therapy was intermediate and not significantly different from any of the other modalities).[22] No differences were evident among the less severely depressed outpatients and there was little evidence of any reduction of risk following successful treatment.[23]

Finally, Frank and colleagues found that maintenance interpersonal psychotherapy reduced risk for recurrence among recovered depressed outpatients.[24] However, maintenance interpersonal psychotherapy was less effective in that regard than was maintenance pharmacotherapy and appeared to confer little additional protection when added to that modality.

On the whole, interpersonal psychotherapy has generally performed well in controlled comparisons. It appears to be superior to control conditions and comparable to tricyclic pharmacotherapy with respect to the treatment of the acute episode, with some indication that combined treatment may be superior to either modality alone. It appears to be more likely to produce changes in social functioning than pharmacotherapy alone. However, although it does appear to have some prophylactic capacity, it does not appear to be as effective as continuation or maintenance pharmacotherapy.

Interpersonal psychotherapy appears to be appropriate for most depressed outpatients. At least one study has suggested that it may be less effective than pharmacotherapy alone with endogenous depressions,[20] but it is not clear that this finding has been replicated in the larger NIMH TDCRP.[22] Although it might appear by its nature to be most appropriate for those patients who have clear difficulties in their interpersonal relationships, it is sufficiently broadly defined so as to be appropriate for virtually any depressed individual. In most respects, interpersonal psychotherapy is a prototype of the more successful, targeted psychosocial interventions that have been developed in the last two decades.

BEHAVIOR THERAPY

Behavioral theories of depression typically emphasize the role of insufficient reinforcement in the etiology and maintenance of the disorder.[25] Insufficient reinforcement can be either the consequence of a skills deficit (which renders the individual incapable of eliciting available reinforcement from the environment) or of a nonresponsive environment. Interventions based on contingency management or social skills training[26] have predominated. Closely

related is a self-control approach, which views depression as a consequence of a deficit in self-reinforcement.[27] Although self-control therapy contains some cognitive elements, it is typically classified as a behavioral intervention.

McLean and Hakstian found behavior therapy, based on contingency management procedures, superior to tricyclic pharmacotherapy and several control conditions.[28] However, questions have been raised about the adequacy of the pharmacotherapy.[29] Hersen et al. found no differences among combined treatment involving behavioral social skills training, behavioral social skills training plus a pill placebo, pharmacotherapy alone, and dynamic therapy plus a pill placebo, either at the end of 12 weeks of active treatment or following 6 months of additional maintenance.[30] Social skills training (either alone or in combination) was associated with greater improvement in social functioning than was pharmacotherapy alone.[31] Wilson found no differences between combined treatment, behavior therapy (with pill placebo), pharmacotherapy alone, and pill placebo alone either at the end of 8 weeks or after a 6-month follow-up, although pharmacotherapy was associated with more rapid responses.[32] Finally, Roth and colleagues found no differences between combined treatment including self-control therapy versus self-control therapy alone, either at the end of 12 weeks of active treatment or after a 3-month follow-up.[33]

On the whole, the controlled studies involving behavior therapy have been too few and too weak to serve as the basis for any firm conclusions. Significant differences have been few, even relative to control conditions, and open to multiple interpretations even when evident. Several of the studies have relied on community volunteers, rather than bona fide clinical populations. At the same time, response was more rapid to combined treatment than to behavior therapy alone in two of the three trials,[32,33] whereas skills training was associated with greater improvement in interpersonal functioning in the only trial in which it was assessed.[31] Finally, there was no indication of any preventive effect for behavior therapy (either alone or in combination) in any of the trials, although the brevity of the follow-ups and reliance on cross-sectional assessments may well have precluded finding any such effect even if it did exist.

At this point, it would be premature to speculate about the indications for behavior therapy. Not only has there been no evidence of any differential response as a function of subtype of depression in any of the existing trials, the larger question still remains as to whether the approach can be said to be clinically effective in any general sense. At the same time, behavioral interventions are integral components of the cognitive interventions and do lend themselves to application to more severely depressed patients. Whether they can be said to be clinically effective, and for whom, will have to await further controlled clinical trials.

COGNITIVE THERAPY

Beck and colleagues have put forward a cognitive theory of depression which suggests that the way an individual interprets life events has a profound effect on his or her affective and behavioral responses to those events.[34] Individuals who adopt maladaptive information processing strategies in the face of negative life events are at particular risk for depression. This propensity is manifested by the emergence of beliefs about the self, the world, and the future that interfere with adaptive functioning in the face of stress.

Cognitive therapy is predicated on the notion that the systematic correction of those problems in thinking can reduce dysphoric affect and facilitate efforts to cope behaviorally.[34] In cognitive therapy, the client is trained to identify his or her beliefs and their relations to both affect and behavior, and to systematically evaluate their accuracy by means of both the application of reason and empirical hypothesis testing. As previously noted, behavioral interventions play an important role in cognitive therapy, particularly in the early sessions and with more severely depressed patients, so that cognitive therapy might more accurately be considered a cognitive-behavioral intervention.

Cognitive therapy has generally fared well in comparisons to tricyclic pharmacotherapy, but many of these studies have been criticized on methodological grounds.[2,29] Rush and colleagues found cognitive therapy superior to imipramine pharmacotherapy after 12 weeks of active treatment, but discontinued medication 2 weeks before the post-treatment evaluation.[35] Blackburn and colleagues found both cognitive therapy and combined treatment superior to tricyclic pharmacotherapy in a general practice sample (no differences were observed in a psychiatric outpatient sample), but had such poor response to drugs in the general practice sample as to call into question the adequacy with which it was implemented.[36] Murphy and colleagues and Hollon and colleagues found no differences between cognitive therapy and tricyclic pharmacotherapy in studies that appeared to provide adequate pharmacotherapy.[37,38] Although these latter two studies would appear to suggest at least comparability to tricyclic pharmacotherapy, the absence of pill-placebo controls precludes determining whether the samples were truly drug responsive.

Cognitive therapy's worst performance to date has come in the NIMH TDCRP, the only such trial to include a placebo control.[22] In that trial, although cognitive therapy was not significantly less effective than either imipramine pharmacotherapy or interpersonal psychotherapy, it was the only one of the three active interventions which was not demonstrably superior to pill placebo among more severely depressed outpatients. This project, the most ambitious yet conducted, might suggest a lesser efficacy for cognitive therapy than had previously been evident. At the same time, other similar trials have noted no particular advantage for tricyclic pharmacotherapy over cognitive therapy among more severely depressed outpatients[38] and questions have been raised regarding the adequacy with which cognitive therapy was implemented, particularly with respect to the frequency of supervision provided, in the NIMH trial.[2] Clearly, additional research is needed which incorporates the rigor of a placebo control while simultaneously ensuring that cognitive therapy is adequately implemented before any firm conclusions can be drawn about either the efficacy of cognitive therapy or the indications for its use.

There are some indications that combined cognitive-pharmacotherapy might be superior to either modality alone.[2] However, these differences have typically not been large in magnitude and have only rarely met conventional levels of statistical significance. Among the studies already described, only Blackburn and colleagues found a significant advantage for combined treatment over either single modality, and that only in the sample (the general practice patients) that received pharmacotherapy of questionable quality.[36] Teasdale and colleagues and Miller and colleagues both found an advantage for combined treatment relative to "treatment-as-usual" conditions involving pharmacotherapy (Miller et al. in an inpatient sample), but in each instance, only some of the patients in the "treatment-as-usual" conditions received medications.[39,40] Beck and colleagues found no difference between combined treatment versus cognitive therapy alone, but provided only marginal pharmacotherapy,[41] whereas Covi and Lipman found no differences between combined treatment and cognitive therapy alone, both provided in a group format (as previously noted, each outperformed a dynamic intervention of questionable quality).[9]

What does appear to be more robust is cognitive therapy's apparent capacity to reduce subsequent risk following successful treatment. The majority of the studies just described have conducted naturalistic follow-ups of up to 2 years duration following the acute treatment comparisons. In the majority of these trials, prior cognitive therapy, either alone or in combination with medication, has typically reduced rates of subsequent relapse by over 50 per cent relative to medication discontinuation.[23,42–45] In the only trial in which they have been directly compared, prior cognitive therapy did at least as well as continuation medication in preventing subsequent relapse.[45]

Although encouraging, it is by no means certain that cognitive therapy has any true preventive effect. In many of these studies, relapse was defined as either renewed symptomaticity or return to treatment. In two studies, differences between the conditions were largely limited to return to treatment[23,44] and in one other study no differentiation between the two indices was presented.[43] It is possible that receiving cognitive therapy may render remitted patients less likely to seek *unnecessary* additional treatment without actually reducing risk for subsequent relapse.

Further, these naturalistic follow-ups have typically studied only a fraction of the samples initially randomized to treatment. Since only about 70 per cent of all patients initially assigned actually complete treatment and only about 70 per cent of those treatment completers actually respond, the samples of responding completers studied in these follow-ups typically represent only about half of the sample initially randomized. With such massive attrition, it is quite possible that treatment has acted as a "differential sieve." That is, if patients with more severe disorders are more likely to complete or respond to pharmacotherapy than cognitive therapy, then the sample of responding completers entering the follow-up would contain a higher proportion of high-risk patients previously treated with pharmacotherapy than with cognitive therapy. Thus, cognitive therapy's apparent preventive effect might be nothing more than an artifact of differential retention.

Finally, it has become customary to distinguish between *relapse*, the return of symptoms associated with the treated episode, and *recurrence*, the onset of a wholly new episode. Indeed, Frank and colleagues have recently proposed using the term *remission* to describe those patients in whom manifest symptoms have been ameliorated without any resolution in the underlying episode, and reserving the term *recovery* for those patients in whom the underlying episode has actually resolved.[46] In a review of the continuation literature, Prien and Kupfer suggested that pharmacologically-treated patients demonstrate at least 4 months free of symptoms before medications are discontinued,[47] and Hollon and colleagues noted that this period of elevated risk for relapse coincides with the length of the period needed for the episode to run its course if left untreated.[48] Given that the bulk of the naturalistic follow-ups involving cognitive therapy have involved short-term treatment (typically 3–to–5 months) and relatively brief follow-ups (12–to–24 months), it is quite likely that what has been documented has largely involved differences in relapse, rather than recurrence. Thus, even if cognitive therapy's apparent advantage over prior pharmacotherapy were to prove to be genuine, there is no guarantee that it would extend to the prevention of new episodes.

CONCLUSIONS

Several of these newly articulated interventions, particularly interpersonal psychotherapy and cognitive therapy, appear to approach the efficacy of tricyclic pharmacotherapy, the current standard of treatment. There are as yet unsubstantiated indications that combined treatment may enhance the overall rate of response even further. Even if combined treatment were no more effective than pharmacotherapy alone in reducing acute symptoms, combined treatment might still be preferable, since each single modality appears to possess advantages not found in the other. Pharmacotherapy appears to work more rapidly than most of the psychosocial interventions, interpersonal psychotherapy (and possibly some of the marital and behavioral interventions) appears to produce greater change in social functioning, and cognitive therapy appears to be associated with a reduction in subsequent risk. The available literature suggests that each of these advantages are maintained when drugs and psychotherapy are combined.

It is less clear whether other types of psychosocial interventions have a useful role to play in the treatment of depression. There is little good evidence that traditional dynamic psychotherapy has much to contribute, but existing studies have been particularly poorly done and no effort has yet been made to test some of its newer short-term modifications. Behavior therapy has similarly not been all that adequately tested, but it has not fared poorly in those tests that have been conducted. If any intervention is likely to have an immediate impact on very severe depressions, it is likely to be behavior therapy. The newer marital and family systems interventions are just beginning to be explored, but initial indications suggest that they may prove to be particularly useful adjunctive interventions for bipolar and severe unipolar populations.

Aside from the exceptions just noted, the bulk of the existing literature has focused on nonpsychotic, nonbipolar depressed outpatients. Whether the psychosocial interventions have any particular advantage to confer beyond the nonspecific benefits afforded by supportive clinical management for more severe populations (e.g., psychotic, bipolar, or inpatient depression) remains an open question, but it is clear that pharmacotherapy and somatic therapy remain the treatments of choice for those populations.

Finally, it should be clear that conclusions regarding the efficacy of the pharmacotherapies can be drawn with far greater certainty than can conclusions regarding the psychotherapies. Controlled trials involving the former number in the hundreds, whereas controlled trials involving the latter probably number less than 25. Clearly, the pharmacological interventions have been subjected to far more rigorous scrutiny than have the psychotherapies. Although this may, in part, reflect a greater complexity in researching the psychosocial interventions, it may also reflect a willingness to accept unsubstantiated clinical experience in lieu of more rigorous standards of proof on the part of advocates of these latter approaches. Recent trends in the research literature suggest that this may well be changing, but it is an unfortunate tendency that has retarded the acquisition of knowledge and slowed progress in the development of effective clinical interventions.

SUMMARY

It is clear that considerable progress has been made over the last two decades in developing and testing psychosocial interventions specifically targeted for the treatment of depression. Interpersonal psychotherapy and cognitive therapy appear to be particularly promising interventions, and there is reason to think that a variety of other interventions may prove to have merit as well. Although the existing research literature is not as extensive and rigorous as might be desired, there are clear indications of a qualitative improvement in that regard as well. Although the various pharmacological and somatic interventions remain the standard of treatment, particularly for the more severe depressions, there is growing evidence that the psychosocial interventions may have a useful role to play, either as alternative or complementary interventions in the outpatient depressions and as adjunctive treatments for the more severe disorders.

REFERENCES

1. Hollon SD, Beck AT: Psychotherapy and drug therapy: Comparison and combinations. In Garfield SL, Bergin AE, eds. Handbook of Psychotherapy and Behavior Change: An Empirical Analysis. 2nd ed. New York: John Wiley, 1978:437.
2. Hollon SD, Shelton RC, Loosen PT: Cognitive therapy in relation to pharmacotherapy for depression. J Consult Clin Psychol 59:88–99, 1991.
3. Hollon SD, Haman K: Combined drugs and psychotherapy for depression: A review and methodological critique. In Blumenthal SJ, ed. Combined Psychopharmacologic and Psychosocial Treatments for Psychiatric Disorders. Washington DC: American Psychiatric Press, in press.
4. Karasu TB: Toward a clinical model of psychotherapy for depression. I. Systematic comparison of three psychotherapies. Am J Psychiatry 147:133–147, 1990.
5. Strupp HH, Binder JL: Psychotherapy in a New Key: A Guide to Time-limited Dynamic Psychotherapy. New York: Basic Books, 1984.
6. Luborsky L: Principles of Psychoanalytic Psychotherapy: A Manual for Supportive-Expressive Treatment. New York: Basic Books, 1984.
7. Daneman EA: Imipramine in office management of depressive reactions (a double-blind study). Dis Nerv Syst 22:213–217, 1961.
8. Covi L, Lipman RS, Derogatis LR, et al: Drugs and group psychotherapy in neurotic depression. Am J Psychiatry 131:191–198, 1974.
9. Covi L, Lipman RS: Cognitive-behavioral group psychotherapy combined with imipramine in major depression. Psychopharmacol Bull 23:173–176, 1987.
10. Hollon SD, DeRubeis RJ: Placebo-psychotherapy combinations: Inappropriate representations of psychotherapy in drug psychotherapy comparative trials. Psychol Bull 90:467–477, 1981.
11. Klerman GL: The psychiatric patient's right to effective treatment: Implications of Osheroff v. Chestnut Lodge. Am J Psychiatry 147:409–418, 1990.
12. Ackerman N: The Psychodynamics of Family Life. New York: Basic Books, 1958.
13. Friedman A: Interaction of drug therapy with marital therapy in depressed patients. Arch Gen Psychiatry 32:619–637, 1975.
14. Clarkin JF, Glick ID, Haas GL, et al: A randomized clinical trial of inpatient family intervention: V. Results for affective disorders. J Affective Disord 18:17–28, 1990.
15. Klerman GL, Weissman MM, Rounsaville B, et al: Interpersonal Psychotherapy of Depression. New York: Basic Books, 1984.
16. Weissman MM, Klerman GL, Paykel ES, et al: Treatment effects on the social adjustment of depressed patients. Arch Gen Psychiatry 30:771–778, 1974.
17. Klerman GL, DiMascio A, Weissman M, et al: Treatment of depression by drugs and psychotherapy. Am J Psychiatry 131:186–191, 1974.
18. Weissman MM, Prusoff BA, DiMascio A, et al: The efficacy of drugs and psychotherapy in the treatment of acute depressive disorders. Am J Psychiatry 136:555–558, 1979.
19. DiMascio A, Weissman MM, Prusoff BA, et al: Differential symptom reduction by drugs and psychotherapy in acute depression. Arch Gen Psychiatry 36:1450–1456, 1979.
20. Prusoff BA, Weissman MM, Klerman GL, et al: Research diagnostic criteria subtypes of depression: Their role as predictors of differential response to psychotherapy and drug treatment. Arch Gen Psychiatry 37:796–801, 1980.
21. Weissman MM, Klerman GL, Prusoff BA, et al: Depressed outpatients: Results one year after treatment with drugs and/or interpersonal psychotherapy. Arch Gen Psychiatry 38:51–55, 1981.
22. Elkin I, Shea MT, Watkins JT, et al: NIMH Treatment of Depression Collaborative Research Program. I. General effectiveness of treatments. Arch Gen Psychiatry 46:971–982, 1989.
23. Shea MT, Elkin I, Imber SD, et al: Course of depressive symptoms over follow-up: Findings from the National Institute of Mental Health Treatment of Depression Collaborative Research Program. Manuscript submitted for publication, 1990.
24. Frank E, Kupfer DJ, Perel JM, et al: Three-year outcomes for maintenance therapies in recurrent depression. Arch Gen Psychiatry 47:1093–1099, 1990.
25. Lewinsohn PM: A behavioral approach to depression. In Friedman RM, Katz MM, eds. The Psychology of Depression: Contemporary Theory and Research. Washington, DC: Winston/Wiley, 1974:157.
26. Becker RE, Heimberg RG, Bellack AS: Social Skills Training Treatment for Depression. New York: Pergamon Press, 1987.
27. Rehm LP: A self-control model of depression. Behav Ther 8:787–804, 1977.
28. McLean PD, Hakstian AR: Clinical depression: Comparative efficacy of outpatient treatments. J Consult Clin Psychol 47:818–836, 1979.
29. Meterissian GB, Bradwejn J: Comparative studies on the efficacy of psychotherapy, pharmacotherapy, and their combination in depression: Was adequate pharmacotherapy provided? J Clin Psychopharmacol 9:334–339, 1989.
30. Hersen M, Bellack AS, Himmelhoch JM, et al: Effects of social skill training, amitriptyline, and psychotherapy in unipolar depressed women. Behav Ther 15:21–40, 1984.
31. Bellack AS, Hersen M, Himmelhoch JM: A comparison of social-skills training, pharmacotherapy and psychotherapy for depression. Behav Res Ther 21:101–107, 1983.
32. Wilson PH: Combined pharmacological and behavioral treatment of depression. Behav Res Ther 20:173–184, 1982.
33. Roth D, Bielski R, Jones M, et al: A comparison of self-control therapy and combined self-control therapy and antidepressant medication in the treatment of depression. Behav Ther 13:133–144,1982.
34. Beck AT, Rush AJ, Shaw BF, et al: Cognitive Therapy of Depression: A Treatment Manual. New York: Guilford Press, 1979.

35. Rush AJ, Beck AT, Kovacs M, et al: Comparative efficacy of cognitive therapy versus pharmacotherapy in outpatient depressives. Cog Ther Res 1:17–37, 1977.

36. Blackburn IM, Bishop S, Glen AIM, et al: The efficacy of cognitive therapy in depression: A treatment trial using cognitive therapy and pharmacotherapy, each alone and in combination. Br J Psychiatry 139:181–189, 1981.

37. Murphy GE, Simons AD, Wetzel RD, et al: Cognitive therapy and pharmacotherapy, singly and together in the treatment of depression. Arch Gen Psychiatry 41:33–41, 1984.

38. Hollon SD, DeRubeis RJ, Evans MD, et al: Cognitive therapy, pharmacotherapy, and combined cognitive-pharmacotherapy in the treatment of depression. Manuscript submitted for publication, 1991.

39. Teasdale JD, Fennell MJV, Hibbert GA, et al: Cognitive therapy for major depressive disorder in primary care. Br J Psychiatry 144:400–406, 1984.

40. Miller IW, Norman WH, Keitner GI, et al: Cognitive-behavioral treatment of depressed inpatients. Behav Ther 20:25–47, 1989.

41. Beck AT, Hollon SD, Young JE, et al: Treatment of depression with cognitive therapy and amitriptyline. Arch Gen Psychiatry 42:142–148, 1985.

42. Kovacs M, Rush AT, Beck AT, et al: Depressed outpatients treated with cognitive therapy or pharmacotherapy: A one-year follow-up. Arch Gen Psychiatry 38:33–39, 1981.

43. Blackburn IM, Eunson KM, Bishop S: A two-year naturalistic follow-up of depressed patients treated with cognitive therapy, pharmacotherapy and a combination of both. J Affective Disord 10:67–75, 1986.

44. Simons AD, Murphy GE, Levine JE, et al: Cognitive therapy and pharmacotherapy for depression: Sustained improvement over one year. Arch Gen Psychiatry 43:43–49, 1986.

45. Evans MD, Hollon SD, DeRubeis RJ, et al: Differential relapse following cognitive therapy, pharmacotherapy, and combined cognitive-pharmacotherapy for depression. Manuscript submitted for publication, 1991.

46. Frank E, Prien R, Jarrett RB, et al: Conceptualization and rationale for consensus definitions of terms in major depressive disorder: Response, remission, recovery, relapse, and recurrence. Arch Gen Psychiatry 48:851–855, 1991.

47. Prien RF, Kupfer DJ: Continuation drug therapy for major depressive episodes: How long should it be maintained? Am J Psychiatry 143:18–23, 1986.

48. Hollon SD, Evans MD, DeRubeis RJ: Preventing relapse following treatment for depression: Cognitive mediation and the implications of differential risk. In Ingram RE, ed. Psychological Aspects of Depression. New York: Guilford Press, 1990:117.

39

MOOD STABILIZERS: A Review

JAMES W. JEFFERSON, M.D.

To discuss bipolar disorder and its treatments without immediate reference to the encyclopedic text of Goodwin and Jamison would be heresy.[1] This 1990 publication provides a comprehensive overview and in-depth examination of all aspects of the illness with extensive and remarkably up-to-date references. Since the field is expanding rapidly, a service to be considered for timely, "cutting-edge" information is the Lithium Information Center,[a] a comprehensive computer-based information service on lithium and its alternatives available to professionals and lay persons.

Bipolar disorder is a mood disorder characterized by one or more manic or hypomanic episodes, usually in association with episodes of depression. Since it is usually a recurrent condition, treatment strategies must deal not only with acute mania and

depression, but also with the prevention of future episodes. In addition, the spectrum of bipolar disorder includes conditions such as cyclothymia, schizoaffective disorder, bipolar II disorder (recurrent episodes of major depression and hypomania), and mixed or dysphoric states in which manic and depressive symptoms coexist. Finally, organic mood disorders (". . . a prominent and persistent depressed, elevated, or expansive mood, resembling either a Manic Episode or a Major Depressive Episode, that is due to a specific organic factor")[2] must be considered part of a differential diagnosis.

Lithium

Lithium is the king of mood stabilizers against which challengers to the throne must be compared. It is the only drug with Food and Drug Administration (FDA) labeling approval for ". . . the treatment of the manic episodes of manic-depressive illness and for maintenance therapy to prevent or diminish

[a] Department of Psychiatry, University of Wisconsin, 600 Highland Avenue, Madison, WI 53792, (608) 263-6171.

the intensity of subsequent episodes in those manic-depressive patients with a history of mania" (PDR, page 2110).[3]

Mania

The antimanic effectiveness of lithium has been established in comparison with placebo, antipsychotic drugs, and anticonvulsants.[1] The placebo-controlled lithium studies involved a total of only 116 patients, were a crossover design, and involved relatively brief treatment periods. Their outcomes, nonetheless, were consistently positive, with an overall response rate of 78 per cent. Since lithium has a slow onset of action, acute mania, especially when severe, usually requires the adjunctive use of a neuroleptic or a benzodiazepine or both for more immediate behavior control.

Depression

While lithium is not FDA approved as an antidepressant, most studies have found it to be more effective than placebo and as effective as tricyclics.[1] The response rate in bipolar depression (79 per cent) was more robust than in unipolar depression (36 per cent). Small sample sizes and other study inconsistencies leave the antidepressant effectiveness of lithium somewhat less than firmly established. Nonetheless, lithium alone or in combination with a traditional antidepressant is often recommended as the treatment of first choice for bipolar depression. While tricyclics have been the most commonly used antidepressants, there is growing evidence that other drugs may be more effective (e.g., monoamine oxidase inhibitors, fluoxetine, bupropion). Concerns with the use of antidepressants (especially alone) in the treatment of bipolar depression include drug-induced mania and the induction of rapid cycling.

Maintenance

The effectiveness of long-term lithium for preventing recurrences of mania and depression is well established. According to Goodwin and Jamison: "That lithium has profound prophylactic effects in bipolar illness is now incontrovertible."[1] They cite the results of ten double-blind placebo-controlled studies in which the overall percentage of patients relapsing on lithium was 34 per cent as compared to 81 per cent on placebo.[1] Lithium reduces frequency, duration, and intensity of both manic and depressive episodes with a somewhat more complete effect in mania. Most patients who benefit have a less than complete response, and a certain amount of "fire-fighting" must be done to deal with manic and depressive breakthroughs. In addition, there is growing concern that bipolar patients of today are different from those of yesteryear, whose robust response to lithium prophylaxis was "incontrovertible." For unclear reasons, which may involve changes in the intrinsic nature of the illness, differences in patient selection, and the effects of prior treatments, there appears to be an increasing number of lithium nonresponders (see later in chapter). Nonetheless, lithium remains the drug of choice for the long-term treatment of bipolar disorder.

Using Lithium

Prior to initiating treatment with lithium, laboratory studies of kidney and thyroid function should be obtained. Lithium is excreted almost entirely by the kidney and it can also have adverse effects on kidney function. Thyroid disorders can cause mood disturbances and lithium can cause thyroid dysfunction. Consequently, measurement of serum creatinine and sensitive thyroid-stimulating hormone (TSH) should be an essential part of a prelithium evaluation. Depending on the age and medical history of the patient and the preferences of the treating physician, additional testing may include complete blood count (CBC), chemistry panel, electrolytes, more complete studies of renal and thyroid function, and an electrocardiogram (ECG).

In the United States, lithium carbonate is available in 150-, 300-, 450-, and 600-mg dosage forms (some of these are standard, and some are slow or controlled-release preparations). Lithium citrate syrup contains the same amount of lithium in 5 ml as does 300 mg of the carbonate. Regardless of form, lithium is usually administered in divided doses (although single daily dosing of at least moderate amounts is both effective and safe), with the ultimate dose determined by clinical response and serum lithium level. To be meaningful, serum lithium levels must be determined on blood samples drawn in the morning as close as possible to 12 hours after the last dose. In addition, at least 4 to 5 days on a given dose is necessary before steady-state blood levels are attained.

The dose of lithium carbonate used for acute mania usually ranges from 1200 to 2100 mg/day with serum levels of 0.9 to 1.2 mEq/liter. Higher levels may sometimes be necessary, but intolerable side effects often limit this approach. The response rate of mania to levels below 0.9 mEq/liter is less substantial. Considerably less is known about the correlation between dose, blood level, and the antidepressant effect of lithium, but in general a clinical trial should last at least several weeks with serum levels in the range of 0.8 to 1.2 mEq/liter. Maintenance therapy with lithium usually requires a total daily dose of 900 to 1500 mg of lithium carbonate with serum lithium levels in the range of 0.6 to 1.0 mEq/liter. The lower the maintenance level, the fewer the side effects, but the higher the relapse rate. In a 3-year prospective study, Gelenberg et al. found that patients maintained in the range of 0.8 to 1.0 mEq/liter (average 0.83 mEq/liter) had a 2.6 times lower risk of relapse than those maintained between 0.4 and 0.6 mEq/liter (average 0.54 mEq/liter).[4] Unfortunately, the dropout rate from side effects and for administrative reasons was much greater in the higher level group.

In general, the elderly require lower doses to reach a given blood level and are often more sensitive to both side effects and toxicity. Once patients have been stabilized on lithium, the frequency of blood tests (lithium levels, kidney and thyroid function testing) can be reduced, and it is not uncommon to monitor every 3 to 4 months.

Side Effects and Toxicity

Most patients taking lithium have side effects. While it has been estimated that fewer than 20 per cent have no complaints, only about 30 per cent have complaints of moderate or greater severity.[5]

Neurological Effects

Complaints of nontoxic neurological effects from lithium are common, although it is often difficult to know if they are drug related, secondary to the illness itself, or coincidental. These include lack of spontaneity, reduced reactivity, intellectual inefficiency, memory problems, difficulty concentrating, and dysphoria. Treatment approaches include recognition and treatment of breakthrough depression and lithium-induced hypothyroidism, assessing the role of other medications, and a trial of lithium dosage reduction.

How creativity is altered by lithium varies greatly among patients, with some pleased that it improves, others dissatisfied with a decrease, and many unaware of a change. Subjective impressions and objective opinions may differ considerably when assessing the impact of lithium on creativity.

Lithium tremor occurs in 10 to 45 per cent of patients, resembles a physiological or benign essential tremor, and is aggravated during activities requiring fine-motor control. Tremor is more likely at higher serum lithium levels, in the elderly, when antidepressant drugs or caffeine (or both) are also used, and in the presence of anxiety. The tremor is benign, but should it worsen or generalize to involve areas other than the fingers and hands, lithium intoxication should be suspected. A benign tremor that is annoying and does not lessen over time is likely to improve with one or more of the following: dosage reduction, a slow-release preparation, restriction of caffeine intake, anxiety reduction, or the use of a β-blocker or primidone.

Other nontoxic neurological effects that have only rarely been attributed to lithium include extrapyramidal manifestations, peripheral neuropathy, worsening of myasthenia gravis, and benign intracranial hypertension (pseudotumor cerebri).

Lithium intoxication is primarily a neurotoxicity, although gastrointestinal symptoms, cardiac arrhythmias, and renal insufficiency may also occur. The severity of intoxication depends on the magnitude and duration of exposure together with individual susceptibility. While there have been clear-cut cases of intoxication at therapeutic levels (especially in the elderly), a serum level of 1.5 mEq/liter or higher is usually present. In general, acute overdoses are better tolerated than are gradual intoxications in which tissue saturation is greater and clinical manifestations resolve more slowly. In the latter, clinical improvement may lag many days behind the fall in the serum lithium level. Mild intoxications are characterized by coarse tremor, ataxia, dysarthria, and lethargy; whereas more severe intoxications include a worsening of these findings, progressive impairment of consciousness, disorientation, myoclonic jerks, and seizures. The therapeutic index of lithium is relatively narrow, and both death and permanent neurological damage (usually cerebellar) have occurred. Causes of lithium poisoning include excessive intake (deliberate or accidental), reduced excretion (kidney disease, low-salt diets, drug interactions), or reduced volume of distribution (dehydration or weight loss). Treatment of intoxication involves general supportive measures, reducing further drug absorption (activated charcoal is of no value, but a cation-exchange resin may help), and maximizing excretion. Milder intoxications in the presence of normal kidney function usually respond well to hydration. It is unclear whether forced diuresis is of added benefit. More severe intoxication, especially if renal function is compromised, should be treated with hemodialysis. Since lithium is chemically simple (an element with atomic number 3), has no metabolites, is not protein bound, and is water soluble, it is readily removed by dialysis. Following dialysis, the serum level may increase over several hours as reequilibration occurs between plasma and tissues.

Thyroid Effects

Lithium therapy increases the risk of euthyroid and hypothyroid goiter (about 6 per cent) and hypothyroidism (about 5 per cent). These problems can occur anytime during the course of therapy. For unclear reasons, women are at considerably greater risk for developing hypothyroidism. Mild increases of serum TSH usually normalize without treatment, whereas more extreme elevations usually evolve into clinical hypothyroidism unless treated with exogenous thyroxine. While monitoring thyroid function is considered an integral part of long-term lithium treatment, opinion varies with regard to testing at fixed intervals (e.g., every 6 or 12 months) or only when clinically indicated. Autoimmune thyroid disease does not appear to be caused by lithium, but its presence prior to treatment increases the likelihood of lithium-induced hypothyroidism. For this reason, some clinicians obtain antithyroid antibody titers (antithyroglobulin and antimicrosomal) prior to initiation of therapy.

Weight Gain

Approximately 20 per cent of patients gain an average of 10 kg during treatment with lithium. This problem tends to occur early in treatment and is more likely in patients with prior weight-control difficulties. While most weight gain is due to the complex metabolic effects of lithium, occasionally it is associated with lithium-induced hypothyroidism or excessive caloric intake in beverages consumed to combat dehydration from lithium-induced polyuria.

Hematological Effects

By stimulating granulocyte production, lithium may cause a mild leukocytosis of no clinical consequence. Leukopenia associated with carbamazepine use is less likely in the presence of lithium.

Cardiovascular Effects

Lithium often causes benign, reversible T-wave changes on the ECG. Lithium-induced sinus node dysfunction may be associated with bradyarrhythmias and syncopal episodes. While quite rare, this complication is a contraindication to continued lithium use unless a pacemaker is implanted. Lithium has no adverse effects on blood pressure.

Gastrointestinal Effects

Nausea is a common and usually transient complaint, especially during the initial phases of therapy. More severe gastrointestinal symptoms can be prodromata of lithium intoxication. An occasional patient is unable to tolerate lithium because of persistent diarrhea. Changing to a different preparation may be of benefit.

Renal Effects

Impaired renal concentrating ability occurs in 30 to 96 per cent of patients treated with lithium, whereas polyuria (24-hour urine volume over 3 liters) has been reported in as high as 40 per cent. Lithium inhibits the action of antidiuretic hormone (ADH) on renal adenylate cyclase. Mild polyuria is usually well tolerated, but a more substantial urine output places patients at risk for dehydration, interferes with sleep, is socially and vocationally compromising, and may be associated with poor nutrition and dental problems due to a predominately liquid diet. Measures that may minimize polyuria include (1) maintaining the lowest possible serum lithium level, (2) single daily dosage, (3) dietary potassium supplementation (currently investigational), and (4) the use of a thiazide or potassium-sparing diuretic or both. To avoid the hypokalemia often caused by thiazides, a potassium-sparing diuretic such as amiloride (5 to 10 mg b.i.d.) is suggested for initial treatment. Resistant conditions may respond to a combination of the two diuretics. These diuretics reduce renal lithium clearance so that lithium dosage reduction may be necessary to avoid unwanted increases in serum level.

There is some evidence that lithium causes mild morphological changes in the kidneys, but long-term studies of glomerular filtration rate suggest little, if any, deterioration over time. Nonetheless, exceptions may occur and longer term studies are needed; consequently, periodic monitoring of renal function is advised. Rarely, nephrotic syndrome occurs in association with lithium therapy.

Dermatological Effects

Acne and psoriasis may worsen during lithium therapy. While acne often responds to standard therapeutic interventions, it may be necessary to stop lithium before treatment of psoriasis can be effective.

Hair loss has been described during lithium therapy, and while uncommon, is a well-documented side effect. Why this occurs is unknown (most patients are not hypothyroid). Regrowth may or may not occur if lithium is continued.

Pregnancy

Lithium is in FDA pregnancy category D (there is positive evidence of human fetal risk, but potential benefits may warrant use in pregnancy) based on findings of a higher than expected incidence of cardiovascular malformation in babies exposed during the first trimester. Recent findings have challenged this conclusion. Nonetheless, it remains prudent to avoid exposure to lithium during the first trimester. As pregnancy progresses, maternal lithium requirements may vary, so that careful monitoring is necessary. The drug should be discontinued shortly before delivery to reduce the level in the newborn, but restarted shortly thereafter to minimize the risk of a postpartum affective episode. Although the amount of lithium reaching an infant in breast milk is small, breast-feeding is usually discouraged.

Drug Interactions

Clinically important interactions between lithium and other drugs have been substantiated. Whether there is a unique incompatibility between lithium and haloperidol will never be fully resolved. While most authorities feel that the judicious use of the combination is safe, the package insert for lithium carries a warning that an encephalopathy has occurred when lithium and haloperidol were used together.

Diuretic interactions with lithium vary with the class of drug. Xanthine and osmotic diuretics increase renal lithium clearance and decrease serum lithium levels. Thiazide and probably potassium-sparing diuretics do just the opposite. Loop diuretics generally do not alter serum lithium levels, although there have been case reports to the contrary.

Most nonsteroidal anti-inflammatory drugs (aspirin and sulindac are exceptions) reduce renal lithium clearance and may increase serum lithium level. Risk factors include advanced age, higher drug doses, and compromised renal function.

While angiotensin-converting enzyme (ACE) inhibitors do not consistently alter serum lithium levels,[6] there have been several case reports of lithium toxicity following the addition of an ACE inhibitor to a stable lithium regimen. Consequently, serum lithium levels should be carefully monitored if an ACE inhibitor is started or discontinued.

This discussion of interactions is not meant to be comprehensive. Detailed information can be obtained from the Lithium Information Center, regional drug information centers, and other publications.[7]

CARBAMAZEPINE

Effectiveness

The literature on carbamazepine (Tegretol and others) and its use in psychiatry is dwarfed by the data base for lithium. Nonetheless, carbamazepine is currently the best studied alternative to lithium.[8,9] Since many of the carbamazepine studies involved treatment-resistant patients, direct comparisons with lithium are limited.

Mania

According to Small: "There are now at least 13 double-blind, controlled trials of carbamazepine in the treatment of mania."[8] These include comparisons with placebo, lithium, and neuroleptics, but not yet with valproate. In brief, carbamazepine is an effective antimanic drug, with a favorable response occurring in about 60 per cent of patients. It is better than placebo, at least as good as neuroleptics (and with a better side-effects profile), and comparable to lithium (although direct comparisons in patients not previously treated with lithium are few).

Depression

Unlike lithium, the antidepressant effect of carbamazepine is not well established. Post et al.[10] found a response rate of 34 per cent in a group of unipolar and bipolar depressed patients. In a relatively treatment-resistant group of mostly unipolar patients, Small et al. (unpublished, but summarized in [9]) observed a 32 per cent response rate to carbamazepine alone or carbamazepine and lithium, but only a 13 per cent response to lithium alone. Lithium augmentation of carbamazepine in otherwise resistant depression was effective in 8 of 15 (53 per cent of patients).[11]

Maintenance

Five double-blind studies (one with oxcarbazepine) have found carbamazepine useful in maintenance treatment.[9] One was placebo-controlled, whereas the others were comparisons with lithium. Small sample sizes, mixed diagnoses, varying degrees of treatment resistance, and use of ancillary medications do not allow firm conclusions to be reached. Nonetheless, when these results are combined with those from open trials of variable design, there is consistent support for the usefulness of carbamazepine for long-term treatment.[12] Post et al.[13] noted a disturbing loss of prophylactic efficacy in 11 of 24 patients, and discuss concerns about "discontinuation-induced inefficacy" and "contingent tolerance." In summary, while carbamazepine appears to be an effective long-term mood stabilizer, definitive studies remain to be done.

Using Carbamazepine

Despite recognition that the risk of agranulocytosis and aplastic anemia is very low, baseline hematological testing is still recommended prior to starting carbamazepine. Both for baseline and periodic monitoring, truly conservative clinicians will follow package insert guidelines, while others will adopt standards of neurologists in their communities. The package insert for Tegretol brand of carbamazepine (PDR, pages 1015 to 1019)[3] advises: "Complete pretreatment blood counts, including platelets and possibly reticulocytes and serum iron . . . . Baseline and periodic monitoring of liver function . . . . Baseline and periodic complete urinalysis and BUN determinations." Interestingly, the package insert no longer has specific recommendations regarding periodic hematological testing but rather states: "If a patient in the course of treatment exhibits low or decreased white blood cell or platelet counts, the patient should be monitored closely."

In the United States, carbamazepine is available as 100 and 200 mg, scored tablets, and a 100 mg per 5 ml suspension. The drug is administered in divided dose (the effectiveness of single daily dosing has not been studied in psychiatry) starting with 100 to 200 mg b.i.d. with appropriate modifications for age, associated illness, and possible drug interactions. Dosage is gradually increased until symptoms are controlled, side effects become troublesome, or blood levels become excessive. Therapeutic ranges have not been established for psychiatric indications; rather, the usual adult serum level in neurology (4 to 12 μg/ml) has been adopted. Like lithium, blood levels are determined on morning samples drawn before the first dose of the day. Carbamazepine induces its own metabolism (autoinduction) and there may be a decrease in serum level during the first few weeks of treatment. The dose of carbamazepine necessary to attain a given blood level varies widely among individuals.

Side Effects and Toxicity

Neurological Effects

Neurological complaints are common and represent half of all reported carbamazepine side effects.[5] They include drowsiness, dizziness, diplopia, blurred vision, ataxia, and nystagmus. They usually occur early in treatment, often resolve over time, and can be minimized by following the principle of "start low and go slow."

Overdose

Carbamazepine is structurally similar to tricyclic antidepressants and overdose manifestations are similar (although the lethality of carbamazepine relative to tricyclics has not been established). Common findings are neurological (coma, abnormal movements, and seizures), cardiovascular (hypotension, heart block, and other arrhythmias), and respiratory (depression). There is no specific treatment for carbamazepine intoxication, but measures such as lavage, activated charcoal, cathartics (controversial), and supportive medical and nursing care are recommended. Hemoperfusion may be of value.[14]

Thyroid Effects

Thyroid effects of carbamazepine are unlikely to be of clinical importance. Statistically significant decreases in serum levels of T_3 and T_4 occur but tend to remain within the range of normal and serum TSH levels do not increase. Routine thyroid function testing is not necessary. Whether the combination of lithium and carbamazepine increases the risk of lithium-induced hypothyroidism is not known.

Hematological Effects

The spectre of death from aplastic anemia or agranulocytosis hovers over patients receiving carbamazepine, but the rarity of such events is quite reassuring. Aplastic anemia from carbamazepine occurs at a rate of about two per million per year while agranulocytosis is found in six per million per year. These events are idiosyncratic and, hence, unpredictable. A more benign leukopenia occurs transiently in about 10 per cent of patients and persists in about 2 per cent. While recommendations vary, one set of guidelines suggests that total WBC levels below 2500 to 3000/μl or neutrophiles below 1500/μl be considered reason for drug discontinuation. Thrombocytopenia occurs in about 2 per cent of patients and may present clinically as petechiae, epistaxis, or easy bruising. Platelet counts below 100,000/μl are cause for concern, although improvement occurs rapidly once the drug is stopped.

The frequency with which hematological parameters are monitored varies with the stage of treatment (more often in the beginning) and the conservativeness of the physician. A practical approach would be to adopt the schedule used by neurologists in the community.

Cardiovascular Effects

Unlike tricyclic antidepressants, therapeutic amounts of carbamazepine have little, if any, effect on blood pressure. Its arrhythmogenic potential does not appear great, although there have been reports of sinus node dysfunction and atrioventricular block. These problems are more likely to occur in predisposed individuals, especially the elderly with coexisting cardiac disorders.

Gastrointestinal Effects

Transient complaints of nausea are common, and vomiting occasionally occurs early in treatment, especially if dosage is increased too rapidly. Taking the medication with meals may be helpful.

Hepatotoxicity has been attributed to carbamazepine. While mild increases in liver function tests are common, they often resolve despite continued treatment. Increases above two to three times normal should be reason to consider stopping the drug.

Severe, sometimes fatal, hepatotoxicity is rare, unpredictable, and usually occurs during the first month of treatment. It tends to be cholestatic although hepatocellular hepatitis has also been reported. Clinical symptoms suggestive of hepatitis should be evaluated promptly with physical examination and liver function studies.

Hyponatremic Effects

Carbamazepine causes hyponatremia by either directly or indirectly enhancing the effect of antidiuretic hormone on the kidney, thus impairing free-water clearance. About 20 per cent of patients taking carbamazepine have a mild decrease in serum sodium (130 to 135 mmol/liter), while lower levels are far less common. Factors which increase the risk of severe hyponatremia include advanced age, higher carbamazepine serum levels, lower initial sodium levels, and the use of diuretics. While routine monitoring of the serum electrolytes is not necessary, symptoms suggestive of hyponatremia (such as lethargy, weakness, confusion, or seizures) should be promptly evaluated.

Dermatological Effects

While rare, carbamazepine-associated life-threatening dermatological conditions such as Stevens-Johnson syndrome, exfoliative dermatitis, and toxic epidermal necrolysis have occurred. In such cases, drug discontinuation is essential and rechallenge is not advised. Mild, benign rashes have been described in about 3 per cent of patients taking carbamazepine.

Pregnancy

Carbamazepine teratogenicity was reported by Jones et al. to consist of cranial facial defects (11 per cent), fingernail hypoplasia (26 per cent), and developmental delay (20 per cent).[15] Also, the risk of spina bifida from in utero exposure to carbamazepine is about 1 per cent (13.7 times greater than in the general population).[16] The drug is in FDA pregnancy category C (animal studies have shown adverse effects, but well-controlled studies in humans are lacking), which is one level less ominous than for lithium and valproate. Carbamazepine appears in breast milk, but whether there are adverse consequences from breast-feeding is not known.

Drug Interactions

Not only does carbamazepine interact with itself (it induces its own metabolism) but it interacts in clinically important ways with a number of other drugs. For example, substantial increases in carbamazepine blood levels occur during treatment with fluoxetine (Prozac), cimetidine (but not ranitidine), propoxyphene (Darvon), danazol (a synthetic androgen), the calcium channel blockers verapamil and diltiazem (but not nifedipine), erythromycin, and isoniazid.[17]

Carbamazepine, on the other hand, causes a decrease in blood level of haloperidol (by as much as two- to threefold), valproate, oral contraceptives (with breakthrough bleeding and contraception failure), alprazolam and clonazepam, theophylline, and tricyclic antidepressants. It is likely that other interactions occur but have not been recognized.

VALPROATE

Effectiveness

Interest in valproate as a mood stabilizer has increased greatly in recent years, and ongoing research promises to more clearly define its role. A recent review of open and controlled studies involving bipolar and schizoaffective patients reported that 57 per cent responded favorably to valproate.[18]

Mania

Until recently there were only three double-blind, placebo-controlled trials of valproate for mania, involving a total of 14 patients.[8] Ten (71 per cent) had a favorable response, but five of six responders in one study did not relapse when switched to placebo after only 2 weeks of valproate. This data base was expanded by Pope et al.,[19] who treated 36 lithium treatment failures for 3 weeks in an inpatient setting with either valproate or placebo under double-blind conditions. An antimanic response occurred in 53 per cent (9 of 17) on valproate and only 11 per cent (2 of 19) on placebo. Freeman et al. compared valproate with lithium in a 3-week, double-blind study (N = 27) and found a positive response to lithium in 92 per cent (12 of 13) and to valproate in 64 per cent (9 of 14). Dysphoric features predicted the valproate responders.[20]

Depression

There are no controlled studies of valproate for acute depression, and open studies have not been impressive (an estimated response rate of less than 30 per cent).

Maintenance

Controlled studies of valproate maintenance are lacking, although several open studies have described a beneficial effect from long-term treatment.[12,18] These favorable reports vary considerably with regard to diagnoses, duration of treatment, outcome measures, and use of ancillary medications such as lithium, antipsychotics, and antidepressants. In an open study of 55 rapid-cycling bipolar patients, the majority of whom were unresponsive to lithium or carbamazepine, Calabrese and Delucchi found a moderate to marked response to valproate with regard to prophylaxis against manic, mixed, and depressed episodes.[21] Mean treatment duration was 7.8 ± 5.9 months, and most patients (64 per cent) were also on other medications.

In brief, valproate shows promise as an antimanic agent and for the long-term management of bipolar disorder. Studies in mania, when completed, should be among the most definitive done for this condition. On the other hand, controlled long-term studies are considerably more difficult and expensive to conduct and, for the time being, the merits of maintenance valproate rest on clinical impression and open reports. Of great interest would be a direct comparison of valproate and carbamazepine in bipolar disorder to address issues of relative efficacy, adverse reactions, and drug interactions.

Using Valproate

Laboratory evaluation recommended prior to and during valproate therapy includes liver function tests, platelet counts, and coagulation tests (PDR, pages 509 to 513).[3] The frequency of testing is not specified, but rather left to the physician's clinical judgment as evidenced by terms such as "frequent," especially during the first 6 months (liver) and "periodic" (platelets). For many clinicians, testing will consist of a complete blood count with platelet count and a chemistry panel. Additional laboratory testing should be obtained as indicated by the clinical state of the patient.

Valproate is available in the United States as valproic acid (Depakene and others) in 250-mg capsules and a syrup (250 mg/5 ml), and divalproex sodium (Depakote) is available in 125-, 250-, and

500-mg enteric-coated tablets and a 125-mg capsule (which can be swallowed whole or opened and sprinkled over food).

While valproic acid is more rapidly absorbed and, hence, preferred for pharmacokinetic studies, the gentler gastrointestinal side-effects profile of divalproex sodium (Depakote) makes it preferred for general clinical use. The usual starting dose is 250 mg b.i.d., with subsequent increases based on clinical response, side effects, and blood levels. The therapeutic range in neurology (50 to 100 or 120 μg/ml) has been adopted by psychiatry, although there are no studies establishing a relationship between blood level and efficacy. The drug is highly protein bound (greater than 90 per cent) and there is evidence that at higher concentrations, the amount of free drug increases substantially in a nonlinear fashion. The dose necessary to obtain a given blood level varies widely among individuals. Elimination half-life ranges between 8 and 19 hours.

Side Effects and Toxicity

Neurological Effects

While valproate may have subtle adverse effects on cognitive function, it is generally well tolerated. Sedation may occur early in treatment, especially if dose escalation is too rapid. A mild tremor that resembles a benign essential tremor is not uncommon, and is more likely to occur at higher blood levels.

Overdose

Valproate overdose can cause severe coma and death. Treatment is primarily symptomatic and supportive. Naloxone has been used to reverse coma, although it may also reverse the anticonvulsant effect of the drug.

Hematological Effects

Thrombocytopenia occurs occasionally during the course of valproate therapy. In addition, valproate may impair platelet function, even in the presence of a normal platelet count. Because of this, both a platelet count and a measure of function platelet integrity is indicated prior to surgical or dental procedures. Similarly, easy bruising, epistaxis, petechiae, or hematomas should initiate appropriate testing and consideration of drug discontinuation.

Gastrointestinal Effects

Nausea, appetite loss, and vomiting are common side effects of valproic acid (Depakene) but are less likely to be problematic with divalproex sodium (Depakote). Pancreatitis is a rare complication of valproate treatment, and measurement of pancreatic enzymes is essential if a patient presents with abdominal pain and vomiting.

Hepatic dysfunction has been the major concern regarding the use of valproate. Mild and often transient elevations in hepatic enzymes occur in 20 to 40 per cent of patients. Unless enzyme levels double or triple, the drug can usually be continued with periodic monitoring. Fatal hepatotoxicity is rare, idiosyncratic, and unrelated to dose. At greater risk are children with severe epilepsy and related disorders under the age of 2 on polypharmacy (1 of 500). Periodic assessment of liver function is recommended, especially during the first 6 months of therapy. Symptoms suggestive of hepatic dysfunction should be pursued with appropriate physical examination and laboratory testing.

Dermatological Effects

Hair loss and rash have been attributed to valproate. Hair loss occurs in 0.5 to 4 per cent of patients, is usually mild, and seldom requires drug discontinuation. Regrowth is sometimes associated with curlier hair. Unlike carbamazepine, life-threatening dermatological complications have not been a particular problem with valproate.

Weight Gain

Weight gain is common (7 to 57 per cent), is sometimes substantial, and may lead to noncompliance. Its cause is unknown and there are no treatments other than conventional weight reduction measures.

Pregnancy

Valproate crosses the placenta, and neural tube defects such as spina bifida have occurred in 1 to 2 per cent of children exposed in utero. If at all possible, the drug should be avoided during the first trimester of pregnancy. Valproate is excreted in breast milk, but the implications of breast-feeding are unknown. The drug share swith lithium a classification in FDA pregnancy category D.

Drug Interactions

Valproate increases serum levels of phenobarbital and primidone in many, but not all, patients. Its interactions with phenytoin are complex, since it lowers phenytoin blood levels but also increases free drug levels by displacement from protein binding sites. Valproate increases the serum level of the epoxide metabolite of carbamazepine and may also increase free carbamazepine levels through displacement from serum proteins. Plasma concentrations of amitriptyline and its metabolite nortriptyline were increased in the presence of valproate.

Because of hepatic enzyme induction, valproate blood levels tend to be lower in the presence of carbamazepine, phenytoin, and phenobarbital. Overall, there appear to be fewer interactions between valproate and other drugs than between carbamazepine and other drugs.[22]

OTHER MOOD STABILIZERS

Benzodiazepines

These drugs have been useful for treating mania, but whether they function only as sedatives or have a more specific antimanic effect has not been resolved. The benzodiazepines are also commonly used in conjunction with low doses of neuroleptics during the treatment of mania. Whether these drugs will be useful for long-term treatment remains to be established.[8,9,12]

Calcium Channel Blockers

Open and double-blind studies have shown verapamil to have antimanic properties.[8] These studies involved relatively few patients, lacked consistency in design, used ancillary drugs, and suffered from other flaws. Consequently, calcium channel blockers do not have a firmly established role as mood stabilizers.

Electroconvulsive Therapy

Electroconvulsive therapy (ECT) is an effective treatment for mania. This statement is supported by retrospective studies as well as by a prospective comparison with lithium.[8,9] Anecdotal reports suggest a role for ECT in treating rapid cycling. Maintenance ECT may be of value in preventing recurrent episodes of mania and depression. Lithium should be at least temporarily discontinued during ECT, since the combination appears to cause greater short-term neurological side effects.

Miscellaneous

Many other drugs have been studied as potential antimanic agents, but none have shown consistent promise. These include fenfluramine, clonidine, methysergide, tryptophan, bromocriptine, phenytoin, carbonic anhydrase inhibitors, digoxin, piribedil, and methylene blue.

CONCLUSIONS

While lithium remains the preferred treatment for bipolar disorder, there are a substantial number of patients who are nonresponders or are intolerant of the drug. In recent years, both carbamazepine and valproate have gained acceptance as alternatives to lithium or for use in combination with lithium. These and other less well-established mood stabilizers suggest a bright future for the effective acute and long-term treatment of bipolar disorder.

REFERENCES

1. Goodwin FK, Jamison KR: Manic-Depressive Illness. New York: Oxford University Press, 1990:909.
2. American Psychiatric Association: Diagnostic and Statistical Manual of Mental Disorders (DSM-III-R). 3rd ed. Revised. Washington, DC: American Psychiatric Association, 1987:111–112.
3. Physicians' Desk Reference (PDR). 45th ed. Oradell, NJ: Medical Economics, 1991.
4. Gelenberg AJ, Kane JM, Keller MB, et al: Comparison of standard and low serum levels of lithium for maintenance treatment of bipolar disorder. N Engl J Med 321:1489–1493, 1989.
5. Jefferson JW, Greist JH: Lithium carbonate and carbamazepine side effects. In Hales RE, Frances AJ, eds. American Psychiatric Association Annual Review, Vol. 6. Washington, DC: American Psychiatric Press, 1987:746–780.
6. DasGupta K, Jefferson JW, Kobak KA, et al: The effect of enalapril on serum lithium levels in healthy men. (in press).
7. Creelman W, Ciraulo DA, Shader RI: Lithium drug interactions. In Ciraulo DA, Shader RI, Greenblatt DJ, Creelman W, eds. Drug Interactions in Psychiatry. Baltimore: Williams and Wilkins, 1989:127–157.
8. Chou JCY: Recent advances in treatment of acute mania. J Clin Psychopharmacol 11:3–21, 1991.
9. Small JG: Anticonvulsants in affective disorders. Psychopharmacol Bull 26:25–36, 1990.
10. Post RM, Uhde TW, Roy-Byrne PP, et al: Antidepressant effects of carbamazepine. Am J Psychiatry 143:29–34, 1986.
11. Kramlinger KG, Post RM: The addition of lithium to carbamazepine: Antidepressant efficacy in treatment-resistant depression. Arch Gen Psychiatry 46:794–800, 1989.
12. Prien RF, Gelenberg AJ: Alternatives to lithium for preventive treatment of bipolar disorder. Am J Psychiatry 146:840–848, 1989.
13. Post RM, Leverich GS, Rosoff AS, et al: Carbamazepine prophylaxis in refractory affective disorders: A focus on long-term follow-up. J Clin Psychopharmacol 10:318–327, 1990.
14. Nilsson C, Sterner G, Idvall J: Charcoal hemoperfusion for treatment of serious carbamazepine poisoning. Acta Med Scand 216:137–140, 1984.
15. Jones KL, Lacro RV, Johnson KA, et al: Pattern of malformations in children of women treated with carbamazepine during pregnancy. N Engl J Med 320:1661–1666, 1989.
16. Rosa FW: Spina bifida in infants of women treated with carbamazepine during pregnancy. N Engl J Med 324:674–677, 1991.
17. Ciraulo DA, Slattery M, Shader RI: An overview of drug interactions of anticonvulsants commonly used in psychiatry. In Ciraulo DA, Shader RI, Greenblatt DJ, Creelman W, eds. Drug Interactions in Psychiatry. Baltimore: Williams and Wilkins, 1989:181–233.
18. McElroy SL, Keck PE, Pope HG, et al: Valproate in psychiatric disorders: Literature review and clinical guidelines. J Clin Psychiatry 50(suppl 3):23–29, 1989.
19. Pope HG, McElroy SL, Keck PE, et al: Valproate in the treatment of acute mania. Arch Gen Psychiatry 48:62–68, 1991.
20. Freeman TW, Clothier JL, Pazzaglia P, et al: Valproate in mania: A double-blind study. New Research Program and Abstracts, 143rd Annual Meeting of the American Psychiatric Association (NR 393), 1990:198.
21. Calabrese JR, Delucchi GA: Spectrum of efficacy of valproate in 55 patients with rapid-cycling bipolar disorder. Am J Psychiatry 147:431–434, 1990.
22. Mattson RH, Cramer JA: Valproate interactions with other drugs. In Levy R, Mattson R, Meldrum B, et al., eds. Antiepileptic Drugs. 3rd ed. New York: Raven Press, 1989:621–632.

40

MAINTENANCE TREATMENT FOR MOOD DISORDERS

ROBERT F. PRIEN, Ph.D. and WILLIAM Z. POTTER, M.D., Ph.D.

This chapter deals with maintenance treatment of both unipolar and bipolar disorders. The term "unipolar disorder" refers to a depressive disorder with no history of a manic or unequivocal hypomanic episode. The chapter focuses on two phases of maintenance treatment: continuation therapy and prophylactic therapy.

The longitudinal course of mood disorders has major implications for treatment planning. It is estimated that at least 50 per cent of individuals who have an initial episode of major depression and over 80 per cent who have an episode of mania will have one or more additional episodes.[1] In addition, about one fifth of patients fail to recover fully from a given episode. The incomplete recovery may be due to inadequate treatment of the episode, a preexisting chronic disorder, or the progressive deteriorative effects of recurring episodes. These episodes are not only disruptive, but may be fatal, as an estimated 15 per cent of depressed patients commit suicide.

PHASES OF TREATMENT

The concepts of acute, continuation, and prophylactic treatment are used frequently to classify stages of pharmacological treatment for mood disorders. Acute therapy is treatment directed at the initial control of acute symptoms. Continuation therapy refers to the continuation of treatment after the medication-induced remission of acute symptoms for the purpose of maintaining control over the episode. Prophylactic therapy represents long-term treatment for the purpose of preventing or attenuating new episodes. These phases may be blurred in clinical practice. However, they provide the theoretical underpinning for much of the research-generated guidelines for maintenance treatment and will be discussed in this context.

Continuation Treatment

It is accepted practice to continue treatment of the acute episode for several months after the disappearance of symptoms to ensure that the episode is over. The rationale is that antidepressant and antimanic drugs may suppress symptoms without immediately correcting the biological process or pathophysiology underlying the episode. As a result, even with successful treatment there is likely to be a gap of months between the disappearance of overt symptoms and the end of the episode. When a medication does suppress symptoms, it is difficult to determine when the episode is over and continuation treatment is no longer required.

Nearly a dozen placebo-controlled trials support the need for continuation treatment.[2] In each of these studies, an antidepressant or lithium was used to control acute symptoms, after which approximately one half of the sample was switched, double-blind, to a placebo and the other half continued to receive medication. An average of 50 per cent of the individuals treated with a placebo relapsed within 6 months compared to only 20 per cent receiving medication. Most of the relapses on placebo occurred within the first 3 months. This relatively rapid return of symptoms following withdrawal of medication suggests that the medication was controlling symptoms of an episode that had not run its course. Studies of electroconvulsive therapy (ECT) report a similar pattern of relapse following discontinuation.[3]

A rule of thumb for maintaining control over the episode is to continue medication for 6 to 12 months following initial remission of symptoms and then gradually withdraw the drug over a period of weeks or months. The problem with this plan is that some patients may require a longer period of continuation treatment and may relapse repeatedly during or shortly after medication tapering. Other patients may not need 6 to 12 months of medication. A more precise criterion for determining the length of treatment is provided by recent maintenance therapy studies with depressed patients.[4–7] The studies indicate that it is safe to withdraw medication after the patient has remained in remission for at least 4 months. For patients who have a history of good recovery between episodes, even mild residual symptoms may be an indication that the episode has not run its course.

Care should be taken in withdrawing medication following completion of the episode. Discontinuation of antidepressants can produce withdrawal effects such as sleep disturbance and irritability. There should be gradual tapering of the drug over a period of a month or more. Because of the disruptive effects of a relapse, there should be continued contact with the patient during the first few months following withdrawal of medication. The patient and, where appropriate, his or her family, should be warned that further medication may be required and to report any signs of an emerging episode. Similar considerations should be applied to the management of mania with lithium. Psychotherapy, including interpersonal, cognitive, marital/family, and supportive therapies, should be considered in the planning of continuation treatment, particularly if the patient has a history of significant mood disturbance and poor functioning between episodes.

Prophylactic Treatment

Selection of Patients

There are numerous factors to be considered in determining whether or not to initiate prophylactic treatment. Perhaps the foremost consideration is the likelihood of a recurrence in the near future and the impact that it might have on the patient's career, family, marriage, and interpersonal functioning. Opinions differ as to how many episodes a patient should have to warrant prophylactic treatment. However, most clinicians with a published opinion advise that the patient have two or three episodes before receiving prophylactic therapy. In general, bipolar disorder is viewed with more urgency for early intervention than unipolar disorder. Guidelines from the World Health Organization recommend that prophylactic treatment be initiated with unipolar patients after three episodes, particularly if there have been two episodes, excluding the current episode, within the last 5 years. For bipolar patients, prophylactic treatment is recommended after the second episode. Goodwin and Jamison[8] recommend that prophylactic treatment be considered after the initial manic episode if the episode has a sudden onset, is highly disruptive, involves a high risk of suicide, or occurs in an adolescent, especially one with a substantial genetic loading. For unipolar disorder, there is general agreement that patients who have only a single episode, mild episodes, or a relatively long interval between attacks (e.g., 5 years or more) should not be started on prophylactic treatment unless a subsequent episode would have severely disruptive or life-threatening consequences.

In determining whether or not to start prophylactic treatment, it is necessary to evaluate not only the number, frequency, and severity of prior episodes, but also the rapidity of onset of episodes, potential contraindications to treatment, and the patient's response to prior treatments. Other critical factors are the patient's life situation, extenuating circumstances that may have contributed to prior attacks, and the patient's willingness to commit himself or herself to the treatment program. It is important that the decision to initiate long-term treatment be a collaborative effort between the physician, patient, and available family. Patients and family should be well informed about the treatment and understand its benefits and risks and the importance of complying with the medication schedule. A concerned family member is particularly important for the early detection of a manic or hypomanic episode because many patients do not view this state as a problem and may not seek help on their own.

CHOICE OF TREATMENT FOR BIPOLAR DISORDER

Lithium is the treatment of choice for bipolar disorder, but is not a panacea. The average failure rate for lithium in prophylactic treatment studies is approximately 33 per cent. In most studies, failure is defined as the occurrence of a manic or depressive episode severe enough to require hospitalization or treatment other than the study medication. From another perspective, Schou[10] estimates that with carefully selected patients who are adequately treated with lithium, 30 to 60 per cent will have a complete response, 30 to 50 per cent a partial response, and 10 to 20 per cent a poor response. Generally, complete response means that the patient will not require additional medication or further hospitalization. With partial response, patients show varying outcomes ranging from a modest decrease in the frequency and severity of attacks, to only rare and mild symptoms. Poor response indicates no significant change or worsening.

Predictors of poor lithium response include a recent history of noncompliance in taking medication, rapid cycling (defined as four or more episodes per year) or progression of cycle frequency over time, episodes with mixed manic and dysphoric features, alcohol or drug abuse not associated with mood change, and poor interepisode functioning.[8,11] Classical bipolar disorder characterized by a history of clear-cut onset and recovery of episodes and absence of comorbid complications is a good predictor of positive lithium response.

The most promising and best evaluated of the alternatives to lithium are the anticonvulsants carbamazepine and, more recently, valproate. The results from several maintenance studies of carbamazepine have been generally positive and suggest that the drug may be beneficial with patients who fail to respond adequately to lithium.[9,11] The majority of patients in these studies had carbamazepine added to a previously ineffective regimen, usually lithium. Thus, the efficacy of carbamazepine alone remains an issue. Acute antimanic properties of valproate alone have been demonstrated, even in a lithium nonresponder.[12] Although its efficacy as a prophylactic treatment has not been adequately evaluated, clinical reports are encouraging and include patients in whom valproate and lithium are combined.[13]

The clearest indication for an anticonvulsant is failure to respond to lithium. Carbamazepine has been suggested to be a particularly effective adjunct or alternative to lithium for patients who have a pattern of rapid or continuous cycling, and a similar claim is being made for valproate. Some studies suggest that anticonvulsants are as effective as lithium in bipolar patients without rapid cycles.[11,13] However, more research is needed before either carbamazepine or valproate can be recommended as an across-the-board alternative to lithium. The possibility of rare idiosyncratic agranulocytosis or aplastic anemia with carbamazepine warrants initial hematological and electrolyte monitoring and periodic monitoring thereafter. Carbamazepine may also induce rashes that may warrant discontinuation of medication and synergistic neurotoxic reactions in combination with lithium.[14] Valproate can produce dose-related gastrointestinal symptoms of nausea, vomiting, and diarrhea, as well as central nervous system (CNS)-mediated sedation, tremor, and ataxia. Weight gain and transient (reversible) hair loss are observed during chronic administration. A rare but severe side effect is pancreatitis. As is the case with lithium and carbamazepine, blood level monitoring is used in establishing a safe therapeutic dose.[13]

The most frequently used drugs other than lithium for the treatment of bipolar disorder are the neuroleptics. However, the risk of tardive dyskinesia and the possibility of exacerbating a subsequent episode of depression limit their usefulness as a prophylactic treatment,[15,16] although they are often added to lithium for rapid control of "breakthrough" manias that occur during lithium maintenance therapy. There are numerous other treatments identified in the literature as potential alternatives or adjuncts to lithium for maintenance treatment. None have been carefully studied for this indication. The treatments include the type A monoamine oxidase inhibitor clorgyline, verapamil and other calcium channel blockers, thyroid medications such as L-thyroxine and triiodothyronine, maintenance ECT, and periodic sleep deprivation.

Treatment of Breakthrough Depression in Bipolar Disorder

Breakthrough depressions that occur during lithium prophylactic treatment may be difficult to control. The first response to the occurrence of depressive symptoms should include a reevaluation of the lithium level and thyroid function, and assessment of the patient's life situation for factors that may be contributing to the clinical course. The possibility of noncompliance in taking medication should be explored before progressing to other stages of treatment. Although some breakthrough depressions can be treated successfully by enhancing thyroid function or increasing the dose of lithium (to levels of 1.2 mEq/liter or higher),[8] the standard practice is to add an antidepressant to the lithium regimen. This practice has been criticized by some investigators, who report that antidepressants can precipitate rapid or continuous cycling or mania in some patients.[17] However, the absence of systematic studies on the treatment of breakthrough depressions during lithium maintenance therapy leave the clinician with few options other than adding an antidepressant, particularly if thyroid function, low lithium levels, and noncompliance in taking medication are not problems. Electroconvulsive therapy should also be considered, especially for severe and life-threatening depression. However, ECT administered to patients receiving lithium has been reported to cause memory loss and neurological abnormalities and should be used with caution if the patient remains on lithium therapy.[18] The effectiveness of newer antidepressants for breakthrough depressions has not been established. Bupropion, in particular, is a promising research candidate for this phase of treatment.[19]

Rapid Cycling and Dysphoric Mania

Patients who develop dysphoric mania (a full manic syndrome with concomitant depression) or rapid cycling during lithium maintenance therapy present unique difficulties for treatment. The use of antidepressants may convert the disorders to a continuous cycling form. Thus, if patients are receiving an antidepressant or neuroleptic drug when they develop rapid cycling or mixed states, the withdrawal of these "cycle-inducing" drugs may make the patient more responsive to lithium.[16,17] However, this strategy has not been studied prospectively and raises ethical concerns about withholding antidepressant medication from patients with severe depression. Substance abuse may be an added complication in patients with rapid cycling or mixed states and needs to be dealt with aggressively in treating the disorder.

The anticonvulsants carbamazepine and valproate alone or in combination with lithium are emerging as promising treatments for both dysphoric mania and rapid cycling.[11] With rapid cycling, other treatments reported to be at least partially effective in stabilizing the course of illness include the combination of clorgyline and lithium, haloperidol decanoate, and repetitive sleep deprivation. However, none have been extensively studied in this capacity.

CHOICE OF TREATMENT FOR UNIPOLAR DISORDER

There have been several placebo-controlled studies evaluating prophylactic drug treatment in unipolar disorder. Drugs reported to be more effective than placebo are lithium, imipramine, amitriptyline, fluoxetine, nomifesine, and zimelidine. The latter two drugs have been withdrawn from the market because of adverse effects. A consensus conference on prevention of recurrences in mood disorders convened by the National Institute of Mental Health (NIMH) and the National Institutes of Health[1] reviewed the issue of the comparative efficacy of lithium and tricyclic antidepressants (TCAs) and concluded that both were effective, each with advantages for certain patients. Lithium has potent antimanic properties, whereas the TCAs are relatively ineffective in preventing manic episodes[20,21] and, as noted above, may even precipitate mania or continuous cycling in vulnerable patients. It is estimated that 10 to 15 per cent of patients originally diagnosed as unipolar will have one or more manic episodes. Because of the devastating effects of unexpected manic attacks, lithium may be the preferred treatment where there is suspicion of a latent bipolar disorder.[1] A major risk factor for development of a manic attack is a personal history of hypomania. Although our definition of unipolar disorder excludes patients with an unequivocal episode of hypomania, past episodes of hypomania can be easily missed in the evaluation of a depressed patient, especially if the patient is the sole source of information. Other risk factors are a family history of mania, a high frequency of recurrences, and early age of onset.

The advantage of the TCAs and other antidepressants over lithium for prophylactic treatment is that they are more likely to have been used to treat the acute episode. The clinician who wants to use lithium for prophylaxis either has to discontinue the antidepressant and substitute lithium or add lithium to the antidepressant regimen. Taking away a drug that is effective and well tolerated can create logistical, compliance, and ethical problems. There may also be a loss of control over symptoms if the antidepressant is withdrawn before the episode has run its course. The addition of lithium to an antidepressant regimen presents all the problems associated with drug combinations (risk of adverse reactions, increased noncompliance in taking medication, and the difficulty in identifying which treatment is producing the therapeutic effect). Also, prophylactic studies evaluating the combination of imipramine and lithium demonstrate no significant advantage of the combination over lithium alone.[20,21] Finally, there is evidence that an antidepressant may be more effective than lithium in preventing severe depressions.[21]

In summary, the option of continuing the drug that produced initial control of depressive symptoms should be given serious consideration. A problem is that relatively few antidepressants have been evaluated as prophylactic treatments. However, studies of the use of newer antidepressants for maintenance therapy have provided generally positive results and suggest that the effectiveness of a drug during acute and continuation treatment is a good predictor of its effectiveness in prophylaxis. Unless a drug presents special risks for long-term safety, the advantages of continuing the drug would seem to outweigh the disadvantages. The side-effects profile of a drug and its anticipated effect on the patient's functioning during well periods obviously should be considered in the choice of the long-term treatment. The most cautionary statement may apply to amoxapine and neuroleptics because of the risk of tardive dyskinesia and extrapyramidal reactions. Lithium has teratogenic effects that may complicate its use in women who are (or may become) pregnant. Medication and dietary restrictions with monoamine oxidase inhibitors may pose difficulties for long-term treatment, although a recent long-term trial with phenelzine indicates that with careful monitoring the drug can be used safely.[22] With tertiary amine TCAs in particular, cognitive dysfunction and orthostatic hypotension can cause problems for the elderly. Finally, with newly marketed drugs, there is always the possibility that rare adverse reactions may not have been detected in the carefully screened patient sample used in investigational drug safety trials and may appear only after the drug reaches a broader spectrum of patients.

DOSE

With the exception of lithium, systematic dose-response studies for prophylactic drug treatment are practically nonexistent. Many of the textbook guidelines for pharmacological treatment of mood disorders recommend that the physician use the "lowest effective dose" for prophylactic treatment without indicating how this can be achieved without exposing the patient to a recurrence. A standard practice derived from procedures used in earlier long-term studies with antidepressants is to maintain the patient on a dose equivalent to 75 to 150 mg/day of imipramine. A recent 3-year study by Frank et al.[4] offers another dosing strategy that warrants careful examination—the maintenance of prophylactic dosage at or near the level that initially controlled acute symptoms. The investigators report a high rate of success with imipramine prophylactic treatment using an average dose exceeding 200 mg/day. Relatively good results were also obtained in a premarketing 12-month study of fluoxetine that used a 40-mg/day dose, double the dose subsequently approved for the treatment of acute episodes.[6] These results underscore the need for well-designed dose-response studies for maintenance treatment.

There is better agreement regarding the prophylactic dose range for lithium. The dose generally is targeted at 0.6 to 0.8 mEq/liter, with a level of 0.5 not uncommon for elderly patients.[1,8,10] Occasional patients with troublesome side effects may be treated with levels as low as 0.4,[10] but this is not a generally recognized effective dose. Some patients may benefit from high levels. A study by Gelenberg et al.[23] demonstrates that bipolar patients with a history of fewer than three episodes tend to have a lower rate of recurrence at levels of 0.8 to 1.0 mEq/liter than at levels of 0.4 to 0.6. Patients with a history of three or more episodes respond poorly at both levels. It is possible that higher levels may benefit the latter patients, but there has not been study of this option.

The dosage requirements for prophylactic treatment vary for different patients and may change for a given patient over time, depending upon the patient's clinical response, medical state, psychological complications, adverse reactions, and acceptance of the treatment. It is necessary that the clinician be aware of these developments. The clinician should be particularly alert for side effects that can adversely affect compliance. Reactions that may be viewed by the clinician as being relatively mild may be troublesome enough for the patient to stop treatment. Examples include hand tremor, cognitive impairment, weight gain, and polyuria with lithium; and weight gain, dry mouth, and sexual dysfunction with antidepressants. Numerous other reasons may contribute to noncompliance, such as dislike of having one's mood controlled by a drug, feeling well and seeing no further need for medication, and the hassle in remembering to take medication. The patient and clinician should discuss these and any other problems that might interfere with treatment and arrive at some agreement as to how they may best be handled.

SCHEDULE FOR MONITORING

Goodwin and Jamison, in a review of procedures for monitoring of lithium therapy,[8] suggest that when maintenance treatment is initiated, the patient should be evaluated weekly until the dose and blood level have been stabilized. Thereafter, most patients can be adequately monitored every 4 to 8 weeks during the first year and at less frequent intervals thereafter. The frequency of visits depends upon the patient's reliability in self-monitoring of side effects, compliance in taking medication, and the capability of a significant other to recognize and report signs of an emerging recurrence.

DURATION OF TREATMENT

There is evidence that some patients with a long duration of illness who have been free of recurrences for several years may no longer require prophylactic treatment. Angst et al.[24] found that approximately one of three patients with bipolar disorder and one of eight patients with unipolar disorder over age 65, with a long history of illness, appear to stop having episodes. Unfortunately, there are no valid predictors for identifying these patients. The only way of determining whether the patient still needs medication is to withdraw the treatment and follow the patient for signs of a recurrence. Schou recommends that after the patient has remained well for 3 or 4 years, the clinician and patient should discuss whether medication should be continued, taking

into account the course of illness before and during treatment, the presence of side effects, and the potential consequences of a new episode.[25] If the prior course of illness is characterized by suicide attempts, hospitalization, or serious disruption of career or family functioning, there should be reasonable assurance that if medication is withdrawn a subsequent episode can be detected early enough to prevent development of a full-blown attack.

PSYCHOTHERAPY

Individual psychotherapies (interpersonal, cognitive, and behavioral) and group and marital/family therapies have been used effectively to alleviate depressive symptoms in unipolar disorder. However, the application of these therapies for maintenance treatment has been slow in developing. The only study evaluating psychotherapy as a preventive treatment found that monthly sessions of interpersonal therapy (IPT) administered over a 2-year period served to lengthen the time between episodes in patients not receiving medication.[4] However, the monthly sessions were not as effective as medication in preventing recurrences, nor was there any clear advantage in combining the two modalities. The investigators suggest that the maintenance IPT may be of value to the patient with unipolar disorder who cannot tolerate or chooses not to continue pharmacotherapy.

With bipolar disorder, psychosocial treatments have been used as adjuncts to medication, usually lithium. There are numerous reports citing the value of psychoeducational management techniques for enhancing the retention of patients in treatment programs and for improving compliance in taking medication. Techniques may include psychoeducational sessions with mental health professionals, and education models that convey information about the disorder and its treatments through lectures, handouts, and films. Individual cognitive-behavioral therapies and group and family therapies may also be of value as adjuncts to maintenance treatment for selected patients. Last but not least, support associations such as the National Depressive and Manic Depressive Association and the National Alliance for the Mentally Ill provide excellent educational self-help programs for patients and their families. These programs provide better understanding of the disorder and its management and enhance the therapeutic alliance by encouraging better collaboration with the clinician in the treatment program.

REFERENCES

1. NIMH/NIH Consensus Development Conference Statement. Mood disorders: Prevention of recurrences. Am J Psychiatry 142:469–472, 1985.
2. Prien RF: Maintenance treatment of depressive and manic states. In Georgotis A, Cancro R, eds. Depression and Mania. New York: Elsevier, 1988:439–451.

3. Sackeim H, Prudic J, Devanand DP, et al: The impact of medication resistance and continuation pharmacotherapy on relapse following responses to electroconvulsive therapy in major depression. J Clin Psychopharmacol 10:96–104, 1990.

4. Frank E, Kupfer DJ, Perel JM, et al: Three-year outcomes for maintenance therapies in recurrent depression. Arch Gen Psychiatry 47:1093–1099, 1990.

5. Georgotis A, McCue RE: Relapse of depressed patients after effective continuation therapy. J Affective Disord 17:159–164, 1989.

6. Montgomery SA, Dufour H, Brion S, et al: The prophylactic efficacy of fluoxetine in unipolar depression. Br J Psychiatry 153(suppl 3):69–76, 1988.

7. Prien RF, Kupfer DJ: Continuation drug therapy for major depressive episodes: How long should it be maintained? Am J Psychiatry 143:18–23, 1986.

8. Goodwin FJ, Jamison KR: Manic-Depressive Illness. New York: Oxford University Press, 1990:665–745.

9. Prien RF, Gelenberg AJ: Alternatives to lithium for preventive treatment of bipolar disorders. Am J Psychiatry 146:840–848, 1989.

10. Shou M: Practical problems of lithium maintenance treatment. Adv Biochem Psychopharmacol 40:131–138, 1985.

11. Prien RF, Potter WZ: NIMH workshop on treatment of bipolar disorder. Psychopharmacol Bull 26:409–427, 1990.

12. Pope HG, EcElroy SL, Keck PE, et al: Valproate in the treatment of acute mania: A placebo controlled study. Arch Gen Psychiatry 48:62–68, 1991.

13. McElroy SL, Keck PE, Pope HG, et al: Valproate in psychiatric disorders: Literature review and clinical guidelines. J Clin Psychiatry 50(suppl 3):23–29, 1989.

14. Post RM, Uhde TW: Clinical approaches to treatment-resistant bipolar illness. In Hales RE, Frances AJ, eds. American Psychiatric Association Annual Review, Vol 6. Washington, DC: American Psychiatric Association Press, 1987:125–150.

15. Esparon J, Kollooci J, Naylor GJ, et al: Comparison of the prophylactic action of flupenthixol with placebo in lithium treated manic depressive patients. Br J Psychiatry 148:723–725, 1986.

16. Kukopulos A, Tondo L: Lithium nonresponders and their treatment. In Johnson FN, ed. Handbook of Lithium Therapy. Lancaster, England: MTP Press, 1980:143–149.

17. Wehr TA, Goodwin FK: Can antidepressants cause mania and worsen the course of affective illness? Am J Psychiatry 144:1403–1411, 1987.

18. Rudorfer MV, Linnoila M: Electroconvulsive therapy. In Johnson FN, ed. Lithium Combination Treatment. Basel: S Karger, 1987:164–178.

19. Haykal RF, Akiskal HS: Bupropion as a promising approach to rapid cycling bipolar II patients. J Clin Psychiatry 51:450–455, 1990.

20. Kane JM, Quitkin FM, Rifkin A, et al: Lithium carbonate and imipramine in the prophylaxis of unipolar and bipolar II illness. Arch Gen Psychiatry 39:1065–1069, 1982.

21. Prien RF, Kupfer DJ, Mansky PA, et al: Drug therapy in the prevention of recurrences in unipolar and bipolar affective disorders. Arch Gen Psychiatry 41:1096–1104, 1984.

22. Robinson D, Lerfald SC, Binnett B, et al: Continuation and maintenance treatment of major depression with the monoamine oxidase inhibitor phenelzine: A double-blind placebo-controlled study. Psychopharmacol Bull 27:31–40, 1991.

23. Gelenberg A, Kane J, Keller M, et al: Comparison of standard and low serum levels of lithium for maintenance treatment of bipolar disorder. N Engl J Med 321:1489–1493, 1989.

24. Angst J, Grof P: The course of monopolar depressions and bipolar psychosis. In Vialleneuve A, ed. Lithium in Psychiatry: A Synopsis. Quebec: Les Presses de L'University Laval, 1976.

25. Schou M: Lithium Treatment of Manic-Depressive Illness. A Practical Guide. 4th ed. Basal: S Karger, 1989.

Section E

ANXIETY DISORDERS

41

PROPOSED CHANGES IN DSM-IV FOR ANXIETY DISORDERS

MICHAEL R. LIEBOWITZ, M.D.

The DSM-III and III-R anxiety disorder classifications represented a major conceptual advance by providing the field with a set of diagnostic criteria that appear to be quite treatment relevant. For this reason alone the DSM-IV Anxiety Disorders Work Group would have approached the task of further revision with a conservative bent. In addition, however, the whole DSM-IV process is being guided by the principal of making changes on the basis of empirical evidence, derived from reviews of published studies, reanalyses of unpublished data, and recently begun field trials.

As this process is now underway and not yet completed, the final form of the DSM-IV anxiety disorders criteria cannot yet be fully discerned. Nevertheless, the directions in which things are moving can be highlighted, and their treatment implications discussed. This will be done by disorder, beginning with panic disorder and agoraphobia, and following with social phobia, simple (specific) phobia, obsessive compulsive disorder (OCD), post-traumatic stress disorder (PTSD), generalized anxiety disorder (GAD), and the possible new category of mixed anxiety and depression.

With regard to panic disorder, the issues being considered involve the minimum number of symptoms (threshold) for defining a panic attack, the minimum number of attacks and associated features to meet criteria for panic disorder, and the boundaries of panic disorder with social and simple phobia. This last issue involves consideration of the type of panic attacks experienced by panic disorder and ago-

raphobic patients as opposed to those with social or simple phobia.

The minimum thresholds for defining panic attacks and panic disorder in DSM-III and III-R were derived by consensus rather than empirical study. As we begin to study these issues in clinical and community samples, we have become aware that there may be no absolutely valid minimum threshold for a panic attack or for panic disorder. A low threshold brings in all real cases, but also a high number of false-positives. Too high a threshold, on the other hand, minimizes false-positives but increases the frequency of false-negatives. It appears that the best one can do at this time is to find the thresholds that minimize the combination of false-positives and false-negatives, using some parameter like impairment or help-seeking as a validating measure. Clinicians will at times thus be faced with false-negatives—patients whose symptoms fall short of meeting criteria, but who clinically, and most likely pathophysiologically, in fact have the disorder and should be treated as such. An example would be a patient with limited symptom attacks (panic-like attacks with one, two, or three symptoms) that had resulted in agoraphobia.

While panic attacks were central to panic disorder in DSM-III and III-R, there was the implication that social and simple phobic patients might also suffer panic attacks, although not of the unexpected type. However, many clinicians use the phrase "panic attacks" without a qualifier to indicate the kinds of panic attacks experienced by panic disorder pa-

261

tients. The DSM-IV Anxiety Disorders Work Group is considering making these distinctions explicit by more clearly defining the types of panic attacks that are central to panic disorder with and without agoraphobia, and how they differ from the panic or anxiety episodes of social or specific phobias. This should facilitate differential diagnosis and in turn help guide treatment.

With regard to social phobia, there is an increasing conviction that it can be divided into two or more subtypes. One subtype is represented by the individual with pure performance anxiety who is otherwise socially comfortable. The other type is the individual with widespread or generalized social discomfort and avoidance, who would in most cases also meet criteria for avoidant personality disorder. There may also be an intermediary third group with some performance and limited social anxiety. The monoamine oxidase inhibitors (MAOIs) have been found helpful for patients with the generalized form of social phobia, whether or not they also meet criteria for avoidant personality disorder. This also applies to individuals whose social anxiety seems secondary to minor medical disabilities that are the source of excessive embarrassment, a group that was excluded from social phobia in previous DSM editions.

Simple phobia will also probably undergo some form of subtyping, following the recognition that animal phobics, blood-injection-injury phobics, and situation phobics (closed spaces, airplanes) differ in age of onset, pattern of autonomic arousal, and perhaps also in mode of acquisition. Except for their narrower focus of fear and avoidance, the third group appears more similar to agoraphobics. Further study is needed to see if this has treatment relevance.

Previous DSM versions have been inconsistent in their definitions of obsessions and compulsions. Specifically, it has not been fully appreciated that the mental activity that many OCD patients use to alleviate the anxiety generated by an obsessive thought in fact represents a compulsive activity, albeit of a cognitive sort. Recognition of cognitive compulsions may have treatment relevance both for behavioral and pharmacological approaches, as may the growing sense that some OCD patients have psychotic-like aspects to their illness and still benefit from classical anti-OCD treatment.

There is also a growing awareness of the similarities of OCD to some cases of GAD, hypochondriasis, body dysmorphic disorder, trichotillomania, and Tourette's syndrome. While this creates headaches for the nosologist trying to establish precise language to facilitate differential diagnosis, it also suggests that some of the treatments recently found effective for OCD may have relevance for these other conditions.

There are two important foci for the DSM-IV efforts in the area of PTSD. The first involves study of the criteria themselves, particularly the definition of the stressor. The tenth revision of the International Classification of Diseases (ICD 10) proposes a broader stressor criterion than DSM-III-R, which requires an event outside the realm of normal experience. Loosening the stressor definition might allow inclusion of individuals who suffer PTSD-like features following experiences that do not now qualify for the diagnosis. On the other hand, in a litigous society such as ours, this could open the way for many additional law suits. The clinician in a setting where medicolegal issues are not primary, however, can focus on pathophysiology and might elect to treat someone for a PTSD-like syndrome even if the full DSM-IV criteria are not met.

The other PTSD-related issue that DSM-IV will address is the growing sense that many Axis I and Axis II adult psychopathological features derive from, or at least are influenced by, childhood experiences of physical or sexual abuse. While precise etiological relationships are hard to determine, the underrecognition of the prevalence and detrimental influence of childhood sexual and physical abuse has to be addressed both diagnostically and therapeutically.

Generalized anxiety disorder is in some ways the hardest DSM-III/III-R anxiety disorder to get a handle on. Its boundaries with both the other anxiety disorders and normal anxiety need to be validated, given the high comorbidity seen with GAD in clinical samples and its high prevalence in community samples.

A related issue is the proposed category of mixed anxiety and depression. The DSM-IV Task Force feels compelled to examine this for several reasons. It is included in ICD 10 as a subsyndromal category; that is, for patients with anxiety and depressive features that do not meet criteria for an established anxiety or depressive disorder. Primary care practitioners also report a high frequency of such patients without having a convenient DSM diagnosis for them. Weighing against consideration of such a category for DSM-IV is the fear of creating a "wastebasket" diagnosis that clinicians will use in lieu of attempting more precise differential diagnosis. A collaborative psychiatric–primary care field trial is underway to study this issue.

Other related issues involve ongoing attempts to clarify the interrelationships of adult and child anxiety disorders, and of substance abuse and anxiety disorders, and to further understand cross-cultural influences on the presentation of anxiety disorders. Overall, the efforts are to establish demarcations as well as to highlight continuities where appropriate, both in the service of increasing therapeutic effectiveness.

42

GENERALIZED ANXIETY DISORDER

DEBORAH S. COWLEY, M.D.

Generalized anxiety disorder (GAD) was first defined as a separate entity only 12 years ago, and the diagnostic criteria have been changed significantly since then. Before this, patients with severe, chronic anxiety and panic attacks were recognized as having a significant psychiatric problem and were given the diagnosis of anxiety neurosis, a term introduced over 100 years ago by Freud. In 1980, with DSM-III, panic disorder, previously included in anxiety neurosis, was recognized as a distinct syndrome, leaving a residual collection of anxious patients without frequent panic attacks, who were given the diagnosis of GAD.

DSM-III GAD was apparently quite common, with an estimated 1-month to 1-year general population prevalence of 2.5 to 6.4 per cent,[1] and was equally prevalent in men and women. The drawback of the DSM-III definition, however, was that it required only 1 month of excessive anxiety, and thus included both patients with a lifelong disorder and those with transient episodes of increased anxiety, which might more appropriately be viewed as stress reactions or adjustment disorders. The DSM-III-R attempted to correct this problem by requiring at least 6 months of excessive or unrealistic worry. In addition, patients must have six symptoms of motor tension (e.g., muscle tension, restlessness, shaking, or easy fatigability), autonomic hyperactivity (e.g., palpitations, sweating, diarrhea, shortness of breath), or vigilance and scanning (e.g., feeling on edge, insomnia, increased startle response). The anxiety cannot occur only during a mood or psychotic disorder and cannot be due solely to concerns about the symptoms of another disorder, such as panic attacks or social scrutiny.

Even with these changes, GAD remains quite an imprecise category and includes a heterogeneous group of patients. Diagnostic inter-rater reliability for GAD is lower than for other anxiety disorders, largely because although it may be clear that someone meets the diagnostic criteria, clinicians disagree as to when anxiety is severe enough to be considered pathological and thus warranting psychiatric diagnosis and treatment.[2] In addition, patients given the diagnosis of GAD at one point in time may actually have a residual or prodromal form of major depression or panic disorder. They may have infrequent panic attacks and so not quite meet criteria for panic

disorder, or may have subthreshold forms of other disorders such as obsessive-compulsive disorder, social phobia, or adult forms of attention deficit disorder. In many ways, then, GAD represents a "wastebasket" category used for anxious patients not clearly meeting criteria for other disorders. In addition, patients with alcohol or substance abuse or dependence often present complaining of anxiety and may mistakenly be diagnosed as having GAD.

There are no pathognomonic biological findings of GAD that have been identified as yet. Although an extensive literature suggests that traits of nervousness and emotionality may be heritable, only one family study has examined familial transmission of GAD.[3] Twenty-four of one hundred twenty-three (19.5 per cent) first-degree relatives of patients with DSM-III GAD met criteria for GAD, as opposed to 4 of 113 (3.5 per cent) of relatives of controls. However, relatives of patients with GAD had mild and often stress-related forms of GAD which might now be diagnosed as adjustment disorders. This may be in part because the probands studied had DSM-III GAD, which included more acute and milder forms of anxiety. Further studies are needed to determine the extent to which GAD is familial or heritable.

Frequently changing diagnostic criteria and the heterogeneity of GAD patients makes it difficult to interpret not only the results of biological testing and family studies, but also the outcome and applicability of treatment trials. The inclusion of patients with coexisting panic attacks, depressive symptoms, or differing degrees of illness severity and chronicity may have important effects on treatment outcome data and limit the generalizability of findings to other clinical populations.

Nevertheless, clinicians frequently encounter patients with generalized anxiety, especially in primary care settings, and must often recommend treatment. In this chapter, we will review the available information about specific therapeutic modalities tested in GAD. Before initiating treatment, it is important, however, to rule out anxiety due to medical conditions, and especially due to prescribed or illicit drugs (Table 42–1). A thorough psychiatric assessment should also be performed to rule out coexisting depression, psychosis, or other conditions requiring different types of treatment.

TABLE 42–1. DIFFERENTIAL DIAGNOSIS
OF GENERALIZED ANXIETY

Psychiatric conditions
  Other anxiety disorders, mania, psychotic disorders, delirium
Medications and drugs
  Caffeine, stimulants, alcohol or sedative withdrawal, opiates,
    cocaine, marijuana, hallucinogens, steroids, theophylline,
    sympathomimetics, thyroid replacement, lidocaine, do-
    pamine
Cardiovascular disease
  Arrhythmias, congestive heart failure, pulmonary edema,
    coronary artery disease
Respiratory disease
  Asthma, COPD,[a] pulmonary embolism, hyperventilation,
    pneumothorax
Endocrine and metabolic disorders
  Hyperthyroidism, hypothyroidism, hypoglycemia, Cushing's,
    anemia, hypercalcemia or hypocalcemia, carcinoid, insulin-
    oma, hyperkalemia, hyponatremia
Neurological disorders
  Seizure disorders (especially temporal lobe epilepsy), vertigo,
    tumor, akathisia
Other
  Systemic lupus erythematosis, peptic ulcer disease

[a] COPD, Chronic obstructive pulmonary disease.

PHARMACOLOGICAL TREATMENT

In some patients, generalized anxiety is suffi-ciently severe and disabling that medication treat-ment is necessary. The major medication treatments now in use for GAD are benzodiazepines and bu-spirone. The use of other agents, such as tricyclic antidepressants and β-blockers, will also be dis-cussed here.

Benzodiazepines

Benzodiazepines have long been the pharmacolog-ical treatment of choice for chronic anxiety, with numerous clinical trials attesting to their efficacy.[4] Compared with earlier antianxiety agents such as barbiturates and methaqualone (Quaaludes), benzo-diazepines have less side effects and are less lethal in overdose, thus representing a definite improve-ment. However, there are increasing concerns about risks of long-term use of benzodiazepines, especially tolerance and withdrawal syndromes. In addition, although benzodiazepines are the most widely pre-scribed psychotropic medications in the United States, both patients and physicians often feel strongly that they are harmful, that they are a "crutch" used to avoid really dealing with problems, and that taking them is a sign of emotional and even moral weakness. These attitudes lead to complicated and ambivalent feelings in most anxious patients taking and physicians prescribing these drugs, and often interfere with their prudent and rational use.

Benzodiazepines exert their clinical effects by binding to specific, high-affinity receptor sites asso-ciated with the macromolecular receptor complex for gamma-aminobutyric acid (GABA), the major in-hibitory neurotransmitter in the mammalian central nervous system (CNS).[5] They enhance the actions of GABA, resulting in their anxiolytic, sedative-hyp-notic, anticonvulsant, and muscle relaxant proper-ties.

Efficacy

Benzodiazepines are clearly effective in the acute treatment of generalized anxiety, yielding rapid re-lief of symptoms. Since most medication trials are designed to test safety and initial efficacy, there is less information available about longer term treat-ment with benzodiazepines.

Existing data regarding more chronic benzodiaze-pine use in GAD suggest that many patients may need prolonged treatment. Rickels et al.[6] found that about 50 per cent of 138 GAD patients treated with diazepam for 6 weeks were symptom-free 3 months later, while the relapse rate after a year was 63 per cent. In another study by the same group,[7] 45 chroni-cally anxious GAD patients who completed 6 months of treatment with clorazepate or buspirone were followed up 6 and 40 months after the end of the medication trial. At 6 months, moderate to severe anxiety was reported by 55 per cent of the subjects who had been treated with clorazepate and by 38 per cent of those who had taken buspirone. At 40 months, 34 patients were contacted, and 57 per cent of clorazepate-treated subjects reported moderate to severe anxiety, as opposed to 25 per cent of subjects who had received buspirone. These results suggest that, at least in some patients, GAD is a chronic ill-ness which may require treatment for significantly longer than 6 months. In addition, the observation of apparent longer term gains in buspirone-treated subjects is interesting, although it may be partially explained by the greater number of dropouts in the buspirone group during the 6 months of initial treat-ment, with only the most treatment-responsive pa-tients in the buspirone group remaining in the study.

Other authors have questioned the necessity for chronic anxiolytic, and specifically benzodiazepine, treatment for generalized anxiety. For example, Sha-piro et al.[8] performed a 6-week, double-blind study comparing diazepam (mean dose 21.4 mg/d; range 10 to 40 mg/day) to placebo and brief psychotherapy in 224 anxious outpatients, most of whom were ret-rospectively diagnosed as having DSM-III GAD. Diazepam was superior to placebo only during the first week of treatment. However, many of the sub-jects in this study had anxiety of shorter duration and lesser severity than the patients studied by Rick-els and Schweizer. In Shapiro et al.'s more severely anxious patients, diazepam was superior to placebo on some measures at the end of 6 weeks. Thus, milder and less chronic GAD may not require medi-cation treatment at all, at least beyond the first week, while for some more chronically and severely anx-ious patients, prolonged medication treatment may be necessary.

Although individual benzodiazepines are marketed specifically as sedative-hypnotics or anxiolytics, all available medications in this class have comparable anxiolytic effects when given at comparable doses, with the possible exception of quazepam, which is purported to be a selective hypnotic on the basis of animal studies. In choosing a benzodiazepine for treatment of GAD, pharmacokinetic properties such as half-life, metabolism, and onset of action are the most important factors.[9]

Side Effects

Compared with other psychotropic drugs, benzodiazepines have relatively few side effects. The most common include sedation, incoordination, slowed reflexes, and impaired ability to learn new information.[10] Tolerance to sedation usually develops within the first week of treatment. Mood changes, including depression, mania, paradoxical excitement, and aggression, have been reported with benzodiazepine use. Behavioral disinhibition may be more common with the use of these medications in individuals with poor impulse control, severe personality disorders such as borderline personality disorder, dissociative states, and organic brain syndromes, including acquired immune deficiency syndrome (AIDS).

Important psychomotor effects of benzodiazepines include the documented impairment in driving performance associated with acute administration of benzodiazepines and the increase in falls and hip fractures in elderly patients taking these drugs.[11] Although tolerance to psychomotor effects develops after the first few weeks of treatment, patients must be warned not to drive or attempt complex or dangerous psychomotor tasks at any time when they feel sleepy. Alcohol or any other sedating drug, including such easily overlooked drugs as over-the-counter cold remedies, may potentiate psychomotor side effects and difficulty driving.

Memory effects of benzodiazepines primarily include impaired ability to learn new information, or anterograde amnesia. Anterograde amnesia occurs with all benzodiazepines but may be more common with high-potency compounds such as triazolam. Tolerance may not develop to amnestic side effects and the patient may be unaware of the problem. The clinician must therefore be vigilant in looking for any signs of short-term memory impairment during chronic benzodiazepine treatment.

Benzodiazepines have been widely prescribed for over 30 years without clear-cut evidence of significant long-term medical complications persisting after discontinuation of the drug. Increased ventricular:brain ratios and persistent cognitive and psychomotor side effects with long-term benzodiazepine treatment have been noted in a few reports but contradicted in an equal number of other studies.[7] Animal studies of state-dependent learning have raised concerns that benzodiazepine treatment may impair the ability to cope with new situations, with the patient instead relying on medication to deal with stress. Whether this is a clinically significant consideration in the treatment of anxious patients remains to be established.

Recently, concerns about benzodiazepines have focused on their well-established risks of dependence and withdrawal symptoms.[12] Dose escalation is rare in patients without coexisting substance abuse, with one study showing no dosage increases in 119 anxious patients after an average of 8 years of benzodiazepine use.[13] Benzodiazepines are best avoided in patients with a history of alcohol or other substance abuse or dependence. In addition, first-degree relatives of substance abusers may be at increased risk for addiction if prescribed these drugs.[14] Withdrawal symptoms are common in patients prescribed benzodiazepines for even a few weeks and seem to be more likely to occur with longer duration of use, higher dosages, abrupt taper of short–half-life agents, and in patients with dependent personality traits.[12] To minimize chances of uncomfortable withdrawal symptoms and, most importantly, of the rare risk of withdrawal seizures, benzodiazepines should be tapered no faster than by 25 per cent of the dose every week.

Prescribing Benzodiazepines

Treatment of GAD with benzodiazepines usually requires daily doses of the equivalent of 10 to 40 mg of diazepam. A lower dose may be necessary for the first week until the patient develops tolerance to sedative and psychomotor side effects. It is prudent and may be reassuring to patients to instruct them to take their first dose at home when they do not need to drive, go to work, or perform complex tasks. Patients should be alerted to the risks of enhanced CNS depression with alcohol and other sedatives, of dependence and withdrawal, and of seizures with abrupt discontinuation. It is often helpful to both the physician and the patient to have a clear idea at the outset of the diagnosis and specific symptoms being treated with the medication and the approximate expected length of treatment. With benzodiazepine treatment of GAD, it is especially important to have an idea of whether the medication is designed specifically to treat a temporary exacerbation of symptoms or is being used as a more chronic treatment of a long-lasting condition (see Appendix III).

Buspirone

Buspirone is a new azapirone anxiolytic, which appears comparable in efficacy to benzodiazepines for GAD.[15] It does not interact with benzodiazepine receptors, but instead is a 5-HT$_{1A}$ receptor partial agonist that may also increase CNS noradrenergic and dopaminergic activity. Its apparent lack of sedative and psychomotor effects, dependence, and withdrawal symptoms make it a very attractive alternative to benzodiazepines in the pharmacological treatment of GAD.

Several double-blind studies have now demonstrated that buspirone is superior to placebo and as effective as benzodiazepines in the acute treatment of GAD. Buspirone is equivalent in efficacy to diazepam, lorazepam, clorazepate, and alprazolam, with mean reductions in Hamilton Anxiety Scale scores of 30 to 50 per cent over 2- to 6-week trials. In a primary care setting, a double-blind trial of buspirone versus oxazepam showed comparable results of the two medications in treating anxious patients with a Hamilton Anxiety Scale score of 18 or more, and a 4-week or greater duration of illness.[16] The effects of buspirone, however, build gradually over 2 to 4 weeks in contrast to benzodiazepines, which have immediate results.

A 4-week study by Rickels et al.[17] showed more improvement in psychic anxiety symptoms with buspirone and greater effects on somatic symptoms with diazepam. Feighner and Cohn[18] demonstrated earlier effects of buspirone on psychic than on somatic symptoms of GAD. Thus, buspirone may be particularly effective in patients with prominent cognitive and psychic anxiety, at least in the first few weeks of treatment.

Buspirone also appears effective in long-term treatment of GAD. In the 6-month trial by Rickels et al. mentioned earlier, buspirone was as effective as clorazepate both after the first 4 weeks and for the 6-month maintenance treatment phase.[7] In fact, there was a suggestion of greater therapeutic gains with buspirone. However, there were more dropouts in the buspirone group during treatment, indicating less overall patient satisfaction with this medication.

Buspirone has a half-life of from 2 or 3 to 11 hours and thus requires b.i.d. or t.i.d. dosing. The usual starting dose is 5 mg t.i.d. Average daily doses for GAD are 20 to 30 mg, with doses above 60 mg reported to cause dysphoria. Buspirone is oxidized in the liver and excreted in urine.

Cimetidine increases levels of the major buspirone metabolite, while buspirone may increase blood levels of desmethyldiazepam and haloperidol. Although preliminary reports suggest that buspirone is well tolerated in the elderly, the effects of age and hepatic and renal disease on buspirone metabolism are not yet known. There have been reports of hypertensive reactions in patients taking buspirone with monoamine oxidase inhibitor (MAOI) antidepressants.

Patients withdrawn from prior benzodiazepine treatment have not responded well to buspirone. This is probably a result of several factors. These may be among the most severely ill patients with GAD, since they have required chronic benzodiazepine treatment. Patients accustomed to the rapid relief and sedation produced by benzodiazepines may be less satisfied with buspirone's gradual onset of action. In addition, buspirone does not show cross-tolerance with benzodiazepines and does not treat benzodiazepine withdrawal symptoms.[19] Patients taken off benzodiazepines may be undergoing withdrawal and thus appear not to respond as well to buspirone. To switch medications, a therapeutic dose of buspirone should be added to the benzodiazepine for 2 to 4 weeks before the benzodiazepine is tapered.

Common side effects of buspirone include nausea, dizziness, and headaches. Unlike benzodiazepines, buspirone has not been shown to be sedating, to increase the effects of CNS depressants, or to cause psychomotor impairment. There is no evidence to date of any risk of tolerance, withdrawal symptoms, or rebound anxiety after discontinuation of buspirone. These factors make buspirone now the first-line pharmacological treatment of GAD except in cases where immediate relief of disabling symptoms is essential. Buspirone is particularly attractive in the treatment of elderly patients, those with a history of substance abuse, and those taking CNS depressants or in whom sedation would be dangerous (e.g., truck drivers, pilots, patients with severe respiratory disease).[10]

Other Medication Treatments

One of the features initially used to differentiate GAD from panic disorder was treatment response. While panic disorder was treatable with antidepressants, GAD was thought to respond only to benzodiazepines. This view of GAD has been challenged by recent studies suggesting that tricyclic antidepressants may alleviate GAD symptoms. Kahn et al.[20] found that imipramine was superior to chlordiazepoxide in the treatment of nondepressed outpatients retrospectively diagnosed as having GAD. Hoehn-Saric et al.,[21] in a prospective study of nondepressed patients meeting DSM-III-R criteria for GAD, showed differential effects of alprazolam and imipramine. Overall, alprazolam was more effective in the first 2 weeks, but the two medications were comparable after this period. Imipramine was more effective in treating psychic anxiety symptoms such as dysphoria, obsessionality, interpersonal sensitivity, and negative anticipatory thinking, while alprazolam yielded greater improvements in somatic, especially cardiovascular and autonomic, anxiety symptoms.

β-Blockers have also been studied as a treatment for chronic anxiety.[22] Although some studies have shown superiority of β-blockers over placebo in GAD, others have not, and the literature is inconclusive. It appears that β-blockers may be helpful for patients with prominent cardiovascular complaints, such as tachycardia and palpitations, or for performance anxiety, but that they are not clearly effective for patients with GAD as a group.

Several anxiolytics are now under study and will probably become available in the next few years. These include newer azapirones, such as gepirone and ipsaparone, and adinazolam, another triazolobenzodiazepine. Alpidem and zolpidem are both compounds specifically interacting with limbic benzodiazepine receptors, and thus having less sedative, psychomotor, and cognitive side effects as well as, possibly, less potential for tolerance and withdrawal.

PSYCHOLOGICAL TREATMENTS

In contrast with pharmacological treatments, psychotherapeutic approaches to GAD have been the subject of few systematic studies. However, data now available suggest that psychological approaches can be quite successful in the treatment of many patients, especially those with milder or less chronic forms of GAD.

The oldest psychological treatments for anxiety include relaxation training and biofeedback.[2] Early studies of the efficacy of these treatments used primarily nonclinical populations, such as anxious undergraduates, with only a few studies including subjects with anxiety neurosis. Biofeedback demonstrated consistent benefit only with frontal electromyographic (EMG) biofeedback, which was comparable to relaxation training. Relaxation techniques were generally superior to waiting-list control or placebo conditions. However, only a small minority of subjects treated with relaxation reported significant reductions in anxiety. Relaxation training and biofeedback appear to be relatively nonspecific treatments that may be useful as an adjunct to other treatments, but which are unlikely to suffice as sole or primary treatments of GAD.

A study by Tarrier and Main[23] of 50 patients with panic attacks or generalized anxiety supports this view. In a 6-week trial, they assessed the effects of a treatment package based primarily on progressive muscle relaxation, with the addition of breathing exercises, self-monitoring of anxiety, and positive mental imagery. Treated patients fared better than waiting-list controls, who did not change. Seventy per cent of the treated patients reported some benefit, especially in somatic anxiety symptoms. However, only 20 per cent reported marked improvement and 60 per cent required further treatment after the end of the study.

In recent years, more specific psychological treatments for GAD have been developed. These fall into the two broad categories of anxiety management and cognitive-behavioral therapy. As early as 1974, Beck et al.[24] identified characteristic cognitions associated with free-floating anxiety states. In GAD, patients frequently have fears (which they recognize as irrational or exaggerated) of losing control, being unable to cope, or being publicly embarassed. Anxiety management strategies generally aim to teach ways of coping with anxiety symptoms associated with these fears, while cognitive-behavioral therapy involves examination and change of patients' anxiety-related cognitions and behavior.

Butler et al.[25] used a form of anxiety management to treat 45 patients with Research Diagnostic Criteria (RDC) GAD. Research diagnostic criteria are similar to DSM-III-R criteria for GAD, but patients with panic attacks were included and 13 met criteria for panic disorder. Patients were treated for 4 to 12 1-hour sessions (mean 8.7 sessions) with a treatment combining education regarding anxiety symptoms, instructions in progressive muscle relaxation, identification of factors precipitating or maintaining anxiety, control of upsetting thoughts by examination of how realistic they are, encouraging pleasurable activities, focusing on the patient's strengths, and encouraging exposure to feared situations. This latter measure is interesting, since although patients with GAD do not meet criteria for agoraphobia, they often have fears or mild avoidance as a result of their anxiety and limit their activities without developing disabling phobias or even being conscious of their avoidance behavior.

Treated patients in this study improved significantly in comparison to waiting-list controls. Furthermore, waiting-list controls were then treated, showing comparable treatment responses. Both groups demonstrated decreases in mean Hamilton Anxiety Scale scores from about 16 before treatment, to about 7 after treatment. With treatment, 51 per cent fell below the cutoff used to define a clinical "case" using the Leeds scales. Treatment gains were maintained or increased during 6 months of follow-up. Treatment response was similar in patients with and without a history of panic attacks.

These results were promising, although the treatment package used included a large number of components. It was not clear which measures were the most effective. In addition, patients in this study had been symptomatic for 2 years or less and thus were not among the most chronic and severely affected patients with GAD. Their initial Hamilton Anxiety Scale ratings were lower than those required for most pharmacotherapy trials for GAD, which may indicate differences in rating patterns or milder GAD. A later analysis of this study[26] identified three factors predicting treatment success. Patients with lower initial levels of anxiety, less demoralization about their condition, and more dysphoria had a better treatment outcome. These findings reinforce the view that this type of treatment may be most effective for less severely anxious patients with GAD.

A recent controlled trial by the same group[27] separated the behavioral and cognitive components of anxiety management. Fifty-seven subjects with DSM-III-R GAD were assigned to behavioral treatment, teaching control of anxiety symptoms through relaxation, graded exposure, and participation in pleasurable or rewarding activities, to cognitive therapy focusing on changing dysfunctional thoughts, or to a waiting-list control group. Cognitive therapy was clearly superior to behavior therapy in this study.

These findings confirm observations of other investigators of the efficacy of cognitive therapy in GAD. In 1984, Barlow et al.[28] showed significant improvements in clinical ratings, self-ratings, questionnaire scores, and psychophysiological measures in patients with panic disorder or GAD treated with relaxation and cognitive-behavioral treatment. A waiting-list control group was unchanged. Encouragingly, treated patients continued to improve during the 6-month follow-up period. Preliminary results of a study by this same group of cognitive-behavioral treatment versus relaxation versus a combination of both treatments versus a waiting-list control condition for GAD indicates superior results using cognitive-behavioral therapy for GAD.[2]

Another study of 30 nondepressed patients with DSM-III GAD compared the effects of adding either cognitive-behavioral or nondirective psychotherapy to progressive muscle relaxation.[29] Both groups improved, but cognitive-behavioral therapy was superior to nondirective therapy as assessed by multiple questionnaires. Several patients who developed anxiety with relaxation had a poorer treatment outcome.

Although psychodynamic psychotherapy may be helpful for some anxious patients, no systematic trials of this type of therapy have been performed. As yet, the effects of combined medication and psychological treatment of GAD also have not been assessed. This is an important issue. Although studies of antidepressant and cognitive-behavioral treatment have shown advantages of combined treatment in major depression and panic disorder with agoraphobia, reports of impaired desensitization treatment in simple phobics taking benzodiazepines raise concerns about combined therapy, at least with these medications.

CONCLUSION

There are now several effective treatments available for chronic generalized anxiety. The benzodiazepines provide rapid and dramatic relief of anxiety symptoms and are thus ideal for patients suffering from disabling GAD. The major drawbacks of benzodiazepine use have included sedation, psychomotor impairment, and risks of dependence and withdrawal. Buspirone, which has none of these effects, is a very promising new pharmacological treatment for GAD. In addition, recent studies suggest that many patients may benefit from tricyclic antidepressants.

The development of specific psychotherapies tailored for GAD is an exciting advance. Although patients included in trials of psychological treatments may be less severely or chronically ill, anxiety management and especially cognitive-behavioral treatments are a desirable alternative to medication in what is often a persistent, waxing and waning condition.

The major difficulty in discussing treatment for GAD is still the heterogeneity of this disorder. Identi-

fication of clinically or biologically more homogeneous subgroups of anxious patients may facilitate the performance and interpretation of clinical trials. For now, though, many patients with chronic anxiety diagnosed as having GAD do require treatment.

In most cases, unless immediate symptomatic relief is essential, a trial of psychotherapy is the initial treatment of choice. This should include cognitive-behavioral techniques. Psychotherapy alone may suffice for many more acutely and less severely ill patients. Some patients will also require pharmacotherapy. At this point, buspirone is probably the treatment of choice. Benzodiazepines remain useful for patients needing immediate relief in order to function, especially in the first few weeks of treatment, when they may also be combined with other therapies. Those patients not responding to buspirone may be treated with benzodiazepines or tricyclic antidepressants.

In cases of longstanding GAD, medication can be prescribed on an ongoing basis or used to treat exacerbations of anxiety, with "drug holidays" when symptoms are less severe. It is important to recognize that in some people, GAD is a severe, lifelong, and disabling condition. Despite the clinician and patient's best efforts, long-term medication treatment may be needed and prove very effective for these individuals. This should not be viewed as a failure, but rather as a necessary part of the management of a chronic illness.

Presently, several new antianxiety medications and more specific psychotherapies for GAD are under active investigation. Further development of these agents, as well as investigation of the effects of combining pharmacotherapy with psychological treatments, promises to increase and improve treatment options for patients with GAD.

REFERENCES

1. Weissman MM, Merikangas KR: The epidemiology of anxiety and panic disorders: An update. J Clin Psychopharmacol 46(suppl 6):11–17, 1986.
2. Barlow DH: Anxiety and its Disorders. New York, Guilford Press, 1988.
3. Noyes R, Clarkson C, Crowe RR, et al: A family study of generalized anxiety disorder. Am J Psychiatry 144:1019–1024, 1987.
4. Greenblatt DJ, Shader RI, Abernethy DR: Current status of benzodiazepines (second of two parts). N Engl J Med 309:410–416, 1983.
5. Tallman JF, Paul SM, Skolnick P, et al: Receptors for the age of anxiety: Pharmacology of the benzodiazepines. Science 207:274–281, 1980.
6. Rickels K, Schweizer E, Csanalosi I, et al: Long-term treatment of anxiety and risk of withdrawal: Prospective comparison of clorazepate and buspirone. Arch Gen Psychiatry 45:444–450, 1988.
7. Rickels K, Schweizer E: The clinical course and long-term management of generalized anxiety disorder. J Clin Psychopharmacol 10:101S–110S, 1990.
8. Shapiro AK, Struening EL, Shapiro E, et al: Diazepam: How much better than placebo? J Psychiatr Res 17:51–73, 1983.
9. Cowley DS, Roy-Byrne PP, Greenblatt DJ: Benzodiazepines: Pharmacokinetics and pharmacodynamics. *In* Roy-Byrne

PP, Cowley DS, eds. Benzodiazepines in Clinical Practice: Risks and Benefits. Washington, DC: American Psychiatric Association Press, 1991.

10. Dubovsky SL: Generalized anxiety disorder: New concepts and psychopharmacologic therapies. J Clin Psychiatry 51(suppl 1):3–10, 1990.

11. Hommer DW: Benzodiazepines: Cognitive and psychomotor effects. In Roy-Byrne PP, Cowley DS, eds. Benzodiazepines in Clinical Practice: Risks and Benefits. Washington, DC: American Psychiatric Association Press, 1991.

12. Roy-Byrne PP, Hommer DW: Benzodiazepine withdrawal: Overview and implications for the treatment of anxiety. Am J Med 84:1041–1051, 1988.

13. Rickels K, Case WG, Schweizer E, et al: Low-dose dependence in chronic benzodiazepine users: A preliminary report on 119 patients. Psychopharmacol Bull 22:407–415, 1986.

14. Ciraulo DA, Barnhill JG, Ciraulo AM, et al: Parental alcoholism as a risk factor in benzodiazepine abuse: A pilot study. Am J Psychiatry 146:1333–1335, 1989.

15. Petracca A, Nisita C, McNair D, et al: Treatment of generalized anxiety disorder: Preliminary clinical experience with buspirone. J Clin Psychiatry 51(suppl 9):31–39, 1990.

16. Strand M, Hetta J, Rosen A, et al: A double-blind, controlled trial in primary care patients with generalized anxiety: A comparison between buspirone and oxazepam. J Clin Psychiatry 51(suppl 9):40–45, 1990.

17. Rickels K, Weisman K, Norstad N, et al: Buspirone and diazepam in anxiety: A controlled study. J Clin Psychiatry 43:81–86, 1982.

18. Feighner JP, Cohn JB: Analysis of individual symptoms in generalized anxiety—a pooled, multistudy, double-blind evaluation of buspirone. Neuropsychobiology 21:124–130, 1989.

19. Lader M, Olajide D: A comparison of buspirone and placebo in relieving benzodiazepine withdrawal symptoms. J Clin Psychopharmacol 7:11–15, 1987.

20. Kahn RJ, McNair DM, Lipman RS, et al: Imipramine and chlordiazepoxide in depressive and anxiety disorders. II. Efficacy in anxious outpatients. Arch Gen Psychiatry 43:79–85, 1986.

21. Hoehn-Saric R, McLeod DR, Zimmerli WD: Differential effects of alprazolam and imipramine in generalized anxiety disorder: Somatic versus psychic symptoms. J Clin Psychiatry 49:293–301, 1988.

22. Hayes PE, Schulz SC: Beta-blockers in anxiety disorders. J Affective Disord 13:119–130, 1987.

23. Tarrier N, Main CJ: Applied relaxation training for generalised anxiety and panic attacks: The efficacy of a learnt coping strategy on subjective reports. Br J Psychiatry 149:330–336, 1986.

24. Beck AT, Laude R, Bohnert M: Ideational components of anxiety neurosis. Arch Gen Psychiatry 31:319–325, 1974.

25. Butler G, Cullington A, Hibbert G, et al: Anxiety management for persistent generalised anxiety. Br J Psychiatry 151:535–542, 1987.

26. Butler G, Anastasiades P: Predicting response to anxiety management in patients with generalised anxiety disorders. Behav Res Ther 26:531–534, 1988.

27. Butler G, Fennell M, Robson P, et al: Comparison of behavior therapy and cognitive behavior therapy in the treatment of generalized anxiety disorder. J Consult Clin Psychol 59:167–175, 1991.

28. Barlow DH, Cohen AS, Waddell MT, et al: Panic and generalized anxiety disorders: Nature and treatment. Behav Ther 15:431–449, 1984.

29. Borkovec TD, Mathews AM, Chambers A, et al: The effects of relaxation training with cognitive or nondirective therapy and the role of relaxation-induced anxiety in the treatment of generalized anxiety. J Consult Clin Psychol 55:883–888, 1987.

43

SIMPLE AND SOCIAL PHOBIA

JOHN E. CARR, PH.D.

There is a body of research devoted to demonstrating that the various anxiety disorders are diagnostically distinct disease entities. However, differential diagnoses of these disorders are made largely on the basis of the situation that precipitates the anxiety, to the exclusion of almost all other variables. If the fear is of a circumscribed stimulus, object, or situation, such as animals, heights, darkness, or driving, then the disorder qualifies as a simple phobia, but only if the clinician can exclude the fear of having a panic attack (as in panic disorder) or the fear of social embarrassment (as in social phobias). If the fear is of a social situation in which the patient feels likely to manifest anxiety or behave in a humiliating or embarrassing manner, or is subject to the evaluative scrutiny of others, then the disorder qualifies as a social phobia, but only if the clinician can exclude the fear of having a panic attack or of some specific characteristic of the situation. If the patient experiences a panic attack, with a discrete period of intense fear or discomfort that occurs "unexpectedly" (i.e., does not appear to occur in conjunction with either a social situation or a specific object or event), then the event qualifies as a panic attack. Thus, differentiating between a simple phobia, social phobia, agoraphobia, or panic attack is largely a function of determining the precipitating circumstance, and whether or not it is a specific cue, socially evaluative circumstance, cognitive set, or unknown and unexplained precipitant. The Epidemiologic Catchment Area (ECA) program found phobias to be the most common psychiatric disorder in the community, "more common than major depression or alcohol abuse or dependence."[1] According to this study, the 1-month prevalence is between 4 and 11.1 per cent, with the estimated prevalence in the United States being 6.2 per cent. There appears to be a tendency for prevalence rates to be higher in urban areas versus rural areas, and a slight trend in favor of higher rates among lower socioeconomic classes.

Simple phobia, like agoraphobia, is found to occur in significantly higher rates among women, whereas social phobia, which is less prevalent, appears to occur in equal rates among males and females. Social phobia is estimated to occur in 1.3 per cent of the population. However, social phobia, when cases of agoraphobia are excluded, represents only an estimated 0.6 per cent of the U.S. population. Similarly, simple phobia is estimated to occur in 5.1 per cent of the population, but when cases of agoraphobia or social phobia are excluded, may account for only 2.8 per cent of the U.S. population.[1]

While phobias are among the most commonly diagnosed psychiatric disorders, they are not the most frequently treated. Low treatment rates have been attributed to (1) the tendency to avoid dealing with distressing emotional issues, which is a characteristic of the disorder; and (2) the severity of the disorder and the relative ease with which some phobics may avoid anxiety-inducing situations without significantly impairing their lives.[1] Phobias are also found to be common among persons with other psychiatric disorders.

According to the ECA program the mean age of onset in all phobic disorders is 11 to 17 years, with a duration of 24 to 31 years.[1] However, the age-of-onset curve is highly skewed, the modal onset being in early childhood and the age-of-onset curve decreasing steeply with age. Age of onset of phobia may vary widely depending upon a multiplicity of factors: developmental course, personality, life events, precipitating events, all of which may have an impact across the entire lifespan.

Thus, phobias can develop at any age. The tendency for age of onset to vary with type of phobia is, in large part, a byproduct of the precipitating condition and onset experience. Animal phobias arise largely in the early childhood years, reflecting early encounters with animals (or teasing peers). They are less prevalent in later years, although adult fearful experiences with animals still occur (e.g., dog attacks). Social phobias tend to appear during adolescence, reflecting the increasing importance assigned to social approval by peers reinforced by family of origin. Agoraphobic disorders tend to have a later onset, reflecting the impact of stressful life change on self-esteem, sense of self-control, and perceived ability to handle anxiety and "panic."

Etiology

Phobic disorders tend to occur in greater frequencies in some families than in others. Twin studies reflect a higher rate of concordance for phobic disorders among monozygotic twins than in dizygotic twins.[2] At the same time, developmental history, socialization practice, and learning experiences obviously contribute to the acquisition and maintenance of phobic avoidant behavior. The most parsimonious explanation for these findings is that biological factors contribute to a certain susceptibility or sensitivity within biochemical or neurophysiological functioning. This biological vulnerability may lead to subtle personality differences, which in response to differential learning conditions and environmental precipitants, can lead to the development of maladaptive (avoidant) coping behaviors.[2] We have observed that phobic patients (1) appear to come from families that are somewhat conceptually naive regarding emotion, and (2) have experienced a precipitating event of severe intensity at a particular time in their lives when they were psychologically vulnerable.[3] Hence, cognitive and affective aspects of the learning history, interacting with genetic vulnerabilities, appear to play a significant role.

In the case of the simple phobic, the precipitating experience is generally tied to a specific event (e.g., being bitten by a dog, an encounter with a snake, an auto accident, an extremely rough airline flight, a visit to the dentist). The precipitating situation results in an intense surge of seemingly overwhelming anxiety and fear in an individual ill prepared conceptually or experientially to deal with this phenomenon. The very nature of the phenomenon, being so strange and alien, adds to its fearfulness. The patient concludes that this experience (intense fear) is not to be repeated, and develops an anticipatory dread that leads to avoidance of any situation or condition likely to generate the same fear response. Thus, the phenomenon in question is an anticipatory fear of the original fear. "Fear of the fear," an expectation of fear rather than an expectation of physical harm, is the primary factor in the maintenance of simple phobias.[4] The anxiety and its intensity is not only conditioned to the precipitating situation, but in large part is also identified closely with the physical symptomatology of the fear itself.

The patient may conclude that at any time somatic anxiety symptoms occur they are indicative of the onset of an anxiety attack. Thus, even symptoms precipitated by any number of other etiological factors (e.g., side effects of medication, diet, physiological response to other illnesses, or physical activity) may be interpreted as signs of phobic fear. These erroneous attributions, in turn, may lead the patient to associate the phobia with yet another environmental condition, and so on. Thus, it is not difficult to see how phobic avoidance can generalize progressively, given the dynamic interplay between biological response, cognitive attributions, environmental setting, and behavior.

Simple Phobias

Himle et al.[5] have identified four subtypes of simple phobia: (1) situational, (2) animal-insect, (3) blood-injury, (4) and choking-vomiting. Animal-insect and blood-injury phobias appear to have an age of onset in early adolescence, whereas situational phobias appear to come on in the patient's late twenties. Choking-vomiting phobias make their appearance across the age span, which is not surprising, since they are associated with a behavior (eating) that is more uniformly distributed across the developmental lifespan.

The course and outcome of simple phobia, as with all phobic conditions, is largely dependent upon the same factors that contributed to its etiology. Popular wisdom maintains that simple phobias tend to "remit spontaneously." By this it is meant that either intentionally or serendipitously, circumstances may occur that enable the individual to confront and master the fear (a child falls from a bicycle, but encouraged by peers and parents, gets back on). Thus, course and outcome will be a function of time since the onset, and the degree to which the fear and a repertoire of avoidant responses has had time and opportunity to generalize before remedial action is taken. Opportunity will, in part, be determined by the patient's life situation. (It has been 5 years since a frightening airline incident, yet a passenger's fear and avoidance of flying has never been addressed, since the passenger has had no opportunity, need, or desire to fly. By the same token, the experienced clinician will recognize that despite its 5-year duration, for the same reasons, the fear remains relatively ungeneralized and therefore easier to treat.)

For the simple phobic, the feared consequence is the fear response itself. For the social phobic, the feared consequence is less the fear response per se (although this is clearly a condition of great discomfort for the patient), but rather the resultant embarrassment and humiliation that he or she will experience with the realization that others in the social situation have observed his or her anxiety. Agoraphobia, by comparison, appears to take the social evaluation of the social phobic one step further. The onset of the feared anxiety attack implies for the agoraphobic a loss of control and inability to function, not simply social embarrassment but social and personal incompetence. For the agoraphobic, each successive attack of anxiety represents a progressive diminution in confidence and self-esteem.

Social Phobia

Social phobia is generally characterized by a somewhat greater degree of severity of symptomatology, physiological distress, and life impairment than simple phobia, but less than agoraphobia and panic disorder.[6] Some evidence suggests that social phobia may be composed of two subgroups: "generalized social phobics" and "specific social phobics." The usual distinction between these subcategories is that the generalized social phobic is an individual who possesses fewer social skills in general, covering a wider number of situations, whereas specific social phobics may possess acceptable generalized social skills, but find themselves immobilized in specific situations; for example, public speaking. General social phobias are more likely to develop slowly and to be more chronic in nature. This reflects both the social reticence of the patient and the tendency of friends and family to disregard what is perceived as simply shyness. As with simple phobia, however, where more timely efforts are made to encourage confrontation and mastery of the fear, the phobic disorder can have a shorter course. The situation-specific social phobic is more likely to seek professional assistance or undertake remedial actions (e.g., Toastmasters), especially where the more focal difficulty impinges upon the patients occupation or other important life circumstance.

Differential diagnosis between social phobia and avoidant personality is problematic. Three of eight DSM-III-R criteria for avoidant personality are identical with criteria for social phobia. Avoidant personalities appear to be equally anxious, but have fewer social skills than social phobics, whose anxiety is more limited to specific situations and discrete in its onset. Whereas social phobia and avoidant personality are equally prevalent among males and females, avoidant personalities consistently demonstrate significantly poorer eye contact, poorer voice tone in social situations, and poorer overall skill in same-sex and opposite-sex social interactions than social phobics.

Differential diagnosis between social phobia and schizoid personality hinges on the nature of the social withdrawal. Whereas the social phobic has a pronounced desire to function in social settings but is impaired in so doing by severe anxiety, the schizoid personality appears to have little or no interest in social interaction and is characterized by a profound anhedonia and lack of social responsiveness as opposed to severe anxiety.

There is evidence to suggest that simple phobia, social phobia, and agoraphobia lie along a continuum of increasing severity, general distress, and debilitation.[6] The disorders can also be distinguished along cognitive dimensions as well. Simple phobia seems primarily concerned with the nature of the fear response, social phobia with the negative evaluation of others, and agoraphobia with the implications regarding personal control and confidence. Our clinical observations in this regard are confirmed by those of Turner and Beidel.[7]

Assessment

As variability in definition, differential diagnosis, estimates of prevalence, and age of onset suggest, phobic disorders are difficult to measure objectively. For example, although designed to provide a reasonably objective assessment of DSM-III-R–defined phobic disorder by even nonprofessional staff, the Diagnostic Interview Schedule suffers from relatively poor inter-rater reliability (k = .47) when used to measure phobia.[8] DiNardo et al.[9] developed the Anxiety Disorders Interview Schedule (ADIS) designed to yield differential diagnoses among the DSM-III-R anxiety categories. Interrator reliability was quite high for agoraphobia (k = .85) and social phobia (k = .91), but low for simple phobia (k = .56)

PHARMACOTHERAPY OF SIMPLE AND SOCIAL PHOBIA

Simple Phobia

Controlled studies of the pharmacotherapy of simple phobias are conspicuous by their rarity in the literature. In an early study, Marks et al.[10] administered a single dose of diazepam to simple phobics randomly assigned to 2-hour live-exposure sessions starting (1) 1 hour after oral diazepam 0.1 mg/kg, (2) 4 hours after the same dose, or (3) 1 to 4 hours after oral placebo. Two to three days after treatment, improvement was observed in all three conditions, but was greatest when exposure followed 4 hours after medication ingestion, and least under placebo conditions.

Simple phobics were exposed to a feared stimulus 1.5 hours after a single dose of tolamolol (20 mg), diazepam (10 mg), or placebo.[11] During the exposure test, tolamolol abolished the fear-induced tachycardia but not the avoidance or anxiety, while diazepam reduced avoidance but not tachycardia. Neither medication appeared to have any significant effect upon subjective fear.

Several studies have addressed the question of whether β-blocking drugs might enhance the effects of behavioral treatments of simple phobias. When administered in single doses, β-blocking drugs do not appear to enhance the outcome of behavior therapy. In some instances, selected symptomatic relief has been observed within individual treatment sessions, but this did not lead to sustained improved treatment outcome. In this regard, the effects appear to be similar to those of benzodiazepines.[12]

A distinct absence of effect for imipramine has been reported in the treatment of simple phobias.[13] Imipramine does appear to be effective in the treatment of school phobia in children who have been out of school 2 or more weeks. No improvement was observed after 3 weeks' of treatment, but by 6 weeks, children on imipramine showed definite improvement contrasted to children on placebo. However, the imipramine group had more side effects and more dropouts than the placebo group.[14] In summary, there appears to be little evidence that any of the psychotropic medications are notably effective in the treatment of simple phobias.[15,16]

Social Phobia

Although long overlooked by researchers, there has been a recent upturn in investigations of social phobia, and especially, the central neurobiological mechanisms involved in social anxiety.

Benzodiazepines

There are few controlled studies that specifically address the therapeutic effects of benzodiazepines in social phobia. Social phobics treated with clonazepam demonstrated significant improvement over nontreatment controls on overall anxiety, phobic avoidance, and social phobic symptoms.[17,18]

β-Adrenergic Blockers

The potential efficacy of β-blockers in treating social phobias was suggested in the early literature on performance anxiety. In two clinical trials. Liebowitz et al.[19] administered atenolol (50 to 100 mg/day) to ten social phobic patients for 8 weeks and the monoamine oxidase inhibitor (MAOI) phenelzine (30 to 90 mg/day) to 11 patients for 8 weeks. All patients were seen weekly but received no other therapy. Five of the ten atenolol patients improved markedly, four moderately, and one did not improve. Seven of the phenelzine patients improved markedly; four moderately.

Tricyclic Antidepressants

It is generally concluded that tricyclic antidepressants are effective in treating panic disorder, agoraphobia, generalized anxiety, and obsessive-compulsive disorder, but lack efficacy in the treatment of simple or social phobia. However, very few studies appear in the literature in which tricyclic antidepressants have been administered to social phobics.

Monoamine Oxidase Inhibitors

In a study of 41 social phobics administered phenelzine (MAOI), atenolol (β-blocker), or placebo, no significant differences were found after 4 weeks. However, after 8 weeks, phenelzine demonstrated greater efficacy than either atenolol or placebo, which did not differ significantly in their effects. In a post hoc analysis, the authors concluded that phenelzine appears to be more effective for generalized social phobia, whereas atenolol is more effective with specific social phobia.[20]

Thirty-two DSM-III–diagnosed social phobics were treated over 1 year with tranylcypromine (a nonhydrazine MAOI) in dosages of 40 to 60 mg/day. Sixty-two per cent of the patients were rated as markedly improved, and 17 per cent were moderately improved. Side effects were frequent and delayed some cases from reaching optimal dose levels until the third month of treatment.[21]

In summary, both β-blockers and MAOIs have been found effective in treatment social phobia. β-Blockers appear to reduce autonomic symptomatology. The MAOIs appear to have an effect on the cognitive as well as physiological dysfunction of social phobics and would thus make them applicable to a broader range of social phobics. β-Blockers are generally viewed as more applicable in the treatment of a specific social phobia, whereas MAOIs seem more useful in treating the generalized social phobic.

PSYCHOLOGICAL TREATMENT

Simple Phobia

The efficacy of the behavioral therapies was presumably established in treating simple phobia. The primary component of systematic desensitization, controlled exposure, has come to be recognized as the essential feature of all successful fear-reduction behavioral therapies.[22] Exposure may be accomplished through imagery or in vivo situations, over short or prolonged (flooding) periods of time, may be facilitated by modeling, and dose involve some use of cognitive techniques, albeit not to the extent required in other anxiety disorders. There are numerous variations on exposure techniques that have been developed in response to a wide range of specific phobias and are described extensively elsewhere.[23,24] Whereas research studies have been conducted to contrast the relative efficacy of these various approaches and conditions, the following general principles generally guide experienced therapists:

1. The treatment program must be based upon careful analysis of the patient's history, with careful attention paid to the complex interdependency of physiological, cognitive, and behavioral response systems.
2. The optimal procedure appears to be extended sessions of in vivo exposure (flooding) until anxiety dissipates, with practice in cognitive and behavioral coping skills carried out in conjunction with the exposure and especially during the anxiety-free period following dissipation of anxiety. Under these conditions, successful treatment has been reported in as few as three to six sessions.
3. The treatment must involve opportunities not only for the patient to be exposed to the feared situation, but also provide opportunity for "emotional education," and the development of coping skills.[3]

Social Phobia

In recent years, research interest in the simple phobias has waned as interest in school phobias has increased. Reviews of the social phobia treatment-outcome literature suggest that there are a limited number of well-controlled studies; that diagnostic definitions of the disorders have not been uniform; and that treatments vary from one study to the other.[25] Four categories of treatments are described: social skills training, relaxation training, exposure therapy, and cognitive-behavioral therapy.

Social skills training (SST) would appear to have "face validity" in the treatment of social phobia, es-

pecially in situations where social skills deficits are believed to contribute to the patient's discomfort. Ost et al.[26] found SST effective in the treatment if "behavioral reactors" (i.e., patients who demonstrated poor or inappropriate reactivity or minimal autonomic stress response). Relaxation training appeared to be more effective for "physiological reactors" (i.e., patients who manifested greater autonomic response).

Stravynski et al.[27] have questioned whether SST is effective for social phobics, or simply effective for avoidant personality disorders misdiagnosed as social phobics. According to these authors, the treatment effect does not appear to represent a "skills acquisition" process, but rather anxiety reduction, which in turn mediates behavior change. Thus, the effect of SST may be attributable to an exposure (to the fear-inducing situation) effect inherent in SST procedures and work assignments.[28]

Similarly, the vaguely defined standard relaxation training procedure per se does not appear to be effective as a treatment for social phobia. However, where it is designed to aid in developing relaxation skills that can be used in actual phobia situations, it appears to be effective to the extent that it provides a structure by which patients are encouraged to rehearse relaxation skills in role play and in vivo situations, thus incorporating other coping and exposure processes generally absent from standard relaxation training.[28] Also, where it is designed to focus attention on and familiarize the patient with his or her physiological concomitants of anxiety, it appears to be effective, again to the extent that it provides a structure by which exposure and coping exercises are encouraged and rehearsed.[3]

Although there is evidence that exposure to the feared situation is an essential component of the treatment process,[22,28] several studies suggest that patients undergoing exposure per se are more likely to demonstrate some deterioration upon long-term follow-up assessment. Thus, whereas exposure appears to lead to more immediate behavioral change, it seems to have less effect upon cognitive change, which may be especially important in long-term maintenance and relapse prevention. The combining of cognitive and exposure techniques, by design or by serendipity, appears to have addressed this problem. Exposure plus cognitive therapy shows greater long-term improvement than exposure alone or waiting-list control. The addition of cognitive restructuring to exposure therapy appears to combine immediate improvement in behavioral response with the longer term cognitive changes required for successful coping and increased relapse prevention.

In summary, the key to the combined therapy is the integration of the cognitive and exposure components (i.e., cognitive techniques must accompany and be incorporated into the exposure procedure). When this is done, patients in combined therapies evidence greater overall improvement following therapy, which is maintained at follow-up; in contrast to exposure alone, which shows selective behavioral change but less overall improvement and greater likelihood of deterioration at follow-up.

REFERENCES

1. Boyd JH, Rae DS, Thompson JW, et al: Phobia: Prevalence and risk factors. Soc Psychiatry Epidemiol 25:314–323, 1990.
2. Torgersen S: The nature and origin of common phobic fears. Br J Psychiatry 134:343–351, 1979.
3. Carr JE: Biobehavioral interactions in the treatment of phobic anxiety. *In* Roy-Byrne P, ed. Anxiety: New Findings for the Clinician. Washington, DC: American Psychiatry Association Press, 1989:181–204.
4. Di Nardo PA, Guzy LT, Jenkins JA, et al: Etiology and maintenance of dog fear. Behav Res Ther 26:241–244, 1988.
5. Himle JA, McPhee K, Cameron OG, et al: Simple phobia: Evidence for heterogeneity. Psychiatry Res 28:25–30, 1989.
6. Turner MS, McCann BS, Beidel DC, et al: DSM-III classification of the anxiety disorders: A psychometric study. J Abnorm Psychol 95:168–172, 1986.
7. Turner SM, Beidel DC: Social phobia: Clinical syndrome, diagnosis, and comorbidity. Clin Psychol Rev 9:3–18, 1989.
8. Robins LN, Helzer JE, Croughan J, et al: National Institute of Health Diagnostic Interview Schedule, its history, characteristics, and validity. Arch Gen Psychiatry 38:381–389, 1981.
9. Di Nardo PA, O'Brien GT, Barkow DH, et al: Reliability of DSM-III anxiety disorder categories using a new structured interview. Arch Gen Psychiatry 40:1070–1075, 1983.
10. Marks IM, Viswanathan R, Lipsedge MS, et al: Enhances relief of phobias by flooding during waning diazepam. Br J Psychiatry 121:493–505, 1972.
11. Bernadt MW, Silverstone T, Singleton W: Beta adrenergic blockade in phobic subjects. Br J Psychiatry 137:452–457, 1980.
12. Noyes R: Beta-adrenergic blockers. *In* Last CG, Hersen M, eds. Handbook of Anxiety Disorders. New York: Pergamon Press, 1988:445–459.
13. Zitrin CM, Klein DF, Woerner MG, et al: Treatment of phobias: I. Imipramine and placebo. Arch Gen Psychiatry 40:125–138, 1983.
14. Gittelman-Klein R, Klein DF: Controlled imipramine treatment of school phobia. Arch Gen Psychiatry 25:204–207, 1971.
15. Klein DF, Rabkin JG, Gorman JM: Etiological and pathophysiological inferences from the pharmacological treatment of anxiety. *In* Tuma AH, Maser J, eds. Anxiety and the Anxiety Disorders. Hillsdale, NJ: Lawrence Erlbaum, 1985:501–532.
16. Roy-Byrne PP, Lydiard RB: New developments in the psychopharmacologic treatment of anxiety. *In* Roy-Byrne PP, ed. Anxiety: New Findings for the Clinician. Washington, DC: American Psychiatry Association Press, 1989:151–178.
17. Munjack DJ, Baltazar PL, Bohn PB, et al: Clonazepam in the treatment of social phobia: A pilot study. J Clin Psychiatry 51(suppl 5):35–40, 1990.
18. Ontiveros A, Fontaine R: Social phobia and clonazepam. Can J Psychiatry 35:439–441, 1990.
19. Liebowitz MR, Campeas R, Levin A, et al: Pharmacotherapy of social phobia. Psychosomatics 28:305–308, 1987.
20. Liebowitz MR, Gorman JM, Fyer AJ, et al: Pharmacotherapy of social phobia: An interim report of a placebo controlled comparison of phenelzine and atenolol. J Clin Psychiatry 49:252–257, 1988.
21. Versiana M, Mundim FD, Nardi AE, et al: Tranylcypromine in social phobia. J Clin Psychopharmacol 8:279–283, 1988.
22. Marks IM: Fears, phobias and rituals. New York: Oxford University Press, 1987.
23. Sturgis ET, Scott R: Simple phobia. *In* Turner AM, ed. Behavioral Theories and Treatment of Anxiety. New York: Plenum, 1984:91–141.
24. O'Brien GT: Clinical treatment of specific phobias. *In* Mavissakalian M, Barlow DH, eds. Phobia: Psychological and Pharmacological Treatment. New York: Guilford Press, 1981.
25. Agras WS: Treatment of social phobias. J Clin Psychiatry 51(suppl):52–58, 1990.
26. Ost LG, Jerremalm A, Johnasson J: Individual response patterns and the effects of differential behavioral methods in the treatment of social phobia. Behav Res Ther 19:1–16, 1981.
27. Stravynski A, Grey S, Elie R: Outline of the therapeutic process in social skills training with socially dysfunctional patients. J Consult Clin Psychol 55:224–228, 1987.
28. Heimberg RG: Cognitive and behavioral treatments for social phobia: A critical analysis. Clin Psychol Rev 9:107–128, 1989.

44

PANIC DISORDER

DAVID V. SHEEHAN, M.D., and B. ASHOK RAJ, M.D.

CLINICAL DESCRIPTION

Although panic disorder as a diagnostic label was first used in 1980 in the DSM-III, a similar cluster of symptoms has been described in considerable detail by clinicians in earlier centuries. The essential clinical nature of panic disorder is the occurrence of unexpected panic attacks at some point in the patient's history. A panic attack is defined as any attack with at least 4 of 13 characteristic symptoms (see Table 44–1). The patient does not need to have an intense, cognitive feeling of panic to define an attack as a panic attack. A panic attack occurs when four or more of the symptoms in criterion C are present and not by any judgment of the intensity of the attack. To meet criteria for panic disorder, the patient must also have four such attacks within a 4-week period at some point in the history, or one or more such attacks followed by at least a month of persistent fear of having another such attack. It is not necessary, as is commonly assumed, that all four attacks occur in the weeks immediately prior to evaluation.

The majority of patients have two to four unexpected, unprovoked anxiety attacks per week. Typically they last about 15 to 20 minutes, with some lasting only a minute or two and some lasting more than an hour. There is considerable variability in the number of symptoms that occur during each attack; many attacks have only one or two symptoms whereas others have as many as 10 or 12 symptoms. The typical attack will usually have four to eight symptoms and is accompanied by considerable cognitive anxiety.

Approximately half of all cases of panic disorder first begin not with a full-blown panic attack, but with attacks of three or fewer symptoms. Such attacks limited to one, two, or three symptoms have been labeled as subpanic symptom attacks[1] or as limited symptom attacks. Those patients who initially experience a full-blown panic attack usually experience many limited symptom attacks in the weeks that follow their first panic attack.

It has been widely assumed that cognitive anxiety is always present during the attacks in panic disorder. However, approximately 20 per cent of all of the attacks in this disorder occur in the absence of any subjective, cognitive sense of anxiety. Limited symptom attacks are more likely than panic attacks not to be associated with cognitive anxiety.

EPIDEMIOLOGY

The Epidemiological Catchment Area (ECA) study[2] identified anxiety and phobic disorders as the most common disabling psychiatric disorders in the United States. Lifetime prevalence of these disorders is 8.3 per cent of the general adult population.[2] Panic disorder was found to have a lifetime prevalence of approximately 1.5 per cent of the general population.[2] The sex-specific rates are approximately 2.1 per cent for females and 0.6 per cent for males.[2] The criteria used in the ECA study to identify panic disorder were the Research Diagnostic Criteria (RDC), which are more restrictive than the criteria of DSM-III-R.[3] The DSM-III-R liberalized the diagnostic criteria for panic disorder to accommodate some cases that previously would have been diagnosed as generalized anxiety disorder and most cases of agoraphobia. As a result, many of those cases identified as agoraphobia and some of those identified as generalized anxiety disorder in the ECA study would now be counted among those having panic disorder. It is now estimated that the lifetime prevalence of panic disorder as identified by the DSM-III-R is approximately 3 or 4 per cent of the general population. It is estimated that approximately 2.6 million people in the United States have panic disorder using the conservative ECA findings, whereas approximately 6 million people are affected using the broader definition of panic disorder in the DSM-III-R.[4]

Age of Onset

Panic disorder has a uniform, unimodal age of onset distribution, with a peak in the 20s.[5] The mean age of onset is 23 years. It is rare for this disorder to start before the age of 15 or after the age of 40. Lifetime prevalence data from the ECA study reveal that the disorder becomes less common after the mid-40s.[2] It is twice as common in the 25- to 44-year age group as it is in the 45- to 64-year age group. After the age of 65 its prevalence drops to approximately 1/12th that of the 18- to 45-year age group. The uni-

TABLE 44–1. DIAGNOSTIC CRITERIA FOR PANIC DISORDER[a,b]

A. At some time during the disturbance, one or more panic attacks (discrete periods of intense fear or discomfort) have occurred that were (1) unexpected, i.e., did not occur immediately before or on exposure to a situation that almost always caused anxiety, and (2) not triggered by situations in which the person was the focus of others' attention.

B. Either four attacks, as defined in criterion A, have occurred within a 4-week period, or one or more attacks have been followed by a period of at least a month of persistent fear of having another attack.

C. At least four of the following symptoms developed during at least one of the attacks:
  (1) shortness of breath (dyspnea) or smothering sensations
  (2) dizziness, unsteady feelings, or faintness
  (3) palpitations or accelerated heart rate (tachycardia)
  (4) trembling or shaking
  (5) sweating
  (6) choking
  (7) nausea or abdominal distress
  (8) depersonalization or derealization
  (9) numbness or tingling sensations (paresthesias)
  (10) flushes (hot flashes) or chills
  (11) chest pain or discomfort
  (12) fear of dying
  (13) fear of going crazy or of doing something uncontrolled

D. During at least some of the attacks, at least four of the C symptoms developed suddenly and increased in intensity within 10 minutes of the beginning of the first C symptom noticed in the attack.

E. It cannot be established that an organic factor initiated and maintained the disturbance, e.g., amphetamine or caffeine intoxication, hyperthyroidism.

[a] Reprinted with permission from American Psychiatric Association: Diagnostic and Statistical Manual of Mental Disorders. 3rd ed. Revised. Washington, DC: American Psychiatric Association, 1987:237–238.
[b] Note: Mitral valve prolapse may be an associated condition, but does not preclude a diagnosis of panic disorder.

model age of onset distribution is difficult to explain in psychological terms but is consistent with the biological illness model of panic disorder, in which the disorder appears to afflict women in their childbearing years preferentially.

Life Course

Panic disorder has a chronic fluctuating course during the middle years of life. Approximately 50 per cent of patients are disabled to some degree and 73 to 92 per cent are symptomatic when reevaluated up to 20 years after initial diagnosis.[6,7] Patients with panic disorder have an excess mortality from suicide, and among males from cardiovascular disease, when compared with controls matched for age and sex.[8]

Gender Distribution

Seventy-five to 80 per cent of the victims of panic disorder are women.[5,7] This appears to be unrelated to educational status, ethnic background, or social status. The observation that women are at increased risk for panic disorder is in contrast to the gender distribution in some other anxiety disorders, such as obsessive-compulsive disorder, in which the gender distribution is equal.

GENETICS

Panic disorder is believed to be genetically inherited. Lifetime morbidity risk among first-degree relatives is 15 to 25 per cent.[9] There is an increased concordance in monozygotic as compared to dizygotic twins. The transmission pattern within families is consistent with the inheritance pattern for an autosomal dominant gene or with single-locus genetics.[10] A recent preliminary genetic linkage study suggested that panic disorder may be coded by a gene on chromosome 16, position Q22.[10]

SYMPTOM PROGRESSION OVER TIME

The symptoms of this illness appear to follow an orderly progression over time and do not appear to occur in the random haphazard fashion that was previously believed. The disorder first begins in about 50 per cent of cases with unexpected panic symptom attacks without any feeling of cognitive anxiety or panic (limited symptom attacks). Later an attack may occur with four or more symptoms during the same attack. Because the attacks often occur in an unexpected, unprovoked manner, the patient may be at a loss to explain any psychosocial reason for their symptoms. He or she interprets the events as an expression of a medical illness, and usually first seeks evaluation from an internist or a family physician rather than a psychiatrist. Every specialist evaluating the patient usually finds no serious medical illness to explain the symptoms. The clinician then reassures the patient that "there is nothing seriously wrong," that the disorder is "just stress and nerves." Use of a stress/conflict model to conceptualize this disorder and the physician's reassurance that there is "nothing wrong" rarely helps.

Within weeks the patient usually has another unexpected panic attack and is at a loss to explain why the attack occurred in the absence of any stress or conflict. Because the physician used a stress/conflict model to identify it as an anxiety disorder and the attack occurred in the absence of stress or conflict, the patient interprets this to mean that he or she does not have an anxiety disorder. The patient then assumes he or she has an exotic medical illness and begins to search for a specialist who has the diagnostic sophistication or the appropriate technology to make an accurate diagnosis. Each specialty has a different technology and often a different examination routine in evaluating some dimension of this disorder. The patient engages in excessive health worries and goes doctor shopping in search of a solution.

The majority of patients continue to have attacks unexpectedly in a variety of situations. Patients begin to fear and avoid situations they associate with their bad attacks. If the unexpected attacks continue, the phobias begin to generalize. Patients often progress to the stage of extensive phobic avoidance behavior, and some even become housebound. At this stage they are often labeled as agoraphobic, which means literally a fear of the marketplace or of places where crowds assemble. Extensive phobic avoidance behavior seems to be related to how chronic and how frequently the unexpected anxiety attacks occur.

As they become progressively disabled by their symptoms, patients are given many interpretations of their disorder. Approximately 50 to 60 per cent of patients develop a secondary demoralization depression. The more socially isolated and alienated they feel, and the more misunderstood their symptoms, the more depressed they usually become. Twenty per cent of patients with panic disorder report suicide attempts, and 12 per cent of patients with panic attacks report suicide attempts.[11]

Not all of the patients progress in an orderly manner through these stages as described. In the majority of cases, however, there is a pattern of progression from unexpected attacks to progressive phobic avoidance behavior and increasing depression over time.

DIFFERENTIAL DIAGNOSIS

Psychiatric Differential Diagnosis

Several other anxiety disorders have symptoms in common with panic disorder. If a patient meets criteria for hypochondriasis or somatization disorder, these diagnoses should be made in addition to panic disorder. A suspicion of panic disorder should be present in any patient in whom one suspects either hypochondriasis, depersonalization, or somatization disorder. Before making a diagnosis of agoraphobia without panic attacks, it is important to rule out a past history of panic disorder, even if the patient does not currently meet criteria for this condition. It is also wise not to give a diagnosis of simple or social phobia without first being careful to ensure that at no stage in the natural history of the disorder did the patient ever meet criteria for panic disorder. Many patients with panic disorder have low-grade obsessions or compulsions. However, it is unusual for patients with panic disorder to engage in rituals of an hour or more per day, such as are necessary to meet full criteria for obsessive-compulsive disorder (OCD).

Approximately 50 per cent of patients with panic disorder have a secondary demoralization depression at the time of evaluation, and 70 per cent give a history of past depressive episodes. It has been estimated that 15 per cent of patients with primary major depressive disorder may have panic attacks. Both diagnoses should be made if the patient meets criteria for both major depressive episode and panic disorder. In assessing which is the primary disorder, one should assess which disorder came first in the natural history and which cluster of symptoms is more prominent in the presenting symptom cluster.

A majority of panic disorder patients meet criteria for generalized anxiety disorder (GAD). Many patients who meet criteria for GAD have had one or more panic attacks at some stage in the course of their disorder. In psychiatric practice pure cases of DSM-III-R GAD (who do not meet criteria for any other anxiety disorder) are rare when structured interviews are used to make the diagnosis.

Panic attacks may occur as part of a withdrawal syndrome from alcohol, barbiturates, and benzodiazepines. Between 10 and 20 per cent of agoraphobic/anxious neurotic outpatients are alcohol dependent.[12] Panic disorder should not be diagnosed when panic attacks are associated with abuse of drugs such as marijuana, caffeine, cocaine, or amphetamine-like stimulants, all of which are associated with high panic rates.

The other major psychiatric syndromes, including bipolar disorder, are usually not difficult to distinguish from panic disorder. However, some cases of bipolar II disorder and rapid cycling bipolar mood disorder may present with complaints of agitation, restlessness, anxiety, and even panic symptoms. Sometimes these patients are referred because there is a history of failure to respond to the usual antipanic drugs. Several such patients seen by these authors responded to carbamazepine.

Medical Differential Diagnosis

Because panic disorder presents with symptoms that affect almost every body system, the clinician is tempted to do costly medical and laboratory evaluations on these patients. Without sensible guidelines, clinicians vacillate between excessive and obsessive laboratory work-ups and failure to properly consider the medical illnesses that can mimic panic disorder. We have suggested an approach to the medical evaluation of the anxious patient.[13] The first step is to take a proper medical history and to do a systematic medical review of systems and past medical illnesses. If this questioning elicits responses of concern to the clinician, a physical exam may be necessary. Positive findings in the history and on physical exam warrant routine laboratory investigation. After these routine tests the clinician is better able to judge the need for more sophisticated levels of laboratory investigation. Table 44–2 lists medical illnesses often associated with anxiety disorders.

TREATMENT

Panic disorder is now usually treated with a sequence of distinct approaches. The first and most

TABLE 44–2.   MEDICAL DISORDERS ASSOCIATED WITH ANXIETY[a]

A. *Cardiovascular/Respiratory*
   Asthma
   Cardiac arrhythmias
   Chronic obstructive pulmonary disease
   Congestive heart failure
   Coronary insufficiency
   Hypertension
   Hyperventilation syndrome
   Hyperdynamic beta-adrenergic state
   Hypoxia, embolus, infections
B. *Endocrine*
   Carcinoid
   Cushing's syndrome
   Hyperthyroidism
   Hypothyroidism
   Hypoparathyroidisms
   Hypoglycemia
   Menopause
   Pheochromocytoma
   Premenstrual syndrome
   Pregnancy
C. *Neurologic*
   Collagen vascular disease
   Epilepsy
   Huntington's disease
   Multiple sclerosis
   Organic brain syndrome—delirium, dementia
   Parkinson's disease
   Vestibular dysfunction
   Wilson's disease
D. *Substance Related*
   Intoxications:
      Anticholinergic drugs
      Aspirin
      Caffeine
      Cocaine
      Hallucinogens—including phencyclidine ("angel dust")
      Steroids
      Sympathomimetics
      THC
   Withdrawal Syndromes:
      Alcohol
      Narcotics
      Sedative hypnotics

[a] Reproduced with permission from Raj BA, Sheehan DV: Medical evaluation of panic attacks. J Clin Psychiatry 48(8):309–313, 1987.

critical of these is the use of antipanic medication to control the unexpected attacks. Because antipanic medications rarely lead to complete, timely resolution of phobic avoidance, in vivo exposure behavior therapy is then usually necessary to reduce phobic avoidance and anticipatory anxiety. If there are psychosocial problems complicating recovery, psychotherapy is indicated, but it is not routinely imposed on all patients with panic disorder. Finally, to protect patients against future relapse or to equip them if they do relapse, and to ensure good compliance to the other treatment steps, it is important to educate patients about their illness and the rationale for the treatments used. This treatment strategy is outlined in Figure 44–1.

Medication Choices

Although only one medication (alprazolam) has been formally approved by the US Food and Drug Administration for the treatment of panic disorder, there is good evidence suggesting that several classes of medications may be effective. Several studies suggest that benzodiazepines,[14–18] tricyclic antidepressants,[19–21] and monoamine oxidase inhibitors (MAOI)[22,23] are effective.

Although not all benzodiazepines, tricyclices, or MAOI have been systematically studied for panic disorder, clinical experience and case reports suggest that most, if not all, the drugs within these classes are usually effective when appropriately dosed. Neither is there evidence that any one drug within any of these classes is superior to other members of the same drug class, although this question has not been systematically studied. There is conflicting evidence on the value of trazodone in panic disorder, with Charney et al.[24] finding it ineffective (albeit using low doses) whereas in our experience, when properly dosed, it is frequently effective. The newest class of "antidepressants," the selective serotonin uptake inhibitors (SSUI); e.g., fluoxetine and fluvoxamine) are also frequently effective for panic disorder.[25] There is considerable evidence for the efficacy in panic disorder of clomipramine (a tricyclic with serotonin uptake inhibiting properties). Mianserin, a tetracyclic antidepressant available in several countries but not in the United States, is said to be effective in the treatment of panic disorder (G. Burrows, personal communication, 1988). Not all antidepressants have been found to be effective in panic disorder—bupropion hydrochloride and amoxapine hydrochloride are the exceptions.

Buspirone is a nonbenzodiazepine anxiolytic that is not better than placebo in the treatment of panic disorder.[26]

Medication Comparisons

Although alprazolam is the most thoroughly studied and most widely prescribed medication for panic disorder, the preliminary evidence suggests that it may not be unique among benzodiazepines in this regard. Alprazolam and diazepam are equally efficacious, as is clonazepam.[27,28] We have used almost every available (nonhypnotic) benzodiazepine clinically in the treatment of panic disorder and all appear to have some antipanic effects if correctly dosed. Oxazepam may be less potent than alprazolam or clonazepam, but this is a clinical impression not scientifically documented. More recently we have been using sustained-release formulations of benzodiazepines to minimize the need for frequent dosing and to circumvent the "clock watching—symptom breakthrough" syndrome sometimes seen with the widely prescribed antipanic benzodiazepines. We have found that Tranxene-SD, Valrelease, and adinazolam-SR (all sustained-release formula-

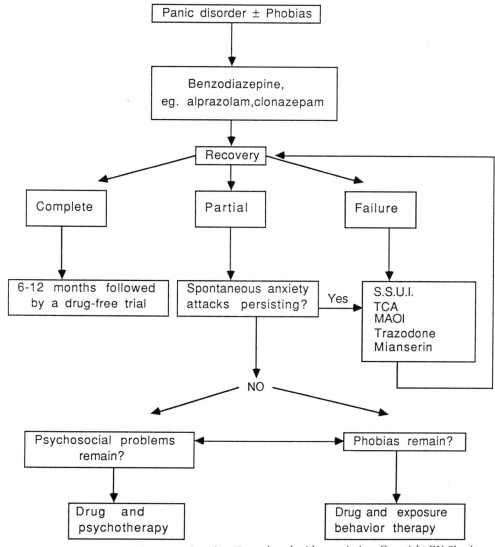

Figure 44–1. Treatment strategy for panic disorder. (Reproduced with permission. Copyright DV Sheehan, 1987.)

tions of benzodiazepines) are frequently effective for panic disorder while providing approximately a 12-hour duration of antipanic effect (not 24-hour effects, as sometimes claimed).[29]

Although imipramine is the most extensively studied tricyclic antidepressant prescribed for panic disorder, there is no evidence that it is superior (or inferior) to any other tricyclic for panic disorder. They are all equally good in our clinical experience over large numbers of patients, although there are sometimes individual variations in sensitivity to one or another. However, this assumption has never been studied in a properly controlled scientific study. It is widely assumed that clomipramine is more effective than other tricyclics for panic disorder, and it is the tricyclic of first choice among European and Australian colleagues for this disorder (G. Burrows, personal communication, 1988). Milligram for milligram it may be more potent than other tricyclics (except nortriptyline), but when an adjustment in

dose is made to compensate for this, it is unclear if clomipramine retains its superiority over other tricyclics. However, this assumption merits serious study.

Phenelzine is the most thoroughly studied MAOI prescribed for panic disorder. We have treated patients successfully with both tranylcypromine and isocarboxazid. Isocarboxazid is a hydrazine MAOI like phenelzine and unlike the nonhydrazine tranylcypromine. We have seen patients fail on tranylcypromine who subsequently responded well to phenelzine, but it is very unusual to find a failure on phenelzine who later responds to tranylcypromine. Our impression is that tranylcypromine is both subjectively better tolerated and slightly less potent overall in severe panic disorder than phenelzine.

The different classes of antipanic drugs have not all been systematically compared with each other. The study comparing phenelzine, imipramine, and placebo found evidence that phenelzine was superior to imipramine on a few but not all outcome measures.[30] A later study replicated this difference and found alprazolam overall not statistically different from either phenelzine or imipramine, although it was less effective in controlling the depressive dimension of the disorder.[19] Phenelzine had a greater effect on disability measures and appeared to be a more potent rehabilitator with its energizing, mood-elevating, confidence-enhancing effects. Overall, phenelzine appears to have a margin of superiority over other antipanic drugs. This is most apparent in severe and chronic cases. In mild to moderate cases the differences in potency are less apparent, and in such cases any of the antipanic drugs usually works well. In panic disorder associated with significant depression the benzodiazepines are not as good as the antidepressants.[19]

There are no double-blind, placebo-controlled studies available yet comparing the SSUIs with the other classes of antipanic drugs. Preliminary clinical impressions of those available suggest they are similar in potency to the tricyclics, but perhaps a little less potent than the hydrazine MAOIs.

Medication Use

The majority of failures on antipanic drugs seen by us occur because the doses used were too low, and the trials for which they were used were too short in duration. Attention to these two issues is critical to good dosage management.

With the most widely prescribed antipanic benzodiazepines, alprazolam and clonazepam, we initiate treatment and titrate the dose over time. Alprazolam has a duration of therapeutic action of 4 to 6 hours, clonazepam 6 to 8 hours, and Tranxene-SD, Valrelease, and adinazolam-SR 12 hours, although all their elimination half-lives are quite different from those figures. Outside these windows of therapeutic benefit, patients begin to experience at least a little symptom recurrence. Consequently, the doses of each benzodiazepine must be spaced differently throughout the day to maintain a plateau of benefit without either troughs of recurrence or peaks of side effects. Most patients achieve optimal benefit after 8 to 10 weeks at between 4 to 6 mg/day alprazolam or 2 to 5 mg/day clonazepam.

With the tricyclic antidepressants we initiate treatment and also titrate the dose. Most patients get worse (more symptomatic) in the first 1 to 2 weeks on tricyclics before this reverses and they improve. This is not a bad omen and not a reason to discontinue the tricyclics. Many patients prematurely stop trials of tricyclics for this reason but might have continued on the trial if they had been warned of this before it happened. Most patients do not achieve good stable clinical benefit until they have been on the tricyclic 4 to 6 weeks. It is wise to warn patients of this lest they stop the drug in the first 3 weeks "because it is not working." Some patients may take as long as 8 to 10 weeks before obtaining significant

benefit. If possible, never abandon a trial of an antidepressant in panic disorder until the patient has been on the maximum dose he or she can tolerate for at least 10 weeks. Some patients are consistently slow responders. The minimum effective therapeutic dose of most tricyclics is 150 mg/day. The average final effective dose after 10 weeks of treatment in most specialty disorder clinics is about 225 mg/day, with some patients needing up to 300 mg/day. The exceptions are nortriptyline and clomipramine whose final doses are one half and two thirds those of imipramine and doxepin, whose doses are 25 to 50 mg/day higher (these are clinical approximations).

With the MAOI we give patients a dose-adjustment schedule with printed food and drug restrictions and have a careful discussion with them of the dietary and drug restrictions and the rationale for those, in addition to guidelines on managing the complications. We have reviewed the practical guidelines for MAOI use in panic disorder in detail elsewhere.[31] They are more widely used than a decade ago, and there is growing acceptance and awareness that, with proper dietary precautions, they are usually well tolerated. With phenelzine most patients respond to either 45 or 60 mg/day (outer range 45 to 90 mg/day), whereas most patients on tranylcypromine or isocarboxazid need 40 to 60 mg/day (outer range 29 to 90 mg/day). Sometimes half-tablet doses need to be used, particularly with phenelzine, to strike the best balance between side effects and benefit. On hydrazine MAOIs, vitamin B_6 deficiency may begin after 3 to 4 months, so supplements of 200 to 300 mg/day of vitamin B_6 are recommended to minimize "shock sensations" and carpal tunnel syndrome. In long-term use, weight gain is a problem on hydrazine MAOIs, and this can lead to tolerance to the benefits of the drug and cosmetic unhappiness. Patients usually lose the weight readily after coming off the phenelzine.

With the SSUIs the usual antidepressant doses are effective in panic disorder after 4 to 6 weeks. With fluoxetine the range of effective therapeutic dose is 10 to 60 mg/day, with occasional patients needing 80 mg/day and most patients responding to 20 or 40 mg/day. Some panic patients experience agitation, tremor, restlessness, and insomnia in the initial weeks of treatment, and this accentuates their anxiety. This is usually transient, and by week 6 to 8 this class of drugs is probably the best tolerated of all the antidepressants and interferes least long term with the quality of life. Five years from now it is likely that this class of drugs will be the most widely prescribed class for panic disorder. Those currently under study include paroxetine, sertraline, fluvoxamine, and venlafaxine.

Treatment of Residual Phobic Avoidance

After the medication has been adjusted correctly, some patients continue to have residual phobias that are a learned complication of having panic attacks. In vivo exposure behavior therapy is the most effective type of behavior therapy for these phobias once the unexpected panic and limited symptom attacks are blocked. Relaxation training is unnecessary. Gradual exposure is usually more acceptable to the patient. Exposure treatment is effective to the extent that the patient is brought in direct contact with the phobia, is kept in contact with the phobia for more than 2 hours, does not make the usual avoidance response, and practices this exposure repeatedly. Of these the most important is the duration of direct exposure. Durations of exposure of more than 1.5 hours per session are usually necessary, and the longer the exposure the greater the extinction effect on the phobia. Patients and their families can be given instructions on how to implement this effectively. When that is not effective, therapist-assisted exposure may be necessary. In treatment-resistant patients, "megadoses" of exposure treatment may be effective.[32]

Long-Term Treatment

If psychosocial problems complicate recovery, then psycotherapy is indicated. After a year of doing well on medication treatment, we tapered 106 patients from their antipanic medications. The relapse rate was in excess of 70 per cent. This is a chronic relapsing disorder, and many more patients than we are now willing to acknowledge will require long-term medication management. However, it is useful to give patients an opportunity every 12 months to see if they need to continue with their antipanic drug. If they suffer a recurrence, it is wise to quickly restart the antipanic drug and maintain them on it for at least another year.

CONCLUSION

There has been a greater proliferation of knowledge and a greater change in the treatment of panic disorder in the past decade than perhaps for any other disorder in psychiatry. This new reconceptualization is likely to continue to be an important stimulus to further understanding and improved treatment approaches.

REFERENCES

1. Sheehan DV, Sheehan KH: The classification of phobic disorders. Int J Psychiatry Med 12(4):243–264, 1982–1983.
2. Robins LN, Helzer JE, Weissman MM, et al: Lifetime prevalence of psychiatric disorders at three sites. Arch Gen Psychiatry 41:949–959, 1984.
3. American Psychiatric Association: Diagnostic and Statistical Manual of Mental Disorders. 3rd ed. Revised. Washington, DC: American Psychiatric Association, 1987.
4. McGlynn TJ, Metcalf HL: Diagnosis and Treatment of Anxi-
ety Disorders: A Physician's Handbook. Washington, DC: American Psychiatric Press, 1989.
5. Sheehan DV, Sheehan KE, Minichello WE: Age of onset of phobic disorders: A re-evaluation. Compr Psychiatry 22(6):544–553, 1981.
6. Greer S: The prognosis of anxiety states. In Lader MH, ed. Studies of Anxiety. London: Royal Medical Psychological Association, 1969:151–157.
7. Marks IM, Lader M: Anxiety states (anxiety neurosis): A review. J Nerv Ment Dis 156:3–18, 1973.
8. Coryell W, Noyes R, Clancy J: Excess mortality in panic disorder: A comparison with primary unipolar depression. Arch Gen Psychiatry 39:701–703, 1982.
9. Crowe RR, Noyes R, Pauls DL, et al: A family study of panic disorder. Arch Gen Psychiatry 40:1065–1069, 1983.
10. Crowe RR, Noyes R, Wilson AF, et al: Linkage study of panic disorder. Arch Gen Psychiatry 44:933–937, 1987.
11. Weissman MM, Klerman GL, Markowitz JS, et al: Suicidal ideation and suicide attempts in panic disorder and panic attacks. N Engl J Med 321(18):1209–1214, 1990.
12. Bibb JL, Chambless DL: Alcohol use and abuse among diagnosed agoraphobics. Behav Res Ther 24:49–58, 1986.
13. Raj A, Sheehan DV: Medical evaluation of panic attacks. J Clin Psychiatry 48(8):309–313, 1987.
14. Sheehan DV, Coleman JH, Greenblatt D, et al: Some biochemical correlates of panic attacks with agoraphobia and their response to a new treatment. J Clin Psychopharmacol 4(2):66–75, 1984.
15. Chouinard G, Annable L, Fontaine R, et al: Alprazolam in the treatment of generalized anxiety and panic disorders: A double-blind placebo-controlled study. Psychopharmacology 77:229–233, 1982.
16. Ballenger JC, Burrows GD, DuPont RL, et al: Alprazolam in panic disorder and agoraphobia: results from a multicenter trial: I. Efficacy in short-term treatment. Arch Gen Psychiatry 45:413–422, 1988.
17. Noyes R, Anderson DJ, Clancy J, et al: Diazepam and propranolol in panic disorder and agoraphobia. Arch Gen Psychiatry 41:287–292, 1984.
18. Dunner DL, Ishiki D, Avery DH, et al: Effect of alprazolam and diazepam on anxiety and panic attacks in panic disorder: a controlled study. J Clin Psychiatry 47(9):458–460, 1986.
19. Sheehan DV, Claycomb JB, Surman OS: The relative efficacy of alprazolam, phenelzine and imipramine in treating panic attacks and phobias. In Scientific Proceedings of the 137th Annual Meeting of the American Psychiatric Association, Los Angeles (abstr), 1984.
20. Klein DF: Delineation of two drug responsive anxiety syndromes. Psychopharmacologia 5:397–408, 1964.
21. Klein DF: Importance of psychiatric diagnosis and prediction of clinical drug effects. Arch Gen Psychiatry 16:118–126, 1967.
22. Tyrer P, Candy J, Kelly DA: A study of the clinical effects of phenelzine and placebo in the treatment of phobic anxiety. Psychopharmacologia 32:237–254, 1973.
23. Solyom L, Heseltine GFD, McClure DJ, Solyom C, Ledwidge B, Steinberg G: Behavior therapy versus drug therapy in the treatment of phobic neurosis. Can Psychiatric Assoc Journal 18:25–31, 1973.
24. Charney DS, Woods SW, Goodman WK, et al: Drug treatment of panic disorder: The comparative efficacy of imipramine, alprazolam, and trazodone. J Clin Psychiatry 47(12):580–586, 1986.
25. Sheehan DV, Zak JP, Miller JA, et al: Panic disorder: The potential role of serotonin reuptake inhibitors. J Clin Psychiatry 49(suppl):23–29, 1988.
26. Sheehan DV, Raj BA, Sheehan KH, et al: Is buspirone effective for panic disorder? J Clin Psychopharmacol 10(1):3–11, 1990.
27. Noyes R, DuPont R, Pecknold JC: Alprazolam in panic disorder and agoraphobia: Results from a multicenter trial. II. Patient acceptance, side effects, and safety. Arch Gen Psychiatry 45(5):423–428, 1900.

28. Tesar GE, Rosenbaum JF, Pollack MH, et al: Double-blind placebo-controlled comparison of clonazepam and alprazolam for panic disorder. J Clin Psychiatry 52(2):69–76, 1991.

29. Sheehan DV, Raj BA, Sheehan KH, et al: Adinazolam sustained release formulation in the treatment of panic disorder: A pilot study. Ir J Psychol Med 7(2):124–128, 1990.

30. Sheehan DV, Ballenger JC, Jacobson G: Treatment of endogenous anxiety with phobic, hysterical and hypochondriacal symptoms. Arch Gen Psychiatry 37:51–59, 1980.

31. Sheehan DV, Raj A: Monoamine oxidase inhibitors. In Last CG, Hersen M, eds. Handbook of Anxiety Disorders. London, Pergamon Press, 1988:478–503.

32. Rapp MS, Thomas MR, Reyes EC: Mega doses of behavior therapy for treatment resistant agoraphobics. Can J Psychiatry 28:105–109, 1983.

45

OBSESSIVE-COMPULSIVE DISORDER AND TRICHOTILLOMANIA

TERESA A. PIGOTT, M.D., TANA A. GRADY, M.D., and
CHERYL S. RUBENSTEIN, M.A.

OBSESSIVE-COMPULSIVE DISORDER

Epidemiology, Phenomenology, and Clinical Characteristics

Obsessive-compulsive disorder (OCD) is an illness that has been recognized for centuries, but until recently has been thought to be rare and largely resistant to standard psychiatric interventions. The cardinal manifestations of OCD are recurrent, intrusive thoughts (obsessions) and perseverative, ritualistic behaviors (compulsions) that are accompanied by anxiety, especially when the patient attempts to resist these symptoms. Obsessive-compulsive disorder is currently classified as an anxiety disorder in DSM-III-R.[1] In most cases, the obsessions and compulsions are regarded as irrational by the patient and often serve as a substantial source of embarrassment with subsequent, often heroic, attempts utilized to conceal the nature and severity of their OCD symptoms.

Perhaps the most surprising result to arise from the 1982 National Institute of Mental Health Epidemiological Catchment Area (ECA) study was the finding that OCD was estimated to have a lifetime prevalence of 2.5%[2]; this is approximately 40 times higher than previous estimates. Obsessive-compulsive disorder has also been noted to have an early age of onset, with over 50 per cent of patients noting substantial OCD symptomatology before the age of 15; for ECA respondents, the median age at onset was 23 years.[2] There is an equal gender distribution in adolescents and adults.

Obsessive-compulsive disorder is currently classified as an anxiety disorder in DSM-III-R, although this is somewhat controversial. There have been a number of attempts to categorize OCD into phenomenological subtypes based upon the predominant symptom manifestation, but no specific categorization has been universally accepted. Common obsessions include excessive fears of contamination, aggression, harm, sin, and loss of control and/or repetitive thoughts concerning order, numbers, or information. Common compulsions include excessive washing, cleaning, checking, repeating, counting, and arranging, and compulsive hoarding. From a clinical standpoint, one way to categorize OCD patients is to divide them into five clusters based upon their predominant symptom(s): (1) washers, (2) checkers, (3) sinners/doubters, (4) counters/arrangers, and (5) hoarders.

Washers are focally preoccupied with cleanliness, including contamination concerns, germs, and/or cleaning compulsions. Checkers have prominent repeating and checking rituals designed to avoid accidents and harm during certain, often routine, tasks. Sinners/doubters become preoccupied with religious or moral concerns and practices. They also are frequently characterized by extreme procrastination and often paralyzing indecisiveness. Counters/arrangers are excessively preoccupied with order, symmetry, and numbers. Finally, some patients with OCD are compulsive hoarders.

Most patients have both obsessions and compulsions, although approximately 25 per cent of OCD patients will be "pure" obsessionals and some manifest solely compulsive behaviors. Many patients with OCD will exhibit different types of symptoms at different times in their lives, and in most cases OCD represents a chronic disorder. There have been few long-term studies of patients with OCD, but most have suggested a guarded prognosis with at least 50 per cent of patients continuing to have symptoms of OCD despite treatment.

The most common complication of OCD is affective disorder, with major depressive episodes occurring in at least 50 per cent of patients with OCD. There is considerable comorbidity between OCD and other anxiety disorders, including phobias and panic disorder. Children and adolescents with OCD have been reported frequently to have other psychiatric disorders, including other anxiety disorders, mood disorders, and tics. There may also be considerable comorbidity between OCD and alcoholism.

Historically, premorbid compulsive personality disorder was hypothesized to be implemental, and indeed critical, to the development of OCD. However, although most studies have reported that more than 50 per cent of OCD patients have a concomitant personality disorder, only 4 to 6 per cent have met criteria for compulsive personality disorder. Instead, the most frequent personality disorder diagnoses have been avoidant, dependent, and histrionic. Schizotypal personality disorder appears to be associated with poorer treatment outcome in patients with OCD; additional evidence suggests that OCD patients with paranoid or schizoid personality disorder may also have a poorer treatment outcome than those with other personality disorders.

Family History and Genetic Studies

Obsessive-compulsive disorder appears to have a familial/genetic component. Recent family studies have demonstrated that 30 to 70 per cent of children or adolescents with OCD have at least one first-degree relative with OCD or OCD symptoms,[3] and there may also be a significant increase of overall psychiatric morbidity among first-degree relatives of patients with OCD. Interestingly, it is relatively rare for similar symptom manifestations of OCD to occur in the same family;[3] suggesting a genetic rather than a learning or modeling phenomenon. Twin studies comparing concordance rates of OCD, anxiety disorders (in general), and "neuroses" have reported a significantly greater concordance among monozygotic twin pairs than in dizygotic twin pairs.[4]

There is substantial evidence that OCD is linked to the neurological disorder, Tourette's syndrome (TS), which is characterized by complex motor and vocal tics. In fact, from 50 to 75 per cent of patients with TS exhibit OCD symptoms, and a much smaller portion of patients with OCD meet criteria for TS (5 to 7 per cent) and motor tics. The first-degree relatives of TS patients have been reported to have substantial rates of TS (11 per cent), chronic multiple tics (18 per cent), and OCD (23 per cent). Pauls and colleagues[5] reported a 7 per cent incidence of OCD among first-degree relatives of patients with TS and noted that the presence of TS was significantly greater in male relatives, but OCD was more common in female relatives. These recent studies provide strong evidence for genetic and familial components to OCD.

Neurobiological and Neuroimaging Studies

There are no specific laboratory or blood tests that are pathognomonic for the diagnosis of OCD. A number of studies have involved central and peripheral measurements of serotonin (5-hydroxytryptamine) in patients with OCD. There have also been attempts to correlate measures of serotonin with eventual treatment response in patients with OCD. Good responses to clomipramine treatment have been correlated with: (1) higher pretreatment levels of cerebrospinal fluid 5-hydroxyinodeacetic acid and (2) higher pretreatment platelet serotonin concentrations, but these have not been replicated.

Psychobiological responses to pharmacological agents have also been extensively utilized in patients with OCD in an attempt to characterize potential behavioral, neurobiological, and physiological responses that might differentiate patients with OCD from controls. Responses to acute sodium lactate, caffeine, clonidine, and fenfluramine administration have not differentiated patients with OCD from controls. However, several agents that selectively affect serotonin have been associated with differential behavioral or neuroendocrine responses or both in patients with OCD, in comparison to controls.

Despite a number of attempts to characterize neuropsychological functioning in patients with OCD, no specific abnormalities have been consistently demonstrated. Positron emission tomography (PET) scans have been particularly invaluable in demonstrating evidence of specific neurobiological dysfunction in patients with OCD in comparison to controls. Baxter and colleagues[6] were the first to report increased metabolic rates in the left orbital gyrus and bilaterally in the caudate nuclei in patients with OCD in comparison to controls; subsequent studies have replicated this finding and have reported that patients with OCD and TS have higher metabolic rates in the orbital prefrontal cortex and striatum and that depressed OCD patients have additional abnormalities in the anterolateral prefrontal cortex.[7]

Differential Diagnosis and OCD Spectrum Disorders

Approximately 20 per cent of patients with affective illness, particularly melancholic or psychotic depression or both, exhibit OCD symptoms. However, the obsessional symptoms or compulsive behaviors that complicate depression occur in the context of a depressed mood and represent secondary features that resolve as the affective disturbance improves. At times, OCD and phobic anxiety can be difficult to differentiate, but phobias are characterized by certain external stimuli, whereas OCD is characterized often by internal stimuli; in addition, phobics can allay their anxiety through avoidance of the feared stimuli, but the anxiety associated with OCD is alleviated through compulsive rituals or "undoing behaviors." Obsessive-compulsive disorder symptoms have been described in 3.5 per cent of patients with schizophrenia, and persistent OCD symptoms in patients with schizophrenia have been reported to be associated with a poorer prognosis. However, schizophrenia can be differentiated from OCD by its pervasive thought disturbance rather than just focal bizarre ideation. Finally, behaviors such as kleptomania, pyromania, pathological gambling, and substance abuse are often labeled "compulsive," but the performance of these behaviors is generally associated with pleasure or reward, whereas OCD behaviors are generally senseless and associated with negative affect.

There has been increasing speculation concerning links between OCD and other potential OCD spectrum disorders. For example, trichotillomania, anorexia nervosa, bulimia nervosa, hypochondriasis, and monosymptomatic hypochondriasis are all characterized by focal preoccupations or compulsive behaviors. Trichotillomania is discussed in detail later in this chapter. Hypochondriasis and monosymptomatic hypochondriasis are both characterized by an excessive preoccupation with physical symptoms or appearance, but this preoccupation is not considered excessive or irrational by the patient. Both of these disorders are generally refractory to most psychiatric interventions, especially since the patient is rarely motivated to seek psychiatric treatment. Both anorexia nervosa and bulimia nervosa are characterized by excessive preoccupations with food, weight, and appearance; in addition, patients with anorexia and bulimia nervosa have been noted to exhibit evidence of classic OCD symptoms, as well as elaborate and repetitive behaviors including calorie counting, repeated weigh-ins, and exercising rituals. A substantial number of patients with OCD have been reported to have a history of anorexia or bulimia nervosa.

Treatment

Pharmacological Treatment

In controlled trials, patients with OCD have been demonstrated to be markedly more responsive to treatment with serotonin-selective uptake inhibitors than to treatment with norepinephrine-selective or nonselective uptake inhibitors or other psychoactive medications. This pattern of treatment response is in marked contrast to that for affective disorders and anxiety disorders, which do not exhibit evidence of preferential efficacy to certain antidepressants or psychotropic medications. The antidepressants clomipramine, fluvoxamine, fluoxetine, and sertraline represent the only agents that have been demonstrated in controlled trials to possess significant antiobsessive effects. All of these agents share a high potency for the blockade of serotonin reuptake, supporting a serotonergic mechanism for antiobsessional drug action.

There are several features that appear to be shared by all effective antiobsessive agents in the treatment of OCD:

1. Antiobsessive agents require an extended duration of treatment (4 to 12 weeks) before substantial benefits are attained.
2. OCD symptom reduction is generally partial, averaging approximately a 40 per cent improvement from baseline.
3. Improvement in OCD symptoms is independent of, and occurs despite the presence of, depressive symptoms.
4. Rapid relapse in OCD symptoms is common after drug discontinuation.

Clomipramine has been the most well-studied antiobsessive agent to date; it has been demonstrated to be superior to placebo in multiple controlled trials.[8] Clomipramine has also been found to be superior to several other antidepressants in controlled trials, including desipramine, amitriptyline, clorgyline, zimelidine, and imipramine. Buspirone was found similar to clomipramine in reducing OCD symptoms in a controlled trial,[9] and nortriptyline treatment was not significantly different than clomipramine treatment in another study.[8] There have been a number of attempts to correlate plasma clomipramine levels with clinical response in patients with OCD, but there have not been consistent correlations.

There are often considerable side effects associated with clomipramine treatment, including sedation, dry mouth, blurred vision, tremor, weight gain, and sexual dysfunction. Clomipramine treatment is generally initiated at 25 to 50 mg/day, with gradual increases to the usual daily dose of 150 to 250 mg; it is generally well tolerated in a single nighttime dosage regimen. The maximum daily recommended dose for clomipramine is 250 mg, because higher doses are associated with an increased incidence of seizures.

Fluvoxamine, a highly serotonin-selective uptake inhibitor, has been shown to have significant therapeutic efficacy in the treatment of OCD in several comparisons with placebo, and also exhibited significant antiobsessional superiority in comparison to desipramine.[10] Fluvoxamine's main side effects are sedation, tremor, nausea, sexual dysfunction, and weight loss. Fluvoxamine treatment is generally initiated at 50 mg/day, with gradual increases to the usual daily dose of 150 to 300 mg.

Fluoxetine has been reported to be significantly effective in OCD in a single-blind trial and in a number of open trials. Our group conducted the first double-blind comparison of fluoxetine and clomipramine in the treatment of OCD; both drugs were associated with significant and similar reductions in OCD and depressive symptoms. In addition, there were significantly fewer total side effects reported during fluoxetine than clomipramine treatment.[11] Jenike and colleagues[12] performed a meta-analysis of previous studies of clomipramine (controlled trials) and fluoxetine (open trials) in OCD patients and concluded that both drugs were effective, but clomipramine treatment was associated with a somewhat larger treatment effect and fluoxetine treatment was associated with a more favorable side-effect profile. The most common side effects reported during fluoxetine treatment are sexual dysfunction, nausea, agitation, headache, and insomnia. Although fluoxetine plasma concentration monitoring is available, correlations with clinical response or effective plasma concentration levels or both have not been determined. The optimal daily dose of fluoxetine for patients with OCD has not been determined, although most studies have utilized doses from 40 to 80 mg/day.

Sertraline has been reported to be superior to placebo in patients with OCD; however, reductions in OCD symptoms were somewhat modest in comparison to the percentage reduction generally associated with clomipramine,[13] fluoxetine, and fluvoxamine treatment. The most common side effects noted with sertraline are nausea, headache, and dizziness.

Many psychotropic medications have been reported in controlled and open trials to lack significant antiobsessive properties, including lithium carbonate and carbamazepine. There have been numerous open studies and case reports suggesting the efficacy of a variety of agents in the treatment of OCD, including trazodone, zimelidine, tranylcypromine, phenelzine, venlafaxine, clonazepam, alprazolam, clonidine, L-tryptophan, and dextroamphetamine. Intravenous clomipramine in open reports has been reported to be efficacious in the treatment of OCD, especially in those patients who have not responded to oral clomipramine. Because of the uncontrolled nature and small sample size of these reports, extreme caution appears to be indicated in interpreting and extrapolating these results in most patients with OCD. Consequently, clomipramine, fluoxetine, fluvoxamine, and perhaps sertraline remain the cornerstone of pharmacological treatment for patients with OCD.

Since effective antiobsessive agents are generally associated with only partial improvement in OCD symptoms, augmentation strategies have become an important part of the pharmacological treatment of OCD. Controlled trials of adjuvant medication in the treatment of OCD have been very limited, but include a trial of adjuvant lithium carbonate in fluvoxamine-treated patients and a sequential trial of adjuvant thyroid hormone and lithium carbonate in clomipramine-treated patients with OCD; neither study was associated with significant additional

antiobsessive benefit.[14] A controlled trial of adjuvant buspirone treatment in clomipramine-treated patients with OCD also was not associated with additional antiobsessive benefit in another study by our group.

Additional reports of adjuvant medication in the treatment of OCD have been reported but must be viewed with some degree of caution since they are largely case reports or uncontrolled trials or both. Fluoxetine has been successfully augmented with buspirone and fenfluramine in patients with OCD. Clomipramine has been successfully augmented with lithium, clonidine, fenfluramine, and L-tryptophan. There is also some preliminary evidence that the addition of pimozide, a dopamine antagonist, in fluvoxamine-refractory patients with OCD may be associated with significant additional decreases in OCD symptoms, particularly in those patients with comorbid tic spectrum disorders or schizotypal personality disorders.

Nonpharmacological treatments have also been utilized in patients with OCD, including electroconvulsive therapy[15] and psychosurgery, especially stereotactic limbic leucotomy; they have been reported to be associated with improvement in OCD symptoms.[16] However, these modalities are generally reserved for the most treatment-resistant patients with OCD.

Behavioral Therapy

Traditional psychotherapy has not proven to be effective in significantly reducing OCD symptoms. Behavioral therapy, however, has been demonstrated to be effective in many patients with OCD.[17–20] Behavioral treatment of OCD consists of two basic components: (1) in vivo exposure to anxiety-evoking stimuli (i.e., placing the patient in the "real life" feared situation); and (2) response prevention (i.e., blocking the expression or performance of the compulsive behaviors). Prolonged imaginal exposure to anxiety-evoking scenes ("implosive therapy") has also been reported as efficacious in OCD.[21] In addition, patient self-exposure with response prevention can be as effective as therapist-assisted exposure with response prevention.[22]

Estimates of the efficacy of exposure plus response prevention range between 50 and 90 per cent. Although most patients begin to habituate to anxiety during the first session, it can take weeks or months for patients to complete the anxiety reduction process. Several studies have indicated that behavior therapy is associated with long-term results. Psychological treatments that do not include exposure and response prevention have largely proven unsuccessful in treating OCD.

Several factors are associated with a poor prognosis for the behavioral treatment of patients with OCD, including noncompliance with treatment, concomitant severe depression, absence of rituals, and the presence of concomitant personality disorder. In-

terestingly, treatment refusal/noncompliance and severe personality disorders are also associated with
poor response to pharmacological treatment.

Noncompliance, either through treatment refusal
or avoidance of anxiogenic stimuli, appears to be the
most frequent cause of behavioral treatment failure,
occurring approximately 25 per cent of the time. Depression also interferes with behavioral therapy with
OCD patients. This may occur, in part, because depressed patients are unable to habituate normally to
anxiogenic or fearful stimuli. For patients who are
purely obsessional, pharmacotherapy appears to be
the treatment of choice. However, if this is ineffective, cognitive-behavioral treatments including
thought stopping, assertiveness training, systematic
desensitization, imaginal flooding, and cognitive restructuring may be helpful.

Combined Behavioral and Pharmacological Therapy

It seems likely that the combination of behavioral
and drug treatment, either sequentially or in tandem,
is the most effective treatment option for patients
with OCD. Unfortunately, a review of the literature
reveals few controlled studies of combined behavioral and pharmacotherapy. Results to date seem to
indicate that augmentation of behavior therapy with
serotonergic reuptake inhibitors is associated with
substantial reductions in OCD and depressive symptoms. In summary, effective pharmacotherapy and
concomitant intensive behavioral treatment seems to
represent the treatment of choice for most patients
with OCD in terms of maximal symptom reduction
and potential symptom remission with less chance
of relapse.

TRICHOTILLOMANIA

Diagnosis and Clinical Features

Trichotillomania is a term coined by the French
dermatologist Hallopeau[23] in 1889 to describe compulsive hair-pulling behavior. The hallmark of trichotillomania is the "irresistable urge" to pull out
one's hair. It is currently classified as an Impulse
Control Disorder in the DSM-III-R, although this
classification is somewhat controversial in that some
believe it is more within an anxiety/obsessive-com-
pulsive spectrum.

The exact incidence of trichotillomania is unknown, but is has generally been considered a rare
disorder. However, increasing physician awareness
may contribute to more accurate prevalence estimates in the near future. Most cases of trichotillomania have a childhood or adolescent onset. Interestingly, it seems to predominantly affect females
rather than males. However, Muller[24] reported a
study in which 70 per cent of the trichotillomanic
subjects were female, except in the pre–school age

population where 62 per cent of affected children
were male.

In addition to the irresistible urge to pull one's
hair, DSM-III-R criteria for the diagnosis of trichotillomania include an increasing sense of tension immediately before pulling out the hair and a sense of
gratification or relief when pulling out the hair. Exclusionary criteria for trichotillomania include an
association with a preexisting inflammation of the
skin or hair pulling as a response to a delusion or
hallucination.[1] The majority of patients with chronic
trichotillomania pull hair predominantly from their
scalps, although it is not limited to this region. For
example, patients may describe pulling out their
eyebrows, eyelashes, facial hair, and/or pubic hair as
their primary or secondary symptoms.

At times, the diagnosis of trichotillomania is complicated by the patient's hesitancy to admit to the
behavior; adult patients with trichotillomania are often particularly embarrassed or humiliated by their
behavior. Moreover, parents of children with trichotillomania and some adults will deny or rationalize the problem, or both. In such cases, the histopa-
thology of scalp biopsies may be of value in making
or excluding a diagnosis of trichotillomania. Diagnostic histopathological findings for trichotillomania include the presence of catagen hairs, pigment
casts, and traumatized hair bulbs. Of note is the absence of bulbar inflammation and atrophic anagen
hairs in the patients' scalp biopsies.

There appears to be substantial comorbidity between trichotillomania and other psychiatric disorders. For example, a recent study of patients with
trichotillomania reported that mood disorders, primarily major depression, were the most common
comorbid psychiatric diagnoses, with a reported lifetime prevalence of 65 per cent; in addition, there was
a 57 per cent lifetime prevalence of anxiety disorders
and 10 per cent reported symptoms consistent with a
diagnosis of current obsessive-compulsive disorder.
Additional findings included the presence of eating
disorders (past or present) and psychoactive substance abuse disorders (present) in 20 per cent and
22 per cent of the subjects, respectively.[25]

Trichotillomania can also be associated with several serious medical complications. These medical
problems typically result from trichophagy (hair eating), which often accompanies trichotillomania. Trichophagy can lead to the development of trichobezoars in the stomach or intestines, particularly in
women under 30 years of age. Trichobezoars in turn
can result in gastrointestinal bleeding, intestinal obstruction, perforation, or acute pancreatitis.

Treatment

A variety of treatment modalities have been advocated for trichotillomania. Psychoanalytically oriented psychotherapies (individual, group, or family)
have been associated with only limited success. Cognitive-behavioral or behavioral therapy approaches

have been reported to be of benefit in some studies. However, to date, there is a lack of controlled behavior or psychological studies designed to assess treatment efficacy in patients with trichotillomania. Instead, there are a number of case reports and open trials suggesting that such techniques as relaxation training, habit reversal, and hypnosis may be helpful in substantially reducing trichotillomanic behaviors.[26–30]

In contrast to previous pharmacological approaches to the treatment of trichotillomania, which have been largely anecdotal, Swedo et al.[31] conducted the only controlled double-blind study of pharmacotherapy in trichotillomania. They compared the antidepressants clomipramine and desipramine in a group of patients with trichotillomania. Based upon shared compulsive features, Swedo and colleagues hypothesized that trichotillomania might represent an OCD spectrum disorder and thereby respond preferentially to a serotonin-selective agent such as clomipramine rather than a nonselective serotonergic agent such as desipramine. Interestingly, clomipramine treatment was associated with significant reductions in trichotillomanic behaviors in comparison to desipramine treatment, suggesting that trichotillomania may, indeed, share important characteristics with OCD. While further controlled studies are indicated, this initial study provides compelling evidence for the potential categorization of trichotillomania as an OCD variant disorder.

REFERENCES

1. American Psychiatric Association: Diagnostic and Statistical Manual of Mental Disorders. 3rd ed. Revised. Washington, DC: American Psychiatric Association, 1987.
2. Karno M, Golding SB, Sorenson SB, et al: The epidemiology of obsessive-compulsive disorder in five US communities. Arch Gen Psychiatry 45:1094, 1988.
3. Riddle MA, Scahill L, King R, et al: Obsessive compulsive disorder in children and adolescents: Phenomenology and family history. J Am Acad Child Adolesc Psychiatry 29:766, 1990.
4. Andrews G, Stewart G, Allen R, et al: The genetics of six neurotic disorders: A twin study. J Affective Disord 19:23, 1990.
5. Pauls DL, Raymond CL, Stevenson JM, et al: A family study of Gilles de la Tourette syndrome. AM J Hum Genet 48:154, 1991.
6. Baxter L, Phelps M, Mazziotta J, et al: Local cerebral glucose metabolic rates in obsessive-compulsive disorder. Arch Gen Psychiatry 44:211–218, 1987.
7. Baxter LR Jr, Schwartz JM, Guze BH, et al: PET imaging in obsessive-compulsive disorder with and without depression. J Clin Psychiatry 51(suppl):61, 1990.
8. Thoren PM, Asberg B, Cronholm L, et al: Clomipramine treatment of obsessive-compulsive disorder: I. A controlled clinical trial. Arch Gen Psychiatry 37:1281, 1980.
9. Pato MT, Pigott TA, Hill JL, et al: Controlled comparison of buspirone and clomipramine in obsessive-compulsive disorder. Am J Psychiatry 148:127–129, 1991.
10. Goodman WK, Delgado PL, Price LH, et al: Comparison of fluvoxamine and desipramine in OCD. Arch Gen Psychiatry 47:577–585, 1990.
11. Pigott TA, Pato MT, Bernstein SE, et al: Controlled comparisons of clomipramine and fluoxetine in the treatment of obsessive-compulsive disorder. Arch Gen Psychiatry 47:926–932, 1990.
12. Jenike MA, Baer L, Greist JH: Clomipramine versus fluoxetine in obsessive-compulsive disorder: A retrospective comparison of side effects and efficacy. J Clin Psychopharmacol 10:122–124, 1990.
13. Jenike MA, Baer L, Summergrad P, et al: Sertraline in obsessive compulsive disorder: A double blind comparison with placebo. Am J Psychiatry 147:923–928, 1990.
14. Pigott TA, Pato MT, L'Heureux F, et al: A controlled comparison of adjuvant lithium carbonate or thyroid hormone in clomipramine-treated OCD patients. J Clin Psychopharmacol 11:242–248, 1991.
15. Mellman LA, Gorman TM: Successful treatment of obsessive compulsive disorder with ECT. J Clin Psychiatry 4:131–132, 1983.
16. Kelly D: Anxiety and Emotions: Physiological Basis and Treatment. Springfield, IL: Charles C Thomas, 1980.
17. Emmelkamp PMG: Phobic and Obsessive-Compulsive Disorders: Theory, Research, and Practice. New York: Plenum, 1982.
18. Foa EB, Steketee GS, Ozarow BJ: Behavior therapy with obsessive-compulsives: From theory to treatment. In Mavissakalian M, ed. Obsessive-Compulsive Disorder: Psychological and Pharmacological Treatment. New York: Plenum, 1985:188–200.
19. Marks IM, Hodgson R, Rachman S: Treatment of chronic obsessive-compulsive disorder by in vivo exposure. Br J Psychiatry 127:349–364, 1975.
20. Steketee GS, Foa EB: Obsessive-compulsive disorder. In Barlow D, ed. Clinical Handbook of Psychological Disorders: A Step-by-Step Treatment Manual. New York: Guilford Press, 1985:56–80.
21. Stamfl TG, Levis DJ: Essentials of implosive therapy: A learning-theory-based psychodynamic behavioral therapy. J Abnorm Psychol 72:496–503, 1967.
22. Marks IM, Lelliott P, Basoglu M, et al: Clomipramine, self-exposure, and therapist-aided exposure of obsessive-compulsive ritualizers. Br J Psychiatry 152:522, 1988.
23. Hallopeau M: Alopecie par grattage (trichomanie ou trichotillomanie). Ann Dermatol Venereol 10:440–441, 1889.
24. Muller SA: Trichotillomania. Dermatol Clin 5:595–601, 1987.
25. Christenson GA, Mackenzie TB, Mitchell JE: Characteristics of 60 adult chronic hair pullers. Am J Psychiatry 148:365–370, 1991.
26. DeLuca RV, Holborn SW: A comparison of relaxation training and competing response training to eliminate hair-pulling and nail biting. J Behav Ther Exp Psychiatry 15:67–70, 1984.
27. Azrin NH, Nunn RG, Franz SE: Treatment of hair pulling (trichotillomania): A comparative study of habit reversal and negative practice training. J Behav Ther Exp Psychiatry 11:13–20, 1980.
28. Greenberg D, Marks S: Behavioral psychotherapy of uncommon referrals. Br J Psychiatry 141:148–153, 1982.
29. Rowen R: Hypnotic age regression in the treatment of a self-destructive habit: Trichotillomania. Am J Clin Hypn 23:195–197, 1981.
30. Barabasz M: Trichotillomania: A new treatment. Int J Clin Exp Hypn 35:146–154, 1987.
31. Swedo SE, Leonard H, Rapoport JL, et al: A double-blind comparison of clomipramine and desipramine in the treatment of trichotillomania (hair pulling). N Engl J Med 321:497–501, 1989.

POST-TRAUMATIC STRESS DISORDER

KENRIC W. HAMMOND, M.D., RAYMOND M. SCURFIELD, D.S.W.,
and STEVEN C. RISSE, M.D.

Post-traumatic stress disorder (PTSD) is based on the concept that a psychiatric disorder can occur as the result of severe emotional stress. The history of this diagnosis began with recognition of the emotional sequelae of combat, classified as acute and chronic manifestations of traumatic war neurosis and given a variety of names such as "shell shock," "battle fatigue," and "compensation neurosis."[1] Later, post-traumatic mental disorders of nonmilitary origin with similar symptoms were recognized, including the "rape-trauma syndrome" and residuals of child abuse. In 1980 the DSM-III articulated a conceptual unification of the trauma response syndrome and established an operational definition of acute and chronic PTSD.

CLINICAL DESCRIPTION

Post-traumatic stress disorder describes the pathological emotional and behavioral condition that can follow exposure to a traumatic stressor severe enough to be "outside the range of usual human experience and . . . markedly distressing to almost anyone."[2] The causative trauma may be physical or emotional, isolated or repeated, and may range from natural disaster or accident to criminal violence, torture, or war. The trauma may be experienced directly, as in being wounded, or indirectly, as in witnessing the injury or death of another person. Familiarity with responses to extreme stress provides a useful context for understanding treatment of PTSD. Adaptive and pathological responses to stress follow the same general form and mechanisms; the final outcome depends on interactions between the stressor, the survivor, and the surrounding environment.

Severe trauma activates multiple responses directed toward the task of survival. Physiologically, intense adrenergic outflow occurs, with activation of the central and autonomic nervous system and manifestation of the "fight or flight" response.[3] Subjectively, during trauma one is faced with a potentially overwhelming array of sensory stimuli, including pain and suffering; cognitions of threats to self and significant others; and feelings commonly dominated by rage, grief, and helplessness. Threatened organisms take action to survive, either by attacking the threat or by withdrawing to safety. One of the most immediate and adaptive responses to trauma involves suppression and detachment from feelings of terror and grief. Second, there is selective attention, whereby the survivor focuses on an object to the exclusion of other factors. Third, there may be channeling of terror and grief into rage and action. Obviously, rageful expression is only conducive to survival in some circumstances, such as during combat by an armed soldier, and may not be a realistic option in other situations, such as a sexual assault where the perpetrator is armed, or a natural disaster.[4]

Following the trauma, there initially tends to be a phase that includes shock, continued deadening of affect, disbelief, and minimization of the reality and impact of what has occurred. The physiological counterpart of this is a state of exhaustion and neural refractoriness. Later there emerges a repetitive psychological and sensory reexperiencing of aspects of the trauma through intrusive memories, mental pictures, and accompanying intense emotions of rage, grief, terror, blame, and guilt. Trauma memories range in severity from momentary thoughts and impressions to persistent auditory hallucinations, and arise both spontaneously and in response to environmental cues. For example, tree lines may be seen as harboring snipers, men in tennis shoes may be seen as rapists, and loud noises may be heard as gunfire. Reexperiencing, a manifestation that does not overlap with symptoms of any other psychiatric disorder, is accompanied by autonomic and mental "arousal" symptoms such as tachycardia, sweating, hyperalertness, and sleep disturbance. These symptoms may also be present when survivors are unaware of thinking about their trauma, and only on specific questioning can a clear connection with a trauma be established.

To counteract intrusive and arousal symptoms, survivors tend to activate coping mechanisms of denial, numbing, detachment, and isolation to suppress or avoid the reexperiencing. Typically there follows a pattern where periods of intrusion and arousal alternate with periods of numbing. This pattern diminishes as the person recovers from trauma or persists for months, years, or decades if the underlying trauma-related issues are not resolved.

In a trauma *recovery* process the intrusive symptoms will be painful and may be occasionally, but not repetitively, overwhelming. The survivor is able to allow expression and reflection, followed by a degree of detachment sufficient to compartmentalize the painful intrusive symptoms but mild enough to permit life functioning to proceed. The modulation process between intrusion and detachment may then continue over a considerable period of time, and gradually the impact of the trauma is manageably resolved and integrated into the survivor's ongoing life. Subsequent temporary exacerbations of intrusive and arousal symptoms are relatively contained and resolved without deterioration of life functioning.

In contrast, in a *disordered* post-trauma process, the intrusive and arousal symptoms are powerful and threatening, overwhelming the survivor's ability to function day to day and evoking detachment mechanisms to suppress symptoms. Detachment (including substance abuse) presents a stubborn obstacle to recovery, interfering with life activity and adequate processing of the trauma experience. Avoidance of reminders of trauma may range from conscious suppression of thoughts to behavioral activity (e.g., choosing to live in Arizona to avoid thinking of the Vietnam jungle). These repeated efforts to avoid reminders rarely succeed. Failure to suppress intrusive images, ideas, and feelings is frequently manifested in recurrent nightmares or multiple abrupt awakenings without dream recall but accompanied by anxiety, tachycardia, and sweating. Sudden and usually transitory actions or feelings consistent with a sensation that the event is reoccurring may catch the survivor off guard, and provoke episodes of fear or dissociation lasting from minutes to hours. These episodes are often termed flashbacks. While usually brief, flashbacks may involve complex dissociative episodes with acting out. The intense anxiety, dissociation, depression, rage, or guilt and other reactions evoked by reminders may resemble features of other psychiatric disorders. Even when reminders are absent, nonspecific arousal symptoms such as insomnia, hostility, irritability, distractibility, hypervigilance, and an exaggerated startle response are common. Patients may appear depressed, antisocial, or psychotic. If denial and numbing are extremely strong, patients may not even report the traumatic origin of their symptoms. Detachment becomes ingrained and either stabilizes in chronic dysfunction or worsens over time as subsequent life stressors and aging occur.

Thus, the essential determinants of a DSM-III-R diagnosis of PTSD include: a verified stressor; an anxiety syndrome manifested by autonomic arousal, hypervigilance, insomnia, and irritability; persistent emotional responses of reexperiencing the stressor via intrusive memories, imagery, and affects; and efforts to avoid reminders of the trauma through numbing of emotional responsiveness, psychogenic amnesia, and restriction of social attachment behavior. Post-traumatic stress disorder is classified as "delayed" type when the onset of the disorder follows the trauma by more than 6 months.

Clinicians treating PTSD see other important symptoms that are not included in the DSM-III-R criteria.[4,5] Diminished self-worth, damaged identity, rage, and excessive fear of loss of control are often found. A complex of blame, guilt, and shame that can stem from actions taken or not taken at the time of the trauma may completely dominate a patient's current thinking and feeling. Existential despair, with disillusionment over what is meaningful in life, and a profound sense of alienation and disconnection from others and society are common. Post-traumatic stress disorder may affect most aspects of a person's perceptual, social, and vocational functioning and be completely disabling. Family members and close friends of PTSD patients can be adversely affected by the patient's isolation, numbing, tenseness, anger, blaming, and low self-esteem, further damaging the survivor's social network.

EPIDEMIOLOGY

The best estimate of the lifetime prevalence of PTSD in the U.S. general population is 1 per cent (1.3 per cent in women, 0.5 per cent in men) based on 2493 structured interviews conducted in the Epidemiological Catchment Area (ECA) study.[6] In women, a threat or close call and seeing someone hurt or die were the most likely antecedent of symptoms (about 40 per cent). In men, over half the cases were combat related. Over half of the combat-related PTSD episodes lasted more than 3 years, whereas most other cases lasted 6 months or less. Exposure to natural disasters precipitated symptoms in only 3 per cent of cases. Another large study, the 1987 National Readjustment Study of Vietnam Veterans (NRSVV), which examined 1632 Vietnam-theater veterans, indicated a lifetime prevalence of PTSD of 30 per cent, of whom fully half currently qualified for a PTSD diagnosis. The prevalence of PTSD among 716 male veterans of the same era who did not serve in Vietnam was found to be 2.5 per cent, and that among 668 nonveteran males 1.2 per cent.[7]

Numerous studies documenting rates of PTSD in traumatized populations support the concept that prevalence rates increase with the severity and duration of trauma exposure. Twins exposed to intense, prolonged combat in Vietnam showed a 47 per cent lifetime prevalence of PTSD, 9.2 times the rate among their noncombatant brothers.[8] The NRSVV showed greater rates of PTSD among those who had more than one combat tour of duty compared to those with shorter exposure.[7] Other lifetime prevalences of PTSD include: 75 per cent of Indochinese refugees,[9] 40 per cent of wounded Vietnam veterans,[10] and 22 per cent of survivors interviewed within 6 weeks of an airplane crash.[11] The widely circulated assertion that 50,000 or more Vietnam veterans had committed suicide by the mid-1980s is not substantiated. Analysis of Centers for Disease Control and State of Wisconsin cohorts indicates that fewer than 9000 Vietnam veteran suicides occurred prior to 1985, an incidence 27 per cent higher than comparable veterans and nonveterans.[12]

FAMILY STUDIES

Post-traumatic stress disorder is an environmentally induced disorder. The 1990 Veterans Administration cooperative study of 2092 Vietnam veteran monozygotic twin pairs (including 715 monozygotic pairs discordant for military service in Southeast Asia) found that 17 per cent of twins serving in the war zone qualified for a diagnosis of PTSD within the previous 6 months, compared to 5 per cent of their brothers who served elsewhere.[8] The twin design, which controlled for premorbid family environment, socioeconomic status, and genetic variability, demonstrated that the impact of trauma dwarfed any other preexisting factor. Some investigations have tried to find predisposing factors for development of PTSD, such as family history of psychiatric disorders. Davidson found that 24 of 36 patients with chronic PTSD had first-degree relatives with psychiatric illness, including alcohol and drug abuse, anxiety disorder, and depression.[13]

LABORATORY STUDIES

Diagnostic laboratory tests are not yet clinically useful in PTSD. Various studies have suggested PTSD may be diagnosed through physiological reactivity or elevated circulating catecholamines upon exposure to trauma-specific stimuli, altered urinary norepinephrine/cortisol ratios, decreased urinary cortisol excretion, and Minnesota Multiphasic Personality Inventory subscales.[14] To date, none of these methods has proven superior to a clinical history and examination for diagnosing PTSD. Clinically, the most useful laboratory test is urine toxicological testing to detect active coexisting substance abuse problems requiring treatment, given the high comorbidity rate of PTSD and substance abuse.

DIFFERENTIAL DIAGNOSIS AND COMORBIDITY

The hallmark of the diagnosis of PTSD is a history of a major stressor, "e.g., serious threat to one's life or physical integrity; serious threat or harm to one's children, [or] spouse, . . . sudden destruction of one's home or community; or seeing another person who has recently been, or is being, seriously injured or killed . . . as the result of an accident or physical violence."[2] Other events such as job loss, bereavement, and divorce can be stressful and lead to loss of social and occupational function but not meet this criterion. Adjustment disorder should be used to diagnose PTSD-like psychopathology following such events. Post-traumatic stress disorder is not the only psychiatric consequence of trauma. Among Mount St. Helens eruption survivors, increased incidence of generalized anxiety disorder and major depressive episodes as well as PTSD was found, compared to a control community, and these rates were highest among the subgroup most heavily affected by the disaster.[15] Clinical reports of childhood trauma sequelae describe intrusive imagery and rumination symptoms in survivors of isolated trauma events, and when repeated, severe childhood trauma occurred, pervasive personality disorder, dissociation, rage, and emotional numbing predominated among survivors.[16]

Because the nonspecific arousal and numbing symptoms of PTSD are seen in other anxiety disorders, depression, and substance abuse, as well as Axis II disorders such as antisocial, histrionic, and borderline personality, a careful history of childhood, adolescent, and pretrauma functioning, including sources other than the patient, is required to separate pretrauma pathology from dysfunctional sequelae that are specifically trauma related.

One of the confounding factors in diagnosis and treatment is that many cases of PTSD coexist with other psychiatric illness that may or may not be related to the trauma as well. Compared to controls, PTSD patients are twice as likely to carry another psychiatric diagnosis.[6] Because psychiatric comorbidity is so common, diagnosing and addressing coexisting psychiatric illness is an essential step in planning PTSD treatment. Clinicians should not withhold treatment on the basis of secondary versus primary status of the codiagnosis.[17] Epidemiological studies demonstrate rates of increased risk of several comorbidities among patients diagnosed with PTSD compared to age- and sex-matched controls.[6] Drug and alcohol abuse is the most common comorbidity seen in 20 to 80 per cent of PTSD cases, followed by dysthymia and major affective disorders in 10 to 50 per cent, depending on the sample. A very high relative risk of obsessive-compulsive disorder has been found and is consistent with the trauma rumination and ritual checking often seen in PTSD. Other conditions with increased risk of co-occurrence include antisocial personality, panic disorder, and phobia. Comparing the timing of the trauma and the onset of anxiety symptoms and assessing whether the anxiety is related in any way to reexperiencing a trauma are usually required to differentiate the nonspecific arousal of PTSD from panic, phobia, and generalized anxiety.

Drug and alcohol abusers have an increased risk of developing PTSD through accidents or violence related to intoxication and their life-style. Also, it is common for PTSD patients to increase drug and alcohol usage in efforts to induce detachment and reduce hyperarousal, irritability, and insomnia. An ongoing substance abuse recovery program is essential for patients with PTSD to benefit from psychological and pharmacological treatment.

Organic mental disorder may also coexist with PTSD. Some circumstances that produce brain trauma are capable of producing psychic trauma as well, and if brain injury is suggested by the history, one must consider organic factors in personality change following exposure to a stressor. Severe dementia is easily recognized, but symptoms secondary to mild post-trauma dementia may be harder to differentiate from those due to PTSD. Symptom patterns suggesting an ictal component include a brooding, ruminative depressive syndrome, sudden explosive episodes followed by deep regret, olfactory hallucinations, and paradoxical worsening of behavioral control with drugs that lower seizure thresholds. In addition to a complete mental status exam, neurological examination, electroencephalography, and computed tomography are advisable when organicity is suspected. Eliminating effects of psychotropic medication and substance use may be required prior to extensive neuropsychiatric testing. The organic patient with PTSD may also suffer psychological trauma. Prognosis for amelioration of the PTSD component via psychotherapy is directly related to the capacity to learn to process affects and ideation. The presence of dementia or short-term memory deficit requires setting more modest goals in psychotherapy than would be the case in a cognitively intact patient.

DRUG THERAPY ADJUNCT TO PTSD

Psychological interventions that assist patients to assimilate the trauma experience are the main component of effective treatment for PTSD. Psychotropic medication cannot substitute for active psychotherapy, especially for the treatment of avoidance, isolation, and emotional numbing, which respond poorly to medication. Still, drug treatment may be important to therapeutic progress. In particular, optimal treatment of a comorbid condition may be a prerequisite to effective psychotherapy. The limited current literature supports a flexible rather than a dogmatic approach to pharmacotherapy.

Antidepressants

In PTSD drug therapy, antidepressants are the most extensively used and studied agents. Amitriptyline in doses up to 300 mg/day was found superior to placebo in treatment of chronic PTSD in combat veterans. At 4 weeks amitriptyline was superior to placebo for depressive symptoms, and at 8 weeks it was superior on measures of depression, anxiety, intrusiveness, avoidance, and clinical global impression. The recovery rate was modest: at the end of the trial 64 per cent of the amitriptyline group and 72 per cent of the placebo group still met criteria for an active diagnosis of PTSD. Patients diagnosed with another psychiatric illness showed greater drug-placebo differences, but were also less likely to improve than those diagnosed with PTSD alone.[18] Imipramine (up to 300 mg/day) and phenelzine (up to 75 mg/day) were found equivalent and superior to placebo after 8 weeks for treatment of PTSD-specific intrusiveness symptoms in Vietnam combat veterans. Avoidance, nonspecific anxiety, and depressive symptomatology (which was at a low level in this nondepressed sample) did not significantly differ across the groups.[19] In another study, no difference was found between phenelzine (up to 90 mg/day) and placebo in a group of 10 Israeli veterans and civilians treated for 5 weeks.[20] Desipramine (up to 200 mg/day) was found superior to placebo in treating depressive symptoms, but not PTSD-specific symptoms, in a group of combat veterans.[21] These and other uncontrolled studies indicate that antidepressants are predictably effective for significant depressive symptomatology in PTSD, sometimes effective for intrusion and arousal symptoms, and of little effect on avoidant symptomatology.

Antianxiety Agents

The prominence of anxiety symptoms in PTSD has prompted usage of anxiolytic agents, and some of the antidepressant studies reported concurrent treatment with benzodiazepines. The only controlled study reports that, after 5 weeks' therapy of chronic PTSD with alprazolam (up to 6 mg/day), significant improvement occurred for nonspecific anxiety symptoms, but not depression, intrusiveness, or avoidance, when compared to placebo.[22] Anxiolytic treatment of acute combat stress reactions has been used, but current thinking discourages the approach, citing better results with timely psychological support and rest.[1] All benzodiazepines should be used with great caution because they potentially produce tolerance, dependence, and withdrawal, and PTSD patients face a particular risk of benzodiazepine dependence because of a high substance abuse comorbidity. Risse et al. have reported severe reactions after withdrawal of alprazolam in patients with chronic combat-induced PTSD despite very gradual dosage reduction.[23] Buspirone, which reduces anxiety symptoms without sedation or drug dependence, has a theoretical advantage over benzodiazepines in treatment of PTSD-related anxiety in patients at risk for substance misuse. Divided doses of 15 to 60 mg/day benefit the attention-deficit and irritability components of PTSD anxiety. The overlap of PTSD and obsessive-compulsive diagnoses noted in the ECA study and an anti–obsessive-compulsive activity of buspirone provide another rationale for this therapy.[6] Patients receiving buspirone must be prepared to expect a several-week delay before antianxiety effects become apparent, and may be more compliant if taught to identify and monitor target symptoms.

Neuroleptic Therapy

If hallucinations relating to PTSD are experienced, symptomatic treatment of PTSD-specific hallucinosis with neuroleptics is justified.

Other Drugs

Propranolol reduced intrusive and arousal symptoms among children with acute PTSD.[24] In uncontrolled series with adult chronic PTSD, clonidine and propranolol have been used alone and in conjunction with antidepressants to modulate the startle response, nightmares, intrusive thoughts, and other hyperarousal symptoms of PTSD.[25] Carbamazepine accounted for improvement in intrusive symptoms, hostility, and impulsivity in 70 per cent of patients in an uncontrolled study.[26] Lithium-mediated improvement for arousal and intrusive symptoms of PTSD has been reported.[27] The anti–obsessive-compulsive properties of the serotonergic antidepressants clomipramine and fluoxetine may be useful in treating cases of PTSD that overlap with obsessive-compulsive disorder.

Given the lack of a definitive pharmacological treatment of PTSD, we suggest these guidelines:

1. Do not rely on medication as a primary treatment modality; integrate drug therapy for specific symptoms with an overall psychosocial treatment plan.
2. Avoid iatrogenic drug dependency.
3. Treat coexisting diagnosed illness appropriately.

The clearest treatment indications occur when another major mental illness coexists with PTSD. Using appropriate agents to treat the coexisting disorder is almost always indicated, and usually facilitates the overall treatment of PTSD.[14] Active substance abuse or dependence is best treated vigorously before instituting pharmacotherapy or psychosocial treatment. Most studies have shown that optimal response to therapy takes at least 8 weeks. Silver et al. have suggested beginning treatment with a tricyclic antidepressant, and progressing to a monoamine oxidase inhibitor or adding lithium if depression or anger proves refractory. Adding a second drug (clonidine, a β-blocker, carbamazepine, buspirone, or benzodiazepine) may be useful to manage specific arousal or intrusiveness symptoms. If sleep disturbance is prominent, trazodone or short-term benzodiazepines for acute usage may be beneficial.[28]

PSYCHODYNAMIC TREATMENT INTERVENTIONS FOR ACUTE AND CHRONIC PTSD

Psychotherapeutic interventions are the mainstay of PTSD treatment. Some aspects of treatment are generic to both acute and chronic manifestations of PTSD. Establishment of a positive therapeutic bond between patient and therapist and the establishment of trust are critical.[5,29] It is important that the patient be assisted to recount the objective factors surrounding the trauma and his or her reactions prior, during, and following the event. The recounting of the objective factors is necessary to clarify issues and possible distortions in memory and may occur in a very detached, numbed manner. In contrast, the patient may be unable to give an objective account without frequent and profound emotional outbursts. "Dosing," or modulating the patient's ability both to be detached sufficiently to provide objective details and to be able to feel and express associated emotive reactions, is a challenging task. Such abreaction or emotional catharsis is considered central to trauma recovery with various survivor populations.[29,30]

In addition, preoccupation with or actual loss of control over various symptoms may require specific behavioral strategies, using techniques such as "time out," stress management, and sleep disturbance and dream disorder education. Cognitive reappraisal usually is required in order to correct distortions of attribution, altered reality factors about the trauma, and unfair judgments about self and others.[31] Finally, the patient may have a very bleak perspective of the future and of his or her ability ever to move beyond the terrible psychological pain. The presence of trauma-related physical injuries or disabilities causes a further complication: the tendency for both the patient and the health care provider to attend to physical recovery to the exclusion of accompanying emotional issues and dynamics. The process of emotive and cognitive expression and reappraisal, necessary revisions of self-concept and the world, and practice and successful integration of new (or re-emergent pretrauma) behavior and attitudinal patterns may have to be repeated and deepened time and again.[31] The rate of progress of this repetitive process depends on the preexisting strengths and weakness of the survivor prior to the trauma, the nature and severity of the trauma, coping mechanisms utilized during and following, and the social support and post-trauma environment. The therapist will have to alternate among being emotionally supportive, gentle, and nurturing, being task and behavior oriented, being confrontive and demanding, and being attentive to the uncovering and expression of aspects of the trauma per se and the requirement to deal with here-and-now life issues.[32]

Early intervention during the first several days and weeks (or in some cases months) following the trauma has a considerable advantage over longer delay in intervention.[31] Crisis or short-term intervention may be all that is required to reduce acute distress, provide a therapeutic processing of the trauma and its impact, and return a patient relatively quickly to a pretrauma level of functioning. Chronic or delayed PTSD also may be prevented and chronic maladaptive behaviors and attitudes and accompanying psychiatric disorders averted.[31] Military psychiatry principles for treatment of acute battlefield casualties have been effective in reducing the rates of acute casualties[1]; there is some evidence that early interventions are helpful in reducing the emergence of chronic PTSD.[33] However, there is no convincing evidence that returning a trauma survivor to a traumatic environment is helpful to longer term mental health.

In contrast, in cases of delayed or chronic PTSD where knowledgeable trauma-specific interventions do not occur until considerable time has elapsed following the trauma, the patient may or may not be amenable to the same type of abbreviated, crisis-oriented therapy. Relatively quick and simple intervention may still be possible when the patient has been able to maintain a relatively healthy level of functioning and has had a relatively recent exacerbation or onset of latent PTSD symptoms. Oftentimes, such exacerbation is triggered by severe current life stressors such as death, loss, or exposure to other trauma.

Alternatively, the survivor's life course may have been substantially altered in a dysfunctional manner since or relatively soon following the trauma. In such cases, trauma survivors may have developed an ever-spreading symptom picture that could include substance abuse; dysfunctional social, familial, and/or work roles; affective disorders; or other Axis I and II disorders and traits; or some combination of these. Therapeutic attention to both the trauma-derived symptoms and the associated maladaptive behavior patterns and mental disorders is required. In the example of substance abuse, sequential and concurrent treatment efforts are required to address both disorders to prevent relapse of one or both.

Treatment becomes particularly complex when the patient's life course has included several experiences of trauma subsequent or antecedent to the identified trauma, or both. There is a complex relationship between various trauma experiences that may have been experienced at various times throughout the life cycle. There may be a convergence of such issues as rage, blame, terror, and self-denigration that requires therapeutic processing of aspects of each of the traumas that have been experienced. For example, a war veteran with considerable unresolved war trauma issues who was severely abused as a child had an emergence of war trauma issues following a recent automobile accident in which his brother was killed. Required therapeutic processing alternated among the three identified trauma experiences.

Peer group treatment with others who have survived the same or a similar type of trauma has distinctive therapeutic advantages in the resolution of PTSD, both acute and chronic. These advantages can occur both in self-help and in professionally led treatment groups.[5,29] Peer group treatment provides a unique opportunity for direct intercession regarding the dynamics of isolation, denial, exaggeration of self-blame, feelings of abnormality, self-denigration and shame, and inability to forgive or seek absolution. Peers who "have been there" frequently can have an impact in a way that others may not be able to achieve or may only achieve after a much longer period of time has elapsed.

Some trauma survivors may have such deep-seated issues of low self-esteem, shame, negative identity, or fear of loss of control that significant individual therapy prior to or concurrent with peer group treatment may be necessary to prepare the patient to optimally utilize a peer group modality. Finally, there is a considerable array of special challenges in facilitating peer group treatment for trauma survivors: peers are quick to attempt to "rescue" and help each other to deny feelings and issues they cannot yet admit about themselves; "advice giving" that occurs may help or interfere with the processing required by the patient before he or she is able to accept and utilize such advice; some patients may require specific "rehearsal" of issues in individual sessions before they can be brought to the group; and authority-transference reactions to the group therapist with group contagion of the same can be quite threatening and difficult for the clinician. Intense inpatient peer group therapy has been demonstrated to have substantial beneficial impact on low self-esteem, numbing, avoidance, denial, and impaired relationships, a set of symptoms essentially unaffected by psychotropic medication.[34]

Therapy of PTSD often has profound effect on the therapist, and countertransference dynamics encountered in treating survivors of trauma will be significant and ever-present. Attending to such issues is integral to successful interventions with trauma survivors; these issues may be related to the clinician's reactions to aspects of the trauma (e.g., rape, sexual assault) or to his or her own unresolved attitudes about rage, violence, and helplessness.[5,29,35] The clinician's countertransference represents a reaction not only to the survivor per se but also typically to the trauma reported. A common therapist's reaction of detachment and numbing, with adoption of a distant, coldly objective, or impersonal stance, is the last thing that a trauma survivor needs to be able to engage in a trusting relationship.

It is not unusual for "secondary traumatization" to occur in the health care provider frequently exposed to trauma survivors.[35] Indeed, there is a growing recognition of the normalcy of stress reactions among clinicians and other service providers regularly exposed to trauma survivors.[36] Salient risk factors among clinicians who treat trauma survivors include solo practice, a caseload with a preponderance of trauma survivors, and absence of peer support and feedback. Active and ongoing strategies to ensure that therapist stress reactions are appropriately and expeditiously recognized and given attention are recommended, such as establishment of regular peer consultation, support, and debriefing.[29]

Finally, successful recovery from trauma extends beyond therapeutic attention to the relief of painful symptoms. There is also a requirement to guide the survivor toward awareness and enhancement of the latent positive ramifications and perspectives of the survivor experience, although such acknowledgment typically is not possible in the early phases of treatment. Examples of positive aspects of the survival experience include the heroic courage and strength necessary to survive trauma and its aftermath, or development of expanded perspectives and world view.[5,29,37] Another example is progress from morbid rumination about a near-death experience toward a perception that one's post-trauma life is "bonus time," to be cherished and appreciated all the more because one "should" have died. It cannot be overemphasized that recognition and appreciation of such positive effects is as important to the recovery process as the alleviation or mitigation of painful aspects; this is especially relevant in the middle and later phases of treatment.

REFERENCES

1. Rahe RH: Acute versus chronic psychological reactions to combat. Milit Med 153:365–372, 1988.
2. American Psychiatric Association: Diagnostic and Statistical Manual of Mental Disorders. 3rd ed. Revised. Washington, DC: American Psychiatric Association, 1987:250–251.
3. Kolb LC: A neuropsychological hypothesis explaining posttraumatic stress disorders. Am J Psychiatry 144:989–995, 1987.
4. Scurfield RM: PTSD in Vietnam veterans. In Wilson JP, Raphael B, eds. The International Handbook of Traumatic Stress Syndromes, Vol I. New York: Plenum Press, (in press, 1992).
5. Scurfield RM: Post-traumatic stress: Issues, etiology and treatment. In Figley C, ed. Trauma and Its Wake, Vol I. New York: Brunner Mazel, 1985:219–256.
6. Helzer JE, Robins LN, McEvoy E: Post-traumatic stress disorder in the general population: Findings of the epidemiologic catchment area survey. N Engl J Med 317:1630–1634, 1987.
7. Kulka RA, Schlenger WE, Fairbank JA, Hough RL, Jordan BK, Marmar CR, Weiss DS: Trauma and the Vietnam War Generation. Report of Findings from the National Vietnam Veterans Readjustment Study. New York: Brunner Mazel, 1990.
8. Goldberg J, True WT, Eisen SA, Henderson WG: A twin study of the effects of the Vietnam war on posttraumatic stress disorder. JAMA 263:1227–1232, 1990.
9. Kinzie JD, Boehnlein JK, Leung PK, et al: The prevalence of posttraumatic stress disorder and its clinical significance among Southeast Asian refugees. Am J Psychiatry 147:913–917, 1990.
10. Pitman RK, Altman B, Macklin ML: Prevalence of posttraumatic stress disorder in wounded Vietnam veterans. Am J Psychiatry 146:667–669, 1989.
11. Smith EM, North CS, McCool RE, Shea JM: Acute postdisas-

ter psychiatric disorders: Identification of persons at risk. Am J Psychiatry 147:202–206, 1990.
12. Pollock DA, Rhodes P, Boyle CA, et al: Estimating the number of suicides among Vietnam veterans. Am J Psychiatry 147:772–776, 1990.
13. Davidson J, Swartz M, Storck M, et al: A diagnostic and family study of posttraumatic stress disorder. Am J Psychiatry 142:90–93, 1985.
14. Friedman MJ: Biological approaches to the diagnosis and treatment of posttraumatic stress disorder. J Traumatic Stress 4:67–91, 1991.
15. Shore JH, Tatum EL, Vollmer WM: Psychiatric reactions to disaster: The Mt. St. Helens experience. Am J Psychiatry 143:590–595, 1986.
16. Terr L: Childhood traumas: An outline and overview. Am J Psychiatry 148:10–20, 1991.
17. Sierles FS, Chen J, McFarland RE, Taylor MA: Posttraumatic stress disorder and concurrent psychiatric illness: A preliminary report. Am J Psychiatry 140:1177–1179, 1983.
18. Davidson J, Kudler H, Smith R, et al: Treatment of posttraumatic stress disorder with amitriptyline and placebo. Arch Gen Psychiatry 47:259–266, 1990.
19. Frank JB, Kosten TR, Giller EL, Dan E: A randomized clinical trial of phenelzine and imipramine for posttraumatic stress disorder. Am J Psychiatry 145:1289–1291, 1989.
20. Shestazky M, Greenberg D, Lerer B: A controlled trial of phenelzine in posttraumatic stress disorder. Psychiatry Res 24:149–155, 1987.
21. Reist C, Kauffmann CD, Haier RJ, et al: A controlled trial of desipramine in 18 men with posttraumatic stress disorder. Am J Psychiatry 146:513–516, 1989.
22. Braun P, Greenberg D, Dasberg H, Lerer B: Core symptoms of posttraumatic stress disorder unimproved by alprazolam treatment. J Clin Psychiatry 51:236–238, 1990.
23. Risse SC, Whitters A, Burke J, et al: Severe withdrawal symptoms after discontinuation of alprazolam in eight patients with combat-induced posttraumatic stress disorder. J Clin Psychiatry 51:206–209, 1990.
24. Famularo R, Kinscherff R, Fenton T: Propranolol treatment for childhood posttraumatic stress disorder, acute type: A pilot study. Am J Dis Child 142:1244–1247, 1988.
25. Kolb LC, Burris BC, Griffiths S: Propranolol and clonidine in the treatment of post-traumatic stress disorders of war. In Van der Kolk BA, ed. Posttraumatic Stress Disorder: Psychological and Biological Sequelae. Washington DC: American Psychiatric Press, 1984:97–105.
26. Lipper S, Davidson JRT, Grady TA, et al: Preliminary study of carbamazepine in post-traumatic stress disorder. Psychosomatics 27:849–854, 1986.
27. Kitchner I, Greenstein R: Low dose lithium carbonate in the treatment of posttraumatic stress disorder: Brief communication. Milit Med 150:378–381, 1985.
28. Silver JM, Sandberg DP, Hales RE: New approaches in the pharmacotherapy of posttraumatic stress disorder. J Clin Psychiatry 51(suppl):33–38, 1990.
29. Scurfield RM: Treatment of PTSD in Vietnam veterans. In Wilson JP, Raphael B, eds. The International Handbook of Traumatic Stress Syndromes, Vol II. New York: Plenum Press, (in press, 1992).
30. Fairbank JA, Nicholson RA: Theoretical and empirical issues in the treatment of post-traumatic stress disorder in Vietnam veterans. J Clin Psychology 43:44–55, 1987.
31. Horowitz MJ: Stress-response syndromes: A review of posttraumatic and adjustment disorders. Hosp Community Psychiatry 37:241–248, 1986.
32. Scurfield RM, Corker TM, Gongla PA, Hough R: Three post-Vietnam "rap/therapy" groups: An analysis. Group 8:3–21, 1984.
33. Solomon A, Benbenishty R: The role of proximity, immediacy and expectancy in frontline treatment of combat stress reaction among Israelis in the Lebanon war. Am J Psychiatry 143:613–621, 1986.
34. Scurfield RM, Kenderine SK, Pollard RJ: Inpatient treatment for war-related posttraumatic stress disorder: Initial

findings of a longer-term outcome study. J Traumatic Stress 3:185–201, 1990.

35. McCann IL, Pearlman LA: Vicarious traumatization: A framework for understanding the psychological effects of working with victims. J Traumatic Stress 3:131–149, 1990.

36. Mitchell JT, Dyregrov A: Traumatic stress in disaster workers and emergency personnel: Prevention and intervention. *In* Wilson JP, Raphael B, eds. The International Handbook of Traumatic Stress Syndromes, Vol II. New York: Plenum Press, 1991.

37. Frankl V: Man's Search for Meaning: An Introduction to Logotherapy. Boston: Beacon Press, 1990.

47

REVIEW OF ANXIOLYTIC DRUGS

DANE WINGERSON, M.D., and PETER P. ROY-BYRNE, M.D.

Pharmacotherapy has become a standard component in the treatment of many of the anxiety disorders. Recent research has increased our knowledge of the efficacy, risks, and benefits of many of the anxiolytic medications. In this chapter we review the multiple medications with anxiolytic effects, focusing on indications and relative contraindications, absorption and pharmacokinetics, dosing and titration, side effects, and drug interactions.

PRIOR TO INITIATION OF ANXIOLYTIC MEDICATION THERAPY

Prior to starting an anxious patient on anxiolytic medication, the clinician needs to adequately "prepare" the patient. A trusting therapeutic alliance must be established between the clinician and patient. Because of their anxiety and fear, these patients may initially be reluctant to begin a medication unless questions regarding the nature of their illness and the rationale for pharmacotherapy have been adequately answered. Many anxious patients fear that they are "emotionally weak" or deficient in some way. Because of this, it is frequently helpful to present a medical model and emphasize the biological component of their illness, thus relieving their guilt about being responsible for the illness, decreasing resistance toward pharmacotherapy, and reassuring them that help is available to decrease their symptoms. Simultaneously, it is important to note that cognitive and environmental factors frequently play an important role in the anxiety disorders, thereby indicating that psychotherapeutic modalities may also play an important treatment role, and that the patient, through his or her own effort and work, will be able to gain some mastery over the illness.

Although it is helpful to emphasize the "medical model," care must be taken not to give patients the expectation of a "cure" for their illness. The anxiety disorders are chronic illnesses that wax and wane. Patients need to be aware that anxiolytic medications likely will not eliminate all of their symptoms but will help to decrease overall anxiety and improve global functioning.

In the early stages of treatment, it is important for the clinician to be readily available to the patient. Anxious patients need to feel that they can reach their clinician quickly if necessary. Taking the time to give reassurance or to answer questions early on may reap increased compliance, improved outcome, and ultimately decreased phone calls from the patient later.

It is frequently advisable to involve the patient's spouse or significant other in treatment. If cooperation of the spouse can be enlisted, additional reassurance and support are available to the patient. If the spouse is not involved, the spouse may instead inadvertently interfere with treatment by voicing his or her own concerns about the medication, thus increasing the patient's fear and perhaps decreasing compliance.

The clinician should anticipate possible difficulties in the treatment course and share these with the patient early on. It is important to discuss the likely time course of treatment, possible medication side effects, and even the possibility of nonresponse or the need to switch medications. Care must be exercised, however, in the discussion of medication side effects, because many anxious patients are hypersuggestible and may focus unduly on certain bodily sensations to which they have been alerted.

Accurate assessment of response to pharmacotherapy requires a detailed history of the patient's anxiety symptoms and the associated degree of social, occupational, or interpersonal disability. It is frequently helpful to have patients keep a daily symptom diary as a method of charting illness progression and, if possible, to begin the diary prior to the introduction of medications in order to obtain a baseline upon which treatment can be measured. It is important to note that patients may improve in terms of social or occupational functioning without dramatic reduction in symptoms, suggesting that several measures are needed when evaluating effectiveness of treatment.

BENZODIAZEPINES

Description and Mechanism of Action

The benzodiazepines are a group of closely related compounds whose basic structure consists of two benzene rings connected by a seven-sided ring containing two nitrogen atoms. Benzodiazepines act by facilitating inhibitor neurotransmission via potentiation of the action of gamma-aminobutyric acid (GABA). They bind stereospecifically to GABA receptor subunits, which have their highest density in limbic brain areas controlling affect, arousal, and visceral/autonomic function.

Indications

The high-potency benzodiazepines alprazolam, lorazepam, and clonazepam have been shown to be effective in multiple double-blind, placebo-controlled trials of panic disorder patients. Benzodiazepines of all potencies have been shown to be effective in the treatment of generalized anxiety disorder. Limited evidence suggests that high-potency benzodiazepines may work in social phobia. Benzodiazepines have not been shown to be effective in obsessive-compulsive disorder, and their use in patients with post-traumatic stress disorder (PTSD) has been fraught with problems because of the high comorbid alcohol and drug abuse in some individuals with PTSD. In fact, one recent report[1] documented severe withdrawal symptoms in chronic PTSD veterans following discontinuation of alprazolam, with sleep disturbances, rage reactions, intrusive thoughts, and homicidal ideation. These medications, because of the risks of abuse, dependence, and cognitive-psychomotor impairment, have not been traditionally considered first-line antianxiety drugs. However, for nonresponders to other psychopharmacological interventions such as antidepressants (possibly a quarter to a third of panic patients), the benefits of these medications clearly outweigh the risks. In addition, for patients whose acute symptoms are producing significant disability, benzodiazepines, because of their far more rapid onset of effect, are the first-line

treatment of choice. In such cases, traditional antidepressant drugs whose long-term use is not associated with dependence can be added on after the initial symptoms resolve in 1 to 3 weeks, and the benzodiazepine slowly tapered and discontinued following 12 weeks of antidepressant treatment.

Pharmacokinetics and Dose Titration

Benzodiazepines are well absorbed on an empty stomach. Antacids interfere with the absorptive phase of benzodiazepines and, hence, should not be given within several hours of dosing. Intramuscular injection of benzodiazepines often results in unpredictable and erratic absorption. In intramuscular dosing, lorazepam is probably the most reliably absorbed benzodiazepine; however, its use should be confined to emergent situations in inpatient settings where other symptoms, such as dangerous agitation, are being treated. Lorazepam, triazolam, temazepam, and oxazepam are metabolized in the liver by direct conjugation and have no active metabolites. Other benzodiazepines, alprazolam, diazepam, chlorazepate, chlordiazepoxide, and flurazepam, are oxidized by microsomal enzymes in the liver to other active metabolites, which in turn are conjugated in the liver and excreted in the urine. These benzodiazepines are less likely to be cleared effectively in patients with liver disease. Clonazepam is metabolized by both oxidation and nitroreduction and has no active metabolites. The various benzodiazepines do differ significantly in rate of absorption, distribution into fat, and elimination half-life. Therefore, pharmacokinetics are a more important determinant of drug selection with benzodiazepines than with any other class of psychotropic drugs.

Benzodiazepines are all lipophilic, rapidly cross the blood-brain barrier and reach equilibrium in the CNS relatively quickly. For chronic benzodiazepine dosing (i.e., more than a p.r.n. basis), achievement of steady-state drug levels depends upon the drug's half-life, with approximately four to five half-lives needed to achieve steady-state levels. The longer the half-life, the longer time necessary to reach steady-state blood levels. The individual benzodiazepines have variable half-lives based upon individual differences in metabolism. For example, alprazolam, clonazepam, and lorazepam have half-lives of 6 to 20 hours, 18 to 50 hours, and 10 to 20 hours, respectively. Half-life duration dictates dosage intervals, because interdose fluctuation in blood concentration varies with elimination. In general, a dosage interval equal to the elimination half-life yields fluctuations in blood concentration reasonably close to average steady-state concentration.

Individual benzodiazepines differ in milligram doses required to produce similar therapeutic effects. These differences are thought to be secondary to the extent of entry into the CNS and to result from differences in receptor binding. Alprazolam is a "high-potency" benzodiazepine because it binds to the GABA-benzodiazepine receptor with higher affinity as compared to the "low-potency" benzodiazepine diazepam, which binds with lower affinity.

In clinical practice the two most frequently used benzodiazepines at this time appear to be two of the high-potency benzodiazepines, alprazolam and clonazepam. Although the short half-life of alprazolam may result in breakthrough anxiety between doses, clonazepam may be associated more often with emergent depression. Individual patient differences will dictate the most appropriate choice of treatment. Clonazepam is twice as potent as alprazolam, and lorazepam is half as potent as alprazolam. Doses are given for alprazolam, but appropriate translations can be easily made.

In the treatment of panic disorder, alprazolam can be initiated at a dosage of 0.25 to 0.5 mg q.i.d. (lorazepam may be used t.i.d. and clonazepam on a b.i.d. basis). Titration of alprazolam can be increased slowly to the desired effect. Although Food and Drug Administration approval now supports dosing of up to 10 mg/day for alprazolam in panic, we rarely use more than 6 mg/day in our clinic. Generally, 2 mg/day works for some patients, and 4 mg/day is usually adequate for many others. This is not inconsistent with the mean daily dose of 4.8 mg total per day reported in a large study.[2] The initiation and titration of benzodiazepines for the treatment of generalized anxiety disorder is similar to that for panic disorder, although the total daily dose is usually only one half as much. Limited data in benzodiazepine treatment of social phobia have shown that doses of 1.5 mg of clonazepam and 3 mg of alprazolam total per day have been effective.[3,4] Anecdotal reports have suggested that benzodiazepines can also be used on a p.r.n. basis for discrete performance anxiety, although their effects on cognition and psychomotor performance can make them more problematic for this purpose.

Side Effects and Drug Interactions

The major side effects of benzodiazepines are sedation and psychomotor impairment. Sedation usually disappears within 1 to 2 weeks of treatment, although psychomotor impairment may persist to a subtle degree, especially in the first few hours after dosing when levels are at their peak. Patients need to be cautioned regarding these psychomotor effects if they are to perform complex psychomotor tasks such as driving. There is some effect on recent memory that also may persist.[5] The major "toxicity" of benzodiazepines is the well-publicized tendency of patients to abuse them and develop dependence. Clearcut risk of abuse with dose escalation and tolerance is confined to patients with personal histories of alcohol or chemical dependency, although some patients with no personal history, but a substance abuse history in first-degree relatives, may be at relatively greater risk for abuse.[6] The best long-term study to date clearly shows that panic patients

treated with alprazolam followed up 2.5 years later are taking on the average considerably lower doses, and despite the lower dose are less symptomatic.[7] Hence, there is little evidence for dose escalation or tolerance in anxiety patients, most of whom do well on long-term benzodiazepine treatment. The greatest problem, for which there are fewer solutions, is dependence, defined by the withdrawal symptoms that occur on discontinuation of medication.[8] Dependence will develop in a large number of individuals treated for several months. It is extremely difficult to distinguish between reemergence of underlying anxiety symptoms and physiological withdrawal symptoms. The reemergence of anxiety symptoms in previously symptom-free patients may be so frightening that a drug-free interval cannot be tolerated, and patients often restart their benzodiazepines despite the risk of dependence. Benzodiazepines should not be discontinued abruptly, particularly because of the risk of withdrawal symptoms, including seizures. Benzodiazepine taper should be tailored to the individual patient. A reasonable dosage reduction of alprazolam is 0.5 mg/week until a dose of 1 mg is reached and then 0.25 mg/week.

Benzodiazepines do not induce liver enzymes and generate few adverse drug reactions. The major problematic drug interaction is potentiation of alcohol, a vitally important, yet frequently ignored, problem. Cimetidine, isoniazid, and fluoxetine may slightly raise the blood level of benzodiazepines that undergo oxidation in the liver.

Comparison of Effectiveness of Various Benzodiazepines

There may not be absolute equivalence between benzodiazepines. For example, some patients are highly responsive to clonazepam after failing to respond to alprazolam and vice versa. Not infrequently, the choice of benzodiazepine rests with pharmacokinetic differences. Benzodiazepines with long elimination half-lives take longer to reach steady-state blood levels, take longer to be eliminated from the body (which may be important in cases of overdose or severe side effects), and result in extensive drug accumulation. However, long half-lives also minimize interdose fluctuations and may be convenient because of relatively infrequent dosing schedules. Benzodiazepines with short half-lives have the opposite consequences, with a shorter time needed to reach steady-state blood levels, faster elimination, and less drug accumulation. With short half-lives come the difficulties of interdose fluctuations, increased likelihood of withdrawal reactions with missed doses, and the need for more frequent dosing. The use of benzodiazepines on a p.r.n. basis for chronic anxiety symptoms is to be avoided, because patients come to associate "the pill" with symptom relief, which in turn may lead to psychological dependence. It is preferable to give benzodiazepines on a regularly scheduled basis in order to block anxiety symptoms totally before they occur.

Duration of Treatment

Response to treatment with benzodiazepines is rapid, occurring in 1 to 2 weeks and peaking at 4 to 8 weeks. Although there have been no studies directed at duration of treatment for benzodiazepines in patients with anxiety disorders, the overall evidence suggests that the use of benzodiazepines should be short, generally less than 6 months. There may be indications, however, for long-term benzodiazepine use, especially in panic disorder patients or in other chronically ill patients with anxiety symptoms who fail to respond to other interventions. By limiting the duration of treatment, difficulties of benzodiazepine dependence and rebound anxiety may be avoided more successfully.

AZASPIRONES

Description and Mechanism of Action

Buspirone is an azaspirone that is not chemically or pharmacologically related to benzodiazepines or other anxiolytic drugs. Buspirone has a high affinity for serotonin 5-HT_{1A} receptors, as well as a more modest affinity for D_2 dopamine receptors. Its serotonergic properties are assumed to underlie its anxiolytic activity. Buspirone does not bind at a GABA binding site as do benzodiazepines.

Indications

Double-blind placebo-controlled studies have shown that buspirone is as effective as several benzodiazepines in the treatment of generalized anxiety disorder. The few investigations of buspirone in the treatment of panic disorder have yielded negative results. A preliminary report suggests that buspirone may have efficacy in social phobia,[9] as well as possibly comparable efficacy when compared with clomipramine in obsessive-compulsive disorder.[10] Clearly, more studies need to be done regarding the efficacy of buspirone in disorders other than generalized anxiety disorder.

Buspirone has absolutely no abuse liability, has no effect on cognition or psychomotor function, and does not produce a withdrawal syndrome when it is abruptly discontinued. There is no cross-tolerance with alcohol. In generalized anxiety disorder, it is probably the drug of choice for patients prone to alcohol or drug abuse, or those likely to require long-term anxiolytic therapy, since these patients are at risk for developing benzodiazepine dependence. Some reports suggest that patients who have formerly used benzodiazepines respond less well to buspirone although their response is still better than that to placebo.

Although buspirone seems to be comparable to the benzodiazepines for treatment of generalized anxiety disorder, a significantly larger dropout rate in one 6-month study[11] suggests that for some of these patients buspirone may be less acceptable than benzodiazepines. Buspirone may be particularly ideal for a patient with prominent ruminative cognitive symptoms as opposed to somatic symptoms of generalized anxiety, although somatic symptoms also are clearly responsive.

Pharmacokinetics and Dose Titration

Buspirone is rapidly absorbed and undergoes extensive first-pass metabolism. The average elimination half-life of unchanged buspirone after single doses is about 2 to 3 hours. The onset of action of buspirone is delayed, and this is often a key point not appreciated by clinicians or patients eager for quick results. The initial dose is 5 mg t.i.d. The dose can be increased as tolerated by 5 mg every 2 days to 10 mg t.i.d. At this point the clinician should wait about 2 weeks before raising the dose to 15 mg t.i.d. if there is no response. The maximum dose is 20 mg t.i.d. Initial beneficial effects may not occur for several weeks, similar to results obtained for anxiolytic treatment with tricyclic antidepressants. A likely response rate as measured by a 50 per cent reduction in the Hamilton anxiety score is between 60 and 80 per cent. Many anxious patients will do well on 30 to 45 mg of buspirone per day. Higher doses may be helpful in patients with additional symptoms of depression.

Side Effects and Drug Interactions

The most common side effects of buspirone are dizziness, nausea, insomnia, restlessness, and agitation. No toxicity has been reported with clinically relevant doses. There are few significant drug interactions. Buspirone may slightly elevate digoxin levels. Occasionally dose reduction will reduce side effects. Depending on the timing of these symptoms, clinicians can reduce one or two of the three doses.

Duration of Treatment

There are no clear indications for duration of treatment with buspirone in generalized anxiety disorder; however, buspirone's efficacy is supported in short-term 6- to 12-week studies, as well as in longer term 6-month studies.

SEROTONIN REUPTAKE BLOCKERS

Description and Mechanism of Action

Clomipramine is a chlorinated derivative of imipramine. It has in general the same metabolic, kinetic, and side-effect profile as the other tricyclic antidepressant medications. However, clomipramine has a relatively selective capacity to inhibit the reuptake of serotonin as compared to the other tricyclic antidepressants. Fluoxetine is an atypical antidepressant that is chemically unrelated to tricyclic medications. Its action is also presumed to be secondary to its potent serotonin reuptake inhibition capability.

Indications

Placebo-controlled studies have conclusively demonstrated that clomipramine is effective for obsessive-compulsive disorder. Other reports suggest that fluoxetine is probably comparable in effectiveness to clomipramine for this disorder. (Interestingly, recent studies of the investigational serotonin reuptake blocker sertraline have shown mixed efficacy results, thus confusing the "serotonin hypothesis" for obsessive-compulsive disorder.[12,13]) More limited evidence suggests that clomipramine and fluoxetine are effective for panic disorder. There are few data regarding the usage of serotonin reuptake blockers in generalized anxiety disorder or PTSD. One report has suggested that fluoxetine may be particularly effective in social phobia.[14]

Pharmacokinetics and Dose Titration

Clomipramine is well tolerated in doses of up to 3 mg/kg or 250 mg/day. Titration of clomipramine can be done fairly rapidly, although it must be remembered that some panic disorder patients will show early aggravation of their symptoms, suggesting that low doses may be required initially. We usually begin with 25 mg at bedtime, although the medication should be titrated up to 100 mg in the first 1 to 2 weeks. Further titration should continue to maximum dosage or toleration of side effects. Some reports suggest that lower doses (25 mg/day) may be effective for panic disorder.

Fluoxetine is metabolized in the liver and excreted by the kidney. Fluoxetine and its active metabolites have extremely long half-lives of up to 9 days. For panic disorder, an initial dose of 20 mg/day of fluoxetine often produces overstimulation and a high dropout rate of approximately 50 per cent.[15] Beginning at 5 mg rather than 20 mg/day results in fewer dropouts and a higher response rate.[16] Dosing may start at 2 mg, particularly if there is a history of hypersensitivity to the stimulatory effects of tricyclic medications. With this strategy the dose can be increased slowly at first and, if there are no initial problems, more rapidly increased to 20 mg/day. An elixer preparation (4 mg/ml) is available now to facilitate such strategies. Fluoxetine's broader spectrum of action suggests that it ultimately may become a viable alternative to monoamine oxidase inhibitors (MAOIs) as a second-line treatment for panic. We have seen several patients with purported hypersensitivity to every tricyclic antidepressant, MAOIs, and even benzodiazepines who are able to tolerate extremely low doses (1 mg) of fluoxetine and with upward titration to doses of around 5 mg had amelioration of panic.

For patients with obsessive-compulsive disorder, fluoxetine should probably be started at 20 mg/day and titrated up to reach a dose of 60 to 80 mg/day within the first 1 to 2 weeks of treatment.

Side Effects and Drug Interactions

Clomipramine has strongly anticholinergic and sedative effects and also causes orthostatic hypotension. In contrast, fluoxetine has been widely embraced because of its limited side-effect profile, which includes increased anxiety and insomnia and in some cases decreased appetite and weight loss. At higher dosages, patients may experience additional side effects, including headache, nausea, and gastrointestinal upset.

Clomipramine has drug interactions similar to those of tricyclic antidepressants. Fluoxetine can potentially cause hypertensive crisis in patients treated with MAOIs and should not be used concomitantly with them. Monoamine oxidase inhibitors should not be started within 5 weeks of discontinuation of fluoxetine, and fluoxetine should not be started within 14 days of discontinuation of an MAOI. Fluoxetine may also increase plasma levels of tricyclic antidepressants by twofold. Because fluoxetine is tightly bound to plasma proteins, concomitant administration with other drugs that are protein bound, such as Coumadin or digoxin, may result in increased plasma concentrations potentially leading to adverse effects.

Duration of Treatment

For obsessive-compulsive disorder, time course of response with serotonin reuptake blockers suggests that initial effects will appear within the first 2 weeks, but full response may take up to 16 weeks. No clear current evidence exists that correlates blood levels and treatment response. It is important to note that in clomipramine treatment of obsessive-compulsive disorder patients, response rate is considerably higher than placebo, although one third of patients may show little if any response and another third, although showing some modest response, still remain substantially symptomatic. Fluoxetine, because of its side effect profile, may be tolerated better than clomipramine, although this has not been demonstrated in this particular population.

TRICYCLIC AND STRUCTURALLY RELATED ANTIDEPRESSANTS

Description

Tricyclic compounds, first developed in the 1950s as possible antipsychotic medications, were serendipitously found to have antidepressant effects. Tricyclics have the general chemical structure of two benzene rings joined by a seven-member ring that may consist entirely of carbon atoms or may have one nitrogen substitution. The more recently discovered heterocyclic medications consist of variations of this general chemical structure. For a detailed discussion of the mechanism of action and pharmacokinetics of these medicines, see Chapter 37.

Indications

Extensive evidence supports the efficacy of tricyclic antidepressants for panic disorder, generalized anxiety disorder, and, to a limited extent, PTSD. They are not effective for social phobia or obsessive-compulsive disorder. (See the section on serotonin reuptake blockers for a discussion of clomipramine.)

Pharmacokinetics and Dose Titration

All of these medications are clinically equipotent, with the exception of nortriptyline, which is twice as potent, and trazodone and amoxapine, which are half as potent. Because of the danger of early amphetamine-like side effects in some patients, treatment should begin with small doses (i.e., 10 mg of imipramine or desipramine and 5 mg of nortriptyline) with slow titration, increasing by 10 mg every 2 to 4 days. If no initial problems are encountered, further titration to full doses can be more rapid (25 mg every 2 to 3 days). Dosages should be titrated to side effects or 150 to 300 mg (3 mg/kg) for the average 70-kg individual (75 to 150 mg for nortriptyline). Elderly patients will not usually require such high doses, with a range of 75 to 150 mg being adequate. Because the half-life of all these drugs is approximately 24 hours, once-a-day doses are sufficient; divided doses are useful only to attenuate side effects or, perhaps in anxious patients, to produce sedating cues that may be somewhat comforting or calming. Patient dosages should be titrated upward until the troubling symptoms have been ameliorated. Full therapeutic effect may take up to 8 to 12 weeks. Some patients may show substantial improvement in 1 to 2 weeks, although this phenomenon often represents a placebo effect. Nonresponse should prompt the clinician to check the antidepressant blood level.

Side Effects

In anxious patients, particularly those with panic disorder, tricyclic medication may cause early stimulation with resultant increased anxiety and decreased compliance. This is the side effect most responsible for early discontinuation of antidepressants.[17] Other common side effects are postural hypotension and anticholinergic effects such as dry mouth, constipation, urinary retention, and blurred vision. (See Chapter 37 for further information regarding the side effects and drug interactions of these medications.)

Comparison of Effectiveness of Various Tricyclics and Related Antidepressants

Of all the anxiety disorders, panic disorder has been the most thoroughly studied with respect to treatment with various tricyclic antidepressants. Imipramine has been the prototypically studied drug, with several studies showing that it is highly effective. Uncontrolled reports suggest that desipramine, nortriptyline, amitriptyline, and doxepin are also effective. Although they are probably effective, some panic disorder patients may have problems with the more strongly anticholinergic medications, such as amitriptyline and doxepin, because their side effects may aggravate the patient's already excessive focus on internal physical sensations. Controlled studies have shown that maprotiline and trazodone are inferior to other antidepressants. In addition, the occurrence of priapism, although rare, suggests that trazodone should not be a first-line drug in males. Amoxapine, because it is metabolized in the liver to a neuroleptic (loxapine), poses a theoretical risk of tardive dyskinesia and should not be used. We have used nortriptyline with good effect in many patients.

Duration of Treatment

The optimal duration of treatment, as well as the ability to predict relapse, depends on accurate information regarding the natural course or outcome of the various anxiety disorders. Few if any data are available from the prepharmacological era, so that most of the information we have is based on patients who are already being naturalistically treated with various pharmacological agents. Very few data exist regarding the long-term outcome for treated patients with generalized anxiety disorder or PTSD. For panic disorder, evidence suggests that it is a chronic illness that, however, has a relatively good outcome, with many individuals maintaining a mild level of symptomatology at follow-up.

In our clinical practice, we treat patients for a 6- to 12-month period, as often recommended for major depression, and discourage discontinuation at times of major life stress or change. Relapse of from 50 to 70 per cent for anxiety disorder patients is common within 6 to 12 months of medication discontinuation. Although the more chronic versus episodic nature of the anxiety disorders suggests that fewer patients are able to discontinue drugs and do well than depressed patients, a third to a half may be able to remain in a relatively healthy state with only mild symptoms after medication discontinuation.

MONOAMINE OXIDASE INHIBITORS

Description

Monoamine oxidase inhibitors were first synthesized as antitubercular drugs in the 1950s and fortuitously were noted to have antidepressant properties. Chemically the MAOIs consists of a benzene ring with a single carbon/nitrogen side chain that differentiates between the individual compounds. (For a detailed discussion of the mechanism of action and pharmacokinetics of these medicines, see Chapter 37.)

Indications

Monoamine oxidase inhibitors are probably underutilized in the United States. There is good evidence that MAOIs are effective in the treatment of panic disorder and social phobia. Anecdotal reports[18] also indicate possible effectiveness in PTSD. There is limited information regarding the usage of MAOIs in generalized anxiety disorder. MAOIs are usually not effective in treating obsessive-compulsive disorder uncomplicated by panic attacks.

Dose Titration

Because MAO inhibition, once established, takes 2 weeks to reverse for phenelzine and isocarboxazid and 3 to 4 days for reversal with tranylcypromine, administration need not be in divided doses for efficacy. However, a t.i.d. schedule is routinely recommended to minimize side effects.

For phenelzine, patients should begin by taking 15 mg once a day for 2 days, then 15 mg twice a day for 3 days, and then 15 mg three times a day for 1 week. The dose can then be raised to 60 mg daily, perhaps 30 mg in the morning and 15 mg twice during the day. The dosage ceiling is 90 to 105 mg. After 105 mg, the dose can be increased if there is no efficacy or there are no side effects. Doses of approximately 1 mg/kg of phenelzine are probably required for full therapeutic effect. For tranylcypromine, 10-mg doses are comparable to 15-mg doses of phenelzine, and escalation of dose is similar. There is little published experience using isocarboxazid in the anxiety disorders, although it likely would be effective.

Side Effects and Drug Interactions

These drugs, particularly phenelzine, do not produce the amphetamine-like reactions caused by tricyclic antidepressants in anxious patients. They also, particularly tranylcypromine, have fewer anticholinergic effects. Insomnia is the most common problem and can be avoided by moving the dose earlier or by doubling up the morning dose so that patients take the last dose by 2:00 or 3:00 in the afternoon. Some patients may even be able to tolerate their entire dose at one time in the morning. An initial paradoxical effect of MAOIs is daytime lethargy or sleepiness, not apparently associated with the timing of the dose. Patients may grow tolerant to this over time. (See Chapter 37 for further information on MAOI side effects and drug interactions, particularly the potentially fatal "cheese reaction.")

Comparison of Effectiveness of the MAOIs

Among the MAOIs, no single agent has been found to be more effective than another in the treatment of anxiety disorders. In general, the choice of MAOI depends on the side-effect profile. Patients who would benefit from sedation may do well on phenelzine, whereas patients intolerant to anticholinergic or sedative side effects may be treated better with tranylcypromine.

Duration of Treatment

As with tricyclics, drug treatment should be from 6 to 12 months with gradual discontinuation thereafter, reducing dose by 15 mg every 1 to 2 weeks for phenelzine. Although it is likely that, as in depression, maximal MAO inhibition is required for antianxiety efficacy, no studies have conclusively shown a correlation between percentage MAO inhibition and effect in anxiety disorders or depression. In our experience, many anxiety patients resistant to treatment with tricyclic antidepressants are highly responsive to MAOIs.

β-BLOCKERS

Description and Mechanism of Action

β-Blockers are agents that block the effects of β-adrenergic receptors. Two types of β receptors exist: β_1 receptors, the predominant noradrenergic receptors in the brain, which also regulate heart rate and contractility peripherally, and β_2 receptors, which act primarily on bronchodilation and vasodilation. In the treatment of anxiety, β-blockers are most likely effective by decreasing peripheral symptoms such as tachycardia and tremor.

Indications

With the proven efficacy of tricyclics, MAOIs, buspirone, and benzodiazepines, there is relatively little indication for the usage of β-blockers in the treatment of anxiety disorders. Evidence clearly shows that β-blockers are ineffective for panic attacks,[19] and controlled studies in generalized anxiety disorder show only modest evidence for their efficacy, with significant changes in symptoms often being clinically insubstantial.[20] β-Blockers are not effective in obsessive-compulsive disorder, and propranolol at doses ranging from 120 to 160 mg/day has only anecdotally been noted to decrease hyperarousal symptoms in PTSD patients. β-Blockers may be quite effective in treating symptoms of a performance anxiety subtype of social phobia. Because symptoms of palpitations and tremor are prominent in discrete performance anxiety, β-blockers are well suited for symptom reduction in this disorder. These symptoms serve as a positive feedback cue that intensifies the performance anxiety. Thus, eliminating the troubling symptoms may effectively eliminate the syndrome.

Pharmacokinetics and Dose Titration

β-Blockers are reasonably well absorbed but vary greatly in metabolism and half-life. Propranolol and metoprolol are primarily metabolized in the liver and have short half-lives of from 3 to 6 hours. Atenolol and nadolol are primarily excreted through the kidney, with atenolol having a half-life of 6 to 9 hours and nadolol 14 to 24 hours.

If β-blockers are to be used in the treatment of performance anxiety, a single dose of 10 to 40 mg of propranolol, 50 mg of atenolol or metoprolol, or 40 mg of nadolol given 30 minutes prior to the anxiety-provoking event is usually sufficient. It is often useful to try a test dose at some point prior to the anxiogenic event.

Side Effects and Drug Interactions

β-Blockers have multiple possible side effects. Because of the potential for bronchospasm, they are contraindicated in patients with asthma and relatively contraindicated in patients with other obstructive pulmonary disorders. They may interfere with the normal response to hypoglycemia and therefore must be used cautiously in patients with diabetes. Other common side effects include hypotension, bradycardia, dizziness, and congestive heart failure in patients with poor myocardial function. They may cause numerous gastrointestinal side effects, including nausea, diarrhea, and abdominal pain. Impotence is not uncommon. β-Blockers are thought to sometimes cause depression, as well as depressive symptoms such as fatigue and insomnia. Preexisting angina symptoms may be exacerbated when β-blockers are stopped.

β-Blockers also have multiple drug interactions. Theophylline clearance is reduced when used with propranolol. Chlorpromazine and cimetidine both lead to increased propranolol blood levels. β-Blockers must be used with caution in patients treated with catecholamine-depleting agents such as reserpine because of possible hypotension. Also, β-blockers may mask thyrotoxicosis, and abrupt withdrawal can precipitate thyroid storm.

Comparison of Effectiveness of the Various β-Blockers

Aside from half-life, the β-blockers differ from each other based on lipophilicity and ability to interact with the CNS. Propranolol is highly lipophilic, whereas metoprolol is moderately lipophilic and atenolol and nadolol are both relatively nonlipophilic. Although more lipophilic drugs are thought to cause more prominent CNS effects, recent studies cast doubt on this theory, suggesting that some process other than just diffusion controls their rate of CNS entry. No single β-blocker has proven to be superior in treatment of performance anxiety.

SUMMARY

In review, multiple pharmacological treatments are available for the various anxiety disorders. The multiple risks and benefits must be carefully considered before choosing a particular pharmacological agent as a treatment modality. The benzodiazepines are effective and treat symptoms rapidly in panic and generalized anxiety disorder; however, the side effects of sedation, psychomotor impairment, and possible physiological dependence are significant concerns. Buspirone is relatively safe and effective in treatment of generalized anxiety disorder, although it usually takes several weeks before beneficial effects are seen. Serotonin reuptake blockers are currently the best treatment forms available for obsessive-compulsive disorder, although they also have some side effects to be considered. Tricyclic and structurally related antidepressants are quite effective for panic and generalized anxiety disorder. However, early overstimulation and anticholinergic side effects may interfere with treatment. Monoamine oxidase inhibitor medications are effective in panic disorder and social phobia, although side effects, including significant dietary restrictions, influence treatment decisions. Finally, β-blockers, once a frequent choice in pharmacotherapy of anxiety disorders, now appear to be appropriate only in the treatment of performance anxiety. Whatever pharmacological intervention is chosen, it is important to recognize that a trusting, therapeutic relationship between patient and clinician is a requirement for successful treatment outcome in these serious and debilitating psychiatric disorders.

REFERENCES

1. Risse SC, Whitters A, Burke J, et al: Severe withdrawal symptoms after discontinuation of alprazolam in eight patients with combat-induced post-traumatic stress disorder. J Clin Psychiatry 51:206–209, 1990.
2. Ballenger JC, Burrows GD, DuPont R, et al: Alprazolam in panic disorder and agoraphobia: Results from a multicenter trial, I: Efficacy in short-term treatment. Arch Gen Psychiatry 45:413–422, 1988.

3. Reich J, Yates W: A pilot study of treatment of social phobia with alprazolam. Am J Psychiatry 145:590–594, 1988.

4. Munjack DJ, Baltazar PL, Bohn PB, et al: Clonazepam in the treatment of social phobia: A pilot study. J Clin Psychiatry 51(suppl 5):35–40, discussion 50–53, 1990.

5. Hommer DW: Benzodiazepines: Cognitive and psychomotor effects. In Roy-Byrne PP, Cowley DC, eds. Benzodiazepines in Clinical Practice: Risks and Benefits. Washington, DC: APA Press, 1991:111–130.

6. Ciraulo DA, Barnhill JG, Ciraulo AM, et al: Parental alcoholism as a risk factor in benzodiazepine abuse: A pilot study. Am J Psychiatry 146:1333–1335, 1989.

7. Nagy LM, Kristal JH, Woods SW, et al: Clinical and medication outcome after short-term aprazolam and behavioral group treatment in panic disorder. Arch Gen Psychiatry 46:993–999, 1989.

8. Roy-Byrne PP, Hommer D: Benzodiazepine withdrawal: Overview and implications for the treatment of anxiety. Am J Med 84:1041–1052, 1988.

9. Bruns JR, Munjack DJ, Baltazar PL, et al: Buspirone in the treatment of social phobia. CL22 Selective Therapeutic Index, Family Practice Recertification 115:46–52, 1989.

10. Murphy DL, Pigott TA: A comparative examination of a role for serotonin in obsessive-compulsive disorder, panic disorder, and anxiety. J Clin Psychiatry 51(suppl):53–58, discussion 59–60, 1990.

11. Rickels K, Schweizer E, Csanalos I, et al: Long-term treatment of anxiety and risk of withdrawal: Prospective comparison of chlorazepate and buspirone. Arch Gen Psychiatry 45:444–450, 1988.

12. Jenike MA, Baer L: Summergrad P, et al: Sertraline in obsessive-compulsive disorder: A double-blind comparison with placebo. Am J Psychiatry 147:923–928, 1990.

13. Chouinard G, Goodman W, Greist J, et al: Results of a double-blind placebo-controlled trial of a new serotonin uptake inhibitor, sertraline, in the treatment of obsessive-compulsive disorder. Psychopharmacol Bull 26:279–284, 1990.

14. Sternbach H: Fluoxetine treatment of social phobia. J Clin Psychopharmacol 10:230–231, 1990.

15. Gorman J, Liebowitz MR, Fuger AJ, et al: An open trial of fluoxetine in the treatment of panic attacks. J Clin Psychopharmacol 7:329–332, 1987.

16. Schneier FR, Liebowitz MR, Davies SO, et al: Fluoxetine in panic disorder. J Clin Psychopharmacol 10:119–121, 1990.

17. Noyes R, Garvey MJ, Cook BL: Problems with tricyclic antidepressant use in patients with panic disorder or agoraphobia: Results of a naturalistic follow-up study. J Clin Psychiatry 50:163–169, 1989.

18. Silver JM, Sandberg DP, Haler RE: New approaches in the pharmacotherapy of post-traumatic stress disorder. J Clin Psychiatry 51(suppl):33–38, 1990.

19. Munjack DJ, Clacker B, Cabe D, et al: Alprazolam, propranolol and placebo in the treatment of panic disorder and agoraphobia with panic attacks. J Clin Psychopharmacol 9:22–27, 1989.

20. Meibach RC, Mullane JF, Binstok G: A placebo-controlled multicenter trial of propranolol and chlordiazepoxide in the treatment of anxiety. Curr Ther Res 41:65–76, 1987.

48

REVIEW OF PSYCHOSOCIAL TREATMENTS FOR ANXIETY DISORDERS

ROBERT M. HERTZ, M.D., ANNE MARIE ALBANO, Ph.D.,
TIMOTHY A. BROWN, Psy.D., and DAVID H. BARLOW, Ph.D.

In the last several years, substantial advances have been made in the development of specific psychosocial treatments for anxiety disorders. One of the most remarkable advances that has been achieved is the establishment of detailed therapeutic protocols specifically tailored to each disorder. In addition to the obvious experimental benefits (e.g., replicability of treatment outcome studies), the existence of these protocols allows for their dissemination and subsequent use by psychotherapists serving to mitigate the split that has previously existed between science and clinical practice.

Although great specificity now exists in the extant treatments for the variety of anxiety disorders, it will become apparent that almost all of the procedures have some common elements. For example, the study of anxiety, as well as other emotions, has produced wide agreement that anxiety is expressed in a set of response systems (the tripartite model): subjective/cognitive, physiological, and behavioral.[1] Hence, virtually all treatments for anxiety are designed to have an impact on one or all of these response systems. Central to most approaches is the necessity to arrange for the individual to be exposed somehow to the anxiety-provoking situations, either external or internal (e.g., somatic), to eliminate escape or avoidance behaviors serving, in part, to maintain the disorder (behavioral component). In addition, almost all approaches involve some sort of restructuring of attitudes, beliefs, and cognitions associated with the anxiety-evoking situations (cognitive component). Finally, many of these treatments incorporate techniques for managing physiological symptoms of anxiety. These techniques include progressive relaxation and breathing retraining.

In this chapter, we review current cognitive-behavioral treatments for the anxiety disorders. Because space limitations mitigate detailed discussion of some of these treatments and disorders (e.g., posttraumatic stress disorder, simple phobia), the reader is referred to Brown et al.[2] for a comprehensive review.

PANIC DISORDER WITH AND WITHOUT AGORAPHOBIA

Whereas behavioral treatments of panic disorder and panic disorder with agoraphobia (PDA) traditionally have focused on the situational avoidance component of the disorder, more recently, cognitive-behavioral treatments have been developed to target panic attacks themselves. Regardless of whether the intervention is aimed at panic control or at situational avoidance, assessment and treatment follow along the lines of the tripartite model described above.

Panic Control Treatments

Several recent studies have demonstrated marked success in reducing and, in some cases, eliminating panic attacks in patients with PD using cognitive-behavioral treatments.[3–5] A brief elaboration of the panic control treatment (PCT) designed by Barlow et al.[3] will serve as an example of a multimodal treatment of panic. A central underlying assumption of PCT is that panic is qualitatively distinct from anxiety. Indeed, panic is conceived as representing a very appropriate and adaptive alarm mechanism (i.e., the fight or flight response) that is fired at inappropriate times (i.e., when no real threat is present). These "misfirings" (false alarms), which typically emerge during stressful life periods (e.g., following childbirth or divorce), may lead to the development of intercurrent anxiety over the fear of having another attack (anxious apprehension). In fact, anxious apprehension is considered to be the primary factor serving to maintain the disorder (i.e., panics "spike" off of heightened anxiety and hypervigilance for potential signs/symptoms of an imminent attack).

Panic control treatment was designed to have an impact directly on the three components of panic and its associated intercurrent anxiety. The cognitive component is addressed initially by providing accurate information as to the nature of anxiety and panic (including the role of hyperventilation), stressing the nonpathological nature of the symptoms (e.g., fight or flight model), and presenting the tripartite model of anxiety. Second, the client is taught cognitive techniques aimed at identifying and challenging anxiogenic thoughts, such as probability overestimation (i.e., overestimating the likelihood of negative consequences of panic: "I will have a heart attack") and catastrophization (i.e., viewing the effects of panic as dangerous or insufferable: "If I panic in front of these people, I'll never be able to face them again"). The physical component of panic and anxiety is addressed by teaching the client the technique of breathing retraining to counteract panic attack symptoms elicited by hyperventilation. The technique of interoceptive exposure is designed to have an impact on the behavioral component of panic. Interoceptive exposure involves repeated exposure to internal somatic cues in order to eliminate conditioned fear reactions to, and avoidance of, these sensations. This is achieved via specific symptom induction exercises (e.g., spinning in a chair, step ups, breathing through a straw) and exposure to naturalistic activities (e.g., caffeine consumption, watching thrilling movies).

Craske et al.[6] have reported on the long-term follow-up results of a study examining the efficacy of PCT conducted by Barlow et al.[3] In the earlier report, three treatments were compared to a wait-listed control group. These three treatments were the PCT treatment, consisting of interoceptive exposure plus cognitive restructuring (E&C), progressive muscle relaxation (R), and combination treatment of R and E&C (COMB). At post-treatment evaluation, over 85 per cent of patients in the two groups containing exposure and cognitive restructuring were panic free. The R condition, in contrast, was associated with greater reductions in generalized anxiety but also was associated with greater attrition (33 per cent). At 24-month follow-up, when dropouts were included into the analyses and were assumed to be continuing to panic, Craske et al. observed panic-free rates of 81 per cent for the E&C condition, compared with 43 and 36 per cent for the COMB and R groups, respectively. The authors speculated that a dilution effect, or perhaps a detrimental effect of the addition of relaxation procedures, accounted for the lower success rate of the COMB group. The PCT treatment program is now available in workbook format.[7]

It is noteworthy that these results compare quite favorably against the few studies reporting follow-up results of pharmacological treatments for panic disorder, in which relapse of panic has ranged from 70 to 90 per cent.[8] Nevertheless, Craske et al.[6] observed that, although the majority of E&C subjects were panic free at 24-month follow-up, only 50 per cent met high endstate status criteria. This finding seemed to be due in part to continued mild agoraphobic avoidance in some subjects, suggesting that this feature must be targeted separately in treatment since the elimination of panic alone may not result in the amelioration of agoraphobic avoidance.

More recently, researchers have turned their attention to comparing panic control treatments to pharmacological therapies. For example, Klosko et al.[4] compared PCT to alprazolam, a pill placebo, and a wait-listed control in patients with panic disorder. At post-treatment evaluation, 87 per cent of patients in PCT were panic free, compared to 50, 36, and 33 per cent in the alprazolam, placebo, and wait-listed control groups, respectively.

Treatments for Situational Avoidance

Exposure-based treatments play a central role in the treatment of phobic anxiety and avoidance. Current reviews of the exposure-based treatment literature for PDA indicate that 60 to 75 per cent of patients achieve clinically significant results. These treatments entail exposing the patient to feared and avoided situations until his or her anxiety in, and avoidance of, these situations diminish. A number of variants of exposure-based treatments for PDA have been designed and evaluated (e.g., gradual versus rapid, therapist directed versus self-directed, individual versus group format, in vivo versus imaginal). Based on several reviews of the treatment literature,[8] evidence generally points to the superior efficacy of the format involving therapist-assisted, graduated, in vivo exposure. These treatments begin with the generation of a list of target situations that are arranged hierarchically in terms of current fear and avoidance. Based on this hierarchy, a schedule of exposure or confrontation to these situations is arranged in a graduated fashion. Often, clients are taught to use cognitive coping skills when confronting these feared situations.

Recently, we have found that utilization of the client's spouse in his or her treatment has resulted in enhanced treatment gains beyond the traditional therapist-assisted exposure format. In this format, patients are treated in groups with their spouses in attendance. In addition to learning about the nature and treatment of PDA, spouses serve as cotherapists actively involved in the patient's between-session homework assignments (i.e., situational exposure). This format has the advantage of having a therapeutic agent in the client's own environment, leading to increased compliance with the program, reduction in treatment dropouts, and the facilitation of progress past the point of termination of formal treatment sessions. For example, Cerny et al.[10] found that 86 per cent of PDA patients treated with their spouses were considered treatment responders, in comparison to 43 per cent in the nonspouse group. At 24-month follow-up, the gap between the spouse and nonspouse groups became wider, with patients in the spouse group evidencing continued improvement.[10]

Despite the favorable results of exposure-based treatments, a significant proportion of patients do not fully benefit from exposure or are left with residual symptomatology such as mild anticipatory anxiety or avoidance. This pattern of findings has led several researchers to conclude that exposure therapy, although perhaps a necessary component of treatment, may not be sufficient, in and of itself, to effect full remission of PDA symptomatology. Thus, current research efforts have been directed at examining multimodal treatment packages, including the combination of in vivo exposure and PCT described above.

GENERALIZED ANXIETY DISORDER

The psychosocial treatment of generalized anxiety disorder (GAD) is guided by the rationale that anxiety is maintained by thoughts about symptoms or situations that provoke anxiety, and through reactions to these symptoms by avoidance, loss of control, and physical tension.[11] Early behavioral studies focused on the utilization of progressive muscle relaxation training or biofeedback procedures for the treatment of anxiety states. Although patients showed some improvement with relaxation or biofeedback procedures, these results were marginal and indicated that relaxation alone is insufficient in the treatment of chronic anxiety.[2]

In the DSM-III-R, the criteria for GAD were refined such that the disorder now has chronic and pervasive worry, focused on two or more life circumstances, as its own key symptom. With this symptom in mind, research on GAD has revealed three distinct observations: (1) GAD patients perceive many situations as insurmountable threats and perceive themselves as lacking resources to deal with such threats; (2) GAD patients fear or avoid (or both) a variety of situations as well as thoughts about problems or feelings, and situations that may provoke conflict with others; and (3) demoralized patients, with limited or underused coping resources, respond less well to psychological intervention.[11] Given these observations and the limited utility of relaxation procedures alone, a variety of cognitive-behavioral treatment (CBT) packages have been proposed and currently are being evaluated.

The basic premise of CBT is that specific, discrete thoughts provoke and maintain the person's anxiety. These thoughts are reinforced through avoidance, and through the person's accompanying feelings of demoralization and depression. The goals of CBT are to teach the patient to become aware of these anxious thoughts, to examine the thoughts for distortions or errors, and to replace these thoughts with realistic and adaptive cognitions. These cognitive goals are supplemented with relaxation procedures to decrease general feelings of tension and, with exposure practice, to disrupt the person's pattern of avoidance (e.g., applying relaxation skills to personally relevant everyday anxiety-provoking situations in a graduated manner).

A central component of our CBT protocol for GAD is education on the nature and tripartite model of anxiety. In a program similar to that of Butler and Booth,[11] clients are taught that a realistic goal of treatment is the management of anxiety, as opposed to the elimination of anxiety altogether. Through between-sessions self-monitoring of cognitions, clients learn to identify and challenge anxiogenic thoughts. As noted in the previous section, a common cognitive error is "probability overestimation," which is often quite salient in GAD (e.g., worrying about not meeting job deadlines despite repeated prior success). This type of thought is restructured by having the client examine the evidence for such a prediction and then modify his or her thought in accordance with the realistic probability of the event. Our protocol focuses directly on thoughts associated with chronic worry, and on fostering a greater sense of self-control over management of daily activities and commonplace situations that may provoke anxiety.

Recently, we completed a 24-month follow-up of our GAD protocol, and results indicate maintenance of treatment gains, including decrease in clinical severity, a decline in the amount of time spent worrying, and a significant decline in the number of intense anxiety episodes experienced per week.[12] Similarly, Butler et al.[13] reported a consistent pattern of improvement in GAD clients treated with CBT. These data suggest that CBT results in fewer dropouts, produces greater positive cognitive changes, and reduces depression as well as anxiety in patients with both symptoms. Furthermore, a decline in regular use of anxiolytic and hypnotic medications was reported in both of the aforementioned investigations. Taken together, these results appear to support the major advantage of CBT over traditional or pharmacological interventions: that clients learn something in treatment that allows for both maintenance and consolidation of treatment effects. The latest treatment protocol for GAD is now available in workbook format.[14]

SOCIAL PHOBIA

Several studies have indicated the effective utilization of the monoamine oxidase inhibitor (MAOI) phenelzine and certain β-blockers (atenolol) in the treatment of social phobia.[15] These treatments, however, are not without limitations. For example, some patients do not evidence a therapeutic response, and others relapse upon discontinuation. Pharmacological intervention for social phobics may be complicated further by the contraindications inherent in the use of the MAOIs (e.g., risk of hypertensive crisis, strict dietary restrictions) and by the patient's physical status (e.g., presence of heart or thyroid disease, pregnancy). Given these and other limitations, recent attention has turned toward developing effective psychosocial treatments.

Although researchers in the area of social phobia acknowledge the utility of exposure-based approaches in the treatment of social anxiety, cognitive restructuring is given equal or greater emphasis in light of the postulation that cognitive factors (e.g., fear of negative evaluation) are apt to play a large role in the etiology and maintenance of the disorder. In a controlled study examining the contributions of exposure and cognitive techniques, Mattick and colleagues[16] evaluated the efficacy of three treatments compared to a wait-list control group: exposure only, cognitive restructuring, and combined exposure plus cognitive restructuring. Althogh the combined group was superior to the exposure-only group on only two measures, the authors concluded that treatments involving both exposure and cognitive techniques are superior given the fact that, as in prior studies, exposure alone does not affect attitudinal changes (e.g., fear of negative evaluation). This point is highlighted by the fact that, in several instances, changes in fear of negative evaluation accounted for the majority of variance in treatment outcome.

More recently, Heimberg et al.[17] developed a similar group treatment package that incorporates several cognitive-behavioral strategies. Cognitive-behavioral group therapy (CGBT) is administered by a male and female cotherapist pair to five to six social phobics in 12 weekly, 2-hour sessions. Treatment involves education on the nature of social anxiety and the systematic application of both cognitive restructuring techniques and graduated exposure to feared social situations. The cognitive component consists of training the patient to be able to identify, analyze, and dispute maladaptive thinking, with emphasis on perceptions of negative evaluation by others. Patients are exposed to anxiety-provoking situations through roleplays and self-directed in vivo homework. The cognitive restructuring techniques are woven into the behavioral component of the therapy by employing them before, during, and after the exposures. Recently, Heimberg et al.[17] reported the results comparing CBGT to an educational and supportive control group. Although patients in both groups improved, those in the CBGT improved more at 6-month follow-up. Cognitive-behavioral group therapy patients reported less anxiety before and during a simulation of a personally relevant anxiety-provoking situation. Following this exposure test, they reported fewer negative and more positive self-statements than the patients in the control group.

Several investigators have addressed matching patient characteristics to treatment type.[18] For example, there has been some indication that "discrete" social phobics (e.g., those with public speaking fears only) have been shown to respond more favorably to CBGT than social phobics who fear a wide variety of social situations ("generalized"). In a series of studies investigating differential response to pharmacotherapy, Liebowitz and his colleagues reported that the response rate was higher for generalized social phobics receiving phenelzine than for discrete subjects, whereas discrete social phobics had greater symptom reductions (decreased palpitations, sweating, trembling) with atenolol.[15] However, although no study to date has evaluated the effectiveness of combining psychosocial and pharmacological treatments, Agras[19] has suggested the combined utilization of a β-blocker and a CBT package for discrete social phobics and a combination of an MAOI and CBT for generalized social phobics. It is quite possible, however, that some social phobics (especially discrete phobics) may respond to psychosocial treatment alone and that pharmacological treatment would be better reserved for nonresponders to psychosocial treatment. Currently, Heimberg and his colleagues are evaluating these and other issues by examining the relative effectiveness of CBGT and phenelzine in the treatment of social phobia.

ANXIETY DISORDERS IN CHILDHOOD AND ADOLESCENCE

The assessment and treatment of anxiety disorders in children and adolescents has received increasing attention in recent years. Behavioral treatment approaches for the childhood anxiety disorders have been derived mainly from the adult literature, with adaptation of techniques designed according to age and developmental level. Because fears, worries, and behavioral rituals may become pronounced as a function of normal developmental fluctuations, the persistence, magnitude, and maladaptive interference of such behaviors must be addressed in order to determine if a phobia or anxiety disorder is evident. In this section, we review current behavioral treatments for specific fears and anxieties in children.

Review of the behavioral treatment literature for childhood fears and anxieties reveals effective application of systematic desensitization, exposure-based techniques, contingency management, modeling, and cognitive-behavior modification.[20,21] Selection of a particular treatment technique depends on several factors: knowledge of differential effectiveness (if evidence exists), the nature of the anxiety and its trigger (stimulus), the developmental and cognitive characteristics of the child, parent involvement, cost effectiveness, and ethical considerations.

Systematic Desensitization and Exposure

Barrios and O'Dell[20] reviewed the findings of 41 studies investigating the effectiveness of systematic desensitization procedures with children (age range 11.5 months to 17 years). Results of both case studies and controlled experiments consistently found these procedures to be effective in reducing fears and anxieties, with the most common foci related to school, nighttime, small animals, separation, and test taking. The basic process of systematic desensitization proceeds as with adults (i.e., training in progressive relaxation, establishing a hierarchy of distressing situations, imaginal exposure to each situation while

relaxed), with variations of the procedure with children involving the use of slides, toys, or photographs of the feared stimulus. Whereas older children and adolescents appear to manage these procedures with little difficulty, younger children tend to have problems achieving the muscle relaxation response and adequately imagining the feared stimulus. Various forms of "emotive imagery" include having the child imagine confronting the feared stimulus with support from his or her favorite "superhero," or pairing feelings of self-assertion and pride with the anxiety antagonistic response.

Exposure treatment requires the child to confront the anxiety-provoking stimulus either in vivo or via imaginal representation. Using the hierarchical presentation, the child imagines or is confronted with each anxiety-provoking situation until he or she is no longer frightened in that situation. Treatment effectiveness depends upon the conditioned stimulus (feared object/situation) being presented to the child in absence of the unconditioned stimulus. For example, if a child who was fearful of dogs is treated in vivo, the clinician must ensure that during exposure the dog does not bite the child. Such an event no doubt would augment an extremely strong fear response that would be most resilient to change. Exposure-based techniques have been applied for anxieties including school phobia, social situations, and specific fears (e.g., dark, dentists, noise).

Prolonged exposure has been used most often in combination with response prevention for the treatment of obsessive-compulsive disorder (OCD) in adults. To date, there are limited case reports of such treatment with children[22]; however, the evidence suggests these techniques are effective with children. A typical protocol would involve exposing the child to the feared stimulus, such as touching "contaminated" objects like doorknobs or using imaginal scenes, and then preventing the ritualized response (e.g., removing taps from faucets and monitoring the child's actions). Appropriate washing for daily hygiene would be reintroduced on a schedule. At our center, we are currently evaluating the effectiveness of response prevention and exposure techniques with children with OCD, and the inclusion of parents trained as therapists for enhancing treatment effects.

Reinforcement and Modeling Procedures

Contingency management procedures involve the manipulation of environmental events that follow children's behaviors. Various procedures include setting up reinforcer systems to reward approach or adaptive behavior, with removal of reinforcement for displays of the target behavior (i.e., avoidance responses). Parents usually are trained or educated in the use of delivering reinforcement for desired behavior and ignoring fear or anxiety responses to promote extinction of undesired behavior. For example, with younger children, charts may be used on which "stars" are given as daily reinforcers to be turned in for treats after a specified number are earned. With older children or adolescents, "contracts" are developed that specify the desired behavior and the reinforcer that the parent will deliver. Barrios and O'Dell[20] reviewed the successful application of contingency management in 15 studies, with treatment mainly focused on school and social anxiety.

Modeling procedures involve the child observing another person interacting adaptively with the feared stimulus, and vary according to whether the observation is in vivo, filmed, or imaginal, or involves "guided support" from the model. Treatment effectiveness appears to be enhanced when the model is similar in age and sex to the child and shows similar levels of fear to that initially displayed by the child, and when the child's parent responds with minimal fear toward the stimulus.[20] Modeling techniques appear to be most effective with fears of medical and dental procedures and fears of animals.

Cognitive-Behavioral Treatments

The basic premise underlying the cognitive-behavioral approaches is that the child's negative or maladaptive "self-talk" leads to maladaptive behavior. The focus is on helping the child to develop specific cognitive skills that he or she may apply when confronted with a particular fear or anxiety-producing stimulus.[23] Initially, an assessment of cognitions is conducted to identify negative self-statements, attributions, or images that the child produces during anxiety-provoking situations. In the cognitive-restructuring approach, the child would be taught to replace these negative cognitions with adaptive, realistic coping statements. From this perspective, a socially phobic child who avoids gym or recess because "none of the kids like me; no one will want to play with me" may be taught to restructure the statement to "there may always be some kids with whom I don't get along, but I know there are some kids whom I can play with!" Self-instructional training, another variation of the cognitive-behavioral methods, involves the rehearsal of self-control and competence-based statements, with self-reinforcement and praise for coping.

Although the efficacy of CBT alone (i.e., a program that does not include additional components such as relaxation or modeling) has not been examined in the literature, a great deal of research exists to support the effectiveness of these treatment packages.[23] In a recent study, Kane and Kendall[24] employed a cognitive-behavioral package in the treatment of four children (ages 9 through 13) diagnosed with overanxious disorder. Through self-monitoring of thoughts and reactions, children learned to identify anxious feelings and somatic responses to anxiety, pinpoint negative cognitions that occur in response to anxiety-provoking situations, modify these negative cognitions with coping and problem-solving statements, and evaluate the success of coping as

well as employ self-reinforcement for adaptive responding. In this study, behavioral treatments such as modeling, in vivo exposure, role play, relaxation training, and contingency management also were incorporated. All children showed improvement on parent and independent clinician ratings, and on self-report.

Summary

Various combinations of the aforementioned techniques have been used in clinical practice to treat anxiety disorders in children and adolescents. Although controlled empirical investigations are forthcoming, preliminary reports and the research reviewed suggest that behavioral and cognitive-behavioral techniques are effective across the three components of anxiety: reduction of physiological arousal, decreasing avoidance and related behaviors, and changing anxiogenic cognitions.

CONCLUSIONS

The purpose of this chapter has been to present a brief overview of specific cognitive-behavioral treatments for several anxiety disorders, with identification of the common elements underlying these interventions. In treating the person suffering from an anxiety disorder, modifying and/or combining the various cognitive-behavioral techniques permits the therapist to adjust the treatment to the particular disorder as well as to the unique presentation of the individual client. This point is exemplified most dramatically in the treatment of childhood anxiety, wherein the therapist is further challenged in tailoring the treatment not only to the specific disorder, but also to the degree of social, intellectual, and emotional maturation of the child.

Finally, we are currently witnessing a significant advance in the treatment of anxiety disorders with the initiation of combined and comparative cognitive-behavioral and pharmacological treatment outcome trials.[2] As the results of these studies begin to emerge, so will the explication of patterns of differential effectiveness, thereby facilitating the process of treatment selection and optimal patient-treatment matching.

REFERENCES

1. Lang, PJ: Fear reduction and fear behavior: Problems in treating a construct. In Shlien JM, ed. Research in Psychotherapy, Vol 3. Washington, DC: American Psychological Association, 1968:90–102.
2. Brown TA, Hertz RM, Barlow, DH: New developments in cognitive-behavioral treatment of anxiety disorders. In Tasman A, ed. American Psychiatric Press Review of Psychiatry, Vol 11. Washington, DC: American Psychiatric Press, in press.
3. Barlow DH, Craske MG, Cerny JA, et al: Behavioral treatment of panic disorder. Behav Ther 20:261–282, 1989.

4. Klosko JS, Barlow DH, Tassinari R, et al: A comparison of alprazolam and behavior therapy in treatment of panic disorder. J Consult Clin Psychol 58:77–84, 1990.
5. Ost LG: Applied relaxation in the treatment of panic disorder. Behav Res Ther 26:13–22, 1988.
6. Craske MG, Brown TA, Barlow DH: Behavioral treatment of panic: A two-year follow-up. Behav Ther 22:289–304, 1991.
7. Barlow DH, Craske MG: Mastery of Your Anxiety and Panic. Albany, NY: Graywind Publications, 1989.
8. Barlow DH: Anxiety and its Disorders: The Nature and Treatment of Anxiety and Panic. New York: Guilford Press, 1988.
9. Barlow DH, O'Brien GT, Last CG: Couples treatment of agoraphobia. Behav Ther 15:41–58, 1984.
10. Cerny JA, Barlow DH, Craske MG, et al: Couples treatment of agoraphobia: A two-year follow-up. Behav Ther 18:401–415, 1987.
11. Butler G, Booth RG: Developing psychological treatments for generalized anxiety disorder. In Rapee RM, Barlow DH, eds. Chronic Anxiety, Generalized Anxiety Disorder, and Mixed Anxiety Depression. New York: Guilford Press, in press.
12. Barlow DH, Rapee RM, Brown TA: Behavioral treatment of generalized anxiety disorder. Manuscript submitted for publication.
13. Butler G, Fennell M, Robson P, et al: Comparison of behavior therapy and cognitive behavior therapy in the treatment of generalized anxiety disorder. J Consult Clin Psychol 59:167–175, 1991.
14. Craske MG, Barlow DH, O'Leary, T: Mastery of Your Anx-

iety and Worry. Albany, NY: Graywind Publications, 1991.
15. Levin AP, Schneier FR, Liebowitz MR: Social phobia: Biology and pharmacology. Clin Psychol Rev 9:129–000, 1989.
16. Mattick RP, Peters L, Clarke JC: Exposure and cognitive restructuring for social phobia: A controlled study. Behav Ther 20:3–23, 1989.
17. Heimberg RG, Dodge CS, Hope DA, et al: Cognitive-behavioral group treatment for social phobia: Comparison with a credible placebo control. Cognitive Ther Res 14:1–23, 1990.
18. Heimberg RG: Cognitive and behavioral treatments for social phobia: A critical analysis. Clin Psychol Rev 9:107–128, 1989.
19. Agras WS: Treatment of social phobia. J Clin Psychiatry 51:52–55, 1990.
20. Barrios BA, O'Dell SL: Fears and anxieties. In Mash EJ, Barkley RA, eds. Treatment of Childhood Disorders. New York: Guilford Press, 1989:167–221.
21. Klein RG, Last CG: Anxiety Disorders in Children. Newbury Park, ST: Sage Publications, 1989.
22. Wolff R, Rapoport J: Behavioral treatment of childhood obsessive-compulsive disorder. Behav Modif 12:252–266, 1988.
23. Ramirez SZ, Kratochwill TR, Morris RJ: Childhood anxiety disorders. In Michelson L, Ascher LM, eds. Anxiety and Stress Disorders: Cognitive-Behavioral Assessment and Treatment. New York: Guilford Press, 1987:149–175.
24. Kane MT, Kendall PC: Anxiety disorders in children: A multiple-baseline evaluation of a cognitive-behavioral treatment. Behav Ther 20:499–508, 1989.

Section F

SOMATOFORM AND DISSOCIATIVE DISORDERS

49

SOMATOFORM AND DISSOCIATIVE DISORDERS:
A Summary of Changes for DSM-IV

C. ROBERT CLONINGER, M.D. and SEAN YUTZY, M.D.

One of the most innovative developments of the third edition of the American Psychiatric Association's *Diagnostic and Statistical Manual of Mental Disorders* (DSM-III)[1] was the introduction of the category of somatoform disorders. According to the DSM-III, the essential features of somatoform disorders were "physical symptoms suggesting physical disorder (hence, somatoform) for which there are no demonstrable organic findings or known physiological mechanisms and for which there is positive evidence, or a strong presumption, that the symptoms are linked to psychological factors or conflicts." This definition was controversial because DSM-III was intended to be "atheoretical with regard to etiology or pathophysiological process except for those disorders for which this is well established" (DSM-III, page 7). Changes under consideration for the DSM-IV reveal fundamental doubt about the utility and validity of the assumptions made in the DSM-III regarding the etiology of somatoform disorders. Serious questions remain about the boundaries for the overall diagnostic category of somatoform disorders, as well as about the validity of criteria for some individual somatoform disorders.

BASIC CONCEPTUAL ISSUES

Research and clinical experience with the DSM-III and its revision (the DSM-III-R)[2] revealed widespread uncertainty regarding the utility and validity of the separation of somatoform disorders from other disorders, including dissociative, anxiety, mood, psychotic, personality, and physical disorders. These boundary issues reflect much fundamental uncertainty about the nature and etiology of psychiatric disorders in general.

The most basic issue is the distinction between "organic" and "psychological" causal mechanisms, as reflected in the distinction between somatoform and physical disorders. The DSM-III assumed that somatoform disorders have nonorganic etiology so that, once the pathophysiology became known, the disorder became a physical disorder classified on Axis III. This led to the elimination of psychophysiological disorders as a category in the official nomenclature in the transition from the DSM-II[3] to the DSM-III. Consequently, even though disability from headache is characteristic of somatization disorder, headaches were excluded as diagnostic features of somatization disorder because their pathophysiology was often presumably known.

Nevertheless, adoption studies have shown that the best validated somatoform disorder, somatization disorder, is a heritable disorder.[4,5] This is a crucial observation because heritability necessarily implies at least partial organic causation for somatoform and many other psychological phenomena. This suggests the possibility that the distinction between mind and body (or mental and organic) is illusory and artificial. What characterize psychiatric disorders are their behavioral and cognitive manifestations, and the expertise of psychiatrists in their management.

According to current proposals for the DSM-IV, distinctions are made between somatoform disorders such as somatization disorder and "other non-psychiatric medical disorders," not between organic and psychological causation. In pain disorders, it is recognized that the distinction between psychological conditions and nonpsychiatric medical conditions is frequently ambiguous, and both often contribute to the etiology.

Other questionable boundary issues between somatoform disorders and other categories of psychiatric disorder include the validity of the separation of conversion disorder from dissociative disorders, hypochondriasis from anxiety disorders, and body dysmorphic disorder from psychotic disorders. These are considered in relation to individual disorders.

SOMATIZATION DISORDER

Somatization disorder, or Briquet's syndrome, is an unusual example of a disorder that has been well validated by follow-up and family studies.[5] Nevertheless, this diagnosis has seldom been made by most psychiatrists because of the complexity of the original diagnostic criteria. The original criteria of Guze required elicitation of at least 20 of 59 symptoms in nine of ten groups in addition to a complicated or dramatic medical history of recurrent physical complaints beginning before 30 years of age. In the DSM-III-R these criteria were simplified somewhat to require 13 positive symptoms out of a possible 35. Seven symptoms were also identified to simplify screening for the diagnosis, but the low specificity (high false-positive rate) of the screening items requires use of the full criteria for a final diagnosis.[2] Consequently, most psychiatrists still regard the DSM-III-R criteria as too complex for routine clinical use.

As part of the efforts of the DSM-IV Task Force to improve diagnostic criteria, Cloninger has developed a new diagnostic strategy that markedly simplifies the diagnostic criteria and is usable in routine practice. He found in a study of 500 psychiatric outpatients[6] that somatization disorder could be diagnosed by requiring (1) a history of pain in at least four different body sites, (2) at least two gastrointes-

tinal symptoms other than pain, (3) a history of at least one sexual or reproductive symptom other than pain, and (4) a history of at least one symptom or deficit suggesting a neurological disorder not limited to pain (i.e., conversion or dissociative symptoms). These criteria identified nearly the same patients as either the original Guze criteria for Briquet's syndrome or the DSM-III-R criteria for somatization disorder (kappa = .79, sensitivity = 81 per cent, specificity = 96 per cent). The combination of four or more bodily pains and at least one conversion or dissociative symptom has sensitivity of 96 per cent and specificity of 82 per cent for the diagnosis based on DSM-III-R criteria. Each of these four requirements is necessary for diagnosis, so the diagnosis can be confidently excluded if any one is lacking. In order to confirm the generalizability of these criteria, a field trial is underway now at five sites across the United States.

The June 12, 1991, draft of the proposed DSM-IV somatization criteria is presented in Table 49–1. Note that the symptoms "must not be fully explained by a known non-psychiatric medical condition," which admits the possibility that the pathophysiology of a psychiatric disorder may become known and does not assume the absence of "organic" influences. Also note that "psychophysiological" symptoms such as tension headaches or spastic colon symptoms are included as part of the diagnostic picture if they satisfy the behavioral disability requirements. The specific symptoms are listed as typical

---

TABLE 49–1.   PROPOSED DSM-IV SOMATIZATION DISORDER CRITERIA

A. A history of many physical complaints beginning before the age of 30, occurring over a period of several years, resulting in medical treatment or altering life-style.

B. The following specific pattern of complaints (i.e., (1), (2), (3), and (4)) must be met. To count a symptom as significant, it must not be fully explained by a known non-psychiatric medical condition, or the resulting complaints or impairment are in excess of what would be expected from physical examination or laboratory tests.
  (1) a history of pain in at least four different sites or functions (such as head, abdomen, back, joints, extremities, chest, rectum, during sexual intercourse, menstruation, or urination)
  (2) a history of at least two gastrointestinal symptoms other than pain (such as nausea, bloating, vomiting other than during pregnancy, intolerance of several different foods, or diarrhea)
  (3) a history of at least one sexual or reproductive symptom other than pain (such as sexual indifference, impotence, irregular menses, excessive menstrual bleeding, vomiting throughout pregnancy)
  (4) a history of at least one symptom or deficit suggesting a neurological disorder not limited to pain (conversion symptoms such as blindness, double vision, deafness, loss of touch or pain sensation, aphonia, impaired coordination or balance, paralysis or localized weakness, difficulty swallowing, urinary retention, seizures, dissociative symptoms such as amnesia or loss of consciousness other than fainting)

examples, not as specific requirements, so clinicians need only recall the four basic requirements.

CONVERSION AND DISSOCIATIVE DISORDERS

In the DSM-III-R, conversion disorder was defined as an involuntary psychogenic loss or alteration in physical functioning, suggesting a physical disorder. The only aspect of this definition that is likely to be retained without modification in the DSM-IV is the involuntary aspect, which is specified by the requirements that "the person is not conscious of intentionally producing the symptoms" and that "the symptom is not a culturally sanctioned response pattern" (DSM-III-R, page 259).

The psychogenic assumption about conversion disorder in the DSM-III-R required that "psychological factors are judged to be etiologically related to the symptom because of a temporal relationship between a psychosocial stressor that is apparently related to a psychological conflict or need and initiation or exacerbation of the symptom" (DSM-III-R, page 259). This requirement was retained because the psychogenic assumption was widely accepted, despite the absence of empirical evidence that such judgments were reliable or valid.[5] It has been proposed by the DSM-IV Task Force that this requirement be modified to verifiable judgments about temporal association, not psychogenic causation: "psychological factors are judged to be associated with the symptom because of a temporal relationship between the initiation (or exacerbation) of symptoms and psychosocial stressors, psychological conflicts or needs" (June 12, 1991, draft).

The distinction between psychogenic and organic etiologies is also modified so that "the symptom cannot, after appropriate investigation, be fully explained by a known non-psychiatric medical condition," rather than requiring that it cannot be explained by a known physical disorder.

Furthermore, it is being proposed for the DSM-IV that conversion symptoms be limited to symptoms suggestive of a neurological disorder affecting sensation (e.g., blindness, double vision, deafness, loss of pain or touch sensation) or motor function (e.g., aphonia, ataxia, paralysis, seizures). This is close to the DSM-II, which required loss of function of one of the special senses or voluntary nervous system.[3] This addresses the criticism that the DSM-III and its revision were too inclusive because non-neurological symptoms were more likely to have a known medical etiology or more chronic prognosis than were pseudoneurological symptoms.[5,7]

Finally, conversion disorder and dissociative disorder were types of hysterical neurosis in the DSM-II, but are placed in separate categories in the DSM-III and its revision. Nevertheless, the same patients often have both conversions and dissociations, and the same dissociative mechanism is widely believed

to be involved in the development of both types of disorder. Accordingly some have advocated reuniting conversion and dissociation in one category. However, the definition of somatoform disorders then would be violated because conversion symptoms clearly suggest physical illness such as neurological disorders. Such boundary conflicts reflect the artificial nature of descriptive categorization.

Changes in dissociative disorder criteria that have been proposed for the DSM-IV are largely minor wording changes. There is consideration of addition of criteria for trance, possession, and brief reactive dissociation for compatibility with coverage in the tenth edition of the International Classification of Diseases (ICD-10).

PSYCHOPHYSIOLOGICAL DISORDERS

The DSM-III and its revision eliminated the DSM-II category of psychophysiological disorders, which were defined as "physical symptoms that are caused by emotional factors and involve a single organ system, usually under autonomic nervous system innervation" (DSM-II). In the DSM-III and its revision, such symptoms were classified as "psychological factors affecting physical condition," part of somatization disorder, or a conversion disorder. With the proposed narrowing of conversion symptoms to pseudoneurological symptoms and the recognition of the lack of a clear boundary between physical and mental phenomena, there appears to be some need for a diagnosis like psychophysiological disorders. A diagnosis called "Autonomic Arousal Disorder," consistent with a name proposed for ICD-10, is under consideration. This would include persistent, disabling symptoms, other than pain, that cannot be explained by a known nonpsychiatric medical condition and that are attributable to autonomic arousal in any of the following systems or organs: cardiovascular system (e.g., palpitations, fainting), respiratory system (e.g., dyspnea), gastrointestinal system (e.g., diarrhea), urogenital system (e.g., dysuria), and skin (e.g., flushing, blushing). The validity and utility of such a diagnosis is supported by few data, but desires to facilitate future research and to allow comprehensive coverage have usually overridden such scientific reservations in official nomenclatures.

HYPOCHONDRIASIS

In the DSM-III and its revision, hypochondriasis is defined as a persistent preoccupation with the fear of having, or belief that one has, a serious disease based on the misinterpretation of physical signs or sensations despite medical reassurance. The requirement that the preoccupation was based on the misinterpretation of physical signs and sensations was not made in the DSM-II, and its elimination has been proposed for the DSM-IV. There are certainly clear examples of persistent worry about health in the absence of physical signs and symptoms (e.g., fear of being HIV-positive), but few data are available to evaluate the diagnostic and prognostic significance of alternative criteria. In particular, how does the presence or absence of associated physical signs and symptoms influence comorbidity with anxiety, mood, personality, and other somatoform disorders?

Some have urged consideration of placing hypochondriasis in the anxiety disorder category along with phobic and obsessional disorders. However, there is frequent comorbidity of hypochondriasis with either somatization disorder or anxiety disorders. Also hypochondriacs often present with physical complaints in medical settings, so a change in placement out of the somatoform category would be inconsistent with the current definition of somatoform disorders and would undermine the utility of the category in facilitating differential diagnosis of disorders presenting with physical complaints.

PAIN DISORDERS

The DSM-III and its revision included disorders involving psychogenic pain or disability from pain judged to be in excess of physical causes. These diagnoses have been difficult to make reliably because of the multifactorial influences on pain-related behavior. In accord with the overall conceptual reorientation of the DSM-IV about the mind-body distinction, it has been proposed that the category be renamed "Pain Disorder," omitting the adjectives psychogenic and somatoform. The only requirements are that the pain is a major part of the clinical picture and causes significant occupational/social impairment or distress. Subtypes may be specified according to whether psychological factors, nonpsychological medical factors, or both are thought to be predominant.

OTHER SOMATOFORM DISORDERS

Few data have been accumulated about body dysmorphic disorder since its introduction in the DSM-III-R, but there is concern about its possible overlap with delusional disorders. There is consideration of adding a category for neurasthenia to the DSM-IV for compatibility with ICD-10, but the differential diagnosis from anxiety disorders is uncertain with available data.

DISCUSSION

The proposed changes to the somatoform disorder section of the DSM-III-R are extensive. More remarkable is the fact that the changes involve in several cases a fundamental reconceptualization of the mind-body distinction as it applies to psychiatric diagnosis. Advances in the genetics and treatment of psychiatric disorders by both biological and psychosocial methods have forced psychiatrists to recognize that the mind-body distinction is artificial and at best ambiguous.

Other changes are largely motivated by desire to simplify use of the criteria in clinical practice, as in the case of somatoform disorder and pain disorder. Some changes are being proposed to improve compatibility with ICD-10. Unfortunately, except in the case of somatization disorder, little empirical research has been carried out that justifies data-based changes. This suggests that the frequency of change in the past has been excessive, even though the proposals of the DSM-III-R and the DSM-IV appear to be improvements in the subjective judgment of the committees recommending the changes.

REFERENCES

1. American Psychiatric Association: Diagnostic and Statistical Manual of Mental Disorders. 3rd ed. Washington, DC: American Psychiatric Association, 1980.
2. American Psychiatric Association: Diagnostic and Statistical Manual of Mental Disorders. 3rd ed. Revised. Washington, DC: American Psychiatric Association, 1987.
3. American Psychiatric Association: Diagnostic and Statistical Manual of Mental Disorders. 2nd ed. Washington, DC: American Psychiatric Association, 1968.
4. Bohman M, Cloninger CR, von Knorring AL, Sigvardsson S: An adoption study of somatoform disorders. III. Crossfostering analysis and genetic relationship to alcoholism and criminality. Arch Gen Psychiatry 41:872, 1984.
5. Cloninger CR: Somatoform and dissociative disorders. In Winokur G, Clayton P, eds. The Medical Basis of Psychiatry. Philadelphia: W.B. Saunders Company, 1986:123.
6. Cloninger CR, Martin RL, Guze SB, Clayton PJ: Somatization in men and women: A prospective follow-up and family study. Am J Psychiatry 143:873, 1986.
7. Cloninger CR: Diagnosis of somatoform disorders: A critique of DSM-III. In Tischler GL, Ed. Diagnosis and Classification in Psychiatry. A Critical Appraisal of DSM-III. Cambridge, England: Cambridge University Press, 1987:243.

50

SOMATIZATION DISORDER, HYPOCHONDRIASIS, AND CONVERSION DISORDER

WAYNE KATON, M.D.

Recent epidemiological studies in primary care have determined that 25 to 35 per cent of primary care patients suffer from a DSM-III-R–defined mental illness.[1] Moreover, these studies have found that 50 to 70 per cent of patients with a mental illness initially present with a somatic symptom such as headache, back pain, or fatigue and often receive costly, unnecessary medical work-ups. Researchers have found a high rate of misdiagnosis of mental illness in primary and specialty medical care, and the high rates of misdiagnosis primarily occur in patients who present with somatic complaints as an expression of psychosocial distress.[2]

In these days of escalating medical costs, researchers have found that patients with mental illness use two to three times as many outpatient visits as non-distressed controls.[1] Medical inpatients with coexisting psychiatric illness have also been found to have longer hospital stays compared to patients with medical illness alone, even after controlling for severity of medical illness.[3] A recent study of high utilizers of primary care determined that 10 per cent of patients utilize almost one third of ambulatory visits and half of inpatient hospital days. Approximately one half of these patients were psychologically distressed, and among these distressed high utilizers one fifth had somatization disorder and three quarters met an abridged definition of somatization.[4] Patients with somatization disorder have been estimated to have a per capita expenditure for health care of up to nine times the average per capita amount.[5] The above data on the economic consequences of mental illness in medical patients have stimulated both research in health services and psychiatric consultation interventions in the medical setting.[3-5]

Historically, the presentation by patients of somatic complaints for which no medical pathology could be found and obvious psychosocial precipitants were apparent was one of the key subjects that first attracted physicians to the study of psychiatry.[6] This chapter reviews three of the somatoform syndromes that were historically lumped under the single nosological term "hysteria." These three syndromes include somatization disorder, hypochondriasis, and conversion disorder. These disorders have a rich historical background with excellent descriptions provided prior to the twentieth century.

SOMATIZATION DISORDER

The DSM-III-R describes the patient with somatization disorder as having a history of multiple physical complaints or the belief that he or she was sickly, beginning before the age of 30 and persisting for several years.[7] In addition, the patient must have at least 13 of 37 characteristic symptoms. In order for a symptom to be a positive or medically unexplained symptom, no organic pathology or pathophysiological mechanism accounting for the symptom can be described; it must occur at times other than just during the panic attacks; and it must cause the patient to take medicine, see a doctor, or alter lifestyle.

Typically, somatization disorder occurs in female patients, who begin having significant symptoms at the time of menses. These symptoms usually include dysmenorrhea and taking to bed during periods. These patients characteristically have migratory pains and other symptoms such that if a doctor works up one complaint and finds no pathology, the patient will develop another pain or symptom in months to years. Very commonly the patient has been subjected to multiple work-ups, and oftentimes becomes a polysurgery patient who develops secondary iatrogenic problems from the surgeries.[6,8] These iatrogenic problems occur because of the numerous and vociferous patient complaints to well-meaning doctors who become more and more aggressive in their medical work-ups in trying to find the cause of the patient's complaints. Early hysterectomy (before age 30) should always make the clinician suspicious of this disorder.[6]

History

Somatization disorder has been described since at least 1900 B.C. Both the Egyptians and the Greeks hypothesized that this disorder resulted from a wandering uterus, thus the term "hysteria."[6] In these early reports and in later western publications, there was confusion between a monosymptomatic versus a polysymptomatic form of this disorder.[6] The DSM-III later divided these into the monosymptomatic form—conversion disorder—and a polysymptomatic form—somatization disorder.

The modern concept of "hysteria" as a psychological illness was developed by Sydenham, who considered the disturbance to be due to "antecedent sorrows."[6] The modern concept of the illness as a polysymptomatic disease with a chronic course was formulated by Pierre Briquet in 1859. The concept of somatization disorder that utilized a systematic list of symptoms was developed in the early 1950s by Purtell and coworkers.[6] They recognized the disorder usually began before age 35 and was responsible for 2.2 per cent of all hospital admissions. In the late 1950s, Perley and Guze developed operationalized criteria for this illness and found that 90 per cent of patients still met criteria for the diagnosis at follow-up of 6 to 8 years.[9] Based on Guze's work, 25 symptoms in ten symptomatic groups from a list of 60 symptoms were required for diagnosis. The DSM-III then streamlined these criteria to an operational definition that required 14 positive symptoms in women and 12 in men from a list of 37 symptoms. Finally, the DSM-III-R modified the criteria further to require 13 positive symptoms in both men and women from a similar list of 37 symptoms.

Epidemiology

The Epidemiologic Catchment Area (ECA) study estimated that approximately 1:1000 people in the community suffered from somatization disorder.[10] Prior community estimates had been in the 0.4 to 2 per cent range. A less severe form of somatization (6 to 12 medically unexplained symptoms in a female and 4 to 12 in a male) occurred in an estimated 4 per cent of patients in the ECA study.[11]

Estimated prevalence in primary care has varied between 0.4 and 5 per cent.[6] Hospital inpatient estimates have varied between 1:10 and 1:50 patients.[6]

Patients with somatization disorder are overrepresented among women receiving elective hysterectomies (27 per cent), irritable bowel syndrome (17 to 40 per cent), distressed high utilizers of primary care (20 per cent), chronic pain patients (12 per cent), patients with polycystic ovary disease (13 per cent), and patients with conversion disorder (34 per cent).

The ratio of women to men with somatization disorder has been estimated to be between 5:1 and 10:1. Although the disorder, by definition, must begin before age 30, a recent large series of primary care patients had a mean age of onset of 43 years.[6] In the ECA study, age of onset was under 15 years for 55 per cent of patients.[6,10]

Etiological Theories

There are many theories about the etiology of somatization disorder.

Psychodynamic

Early investigators such as Sydenham suggested that this disorder was an expression of "antecedent sorrows."[6] Freud, in his classic 1895 paper on hysteria, suggested that childhood sexual abuse was present in all patients he analyzed. In recent years, several studies have documented an increased prevalence of childhood sexual abuse in these patients.[6] Anecdotally, histories of childhood neglect and abuse appear to be very common in patients with somatization disorder. In these patients, somatic symptoms may be an expression of underlying psychological pain as well as representing a symbolic means to express emotions and ask for care.

Genetic or Familial Mechanisms

Several studies have found that males in the families of patients with somatization disorder have a higher prevalence of alcoholism and antisocial personality than males from control families.[6,9,12] Females from the families of patients with somatization disorder have an increased risk of somatization disorder compared to controls. Although the familial pattern is established, whether somatization is a learned or genetic pattern, is still controversial.

Women with somatization disorder have a tendency to choose as mates men with problems with alcohol abuse and sociopathy.[13] These have a high risk of being abused by these spouses.

Biological Theory

Abnormalities in auditory evoked potentials, attention to stimuli, and right frontal region electroencephalograms, as well as bifrontal impairment of the cerebral hemispheres, all have been reported in somatization disorder.[6] Few of these studies have been replicated, and with frequent histories of trauma and of substance and prescription drug abuse it is unclear whether these are causes or consequences of somatization disorder.

Social Communication Theory

This notion suggests that many patients with somatization disorder learned in their families of origin and adult families that somatic symptoms are an acceptable way to express distress and to elicit care and support from loved ones.[6,8] These symptoms also may be ways to avoid sex, punish a spouse, and manipulate interpersonal relationships.

Psychiatric Comorbidity

Major depression is exceedingly common in somatization disorder, with lifetime rates reported at 80 to 90 per cent.[6,14,15] Anxiety disorders (generalized anxiety disorder, panic disorder, and obsessive-compulsive disorder) also are frequent in patients with somatization disorder. Liskow et al. found 27 per cent of patients with somatization disorder met criteria for obsessive-compulsive disorder, 45 per cent met criteria for phobic disorders, and 45 per cent met criteria for panic disorder.[15] Smith reported that patients with somatization disorder had the following DSM-III anxiety disorders: generalized anxiety disorder (34 per cent), obsessive-compulsive disorder (18 per cent), and panic disorder (26 per cent).[6]

Alcohol abuse also appears to occur with increased prevalence in patients with somatization disorder, with 15 to 30 per cent of patients affected.[6] Prescription drug abuse also is reported to be an associated risk.

Patients with somatization disorder have an increased risk of having a personality disorder. Psychiatric patients with somatization disorder have been reported to have an increased risk of antisocial and histrionic personality disorder.[6] Patients in primary care with somatization disorder have been reported to have an increased risk of avoidant and paranoid personality disorders.[6]

Treatment

Somatization is a chronic disorder with an unknown etiology; therefore, it is premature to discuss cure. However, there are several time-tested principles in caring for patients with this disorder that do make management possible.[5,6,8] These techniques include:

1. Regularly scheduled visits with the primary physician.
2. Acknowledging that the patient's suffering is important. The patient with somatization disorder often interprets the physician's diagnosis of stress or a psychological condition as meaning that the physician does not believe the patient or thinks the symptom is all in the patient's head. This attitude is considered to be unempathic by the patient, who experiences the symptom primarily as a bodily condition.
3. A brief physical exam on each visit in the selected organ system in which the patient currently has symptoms.
4. Ordering tests or consultations only when there is objective evidence of illness.
5. Choosing preselected conservative specialists with whom the physician has experience and can call before referral to explain the patient's tendency to amplify symptoms.
6. Not prescribing antianxiety medication or opiates, if possible, in order to prevent abuse of prescription medications.
7. Conservativeness in writing disability excuses.
8. Helping the patient over time to become open to mental health referral.
9. Appropriate use of antidepressants for associated panic disorder or major depression.

A key aspect of these principles is developing a trusting relationship with a primary physician.[8] These patients are notorious "doctor shoppers" and frequently present to emergency rooms with a specific symptom. This results in multiple work-ups by physicians who do not recognize the polysymptomatic nature of this illness. Even worse, the continued complaints often result in ever-increasing aggressive treatment (e.g., physical exam, upper gastrointestinal tract series, endoscopy and, finally, exploratory laparotomy for abdominal pain). This treatment may leave the patient with iatrogenic injury and addiction to prescription medications.

To help foster an improved relationship, regularly scheduled visits are very helpful.[5,6,8] To begin, add up the number of times the patient has been seen in the last 3 months, and schedule appointments for this same frequency. Thus, if the patient averages two visits a month (usually for acute symptoms), schedule the patient for bimonthly visits. A statement acknowledging the patient's suffering and the medical need for close follow-up is often appreciated by the patient. These regular visits help place the patient's ambulatory care use under the physician's control and often result in decreased somatization. The patient no longer "needs" a symptom as a ticket of admission to the clinic.

During these visits, a brief physical exam, based on the organ system in which the patient is currently symptomatic, is very reassuring. The ritual of "laying on of hands" allows the patient to believe that the physician has taken the symptom seriously and often makes the patient feel cared for.[6,8]

Limiting testing and consultation are important because these patients' symptoms are usually expressions of psychosocial distress.[6,8] Multiple laboratory examinations often result in positive findings by chance alone, which often lead to more costly invasive testing and consultation. Consultation often occurs when physician and patient are frustrated. Specialists believe that they must be very complete and often will test these patients extensively, not taking into account their chronic pattern of somatization. Carefully choosing specialists who are less aggressive about work-ups and more psychosocially attuned, and discussing the patient with them prior to referral, are helpful tactics.

Patients with somatization disorder often have family and personal histories of alcohol abuse and may be prone to addiction with prescription medications. Avoidance of benzodiazepine and opiate prescriptions is important. In contrast, specific use of antidepressant medications to treat associated major depression and panic disorder may help alleviate some degree of psychological distress. However, antidepressants are not curative. Therefore, it is useful to portray these agents as medications that will help with associated symptoms (i.e., panic attacks, insomnia, chronic pain, depression) but not medicines that will cure all symptoms.

A long-term goal is to help the patient and his or her family develop increased acceptance and openness about discussing psychological problems and readiness to seek mental health care.[6,8] This process often involves helping the patient gradually accept the relationship between "stress" and the symptoms. When these patients are followed closely, inevitably psychological crises will occur (i.e., divorce, teenage behavioral problems, spouse abuse). These crises provide the physician with windows of opportunity to help the patient develop a psychotherapy relationship. As yet, no specific psychotherapies have been developed, but psychodynamic, family system, cognitive-behavioral, and group approaches can all have a place in management.[6,8]

Not surprisingly, the same hostile interactions that can occur with physicians can also occur with work supervisors and lead to vocational problems. Trying to keep the patient as functional as possible is a key goal. It is important to limit disability statements, although at times, when the patient has regressed, that is difficult. Work generally helps the patient's self-esteem and provides structure to an often otherwise chaotic interpersonal life.

CONVERSION DISORDER

The DSM-III-R describes conversion disorder as an involuntary and medically unexplainable loss or alteration in physical functioning.[7] In addition, one of the following conditions must be present:

1. There is a temporal relationship between symptom onset and some external source of psychological conflict.

2. The symptom allows the individual to avoid unpleasant activity.

3. The symptom provides an opportunity for support that otherwise may not be available.

Often inconsistency in the anatomy and physiology of neurological symptoms and signs provides clues to the physician of this diagnosis.[16] Gait disturbance, pseudoepilepsy, tremor, and paralysis make up almost 90 per cent of conversion symptoms.[16] In addition, both right- and left-handed patients experience a higher proportion of left-sided symptoms than would be expected by chance.[17–19]

History

Conversion disorder has been diagnosed for over 3500 years. In the nineteenth century Charcot and Janet both gave classic descriptions of patients with conversion symptoms.[17,18] In the late 1800s, Freud hypothesized that conversion symptom originated in some shock or disagreeable feeling experienced in connection with sexual feelings, usually something that happened in childhood.

Epidemiology

Conversion disorder has been estimated to occur in 0.5 per cent of people in the general population, and in as many as one quarter of psychiatric outpatients, and represents probably 2 to 5 per cent of referrals to a psychiatric consultation service in a general hospital.[17,18] Conversion disorder is more prevalent in women and seems to have dramatically decreased in incidence in the last 100 years in the United States and Western Europe. Patients who are less educated, live in rural areas, and are from less affluent socioeconomic groups probably are more prone to conversion disorder. Conversion symptoms are seen in males in the military and as a result of industrial accidents.

Associated Psychiatric Conditions

Patients with conversion disorder frequently have other DSM-III-R psychiatric disorders. A history of somatization disorder with multiple unexplained somatic symptoms over the course of the patient's lifetime is one of the most frequently associated disorders (up to a third of patients in one series).[17,18] In addition, many other patients with conversion disorder have a history of multiple medically unexplained physical symptoms and would meet criteria for an abridged subsyndromal form of somatization. Other commonly associated psychiatric diagnoses include major depression, panic disorder, and substance abuse. In addition, personality disorders are not uncommon. Hysterical personality disorder, which was formerly believed to have been common in patients with conversion disorder, is now believed to occur in less than 10 per cent of patients.[17,18]

Etiological Theories

Psychoanalytical Theories

Psychoanalytical theories posit that the patient's symptoms often are precipitated by stressful life circumstances that cause severe anxiety due to stimulating intrapsychic conflicts.[17,18] These conflicts may be about aggressive action, sexuality, or dependency.

Systems Theory or Communication Theory

At times, the conversion symptom also can be understood as a form of social communication.[18] The systems theorist would try to understand this symptom in terms of the interactions in the family or larger social unit.

Sociocultural Theories

The incidence of conversion disorder has probably decreased during this century. This disorder was described much more commonly in nineteenth century medical literature. In addition, conversion disorder appears to be much more common in patients from third-world countries and those less acculturated to Western society.[17,18]

Biological Theory

As many as 50 per cent of patients with conversion disorder have a neurological disorder. Thus, conversion disorder may be an amplification of a neurological disorder such as pseudoepilepsy in a patient with documented electroencephalographic abnormalities. Patients with conversion disorder also have a higher prevalence of organic brain conditions, suggesting that brain disease may make a patient more susceptible to this disorder.[17,18] Neuropsychological abnormalities, including increased field dependency, impaired recent memory, decrements in vigilance and attention, and heightened suggestibility, have been interpreted as supporting this hypothesis.[17,18]

Treatment

Conversion disorder is a diagnosis of exclusion, and thus careful neurological examination and testing (often including electroencephalogram, lumbar puncture, and computed tomographic or magnetic resonance scan) should be included in the patient's work-up. Once neurological and other medical disease has been excluded as an etiology, psychiatric consultation should follow immediately. Often it is useful in the patient with changing and inconsistent neurological examination findings and/or findings that do fit known anatomical patterns to proceed with psychiatric consultation and further neurological testing concomitantly. In this case, the patient may be told that the symptoms may be his or her body's way of reacting to stress and thus a psychiatric consultation would be helpful, but that serious medical causes will be ruled out with further testing.

Since cases of conversion disorder tend to be sporadic and large populations on which to test research treatment strategies are difficult to obtain, no specific treatments have been tested in randomized trials. Supportive brief psychotherapy associated with suggestion of rapid recovery has been described anecdotally to be helpful. Clinical experience also suggests that both hypnosis and amobarbital interview often lead to return of function during these treatments. A postamytal or posthypnotic suggestion to the patient that this improvement will sustain and expand after treatment is helpful.[17,18] Rehabilitation wards and psychologists also have reported clinical improvement from behavioral programs that provide reward or reinforcement for gradual stepwise improvement.

Prognosis of the Disorder

One of the key features of conversion disorder is that it is a diagnosis of exclusion. No neurological or other medical problem can be found to explain the symptoms. However, many investigators have noted that between 13 and 30 per cent of patients with a diagnosis of conversion disorder develop a neurological or other organic illness over a 2.5- to 10-year period that explains their original symptoms.[16–18] In addition, many patients with preexisting neurological illness (e.g., epilepsy) also develop conversion symptoms (i.e., pseudoepilepsy). These patients often are more difficult to diagnose since they have proven neurological illness. In these patients, external stress or an internal psychological conflict may provoke elaboration of their original symptoms or worsening of a previously stable condition.

Recent studies have found that the majority of hospitalized patients with conversion disorder had either improvement or complete symptom resolution prior to discharge from the hospital.[19] A minority of subjects develop conversion symptoms that do not improve and lead to chronic disability.

HYPOCHONDRIASIS

History

The Greeks used the term "hypochondriasis" to refer to ailments of the region of the body below the ribs and xiphoid cartilage, and they associated changes in mental status with changes in the organs of the hypochondria.[20] Galen later described a group of disorders that he believed were secondary to disturbance of the viscera below the diaphragm.[20] He believed this region of the body was a source of black bile that was thought to cause melancholic states. In the 1800s Rush and others noted that psychological conditions could play a role in the condition that was still referred to as hypochondriasis.[12]

DSM-III-R Diagnostic Criteria

The essential feature of this disorder is a preoccupation with fear of having, or a strong belief that one has, a disease.[7] This fear or preoccupation with disease is based on the person's interpretation of signs and symptoms, despite an appropriate physical evaluation that does not support the fear or belief. This fear or belief of illness despite medical reassurance must be present for 6 months or more, the symptoms the patient misattributes must not be due to panic attacks, and the belief must not be of delusional intensity. Thus, the person usually can acknowledge the possibility that their worry about illness is exaggerated and that there may be no disease at all.

Patients with hypochondriasis may visit multiple physicians or doctor shop. Often, conflictual doctor-patient relationships result from the patient's inability to accept reassurance.

Epidemiology

Age at onset is believed to be between 20 and 30 years.[21] In the only study that measured the prevalence rate of hypochondriasis by structured interview, between 4.2 and 6.3 per cent of general internal medicine patients met criteria for hypochondriasis.[22] Hypochondriacal symptomatology in this study was similar for men and women and in those over and under 65. Patients with hypochondriasis had significantly higher levels of long-term disability than did clinical controls.[22] Twenty-nine per cent of patients meeting the DSM-III-R criteria for hypochondriasis in this study were not working for reasons of health. The prevalence rates in this study are quite similar to past estimates of 0.4 to 14 per cent.[21,23] The prevalence in the general population would be expected to be quite a bit lower, since hypochondriacal patients are overrepresented in medical systems. The above study also found that hypochondriacal attitudes and somatic symptoms appear to be independent of the number of minor and major medical diagnoses.[22]

Etiological Theories

Relationship to Anxiety and Depression

In the twentieth century, much debate has focused on whether hypochondriasis is an independent entity or a secondary aspect of another psychiatric illness, most commonly depression. Even among those who have proposed that hypochondriasis is a long-term trait independent of affective illness, there has been an acknowledgment that hypochondriasis is associated with extremely high lifetime rates of anxiety and depressive disorders.[21–23] Moreover, psychologists have reported on a trait they label "negative affectivity," which is associated with high distress on psychological measures of anxiety, depression, and hostility.[24] Negative affectivity is highly associated with a tendency to somatize or worry about bodily symptoms. Many patients with recurrent DSM-III-R–specified psychiatric disorders have higher psychological distress or negative affectivity between major episodes of DSM-III-R–specified psychiatric illness.[4] Increased psychological distress often leads to increased physical symptoms through heightened autonomic arousal, which may increase smooth muscle contractions and increase tension in voluntary muscle tone, resulting in symptoms such as headaches and backaches.[23] Increased psychological distress also may upset diurnal sleep-wake rhythms.[4] Recent evidence suggests that short-term disruption of stage IV sleep may result in diffuse muscle aches and pains.[25]

Selective Attention

Worry about illness can influence patients to focus closely on an organ system and misinterpret normal variations in function as signs of disease.[21,23] This often occurs transiently after a serious illness such as a myocardial infarction. After a heart attack, minor cardiac symptoms such as an ectopic beat or a gastrointestinal disturbance such as heartburn may be interpreted as signs of continued serious heart disease. This overconcern may lead to anxiety, which leads to more ectopic beats or more gastrointestinal distress, and thus a vicious cycle ensues.

Medical student syndrome is another example of selective attention.[21,23] Medical students are faced with a great deal of stress because of their workload, long study hours, and being confronted with knowledge about painful, disabling diseases. This often leads to transient hypochondriacal worries about having a particular illness that is currently being studied and misperceiving minor symptoms as being signs of serious illness. In time, more complete knowledge and lessened anxiety about learning about serious illness results in a decrease in this phenomenon. Patients with hypochondriasis also often get symptoms of a disease they have recently read or heard about.

Differential Diagnosis

Hypochondriasis must be differentiated from true organic disease such as early-stage systemic lupus erythematosus, multiple sclerosis, and endocrine disorders.[21,23] However, coexisting organic disease does not exclude a diagnosis of hypochondriasis.

Psychotic disorders such as schizophrenia or psychotic depression can be associated with a delusion of bodily disease.[21,23] Patients with these disorders have other associated signs and symptoms of their primary illness (i.e., insomnia, anorexia, weight loss, poor concentration, depressed mood in major depression) and, unlike hypochondriacs, they have lost the ability to test reality by acknowledging that the feared illness may not be present.

Hypochondriacal states also can be symptoms of other primary illness such as panic disorder, generalized anxiety disorder, dysthymic disorder, obsessive-compulsive disorder, and somatization disorder. In all of these disorders except somatization disorder there is rarely a history of longstanding hypochondriacal traits and behavior. In somatization disorder the patient is preoccupied with somatic symptoms, not excessive worry about a specific disease.[6]

Treatment

Patients with hypochondriasis have a persistent worry and fear of illness despite physician reassurance. It is important to do a careful physical exam and medical work-up, but repeated large-scale work-ups and subspecialty visits can be harmful. Repeated testing can lead the patient to conclude that the physician is unsure of the diagnosis and may be missing a serious disorder.

The same principles of treating somatization disorder often are helpful for hypochondriasis.[6,21,23] These include:

1. Regularly scheduled visits based on the frequency of visits over the previous 2 to 3 months.

2. Accepting the patient as one who is truly suffering, which often decreases patient hostility toward disbelieving physicians.

3. Listening to the patient's symptoms and performing a brief physical exam focusing on the symptomatic organ system, coupled with reassurance based on examination findings.

4. Screening for panic disorder and major depression, which are treatable causes of hypochondriasis. These conditions can be treated with antidepressant medications.

5. Over months to years, helping the patient begin to acknowledge the connection between life stresses, mental distress, and worrying about his or her health. Some of these patients may benefit from psychotherapy, although no specific types of therapy have undergone controlled research trials.

CONCLUSION

The three somatoform disorders covered in this chapter have been described for several thousand years, and in the modern era they have received increased research attention. Patients with two of these disorders, somatization disorder and hypochondriasis, are overrepresented in medical samples because of their high utilization of medical care. Knowledge of the DSM-III-R diagnostic criteria and the frequent coexisting DSM-III-R–specified disorders that accompany these somatoform illnesses may alleviate the need for costly, potentially harmful medical work-ups. Time-tested principles of care can help patients with somatization disorder and hypochondriasis better cope with their disorders and life problems. These treatment principles also may reduce physician frustration, which can lead to premature termination of care and potential overaggressive medical testing.

REFERENCES

1. Katon W: Panic Disorder in the Medical Setting. U.S. Department of Health and Human Services, National Institute of Mental Health. DHHS publ no (ADM)89-1629. Washington DC: U.S. Government Printing Office, 1989.
2. Bridges KW, Goldberg DP: Somatic presentation of DSM-III psychiatric disorders in primary care. J Psychosom Res 29:563–569, 1985.
3. Levenson JL, Hamer RM, Rossiter LF: Relation of psychopathology in general medical inpatients to use and cost of services. Am J Psychiatry 147:1498–1503, 1990.
4. Katon W, Von Korff M, Lin E, et al: Distressed high utilizers for medical care: DSM-III-R diagnoses and treatment needs. Gen Hosp Psychiatry 12:355–362, 1990.
5. Smith GR, Monsson RA, Ray DC: Psychiatric consultation in somatization disorder: A randomized controlled study. N Engl J Med 314:1407–1413, 1986.
6. Smith R: Somatization Disorder in the Medical Setting. U.S. Department of Health and Human Services. DHHS publ no (ADM)90-1631. Washington, DC: U.S. Government Printing Office, 1990.
7. American Psychiatric Association: Diagnostic and Statistical Manual of Mental Disorders. 3rd ed. Revised. Washington, DC: American Psychiatric Association, 1987.
8. Quill TE: Somatization disorder: One of medicine's blind spots. JAMA 254:3075–3079, 1985.
9. Perley MJ, Guze SB: Hysteria—the stability and usefulness of clinical criteria. N Engl J Med 266:421–426, 1962.
10. Robins LN, Helzer JE, Weissman MM, et al: Lifetime prevalence of specific psychiatric disorders in three sites. Arch Gen Psychiatry 41:949–958, 1984.
11. Escobar JI, Burnham A, Karno M, et al: Somatization in the community. Arch Gen Psychiatry 44:713–718, 1987.
12. Sigvardsson S, vonKnorring A, Bohman M, Cloninger R: An adoption study of somatoform disorders: The relationship of somatization to psychiatric disability. Arch Gen Psychiatry 41:853–859, 1984.
13. Zoccolillo M, Cloninger CR: Somatization disorder: Psychological symptoms, social disability and diagnosis. Compr Psychiatry 27:65–73, 1986.
14. Katon W, Lin E, Von Korff M, et al: Somatization: A spectrum of severity. Am J Psychiatry 148:34–40, 1991.
15. Liskow B, Penick EC, Powell BJ, et al: Inpatients with Briquet's syndrome: Presence of additional psychiatric syndromes and MMPI results. Compr Psychiatry 27:461–470, 1986.
16. Marsden CD: Hysteria—a neurologist's view. Psychol Med 16:277–288, 1986.
17. Lazare A: Conversion symptoms. N Engl J Med 305:745–748, 1981.
18. Ford C, Folks DG: Conversion disorders: An overview. Psychosomatics 26:371–383, 1985.
19. Folks DG, Ford CV, Regan WM: Conversion symptoms in a general hospital. Psychosomatics 25:285–295, 1984.
20. Barsky AJ, Wyshak G, Klerman GL: Hypochondriasis: An evaluation of the DSM-III criteria in medical outpatients. Arch Gen Psychiatry 43:493–500, 1986.
21. Barsky AJ, Klerman GL: Overview: Hypochondriasis, bodily complaints and somatic styles. Arch Gen Psychiatry 140:273–283, 1983.
22. Barsky AJ, Wyshak G, Klerman GL, Latham KS: The prevalence of hypochondriasis in medical outpatients. Soc Psychiatry Psychiatr Epidemiol 25:89–94, 1990.
23. Kellner R: Hypochondriasis and somatization. JAMA 258:2718–2721, 1987.
24. Pennebaker JW: The Psychology of Physical Symptoms. New York: Springer-Verlag, 1982.
25. Saskin P, Moldofsky H, Lue FA: Sleep and post-traumatic rheumatic pain modulation disorder (fibrositis syndrome). Psychosom Med 48:319–323, 1986.

51

SOMATOFORM PAIN DISORDER AND ITS TREATMENT

SAMUEL F. DWORKIN, D.D.S., Ph.D. and LEANNE WILSON, Ph.D.

CLINICAL DESCRIPTION AND BASIC CONSIDERATIONS

Somatoform pain disorder is distinguished by the complaint of persistent pain that is unsupported by physical findings adequate to explain either the intensity or the disabling emotional and psychosocial sequelae attributed to the pain.

According to the American Psychiatric Association's classification system, DSM-III-R[1] criteria for somatoform pain disorder are:

A. Preoccupation with pain for at least six months.
B. Either (1) or (2):
   (1) appropriate evaluation uncovers no organic pathology or pathophysiologic mechanism (e.g., a physical disorder or the effects of injury) to account for the pain
   (2) when there is related organic pathology, the complaint of pain or resulting social or occupational impairment is grossly in excess of what would be expected from the physical findings

Essential features include the presentation of subjective pain report that does not conform to known distribution of the nervous system or to dermatomal organization of bodily structures. Additional physical complaints, such as paresthesias, muscle spasm, weakness, and other physical restrictions that compel disuse or avoidance of the affected areas or structures, may also accompany pain. Where pain resembles symptoms accompanying known clinical conditions or diseases (e.g., angina, sciatic neuropathy, peripheral vascular disease), whether those conditions are documented or not, extensive diagnostic evaluation confirms that the pain complaint and accompanying pain behavior are not consistent with the extent of organic pathology. Upon investigation, the pain complaint typically becomes vague and diffuse with regard to location and course. The presence of an adequate pathophysiological mechanism to explain the pain, as in muscle tension headache, rules out the diagnosis of somatoform pain disorder.

The relationship to psychosocial factors that are etiologically involved in the onset or maintenance of somatoform pain disorder is somewhat complex and controversial. Despite the absence of adequate physi-

cal findings, there is often a strong, even rigid conviction on the part of the patient that the pain arises from unknown physical causes and is maintained by a pathological process that is not psychological or emotional, but physical or organic. Moreover, most often there is no clear or confirming temporal relationship between traumatic psychological events and the onset or exacerbation of pain.

However, while denial is typically encountered concerning possible psychogenic origins of the pain experience, there is simultaneous evidence of abundant behavioral changes and dysphoria. Prominent changes in behavior include diminished overall activity levels, reflected primarily as isolation and withdrawal from responsibilities at home, school, or work, and diminished interpersonal or social relationships. These avoidant behaviors in personal and interpersonal domains are accompanied by an excess of treatment-seeking behaviors. High utilization of medical care is common, especially increased doctor visits in pursuit of a physical diagnosis and medical or surgical treatments. Excessive use of medications, especially analgesics, is also common. Abuse of narcotic analgesics and substance abuse are often cause for hospital admission or entry into an inpatient pain management program for purposes of drug detoxification.

While the relationship between chronic pain and depression remains somewhat unclear, despite intensive study, an associated diagnosis of major depression is often warranted. In many cases, however, criteria for a formal diagnosis of major depression are not met, although there is evidence of depressive symptoms: anhedonia, sleep disturbance, and blue mood are common. Heightened anxiety can also be an accompanying feature, and there are some reports indicating that generalized anxiety or panic disorder may be associated diagnoses.

Somatoform pain disorder, as a diagnostic entity, makes its first appearance in DSM-III-R, replacing the DSM-III diagnostic category, psychogenic pain disorder. The principal reason for abandoning psychogenic pain disorder as a diagnostic label is acknowledgment that the pain disorder frequently appears without clear evidence that psychological or psychiatric factors play an etiological role. The earlier diagnosis of psychogenic pain disorder required not only the presence of a persistent pain complaint in the absence of adequate physical findings, but also evidence for the causative role of psychological factors. Competing views, still unresolved, have suggested that the appropriate label be idiopathic pain disorder, reflecting its currently obscure etiology, or that the diagnostic entity be abandoned completely in favor of viewing the pain disorder either as a variant of depression or of somatization disorder and not requiring further specification.[2]

At present it seems most useful to view somatoform pain disorder as a dysfunctional or maladaptive chronic pain condition best understood from a biopsychosocial model of chronic pain. Such a model presumes that chronic pain may emerge as a prepotent clinical condition in its own right, largely independent of bodily site. The prevalent view is that such a chronic pain condition represents the ongoing resolution of physical factors, developmental history, current psychiatric status, and social considerations that include the role of significant others (e.g., spousal and family relationships) as well as cultural influences that shape the sick role for a particular patient.

The presence of severe or persistent pain alone is not sufficient to warrant the label of dysfunctional chronic pain. The combination of a persistent preoccupation with pain that has no justifiable organic basis, together with the marked cognitive, behavioral, and affective changes noted, warrants psychiatric evaluation and inclusion of psychologically based therapies as essential components of the overall management of these patients.

For the sake of completeness, mention is made of an important alternative classification system for pain promulgated by the International Association for the Study of Pain (IASP),[3] the internationally recognized scientific organization of pain researchers and clinicians. The IASP classification provides clinical criteria that allow these persistent pain conditions, at every body site (e.g., head and neck, viscera) to be classified as either:

—Pain of psychological origin with known pathophysiologic mechanism (e.g., muscle tension headaches, myofascial pain syndromes)
—Pain of psychological origin: hysterical or hypochondriacal
—Pain of psychological origin: delusional or hallucinatory

These two different classification systems reveal agreement that dysfunctional chronic pain conditions are valid clinical entities that require multidisciplinary evaluation and integrated treatment methods.

EPIDEMIOLOGICAL FACTORS

There are very few direct epidemiological data concerning the prevalence, sex distribution, age of onset, and familial patterns of this new DSM-III-R diagnostic category. The available data, although scarce, confirm the impression that the disorder has a low prevalence in psychiatric populations but is relatively common in general medical practice. Reasons for the low prevalence in psychiatric populations include the generally accepted notion that chronic pain patients resist a psychological interpretation of their pain problem or a psychiatric referral from medical and surgical specialists. It may also be the case that, while persistent pain is a common symptom in the population, it is often not the only symptom presented for management.

Since somewhat more data are available regarding the epidemiology of the DSM-III-R category somatization disorder, some of those findings are cited with the speculation that they may shed some heuristic light on the population characteristics of somatoform pain disorder. For example, among persons in general medical settings or pain centers presenting with chronic pain, somatization disorders, perhaps including somatoform pain disorder, seem to have a prevalence ranging from 16 per cent to more than 50 per cent—that is, pain not only is a commonly presented symptom in general medical practice but is frequently associated with significant psychiatric disturbance. In general, when chronic pain is present, psychiatric diagnoses (e.g., major depressive disorder, panic disorder, substance [especially alcohol abuse]) are more common in those cases in which chronic pain is not accompanied by consistent findings of organic pathology.

Somatoform pain disorder is most commonly diagnosed in women, in a ratio of about 2 : 1, although for many chronic pain conditions in clinic populations the ratio of women to men is much higher. By contrast, DSM-III-R criteria for somatization disorder are rarely met by men; when men do meet criteria for somatization disorder, their psychiatric profile seems comparable to women with the same disorder.

Age of onset is highly variable and can occur from childhood through senescence. Available data indicate that chronic pain conditions most frequently begin between 30 and 40 years of age, except for chest pain (e.g., mimicking angina), which may have a later age of onset, especially for men. Most chronic pain conditions, especially musculoskeletal pain conditions such as tension headache and myofascial pain, diminish in prevalence with age. An important exception is persistent pain accompanying true joint arthritides.

There is some evidence that somatization disorders, generally, may reveal genetically linked characteristics, but the picture is somewhat confusing and the data relatively scanty.

DIFFERENTIAL DIAGNOSIS

The hallmark of somatoform pain disorder is the preoccupation with persistent pain as the preeminent presenting problem. Other categories of somatoform disorders are not characterized by such an exclusive preoccupation with pain.

In somatization disorder the compelling focus is on a plethora of physical symptoms spread over multiple organ systems. While pain may be among the symptoms reported, an abundant and diffuse symptom presentation readily distinguishes somatization disorder from somatoform pain disorder.

Hypochondriasis is characterized by a preoccupation with disease conviction rather than with specific symptoms per se. The longstanding and intense concern with disease process and not individual symptoms distinguishes hypochondriasis from both somatization disorder and somatoform pain disorder.

Conversion disorder, characterized by a dramatic loss or alteration of function in a bodily part, is not typically accompanied by report of persistent pain. Although some workers have argued that somatoform pain disorder represents a conversion disorder and have therefore suggested that somatoform pain disorder is a redundant DSM-III-R category, for the present there seem to be sufficient differences in the courses of the two disorders and in their treatment, according to the formulators of DSM-III-R, to warrant inclusion of both diagnostic categories.

Those patients with major depressive and anxiety disorders often report pain, but it is not central to the clinical picture.

Psychotic states may include pain complaints, but typically not as a major focus. Bizarre somatic delusions involving preoccupation with pain, especially in the form of delusional systems to account for the pain, are readily detected and differentiated from somatoform pain disorder, which is always a nonpsychotic diagnosis.

Personality disorders, specifically histrionic, narcissistic, and borderline disorders, often include dramatic presentations of physical symptoms, including pain. Similarly, cultural and social factors may influence the manner in which pain is presented as a physical symptom. Thus, the dramatic or excessive presentation of pain, even in the absence of pathological change, is not sufficient for diagnosing somatoform pain disorder, since personality traits or cultural influences may modulate the manner of symptom presentation.

Finally, an additional word about the relationship of somatoform pain disorder to the process of somatization. There is growing evidence that the DSM-III-R criteria for somatization disorder are too rigorous and exclude an appreciable number of patients, typically seen in general medical practice, who present with multiple somatic complaints and associated psychiatric disturbance. However, the reduced number of somatic complaints does not allow for a DSM-III-R diagnosis of somatization disorder, and these cases may not be directed toward appropriate psychiatric (as opposed to medical or surgical) treatment.

Since pain is such a ubiquitous symptom, it is highly likely that such patients will include several pain complaints in their presentation. At present it is not clear in this situation if a diagnosis of somatoform pain disorder is permitted, and if too few symptoms overall are presented, then a diagnosis of somatization disorder is similarly not warranted. The recent literature contains the recommendation that an additional DSM category be created or the present category revised to allow the presentation of fewer pervasive and disruptive somatic symptoms (e.g., between four and nine, instead of 13, as at present in DSM-III-R) for a diagnosis of somatization disorder.[4]

Clinically, such a recommendation seems justified, since the number of pain complaints presented is a potent indicator of concomitant psychiatric disturbance. For example, as identified pain sites increase beyond two, not only is heightened somatization observed, but such persons are likely to be at much greater risk for an associated diagnosis of major depressive disorder compared to the general population and even to persons with a single chronic pain condition.[5] If psychiatric disturbance is more prevalent even with modest increases in numbers of pain conditions, then many patients with persistent pain who now fall between diagnostic cracks, so to speak, would be eligible for this "reduced category" somatization disorder diagnosis.

TREATMENT CONSIDERATIONS

Assessment of Treatment Approach

The treatment approaches available for somatoform pain disorder, which are discussed more fully below, include the wide variety of pharmacological, behavioral, cognitive-behavioral, and psychodynamic psychotherapies currently used for somatization disorders in general and, more specifically, for the management of chronic pain patients.

Central to management of somatoform pain disorder is coordination of treatment and open communication among health care providers. Professionals evaluating and treating these individuals should inquire about and regularly consult with others providing care. These efforts can help prevent the patient from obtaining a potentially iatrogenic combination of medications and repeated treatments. Ideally, one provider is designated as the gatekeeper of care, exerting control over schedules and providing supportive visits so that treatment visits are not contingent solely on symptom presentation. Including the spouse, significant other, and sometimes adult family members in the patient's treatment is considered essential by many workers.

The primary focus of psychiatrically based therapies for this pain disorder is the amelioriation of psychosocial disability, rather than the relief of pain per se. The objectives of psychotherapeutic methods are to restore, as much as possible, earlier adaptive levels of psychosocial functioning by reducing extent of deactivation and to provide relief from affective distress. To accomplish these aims and to assist in the selection of the most appropriate combination of therapeutic modalities (e.g., pharmacological and behavioral), it is essential to conduct a broadly based evaluation of the current level of psychological and behavioral functioning. Romano et al.[6] have provided an excellent guide to conducting such a psychological evaluation, and Keefe and Hiu[7] have similarly developed methods for behavioral assessment.

Psychological assessment should include:

1. *Pain history and pain treatment history* (recommended as a good place to start with these typically somatically focused patients)
   —when pain condition began and perceived etiology
   —description of pain location and presence of concurrent pains
   —pain intensity and course, including relationship to activity and inactivity
   —interference with daily activity, perceived disability
   —treatment history: types and responses
2. *Evaluation of substance abuse and medications history*
3. *Identification of recent and longstanding life stressors*
4. *Psychological disorders:* depression, anxiety, personality disorders
5. *Educational background*
6. *Family history:* including assessment of physical, emotional, or sexual abuse
7. *Vocational history:* including disability status, compensation, and litigation
8. *Cognitive aspects:* explanatory models for the pain, appraisal of its impact on self and family, extent of negative and catastrophizing ideation; intellectual/verbal skills and level of functioning possible
9. *Behavioral assessment:* observation of spousal and significant other interactions, nonverbal pain behaviors (grimacing, guarding, task avoidance), behavioral competencies and skills
10. *Family role models of pain and chronic illness:* evidence for social reinforcement of pain behaviors

Pharmacological Treatment

Pharmacological treatment integrated with psychotherapeutic methods is common and warranted in the management of somatoform pain disorder, but caution is highly warranted. Excessive treatment seeking is common, and with it an attendant risk of iatrogenic complications. The most common non-pharmacological iatrogenic complications arise from excessive use of increasingly complex diagnostic tests and repeated surgeries. The most important complication involving pharmacotherapeutics is the potential for polypharmacy and medication abuse, especially of narcotic analgesics. High rates of complications arise because of: (1) concurrent treatment by several physicians who may be unaware of the pharmacy repertoire the patient has developed; (2) high consumption of ethanol for pain relief; (3) development of psychological and physiological drug dependencies resulting from medication abuse; and (4) attendant drug toxicities associated with incompatible combinations of analgesics, sedatives, and nonprescription substances.

Severe drug abuse problems are common enough with chronic pain patients to have given rise to specialized hospitalization-based protocols for drug detoxification. The general approach described here is taken from a review by Benedetti and Butler[8] and uses a "pain cocktail" tailored to the patient's current drug regimen. For the first 48 hours of hospitalization the patient is allowed access to analgesic and sedative drugs in doses needed to produce pain relief and comfort. Dosages of opiates consumed are converted into equianalgesic doses of methadone, and sedative dosages are converted to equivalent doses of phenobarbital. Hydroxyzine and acetaminophen are added to enhance efficacy of the resulting pain cocktail. Methadone is decreased approximately 10 to 20 per cent daily and phenobarbital is decreased 5 to 10 per cent each day, until detoxification is complete. Subsequently, the patient is reevaluated for alternative medications regimens, if appropriate, but that virtually never contain opioid analgesics.

Currently, the most common classes of drugs used are nonsteroidal anti-inflammatory drugs (NSAIDs) in customary doses and antidepressant medication in somewhat lower doses than is typical for psychopharmacological management of major depressive disorders.

The clinical literature concerning psychotropic medications for chronic pain management, reviewed most recently by Monks and Mersky,[9] reports frequent use of amitriptyline with usual starting dosages of 10 to 25 mg and with typical maintenance doses of 10 to 150 mg. Because of their well-known sedative and anticholinergic effects, use of other antidepressants, including doxepin, impramine, and trazodone, has been frequently reported in managing nonspecific chronic pain states. Use of monoamine oxidase inhibitors (e.g., phenelzine) has also been reported. Maintenance therapy may be instituted for months or even years. The recommendation is frequently made for (1) a single daily dose at bedtime during the maintenance phase of antidepressant use, and (2) efforts made to reduce or discontinue drug therapy gradually after about 6 months.

Antidepressants are currently believed to exert an analgesic as well as antidepressant effect through their action on monoamine neurotransmitters such as serotonin and norepinephrine as well as by acting on monoamine components of the endorphin-mediated analgesia systems. These neurotransmitters have all been implicated as acting through centrifugal pathways increasingly activated during chronic pain states.

Neuroleptics are rarely used alone for management of chronic pain, except where associated with delusional pain or other manifestations of psychotic disorders. Neuroleptics in combination with heterocyclic antidepressants (e.g., fluphenazine and nortiptyline) seem to be used increasingly for chronic pain not responsive to other medications.

Psychological Treatment

Psychological treatment approaches emphasize behavioral and cognitive-behavioral psychotherapeutic modalities. Biofeedback and relaxation methods are commonly employed, most typically as component strategies incorporated into a cognitive-behavioral theoretical framework. Hypnosis directed at management of chronic pain is associated with equivocal results. While an extensive literature is available describing and reviewing these psychological approaches (except hypnosis), a much smaller body of work exists with regard to the application or effectiveness of psychodynamic or insight-oriented psychotherapies. Nevertheless, psychodynamic psychotherapies continue to be advocated by leading pain clinicians for those persons seeking a better understanding of the origins and intrapersonal implications of their pain experience.

Behavioral and cognitive-behavioral modalities seem to have gained a foothold because of their perceived closer relevance to concerns over somatic issues. Generally, resistance to "psychologizing" the pain experience will be high among these organically focused patients when confronted with a psychotherapeutic approach (e.g., insight-oriented talking psychotherapy) that does not deal with their immediate bodily experience, but instead focuses on what is going on inside their heads. Resistance is often strong to any form of psychologically based treatment and heightened by any implications that such a referral is an opportunity by health care providers to deny the patient needed medical, surgical, and pharmacological treatment or to convey that the pain is being made up or is "all in the head."

Acceptance of psychologically based modalities seems enhanced when they are presented as an opportunity to learn pain and stress coping skills. It seems fair to say that less resistance is encountered with biofeedback, relaxation, and even hypnosis therapies, which are typically presented as focusing on acquiring direct control over the body experience. Thus, these latter modalities (including the use of psychoactive medication) are considered by many to be an efficacious method for gaining patient acceptance that pain, as a bodily experience, can in fact be managed through essentially psychological (e.g., behavioral, cognitive-behavioral, and even psychodynamic) methods.

Behavioral Approaches

Fordyce[10] was the first to demonstrate the efficacy of a learning theory–based therapy to modify pain behavior. He conceptualized the prime problem for persons with resistant chronic pain as the inappropriate learning of dysfunctional pain behaviors reinforced, albeit often inadvertently, by health care providers (through continued support of treatment seeking and use of medications) and by significant others (through solicitiousness and reinforcement of excessive deactivation). He introduced an operant model for modifying pain behavior in an inpatient, multidisciplinary pain treatment center and demonstrated that planned contingency management of pain behavior resulted in increased behavioral activation and decreased pain medication and treatment seeking. The basic principles of contingency management—identifying and systematically applying appropriate positive and negative reinforcers to shape pain behavior—have had a profound influence on the understanding and management of chronic pain, and Fordyce's methods have served as a model for multidisciplinary chronic pain treatment programs.

According to this model, the indicators for the presence of operant pain, hence supporting the appropriateness of a contingency management approach, include:

1. Pain behaviors that occur in the absence of supporting physical findings or appear excessive in relation to physical findings.
2. Pain behaviors that are a product of disuse or otherwise overcautious behaviors resulting from excessive concern over anticipated painful effects.
3. Pain behaviors that are systematically reinforced in the immediate environment, typically allowing avoidance of activities that are aversive or that carry responsibility, independent of pain.

The objectives of a behavioral therapy program for chronic pain patients are to identify the appropriate contingencies and then:

1. Modify medication behavior: decrease use of analgesic and psychoactive medications.
2. Increase activity levels: increase the scope and frequency of body movements in deactivated patients through exercise and other pleasurable physical activities.
3. Decrease pain communication in behaviors: reduce verbal and body language behaviors that communicate pain and suffering to others.
4. Improve well behaviors: increase the frequency of positively focused behaviors to be undertaken over the long term, such as vocational activity, activities of daily living, and recreation.
5. Modify environmental responses to pain behavior: involve family members in identification of their own responses that reinforce the patient's maladaptive pain behaviors.

Identification of contingencies to be used in the therapy is accomplished through systematic behavioral evaluation. The relationship of environmental consequences to pain behaviors is evaluated through screening questionnaires, separate interviews with the spouse or significant other, psychological tests, direct observation, and diary forms.

Screening questionnaires can provide demographic information, pain and medication history, and treatment history, particularly sources of dissatisfaction with prior treatment. Interviews with significant others reveal information about responses to the communicated pain and suffering of the patient. These interviews suggest important contingencies in the home that shape the dysfunctional chronic pain behaviors. Psychological testing can provide discriminations with regard to mental, emotional, and behavioral levels of functioning. The Minnesota Multiphasic Personality Inventory (MMPI) is probably the most used instrument for this purpose with chronic pain patients in multidisciplinary pain centers. Pain coping scales[11,12] are very useful for more directly assessing patient coping behaviors.

Direct observation of pain behaviors is now possible through the development of methods for reliably assessing overt nonverbal pain behaviors. These measures focus on gross motor movement and on facial expressions associated with pain. The measures developed by Keefe and Hill,[7] especially for recording extent of guarding, bracing, splinting, and grimacing behaviors under standardized observational conditions, have been very useful in evaluating treatment efficacy.

Patient diaries chart the course of pain intensity and aversiveness over the course of the day and the week. These diaries also can be used to record levels of daily activity—so-called up versus down time—which can then be reviewed by the patient and therapist together in order to identify recurrent patterns in pain intensity, activity levels, and coping behaviors.

Contingency management therapies have proven useful in the management of chronic pain; however, this approach has been criticized for its almost exclusive focus on observable behavior. More recent psychologically based therapies have sought to broaden the scope of therapy for resistant pain patients beyond modification of only observable pain behaviors, to include aspects of the patient's emotional and cognitive functioning.

Cognitive-Behavioral Therapy

Cognitive-behavioral therapies, developed rapidly within the past decade, assume that cognitions (i.e., thoughts, images, "mental scripts") influence both behaviors and emotions. Thus, these therapies look beyond observable behaviors, attending to the influence of attributions, expectancies, appraisals, and mental constructs or images as determinants of psychological as well as behavioral status.[13]

As the name implies, these therapies integrate efforts to modify faulty cognitions and alleviate inappropriate or excessive emotional responses with behavior change. Relaxation strategies, hypnosis, and biofeedback therapies as applied to pain patients are most usefully construed as cognitive-behavioral therapies, and these methods are often used in combination. Barsky et al.[14] integrated relaxation and cognitive strategies more directly; they described the use of relaxation exercises to demonstrate how somatic symptoms can be amplified through attention or attenuated through distraction or reattribution.

Cognitive-behavioral therapy, as it has been applied to pain patients,[15] emphasizes:

1. *Cognitive restructuring*: monitoring and evaluating how beliefs and expectancies determine emotional and behavioral responses to other persons and situations; the relationship between maladaptive or negative cognitions and negative emotions; and the possibility of substituting more adaptive cognitions in the service of decreasing negative feelings and maladaptive behaviors.

2. *Coping skills training*: education concerning the rationale for acquiring and applying cognitive and behavioral skills as methods for coping with pain. These skills include behavioral skills such as relaxation; cognitive restructuring or coping skills (see earlier in chapter); and combined cognitive-behavioral skills including imagery, hypnosis, and effective utilization of biofeedback.

Therapy includes education of the patient with regard to the physical basis for pain and the rationale for use of specific medications. The attempt is made to defuse resistance to over-psychologizing by providing an acceptable explanatory model for the pain and its ensuing disability that is grounded in scientific knowledge and direct personal experience. The patient's complaints are validated and explained as an interaction of physical, emotional, and cognitive processes that have come to yield cycles of emotional upheaval (e.g., anxiety or depression), faulty or maladaptive thoughts (e.g., catastrophizing), and physical changes (e.g., the results of overexertion or prolonged disuse). The patient's somatic explanation (i.e., explanatory model) for etiology of the pain (e.g., injury or disease) is not denied or challenged, at least not initially. Instead, treatment is presented as a way to ameliorate behavioral or emotional factors that may exacerbate pain or that have arisen as sequelae to the pain condition.

Skills training involves, in addition to providing an acceptable rationale, the actual experience, with the therapist, of learning methods such as relaxation and imagery that seem both to divert attention and to decrease levels of muscle tension and physiological arousal. In addition, patients acquire experience with identifying irrational thoughts and feelings and substituting previously developed positive coping self-statements. The objective is to facilitate in the patient a growing self-perception of being armed with a repertoire of personal skills for coping with pain and its attendant aversive sequelae.

Cognitive-behavioral therapies employ homework assignments, elicit the support of family members in the patient's self-help activities, and in general expect more patient participation between therapy sessions, by way of practicing skills, than do most other forms of psychotherapy.

Cognitive-behavioral therapy has been conducted with groups of pain patients, although it is most commonly delivered on an individual basis. The groups usually include either cases with a similar pain problem (e.g., low back pain, headache, arthritis pain) or patients undergoing treatment in multidimensional pain therapy programs. There is no evidence available to indicate whether group or individual therapy is more or less appropriate for cases of somatoform pain disorder.

Family or marital therapy using cognitive-behavioral methods has also been reported successful with resistant pain patients. These approaches are indicated when illness in the family is reflected in disturbed family functioning or the family seems overwhelmed by the patient's pain problem. A further indication is the assessment that the family or spouse can be recruited to influence pain cognitions, thoughts, feelings, and behavior.

Overall, cognitive-behavioral therapy programs have been evaluated as making a significant contribution to the rehabilitation of patients with difficult-to-resolve pain problems. With the exception of relaxation, less attention has been paid to evaluating the efficacy of components of the cognitive-behavioral therapy program. Relaxation methods have been shown to be effective for modifying pain perception and producing increased feelings of well-being. The current consensus, in light of available information, is that broad-based cognitive-behavioral therapy programs that incorporate the multiple elements of patient education, cognitive restructuring, and acquisition of coping skills should continue to be used.

Psychodynamic Psychotherapy

The major impetus for applying psychotherapeutic methods to somatic problems arose from the development of psychoanalytical theory and practice. Early psychoanalytical methods sought to uncover specific unconscious conflicts presumed to be associated with symptoms in particular organ systems. According to these formulations, pain was considered equivalent to anxiety, indicating a conversion of unconscious conflict into a somatic expression. Pain, like anxiety, functioned as a signal of psychological conflict, compelling avoidance of behaviors or relationships that represented unacceptable wishes or needs.

Later formulations have given the same role to depression—that is, that persistent pain associated with dysfunctional behavior and thoughts represents the somatic equivalent of depression. According to this formulation, it is not necessary to observe profound depression in all cases of dysfunctional pain, since the presence of pain is serving the useful psychological function of resolving conflict in a punishing way while allowing the pain patient a seemingly appropriate rationale for the avoidance of difficult situations.

Insight-oriented psychodynamic psychotherapies initially sought to lift the defensive, or dynamic, psychological operations that obscured for the patient the origins of his or her psychological conflict. The relief of dysphoria and pain was presumed to be attendant on obtaining insight into the cause and course of conflict. More recently, there seems to be the recognition that psychodynamic psychotherapies may be indicated in cases in which the patient feels that subjective distress associated with the burden of pain is not receiving adequate attention and is poorly understood, both by the patient and by health care providers.[16] Such patients may seek out opportunities to work out their irrational feelings and maladaptive thoughts and behaviors within the context of a therapy that organizes the understanding of the "entire individual." The latter approach need not focus only on psychodynamic hypotheses concerning the repressed meanings of pain; it can also profitably explore the conditions and settings under which pain behaviors emerge and the defensive function they serve.

It has been recommended that dynamic psychotherapy with chronic pain patients generally be of brief duration (e.g., less than 20 sessions) and that the focus of therapy be on limited psychological issues rather than on transformation of the personality structure.

REFERENCES

1. American Psychiatric Association: Diagnostic and Statistical Manual of Mental Disorders. 3rd ed. Revised. Washington, DC: American Psychiatric Association Press, 1987.
2. Williams JB, Spitzer RL: Idiopathic pain disorder: A critique of pain-prone disorder and a proposal for a revision of DSM-III category psychogenic pain disorder. J Nerv Ment Dis 178:415–419, 1982.
3. International Association for the Study of Pain: Classification of chronic pain. Pain (suppl 3):S1–S222, 1986.
4. Katon W, Lin E, Von Korff M, et al: Somatization: A spectrum of severity. Am J Psychiatry 148:34–40, 1991.
5. Dworkin SF, Von Korff M, LeResche L: Multiple pains and psychiatric disturbance: An epidemiologic investigation. Arch Gen Psychiatry 47:239–244, 1990.
6. Romano JM, Turner JA, Moore JE: Psychological evaluation. In Tollison CD, ed. Handbook of Chronic Pain Management. Baltimore: Williams & Wilkins, 1989:38–51.
7. Keefe FJ, Hill RW: An objective approach to quantifying pain behavior and gait patterns in low back pain patients. Pain 21:153–161, 1985.
8. Benedetti C, Butler SH: Systemic analgesics. In Bonica JJ, ed. The Management of Pain, vol II. Philadelphia: Lea & Febiger, 1990:1640–1675.
9. Monks R, Mersky H: Psychotropic drugs. In Wall PD,

Melzack R, eds. Textbook of Pain. 2nd ed. London: Churchill Livingstone, 1989:702–721.

10. Fordyce WE: Behavioral Methods for Chronic Pain and Illness. St. Louis: CV Mosby, 1976.

11. Rosenstiel AK, Keefe FJ: The use of coping strategies in chronic low back pain patients: Relationship to patient characteristics and current adjustment. Pain 17:33–44, 1983.

12. Brown GK, Nicassio PM: Development of a questionnaire for the assessment of active and passive coping strategies in chronic pain patients. Pain 31:53–64, 1987.

13. Turner JA, Romano JM: Cognitive-behavioral therapy. In Bonica JJ, ed. The Management of Pain, vol II. Philadelphia: Lea & Febiger, 1990:1711–1721.

14. Barsky AJ, Geringer E, Wool CA: A cognitive-educational treatment for hypochondriasis. Gen Hosp Psychiatry 10:1–5, 1988.

15. Turk DC, Meichenbaum M, Genest M: Pain and Behavioral Medicine: A Cognitive-Behavioral Perspective. New York: Guilford Press, 1983.

16. Pilowski I, Basset D: Individual dynamic psychotherapy for chronic pain. In Roy R, Tunks E, eds. Chronic Pain: Psychosocial Factors in Rehabilitation. City: Publisher, 1982:107–124.

52

MULTIPLE PERSONALITY, FUGUE, AND AMNESIA

DAVID DAVIS, M.D., F.R.C. PSYCH., D.P.M.

MULTIPLE PERSONALITY DISORDER

Clinical Description

Multiple personality disorder (MPD) refers to a condition in which there exist within one patient two or more distinct personalities or personality states. There should be at least two fully developed personalities, or there may be one dominant distinct personality and one or more personality states in which the pattern is not as intensely pervasive. These personalities or "alters" have unique memories, patterns of behavior, and social relationships. There may be many more than two personalities. The transition from one personality to another is usually sudden, with some personalities being aware of others and other personalities less aware, but most personalities are cognizant of lost periods of time or distortions in their perceptions of periods of time.

The illness is thought to begin in childhood but may not be diagnosed until the third or fourth decade, with the mean age at diagnosis being 28.5 years. Etiologically, it is thought to be related to physical and/or sexual abuse or other severe emotional trauma, or both, and is therefore regarded as a form of chronic post-traumatic dissociative disorder. There is disagreement about the prevalence of the disorder, and there are even arguments in the literature as to whether it exists at all as a separate entity, although Ross et al.[1] have shown, using the Dissocia-

tive Disorders Interview Schedule (DDIS), that MPD is a condition that can be reliably distinguished from schizophrenia, eating disorders, and panic disorders at a high level of significance. When diagnosed, MPD seems to be more common in women and more common in first-degree biological relatives of those with the disorder, but claims for a ratio of females to males tend to vary from 5 : 1 to 2 : 1.

Ross et al.[2] have gathered structured interview data on 102 cases of MPD from four centers using the Dissociative Experiences Scale (DES) and DDIS. (The DES is a 28-item self-report instrument with a test-retest reliability of .84 and good clinical validity, and is a screening but not a diagnostic tool for dissociative disorders. The DDIS is a structured interview that has an interrater reliability of .68, a sensitivity of 90 per cent, and a specificity of 100 per cent for the diagnosis of MPD.) Ross et al.'s paper yields a great deal of data regarding the epidemiology and diagnosis of MPD. Of the 102 individuals interviewed, 90.2 per cent were female and 9.8 per cent were male. Forty-nine per cent have never married, 31.4 per cent were married, 18.6 per cent were separated or divorced, and 0.9 per cent were widowed. A total of 43.1 per cent were employed. With regard to childhood abuse, 90.2 per cent had experienced sexual abuse and 82.4 per cent physical abuse, for a combined total of 95.1 per cent who had been abused. Of the 102 patients, 33.3 per cent reported having had a drinking problem at some time, 28.4 per cent had used street drugs extensively, 9.8 per cent had injected drugs intravenously, and 15.7 per cent had treatment for drug or alcohol abuse. A total of 95.1 per cent had received treatment for an emotional disorder, and 75.5 per cent knew what diagnoses they had been given in the past. These included depression (72.5 per cent), mania (26.5 per cent), schizophrenia (26.5 per cent), anxiety disorder (46.1 per cent), and MPD (35.3 per cent). These latter figures tend to agree with the past literature, which suggests that depression is the most common presenting symptom in MPD, manifested by mood swings, suicidal attempts, and insomnia. Other presenting symptoms are dissociative symptoms such as amnesia, fugue episodes, depersonalization, or sleepwalking; phobic, anxiety, or panic disorders; substance abuse; hallucinations; thought disorder or catatonic-like states; transsexualism and transvestism; neurological symptoms such as headache, syncope, or seizure-like behavior; and hysterical or motor symptoms.

Ross et al.[3] have examined Schneiderian first-rank symptoms in MPD and schizophrenia. The MPD patients come from the series of 102 cases diagnosed in four centers, and Ross et al. found that Schneiderian first-rank symptoms were equally common in all four centers. The average patient experienced 6.4 Schneiderian symptoms. When these 102 cases are combined with two previously reported series of MPD cases (236 from Ross et al.[4] and 30 from Kluft[5]), the average number of Schneiderian symptoms for the 368 cases is 4.9. This contrasts with an average of 1.3 Schneiderian symptoms acknowledged by 1739 schizophrenics in ten published series. Voices commenting and voices arguing are the two most common symptoms in both series. Multiple personality disorder voices apparently are heard from within the head, whereas in schizophrenia the voices tend to come from outside the head. The authors made the point that any patient with schneiderian symptoms should be assessed for a history of childhood abuse, amnesia in one or more forms, and MPD.

Franklin[6] emphasized the subtle dissociative signs by which MPD may be diagnosed. These are based on sudden fluctuations in transferences and affects; fluctuations in developmental levels; marked inconsistencies in attitudes, viewpoints, memories, and behaviors; signs of transitions between alters; signs of influences of alters on each other; transient changes in body posture, facial expression, voice quality, and vocabulary; atypical references to self-aspects and dissociative experiences; and sudden changes in somatic and psychiatric symptoms. Franklin further stated that in some cases of suspected MPD, if other methods do not clarify the diagnosis and subtle signs and other dissociative symptoms continue to be present, this is an indication for the use of hypnosis to uncover alters, since in normal persons or patients with other psychiatric disorders, hypnosis does not elicit full personalities such as those observed in MPD.

The etiology of MPD may be related to an interplay among a biological capacity to dissociate, the experience of life events that are overwhelming, the development of personalities in response to these life events, and an inability to recover from trauma. Terr,[7] in a review of childhood traumas, stated that, in children in whom periods of time cannot be accounted for, and who have behavioral problems, visual and auditory hallucinations, and complaints of headaches, these symptoms may indicate precursors of MPD, but that those children suffering from type II trauma of the self-hypnosis variety may fall short of the MPD or precursors diagnoses. Brown and Anderson,[8] in examining psychiatric morbidity in 947 adult inpatients, found childhood histories of sexual and physical abuse in 18 per cent overall but pointed out that, although some patients retreat from abusive environments through dissociation, MPD, or somatization, many abused people rely on substance abuse to escape, more so than nonabused patients suffering from other psychiatric illnesses. Sanders and Giolas,[9] in a study of 47 adolescents using the DES, concluded that the phenomenon of MPD, with its origins in early overwhelming physical, sexual, and psychological abuse, should be placed at the extreme end of a continuum of dissociative sequelae of childhood stress.

In an interesting paper, Ross et al.[10] reported on their investigation of a sample of 60 subjects consisting of 20 females with MPD (of whom one had a false-negative diagnosis of MPD on structured interview), 20 female prostitutes, and 20 female exotic dancers. The instruments used were the DDIS and the DES. The subjects with MPD met the criteria for more dissociative disorders than did subjects from the other two groups. Nevertheless, psychogenic amnesia and MPD were common among the prostitutes and exotic dancers. Seven dancers met the diagnostic criteria for MPD and seven prostitutes met the criteria for psychogenic amnesia. One prostitute met the criteria for MPD. The subjects with MPD met DSM-III-R criteria for somatization disorder more often than did the prostitutes. Seven of the MPD subjects had somatization disorder, compared to one of the dancers and more of the prostitutes. The three groups did not differ in rates of depression, borderline personality disorder, or substance abuse, but the MPD group was more dissociative and had more Schneiderian symptoms. This is a first attempt to screen a nonclinical population for dissociative disorders using valid and reliable instruments.

Biological and Psychological Studies

Putnam et al.[11] have investigated differential autonomic nervous system activity across nine subjects with MPD and five controls who produced alter personality states by simulation, hypnosis, or deep relaxation. Eight of the nine MPD subjects consistently manifested physiologically distinct alter personality states. Three of five controls also produced physiologically distinct states, but these differed from those of the MPD subjects. A habituation paradigm demonstrated carryover effects at the autonomic nervous system level from one state to the next for both groups. However, there was failure to find consistent alter personality differences in electrodermal laterality in the MPD group as a whole. Miller[12] has shown that MPD subjects had 4.5 times the average number of changes in optical functioning between alter personalities of control subjects on measures of visual acuity with correction, visual acuity without correction, visual fields, manifest refraction, and eye muscle balance. Mathew et al.[13] have studied regional cerebral blood flow in a patient with MPD and found no significant alterations except for some right temporal hyperperfusion more indicative of functional overactivity.

Armstrong and Loewenstein[14] reported preliminary findings for a unique standardized psychological test procedure for evaluating MPD and dissociative disorders. Their sample was composed of 14 patients of whom 13 were female. More than two thirds of the sample had personality profiles that were intellectualized, obsessive, and introversive but not histrionic nor labile. Testing including the DES, Wechsler Adult Intelligence Scale–Revised (WAIS-R), Exner Rorschach, Thematic Apperception Test (TAT), symptoms checklist–90 (SCL-90), Sentence Completion Test, Figure Drawing Tests, and a new subscale of the Exner that they had developed to measure traumatic associations. Eight patients were diagnosed as having MPD and the remainder as having dissociative reaction not otherwise specified. Twelve per cent of the 14 patients met DSM-III-R criteria for post-traumatic stress disorder (PTSD). Coons and Fine[15] blindly rated the results of 63 Minnesota Multiphasic Personality Inventories (MMPI(s) as representing MPD or not. Overall accuracy for the entire sample was 71.4 per cent, with a 68 per cent accuracy rate for correctly identified patients with MPD. Of the 63 patients, 25 had diagnoses of MPD and 38 had other diagnoses such as borderline personality disorder, depression, and schizophrenia.

Differential Diagnosis

There is a need to distinguish MPD from psychogenic fugue and psychogenic amnesia, which do not show repeated shifts in identity and are usually limited to a single brief episode. In view of the findings concerning Schneiderian first-rank symptoms, schizophrenia needs to be considered. Mood disorders with or without psychotic features, borderline personality disorders, and substance abuse also need to be considered, as well as the conditions that may be represented by the presenting features of MPD. Malingering may need to be included, especially when some obvious legal gain may be a possibility. Possession states occurring in MPD tend to somnambulic, in which the patient is not conscious of his or her usual self and does not have memory for the condition following the episode. In lucid states the person is aware of the self but has no control over the other personality.

Treatment

The best recent information regarding treatment is to be found in two books—those of Ross[16] (which also contains a copy of the DDIS) and Putnam.[17] Ross discussed general considerations for treatment coming from earlier work in the field, such as that by Kluft and Braun, and also described inclusion and exclusion criteria for treatment. The main therapy recommended by both authors is psychotherapeutic in nature. Both books include discussion of indications for and pros and cons of adjunctive treatments, including psychopharmacological agents, although both authors commented on the lack of good medication studies. Ross divided psychotherapy into four phases:

1. *Initial:* encompasses such considerations as establishing trust and safety, developing treatment alliance and discussing diagnosis, developing a stated goal of integration, contacting alter personalities, mapping the personality system, developing treatment contracts, and establishing interpersonality communication.

2. and 3. *Middle and Late:* includes abreacting abuse memories; age-appropriate activities with child alters; working with aggressive and persecutory personalities; cognitive restructuring techniques; negotiating with alters' personalities; using metaphors, rituals, imagery and dreams, hypnosis, and relaxation techniques; age progression and age regression; writing exercises; and use of audiovisual materials.

4. *Postintegration:* dealing with the patient who may be vulnerable to relapse as a result of further trauma.

Putnam discussed the pros and cons of various adjunctive therapies and the special problems of MPD patients: fugues, amnesias, trances, or depersonalized states, which are common expressions of crisis in MPD; rapid switching; development of acute somatic symptoms; discovery of new alters or failure of previous fusions; intrusion or rejection of family of origin; and co-presence crises, which tend to resemble old descriptions of "lucid possession" states. He warned against heterogeneous group therapy, and stated that, although homogeneous group therapy may be helpful, it may also be difficult because group members tend to "out-multiple" each other, display rivalry for the therapist's attention, and be suggestible in the group situation. He recommended internal group therapy in which selected alters of a single MPD patient constitute a formal therapy group for patients who have accepted the MPD diagnosis yet are not making progress. He also discussed the use of videotape techniques and saw a limited adjunctive role for family and marital therapy. Putman's discussion of inpatient management is also very helpful.

Ross and Norton[18] have examined the effects of hypnosis on the features of MPD, comparing a sample of 57 MPD patients who had been hypnotized both before and after diagnosis with 38 MPD patients who had not been hypnotized, and concluded that hypnosis facilitates access to the more heavily dissociated states in those individuals. Those hypnotized were able to provide access to more child personalities, protector personalities, and personalities of different age, sex, and race and were able to report higher rates of sexual and physical abuse during childhood. Bowman and Coons[19] have reported the first case of the use of hypnosis in a prelingually deaf patient with MPD using a finger-spelling technique.

Dell and Eisenhower[20] have reported a preliminary study of 11 cases of adolescent MPD. The MPD occurred in the context of one or more concomitant abuse/trauma-related diagnoses (mood disorder, PTSD, disruptive behavior disorder, and borderline personality disorder). The authors pointed out that careful screening for dissociation in adolescents who show three or more of the following symptoms will frequently uncover a heretofore undiagnosed case of MPD: depression, disruptive behavior, mood swings, the hearing of voices, surprising forgetting, apparent lying, trancing out, and sharp changes of behavior. The treatment was similar to that for the adult MPD patient, but a major predictor of treatment failure was the continuing presence in the house of any form of abuse, including emotional abuse.

Pharmacotherapy

There is a dearth of systematic or controlled suudies of the use of medication in MPD. Both Ross[16] and Putnam[17] agreed that medications may be adjunctive to psychotherapy and may be useful for controlling or ameliorating specific nondissociative symptoms, such as depression and anxiety, that may interfere with psychotherapy. Putnam pointed out that MPD patients tend to give nonspecific placebo-like responses and that different alters may respond differently within the same person. There seems to be a greater risk of disabling side effects with MPD patients than with other psychiatric patients. There may be problems with medication compliance, and there tends to be a high incidence of substance abuse among patients with MPD.

Neuroleptics may have to be used cautiously owing to a high incidence of side effects and undesirable psychological effects, and should only be used in low doses for sedation, which may be preferable to hospitalization of the patient. If the patient has been on neuroleptics for a long time prior to being diagnosed, initial discontinuation may produce a marked increase in anxiety level as well as increased acting out by previously suppressed alters.

Antidepressants also need to be used cautiously because of overdosage problems but may be useful for concurrent depression, agoraphobia, panic attacks, anorexia, bulimia, and chronic pain syndromes. However, polycyclic antidepressants may affect only some of the alters. Monoamine oxidase inhibitors are generally discouraged, and lithium does not seem to be helpful.

Anxiolytics may have a role in the generalized anxiety, panic, and phobic states seen in MPD and may help the patient over anxiety associated with major crises, but care needs to be taken with benzodiazepines because of the possibility of dependency, especially where there has been drug abuse prior to integration. Most MPD patients experience panic attacks, and drug treatment may be especially helpful with these as well as in reducing nightmares and night terrors. For inpatients, lorazepam 2 to 5 mg p.o. or IM up to a maximum of 20 mg in 24 hours given every 30 minutes until effect is recommended by Ross. Intravenous diazepam may also be tried.

With anticonvulsants, there tends to be a higher than normal incidence of abnormal electroencephalographic (EEG) findings in MPD patients and in patients with concurrent epilepsy, but the sustained beneficial effect of carbamazepine without clear EEG evidence of concurrent epilepsy has not been demonstrated. However, Fichtner et al.[21] have reported decreased episodic violence and increased control of dissociation in a carbamazepine-treated case of MPD with the result that spontaneous switching to alters was more easily prevented, manic episodes ceased and the patient became less depressed. An EEG 13 weeks after carbamazepine treatment during complete remission of violent behavior showed no rhythmic midtemporal discharges.

Since sleep disturbances are common in MPD, in general sedatives and hypnotics are not advisable for treatment because they may be used for suicide attempts. Audiotapes are recommended as the best method for dealing with insomnia and in helping the patient deal with it without pharmacological help.

Other medications may cause problems. For example, the use of analgesics for pain syndromes may result in abuse and addiction, and in some MPD patients adequate surgical and dental anesthesia may be difficult. Sometimes a child alter is the first to emerge from an anesthetic.

FUGUE

Clinical Description

According to the DSM-III-R, in a psychogenic fugue there is sudden unexpected travel away from one's home or usual place of work with the assumption of a partial or complete new identity, accompanied by an inability to recall one's past during the state as well as specific events during the fugue, even after it has resolved. There is a state of altered consciousness of a dissociative nature, and the behavior may be a symbolic suicidal equivalent in the course of a depressive illness related to personal rejections, losses, or failures or, more common in the context of psychosocial stress, escaping from a conflictual or intolerable situation, as in a hysterical fugue. Riether and Stoudemire,[22] however, argued that the diagnostic criterion that requires the patient to assume a new identity is not a consistent aspect of the syndrome as described in the psychiatric literature.

Little is known of the epidemiology or prevalence of fugue, although it is thought to be rare in childhood and recurrences are probably rare. When it does occur it may persist for months. The frequency of fugues of epileptic origin is considered to be about 78 per cent in temporal lobe types and 6.4 per cent in unspecified epilepsy samples. The psychogenic form is said to be twice as common in men. The fugue is usually preceded by intense affect that the patient finds overwhelming, and recovery is often rapid and sudden. Stengel[23] was usually able to trace a period of hypomania or depression preceding the fugue, and believed the fugue to be related to an affective illness, possibly bipolar disorder. Only one case has been described in recent years of a fugue occurring in a father and son—that of a 24-year-old serviceman with a history of having left home as a youngster and of being found wandering beginning at age 13 or 14. His father had begun extensive wanderings while hospitalized for amputation of a limb, but there was insufficient information available to truly determine the relationship between their respective fugues.[24]

Differential Diagnosis

Psychogenic amnesia: memory impairment centers around confused wandering with sudden inability to remember important personal material. There may be an overwhelming and panic-inducing impulse or narcissistic rage.

Multiple personality: there are repeated shifts of identity, many episodes tend to occur, and there may be a history of identity disturbance since childhood.

Somnambulism: patient behaves out of the ordinary and tends to act out a specific memory of a traumatic event.

Organic mental disorders: there is unexpected wandering from home that is unusual for the individual and tends to have an aimless quality. In complex partial seizure disorders there is no assumption of a new identity and usually no psychosocial precipitating episode. There tends to be repeated wanderings, and they may be preceded by auras, illusions, or anxiety. The condition usually lasts less than 24 hours, and a sodium amytal interview is unproductive. A sleep-deprived EEG with nasopharyngeal leads often is the best diagnostic tool.

Malingering: a practical motive is more easily discovered, especially in those patients with a tendency to lie or a legal motive for wishing to have a fugue state substantiated.

Other conditions to be considered included metabolic disorders, head trauma, postconcussion syndrome, carbon monoxide poisoning, and alcoholic blackouts. A useful summary of differential diagnosis may be found in Akhtar and Brenner.[25]

Other Pertinent Comments

In psychogenic fugue the behavior and travel are more purposeful; there may be the assumption of a new identity, either partial or complete; it is usually a single episode; and the onset of the identity disturbance usually coincides with that of the fugue. There may be a history of previous concussions, and there tends to be reversal of the amnesia under hypnosis or narcoanalysis. Rice and Fisher[26] have described a case in which they studied a fugue state in sleep and wakefulness. They stated that the dream, the fugue, and some sleep talk are psychological correlates related to the rapid eye movement (REM) period organismic state. They considered the possibility of continuity of and reciprocity between the physiological substrates of psychological phenomena in the three organismic states of wakefulness, non-REM sleep, and REM sleep. The patient they described had two grand mal seizures, although fugues recurred after the implantation of a pacemaker.

Treatment

Treatment of fugue usually involves the use of sodium amytal interviews and pursuit of recovery of the missing memories. Treatment should start as soon as possible. Hypnotherapy is also appropriate, involving questioning, persuasion, or automatic writing. With the psychodynamic therapies, 20 per cent of men with fugues had repeat episodes.

Appropriate pharmacotherapy beyond the short-acting barbiturates would be called for when a fugue occurred in association with such conditions as depression, schizophrenia, alcoholism, or epilepsy.

AMNESIA

Clinical Description

Psychogenic amnesia is the most common symptom of the dissociation disorders. It is essentially an anterograde amnesia consisting of a sudden loss of memory in the absence of an organic lesion or disease, and there is an awareness by the patient that a memory disturbance is present. There is a sudden inability to remember important personal material, and the amnesia occurs most frequently in association with a severe stressor such as a natural disaster or a military conflict, especially in young males or in adolescents or young female adults who have no history of psychiatric illness. During periods of public emergency, psychogenic amnesia may be responsible for 15 per cent of all psychiatric admissions to hospitals. The incidence of new admissions to a psychiatric service has been put at 0.26 per cent. Twenty per cent of combat veterans are amnesic for combat experience, and where soldiers are exposed to prolonged marching and fighting under heavy fire, 35 per cent suffer from amnesia for their experiences.

The amnesia may be precipitated by situations involving threat or injury or death, anticipated loss of an important object, an overwhelming panic-inducing impulse, or narcissistic rage. When there has been an earlier organic amnesia, the patient may be predisposed to psychogenic memory loss in the presence of depressed mood and a severe precipitating stress. In 30 to 40 per cent of cases of homicide, amnesia may be claimed by the accused. Amnesia is classified into localized (lasting a few hours), generalized (lasting years), systematized (relating to a special event), and continous (the loss occurs for each successive event as it occurs, but alertness and awareness are not disturbed). During an amnesic event the patient may be perplexed or wander. After the amnesia the patient can usually recall the events. There is no known family history association.

The mechanisms at work in psychogenic amnesia may involve any of the following processes. There may be faulty encoding of information at initial input, giving rise to consequent defects in retrieval since the amnesia often occurs in states of abnormal mood or extreme arousal, as in amnesia for offenses occurring in situations of extreme emotional arousal or severe intoxication or during a psychotic illness. Impaired attention and motivation also occur in depression, which may give rise to amnesia. Psychogenic amnesia may also be seen as an example of "motivated forgetting" or a form of repression, or there may be a primary retrieval defect in which the amnesia reflects a mood-dependent phenomenon similar to that described in depression. Some state-dependent difficulties may occur, as instances of retrieval difficulty.

Differential Diagnosis

Psychogenic amnesia must be differentiated from other dissociative disorders such as MPD. Amnesia may be a sequel of a fugue, in which the patient may adopt a new identity for a period of time. A key feature helping to distinguish these patients from those with organic amnestic disorders, according to Erickson,[27] is that they are able to learn and acquire new information at a normal rate during an episode. Organic conditions such as an alcoholic blackout, benzodiazepine-induced amnesia, or transient global amnesia need to be considered. In alcohol-related conditions, short-term memory is impaired and there is blunted affect, confabulation, and lack of awareness of memory impairment. In postconcussion states the amnesia tends to be retrograde; in epilepsy the onset is sudden, with motor abnormalities, and repeated EEGs show anomalies. In catatonic stupor there is failure of recall and catatonic symptoms. In transient global amnesia the memory disorder lasts some hours, and registration and recall are impaired, but the patient's behavior seems appropriate and there is no loss of personal identity. There is a retrograde amnesia and recovery tends to be complete. A recent study by Hodges and Warlow[28] did not support a vascular cause for transient global amnesia. In organic amnesia in general there is no obvious relationship to stress, the amnesia is more marked for recent events and disappears slowly if at all, and attention deficits and disturbances of affect are frequently present.

Spanos et al.,[29] in a paper concerning the detection of simulated amnesia, have shown that hypnotically amnesic subjects consistently exhibited above-chance levels of recognition for words that they failed to recall during amnesia testing. Simulators consistently exhibited below-chance recognition for such words. These findings are consistent with the hypothesis that hypnotic amnesia cannot be adequately explained in terms of faking. Consistently below-chance scoring on tests of recognition memory may provide a means of detecting simulated amnesia in clinical samples.

An interesting discussion by Good[30] pointed out that transient amnesias and fugues, among other dissociative-like states, may be brought on by medication or be substance-induced, and that organic and psychogenic dissociative disorders may coexist and be intertwined or indistinguishable. He described a number of instances in which state-dependent learning may play a part in substance-induced dissociative conditions and made a plea for a descriptive delineation of substance-induced alterations in brain states.

Treatment

Psychogenic amnesia may resolve spontaneously when the patient is removed from the stressful situation. Hypnosis may facilitate recall and abreaction. Other psychological treatment techniques involve autohypnosis, hypnotherapy, posthypnotic suggestions, and use of progressive relaxation and visual imagery, suggestion, biofeedback, directed association, and free association. The sodium amytal interview may be useful not only as treatment to facilitate the return of memory but as a diagnostic tool for distinguishing organic from psychogenic amnesia, since in the former the lost memories are not recoverable. Perry and Jacobs[31] gave a detailed description of this procedure. If the amnesia is associated with clinical depression, electroconvulsive therapy may be effective in restoring the memory. Brna and Wilson[32] pointed out that precautions should be taken to prevent suicidal actions during therapy for psychogenic amnesia since such amnesia may be a protective mechanism in suicidal persons.

REFERENCES

1. Ross CA, Heber S, Norton GR, et al: Differences between multiple personality disorder and other diagnostic groups on structured interview. J Nerv Ment Dis 177:487–491, 1989.
2. Ross CA, Miller SD, Reagor P, et al: Structured interview data on 102 cases of multiple personality disorder from four centres. Am J Psychiatry 147(5):596–601, 1990.
3. Ross CA, Miller SD, Reagor P, et al: Schneiderian symptoms in multiple personality disorder and schizophrenia. Compr Psychiatry 31(2):111–118, 1990.
4. Ross CA, et al: Can J Psychiatry 34:413–418, 1989.
5. Kluft RP: An J Psychiatry 144:293–298, 1987.
6. Franklin J: The diagnosis of multiple personality disorder based on subtle dissociative signs. J Nerv Ment Dis 178(1):4–14, 1990.
7. Terr LC: Childhood traumas: An outline and review. Am J Psychiatry 148:10–20, 1991.
8. Brown GR, Anderson B: Psychiatric morbidity in adult inpatients with childhood histories of sexual and physical abuse. Am J Psychiatry 148:55–61, 1991.
9. Sanders B, Giolas MH: Dissociation and childhood trauma in psychologically disturbed adolescents. Am J Psychiatry 148:50–54, 1991.
10. Ross CA, Anderson G, Heber S, et al: Dissociation and abuse among multiple-personality patients, prostitutes, and exotic dancers. Hosp Community Psychiatry 41(3):328–330, 1990.
11. Putnam FW, Zahn TP, Post RM: Differential autonomic nervous system activity in multiple personality disorder. Psychiatry Res 31(3):251–260, 1990.
12. Miller SD: Optical differences in cases of multiple personality disorder. J Nerv Ment Dis 177:480–486, 1989.
13. Mathew RJ, Jack RA, West WS: Regional central blood flow in a patient with multiple personality. Am J Psychiatry 142:504–505, 1985.
14. Armstrong JG, Loewenstein RJ: Characteristics of patients with multiple personality and dissociative disorder on psychological testing. J Nerv Ment Dis 178:448–454, 1990.
15. Coons PM, Fine CG: Accuracy of the MMPI in identifying multiple personality disorder. Psychol Rep 66(3, pt 1):831–834, 1990.
16. Ross CA: Multiple Personality Disorder: Diagnosis, Clinical Features and Treatment: New York: John Wiley & Sons, 1989.
17. Putnam FW: Diagnosis and Treatment of Multiple Personality Disorder. New York: Guilford Press, 1989.
18. Ross CA, Norton GR: Effects of hypnosis on the feature of multiple personality disorder. Am J Clin Hypn 32:(9–106, 1989.
19. Bowman ES, Coons PM: The use of hypnosis in a deaf patient with multiple personality: A case report. Am J Clin Hypn 33:99–104, 1990.
20. Dell PF, Eisenhower JW: Adolescent multiple personality disorder: A preliminary study of eleven cases. J Am Acad Child Adolesc Psychiatry 29(3):359–366, 1990.
21. Fichtner CG, Kuhlman DT, Gruenfeld MJ, et al: Decreased episodic violence and increased control of dissociation in a carbamazepine-treated case of multiple personality. Biol Psychiatry 27(9):1045–1052, 1990.
22. Riether AM, Stoudemire A: Psychogenic fugue states: A review. South Med J 81:568–571, 1988.
23. Stengel E: Further studies on pathological wanderings. J Ment Sci 89:224–241, 1943.
24. McKinney KA, Lange MM: Familial fugue–a case report. Can J Psychiatry 28:654–656, 1983.
25. Akhtar S, Brenner I: Differential diagnosis of fugue-like states. J Clin Psychiatry 40:381–385, 1979.
26. Rice E, Fisher C: Fugue states in sleep and wakefulness: A psychophysiological study. J Nerv Ment Dis 163:79–87, 1976.
27. Erickson KR: Amnestic disorders. Pathophysiology and patterns of memory dysfunction. West J Med 152(2):159–166, 1990.
28. Hodges JR, Warlow CP: The aetiology of transient global amnesia. A case-control study of 114 cases with prospective follow-up. Brain 113(pt 3):639–657, 1990.
29. Spanos NR, James B, de Groot H: Detection of simulated hypnotic amnesia. J Abnorm Psychol 99:179–182, 1990.
30. Good MI: Substance induced dissociative disorders and psychiatric nosology. J Clin Psychopharmacol 9:88–93, 1989.
31. Perry JC, Jacobs D: Overview: Clinical applications of the amytal interview in psychiatric emergency settings. Am J Psychiatry 139:552–559, 1982.
32. Brna TG Jr, Wilson CC: Psychogenic amnesia. Am Fam Physician 41(1):229–234, 1990.

Section G

SEXUAL DISORDERS

REPORT OF DSM-IV WORK GROUP ON SEXUAL DISORDERS

CHESTER W. SCHMIDT, JR., M.D.

SEXUAL DESIRE DISORDERS

The issues identified for hypoactive sexual desire were : (1) Is there empirical evidence to assist in the formulation of a more precise diagnostic criteria set for this dysfunction?; (2) Are there research data to permit operationalizing the diagnosis with frequency criteria for fantasy, desire, and behavior?; and (3) Is there evidence for the formation of subcategories of patients with hypoactive sexual disorder? With regard to sexual aversion, the issue addressed was, are there systematic, empirically gathered data on the clinical utility, validity, and reliability of a "broader" versus "narrower" set of criteria for sexual aversion disorders?

Dr. Schiavi found that there was a paucity of empirical information on sexual desire disorders in general. He noted that few investigators focused on this topic and even fewer studies utilized DSM-III-R criteria for subject selection. He recommended there be no changes in the current criteria sets for either hypoactive sexual desire disorder or sexual aversion disorder because the field would be thrown into scientific chaos with further non–data-supported changes. Several changes have been recommended for future criteria sets that are the result of general editing by the Task Force. The criteria sets would read as follows:

Hypoactive Sexual Desire Disorder

A. Persistently or recurrently deficient (or absent) sexual fantasies and desire for sexual activity.

The judgment of deficiency or absence is made by the clinician, taking into account factors that affect sexual functioning, such as age, sex, and the context of the person's life.

B. Occurrence not exclusively during the course of another Axis I disorder (other than a Sexual Dysfunction), such as Major Depression and not better accounted for by a Secondary Sexual Dysfunction due to an Axis III condition or a Substance-induced Sexual Dysfunction.

C. The disturbance causes marked distress or interpersonal difficulty.

Sexual Aversion Disorder

A. Persistent or recurrent extreme aversion to, and avoidance of all, or almost all, genital sexual contact with a sexual partner.

B. Occurrence not exclusively during the course of another Axis I disorder (other than a Sexual Dysfunction) such as Obsessive-Compulsive Disorder or Major Depression.

C. The disturbance causes marked distress or interpersonal difficulty.

SEXUAL PAIN DISORDERS

Dyspareunia

No specific issues were identified. An editorial change is proposed for the criteria for dyspareunia. The option is to expand the exclusion criteria (which were erroneously left out of DSM-III-R) to include an exclusion for pain during intercourse due to a physical condition or due to a substance. The criteria set would read as follows:

A. Recurrent or persistent genital pain in either a male or female before, during or after sexual intercourse.
B. The disturbance is not caused exclusively by a lack of lubrication or vaginismus, another Axis I disorder (e.g., Somatization Disorder), and is not better accounted for by a Secondary Sexual Dysfunction due to an Axis III condition or Substance-induced Sexual Dysfunction.
C. The disturbance causes marked distress or interpersonal difficulty.

Vaginismus

No issues were identified. The B criterion will be altered to read as follows, and a C criterion will be added.

B. This disturbance is not due to another Axis I disorder (e.g., Somatization Disorder) and is not better accounted for by a Secondary Sexual Dysfunction due to an Axis III condition or a Substance-induced Sexual Dysfunction.
C. The disturbance causes marked distress or interpersonal difficulty.

SEXUAL AROUSAL DISORDERS

Female Arousal Disorders

Dr. Segraves noted the current criteria set is dependent upon a combination of objective and subjective criteria for diagnosis. The issues he identified were (1) vagueness and the extent of clinical judgment required to make the diagnosis, and (2) the requirement of a combination of subjective and objective criteria for the diagnosis in the absence of data that demonstrate these two response systems are correlated and constitute a part of the same syndrome. His literature review assessed the sufficiency of data to (1) operationally define the syndrome, and (2) determine whether the subjective and objective criteria are part of the same syndrome.

Because Dr. Segraves found a paucity of literature concerning these issues, he restated the issue: Is there sufficient research evidence for retaining the diagnostic category Female Sexual Arousal Disorder? He discovered the best data concerning the restated issue came from an unpublished data set. Because of the limited scientific data, he suggested three alternatives: (1) deletion of the term, (2) retention as is, and (3) modification of the diagnostic term to comply fully with tenth edition of the International Classification of Diseases (ICD-10). After much discussion, the majority of the Work Group favored a criteria set that restricts the definition of the disorder to include cases with physiological symptoms. This option provides ICD-10 compatibility parallel to the criteria for male erectile disorder and minimizes the

confusion for future studies. The new criteria set would read as follows:

A. Persistent or recurrent inability to attain or maintain an adequate lubrication-swelling response of sexual excitement until completion of the sexual activity.
B. Occurrence not exclusively during the course of another Axis I disorder (other than a Sexual Dysfunction), such as a Major Depression, and not better accounted for by a Secondary Sexual Dysfunction due to an Axis III condition or Substance-induced Sexual Dysfunction.
C. The disturbance causes marked distress or interpersonal difficulty.

Male Erectile Disorder

The issues identified were: (1) the current criteria set includes both objective and subjective symptoms, and (2) the broad definition of the objective criteria could result in data sets that were heterogeneous. The literature search found no evidence to suggest that the subjective criteria were ever used to make the diagnosis of male erectile disorder. In addition, there are no data to support a more precise definition of the objective criteria. The Work Group's recommendation is to return to the DSM-III criteria wording by deleting the subjective criteria. The criteria set would read as follows:

A. Persistent or recurrent inability to attain or maintain an adequate erection until completion of the sexual activity.
B. Occurrence not exclusively during the course of another Axis I disorder (other than a sexual dysfunction) such as Major Depression and not better account for by a Secondary Sexual Dysfunction due to an Axis III condition or Substance-induced Sexual Dysfunction.
C. The disturbance causes marked distress or interpersonal difficulty.

ORGASM DISORDERS

Inhibited Female Orgasm

The issues identified by Dr. Schover were: (1) Is the name of the disorder acceptable (are there physiological subtypes of female orgasm so that one type may be "inhibited" and another not)?; (2) Are there specific antecedents in terms of personality and behavior that discriminate between women with subtypes of the disorder?; and (3) Does subtyping explain variance in treatment outcome? Dr. Schover's literature reviews suggested that Female Orgasmic Disorder would be a more appropriate category name because the change would conform to the ICD-10 and because the assumption of a psychological "inhibition" of the reflex as causal to the disorder could not be scientifically supported. The research evidence was inadequate to justify subtyping female orgasmic disorders beyond dimensions of lifelong versus acquired, and generalized versus situational. Personality correlates of deficits in orgasmic capacity have not been studied adequately to propose changes for criteria sets.

The principle recommendations are the name of the disorder be changed to female orgasmic disorder. In addition, criterion A has been shortened, acknowledging that situational orgasmic problems can be differentiated from the normal range of female sexual functioning only by skilled clinical judgment. The directive in DSM-III-R, suggesting that a course of sex therapy might be necessary to make the diagnosis, is deleted because of its impracticality and circular nature. The proposed criteria take into account the evidence that women increase their ease of reaching orgasm and the range of sexual stimulation that triggers orgasm with both age and sexual experience. Finally, specific examples for the situational subtype have been proposed. The criteria set would read as follows:

A. Persistent or recurrent delay in or absence of orgasm following a normal sexual excitement phase. Women exhibit wide variability in the type or intensity of stimulation that triggers orgasm. The diagnosis of Situational Female Orgasmic Disorder should be based on the clinician's judgment that the woman's orgasmic capacity is less than would be reasonable for her age, sexual experience, and the adequacy of stimulation she receives.
B. Occurrence not exclusively during the course of another Axis I disorder (other than a sexual dysfunction), such as Major Depression and not better accounted for by a Secondary Sexual Dysfunction due to an Axis III condition or a Substance-induced Sexual Dysfunction.
C. The disturbance causes marked distress or interpersonal difficulty.
   Specified Subtype
   Generalized: Inorgasmic in all situations.
   Situational: E.g., orgasmic with self or vibrator stimulation, orgasmic only with partner noncoital stimulation but not in intercourse, inorgasmic with only a particular current partner.

Inhibited Male Orgasm

The issues associated with the term "inhibited" are similar to those discussed in the above section on female orgasm disorders. The literature review did not reveal empirical evidence to support the concept of psychological inhibition associated with male orgasm. The new term will be compatible with the manner in which clinicians and researchers identify the disorder in the literature and with the ICD-10. Also, it is recommended that criterion A be shortened by deleting an explanatory phase better placed in the text. The criteria set for male orgasm disorder would read as follows:

A. Persistent or recurrent delay in, or absence of, orgasm following a normal sexual excitement phase during sexual activity that is adequate in focus, intensity and duration.

B. Occurrence not exclusively during the course of another Axis I disorder (other than a Sexual Dysfunction), such as a Major Depression and not better accounted for by a Secondary Sexual Dysfunction due to an Axis III condition or Substance-induced Sexual Dysfunction.
C. The disturbance causes marked distress or interpersonal difficulty.

Premature Ejaculation

No issues were identified and a literature search was not done. A B criterion is proposed that reads "The disturbance causes marked distress or interpersonal difficulty."

PARAPHILIAS

No issues were identified with regard to exhibitionism, pedophilia, sexual masochism, sexual sadism, voyeurism, or fetishism. Because transvestic fetishism and gender dysphoria are recognized as common comorbid conditions, the issue of whether individuals with transvestic fetishism and gender dysphoria should be diagnosed as having transvestic fetishism–gender dysphoric type or as having gender identity disorder or receive two diagnoses, transvestic fetishism and gender identity disorder, was reviewed. The literature review revealed a frequent association of transvestic fetishism and gender dysphoria. In addition, the gender dysphoria is noted to be mild to moderate, and it waxes and wanes, and patients do not consistently seek surgical reassignment or make efforts to live in the cross-gender role. A new subcategory of transvestic fetishism is therefore proposed to allow the clinician to note the presence of subthreshold levels of gender dysphoria. If full criteria are met for gender identity disorder, that diagnosis takes precedence. The criteria set would read as follows:

Transvestic Fetishism

A. Over a period of six months, in a heterosexual male, recurrent intense sexual urges and sexually arousing fantasies involving cross dressing.
B. The person has acted upon these urges or is markedly distressed by them.
C. Does not meet the criteria for Gender Identity Disorder.
   Specified: With Gender Dysphoria in a person who is distressed by discomfort with gender role or identity.

Telephone Scatalogia

Because of the increased frequency with which telephone scatalogia (obscene phone calling) is being diagnosed, literature reviews were done to determine whether the diagnostic term should remain on a list of examples of paraphilias not otherwise specified or be listed as a distinct diagnosis with its own criteria set. The review revealed a substantial number of descriptive and anecdotal reports, and suggested that obscene phone callers may have other paraphilias. However, the incidence and prevalence could not be cited, and there are no systematic studies of the disorder. The recommendation is that the category telephone scatalogia be proposed for inclusion in the appendix of new categories needing further study. The criteria set proposed would read as follows:

A. Over a period of at least six months, recurrent and intense sexual urges and sexually arousing fantasies involving telephone calls to a nonconsenting individual in order to verbalize erotic or obscene language or to silently fantasize such material.
B. The individual has acted upon these urges or is markedly distressed by them.
C. The behavior is not restricted to episodic behavior undertaken with a group of peers that occurs during latency or adolescence.

Sexual Addiction

The second example of the criteria set for sexual disorders not otherwise specified currently includes the term "nonparaphilic sexual addiction." A literature review was completed to assess the validity of the concept of sexual addiction. The review revealed abundant clinical evidence of sexual activity that can be characterized as "excessive." However, there is no scientific data base to support the concept of excessive sexual behavior as being in the realm of an addiction. Therefore, it is being recommended that the term "sexual addiction" be deleted. The example would read as follows:

(2) Distress about a pattern of repeated sexual conquests involving a succession of people who exist only as things to be used

MISCELLANEOUS CHANGES

A recommendation is being made to add a diagnostic category, Secondary Sexual Dysfunction Due to an Axis III Disorder. The proposed diagnosis does not appear in DSM-III-R. It is suggested for inclusion in DSM-IV in order to facilitate the differential diagnosis of sexual dysfunctions. The codes will start with the letter N, indicating their placement in the Genitourinary section of the ICD-10. The criteria set will read as follows:

A. Sexual dysfunction that results in impairment in sexual functioning subjective to stress or interpersonal difficulty.
B. There is evidence from the history, physical examination, or laboratory findings of a general medical disorder that is thought to cause the sexual dysfunction.

The specific disorders listed will be secondary male erectile disorder, secondary dyspareunia, secondary vaginismus, other secondary male sexual dysfunction, and other secondary female sexual dysfunction.

The category substance-induced sexual disorder will also be recommended. This proposed diagnosis does not appear in DSM-III-R. It is suggested for inclusion in DSM-IV in order to facilitate the differential diagnosis of sexual dysfunctions. The criteria set will read as follows:

A. Sexual dysfunction that results in impairment in sexual functioning, subjective distress, or interpersonal difficulty.
B. There is evidence from the history, physical examination, or laboratory findings of substance use and that the symptoms in A developed during the use of this substance or within four to six weeks of the cessation of the substance use.
C. The disturbance is not better accounted for by a nonsubstance-induced sexual disorder. Evidence that the symptoms are better accounted for by a nonsubstance-induced sexual disorder might include: The symptoms precede the onset of the substance use, persist for greater than four to six weeks after the cessation of substance use, or are substantially in excess of what would be expected given the character, duration, or amount of the substance used.
Specified: (Specific substance), (Intoxication/Withdrawal/Persisting) Sexual Disorder. A list of specific substances will be included for each sexual dysfunction.

54

PARAPHILIAS

JOSEPH LoPICCOLO, Ph.D.

DEFINITION AND EPIDEMIOLOGY

Paraphilia refers to deviant sexual arousal of a compulsive nature. In one type of paraphilia, fetishism, the patient experiences sexual arousal to objects, persons, or situations that the average person does not find to be intrinsically erotic. Examples of this type of paraphilia include arousal to shoes, leather garments, or, in one of the author's cases, bicycle handlebars. Other fetishes include arousal in response to urination and defecation (urophilia and coprophilia), arousal to corpses (necrophilia), and arousal in situations involving physical restraints, pain, or humiliation (bondage and discipline, sadism, and masochism). Heterosexual transvestism, in which a man is aroused by dressing in women's clothing, is also an example of fetishism. Another type of paraphilia involves sexual behavior that the average person might find arousing but does not engage in because of moral values and the threat of negative social sanctions. Examples of this type of paraphilia include peeping (voyeurism) and exhibitionism. Other paraphilias involve assault, including pedophilia (sexual arousal to children), making obscene phone calls, frotteurism ("accidentally" bumping into or rubbing up against a woman's body in a crowded place), and some types of rape. Some paraphilias do not involve nonconsenting victims or fetishistic objects. For example, troilism involves a man who is aroused by watching his wife have intercourse with another man. Similarly, enough men are aroused by listening to descriptions of sexual activity to make the 900 number phone sex business highly profitable, so this activity qualifies as a paraphilia only if it is compulsively engaged in and preferred to actual sexual activity with a partner.

In all paraphilias, the defining characteristics are the compulsivity and preferential nature of the sexual activity. Exhibitionists, for example, will leave a willing sexual partner at home to go out to exhibit themselves. When the exhibitionist is arrested, the wife cannot believe that he would prefer this activity to sex with her, and, at most, may have only wondered if his absences from home meant he was having an affair with another woman.

Paraphilia is what might be called a "high-fidelity, narrow bandwidth, high-intensity" phenomenon. That is, paraphiliacs have a driven, focused, and compulsive quality to their deviant arousal. Because the probability of being arrested for paraphilia is very low, most paraphiliacs seen in treatment have been engaging in their deviant behavior for many years, and often have literally hundreds of offenses in their history other than the one for which they were finally arrested.[1]

The epidemiology of paraphilias is unknown, because typically only those paraphiliacs who are arrested for public offenses, or who are forced to seek treatment by spouses who are not willing to participate in a paraphiliac ritual, ever come to our attention. For most paraphiliacs, the disorder is ego syntonic, and they rationalize their deviance by considering our society to be extremely sexually repressed. Research has shown that around 15 to 20 per cent of women and 4 to 8 per cent of men report they were molested as children. If there are this many victims of just this one type of paraphilia, there must be many more paraphiliacs than either arrest statistics or clinical experience indicates.[2]

The overwhelming majority of paraphiliacs are men. Examples of fetishistic paraphilia, exhibitionism, or voyeurism in women are so rare as to be worthy of case reports in the professional literature. Over 95 per cent of pedophilia cases involve a male perpetrator.[2] For this reason, male gender pronouns are used to refer to paraphiliac patients throughout this chapter.

CLINICAL DESCRIPTION

The time course of paraphilias is variable in terms of onset. Many paraphiliacs first begin their deviant activity in middle adolescence, either in actual behavior or in masturbation fantasies. However, sudden onset in later life is not unknown, often in response to extreme stress, lack of a "normal" sexual outlet, or simply a new opportunity. For example, there are cases of men who were sexually normal until they discovered the 900 number phone sex service, but who then were so compulsively drawn to this activity that they went deep into debt to support this newly developed paraphilia. Spontaneous remission of paraphilias is extremely rare. Most patients continue until they are arrested or forced to seek treatment by a spouse. Some adolescent

339

paraphilias, such as exhibitionism, voyeurism, or frotteurism, do show spontaneous remission when the boy gains access to a female partner for normal sexual gratification, but other paraphiliacs continue the deviant activity after reaching adulthood and marrying.

The cause of paraphilia remains an area of theoretical speculation more than one founded in large amounts of empirical research data. While a full discussion of etiology is beyond the scope of this paper, a few comments can be made. There is certainly no evidence that there are any familial genetic factors involved in paraphilias. Research has not revealed any sex hormone or neurotransmitter abnormalities in paraphiliacs.[3] However, there is a small but intriguing literature that suggests an elevated rate of temporal lobe abnormalities in paraphiliacs, based on electroencephalography and sophisticated magnetic resonance, positron emission tomography and computed tomography imaging studies.[4] Sociologists and feminists have stressed that our male-dominated, double standard–oriented, and sexually repressive culture leads to paraphilia, as does the availability of pornography.[5] This reasoning ignores the fact that all men are raised in the same culture, but only a small percentage become paraphiliacs. Learning theorists stress the role of early "accidental conditioning" experiences, such as seeing a careless neighbor undressing without drawing the curtains, which are then reinforced by masturbation involving memories and fantasies about the event. Again, because such experiences are common in the life histories of men who do not become paraphiliacs, this explanation is, by itself, inadequate. It seems likely that paraphilias are complex, multiply determined conditions, and that any single-element theory of etiology is oversimplified and incorrect. Rather, we should realize that paraphilias clearly involve a host of factors, including arousal conditioned to inappropriate objects, lack of internalized moral values, inability to weigh long-term negative consequences against short-term sexual pleasure, distorted thinking about sexuality, lack of access to gratifying normal sexual outlets, lack of empathy for victim distress, disinhibition by alcohol or drugs, and, possibly, temporal lobe pathology. In individual cases, various combinations of these factors may be more or less important.

Differential diagnosis is not usually an issue in dealing with paraphiliac cases, with the exception of distinguishing heterosexual fetishistic transvestism from gender identity disturbances such as transsexualism. However, the clinician should be aware that there are co-deviations present in many paraphiliacs. The man who comes for treatment of a minor, "victimless" paraphilia may also be a pedophile or rapist; indeed, virtually all paraphiliacs have more than one deviation.[1] One of the author's recent patients, who came for court-mandated treatment because of making obscene telephone calls, later admitted to being a long-term voyeur, and was eventually arrested and convicted for an undisclosed rape and murder. The possibility of underestimating pathology is very real in dealing with paraphiliacs, because the combination of their behavior being both ego syntonic and illegal leads them invariably not to tell the clinician the whole truth about their deviations. It has become fairly standard to attempt to reduce reliance on patient self-report through psychophysiological assessment of arousal patterns.[1] In this procedure, patients are presented with a wide variety of deviant slide, videotape, or audiotape stimuli while erection responses are recorded with a penile plethysmograph. Penile response to normal adult erotic stimuli is used as a standard of comparison. While this procedure is of some use in identifying deviations the patient is initially unwilling to report, it is not foolproof. Patients can voluntarily suppress penile erection to deviant stimuli that they actually find to be highly arousing, the embarrassment present in the laboratory situation itself may interfere with deviant arousal, and an absence of erection to the normal stimuli may only indicate that the patient is put off by the laboratory situation, rather than that he is lacking in normal arousal. For these reasons, penile plethysmograph assessments should be interpreted with great care, and should never be used as a means of establishing the purported guilt or innocence of someone who is accused of a sex crime.

The ego syntonicity of most paraphilias leads patients to overstate therapeutic gains, and to resist or prematurely terminate treatment. Similarly, paraphilias are highly prone to relapse, even after apparently successful treatment, and need to be reassessed and perhaps retreated periodically following the intensive treatment stage of therapy. In one subtle form of resistance, patients will report, early in therapy, that they are losing their deviant sexual arousal and have become interested only in consensual sex with adult women. The probability of this being true so soon is extremely low. The clinician should be especially suspicious of statements that the patient has lost all interest in his deviant activity since, following his arrest, he has realized how bizarre and self-destructive his behavior is, and he no longer feels any deviant arousal. Even if the patient is telling the truth about his current feelings, this suppression is not lasting. Once the acute life crisis is resolved, deviant arousal typically returns in full force.

TREATMENT OF PARAPHILIAS

Biological Treatments

Paraphilias have been treated with neurosurgery in eastern European countries, primarily via temporal lobe ablations. Historically, castration was used to treat paraphilias, with some occasional usage continuing into the last decade. Both neurosurgery and castration must be considered extreme, imprecise treatments, with virtually no acceptable scientific evidence of their effectiveness.[6]

Neuroleptic agents, because of their effect of reducing sexual arousal (possibly related to elevated prolactin levels seen with these medications), have also been used to treat paraphilias. Thioridazine (Mellaril) has been the agent most commonly prescribed. Effectiveness of this treatment is not established in empirical research, but clinical reports suggest that perhaps 50 to 70 per cent of patients have a moderate reduction in arousal, and hence, reduced interest in paraphiliac activities. The long-term risk of tardive dyskinesia, as well a short-term effects of drowsiness, neuromuscular spasms, tremors, restlessness, dry mouth, constipation, blurred vision, and so forth, are real issues in the use of neuroleptic agents. Additionally, Mellaril does not specifically reduce only deviant arousal, so if a therapeutic response is obtained, the patient's normal sexual functioning with a wife or lover will also be compromised.[6]

More effective, and more commonly used, is treatment with hormones that deplete testosterone levels and, with some agents, also block end-organ response to testosterone. Cyproterone acetate is widely used in Europe and Canada, but is not approved for use in the United States, where medroxyprogesterone acetate (Depo-Provera) is the agent of choice. Typical dosage is 200 to 300 mg intramuscularly every 2 weeks, but testosterone assays must be relied upon to find a dosage that is effective for the individual patient. Some clinicians recommend reduction of testosterone to prepubertal values of less than 100 ng/dl, whereas others suggest a reduction to 50 per cent of the patient's baseline level, provided this is found to be in the normal range.[5,6]

Considerable research evidence indicates that these agents are effective in reducing or suppressing sexual arousal, sexual fantasies, and nocturnal penile tumescence, but somewhat less effective in reducing penile erection in response to laboratory presentation of erotic stimuli such as videotapes or slides. Normal sexual functioning with the wife is also typically disrupted, but some patients report that this is an acceptable trade-off for being freed of the problematic deviant sexual urges. Side effects include an almost universal weight gain and, less commonly, lethargy, depression, headaches, and feminization effects such as breast development and changes in voice pitch and body hair distribution. There is also the possibility that long-term effects in terms of liver damage or elevated rates of steroid-dependent cancer will be discovered in the future, as data become available from patients who have been maintained on these drugs over time. Current thinking is that the best use of hormonal treatment is relatively short term, to reduce the risk of re-offending during the early stages of psychotherapeutic treatment, especially in cases in which a recurrence would involve harm to a victim. Another valid use of Depo-Provera is in cases of sexual compulsivity at very high levels. For example, a patient who is currently masturbating with paraphiliac fantasies several times per day, engaging in paraphiliac acts such as 900 number phone sex at a high rate, or obsessively ruminating with paraphiliac thoughts throughout the day is extremely unlikely to respond to the behavioral and psychotherapeutic techniques to be discussed later in this chapter. While conceptualizing these patients as "sexual addicts"[7] and referring them to a group such as Sexaholics Anonymous or Sex and Love Addicts Anonymous may be useful, there is certainly much more empirical evidence to support the use of Depo-Provera in reducing sexual compulsivity or addiction to a level where other therapeutic interventions become possible.

Recently, there has been considerable interest in the treatment of paraphilias with the new serotonergic antianxiety/antidepressant agents such as Prozac. While double-blind, placebo-controlled studies are lacking, initial clinical results are somewhat encouraging, and further study seems warranted.

Psychological Treatments

It is important to recognize that all of our available treatment outcome research indicates that standard, unfocused psychotherapy is of limited value in treating paraphilia. It does not matter if the approach is Rogerian, existential, psychoanalytical, rational-emotive, or whatever. While this "nontechnological" type of psychotherapy may be *necessary* for most patients, it is not *sufficient* to effect treatment return. The use of specific technology to deal with the issues peculiar to paraphilia is also necessary.

The clinician must always remember that patients coming for treatment of paraphilia are more motivated to remain out of prison or escape from a current life crisis than they are to change their deviant sexuality. Thus, therapy must be prefaced by attempts to build some rapport with the patient, gain the patient's trust, and help him to realize that it is in his own interest to give up his paraphilia. In dealing with patients under legal sanctions, the therapist can point out that by not fully cooperating in treatment, the patient is guaranteeing that treatment will fail, and, with any re-offense, he faces the possibility of years in prison. Patients who are in therapy at the insistence of their wives can be reminded of impending divorces, loss of their children, and the financial and social standing losses to which their paraphilia makes them vulnerable.

In working on an outpatient basis, there is the issue of temporary control of the patient's deviant behavior until psychotherapy begins to take effect. To aid in this temporary control, there are a number of strategies that can be used. If the patient's sexual acting out is associated with alcohol abuse, as is true in many cases, the therapist should use all available resources, such as Antabuse treatment, Alcoholics Anonymous, and monitoring by family members, to keep the patient from drinking. For patients whose offenses are related to psychopathology, appropriate medication should be prescribed. As was previously discussed, in cases of truly compulsive sexual behavior, the use of Depo-Provera should be considered. The clinician should insist on immediate changes in the patient's life structure that reduce the opportunity to engage in deviant activity. This means, for example, that a pedophiliac must immediately terminate any job, social, or recreational activities that give him access to children, and exhibitors and voyeurs must not be allowed unsupervised time away from home and job settings. Obviously, the cooperation of significant others in the patient's life in enforcing these contracted changes is essential, and the patient's typical wish not to have others know of his problem must be challenged. Similarly, in the case of paraphiliac incest, the father must be required to leave the home and reside separately during the initial stages of treatment. These strategies will reduce the risk of a recurrence during the early stages of treatment. Because the therapist is, in a sense, responsible for the patient's behavior, if the paraphilia includes violence, extreme coercion, or other dangerous and harmful behaviors, outpatient treatment is not indicated initially. Rather, an extensive course of therapy should first occur in a secure inpatient facility; for some extreme paraphilias, such as rape-murder, it is debatable whether outpatient treatment is ever appropriate, as opposed to permanent incarceration.

The treatment of paraphilia is multifaceted. Paraphalias are not just operantly reinforced or classically conditioned deviant sexual arousal, nor are they just a lack of social skills with adult women, nor are they merely anxiety- and stress-reducing mechanisms, and so forth. For most cases, all of the treatment technologies described in the following sections will be useful in varying degrees.

Behavioral Reconditioning Procedures

A central element in treatment of paraphilia is the reduction or elimination of deviant sexual arousal through behavioral reconditioning procedures. In the early years of behavior therapy, reconditioning was attempted with electric shock aversion therapy, but this procedure was not found to be very effective. The major techniques currently used are masturbatory satiation and covert sensitization with olfactory aversion.[5,6]

In masturbatory satiation, the paraphiliac arousal is reduced by continuing exposure to the deviant stimuli after the patient is sexually satiated. In this procedure, the patient is instructed to go home and masturbate with normal fantasies and erotic stimuli such as Playboy or Penthouse centerfolds, books of erotic fantasies, and so forth. The patient verbalizes normal fantasies and descriptions of what he is looking at or reading, and uses a cassette tape recorder so the therapist can review the fantasies and make sure

that they do not contain any subtle paraphiliac elements. The patient uses the normal stimulus material, and verbalizes normal fantasies, until he ejaculates and for a minute or so thereafter, until he loses his erection and enters the refractory period, during which further masturbation is unpleasant. At this point, he switches to fantasizing or reading aloud about his paraphiliac behavior, while he continues to masturbate for an additional 45 minutes to 1 hour, with a flaccid penis. His speech during this phase is also tape recorded for therapeutic review. In a typical case, the patient will ejaculate within 5 or 10 minutes of masturbation with normal stimuli, and then have a very unpleasant, boring, and physically uncomfortable experience while focused on his formerly exciting paraphiliac fantasies and memories. If the patient gets a second erection while verbalizing deviant fantasies, he switches back to normal stimuli and fantasies until he ejaculates again, and then returns to masturbation with deviant fantasies.

A complication arises for patients whose paraphilia is very powerful, and who cannot become erect or ejaculate with normal fantasies and stimuli. In these cases, the patient begins to masturbate with his deviant images, but switches to normal fantasies and stimuli as soon as he is aroused. If erection is lost, he can switch back to deviant stimuli until erection is regained, but he must switch again so that his ejaculation always occurs in the context of looking at, reading about, and verbalizing about normal sexual stimuli. Married paraphiliac patients who were not masturbating prior to entering therapy may conduct their satiation by having intercourse with their wives and, following ejaculation, immediately going into another room, turning on their tape recorder, and masturbating with deviant fantasies for an additional 45 minutes or so. Masturbatory satiation is typically carried out by the patient two to five times per week, for 1 to 3 months. This procedure can be discontinued when the patient has no intrusive paraphiliac thoughts or urges for at least 2 successive weeks. If the procedure is working, the patient often becomes mildly depressed, feeling a sense of loss of his previously exciting and gratifying paraphilia.

A second procedure used to eliminate deviant arousal is covert sensitization with olfactory aversion. Covert sensitization is not used to reduce actual arousal and orgasmic responses to paraphiliac stimuli (the satiation procedure accomplishes this), but rather is used to disrupt and suppress paraphiliac urges, thoughts, and images that precede actual paraphiliac sexual arousal and behavior. In this procedure, the patient generates a list of all the situations in which he would be at risk to commit his paraphiliac behavior. A second list of the possible negative consequences of his behavior is also generated, including items such as loss of job, rejection by family and friends, humiliation, and harm to a victim. The patient picks one of the risk situations, closes his eyes, visualizes the situation, and briefly elaborates on it aloud, until he begins to feel some slight arousal. At this point, he exhales fully, and then takes a deep breath while inhaling a noxious substance such as ammonia or valeric acid. The patient then immediately visualizes and verbally elaborates on one of the negative consequence scenarios. This procedure is done during therapy sessions and the patient also does sessions at home, daily. In addition, whenever he finds himself spontaneously experiencing a paraphiliac thought or urge, he immediately inhales an ammonia capsule and visualizes and verbalizes an aversive consequence.

To illustrate a typical use of these techniques, the situations that cue off deviant urges and the list of aversive consequences for Mr. A, a patient with the paraphilia of exhibiting himself to children, are shown in Tables 54–1 and 54–2. In Table 54–1, the situations are listed in descending order of likelihood of him exhibiting himself.

There are several other aversive techniques sometimes used to reduce deviant arousal. In *shame aversion therapy*, the patient actually engages in his paraphiliac behavior in the therapist's office, with the therapist, wife, and other appropriate significant others observing and expressing the revulsion, disgust, and sadness they feel. This procedure is most typically used with exhibitionists and fetishistic transvestites. In *negative practice*, the patient may be required to spend hours repetitiously engaging in his paraphiliac ritual, until extreme boredom is experienced. *Taste aversion*, using foul-tasting or even emetic drugs to produce vomiting, is sometimes used in conjunction with covert sensitization, instead of the ammonia procedure described above. All of these procedures are extreme, and it is difficult to get patients to consent to them. Given that masturbatory satiation and olfactory-aided covert sensitization are effective, these other techniques are not often used.

Relapse Prevention Training

The other major technology that is used in treating paraphilia is relapse prevention training.[8] Relapse prevention training has several elements. One element involves having the patient identify life situations, emotional states, and stimulus cues that elicit his deviant urges. The patient is then taught avoidance and escape strategies for these high-risk situations, and for situations that he cannot avoid or from which he cannot immediately escape, he is taught alternative coping responses to replace the paraphiliac behavior. A second element involves having the patient identify Seemingly Irrelevant Decisions (SIDs) that initially seem unrelated to his paraphilia but actually are the first steps in a chain of events that lead to acting out. For example, one patient's decision to stop for a drink on the way home from work may seem irrelevant to his voyeurism. In this patient's case, however, doing so reliably provokes his wife into an argument with him, leading her to refuse to have sex with him that night. Unable to sleep, he would next make the seemingly irrelevant decision to go out for coffee. During this trip, he would then "impulsively" engage in peeping. Relapse prevention teaches the patient that paraphiliac acts are not engaged in impulsively. Rather, when he decided to stop for a drink on the way home from work, he knew the result would be feelings of resentment about what he sees as his wife's nagging, which, combined with his job stress and his sexual frustration, justify his voyeurism in his own mind.

Another element of relapse prevention training involves what is termed the Abstinence Violation Effect (AVE). During and following treatment, patients will, of course, occasionally experience brief urges or fantasies about their paraphilia. This constitutes only a manageable "lapse," but patients typically

TABLE 54–1. MR. A's RISK SITUATION LIST: CUES FOR EXHIBITING TO CHILDREN

Location	Cues
In the car	Attractive girl with long brown hair, at street corner, about 13 years old wearing a skirt and knee socks. There is no one else around. I am alert and have erection. The girl shows an interest.
In the car	Girl with short blonde hair, at corner, not very attractive, about 13 years old. I am hung over—no erection. There is no one else around. The girl shows an interest.
In the car	Several girls at the corner. I am alert and have an erection. There is no one else around. The girls show an interest.
In the car	Girl with short blonde hair, not very attractive, in middle of block. No one else around. I am alert and have an erection. Girl shows an interest.
In the car	Attractive girl with skirt and knee socks, in middle of block. No one else around. I am alert and have erection. Girl turns away from car.
In the car	Attractive brown-haired girl, at corner, about 13 years old wearing a skirt. There is a car behind me. I am not very alert, no erection.
In the car	Mixed boys and girls in middle of block. No one else around. I am alert and have erection.
In parking lot	Girl about 10–11 years old alone in a car. Space next to her car empty. No one else around. I am alert and have erection. Girl shows an interest.
In parking lot	Girl about 10–11 years old alone in car. Space next to her car empty. No one else around. I am alert and have an erection. Girl runs from her car.
In parking lot	Attractive girl alone by wall. No one else near by. I am hung over, no erection. The girl runs away from the car.
At a party	Attractive young girl about 10 years old near bathroom window (outside). I am alert and have an erection. No one else around. Girl shows an interest.
At a party	Attractive girl about 10 years old wearing a skirt and knee socks, near bathroom door. Other adults in the area.

TABLE 54–2. Mr. A's LIST OF AVERSIVE CONSEQUENCES

At a party

1. Caught by adult—spreads like wildfire to other adults; caught by female adult—somebody I know—by friend's wife; they stone me—throw me out.
2. They call police.
3. Girl's father punches me out.
4. Wife knows. Very embarrassed; gets up and leaves me there—breaks down, weeps and cries, goes in kitchen, cuts her wrists.
5. Girl screams, runs away, weeps.
6. Fear of person telling parent—stomach knots up, but doesn't knot up to the point of me vomiting.

In a parking lot

1. Parent comes back to car during event, my car blocked, can't get away, they get my license number.
2. Child runs from my car and gets hit by car—I see her bleeding.
3. Parent returns and confronts me directly.
4. Security patrol or police catch me—arrested, taken to jail.
5. Run into child again, she points me out as person who exhibited.
6. Car won't go—stuck there.

In my car/street

1. Car breaks down, I'm stuck there—girl complains.
2. She takes down my license number, is clearly going to remember it.
3. Girl runs off frantically, crying—hit by car, I see her die.
4. Parent looking from house, sees event, gets car description and license plate number.
5. Neighborhood group stops the car, attacks the car and gets me.
6. Police get me.

Nonspecifics

1. Final rejection by father/sister/in-laws.
2. Losing job—losing house, having to move.
3. Learn to live at lower economic level.
4. Marital problems—wife leaves.
5. Children problems—cut back on vacations, less good things.
6. Daughter—disappointed in me.
7. Six-year-old son—favorite child—he finds out.
8. Wife kills self—cuts wrists.
9. Children teased at school—"Your old man's a wienie wagger."

feel that they have experienced a major "relapse" and thus are no longer abstinent from their paraphilia. They then reason that since they have already relapsed, there is no hope, and they might as well actually engage in their paraphiliac behavior. This reasoning constitutes the AVE. Relapse prevention training stresses that involuntary thoughts are only lapses, and that actual relapse behavior is subject to voluntary control. Patients are taught to view lapses as an opportunity to learn more about themselves, identify new high-risk situations of which they were not aware, find new coping strategies for dealing with whatever cued the lapse, and not see a lapse as a sign of impending doom or an excuse to act on a deviant urge. It is important for the patient not to allow himself to dwell on deviant thoughts, become highly aroused, or masturbate, because of what is called the Problem of Immediate Gratification (PIG). "Feeding the PIG" refers to the immediate pleasure that occurs when the patient allows himself to have an extended lapse, even if this only involves fantasies and "harmless" masturbation, as opposed to actually going out and peeping, for example. The pleasure is real and immediate, and self-destructive consequences are only future possibilities that may never arrive. Feeding the PIG both reinforces deviant arousal and exacerbates the AVE. Instead of feeding the PIG, the patient is taught self-control strategies such as leaving the situation, calling a friend, using olfactory aversion and covert sensitization, and so forth.

Patients typically write up a Relapse Prevention Manual, listing high-risk situations to be avoided, alternative coping responses, ways to prevent the Abstinence Violation Effect, and strategies for dealing with the Problem of Immediate Gratification. A very brief selection from the Relapse Prevention Manual of a paraphiliac who makes obscene telephone calls to children is shown in Table 54–3.

Other Therapeutic Procedures

As previously noted, paraphilias are complex, multiply determined phenomena. While reducing deviant arousal and relapse prevention constitute the core of current therapy, there are a host of other procedures used to meet individual patients needs. For patients who are too shy, inhibited, and unskilled to be able to make contact with adults for normal sexual relationships, a course of *social skills training* is usually undertaken. This procedure involves modeling and roleplaying of normal social interactions with the client.[9]

Most married sex offenders claim they have an adequate sexual relationship with their wives, and that sexual frustration is not an element in their motivation to commit offenses, but this is generally untrue. Sexual activity with the wife is typically stereotyped, infrequent, narrowly focused on penile-vaginal intercourse, and lacking in playful, erotic, unrestrained activity. For most married paraphiliacs, a course of *sex therapy* is indicated, focusing more on sexual enhancement and reducing sexual inhibitions in both the patient and his wife than on the elimination of a specific dysfunction.[10]

Some paraphiliacs feel a profound relief from tension and feelings of inadequacy when they engage in their paraphiliac ritual. Often, these are men who are lacking in assertive skills, and so feel powerless and abused by others. For example, an exhibitor who feels he is unjustly criticized at work may be especially likely to exhibit later that day. For these patients, a course of *assertiveness training* to increase self-efficacy and a course of *relaxation training* for stress and tension reduction are indicated.[5]

Most paraphiliacs have a variety of *cognitive distortions* that are intimately related to their deviant behavior. Rapists commonly believe a set of "rape

TABLE 54—3. MR. B's RELAPSE PREVENTION MANUAL FOR ONE HIGH-RISK SITUATION[a]

High-Risk Situation

Staying alone too long in my apartment.

Lapse: Problem of Immediate Gratification—Flash Fantasies

Bringing happiness to young girls.
Fantasizing about submissive young girls doing what I tell them to do sexually.

Relapse Action

Calling random phone numbers to talk about sex with teenage girls.

Alternative Coping Behavior

Just simply leaving the dwelling—go play tennis, visit a friend, etc.
Find an AA or NA meeting and go.
Get a *healthy* roommate.
Read.

Problem of Immediate Gratification—Dealing with Flash Fantasies

Try to leave immediate location.
Call my Probation Officer if possible.
Call up friend for tennis match.
Practice hobby immediately.
Use ammonia and think of my legal problems and my divorce.
See the urge as a wave that crests, then resides. I will handle this.
Close my eyes and visualize myself dealing successfully with controlling and not feeding the PIG. See a wave cresting and then disappearing.

Relapse Actions—What To Do if I Start on a Relapse

Do ammonia and negative consequence cards immediately.
Call Probation Officer or therapist, be honest.
Leave environment immediately.
Open notebook, read this manual.
Unplug phone, lock in trunk of car.
Call support network.

Patterns of Abuse

Planned my day's activities to be able to use phone in midafternoon, when kids are home from school but parents are not.
Planned to be alone (always).

Coping Responses for Patterns of Abuse

Visualize myself getting through this temporary urge.
If that fails, take ammonia and do negative consequence visualization.
Organize other activities for afternoons, such as fishing, tennis, library, practice, etc.
See the urge as a wave that has already crested, and is now ready to subside.
Do not feed this PIG; control him.
I am 39 years old. Think about the responsibilities I have to myself and others. Deal with my age. Act it.
Unplug phone or remove myself from room where the phone is.

List of Social Support People To Call

Probation officer, therapist, mother, Alcoholics Anonymous, Narcotics Anonymous, five different friends

---

[a] Mr. B's manual included several other high-risk situations, such that his actual manual was more than 20 pages long.

myths," including beliefs that women want to be raped and enjoy the rape experience. Pedophiles have a similar set of distorted cognitions, such as the belief that sex between an adult and a child is good for the child, and that children can consent to have sex with an adult and thus are not being "molested." Patients with fetishistic arousal often think of themselves merely as sexually liberated, rather than as deviant. In all these cases, the therapist addresses these defensive cognitive distortions and helps the patient to see himself and his paraphilia in a realistic way.[5]

Working on cognitive distortion leads naturally into a *sex education* component of therapy. Most paraphiliacs know very little about the realities of sexual functioning and about emotional and sexual relationships between adult men and women. This education can occur through discussion with the therapist, but is more efficiently done by having the patient enroll in a community college course, read and write summaries of appropriate-level sex education books, and view educational films and videos.

CONCLUSION

It is apparent that the treatment of sex offenders is a complex, multifaceted, and long-term process. For most paraphilias, treatment is indicated for a minimum of 6 months to 1 year, on a weekly basis. After completion of this intensive therapy, follow-up sessions once every 2 weeks or once a month should be conducted for the next year, with "checkups" every 3 to 6 months for the next several years. There is a strong tendency for the patient to underreport his deviation and overreport his social, sexual, and general life adjustment at these follow-ups, so thorough reevaluation with interviewing of significant others in the patient's life, psychophysiological assessment, wife's report on their sexual relationship, and formal psychometric testing will be needed, rather than just relying on patient self-report. Even following comprehensive treatment as described above, there is a significant relapse rate for paraphilias.[11] However, for untreated paraphiliacs, the relapse rate is probably 100 per cent, even following long jail sentences. Paraphiliacs who have been imprisoned report that, without access to adult women, they masturbated using paraphiliac fantasies and memories during the prison term, and, in so doing, intensified and reinforced their deviant arousal. Unless we are willing to tolerate repeated sexual offenses, or to jail our sexually deviant citizens for life, we have no alternative but to provide comprehensive treatment.

REFERENCES

1. Abel GG, Becker JV, Cunningham-Rathner J., et al: Multiple paraphiliac diagnoses among sex offenders. Bull Am Acad Psychiatry 16:153—168, 1988.
2. Finklehor D, Lewis I: An epidemiologic approach to the

study of child molestation. Ann NY Acad Sci 528:64–77, 1988.

3. Hucker SJ, Bain J: Androgenic hormones and sexual assault. *In* Marshal WL, Laws DR, Barbaree HE, eds. Handbook of Sexual Assault. New York: Plenum Press, 1990:93–102.

4. Langevin R: Sexual anomalies and the brain. *In* Marshal WL, Laws DR, Barbaree HE, eds. Handbook of Sexual Assault. New York: Plenum Press, 1990:103–113.

5. Marshal WL, Laws DR, Barbaree HE, eds. Handbook of Sexual Assault. New York: Plenum Press, 1990.

6. Maletzky BM: Treating the Sexual Offender. Newbury Park, CA: Sage Publications, 1991.

7. Carnes P: The Sexual Addiction. Minneapolis: Comp Care, 1984.

8. Laws DR: Relapse Prevention with Sex Offenders. New York: Guilford Press, 1991.

9. Hollon CR, Trower P: Handbook of Social Skills Training. Oxford, England: Pergamon Press, 1986.

10. LoPiccolo J: Treatment of sexual dysfunction. *In* Bellak AS, Hersen M, Kazdin AE, eds: International Handbook of Behavior Modification and Therapy. 2nd. ed. New York: Plenum Press, 1990.

11. Furby L, Weinrott MR, Blackshaw L: Sex offender recidivism: A review. Psychol Bull 105:3–30, 1988.

55

SEXUAL DYSFUNCTIONS

JULIA R. HEIMAN, PH.D.

Sexual dysfunctions can, and do, occur under a wide variety of conditions and to a similarly broad range of individuals. While precise prevalence figures for sexual dysfunctions are impossible to determine because of the inherent bias in research samples composed of people who volunteer to respond to surveys with sexual contents, estimates of prevalence are available and will be mentioned by diagnosis. In general, it appears that a majority of people, at least in Western industrial cultures where such data are available, at some point in their lives experience a transitory sexual dysfunction, and more enduring sexual disorders may affect at least 50 per cent of marriages and an unknown percentage of gay and lesbian relationships. The number of individuals who may complain to a professional of sexual problems is far lower, however.

The sexual dysfunctions discussed here are almost exclusively restricted to those identified in the DSM-III-R.[1] These include primary sexual disorders of desire, arousal, orgasm, and pain, with brief mention of sexual disorders secondary to Axis III (physical disorders and conditions) and substance use. The issue of primary versus secondary disorders raises the general challenge of describing the etiological features of sexual problems. While a multitude of specific factors have been proposed, and several general models offered, there are no conclusive etiological pathways that definitively account for sexual dysfunction. There are, however, several major categories that summarize and organize what is known about determinants of sexual difficulties. These include:

1. *Neurophysiological factors:* Any illness, disease, drug, or medication that affects neurological or vascular functioning can compromise sexual functioning as well. The normal aging process as it affects neurophysiology has some influence on sexual functioning, although usually not leading to a true dysfunction until very late in the life cycle.[2–4]

2. *Psychosocial factors:* Subcultural (religious) and cultural influences, plus personal history events including exposure to traumatic sexual experiences, sexual abuse, family management of affection and intimacy, sexual history, prior relationships, current self-esteem, gender role satisfaction, and sexual orientation comfort, influence the degree to which a person values and enjoys sexual feelings and can tolerate sexual partners. In addition, anxiety and anger appear to have usually negative but occasional facilitative effects on sexual arousal.[5–7]

3. *Interpersonal, relationship factors:* Current degree of interactional fit in attachment, commitment, conflict, and control in a relationship, plus the history of its fortunes and misfortunes, all influence sexual functioning. While not all relationships require an adequate and happy sex life, most people expect some sexual contact as part of an ongoing love relationship.

These general areas should help guide clinical exploration and treatment planning. In asking questions related to sexual functioning, the clinician needs to be direct but aware of possible patient discomfort. Most patients will also detect an interviewer's discomfort or disinterest. The clinician needs to believe that sexual dysfunctions can be important, in some cases because they trouble the patient's sense of adequacy or because they feel threatening to a relationship, and in other cases because, although not life threatening in and of themselves, they may be symptoms or consequences of life-threatening conditions (cardiac problems, depression, drug side effects). In some cases, patients will avoid taking medications (e.g., for blood pressure management, depression) because of their negative sexual side effects, although they may not tell their physician that is the reason.

SEXUAL DESIRE DISORDERS

Hypoactive Sexual Desire

Diagnosis and Evaluation

Hypoactive sexual desire is marked by persistent or recurring lack of sexual fantasies and desire for sexual activities, not accounted for by an Axis III disorder (illness or medication related), substance abuse (alcohol or frequent cannabis use), or an Axis I disorder (most commonly depressive disorders). This disorder can occur with another sexual dysfunction. Age, sex, and context must be taken into account, as should the disorder's global versus situational and lifelong versus not lifelong occurrence. Clearly this diagnosis is very subjective, since there are no norms for sexual desire. Usually patients complain of hypoactive desire because it has become troubling to their current relationship. In most clinical settings desire problems seem to have increased over the past two decades, with 30 to 50 per cent of patient in sex therapy clinics receiving this diagnosis.[8,9] Usually low desire rates are higher in women than in men in the United States and Europe.[10]

The individual psychological aspects of desire that need to be assessed include the patient's sexual script about what he or she "should be" experiencing,[11] as well as any changes accompanying the loss of desire that might have contributed to a decreased sense of self-worth, self-esteem, or well-being. Examples of the latter can include typical social milestones such as retirement or children leaving home, or sudden traumas such as economic hardship, the threat of job loss, unusual or exacerbated stress, sexual abuse or the recovering of memories of sexual abuse, an affair, and death or illness in the immediate or original family. Additionally, the psychological effects of aging can be as significant as the physical facts. Individuals can begin to feel increasingly unattractive with age and thus less comfortable with being and feeling sexual.

Equally important determinants of hypoactive sexual desire are relationship factors, in particular problems with unresolved conflict, attachment issues, territoriality, and trust. The more common relationship scenarios include ongoing resentments over past transgressions (as with a spouse of a recovering alcoholic, the effects of an affair), the gradual erosion of mutual interests and common values, a change in one partner either in a positive (promotion) or negative (passed over for promotion) direction, and ongoing, easily evoked hostility that appears wedded to an inability to solve differences. In these contexts, decreased desire can appear to be a passive-aggressive response in one partner to the angry or controlling moves in the other. Neither person in fact feels powerful enough to change the situation and thus each remains stuck and resentful. Both partners are often equally stuck and equally fearful of giving up their current strategies.

Treatment

Hypoactive sexual desire is not easily treated, and with some exceptions seems to have a somewhat lower treatment success rate than the other sexual dysfunctions. For example, a random survey of sex therapists and counselors reported that fewer than 50 per cent of low sexual desire patients reported a successful treatment outcome.[8] The heterogeneity of this diagnosis in fact seems to preclude any truly confident estimate of treatment outcome. Factors that make improvement easier are (1) the absence of a primary/global sexual desire disorder, (2) a concomitant sexual dysfunction in males who complain of low sexual interest, and (3) strong commitment to the relationship.[12]

The appropriate treatment depends upon the outcome of the evaluation of a patient's developmental, psychosocial, and health history. If a patient is found to have a primary (lifelong) and/or global (cross-situation) low desire, the first step is a medical screening in which endocrine factors (e.g., testosterone, follicle-stimulating hormone, luteinizing hormone, prolactin), disease, and current medications are reviewed and corrected if necessary. Testosterone injections have probably been overused for men; however, they can have a positive effect if testosterone levels are low and a very short-term effect if testosterone levels are normal, probably because of a placebo response. Interestingly, little attention has been given to the use of testosterone (when combined with estrogen to maintain vaginal integrity) on postmenopausal women. Research on surgically hysterectomized and oophorectomized patients has demonstrated testosterone's role in increasing the sexual desire and arousal of these women.[13]

Should there be no medical disorder and the diagnosis is secondary or situational low desire, treatment can proceed with either individual or couple[9,14] therapy. If there is an ongoing additional sexual dysfunction (e.g., dyspareunia or erectile dysfunction) that preceded the desire problem, it may need treatment first. Treatment for low desire cases has included cognitive-behavioral, systemic, and psychodynamic approaches. A controlled treatment study has not been published yet. We can expect that no one treatment approach will emerge as superior given the remarkable heterogeneity included under this disorder. With no subclassification currently available, differential treatment effectiveness is unknown.

Chemical treatments in the form of folk medicine (e.g., rhino horn, yohimbine), recreational substances (e.g., cocaine, alcohol), and more recently medications (antidepressants, dopamine agonists) all seem to carry more of a placebo effect than a true drug effect.[15] Again, there may be a small subgroup, so far not described, for whom some of these options will work.

Sexual Aversion Disorder

Diagnosis and Evaluation

Sexual aversion describes a specific persistent or recurrent extreme aversion to and avoidance of genital sexual contact with a partner. It is differentiated from hypoactive sexual desire disorder by its strong negative emotional valence. It is expected that sexual aversion does not occur secondary to other Axis I disorders, except for other sexual dysfunctions.

This is a rather rare disorder, occurring most often in women, and is usually accompanied by low sexual desire and occasionally by dyspareunia or vaginismus. It normally does not require a medical evaluation unless pain is reported. It does require a thorough individual and relationship history. Typical historical factors include a history of sexual or physical abuse and/or extensive resentment and anger, often unexpressed, in the relationship.

Treatment

The treatment approach is dependent on the factors that the patient and clinician agree are maintaining the pattern. A combination of individual and couple therapy can be useful, with therapeutic ingredients including options for cognitive and behavior relaxation techniques, systematic (imagery and in vivo) desensitization, working through past abuse issues, and understanding the role of the aversion in the past and present. Couple therapy can work out conflict areas, emotional differences, and control issues, while a sex therapy approach permits genitals gradually to become less negative. It is difficult to have an impact on severe aversion, especially if it is of longstanding duration, and this can take longer than other dysfunction to change. Although there are no outcome statistics available on this disorder, it makes sense to estimate the therapy duration and its success to be at least comparable to those for hypoactive sexual desire disorder.

SEXUAL AROUSAL DISORDERS

Female Sexual Arousal Disorder

Diagnosis and Evaluation

Sexual arousal disorder in women is identified as the persistent and recurrent failure to attain or maintain an adequate (genital) lubrication-swelling response of sexual excitement until the completion of sexual activity. One must rule out Axis I (especially mood disorders), Axis III (e.g., menopause), or substance-induced sexual dysfunction that might better account for the condition. However, other sexual dysfunctions may occur simultaneously.

This is a rather rare complaint for women, unless it is secondary to menopause symptoms, dyspareunia, or orgasmic disorder. Although the DSM-IV will not regard the lack of subjective sense of arousal as a criterion for this disorder, it is essential to ask the patient this in order to get a sense as to how much the lack of physical arousal inhibits psychological arousal or vice versa. Physical and self-reported arousal do not necessarily correlate well, especially in women.[6] Also, it is useful to know if the patient's subjective experience is to chase arousal, passively wait, or feel detached.

Special attention must be paid to ruling out possible physical reasons for lubrication problems, the most likely being menopause or medication. To examine psychological factors, a careful sexual history is needed with attention to messages about sex being disgusting, unfeminine, or sinful, as well as experiences that may have encouraged her not to become sexual aroused, including trauma or being abandoned or psychologically abused in prior relationships. Current attitudes toward sex and feelings toward the partner, both positive and negative, need review. A woman who is very fearful, for example, may not lubricate as well. In addition, the relationship satisfaction, the partner's attitude toward sex, sexual behavior, and techniques currently used can be important.

Treatment

The treatment effectiveness for this disorder is essentially unknown because it is so rarely treated in exclusion of orgasm or pain disorders. If the arousal problem *is* secondary to another sexual dysfunction, treatment strategies should deal with arousal in the context of those primary disorders (to be discussed). Occasionally lubrication can be corrected by simply encouraging couples to use a water-soluble lubricant (e.g., K-Y jelly). Many patients do not try this on their own because it feels "unnatural." Reassurance, with respect to differing lubrication capacity, can be helpful.

Cognitive-behavioral techniques can be offered to help the woman relax, accept sexual stimulation, tolerate arousal feelings, and let past experiences lose their power to interfere with becoming aroused, and, with the woman who has a partner, discuss educational issues about variations in arousal techniques and assumptions about each person's role in the sexual interaction.

Male Erectile Disorder

Diagnosis and Evaluation

Erectile disorders refer to the persistent or recurrent inability to attain or maintain an erection until sexual activity is completed. Other Axis I (except for sexual dysfunctions), Axis III, and substance abuse diagnoses must be assessed to see if the erectile disorder is secondary to these conditions. The current incidence and prevalence of this disorder are unknown, although it is one of the most common male sexual problems to present in clinics.[16]

The need for comprehensive evaluation in erectile disorders is based upon recent changes in techniques a well as broadening patient expectations for a satisfying sex life across the life span. A comprehensive exam, usually done by a urology–psychology/psychiatry team, can involve a medical work-up consisting of interview, history, examination, hormone assay (testosterone, luteinizing hormone, prolactin, estradiol), glucose tolerance test, nocturnal penile tumescence exam, pelvic arterial and venous function tests, and penile and nerve conductivity and sensitivity tests. Part or all of the medical procedures may be bypassed if the erectile disorder is very situational (only occurs with one partner, does not occur on vacations or during masturbation) or coincides with a major recent stressor. In addition to the medical evaluation, it is usually necessary to include a psychological assessment of the patient and his partner. Often the patient is seen alone first, more for convenience's sake than format. The purpose of the psychological interview is to evaluate the contextual features of the dysfunction (relationship history, current satisfaction, and problems; sexual function and dysfunction history; presence of other Axis I, Axis III, or substance abuse disorders) and to begin to understand the degree of psychological contribution to the sexual dysfunction. The partner is also interviewed, where possible. The partner's perspective is important in clarifying diagnostic issues and preparing for a collaborative treatment solution.

Finding the cause of the erectile complaint is usually not a matter of isolating the purely physiological from the purely psychological. Both organic and psychogenic factors are usually involved. While some cases respond well to a purely organic treatment, others will require a combination of medical and psychological interventions. Many male patients want to believe in a physical cause and solution, and they sometimes feel defensive and threatened if the solution is other than purely mechanical. It is impor-

tant to get a sense of this during an evaluation in order to more effectively present treatment options. A review of 99 patients completing a comprehensive evaluation at a urology clinic showed that only 30 per cent complied with the treatment recommendation.[17]

Treatment

If a primarily organic problem is identified and the patient/couple is motivated to explore a biomedical approach, medical treatment options can be recommended. In addition, in some cases in which repeated psychotherapy or sex therapy has been so disappointing that there is no patient motivation to explore it, a medical solution may be acceptable.

Endocrine treatments are offered for endocrine disorders such as low testosterone, hyperprolactinemia, or adrenal tumors. Decreasing bad habits, such as smoking, drinking, and selected recreational drug use is good advice, since these substances do affect neurovascular functioning. Heavy consumers of these substances may not recoup their sexual functioning due to sustained damage. Also, a surprising number of alcoholics seem to have worse functioning the first 2 years after abstinence, most likely because of a combination of increased emotional sensitivity and residual relationship bitterness from past drinking. In collaboration with the prescribing physician, medication dosage and type may be altered to decrease effects on potency. Patient and partner need to be "safe" going to a different medication regimen, so that they do not feel their overall health is compromised.

Less invasive treatment is available using a vacuum constriction device.[18] The penis is placed in a plastic tube in which a vacuum is created. The sinusoidal spaces fill with blood and a band is put on the base of the penis. Although "low-tech" and somewhat cumbersome, many patients and partners are drawn to its noninvasive and low side effect appeal. No long-term studies have been done using these devices, and thus unreserved enthusiasm is not warranted.

Over the last 10 years, vasoactive intracavernous pharmacology has been used, also used in conjunction with cavernosography to diagnose venous leaks, primarily as a treatment for irreversible erectile dysfunctions. It is less often recommended for other types of erectile disorders because of the strong possibility of permanent penile tissue scarring. The injection materials most often currently used are papavarine (although Lilly Laboratories disclaim its use for this purpose) or a combination of prostaglandin E and phentalomine. The patient is trained to provide his own injections.[19]

Surgical procedures include correction of venous leaks, which has a moderate but improving success rate.[20] Penile artery defects are rather rare and the surgeries for it are of limited success. By far the most popular surgical procedure, available for over 40 years, is a penile prosthetic implant. Two basic types of prostheses, a semirigid device and a hydraulic inflatable device, are available. According to one survey following patients for 1 to 4 years after their penile implant surgeries, most patients were quite satisfied in spite of a number of difficulties. Partners were less pleased, however, although they felt the treatment choice had been a good one.[21] Interestingly, patients had less frequent intercourse than they had expected. This confirms clinical observations in our own Reproductive and Sexual Medicine clinic, where a few patients are content merely to have the implant, even if they have minimal (or no) sexual activity.

Psychotherapeutic approaches to erectile disorders are particularly useful for men who do not have an organic basis to their problem, but can also benefit men with blended organic and psychogenic factors as well as assist couples to become comfortable with prosthetic or suction devices. The psychological issues surrounding erectile dysfunction typically include some sense of loss of masculine identity accompanied by a sense of failure, decreased confidence, and anxiety. Partners, especially female partners, may feel a parallel rejection of not being attractive enough and often react with increasing anger and hostility or withdrawal.

Treatment approaches to psychogenic impotence now include cognitive-behavioral, psychodynamic, and systems theory elements in individual, couple, or sometimes group formats. The initial focus is on understanding the effects of the dysfunction on both partners and gradually working on individual and couple issues about sex and the relationship. Classical sex therapy techniques have been shown to be quite useful. Sensate focus, assigning couples exercises outside of the session that are designed to gradually replace negative feelings with sensual ones and to decrease fears and worries about sexual performance, has been the mainstay of sex therapy approaches.[22] Primary erectile problems may benefit from some individual therapy prior to couples therapy. Secondary erectile problems are usually best treated in conjoint treatment unless the couple is uncommitted to the relationship continuing, or if no partner is present.

Although Masters and Johnson's original sex therapy work cited highly successful treatment results (only 40 per cent of primary and 26 per cent of secondary erectile disorders failed to improve), later research suggests that improvement may be less dramatic.[10] Erections improve in approximately 50 to 80 per cent of cases of secondary erectile dysfunction. Overall sexual satisfaction, in spite of sometimes modest symptom improvement, often increases in up to 90 per cent of the cases, in part because the overall relationship improves.[10,23,24] Controlled outcome studies of individual or psychoanalytical approaches to erectile dysfunction are not available.

ORGASM DISORDER

Female Orgasm Disorders

Diagnosis and Assessment

Delayed or absent orgasm after an undefined but "normal" excitement phase is subclassified in DSM-III-R and DSM-IV into generalized (inorgasmic across situations); situational, during self-stimulation only; situational, during partner noncoital stimulation; and mixed situational, orgasmic except in intercourse. Again the diagnosis of orgasmic disorder is very dependent on clinical judgment, which needs to evaluate the situation with consideration given to the woman's age, sexual experience, and adequacy of stimulation. The diagnosis presumes the disorder is not exclusively due to another Axis I disorder (excepting another sexual dysfunction) and not better accounted for by an Axis III condition or a substance-induced dysfunction. It is quite important to attend to depressive symptomatology. Depression can lower desire, and use of antidepressant medication can cause anorgasmia in both sexes.

Orgasmic problems are common sexual complaints. A number of women (estimated at around 10 per cent) have never had orgasm, and a majority of women have situational orgasmic problems.[25] It is rare for the origin of the orgasmic problem to be physiological, but this topic must be explored with respect to a careful history covering surgeries, current medications, recreational drugs and alcohol, and other Axis I and III conditions. Psychological and relationship issues that need assessment are sexual history, early family and close relationship history, and current sexual techniques and functioning in both partners. It is essential to ask what the patient, and partner if available, expect from having (more) orgasms since these expectations may be contributing to the nonorgasmic pattern being maintained.

Treatment

Primary orgasmic disorder is quite effectively treated either by standard sex therapy techniques or by a combined masturbation and sex therapy approach with individuals, couples, or groups (see Heiman and Grafton-Becker's[25] review). These therapies deal with issues of body image, relaxation, self-stimulation, education, acceptance of sexual feelings, tolerating arousal, loss of control, partner functioning, and sensual touching. With situational orgasmic dysfunction, additional relationship therapy may be necessary. Group therapy, especially for women who are preorgasmic, has been very effective, although some studies have found that group therapy's emphasis on autoerotic responsiveness does not generalize to partner stimulation. The major issue may relate to how much effort is made to integrate couple issues. Bibliotherapy is also effective for some patients; among the self-help books available for orgasm problems are those by Barbach[26] and Heiman and LoPiccolo.[27]

Male Orgasmic Disorder

Diagnosis and Assessment

This disorder has been called delayed or retarded ejaculation, describing a persistent delaying or absence of orgasm after a "normal" excitement phase. Again other Axis I, Axis III, and substance abuse disorders must be ruled out as etiological factors.

Male inorgasmia is rare, accounting for only 1 to 2 per cent of the clinical sex dysfunction population. A rather convincing case has been made for calling male inorgasmic disorder a masked sexual desire disorder.[28] While this is not the place for a discussion of this point, the issue is worth considering in proposing treatment options. The presenting clinical picture is that the man who has delayed ejaculation is one whose erection is out of phase with his level of desire and subjective arousal. Men will report a feeling of numbness after a few minutes of having an erection during coitus. In some cases, significant marital distress and actual dislike for the partner are present. Some therapists believe that the man with retarded ejaculation is withholding or unable to give, and certainly partners often feel this way. Yet the clinical evidence for this interpretation is in fact minimal.

Treatment

Masters and Johnson's[22] treatment of this disorder is one of forcing ejaculation, a very different approach from that of female orgasmic dysfunction. Typically the woman masturbates the man nearly to orgasm, then rapidly inserts his penis into her vagina. They claimed to have a low failure rate (17.6 per cent). Apfelbaum[28] recommended a much different strategy called "counterbypassing," which involves helping the man express feelings about how difficult and unpleasant sex is, actively voicing his negative feelings during sexual interaction, in order to encourage higher levels of pleasure to erections without the demand to have intercourse until he feels really aroused. However, the majority of cases seen by this clinician have used specially trained "body work therapists" who carry out sexual assignments with patients. Since body work therapists are almost never available and may pose legal complications, the counterbypassing strategy must be carefully modified when working with partners in an ongoing relationship.

Premature Ejaculation

Diagnosis and Assessment

This disorder refers to persistent or recurrent ejaculation that occurs with minimal sexual stimulation before or soon after penetration or before the person wishes it. Younger age, partner novelty, and lowered sexual frequency are some of the conditions to take into account as possibly decreasing the latency to ejaculation. In addition, psychological factors such as tension, anxiety, anger, and performance demands imposed by the man or his partner can influence the length of the excitement phase.

Premature ejaculation is a common complaint and may be nearly universal in men's initial sexual experiences. Up to 50 per cent of men in one nonclinical study complained of ejaculating more rapidly than they wanted to.[29] Female partners may feel used or disregarded and often are unable to reach orgasm during intercourse because the male ejaculates so quickly. However, less is written about premature ejaculation in gay men, so it is not clear what the effect of rapid ejaculation is on gay sexuality. Nevertheless, the techniques to improve ejaculation latency should be effective for homosexuals and heterosexuals.

Treatment

Semans[30] introduced the "stop-start technique" to teach men the point of ejaculatory inevitability first during noncoital stimulation. The penis is stimulated until the man reports he is close to the point of inevitability, then stimulation stops until the sense of inevitability subsides and the stimulation is resumed. This pattern continues two more times and ends in ejaculation. Masters and Johnson[22] used the same concept but accompanied the pause (stop) with a firm squeeze to the glans of the erect penis. After practice of either of these techniques, intercourse without movement is tried and then intercourse with thrusting is gradually included. Other sensate, nondemand exercises are also included, as are methods for decreasing the self-defeating cognitions and anxiety.[31] This procedure is quite successful in at least 90 per cent of the cases, although many men need to practice this behavioral control at certain times throughout their lives. Bibliotherapy may also be useful.

SEXUAL PAIN DISORDERS

Dyspareunia

Diagnosis and Assessment

Dyspareunia refers to pain during or after intercourse that is not caused by vaginismus, lack of lubrication, or another Axis I disorder, and is not accounted for by a secondary sexual dysfunction due to Axis III or substance abuse conditions. Axis III conditions are very common in this disorder, and a very careful gynecological and/or urological exam is required to rule out or treat these physical conditions. Untreated menopausal symptoms are also correlated with dyspareunia.

Among the psychological factors influencing dyspareunia, the most likely according to a recent review by Lazarus[32] are developmental factors (guilt, shame, and taboos surrounding sex), traumatic events (incest, rape, loss of parental figures), and relationship issues (conflicts, anger, anxiety, lack of sexual feelings). These areas need to be carefully assessed over a number of sessions because the sufferer of dyspareunia is often unaware of or unready to face troubled issues in these areas. A very careful assessment is necessary to try to clarify the history of behavior, cognition, affect, and interpersonal experiences that influence the pain symptoms. The partner should be included in part of the assessment.

It is unclear how common this disorder is. Men report dyspareunia far less frequently than women. If a patient has had dyspareunia for many years, the progress of treatment is likely to be more difficult.

Treatment

The treatment depends very much on the outcome of the assessment. If developmental factors appear to be an issue, discussion, reading, and imagery work around sexual feelings are needed. With a traumatic history, usually some time needs to be spent dissecting and retiring these memories, which is often a time-consuming process. With relationship dissatisfaction, each person's feelings about their attachment and sensual attraction to each other need attention. Although sensate focus exercises can be a useful component,[22] a great deal of cognitive preparation is important to begin to imagine various activities as relaxing, pleasurable, or exciting. Through cognitive imagery, the patient is also able to clarify further what factors may be maintaining the psychological aspects of the pain.

Vaginismus

Diagnosis and Assessment

Vaginismus describes a condition of involuntary spasm of the vaginal musculature that interferes with coitus. One must decide whether it is better accounted for by another Axis I disorder, such as somatization or post-traumatic stress disorder, or by Axis III or substance abuse conditions. Again Axis I or III disorders are not uncommon with this diagnosis, and careful medical and psychological histories are necessary, along the lines of those described for dyspareunia.

Care should be taken to evaluate the partner's reactions, since he often feels responsible and guilty for causing pain and may play a role in maintaining it. Most typically vaginismus is conceptualized as a conditioned response to real or expected harm. A number of women present with this diagnosis when they want to become pregnant and coitus has become impossible. Exploration of the possible conflicts around this decision is clearly necessary, as is

the option of artificial insemination to reduce some of the pressure around sex.

Treatment

The most common elements of successful treatment for vaginismus include an emphasis on relaxation, desensitization, and control. A dilation procedure is used, employing a graduated series of dilators or finger insertions first by the woman and then with her partner. Gradual penile insertion is then attempted, at first without thrusting and under the woman's guidance. The woman's desired pace and need for control are encouraged while acknowledging the partner's role as supportive. For very phobic women, additional individual imagery and systematic desensitization may be useful. The prognosis overall is quite good, although symptoms may reappear in some couples if the woman's (and partner's) ambivalence and anxiety about change are not carefully addressed.[33]

SUMMARY

This chapter provides a brief summary of the current diagnosis and treatment issues relevant for sexual dysfunctions. Although there are many areas needing further development, a number of sexual problems have encouraging treatment results. Much more research is needed on the nature of sexual desire, response, pain management, and women's sexual functioning. In addition, more attention should be given to "excesses" of sexual desire response under sexual dysfunction disorders. For the moment hyperactive sexual desire is seen as an obsessive-compulsive disorder, which may not ultimately be most clinically and nosologically useful for understanding the nature of sexual functioning and dysfunctioning.

REFERENCES

1. American Psychiatric Association: Diagnostic and Statistical Manual of Mental Disorders. 3rd ed. Revised. Washington, DC: American Psychiatric Association Press, 1987.
2. Leiblum SR, Segraves RT: Sex therapy with aging adults. In Leiblum SR, Rosen RC, eds. Principles and Practices of Sex Therapy. 2nd ed. New York: Guilford Press, 1989:352–381.
3. Schiavi R: Chronic alcoholism and male sexual dysfunction. J Sex Marital Ther 16:23–33, 1990.
4. Sherwin B: Aging and female sexuality: A biological and psychosocial perspective. Annu Rev Sex Res 2 (in press).
5. Bozman AW, Beck JG: Covariation of sexual desire and sexual arousal. Arch Sexual Behav 20:47–60, 1991.
6. Rosen RC, Beck JG, eds. Patterns of Sexual Arousal: Psychophysiological Processes and Clinical Applications. New York: Guilford Press, 1988.
7. Rowland DL, Heiman JR: Self-reported and genital arousal changes in sexually dysfunctional men following a sex therapy program. J Psychosom Res 35:609–619, 1991.
8. Kilmann PR, Boland JP, Norton SP, et al: Perspectives of sex

therapy outcome: A survey of AASECT providers. J Sex Marital Ther 12:116–138, 1986.

9. LoPiccolo J, Friedman JM: Broad-spectrum treatment of low sexual desire: Integration of cognitive, behavioral and systemic therapy. In Leiblum SR, Rosen RC, eds. Sexual Desire Disorders. New York: Guilford Press, 1988:107–144.

10. Hawton K, Catalan J, Martin P, Fass J: Prognostic factors in sex therapy. Behav Res Ther 24:377–385, 1986.

11. Rosen RC, Leiblum SR: Current approaches to the evaluation of sexual desire disorders. J Sex Res 23:141–162, 1987.

12. Rosen RC, Leiblum SR: Assessment and treatment of desire disorders. In Leiblum SR, Rosen RC, eds. Principles and Practices of Sex Therapy. 2nd ed. New York: Guilford Press, 1989:19–50.

13. Sherwin B, Gelfand M, Brender W: Androgen enhances sexual motivation in females: A prospective, cross-over study of sex steroid administration in the surgical menopause. Psychosom Med 47:339–351, 1985.

14. Verhulst J, Heiman J: A systems perspective on sexual desire. In Leiblum SR, Rosen RC, eds. Perspectives on Sexual Desire. New York: Guilford Press, 1988:168–191.

15. Segraves RT: Drugs and desire. In Leiblum SR, Rosen RC, eds. Sexual Desire Disorders. New York: Guilford Press, 1988:313–347.

16. Tiefer L, Melman A: Comprehensive evaluation of erectile dysfunction and medical treatments. In Leiblum SR, Rosen RC, eds. Principles and Practices of Sex Therapy. 2nd ed. New York: Guilford Press, 1989:207–236.

17. Tiefer L, Melman A: Adherence to recommendations and improvement over time in men with erectile dysfunction. Arch Sexual Behav 16:301–309, 1987.

18. Witherington R: Suction device therapy in the management of erectile impotence. Urol Clin North Am 15:123–128, 1988.

19. Sidi AA: Vasoactive intracavernous pharmacology. Urol Clin North Am 15:95–101, 1988.

20. Lewis RW: Venous surgery for impotence. Urol Clin North Am 15:115–121, 1988.

21. Tiefer L, Pedersen B, Melman A: Psychosocial follow-up of penile prosthesis implant patients and partners. J Sex Marital Ther 14:184–201, 1988.

22. Masters W, Johnson V: Human Sexual Inadequacy. Boston: Little, Brown, 1970.

23. Heiman J, LoPiccolo J: Clinical outcome of sex therapy: Effects of daily v. weekly treatment. Arch Gen Psychiatry 40:443–449, 1983.

24. LoPiccolo J, Heiman J, Hogan D, Roberts C: Effectiveness of single therapists versus co-therapy teams in sex therapy. J Consult Clin Psychol 53:287–294, 1985.

25. Grafton-Becker V: Orgasmic disorders in women. In Leiblum SR, Rosen RC, eds. Principles and Practices of Sex Therapy. 2nd ed. New York: Guilford Press, 1989:51–88.

26. Barbach LG: For Yourself. New York: Doubleday, 1975.

27. Heiman J, LoPiccolo J: Becoming orgasmic: A Sexual and Personal Growth Program for Women. 2nd ed. New York: Prentice-Hall, 1988.

28. Apfelbaum B: Retarded ejaculation: A much misunderstood syndrome. In Leiblum SR, Rosen RC, eds. Principles and Practices of Sex Therapy. 2nd ed. New York: Guilford Press, 1989:168–206.

29. Frank E, Anderson A, Rubinstein D: Frequency of sexual dysfunction in "normal" couples. N Engl J Med 299:111–115, 1978.

30. Semans JH: Premature ejaculation: A new approach. South Med J 49:353–357, 1956.

31. McCarthy BW: Cognitive-behavioral strategies and techniques in the treatment of early ejaculations. In Leiblum SR, Rosen RC, eds. Principles and Practices of Sex Therapy. 2nd ed. New York: Guilford Press, 1989:141–164.

32. Lazarus AA: Dyspareunia: A multimodal psychotherapeutic perspective. In Leiblum SR, Rosen RC, eds. Principles and Practices of Sex Therapy. 2nd ed. New York: Guilford Press, 1989:89–112.

33. Leiblum SR, Pervin LA, Campbell EH: Treatment of vaginismus: Success and failure. In Leiblum SR, Rosen RC, eds. Principles and Practices of Sex Therapy. 2nd ed. New York: Guilford Press, 1989:113–140.

56

PSYCHOTROPIC-INDUCED SEXUAL DYSFUNCTION

NANCY C. NITENSON, M.D. and JONATHAN O. COLE, M.D.

Adverse sexual side effects decrease medication compliance. An effort to reduce such effects requires basic knowledge of specific sexual disorders, sexual physiology, and psychotropic medications most often associated with sexual dysfunction. This chapter focuses on the sexual effects of commonly used psychiatric medications.

TERMINOLOGY

In the male, libido refers to sexual desire; it should be noted that testosterone is important in maintaining libido in both men and women. Impotence, also referred to as erectile dysfunction, is defined as the inability to achieve or maintain an erection. It should be noted that partial erections can occur, and the extent of erectile dysfunction should be clarified with the patient. Premature ejaculation has been defined in various ways, including by the number of thrusts prior to orgasm as well as by time intervals (30 seconds to 2 minutes after intromission, according to different sources). In more general terms, premature ejaculation results when a man is unable to exert voluntary control over his ejaculatory reflex, with a short interval between erection and orgasm. Some men ejaculate immediately upon intromission. Psychotropic medications have not been reported to cause premature ejaculation. Retarded ejaculation is inhibition of the ejaculatory reflex, and can vary in severity from prolonged time to ejaculation to inability to ejaculate entirely. Patients and clinicians may also refer to this as anorgasmia.

Female sexual dysfunction has in the past been referred to as frigidity. Frigidity is a pejorative and general term that is not particularly helpful in a discussion of specific sexual disorders. Libido, as in the male, refers to sexual desire. Desire may be present without the physiological response of lubrication. Lubrication is analogous to erection in the male, Interestingly, impotence is often mentioned as a sexual side effect while failure to lubricate is almost never discussed. Female orgasmic dysfunction is a specific inhibition of the orgasmic reflex without a primary disturbance of sexual arousal. It is also referred to as anorgasmia. Anorgasmia is used not only to describe absolute inability to attain orgasm, but also to describe situations in which there is a very prolonged time to orgasm. Vaginismus is involuntary spastic contraction of the vaginal entrance. Vaginismus has not been associated with the use of psychotropic medications.

ANTIDEPRESSANTS

Nearly all the antidepressants have been associated with sexual side effects. However, it should be noted that much of the data consist of case reports. Double-blind, placebo-controlled trials are desperately needed to determine the incidence, nature, and severity of antidepressant-induced sexual dysfunction. Conversely, because decreased libido is often a symptom of depression, treatment can also result in return of sex drive.

Tricyclics

The tricyclic antidepressants (TCAs) interfere with norepinephrine, serotonin, histamine, and acetylcholine neurotransmission in varying degrees. While the incidence is unknown, all TCAs have been reported to cause sexual side effects. The more commonly reported side effects have been decreased libido, impotence, inhibited ejaculation in men, and anorgasmia in women. There have been occasional reports of increased libido, painful ejaculation, and dry ejaculation. In addition, Rosenbaum and Pollack[1] reported two cases of "anhedonic ejaculation" (ejaculation without orgasm) with desipramine, a potent noradrenergic reuptake blocker. The authors suggest that an adrenergic effect may be responsible. Sexual side effects of TCAs are listed in Table 56–1.

Few controlled trials have been performed focusing on the effects of antidepressants on sexual function. In a double-blind trial using a three-way crossover design, Kowalski et al.[2] studied the effects of amitriptyline, mianserin, and placebo on nocturnal sexual arousal. The amplitude and total duration of nocturnal erections were significantly decreased with both the tricyclic and tetracyclic drugs. The drugs were found to diminish rather than eliminate erectile responses. The investigators suggest increased noradrenaline turnover secondary to presynaptic α_2-adrenoceptor antagonism as a possible explanation.

While the incidence of sexual dysfunction secondary to most TCAs is unknown, clomipramine appears to be commonly associated with anorgasmia. In a double-blind, placebo-controlled study of clomipramine and placebo in men and women with obsessive-compulsive disorder, clomipramine treatment resulted in partial or total anorgasmia in all 24 previously orgasmic patients.[3] None of the nine patients on placebo had difficulty obtaining orgasm. Other sexual side effects encountered during the

TABLE 56–1.   REPORTED SEXUAL SIDE EFFECTS OF TRICYCLIC ANTIDEPRESSANTS[a]

Drug	Increased Libido	Decreased Libido	Impotence	Inhibited Ejaculation	Anorgasmia in Females	Painful Ejaculation
Amitriptyline		X	X	X		
Protriptyline		X	X	X		X
Trimipramine		X		X		
Doxepin		X		X		
Imipramine	X		X	X	X	X
Clomipramine		X	X	X	X	X
Nortriptyline		X	X	X	X	
Amoxapine	X	X	X	X	X	X
Desipramine		X	X	X	X	X

[a] Information obtained from refs. 5, 8, 18, 21, and 23.

study were erectile difficulties, problems with lubrication in females, pain at orgasm, and pain on micturition. The mean dose was 140 mg (range 25 to 200 mg). Anorgasmia occurred within the first few days of treatment with clomipramine. Total anorgasmia was usual after a dose of 100 to 150 mg. Return to normal sexual function occurred within days of discontinuing the drug. The mechanism of anorgasmia induced by clomipramine is unclear. Clomipramine has central serotonin and noradrenaline reuptake blocking as well as anticholinergic effects. It has been suggested that desipramine may cause less anorgasmia because it produces less anticholinergic, α-adrenergic blocking, or serotonergic activity.

The mechanism for antidepressant-induced anorgasmia remains unknown. Segraves summarized possible mechanisms responsible for inhibited orgasm in females treated with antidepressants.[4] Anorgasmia secondary to anticholinergic effects has been suggested; however, there is little evidence to support this. A serotonergic mechanism has been suggested given that the sexual response in animals can be inhibited by drugs that enhance central nervous system serotonergic neurotransmission. This may explain why desipramine, which has less serotonergic activity than imipramine, results in less anorgasmia. In addition, cyproheptadine, which has antiserotonergic, anticholinergic, and antihistaminic properties, has in some cases been helpful in the treatment of antidepressant-induced anorgasmia. Yet another possible mechanism is that orgasmic inhibition is secondary to the α_1-blockade associated with most heterocyclic antidepressants. In men, the erectile dysfunction caused by TCAs may be due to presynaptic α_2-receptor antagonism, resulting in vasoconstriction.[5]

Monoamine Oxidase Inhibitors

Monoamine oxidase inhibitors (MAOIs) block the oxidative deamination of endogenous norepinephrine, epinephrine, dopamine, and serotonin. Little has been written on the sexual dysfunction produced by MAOIs, despite the fact that sexual side effects are more common than the well-known adverse effects of hypotension, liver toxicity, and hypertensive crisis.[6] It has been suggested that MAOI-associated sexual dysfunction may occur in 10 to 30 per cent (or more) of MAOI-treated patients.[6] Phenelzine appears to cause more sexual impairment than other MAOIs. Phenelzine has been associated with decreased libido, impotence, and anorgasmia in both men and women. Sitsen[5] cited a review of 198 depressed outpatients among whom sexual side effects were reported by 22 per cent of phenelzine-treated patients, 5 per cent of imipramine-treated patients, and 2.5 per cent of patients on tranylcypromine. Harrison et al. compared the sexual effects of imipramine, phenelzine, and placebo in a double-blind trial.[7] Both imipramine and phenelzine were associated with a high incidence of sexual side effects in both men and women. Orgasm and ejaculation were impaired to a greater extent than erection. Phenelzine resulted in decreased interest, impaired ejaculation, and anorgasmia more often than did imipramine.

Tranylcypromine has been reported to cause an increase in libido, impotence, spontaneous erections, and anorgasmia.[5] It appears that tranylcypromine causes fewer sexual side effects than phenelzine. Isocarboxazid treatment can result in erectile dysfunction[5] and anorgasmia.[8] L-Deprenyl, a selective inhibitor of MAO-B, has not been reported to cause sexual dysfunction; it may be less serotonergic.[6]

Atypical Antidepressants

The atypical antidepressants fluoxetine, trazodone, and bupropion are now being used more often by clinicians. They differ from the first-generation antidepressants as well as from each other with respect to sexual side effect profiles.

Trazodone and Priapism

Trazodone is a serotonin reuptake inhibitor with α-blocking activity but with minimal anticholinergic activity. Trazodone has been associated with anorgasmia, increased libido, retrograde ejaculation, and priapism. Prolonged erections without priapism have also been reported. There have been no reported cases of clitoral priapism in women treated with trazodone. There is one publication, however, attributing increased libido to treatment with trazodone in three depressed women.[9] Given the lack of understanding of the neurophysiology of the female sexual response, further study is indicated.

By far the most serious sexual side effect of trazodone treatment is priapism. Priapism is a prolonged, painful erection of the penis, unaccompanied by erotic feelings. There is obstructed venous drainage from the corpora cavernosa, while the corpus spongiosum and glans penis are unaffected. Untreated, venous stasis results in thrombosis and ultimately fibrosis of the corpora cavernosa. The result can be irreversible erectile impotence. Trazodone-induced priapism therefore requires rapid diagnosis and treatment. The incidence is believed to be somewhere between 1:10,000 and 1:1000. Priapism is most likely to occur within the first month of treatment; however, it has been reported to occur up to 18 months after the initiation of trazodone. Most cases occur at doses of 150 mg or less, but priapism has been reported with doses as low as 50 mg daily. Prolongation of erections should alert the clinician to the possibility of impending priapism.[10]

Fishbain[11] reported a case in which a fluphenazine-treated patient developed priapism. Intravenous diphenhydramine given to treat acute dystonia resulted in resolution of the priapism. He concluded that perhaps the ratio of α-adrenergic blockade to anticholinergic activity may be important in the ability of psychotropics to cause priapism. Neuroleptics causing α-adrenergic blockade may inhibit sympathetically mediated detumescence. Cholinergic dominance would result, leading to priapism. This would also explain the higher incidence of priapism caused by trazodone, given trazodone's α-adrenergic blocking activity with virtually no anticholinergic activity in comparison to the TCAs.[11]

Men being prescribed trazodone should be warned of this rare but serious side effect. Early identification is important, and treatment should be sought immediately. Classically, treatment has been surgical, but in recent years intracorporal injection of α-adrenergic drugs has been successful in some cases.

Fluoxetine

Fluoxetine is a potent and specific serotonin reuptake blocker with very little antagonism of muscarinic, histaminergic, and α_1-adrenergic receptors compared with the TCAs. Zajecka et al. reported that 6 out of 77 depressed outpatients (7.8 per cent) treated through a humanitarian protocol spontaneously reported orgasmic dysfunction within 6 weeks of initiating fluoxetine on doses ranging from 20 to 80 mg/day.[12] It is likely that the incidence of anorgasmia may be much higher given that many patients may not be volunteering information on sexual function. In fact, the incidence of orgasmic dysfunction was found to be 16 per cent in another study involving 32 individuals. A serotonergic mechanism for fluoxetine-induced orgasmic dysfunction has been suggested. Cyproheptadine 4 to 12 mg taken 1 to 2 hours before sexual activity has been successful treatment in some cases.

Bupropion

Bupropion hydrochloride is pharmacologically and chemically unrelated to other antidepressants. Its mechanism of action is unknown. There is evidence to suggest that bupropion lacks associated sexual dysfunction.[13] Bupropion's lack of serotonin and norepinephrine uptake blockade, with minimal anticholinergic activity and mild dopamine uptake blockade, may account for its low sexual side effect profile. Bupropion may be an important option for patients who are sensitive to the sexual side effects of other antidepressants, especially in the treatment of chronic depression where long-term treatment is required.

MOOD STABILIZERS

Lithium

There have been few reports of sexual impairment related to the use of lithium. However, lithium therapy has been associated with decreased libido and erectile failure in men, and with decreased libido and orgastic dysfunction in women.[8,14] These effects are apparently reversible with discontinuation of lithium. Since bipolar patients may enjoy the hypersexuality that may accompany the hypomanic state, it is possible that they perceive a drop in sexual desire as an adverse effect.[8] Some bipolar patients have also reported a positive influence on sexual functioning that they attributed to lithium's positive influence on their general life situation.[14] Lithium is often prescribed in combination with other psychotropics, including TCAs and neuroleptics. Concurrent medication may increase the likelihood of sexual side effects. Overall, it appears that this widely used mood stabilizer may be relatively benign with respect to sexual function. More controlled data are needed.

Carbamazepine

Carbamazepine is currently used in the treatment of bipolar illness in patients resistant to lithium as well as in other psychiatric disorders. Carbamazepine has been reported to cause decreased libido and impotence in 13 per cent of patients given the medication for treatment of a generalized seizure disorder.[15] Sexual dysfunction in patients has been correlated with the decrease in free testosterone seen with carbamazepine treatment.[5]

ANXIOLYTICS

Benzodiazepines

Benzodiazepines are used as anxiolytics, as well as sedatives and hypnotics. There are rare case reports of benzodiazepine-induced sexual dysfunction. Benzodiazepines have on occasion been associated with erectile disorders, inhibition of sexual desire, and orgasmic dysfunction. Dosage may be a factor, with high doses resulting in central sedative effects. Given the large number of psychiatric patients prescribed these medications and the few reports of adverse sexual side effects, it is likely that benzodiazepines in moderate doses cause little in the way of sexual dysfunction. In addition, because anxiety can greatly affect sexual performance, alleviation of anxiety, particularly in patients with diagnosed anxiety disorders, may positively affect sexual function. As with other medications, a patient's expectations may of course play a role.

Buspirone

Buspirone is an anxiolytic pharmacologically unrelated to the benzodiazepines. While its mechanism of action is unknown, buspirone has high affinity for serotonin receptors and moderate affinity for brain D_2 receptors, while gamma-aminobutyric acid binding is not affected. Othmer and Othmer, in an open label pilot study, reported normalization of sexual function in eight of ten patients with generalized anxiety disorder.[16] The authors suggested that this effect may be due to buspirone's dopaminergic and antiserotonergic effects. Improvement occurred in both sexes and was not correlated with anxiety reduction. Given the small size of this uncontrolled study along with the fact that psychotropics discontinued prior to buspirone treatment may have been the cause of sexual dysfunction, no conclusions can be drawn about this atypical anxiolytic. Of note, there is one case report in the literature of priapism associated with buspirone.[17]

NEUROLEPTICS

This category is composed of several different chemical classes including the phenothiazines, thioxanthines, butyrophenones, and atypical neuroleptics such as loxapine, molindone, and clozapine. The typical antipsychotic drugs all produce dopamine blockade, with varying degrees of α-adrenergic blockade and anticholinergic effects. The most commonly reported sexual side effects are erectile dysfunction and ejaculatory failure in men, and anorgasmia in women. While controlled series are lacking for both sexes, numerous case reports exist describing sexual impairment in men medicated with neuroleptics. It is possible that men treated with antipsychotics may be more susceptible to adverse sexual side effects. However, more likely, women may not be reporting sexual side effects to their physicians.

Phenothiazines

Phenothiazines have been associated with erectile impotence, ejaculatory disorders, decreased libido, and priapism in men. In females, anorgasmia has been reported with thioridazine, trifluoperazine, and fluphenazine.[4,18] Sexual side effects of the commonly used phenothiazines are listed in Table 56–2.

Thioridazine appears to be the neuroleptic most commonly associated with sexual impairment. It has been associated with decreased libido, impotence, priapism, and various ejaculatory difficulties, including delayed, painful, and retrograde ejaculation. Kotin et al. found thioridazine to be associated with sexual dysfunction in 60 per cent of 87 patients taking the drug.[19] Only 25 per cent of patients on other major tranquilizers reported sexual impairment, still a large portion when considering issues such as medication compliance and quality of life. Over one third (35 per cent) of thioridazine-treated patients reported erectile difficulties, and almost half (49 per cent) reported ejaculatory difficulties and changes in quality of orgasm. Pain at orgasm was also reported in a small number of patients. The other phenothiazines are capable of causing sexual effects similar to those seen with thioridazine, but apparently less frequently. Sexual impairment can occur at low to moderate doses and can appear within days. Sexual dysfunction is reversible upon discontinuation of the offending agent.

Thioxanthenes

Sexual side effects have been attributed to the thioxanthenes chlorprothixene and thioxthixene, but to a lesser degree than seen with the phenothiazines. Chlorprothixene has been reported to cause decreased libido, ejaculatory dysfunction, and orgasmic inhibition.[5] Thiothixene has been associated with ejaculatory difficulties, erectile failure, priapism, and spontaneous ejaculations.[5,20,21]

Butyrophenones and Other Neuroleptics

Sexual dysfunction with the butyrophenone haloperidol appears infrequently. It has occasionally been noted to cause decreased libido, impotence, ejaculatory difficulties, and priapism at low to moderate doses (1 to 5 mg/day).[5] In addition, painful ejaculation occurs rarely.[21] Little information is known about the atypical agents with respect to sex-

TABLE 56–2.   REPORTED SEXUAL SIDE EFFECTS OF PHENOTHIAZINES[a,b]

Drug	Erect Dys	Ejac Dys	Anorg Fem	Priapism	Decr Lib	Delay Ejac	Pain Ejac	Retro Ejac
Thioridazine	×	×[c]	×	×	×	×	×	×
Chlorpromazine	×	×		×	×			
Mesoridazine	×	×		×				×
Perphenazine[d]			×[e]					
Trifluoperazine[d]		×	×			×		
Fluphenazine	×	×	×		×			

[a] Information obtained from refs. 4, 20, 21, and 24.
[b] Key: Erect Dys, erectile dysfunction; Ejac Dys, ejaculatory dysfunction; Anorg Fem, anorgasmia in females; Decr Lib, decreased libido; Delay Ejac, delayed ejaculation; Pain Ejac, painful ejaculation; Retro Ejac, retrograde ejaculation.
[c] Ejaculatory disturbance is well documented.
[d] This agent may cause less sexual side effects compared with other phenothiazines.
[e] The combination of amitriptyline and perphenazine may cause anorgasmia in females.

ual function. It is unclear whether the scarce data, including lack of case reports, indicate a lower incidence of drug-induced sexual effects or simply less prescribing of these agents. Molindone, a dihydroindolone, has been associated with prolonged erection and priapism possibly due to peripheral adrenergic blockade, inhibiting sympathetically mediated detumescence.[5,22] Few data exist on the sexual side effects of the dibenzoxazepine loxapine and the dibenzodiazepine clozapine. Clozapine has been reported to cause abnormal ejaculation (package insert). Pimozide, a diphenylbutylpiperidine, has been cited as causing ejaculatory dysfunction and impotence.[5,20]

Mechanisms

Various mechanisms have been proposed to explain antipsychotic-induced sexual impairment based on anticholinergic, antidopaminergic, and endocrine effects. In laboratory animals, dopamine is a stimulator of sexual behavior. Dopamine blockade may be the mechanism by which antipsychotics reduce libido.[20] In addition, dopamine may play a role in the neurotransmission of normal erectile function.[5] Anticholinergic activity may contribute to erectile dysfunction, and strong α-adrenergic blocking action may be responsible for the high incidence of ejaculatory disturbances seen, for instance, with phenothiazines. α-Blockade of varying degrees with different agents may cause problems with emission, priapism, and various ejaculatory disturbances, including delayed, absent, or retrograde ejaculation. It appears that neuroleptics with a high degree of α-blockade are more likely to cause priapism. Finally, not to be ignored is the fact that neuroleptics affect the hypothalamic-pituitary-gonadal axis.[20] Dopamine results in inhibition of prolactin release from the anterior pituitary. Most typical neuroleptics, because of their dopamine blocking properties, result in an increase in prolactin levels. In addition, antipsychotics, particularly thioridazine, may be associated with a slight decrease of testosterone that is not likely to be clinically significant.

MANAGEMENT OF PSYCHOTROPIC-INDUCED SEXUAL DYSFUNCTION

Clinicians have several options when considering the management of psychotropic-induced sexual dysfunction. Spontaneous remission can occur, in which case the clinician need only wait and observe. Some patients may initially prefer this if they have had an otherwise good response to pharmacotherapy. If spontaneous remission does not occur, often dose reduction is effective in alleviating sexual side effects. Obviously, close observation is necessary to avoid undertreating the illness, and a minimal effective dosing strategy should be employed. Discontin-

uation of psychotropic medication almost always results in a return to previous sexual functioning, and therefore patients should be educated to allay fears of permanent dysfunction. For antidepressant-induced side effects, switching to desipramine or bupropion can be useful. As for MAOIs, although not clearly stated in the literature, tranylcypromine may be preferable over phenelzine given phenelzine's high incidence of sexual dysfunction. Regarding neuroleptics, since thioridazine is the major culprit, switching to another neuroleptic in a different class may be useful. Given the high incidence of ejaculatory disturbances, it may be preferable to start with a neuroleptic other than thioridazine when treating men. As with antidepressants, lowering the dose is also worthwhile in an effort to alleviate sexual side effects.

One patient with neuroleptic-induced sexual dysfunction was instructed to take his antipsychotic medication on weekdays, allowing for normal sexual function on weekends (Fr. Frankenburg, personal communication). This type of dosing strategy requires intact patient compliance as well as close follow-up to avoid relapse, and should be reserved for cases in which other treatment strategies have failed.

Specific agents that have been used to treat sexual side effects include bethanecol chloride and cyproheptadine; however, their use consists mainly of anecdotal reports. Studies involving efficacy and safety of these agents are lacking. Bethanecol chloride, a cholinergic agonist, has been useful in treating anorgasmia at a dose of 12.5 to 25 mg in the evening. Bethanecol is contraindicated in cases of asthma, coronary insufficiency, and peptic ulcer. In high doses, flushing of the skin, diarrhea, and cramps can occur.[18] Cyproheptadine 4 to 12 mg taken 1 to 2 hours before sexual activity has been helpful in some cases of drug-induced anorgasmia.[18] The major side effect is drowsiness. A toxic reaction has been reported in a phenothiazine-medicated patient given cyproheptadine.

CONCLUSION

Drug-induced sexual dysfunction occurs within all classes of psychotropic medication. The incidence is probably higher than current estimates would indicate because of patient underreporting. While physicians may be hesitant to discuss adverse sexual side effects with patients, to avoid a self-fulfilling prophecy, it is probably beneficial to outline with patients possible sexual drug effects. Patients should be made aware of the fact that most sexual side effects are reversible shortly after discontinuation of the offending agent. Polypharmacy may increase the likelihood of sexual dysfunction, especially when psychotropics are given concurrently with medications commonly associated with sexual side effects, such as antihypertensives.

More information is needed on the frequency, nature, and severity of adverse sexual side effects based on double-blind, placebo-controlled studies. Without controlled clinical studies, conclusions cannot be drawn. Still, clinicians should remain aware of the possibility of drug-induced sexual disorders.

REFERENCES

1. Rosenbaum JF, Pollack MH: Anhedonic ejaculation with desipramine. Int J Psychiatry Med 18(1):85, 1988.
2. Kowalski A, Stanley RO, Dennerstein L, et al: The sexual side-effects of antidepressant medication: A double-blind comparison of two antidepressants in a non-psychiatric population. Br J Psychiatry 147:413, 1985.
3. Monteiro WO, Noshirvan HF, Marks IM, et al: Anorgasmia from clomipramine in obsessive-compulsive disorder. A controlled trial. Br J Psychiatry 151:107, 1987.
4. Segraves RT: Psychiatric drugs and inhibited female orgasm. J Sex Marital Ther 14(3):202, 1988.
5. Sitsen JMA: Prescription drugs and sexual function. In Sitsen JMA, ed. Handbook of Sexology. New York: Elsevier Science Publishers BV, 1988:425.
6. Nurnberg HG, Levin PE: Spontaneous remission of MAOI-induced anorgasmia. Am J Psychiatry 144(6):805, 1987.
7. Harrison WM, Rabkin JG, Ehrhardt AA, et al: Effects of antidepressant medication on sexual function. J Clin Psychopharmacol 6(3):144, 1986.
8. Buffum J: Pharmacosexology update: Prescription drugs and sexual function. J Psychoactive Drugs 18(2):97, 1986.
9. Gartrell N: Increased libido in women receiving trazodone. Am J Psychiatry 143(6):781, 1986.
10. Warner MD, Peabody CA, Whiteford HA, et al: Trazodone and priapism. J Clin Psychiatry 48(6):244, 1987.
11. Fishbain DA: Priapism resulting from fluphenazine hydrochloride treatment reversed by diphenhydramine. Ann Emerg Med 14(6):600, 1985.
12. Zajecka J, Fawcett J, Schaff M, et al: The role of serotonin in sexual dysfunction: Fluoxetine-associated orgasm dysfunction. J Clin Psychiatry 52(2):66, 1991.
13. Gardner EA, Johnson JA: Bupropion—an antidepressant without sexual pathophysiological action. J Clin Psychopharmacol 5(1):24, 1985.
14. Kristensen E, Jorgensen P: Sexual dysfunction in lithium-treated manic-depressive patients. Pharmacopsychiatry 20:165, 1987.
15. Mattson RH, Cramer JA, Collins JF, et al: Comparison of carbamazepine, phenobarbital, phenytoin, and primidone in partial and secondarily generalized tonic-clonic seizures. N Engl J Med 313(3):145, 1985.
16. Othmer E, Othmer SC: Effect of buspirone on sexual dysfunction in patients with generalized anxiety disorder. J Clin Psychiatry 48(5):201, 1987.
17. Coates NE: Priapism associated with Buspar [letter]. South Med J 83(8):983, 1990.
18. Shen WW, Sata LS: Inhibited female orgasm resulting from psychotropic drugs. A five-year, updated, clinical review. J Reprod Med 35(1):11, 1990.
19. Kotin J, Wilbert DE, Verburg D, et al: Thioridazine and sexual dysfunction. Am J Psychiatry 133(1):82, 1976.
20. Smith PJ, Talbert RL: Sexual dysfunction with antihypertensive and antipsychotic agents. Clin Pharmacy 5:373, 1986.
21. Wein AJ, Van Arsdalen KN: Drug-induced male sexual dysfunction. Urol Clin North Am 15(1):23, 1988.
22. Gomez EA: Neuroleptic-induced priapism. Tex Med 81(9):47, 1985.
23. Jani NN, Wise TN: Antidepressants and inhibited female orgasm: A literature review. J Sex Marital Ther 14(4):279, 1988.
24. Segraves RT: Sexual side-effects of psychiatric drugs. Int J Psychiatry Med 18(3):243, 1988.

Section H

SLEEP DISORDERS

57

CLASSIFICATION OF SLEEP DISORDERS:
A Preview of the DSM-IV

DANIEL J. BUYSSE, M.D., CHARLES F. REYNOLDS III, M.D., and
DAVID J. KUPFER, M.D.

PREVIOUS AND CURRENT CLASSIFICATIONS OF SLEEP DISORDERS

The DSM-III-R was the first edition of the DSM to include a specific section for sleep disorders.[1] The DSM-III-R organizes sleep disorders into dyssomnias (disturbances in the amount, timing, or quality of sleep) and parasomnias (abnormal events occurring during sleep, or at the threshold of sleep and wakefulness, in which the predominant complaint is the disturbance itself). Dyssomnias are further divided into insomnias, hypersomnias, and sleep-wake schedule disturbances. While the DSM-III-R system appears to be usable in most psychiatric settings, it has been criticized by sleep specialists for not specifically including some well-recognized disorders, such as narcolepsy and sleep apnea, and for "lumping" disorders into overly broad categories.

PREVIEW OF DSM-IV

Revision of all disorders in the DSM-IV, including sleep disorders, is based on a three-part process: (1) literature reviews, (2) analysis of unpublished data, and (3) focused field trials. For the sleep disorders section, an overriding question has been whether a more detailed or a more general classification should be adopted.

The literature reviews for the DSM-IV support the clinical utility and validity of some more specific disorders, such as narcolepsy and sleep apnea syndrome, while maintaining a more conservative stance on other disorders such as subtypes of insomnia. The general-specific tension is especially obvious in considering insomnia diagnoses.[2] On the one hand, there is a danger of reifying the general DSM-III-R category "primary insomnia" into a single disorder, and giving insufficient attention to legitimate subtypes of insomnia. On the other hand, while it is clear that many factors can contribute to insomnia disorders, it is less clear whether each of these factors should be conceptualized as a separate disorder.

Analysis of unpublished data supports the notion that the general classification of the DSM-III-R is associated with greater interrater reliability than a more specific system (Buysse, Reynolds, and Kupfer, unpublished data). Other data demonstrate that the use of a structured sleep disorders interview for the DSM-III-R produces very good rates of test-retest and interrater reliability (Schramm and Berger, unpublished data).

The DSM-IV classification will include a larger number of disorders than that in the DSM-III-R, but far fewer than in the International Classification of Sleep Disorders (ICSD).[3] Other possible subtypes of disorders will be discussed in the text. Like the ICSD, the DSM-IV classification will be organized by pathophysiology and presumed etiology, although the general categories will differ. Basically, the DSM-IV will include four general categories: primary sleep disorders, sleep disorders related to another mental disorder, secondary sleep disorders (due to an Axis III disorder), and substance-induced sleep disorders. This organization will make the sleep disorders section compatible with other sections of the DSM-IV. Within the four major categories, the DSM-IV will include subsections for dyssomnias and parasomnias. Specific disorders with well-accepted clinical validity, such as narcolepsy and breathing-related sleep disorder (sleep apnea), will be included. Like the DSM-III-R, the DSM-IV will rely on clinical criteria, and will not require specific polysomnographic criteria except for breathing-related sleep disorder. Polysomnographic characteristics for other disorders will be discussed in the text.

A field trial is currently underway to assess the utility and reliability of proposed DSM-IV diagnoses, both independently and in comparison to ICSD and International Classification of Diseases diagnoses.

The changes proposed for sleep disorders in the DSM-IV represent evolutionary rather than revolutionary changes relative to the DSM-III-R. It is hoped that the new classification will entice clinicians to consider sleep disorders from an etiological and pathophysiological perspective, and to make the most specific appropriate diagnoses. In this sense, the DSM-IV will serve an educational function as well as a communicative one.

ACKNOWLEDGMENTS

Supported in part by grants MH00295, MH37869, MH30915, and MH47200 to Allen Frances, M.D., principal investigator.

REFERENCES

1. American Psychiatric Association: Diagnostic and Statistical Manual of Mental Disorders. 3rd ed. Revised. Washington, DC: American Psychiatric Association, 1987.
2. Reynolds CF, Kupfer DJ, Buysse DJ, et al: Subtyping DSM-III-R "primary" insomnia: a literature review by the DSM-IV work group on sleep disorders. Am J Psychiatry 148:432–438.
3. Diagnostic Classification Steering Committee, Thorpy MJ, Chairman: The International Classification of Sleep Disorders: Diagnostic and Coding Manual. Rochester, MN: American Sleep Disorders Association, 1990.

58

PARASOMNIAS

DONNA E. GILES, Ph.D. and DANIEL J. BUYSSE, M.D.

Parasomnias are disorders characterized by abnormal behavioral or physiological events that occur throughout sleep, during specific sleep stages, or in sleep-wake transitions. The behaviors that occur in parasomnias may be normal in the context of wakefulness, but are abnormal because they occur during sleep. Walking, talking, urinating, rhythmic movements, being frightened, the startle response, reacting to the threat of danger, or moving to avoid harm are all expected behaviors in the appropriate wakeful context. When these behaviors occur in sleep, however, consequences can be painful or dangerous to the individual and/or very disruptive or disturbing to those close to that individual.

Another subset of parasomnias are truly aberrant and range from being annoying (e.g., primary snor-ing) to fatal (sudden infant death syndrome [SIDS]; sudden unexplained nocturnal death).

Most of the parasomnias that occur in childhood, again with the important exception of SIDS, have no implication for maladjustment later, are not volitional, and are most probably a function of an immature and developing central nervous system. Those parasomnias with onset in adulthood tend not to have such a benign prognosis.

Parasomnias can be usefully categorized by sleep stage of origin: parasomnias that occur only in non–rapid eye movement (REM) sleep, those that occur only in REM sleep, those that show no sleep stage preference, and those for which sleep stage of origin has not yet been documented. These categories have implications for treatment intervention and are used here to organize this presentation of parasomnias. In the context of this chapter, we base our description of parasomnias on those recognized in the International Classification of Sleep Disorders (ICSD).[1] The series of parasomnias classified in the ICSD are summarized briefly in Tables 58–1 through 58–4. More detailed focus is presented for those parasomnias that are more common and better understood.

PARASOMNIAS IN NON-REM SLEEP

Parasomnias that have been documented to occur exclusively, or almost exclusively, in non-REM sleep include sleepwalking, sleep terrors, confusional arousals, sleep bruxism, rhythmic movement disorder, sleep starts, sleep-related abnormal swallowing, nocturnal paroxysmal dystonia, and benign neonatal sleep myoclonus. These disorders are outlined in Table 58–1. The most common non-REM parasomnias (sleepwalking, sleep terrors, confusional arousals, sleep bruxism, and rhythmic movement disorder) are described in more detail in this section.

Sleepwalking, Sleep Terrors, and Confusional Arousals

These parasomnias are discussed as a group for several reasons. All arise out of slow wave or deep sleep, all represent partial awakenings, all are more likely to occur in the first third of the night, and manifestation of one is associated with an increased likelihood of expressing the others. Onset in early childhood, which is the most likely time, reflects an underdeveloped central nervous system, and these parasomnias usually disappear with developmental maturation. Nonetheless, these disorders can be dangerous to the patient or terrifying to parents.

Patients who *sleepwalk* are capable of complex and inappropriate behavior varying from simply sitting up in bed to urinating in a closet or walking out a door into the street. Disorientation, difficulty in awakening fully, or both are apparent. The patient can mistake windows for doors, causing serious, if not fatal, personal trauma. Awakened sleepwalkers can become violent toward objects or persons in their vicinity, despite retrograde and anterograde amnesia for this behavior.

The prevalence of sleepwalking, when viewed in the context of one-time occurrences, is estimated to be about 20 per cent. Population prevalence is estimated to vary between 1 and 15 per cent when more frequent occurrences are considered.

With *sleep terrors*, the child utters a blood-curdling scream and is agitated, is usually amnestic for cause, is clearly confused, and has markedly increased heart rate and respiration. If the child has any recall, it is typically vague and image-like, without the story found in a dream. Sleep terrors are very important to distinguish from nightmares. Night-

mares, in contrast to sleep terrors, occur during REM sleep. The patient, while clearly frightened, becomes oriented immediately, has vivid recall for details of the dream, and has more moderate increases in heart rate and respiration.

The prevalence of sleep terrors is difficult to estimate with precision, since parent reports are generally the source of information and sleep terrors are not always distinguished from nightmares. To the best of our knowledge, prevalence ranges between 1.5 and 3 per cent.

Confusional arousal is a diagnostic category that was recently added to the sleep disorders nomenclature (ICSD). As noted in Table 58–1, predisposing factors for confusional arousals include presence of sleepwalking and sleep terrors. Confusional arousals are characterized by several features, consistent with those described in sleepwalking. These features include disorientation, inappropriate behavior in response to environmental events, and complete anterograde and retrograde amnesia for the arousal.

Confusional arousals are most prevalent in children when they are forcibly roused from deep sleep. As noted in Table 58–1, this state occurs in virtually all children at some time if aroused by caretaker prodding. Confusional arousals are rare among adults. When adults present with this complaint, it is often in association with idiopathic hypersomnia or with sleep deprivation.

Sleepwalking, sleep terrors, and confusional arousals tend to be evenly distributed between the sexes, with some evidence that slightly more males than females express sleep terrors. Onset for all three parasomnias is early in childhood, and the conditions tend to be self-limited.

When adults manifest sleepwalking or sleep terrors, these disorders tend to have persisted or recurred from childhood. Unlike the self-limited, childhood form of the disorders, sleepwalking and sleep terrors in adults have been associated with Axis I disorders (schizophrenia, anxiety disorders, major depression). The clinician must also consider alcohol and substance abuse as well as organic brain disorders as potential causes. Results of personality assessment have been variable. Some studies have suggested that patients who sleepwalk tend to score higher on dimensions of hostility/aggression and patients with sleep terrors score higher on anxiety-related scales. Other studies have found no evidence of character differences.

Family history studies indicate that sleepwalking and sleep terrors assort together in families even when probands are identified with only one disorder. Sleepwalking and night terrors appear to be manifestations of a common genetic predisposition, although environmental factors probably influence their expression as well.[2]

Some laboratory studies have found no differences in daytime electroencephalographic (EEG) activity among patients with sleepwalking, sleep terrors, and no sleep disorder,[3] whereas other studies have found a greater prevalence of interictal activity.[4] Based on a single case report, there is a suggestion that patients with confusional arousals do not show normal blood pressure activation in response to arousal.

Successful treatment of sleepwalking and sleep terrors in children includes education on appropriate sleep habits. By providing guidelines for a regular sleep-wake schedule, sleep deprivation and compensatory slow wave sleep rebound can be avoided. Daytime naps also serve to decrease pressure for slow wave sleep at night and can be helpful. Hypnosis as well as the benzodiazepine family of medications have been used in some cases. Efforts to make the environment safe, such as removing sharp objects from bedside tables and ensuring that windows are securely locked, should also be considered. Psychotherapy, non-REM—suppressing psychotropic medications, and anticonvulsants have also been reported to be successful with adults.

Sleep Bruxism

Sleep bruxism is characterized by rhythmic contractions of the masseter muscles, resulting in grinding of the upper and lower teeth. It is considered a disorder because chronic occurrences lead to tooth abrasion, damage to bone and soft tissue surrounding the teeth, facial pain, and possible headaches. Sleep bruxism is separate from bruxism during the day. Bruxism during the day has been associated with increased stress, whereas sleep bruxism has been thought to be unrelated to psychological factors. There is some controversy regarding this distinction, however, since a number of patients who apparently brux only at night have also been found to be characterologically more anxious individuals.

Sleep bruxism is described as a non-REM phenomenon (Table 58–1) because it occurs predominantly in stage 2 sleep, although it can occur in any stage sleep. There is suggestive evidence, however, that severe bruxism may be more often associated with REM sleep.[5]

Sleep bruxism is a common occurrence in many people sporadically at some time and shows no sex preference. It appears to decrease with time except in more severe cases, for which intervention is sought, usually because of jaw pain.

Treatment modes have included mechanical devices designed to prevent bruxism (occlusal splints), behavioral techniques that functionally increase arousal and thereby decrease occurrences, physical therapy, and anxiolytic medication.

Rhythmic Movement Disorder

Rhythmic movement disorder represents an expansion of the former category of sleep disorder loosely described as "headbanging." Headbanging is the most frequently occurring rhythmic movement disorder, but several other stereotyped, repetitive movements, usually involving large muscles of the head, neck, and upper body, are appropriately classified here. These rhythmic movements include rocking, body rolling, and head rolling and can also extend to leg rolling or leg banging.

This parasomnia, like most parasomnias with childhood onset, has a benign and self-limited course, although injuries can occur infrequently. Onset usually occurs by age 5 and the movements usually subside at puberty, although rhythmic movement disorder can persist into adulthood. Boys manifest rhythmic movement disorder much more frequently than girls (the ratio is approximately 4 : 1). Rhythmic movements occur most frequently in drowsiness and into the light stages of sleep. The etiology of these movements is unknown, but they are thought to provide some measure of self-comfort or self-stimulation. An immature or underdeveloped nervous system has been implicated as a cause, in part because of the disorder's childhood onset and in part because it occurs more frequently in children of limited intellectual ability. It should be noted, however, that rhythmic movement disorder is neither diagnostic nor prognostic for intellectual deficiency and occurs frequently in otherwise normal children.

Few studies of rhythmic movement disorder have been performed in the sleep laboratory. This may reflect the low probability of parental complaints to polysomnographers. To the extent the laboratory studies have been completed, rhythmic movement disorder has been documented to be a non-REM sleep phenomenon that occurs largely in sleep-wake transitions. Rhythmic movement disorders have been found in identical twins. It is unclear whether this is an effect of shared genes or shared environment.

Treatment is usually not necessary for rhythmic movement disorder, since movements are confined and occur usually without injury. Among patients for whom personal injury is a risk, padding or a protective helmet may be necessary. In addition, the environment surrounding the bed should be kept safe. Restraints are usually unsuccessful in inhibiting the behavior and serve to exacerbate sleep problems by increasing frustration or anxiety.

PARASOMNIAS IN REM SLEEP

The series of parasomnias identified as occurring in REM sleep are described in Table 58–2. Not all parasomnias that occur in REM sleep necessarily involve dream content, but those that do are quite striking in their clinical presentation. For example, nightmares, sleep paralysis, and REM sleep behavior disorder can be so disturbing that patients fear sleep and develop a secondary insomnia to avoid the fear associated with these disorders. Those REM sleep parasomnias that have received the most research attention are outlined in this section.

TABLE 58–1. PARASOMNIAS IN NON-REM SLEEP

Disorder	Prevalence	Usual Stage of Sleep	Sex Ratio (F:M)	Age of Onset	Course	Predisposing Factors	Family History	Differential Diagnosis
Sleepwalking	1–15%: children <1%: adults	SWS	1:1	4–8 yr	Disappears with adolescence	Fever Sleep deprivation Neuroleptics Chloral hydrate Lithium	Familial 45% affected offspring when one parent affected 60% affected offspring when both parents affected	Sleep terrors REM sleep behavior disorder Sleep-related epilepsy
Sleep terrors	5%: children <1%: adults	SWS	F < M—children 1:1—adults	4–12 yr 20–30 yr	Disappears with adolescence	Fever Sleep deprivation CNS depressants	Familial—genetics unknown	Nightmares Confusional arousals Sleep-related epilepsy Obstructive sleep apnea Nocturnal cardiac ischemia REM sleep behavior disorder
Confusional arousals	Common: children Rare: adults	SWS	1:1	<5 yr	Decrease with age	Young age Sleep deprivation CNS depressants Toxic/metabolic conditions Encephalopathy Sleep terrors Sleepwalking	Familial—genetics unknown	Sleep terrors Sleepwalking REM sleep behavior disorder Sleep-related partial complex seizures
Sleep bruxism	85–90%	2	1:1	10–20 yr	Unknown	Anatomic defects Anxiety	Probable	Partial complex seizures Generalized seizure disorder
Rhythmic movement disorder	4–66%	Drowsiness, 1–2	1:4	<1 yr	66% at 9 mo <50% at 18 mo 4% at 4 yr	Stress? Self-stimulation?	Occurs in identical twins	Bruxism Thumb sucking Periodic limb movement disorder Epilepsy

Disorder	Prevalence	Sleep stage	Sex ratio	Age of onset	Course	Precipitating factors	Genetics	Differential diagnosis
Sleep starts	60–70%	Drowsiness, 1	1:1	Any age	Benign	Caffeine/stimulants Intense physical exercise Emotional stress	Unknown	Hyperexplexia syndrome Epileptic myoclonus Periodic limb movement disorder Restless leg syndrome Fragmentary myoclonus Benign neonatal sleep myoclonus
Sleep-related abnormal swallowing	Rare	Arousals	Unknown	Middle age	Unknown	Hypnotic agents CNS depressants	Unknown	Obstructive sleep apnea Gastroesophageal reflux Sleep terrors Sleep choking syndrome
Nocturnal paroxysmal dystonia	Unknown	2	1:1	Infancy–40s	Chronic	Unknown	Familial	Sleep terrors REM sleep behavior disorder Epilepsy Periodic limb movement disorder
Benign neonatal sleep myoclonus	Rare	Quiet	1:1	<1 wk	Self-limited and benign	None known	Familial?	Seizures Drug withdrawal Infantile spasms Periodic limb movement disorder Fragmentary myoclonus

TABLE 58–2. PARASOMNIAS IN REM SLEEP

Disorder	Prevalence	Sex Ratio (F:M)	Age of Onset	Course	Predisposing Factors	Family History	Differential Diagnosis
Nightmares	20%: children 5–10%: adults	1:1 children 2:1–4:1 adults	3–6 yr	Can persist into adulthood Decrease over decades	Depression PTSD Anxiety disorders Borderline personality Schizophrenia Withdrawal from REM-suppressing drugs	?	Sleep terrors REM sleep behavior disorder PTSD
Sleep paralysis	Once: 40–50% >1:3–6%	1:1 except familial (F > M)	Young adults	Usually isolated unless familial (then chronic)	Irregular sleep Sleep deprivation Stress Supine sleep	Usually none; X-linked dominant when familial	Narcolepsy Atonic generalized seizures
Impaired sleep-related penile erections	10% Increase with age	Males only	>45 yr	Increases with age Seldom improves without treatment	Vascular disease Neurological disease Endocrine disease Depression	As determined by organic cause	—
REM sleep behavior disorder	Rare?	F < M	>50 yr	Progresses over months–years	Increasing age Neurologic disease, especially of brain stem	?	Sleep-related seizures Confusional arousals Sleepwalking Sleep terrors PTSD Nightmares
Sleep-related painful erections	Increase with age	Males only	>40 yr	More severe with age	Trazodone Autonomic medication	?	Peyronie's disease Infections Phimosis Priapism
REM sleep–related sinus arrest	?	?	Young adults	?	?	?	Cardiac arrhythmias secondary to other sleep-related breathing disorders

Nightmares

A nightmare is a frightening or anxiety-provoking dream with complex mental content. Essential features of a nightmare are significant fear or anxiety (subjectively determined) and vivid recall for the details of the dream. Arousals often occur when the dreamer physically tries to escape from the feared stimulus. The dreamer, when aroused, is fully lucid and can recall the nightmare in great detail. Autonomic activity is somewhat increased, but not to the extent observed in sleep terrors; in addition, increased autonomic activity quickly returns to resting levels.

Estimates of prevalence vary depending on the survey, and isolated nightmares occur in the majority of children, especially between the ages of 3 and 6 years. More frequent nightmares occur in approximately 20 per cent of children, although the prevalence ranges from 10 to 50 per cent. In childhood, both boys and girls are affected equivalently. Nightmares in childhood tend to be self-limited and decrease in frequency as the child matures.

In adults, women report more nightmares than men (the ratio varies from 2 : 1 to 4 : 1), although the overall prevalence is only about 5 per cent. When nightmares occur in adulthood, about half the time it is in the context of a major psychiatric disorder, such as anxiety disorder, schizophrenia, post-traumatic stress disorder, or depression, or a major medical disorder, such as emphysema or asthma. Another common condition that disposes to nightmares is withdrawal from REM-suppressing drugs, such as benzodiazepines, amphetamines, or alcohol. Among those individuals with no primary diagnosis, nightmares most frequently occur following very traumatic or stressful life events, such as an assault. In adults, as with children, there tends to be a decrease in the frequency of nightmares with age, at least in women.

Family history studies evaluating the transmission of nightmares have not been done.

Given that nightmares are largely a REM or REM rebound phenomenon, medications that suppress REM sleep have been therapeutic in some instances. Antidepressant and anxiolytic medications have REM-suppressing properties and can be effective in suppressing REM sleep, improving sleep continuity, and reducing anxiety. Behavioral techniques such as relaxation therapy have been effective in some cases. Psychotherapy has been a time-honored, although not necessarily empirically validated, means of addressing anxiety-related issues that may be associated with nightmares.

Sleep Paralysis

Sleep paralysis is a cardinal symptom of narcolepsy but can exist alone without any other disabling features. Paralysis of voluntary muscles in the trunk and limbs occurs for a short period of time at either sleep onset or sleep termination. Extraocular muscles are spared. Typically, sleep paralysis is associated with brief but intense fear, sometimes exacerbated by a sense of breathing difficulty. The patient is lucid, with clear sensorium, and is fully aware of the inability to move. The episode may last for 1 minute or for as long as several minutes. Sleep paralysis can disappear spontaneously or it may be terminated by touch or movement from another person. It is not unusual to experience dream mentation concurrent with the paralytic state, which can serve to make the experience even more frightening.

The prevalence of sleep paralysis has been evaluated cross-culturally. Estimates for isolated sleep paralysis episodes, when not related to narcolepsy, have ranged as high as 50 per cent. Recent surveys of Japanese college students[6] and Nigerian medical students[7] have indicated a prevalence from 26 to 40 per cent. A survey of American medical students found a lifetime prevalence of 16 per cent. Onset is usually in young adulthood. There appears to be no sex preference in the idiopathic form of sleep paralysis.

Sleep paralysis is thought to result from postsynaptic inhibition of alpha motoneurons at the level of the medulla. This is the mechanism for muscle inhibition during REM sleep. Selected individuals have been found to have a genetic basis for sleep paralysis. In these cases, the disorder occurs more frequently, is chronic, and is more likely to be associated with the transition from wakefulness to sleep. In idiopathic cases, sleep paralysis occurs more frequently in the transition from sleep to wakefulness. The genetic variant of sleep paralysis appears to be X-linked dominant, and the disorder occurs more frequently in females.

Most cases of sleep paralysis do not require intervention. While the experience with sleep paralysis is very frightening, the individual quickly learns that the paralysis is time limited. Some patients have reported that vigorous eye movements or repeated attempts to move terminate the episode. Case reports have supported serotonergic agents, such as L-tryptophan, to be efficacious in controlling the disorder. Hypnosis has also been reported to be successful in at least one case. Tricyclic antidepressants, which suppress REM sleep, may also provide relief.

Impaired Sleep-Related Penile Erections

During the normal course of sleep, males have periodic penile erections during REM sleep. When erectile dysfunction occurs in the presence of normal electrophysiological sleep, the condition is described as impaired sleep-related penile erections. Assessing nocturnal penile tumescence during sleep is a critical means of distinguishing between functional and organic impotence. Impaired nocturnal tumescence is considered a defining characteristic of organically mediated erectile dysfunction, whereas relatively normal nocturnal tumescence is seen in psychogenic impotence.

Impaired sleep-related penile erections are unlike other parasomnias inasmuch as this complaint is not directly expressed nor does it, by itself, bring the patient to the attention of the health care system. Most often, impaired tumescence is detected as part of an ongoing evaluation for reported wakeful erectile dysfunction. Polysomnographic and nocturnal penile tumescence studies are requested because the urologist may have found no organic basis or insufficient organic cause for the dysfunction, or there may be reasonable suspicion that the dysfunction is psychogenic in origin. Finally, the evaluation of erectile dysfunction may provide confirmatory evidence prior to corrective surgery.

Prevalence rates depend in part on the concurrent medical disorders. Evaluation of an unselected adult male population suggests a base rate estimate of 10 per cent. This increases with age. Onset can occur at any time in the adult years, but impaired sleep-related erections are most often associated with middle-aged and older men. Sleep-related erectile impairment is most often a complication of diseases that affect the vascular, neural, or endocrine systems. Impaired sleep-related erections have also been found consistently in a subset of depressed males.

To the extent that there is an organic basis to erectile impairment, the condition generally does not improve without treatment. With hypogonadal males, there is a dose-response relationship between testosterone replacement and improved erectile function. In depression, erectile function is improved with symptomatic improvement of depression. In cases of chronic illness such as diabetes mellitus, prostheses have been used with variable success.

REM Sleep Behavior Disorder

REM sleep behavior disorder is a recently described parasomnia characterized by the loss of muscle atonia, which usually occurs in REM sleep. As a result, patients with this disorder manifest a variety of purposeful movements appropriate to the content of their dreams. Unfortunately, their dream content often includes themes of pursuit, violence, or action, so that presenting symptoms may consist of punching, kicking, or running during sleep. Patients with REM sleep behavior disorder often damage furniture or injure themselves or a bedpartner.

Important differential diagnoses for REM sleep behavior disorder include non-REM parasomnias (sleepwalking, night terrors), nocturnal seizures, and nightmares. Unlike non-REM parasomnias or seizures, REM sleep behavior disorder is often associated with rapid arousal and detailed dream recall. Also unlike non-REM parasomnias, which occur almost exclusively in the first third of the night, the behavioral episodes may occur at any time, coincident with the 90 to 110-minute REM cycle. Nightmares, by contrast, do not include the motor activity characteristic of REM sleep behavior disorder.

There are no reliable estimates of the prevalence of REM sleep behavior disorder. Men are affected more often than women, particularly in idiopathic cases. Although onset at any age is possible, REM sleep behavior disorder is most often seen in the sixth or seventh decades. A familial association has been suggested by some case histories.

Neurological disease, including vascular, infectious, degenerative, and neoplastic disorders, can be identified in approximately 40 per cent of cases. Less frequently, patients receiving REM-suppressing medications such as tricyclic antidepressants and monoamine oxidase inhibitors may have loss of REM atonia sufficient to cause behavioral events. Rapid withdrawal from antidepressants, alcohol, or amphetamines may also precipitate REM sleep behavior disorder symptoms. A syndrome essentially identical to REM sleep behavior disorder has been reported in cats with experimental lesions in the peri−locus ceruleus alpha region of the pontine tegmentum.[8]

Polysomnographic studies reveal that the behavioral events arise out of REM sleep. In addition, REM sleep is often marked by a tonic increase in muscle tone, as well as a notable increase in phasic muscle twitches and jerks.

In idiopathic cases, REM sleep behavior disorder may be heralded by a prodrome of minor symptoms, whereas in "symptomatic" cases, the onset is more abrupt. The course is chronic and often progressive in terms of the frequency and severity of behaviors. Treatment is directed at securing the environment, preventing REM sleep rebound (as might occur with alcohol), and the use of medications. Tricyclic medications may suppress behavioral events in some patients, but more reliable results have been reported with low doses of clonazepam. Comparable low doses of other benzodiazepines may also be effective.

PARASOMNIAS IN ANY STAGE SLEEP

Parasomnias that occur in any stage of sleep are thought to occur most frequently in stage transitions. These parasomnias include sleep enuresis, primary snoring, sleep talking, and congenital central hypoventilation syndrome and are briefly described in Table 58−3. Sleep enuresis and primary snoring are the parasomnias most likely to come to the attention of the health care provider and are described in more detail in this section.

Sleep Enuresis

Sleep enuresis is defined as involuntary micturition during sleep. Sleep enuresis is designated as primary or secondary based on whether a bed-wetting−free period preceded the onset of enuresis. The threshold to determine onset of primary enuresis varies from 3 to 6 years. By age 6, approximately 90

TABLE 58–3. PARASOMNIAS IN ANY STAGE SLEEP

Disorder	Prevalence	Sex Ratio (F:M)	Age of Onset	Course	Predisposing Factors	Family History	Differential Diagnosis
Sleep enuresis	4 yr: 30% 6 yr: 10% 10 yr: 5% 12 yr: 3% 18 yr: 1–3%	2:3	Infancy	Resolves before 6 yr May be chronic without intervention	Institutionalization Lower socioeconomic status Metabolic/endocrinological disorders Obstructive sleep apnea Anatomical defects Neuroleptics	Genetic: single recessive gene?	Seizure disorder Sleep apnea
Primary snoring	Increases with age	F < M	Middle age	Predisposition to obstructive sleep apnea?	Enlarged tonsils Retrognathia CNS depressants Supine sleep Nasal congestion/obstruction Obesity	Familial	Obstructive sleep apnea
Sleep talking	Common?	F < M?	Not known	Benign and self-limited	Stress Fever Sleep terrors Confusional arousals Obstructive sleep apnea REM sleep behavior disorder	Possible	Obstructive sleep apnea REM sleep behavior disorder Sleep terrors Nightmares
Congenital central hypoventilation syndrome	Rare	1:1	Birth	Chronic	None known	None	Inborn metabolic errors Brain stem damage Hypothyroidism Primary lung disease
Nocturnal leg cramps	16%	F > M?	Late adult	Wax and wane	Pregnancy Metabolic disorders Endocrine disorders Vigorous exercise Oral contraceptives Electrolyte imbalance Neuromuscular disorders	None known	Chronic myelopathy Peripheral neuropathy Akathisia Restless leg syndrome Muscular pain–fasciculation syndrome Calcium metabolism disorder
Infant sleep apnea Apnea of infancy	Unknown	10:11	4–8 wk to 8 mo	30%—isolated events 50% > 1 per week 7% need resuscitation Remit at 6 months	Apnea of prematurity	Unknown	Hypoxia Acidosis Lung disease Pneumothorax
Apnea of prematurity	<31 wk: 50–80% 34–35 wk: 7%	1:1	<37 wk gestational age	Several/hour—1/wk Inversely related to gestational age	Spontaneous or event-related neck flexion Squirming from pain Hiccup Regurgitation Feeding	None	Respiratory infections Hypo/hyperthermia Hypo/hyperglycemia Anemia Electrolyte imbalance Sepsis

per cent of children have been able to inhibit normal nocturnal urinary discharge. When this capability has not been attained for up to 6 months by age 5, then the disorder is considered primary. If the child has had a period of 6 months or longer when he or she has successfully inhibited nocturnal urinary discharge, then enuresis is described as secondary.

Sleep enuresis occurs more frequently in boys than in girls (the ratio is 3:2). A number of predisposing organic causes have been listed (Table 58–3), but enuresis is most commonly functional in origin. When sleep enuresis is functional in origin, it is self-limited but can persist into the late teen years and is the source of much shame and inconvenience. Patients and their parents should be reassured that enuresis is *not* volitional.

Laboratory studies have indicated that enuresis occurs in each sleep stage in proportion to the amount of sleep in that stage. Most of these studies indicate no evidence of EEG arousal, such as sleep stage lightening or sleep stage transition, with each occurrence. Rhythmic slow wave sleep of longer than age-appropriate duration, evidence of sleep immaturity, has been noted to precede enuretic occurrences.[9] Sleep enuresis is one of the few sleep disorders for which there appears to be reasonable evidence for transmission by a single recessive gene.

Treatment should first be educational. It should be made clear that bed-wetting is not purposeful on the part of the patient. Urological evaluation may be indicated to determine whether there is evidence of anatomical abnormalities or obstructions. Assuming that organic causes have been ruled out, a variety of interventions are possible. These include medications (e.g., imipramine), nocturnal conditioning methods (pad and alarm), daily Kegel exercises to increase bladder control, restriction of fluids in the evening, and rousing the child during the night. Psychotherapy has been suggested in instances in which enuresis is secondary to psychological problems occurring in the home. All of the outlined treatments require time and persistence.

Primary Snoring

Snoring is considered a primary diagnosis when apnea and hypoventilation can be excluded. By definition, snoring is loud inspiratory or expiratory breathing sounds. Usually primary snoring comes to the attention of the health care system because of bedpartner complaints.

Primary snoring usually does not occur until adulthood, and onset usually does not occur prior to middle age. Prevalence increases thereafter across the lifespan. Snoring occurs most frequently in the supine sleeping position. More males are affected than females. The course of primary snoring had been thought to be benign, but it can cause hearing loss and has been found recently to be a vulnerability factor for breathing-related disorders.[10] In a study of 177 male patients ages 16 to 60 years, snoring was the only factor that predicted sleep-related brain infarction.[11]

Primary snoring has been documented in all sleep stages but is much more often a non-REM sleep phenomenon, most often occurring in slow wave sleep. To the extent that anatomy and weight are heritable, snoring has been found to be familial.

Treatment usually includes procedures to change body position during sleep, or to encourage weight loss, if relevant. The patient should be cautioned to avoid alcohol and sleep deprivation. Surgery, including uvulopalatopharyngoplasty and correction of craniofacial abnormalities, may be useful.

PARASOMNIAS: SLEEP STAGE UNKNOWN

Parasomnias for which the sleep stage is unknown (Table 58–4) have not been successfully studied in the laboratory, in part because of the lethality of the disorder, the immaturity of the patient, and the difficulty in documenting sleep staging and in part because of the low prevalence of the disorder.

Sudden Infant Death Syndrome

Sudden infant death syndrome (SIDS) is a devastating parasomnia that takes the lives of one to two babies per 1000 live births in the United States. SIDS is essentially a diagnosis by exclusion and is used only when there is no other apparent cause of death. Sex ratio indicates that males are slightly more vulnerable than females (1.2:1 to 1.5:1). The period of greatest vulnerability occurs when the infant is between 1 week and 12 weeks old; risk greatly diminishes after 6 months and is virtually nonexistent at 12 months. Factors that increase the probability of SIDS are listed in Table 58–4. These factors, singly or cumulatively, account for very little predictive variance. The course is, by definition, fatal.

SIDS has received significant research attention, and a series of mechanisms, operating singly or in concert, have been posited and evaluated. Several studies have evaluated factors as simple as sleeping position and have found that sleeping in the prone position occurs much more frequently. The relative risk with sleeping face down varies from 2.0 to 8.8 in SIDS victims.

It has been noted that the critical period for SIDS coincides directly with the time in infant development when sleep coalesces from brief to more protracted sleep periods. Immaturity in homeostatic mechanisms controlling variability in heart rate, respiration, arousal thresholds, and thermoregulation has been implicated. Although studies on each of these mechanisms do not yield uniform findings, the majority of studies indicate consistent disturbances in arousal threshold,[12] diminished variability in heart rate from sleep stage to sleep stage,[13] increased respiratory pauses or apneic events,[14,15] faulty coupling of cardiac and respiratory rhythms,[16] and dis-

TABLE 58–4. PARASOMNIAS: STAGE OF SLEEP UNKNOWN

Disorder	Prevalence	Sex Ratio (F:M)	Age of Onset	Course	Predisposing Factors	Family History	Differential Diagnosis
Sudden infant death syndrome	1–2/1000 live births	1 : 1.2–1.5	>1 wk <6 months	Fatal	Preterm birth Twins or triplets Sib with SIDS Substance-abusing mother Apnea of infancy Lower socioeconomic status Teenage pregnancy Short interpregnancy interval Birth in winter, spring, fall Smoking during pregnancy	Familial—genetics unknown	Pneumonia Meningitis Myocarditis Intracranial hemorrhage Child abuse Botulism
Sudden unexplained nocturnal death syndrome	0.0006 to 0.0009	Male only	24–44 yr	Fatal	Southeast Asian refugees in United States Laotians	Unknown	Other sudden sleep-related deaths

turbance in thermoregulation.[17] To the extent that these mechanisms have been reliably measured during sleep, several studies implicate active sleep or REM-stage sleep as the sleep stages wherein the dysregulation becomes fatal,[12–15,18] although other studies suggest quiet or non-REM sleep.[19,20] Most of our information on SIDS has been ascertained from infants who have required resuscitation from prolonged apneic events or from siblings of SIDS victims. While the risk to a sibling of a SIDS victim is greater than the risk to the general population, it is unknown whether the mechanism or mechanisms responsible for SIDS are genetic.

Because of the lethality of SIDS, the importance in identifying infants at risk becomes paramount. Home monitoring is the treatment of choice in cases of infants who have been resuscitated from apneic events. It must be cautioned, however, that the number of false-positive alarms is high. Treatment for siblings of SIDS victims is determined on a case-by-case basis.

SUMMARY

Parasomnias represent a subset of sleep disorders occurring episodically during sleep that may disturb the process of sleep, but are generally not associated with subjective complaints of insomnia or excessive daytime sleepiness. The appearance of waking behaviors in sleep underlines the complex interrelationship of sleep and wakefulness and provides clues to endogenous brain processes not yet understood. Causes of parasomnias can vary from fundamental dysregulation of neural mechanisms to benign and expected normal central nervous system development to effects of altered environmental time cues and sleep loss. A cardinal feature of a parasomnia is that it occurs in all cases without conscious control. This feature can be perplexing when behavior suggests deliberate action associated with wakefulness, yet, at a conscious level, the brain sleeps. Parasomnias will be refined and redefined as we learn more about the physiology of sleep and the coordination of endogenous cyclical rhythms.

REFERENCES

1. Thorpy MJ, ed: International Classification of Sleep Disorders: Diagnostic and Coding Manual. Rochester, MN: American Sleep Disorder Association, 1990.

2. Kales A, Soldatos CR, Bixler EO, et al: Hereditary factors in sleepwalking and night terrors. Br J Psychiatry 137:111–118, 1980.

3. Soldatas CR, Vela-Bueno A, Bixler EO, et al: Sleepwalking and night terrors in adulthood: Clinical EEG findings. Clin Electroencephalogr 11:136–139, 1980.

4. Amir N, Navon P, Silverberg-Shalev R: Interictal electroencephalography in night terrors and somnambulism. Isr J Med Sci 21:22–26, 1985.

5. Ware JC, Rugh JD: Destructive bruxism: Sleep stage relationship. Sleep 11:172–181, 1988.

6. Fukuda K, Miyasita A, Inugami M, et al: High prevalence of isolated sleep paralysis: Kanashibari phenomenon in Japan. Sleep 10:279–286, 1987.

7. Ohaeri JU, Odejide AO, Ikuesan BA, et al: The pattern of isolated sleep paralysis among Nigerian medical students. J Natl Med Assoc 81:805–808, 1989.

8. Morrison A, Reiner P: A dissection of paradoxical sleep. Brain Mechanisms of Sleep New York: Raven Press, 1985: 97–110.

9. Inoue M, Shimojima H, Chiba H, et al: Rhythmic slow waves observed on nocturnal sleep encephalogram in children with idiopathic nocturnal enuresis. Sleep 10:570–579, 1987.

10. Bliwise DL, Feldman DE, Bliwise NG, et al: Risk factors for sleep disordered breathing in heterogeneous geriatric populations. J Am Geriatr Soc 35:132–141, 1987.

11. Palomaki H, Partinen M, Juvela S, et al: Snoring as a risk factor for sleep-related brain infarction. Stroke 20:1311–1315, 1989.

12. Coons S, Guilleminault C: Motility and arousal in near miss sudden infant death syndrome. J Pediatr 107:728–732, 1985.

13. Schechtman VL, Harper RM, Kluge KA, et al: Cardiac and respiratory pattern in normal infants and victims of the sudden death syndrome. Sleep 11:413–424, 1988.

14. Watanabe K, Inokuma K, Negoro T: REM sleep prevents sudden infant death syndrome. Eur J Pediatr 140:289–292, 1983.

15. Beary MD, Mintram MK, Crutchfield MB, et al: Sleep apnoea occurring only in REM (possible relevance of the case for some cot deaths). Postgrad Med J 58:235–236, 1982.

16. Kluge KA, Harper RM, Schechtman VL: Spectral analysis assessment of respiratory sinus arrhythmia in normal infants and infants who subsequently died of sudden infant death syndrome. Pediatr Res 24:677–682, 1988.

17. Fleming PJ, Gilbert R, Azaz Y, et al: Interaction between bedding and sleeping position in the sudden infant death syndrome: A population based case-control study. Br Med J 301:85–89, 1990.

18. Harper RM, Frostig Z, Taube D, et al: Development of sleep-waking temporal sequencing in infants at risk for the sudden infant death syndrome. Exp Neurol 79:821–829, 1983.

19. Peirano P, Lacombe J, Kastler B, et al: Night sleep heart rate patterns recorded by cardiopneumography at home in normal and at-risk for SIDS infants. Early Hum Dev 17:175–186, 1988.

20. Guilleminault C, Ariagno R, Coons S, et al: Near-miss sudden infant death syndrome in eight infants with sleep apnea-related cardiac arrhythmias. Pediatrics 76:236–242, 1985.

59

CLINICAL SLEEP-WAKE DISORDERS IN PSYCHIATRIC PRACTICE:
Dyssomnias

J. CHRISTIAN GILLIN, M.D.

INSOMNIA DISORDERS

The diagnosis of insomnia is based upon the subjective complaint of difficulty in initiating or maintaining sleep or of nonrestorative sleep (not feeling well rested after sleep that is apparently adequate in amount).[1] Over 30 per cent of the general population complains of insomnia during the course of a year and about 17 per cent of the population reports that it is "serious." Insomnia is more common in women than men, increases with age, and is often associated with medical and psychiatric disorders, or abuse of alcohol, drugs, and medications. Since chronic insomnia most often occurs as a comorbid diagnosis together with other disorders, the clinician should usually carefully look for other conditions and treat the primary disorder.

In the abbreviated DSM-III-R nosology of sleep disorders, three types of insomnia disorders are identified: insomnia related to another mental disorder (nonorganic), insomnia related to a known organic factor, and primary insomnia. In the present chapter, we provide a somewhat expanded nosology, based partially upon the International Classification of Sleep Disorders (ICSD) Diagnostic and Coding Manual.[2]

Insomnia Associated with Behavioral/Psychophysiological Disorders

Acute stress is probably the most common cause of transient and short-term insomnia. These patients are unlikely to come to the attention of a clinician since the condition is self-limited.

Psychophysiological insomnia is defined as a "disorder of somatized tension and learned sleep-preventing associations that result in a complaint of insomnia."[2] All patients with chronic insomnia probably develop some secondary and learned sleep-preventing associations, such as marked overconcern with their inability to sleep. The frustration, anger, and anxiety associated with trying to sleep only serve to arouse them as they try to go to sleep or maintain sleep. The bed and the bedroom may acquire secondary aversive associations that further arouse them and prevent sleep. These patients often sleep better in places other than the bedroom, such as the TV or living room, hotels and vacations sites, and the sleep laboratory.

Insomnia Associated with Psychiatric Disorders

Table 59–1 presents a summary of the polygraphic sleep studies of depression and other disorders. This table is based upon a meta-analysis of 168 published all-night polygraphic sleeps studies, based upon over 7000 subjects.[3] In the case of depression, short rapid eye movement (REM) latency (time between onsets of sleep and the first REM period), increased duration of the first REM period, and increased REM density (the amount of ocular activity per minute of REM sleep, especially of the first REM period) have now become well-established biological makers of depression, varying roughly with the degree of depression (e.g., worse in delusional than nondelusional depression), and perhaps a weak trait marker for depression. Depressive patients were the only psychiatric group to show a significant elevation of REM percentage.

Surprisingly, total or partial sleep deprivation for one night has temporary antidepressant effects in about half of depressed patients.[4] In addition, selective deprivation of REM sleep by the awakening method for 2 to 3 weeks has been reported to have antidepressant effects.

Short REM latency has been reported commonly in three other psychiatric disorders besides depression: borderline patients, eating disorder patients, and schizophrenics.

Patients with *alcoholism* may suffer from a variety of sleep disturbances: insomnia, hypersomnia, circadian rhythm disturbances, and acute and subacute withdrawal syndromes. Alcohol is probably one of the most common self-administered sleeping medications. In small amounts it does induce sleep, but it

373

TABLE 59–1. SUMMARY OF POLYGRAPHIC SLEEP STUDIES IN VARIOUS DIAGNOSTIC GROUPS COMPARED WITH NORMALS[a]

Groups	TST	SE (%)	SL	SWS Time	NREM	RL	REMD REMP#1	REM%
Depression	↓↓	↓↓	↑↑	↓↓	↓	↓↓	↑	↑↑
Alcoholism[d]	↓	?	○↑	↓	↓	○	○↑	○↑
Anxiety	↓↓	↓↓	↑↑	○	○	○	○	○
Borderline[e]	↓○	↓○	○↑	○	○	○↓	○	○
Dementia[f]	↓↓	↓↓	↑↑	○	○	○↓	○	○
Eating[g]	↓○	↓○	○	○	○	○↓	○↓	○
Schizo[h]	↓	↓	○↑	○	○	○↓	↑	○
Insomnia[i]	↓↓	↓↓	↑↑	↓↓	○↓	○	○	○

[a] Based on meta-analysis of 168 published studies in various psychiatric groups.[3]

[b] TST, total sleep time; SE, sleep efficiency; SL, sleep latency; SWS time, stages 3 and 4 sleep time; NREM, non-REM sleep; RL, REM latency; REMD REMP#1, REM density of the first REM period; REM%, percentage REM sleep.

[c] Down, Long, Short, or Up, significantly decreased, longer, shorter, or increased compared with normal controls; ?, insufficient data; young, younger patients (20–50 years of age).

[d] Mostly alcoholics in prolonged abstinence state.

[e] Borderline personality disorder.

[f] Mostly senile dementia of the Alzheimer's type.

[g] Eating disorders.

[h] Schizophrenia, mostly in a stable chronic psychosis.

[i] Mostly primary insomnia.

Statistical differences: ↓↓, strongly decreased in patients; ↓, decreased in most analysis; ○, same: ↑, increased in patients in some analyses; ↑↑, strongly increased: ○↓, both normal and decreased reports: ○↑, both normal and increased reports.

also often causes difficulty maintaining sleep as blood levels fall over the course of the sleep period, and if somatic symptoms such as gastric irritation or headache awaken the subject. For this reason, clinicians should always inquire about alcohol consumption when evaluating patients with sleep complaints.

During heavy bouts of drinking, alcoholics may show hypersomnia induced by imbibing large amounts of alcohol or marked circadian disturbances of sleep-wakefulness, such as short bouts of sleep and wakefulness. During acute withdrawal, patients may occasionally show "terminal hypersomnia" in association with delirium tremens, but more commonly experience marked agitation without sleep for several days. During prolonged withdrawal, patients with alcoholism show persistent objective and subjective sleep disturbances, including prolonged sleep latency, short total sleep time, reduced delta sleep, and loss of non-REM sleep. These changes may persist for weeks to months; indeed, in some studies they last up to 2 years. Unfortunately, no satisfactory pharmacological treatment can now be recommended for the alcoholic patient in prolonged abstinence. Benzodiazepines should probably not be used because of cross-tolerance. Some clinicians have recommended small doses of sedating antidepressants at bedtime.

Patients with anxiety disorders, post-traumatic stress disorder, obsessive-compulsive disorder, and panic disorder may complain frequently of difficulty falling or staying asleep, or of inadequate sleep. Interestingly, panic attacks may occur during sleep itself.

Insomnia Associated with Drug Dependency

Kales et al. have reported that some chronic insomniac patients on high doses of hypnotic drugs sleep better once the drugs are discontinued.[5] In addition, it is now well recognized that use of benzodiazepines may be followed by withdrawal phenomena, such as "rebound insomnia," particularly following discontinuation of drugs with short half-lives. For these reasons, it is wise to taper patients off of benzodiazepines when possible and to keep the doses as low as possible.[6]

Insomnia and Other Complaints Associated with Sleep-Induced Respiratory Impairment

Complaints of insomnia are not uncommon in patients with *central sleep apnea*, which results when the patient essentially "turns off" the respiratory drive center in the brain stem during sleep. Likewise, patients with *chronic obstructive pulmonary disease* often complain of insomnia, in part because of the respiratory difficulties and in part because of anxiety. In addition, the syndrome of *alveolar hypoventilation* may cause either insomnia or hypersomnia. This syndrome is caused by shallow breathing and may be either idiopathic or secondary to a known disorder, such as poliomyelitis.

Other sleep-related respiratory disorders include *sleep-related asthma* and *altitude insomnia*. Individuals climbing rapidly to high altitudes (3000 m) may develop altitude sickness, which is associated with sleep-induced Cheyne-Stokes respiration or sleep apnea. These persons should probably not be treated with hypnotic medications, which further suppress the respiratory centers, but may benefit from acetazolamide.

Insomnia Associated with Sleep-Related Movement Disorders

Relatively rare cases of insomnia result from different types of movement disorders that occur primarily or exclusively in association with sleep. *Sleep starts (hypnagogic jerks)* are sudden brief jerks at sleep onset, usually of the arms and legs, sometimes associated with a subjective feeling of falling, a sensory flash, or a hypnagogic dream. *Restless legs syndrome* is characterized by disagreeable sensations in the legs, akin to akathisia, usually prior to sleep or any time the patients assumes a recumbent or rest position, which cause an almost irresistible urge to move the legs. *Periodic limb movement disorder (nocturnal myoclonus)* involves highly stereotyped, brief limb muscle movements that occur every 20 to 40 seconds during sleep and are characterized by extension of the big toe in combination with partial flexion of the ankle, knee, and sometimes hip. *Nocturnal leg cramps* are painful sensations of muscular tightness or tension, usually in the calf but occasionally in the foot, that occur during sleep episodes. A recently discovered condition called *REM sleep behavior disorder* is associated with violent or injurious behavior during sleep, limb or body movements during REM sleep associated with dream mentation, and partial preservation of muscle tone during REM sleep so that dreams can be "acted out."

Insomnia (and Other Sleep Disturbances) Associated with Neurological Disorders

Sleep disturbances occur frequently with a variety of neurological disorders, including epilepsy, headache (especially migraine), Parkinson's disease, and cerebral degenerative disorders. In the moderate to severe forms of *Alzheimer's disease* and other dementias, disturbed sleep at night and excessive sleepiness by day, night wandering, disorientation and confusion ("sundowning"), and problems of behavioral management are often major reasons for institutionalization and for disruption of the life of family caregivers. Polygraphic features include sleep fragmentation, prolonged sleep latency, lowered sleep efficiency, and decreased total sleep time, delta sleep, and non-REM sleep.

Insomnia Associated with Medical Conditions

Epidemiological studies suggest that the modal hypnotic user is an older woman with chronic medical conditions. Sleep in these individuals may be disturbed for many reasons, among them pain and physical discomfort, cardiovascular insufficiency, anxiety, and lack of physical activity during the day. The high incidence of sleep disturbance with respiratory diseases has already been mentioned.

Idiopathic (Childhood-Onset) Insomnia

This relatively rare disorder begins in childhood and is a lifelong, relentless condition that shows little variation in severity over time.[7] The cause is unknown, but may involve abnormalities of central sleep regulating systems of the brain.

General Therapeutic Approaches to the Treatment of Insomnia

Treatment of insomnia begins with determination of the underlying diagnostic cause or causes of the insomnia, which should generally be the target of therapy.

Sleeping Pills

Sleeping pills may be beneficial for patients with short-term or transient insomnia, especially if there is documented sleep loss. The indications for use of sleeping pills in chronic insomnia, whether idiopathic (primary) or secondary, are less clear. Finally, there is general agreement that benzodiazepines are currently the preferred hypnotic drugs of choice for most patients. Compared with most other hypnotics, benzodiazepines are unlikely to be addicting, to be fatal in overdose, to be associated with clear pharmacological tolerance with repeated nightly use, or to displace certain other drugs from carrier proteins in blood. In the near future (late 1992), a new nonbenzodiazepine, zolpidem, will probably be released in the United States. It appears to be as safe as or safer than the classical benzodiazepines.[8]

BENZODIAZEPINES

Flurazepam (Dalmane), quazepam (Doral), temezapam (Restoril), estazolam (ProSom), and trizolam (Halcion) are specifically marketed in the United States as hypnotics, but other benzodiazepines are also effective.[1] Diazepam is the most rapidly absorbed of the available benzodiazepines, whereas temazepam and triazolam have intermediate rates of absorption. More slowly absorbed benzodiazepines are probably ineffective for sleep-onset insomnia if they are taken less than an hour before bedtime.

Benzodiazepines are metabolized primarily by microsomal oxidation and glucuronide conjugation. The former system is compromised by liver disease (acute heptatitis, cirrhosis) and old age; thus, normally long-acting benzodiazepines become even longer acting. In addition, certain drugs that compete for metabolism by microsomal enzymes, such as cimetidine, estrogens, disulfiram, and isoniazid, may prolong the half-life of some benzodiazepines. In contrast, conjugative enzymes remain essentially unaffected by liver disease, advancing age, or drugs. Thus, oxazepam, lorazepam, and temezapam, which are metabolized primarily by conjugation, are not affected by liver disease or old age.

There are relative advantages and disadvantages to long- and short-acting benzodiazepines, respectively. Long-acting hypnotics tend to have carryover effects the next day and accumulate when taken on a nighty basis. These effects can be good if daytime sedation is desirable (e.g., in anxious patients) or if continued hypnotic effects are desired for several nights once the drug is stopped. However, daytime carryover effects may be undesirable if full alertness, cognitive skills, or motor coordination are needed. Furthermore, some individuals may be particularly sensitive to the accumulation of active metabolites, such as the elderly or individuals who take other sedating compounds, including alcohol. Short-acting benzodiazepines are therefore advantageous if carryover effects are undesirable either the next day or with continued use. However, rebound insomnia, daytime anxiety, and early morning wakefulness have been associated with short-acting benzodiazepines in some, but not all studies; these undesirable side effects presumably occur because of rapid withdrawal and uncovering of up-regulated receptors.

Lorazepam and triazolam have particularly been associated with amnesia, especially when combined with alcohol, as often occurs during air travel ("traveler's amnesia"), or when subjects are awakened at night after taking a hypnotic. Long-acting hypnotics may also cause amnesia, although apparently less commonly than the short-acting agents.

BARBITUATES

The popularity of secobarbital, nembutol, and other barbituates has declined during the past 15 years, since the introduction of the benzodiazepine hypnotics. They have a lower therapeutic index, induce microsomal enzymes, and produce tolerance and physical dependence.

NON BENZODIAZEPINE, NONBARBITURATE HYPNOTICS

Chloral hydrate, methyprylon, ethchlorvynol, and glutethimide possess clinical, pharmacological, and adverse effects similar to those of the barbiturates. Chloral hydrate is still widely used, especially for the elderly. A small but significant amount becomes trichloracetic acid, which has a half-life of 4 days. This metabolite accumulates with chronic use and can displace acidic drugs from the plasma protein-binding site, which may be hazardous with oral anticoagulants or hypoglycemic agents.

ANTIHISTAMINES

Diphenhydramine hydroxyzine, doxylamine, and other antihistamines are sedating and are often used as hypnotic agents. Tolerance, however, appears to develop rapidly. Moreover, these drugs have anticholinergic effects, causing memory impairment, in-

hibition of bowel and bladder function, and tachycardia, especially in the elderly. In addition, they tend to lower the seizure threshold and should be used cautiously in epileptic patients or during withdrawal from alcohol.

SEDATIVE ANTIDEPRESSANTS

Doxepin, trazodone, trimipramine, and amitriptyline are occasionally prescribed in relatively low doses as hypnotics. They are nonaddicting and unlikely to be abused. However, they have anticholinergic side effects, may cause orthostatic hypotension, and may lower seizure thresholds. Little research has been published on their usefulness and side effects in insomniac patients.

L-TRYPTOPHAN

This essential amino acid appears to be a "natural hypnotic." Because of recent reports of the eosinophilia-myalgia syndrome associated with tryptophan, it should not be used until its safety is established.

OVER-THE-COUNTER SLEEPING PILLS

The effectiveness of these drugs is not well documented, but there are potential sides effects, since they often contain scopolamine, diphenhydramine, or salicylate.

Doctor-Patient Relationship

The doctor-patient relationship is often important not only for its positive benefits, but preventing secondary complications of insomnia, such as psychological dependence on and misuse of hypnotics, alcohol abuse, and chronobiological disturbances.

Counseling and Psychotherapy

Some authorities, such as Kales and his associates,[9] advocate psychotherapy, since they regard the complaint of insomnia as resulting from "internalization of emotions," anxiety, depression, obsessive rumination, and other cognitive and emotional arousal processes.

Sleep Hygiene

For some chronic insomniacs, the bed acquires many secondary unpleasant associations, a place to worry and be frustrated rather than to rest. In order to reduce these factors and to improve general sleep-wake habits, patients may be instructed in several aspects of "sleep hygiene":

1. Wake up and go to bed at the same time every day, even on weekends.
2. Avoid long periods of wakefulness in bed. Use the bed for sleep or marital relations, not as a place to read, watch television, or work. If sleep does not begin within a certain period of time, say 30 minutes, leave the bed and do not return until drowsy.

3. Avoid napping.

4. Exercise regularly three or four times a week, but usually not in the evening if this tends to arouse the body and interfere with sleep.

5. Discontinue or reduce alcohol, caffeine-containing beverages, cigarettes, and other substances that may interfere with sleep.

6. "Wind down" before bed with quiet or relaxing activities.

7. Optimize the sleeping environment by maintaining room temperature at a cool, comfortable level (50° to 70°F), reducing noise, or promoting restful background sounds.

These so-called stimulus control treatment approaches have been shown to be effective in some studies, usually with relatively mild, young insomniacs.

Behavioral and Biofeedback Techniques

A variety of techniques have been advocated in treating chronic insomnia, including autogenic training, progressive muscle relaxation, electromyographic biofeedback, and electroencephalographic feedback. While these treatments appear to be safe, their effectiveness and indications are not well established.

Sleep Restriction Therapy

Since many chronic insomniac patients both underestimate their actual sleep time and have poor sleep efficiency, Spielman et al.[10] have recently proposed that patients limit time in bed to the estimated duration of total sleep; for example, if the patient reports sleeping 6 hours per night, he or she is required to limit time in bed to 6 hours or slightly more. This simple maneuver usually produces mild sleep deprivation, shortens sleep latency, and increases sleep efficiency. As sleep becomes more consolidated, the patient is allowed to gradually increase time in bed.

DISORDERS OF EXCESSIVE DAYTIME SLEEPINESS

Fatigue should not be confused with pathological sleepiness. The former, for example, is a common complaint of patients with insomnia (feelings of lethargy and "tiredness"), but it is not accompanied by a propensity to sleep when offered the opportunity. Pathological excessive daytime sleepiness, in contrast, describes varying degrees of true sleepiness in the absence of obvious causes, such as profound sleep deprivation or heavily sedating medications. Although excessive daytime sleepiness (EDS) is sometimes used synonymously with hypersomnia, this equation can be misleading in the sense that not all patients with EDS have excessive amounts of sleep. In its more severe forms, pathological excessive sleepiness significantly interferes with work, social relationships, hobbies, and family life and may even be a risk for death or serious accident should the individual fall asleep at a critical time.

Patients with suspected EDS should be referred to a sleep disorders clinic for several reasons. First, it is important to establish by objective criteria that the patient really has excessive daytime sleepiness, since the differential diagnosis of EDS almost always includes personality disorders (e.g., passive-aggressive or passive-dependent personality disorders, or "acting out" against norms such as punctuality, attention, and responsibility) and drug-seeking behavior (malingering). The major objective test is the Multiple Sleep Latency Test (MSLT), in which the latency to sleep onset is measured in four or five naps taken at intervals across the day (10:00 A.M. and 12:00, 2:00, 4:00, and 6:00 P.M.). If the mean of these sleep latencies is below 5 minutes, the condition is judged to be severe (normal subjects usually have a sleep latency above 15 minutes). In addition, the specific etiology can be determined in many cases during the clinical evaluation, all-night polysomnography, and MSLT, particularly in cases of sleep apnea or narcolepsy.

The DSM-III-R identifies three types of hypersomnia disorders: related to another mental disorder (nonorganic), related to a known organic disorder, and primary hypersomnia. In this section a more complete classification is presented, based in part upon the International Classification of Sleep Disorders (ICSD). Reference has previously been made to other disorders that may be associated with either insomnia or EDS, such as some forms of depression, periodic leg movements, sleep-related respiratory disorders, and various neurological-medical conditions.

Narcolepsy

This disorder of EDS is associated with cataplexy and, sometimes, hypnagogic hallucinations and sleep paralysis (the narcoleptic "tetrad"). These patients typically experience repeated cycles of brief napping (10 to 20 minutes) or irresistible sleep "attacks" that are refreshing for a few hours but are gradually followed by periods of sleepiness. Cataplexy is the sudden loss of bilateral tone in major antigravity muscles, often provoked by strong emotion, such as laughing, weeping, fright, or surprise. Sleep paralysis is a brief period of muscle atonia at the transitions between wakefulness and sleep, and hypnagogic hallucinations are vivid perceptual experiences ("dreams") that occur at sleep onset. Cataplexy and sleep paralysis are thought to be related to the muscle atonia that normally occurs during REM sleep, whereas the hypnagogic hallucinations are related to the dreaming of REM sleep.

The prevalence of narcolepsy is estimated to be 0.03 to 0.16 per cent. It usually begins in the second decade, often first with the symptom of EDS, and is found equally in men and women. Genetic factors are suggested by the increased risk in relatives. Human leukocyte antigen (HLA) typing indicates a very high prevalence of HLA-DR2 and -DQwl, again suggesting a genetic predisposition.

After ruling out exclusion criteria, the diagnosis is confirmed by all-night polysomnography and both short sleep latency (less than 5 minutes) and short REM latency (less than 20 minutes on two or more naps) in the MSLT. Pharmacological treatment usually involves (1) nonsedating, stimulating tricyclic antidepressants, such as protriptyline or, more recently, fluoxetine, usually in low doses, to control cataplexy, and (2) stimulants, such as methylphenidate, amphetamine, or pemoline, to reduce EDS.

Obstructive Sleep Apnea

Obstructive sleep apnea results from repeated episodes of upper airway obstruction during sleep. It is usually associated with periods of loud snoring and gasping that punctate the apneic periods, frequent brief arousals from sleep, bradytachycardia, arterial oxygen desaturation, hypertension, morning headaches, dry mouth, unrefreshing sleep, and short sleep latencies on the MSLT. Polysomnographic monitoring shows more than five episodes of obstructive apnea, each lasting at least 10 seconds, per hour of sleep (that is, an apnea index of five or greater).

The disorder is most common in overweight, middle-aged men, but can involve any age and gender, especially in forms resulting from mechanical or medical types of upper airway obstruction, such as enlarged tonsils, hypothyroidism, acromegaly, or craniofacial abnormalities such as micrognathia and retrognathia. The prevalence is estimated to be about 1 to 2 per cent in the population. Aside from daytime sleepiness, the major complications are the secondary physiological and psychological consequences: life-threatening cardiovascular arrhythmias, right-sided heart failure, and hypertension; cognitive impairment, including in severe cases neuropathological injury and stroke; depression; impotence; and social and economic impediments.

Some patients with obstructive sleep apnea will respond to tricyclic antidepressants, which apparently increase muscle tone in the upper airway. More commonly, however, nasal continuous positive airway pressure (CPAP) has proven to be a very effective form of therapy. This involves sleeping with a small mask that covers the nose, through which room air is delivered at low pressure (5 to 15 cm H_2O) thus "splinting" the soft tissues of the upper airway and maintaining patency during breathing. Another mechanical aid is the tongue retaining device (RTD), a mouthpiece that holds the tongue forward and keeps the airway open. Finally, a number of surgical operations have been advocated, such as uvulopalatopharyngoplasty (UPPP), a "Rotor Rooter" procedure designed to open up the airway during sleep.

Idiopathic Hypersomnia

Idiopathic hypersomnia is a disorder of prolonged sleep periods, EDS, or excessively "deep sleep," usually beginning insidiously before the age of 25. While these patients do show short sleep latencies on the MSLT, they do not show sleep-onset REM periods or complain of cataplexy, sleep paralysis, or hypnagogic hallucinations.

Recurrent Hypersomnia (Kleine-Levin Syndrome)

Recurrent hypersomnia is characterized by recurrent episodes of hypersomnia (at least 18 hr/day) lasting at least 3 days at a time. These episodes usually occur once or twice a year and may be associated with binge eating, weight gain, hypersexuality, and disinhibited behaviors (irritability, aggression, confusion, hallucinations). Functioning is normal between episodes. The cause and prevalence are unknown. It typically occurs in adolescent boys.

Hypersomnia Associated with Stimulant Withdrawal

During acute withdrawal from cocaine, amphetamine, and other stimulants, substance abusers may show prolonged total sleep time, with short REM latency and elevated REM percentage, for a week to 10 days. During the day, they appear to hypersomnolant.

CIRCADIAN RHYTHM DISORDERS OF THE SLEEP-WAKE CYCLE

Two processes modulate the daily tides of sleep and wakefulness: (1) a homeostatic process—the longer the period of wakefulness, the greater the propensity to sleep (sleep reverses the effect of wakefulness); and (2) a circadian process (circa = about, dian = 1 day) that regulates the propensity to sleep across the 24-hour day—in persons living on a "normal sleep schedule" (11:00 P.M. to 7:00 A.M.), the sleep propensity is greatest at night and, interestingly, in midafternoon (the "siesta hour").[11] The "phase position" of the biological clock or clocks that determine circadian sleep propensity is probably determined primarily by environmental lighting conditions. Information about light reaching the retina is conveyed to the suprachiasmatic nucleus, a small bilateral nucleus in the anterior hypothalamus, thus synchronizing the internal clock with the external world.

The major characteristic of circadian rhythm disturbances is a misalignment between the timing of sleep-wake patterns and the desired or normal pattern. Patients may complain of either insomnia or EDS.

Jet Lag (Time Zone Change) Syndrome

Jet lag is characterized by varying degrees of insomnia, excessive daytime sleepiness, impaired performance, and gastrointestinal and other symptoms that follow rapid travel across multiple time zones. Individuals differ in susceptibility to jet lag; some evidence indicates that it tends to be worse in older people, introverts, and "morning types" ("larks"). The resolution of jet lag involves realigning the circadian clock with the new light-dark cycle. Eastward trips (a phase advance of the endogenous clock) usually take longer to adjust to than westward trips (a phase delay).

Shift Work Sleep Disorder

Shift work sleep disorder consists of symptoms of either insomnia or excessive sleepiness in relationship to certain work schedules (rotating or permanent shift work, roster work, or irregular work hours). Complications include gastrointestinal symptoms, possibly cardiovascular symptoms, increased abuse of alcohol, disruption of family and social life, low morale and productivity, and high absenteeism. Many individuals never completely adjust to the work schedule because they try to maintain a normal sleep-wake schedule on weekends and holidays in order to participate in family and social activities. The prevalence and severity of this disorder are unknown, although about 26 per cent of the working population have a schedule outside the usual 8:00 A.M. to 5:00 P.M. job.

Delayed Sleep Phase Syndrome

Delayed sleep phase syndrome is a disorder in which the major sleep period is delayed in relation to the desired clock time. The major symptom is difficulty in waking up at the desired time in the morning, as well as prolonged sleep latency at night. These individuals are, in essence, extreme "night owls." The general prevalence is unknown, but it appears to be highest in adolescents (7 per cent according to one survey). Complications include difficulties with tardiness and attention for early morning activities, absenteeism, misuse of hypnotics and stimulants, and labeling as lazy or as having a passive-aggressive personality disorder.

A standard method of treatment is to phase-delay the onset of bedtime and arousal by 2 to 3 hours per day each day, and thereby bring the bedtime to a desired time (11:00 P.M., for example) over a period of 5 to 7 days.

Advanced Sleep Phase Syndrome

Advanced sleep phase syndrome is a disorder in which the major sleep period is advanced in relationship to the desired bedtime, resulting in symptoms of early evening sleepiness, early sleep onset, and early morning awakening. The prevalence is unknown. Since normal aging tends to be associated with an "early to bed, early to rise" pattern, this syndrome is probably more common in the elderly than the young.

Non–24-Hour Sleep-Wake Syndrome

Non–24-hour sleep-wake syndrome is a chronic disorder in which the individual shows daily delays of 1 to 2 hours in both sleep onset and wake times under normal environmental conditions. These patients, like normal experimental subjects living in isolation from normal time cues, are living on an approximately 25-hour cycle of rest-activity. This disorder appears to be rare in the general population, but may occur in as many as 40 per cent of blind individuals. It may result from ophthalmological or neurological disorders that interfere with the synchronization of the suprachiasmatic nucleus with the environment, but personality disorders may be paramount (i.e., individuals who willfully or unconsciously disregard environmental cues). In one uncontrolled clinical trial, vitamin B_{12} was helpful.[12]

General Principles in the Treatment of Circadian Rhythm Disorders

The judicious use of short–half-life sleeping pills in short-term circadian rhythm disorders, such as jet lag, may ameliorate the sleep loss, but this benefit must be weighed against the risks of amnesia, hangover effects, and impaired arousal while under the influence of the drug. Their efficacy in long-term disorders, such as shift work, is virtually unknown.

In treating circadian rhythm disorders, it is useful to follow known principles. First, try to synchronize sleep and wakefulness to the underlying phase position of the circadian clock. Second, remember that the natural cycle length of the circadian clock is longer than 24 hours. Thus, going westward (i.e., phase delaying) is usually easier than going eastward (i.e., phase advancing). Shift workers, for example, appear to do better when shifting in a "clockwise direction" (from day to evening to night work schedules) rather than "counterclockwise." Third, make use of appropriated *Zeitgebers* ("time givers") to move and establish the phase position of the biological clock. Although not yet tested extensively in clinical situations, the appropriate manipulation of the light-dark cycle may be helpful. For example, exposure to bright light in the evening, coupled with deprivation of light in the early morning, may permit more rapid adaptation to new sleep-wake schedules when phase delaying.

REFERENCES

1. Gillin JC, Byerly WF: Drug therapy: The diagnosis and management of insomnia. N Engl J Med 322:239–248, 1990.

2. Diagnostic Classification Steering Committee, Thorpy MJ, Chairman: The International Classification of Sleep Disorders: Diagnostic and Coding Manual. Rochester, MN: American Sleep Disorders Association, 1990.

3. Benca RM, Obermeyer WH, Thisted RA, Gillin JC: Sleep and psychiatric disorders: A meta-analysis. Arch Gen Psychiatry, (in press, 1992).

4. Hillman E, Kripke DF, Gillin JC: Sleep restriction, exercise, and bright lights: Alternate therapies for depression. In Tasman A, Kaufman C, Goldfinger S, eds. American Psychiatric Press Review of Psychiatry: Section I: Treatment of Refractory Affective Disorder. Post R, sect ed, vol 9. Washington, DC: American Psychiatric Press, 1990:132–144.

5. Kales A, Bixler EO, Tan TL, et al: Chronic hypnotic drug use: Ineffectiveness, drug withdrawal insomnia, and dependance. JAMA 227:513–517, 1974.

6. Greenblatt D, Harmatz JS, Zinny MA, Shader RI: Effect of gradual withdrawal on the rebound sleep disorder after discontinuation of triazolam. N Engl J Med 317:722–728, 1987.

7. Hauri P: A cluster analysis of insomnia. Sleep 6:326, 1980.

8. Sauvantet JP, Langer SZ, Morselli PL, eds. Imidazopyridines in Sleep Disorders. New York: Raven Press, 1988.

9. Kales A, Kales J: Evaluation and Treatment of Insomnia. New York: Oxford University Press, 1984.

10. Spielman AJ, Saskin P, Thorpy MJ: Treatment of chronic insomnia by restriction of time in bed. Sleep 10:45–56, 1987.

11. Daan S, Beersma DG, Borbely AA: Timing of human sleep: Recovery process gated by a circadian pacemaker. Am J Physiol 246:R161–R183, 1984.

12. Kamgar-Parsi B, Wehr TA, Gillin JC: Successful treatment of human non-24 hour sleep-wake syndrome. Sleep 6:257–264, 1983.

Section I

EATING DISORDERS

60

PROPOSED DSM-IV CRITERIA FOR EATING DISORDERS

B. TIMOTHY WALSH, M.D., and COLLEEN M. HADIGAN, B.A.

The Eating Disorders Work Group of the American Psychiatric Association's Task Force on the DSM-IV identified five questions to be examined:

1. Should anorexia nervosa be subtyped into a group of patients who binge eat and a group of patients who do not?
2. Can it be documented that criterion E for bulimia nervosa ("Persistent overconcern with body shape and weight") was a useful addition to the criteria for bulimia nervosa in DSM-III-R?
3. Is there evidence to suggest that bulimia nervosa should be subtyped, for example, into a group of patients who purge via the use of self-induced vomiting or laxatives and a group of patients who do not?
4. Can any clarification be provided for criterion A of bulimia nervosa, which requires that binges be "rapid" and "large?" Can documentation be provided to justify that binges occur, on average, twice a week for 3 months in order to merit a diagnosis?
5. Are there data to suggest that another diagnostic category is needed for a group of people with overeating disturbances who do not meet current criteria for bulimia nervosa?

Portions of this chapter have appeared in Walsh BT: Diagnostic criteria for eating disorders in DSM-IV: Work in progress. Int J Eating Disord (in press).

ANOREXIA NERVOSA

DaCosta and Halmi[1] found substantial data suggesting that the distinction between bulimic and nonbulimic subtypes of anorexia nervosa is a useful one. For example, patients with anorexia nervosa who binge eat were consistently more likely to exhibit characteristics such as impulsive behavior and mood lability compared to patients with anorexia nervosa who do not engage in binge eating. The Work Group has therefore recommended that anorexia nervosa be subtyped into bulimic and nonbulimic types in DSM-IV using the following criteria:

Bulimic Type: During the episode of Anorexia Nervosa, the person engages in recurrent episodes of binge eating.
Non-bulimic Type: During the episode of Anorexia Nervosa, the person does not engage in recurrent episodes of binge eating.

This recommendation implies that individuals with anorexia nervosa who have bulimia will receive a diagnosis of "anorexia nervosa, bulimic type" rather than simultaneous diagnoses of anorexia nervosa and bulimia nervosa.

In addition to the recommendation to subtype anorexia nervosa, the Work Group felt that the examples in criterion C for anorexia nervosa were not typical of many patients with this illness, and therefore has suggested that the criterion be broadened to identify additional manifestations of a disturbance of body shape and weight. According to the proposed wording for criterion C, the patient must evidence a "disturbance in the way in which one's body weight or shape is experienced, undue influence of body shape or weight on self-evaluation, or denial of the seriousness of the current low body weight."

BULIMIA NERVOSA

Regarding bulimia nervosa, the review concerning the utility of overconcern with shape and weight clearly documented that this was a relatively specific and highly characteristic feature of patients with this disorder.[2] For example, in a sample of 107 women seeking treatment for eating problems at Toronto Hospital, only 3 per cent did not evidence overconcern with shape or weight as determined by the Eating Disorder Examination. The Work Group believes that this clinical feature should be retained as a diagnostic criterion in DSM-IV. However, the Work Group recommended that the criterion regarding overconcern with shape and weight be reworded to emphasize that the critical disturbance is the undue influence of body shape and weight on self-esteem.

The question of whether bulimia nervosa should be subtyped into a group of patients who purge via the use of self-induced vomiting or laxatives and a group of patients who do not purge has raised considerable debate and resulted in the following two alternatives. The first alternative is to confine the diagnosis to those patients who binge eat and use either self-induced vomiting or laxatives in order to avoid weight gain. One rationale for this recommendation is that the overwhelming majority of patients in treatment studies of bulimia nervosa use these forms of purging,[3] so that the data being accumulated concerning treatment response apply only to this group of individuals. In addition, there are indications that individuals who binge and use active methods of purging comprise a more homogeneous and distinct group. Several studies suggest that individuals who regularly purge after binge eating exhibit greater eating-related psychopathology than individuals with bulimia nervosa who do not purge. The second alternative would be to retain the current DSM-III-R criterion but to add a subtyping scheme to distinguish those individuals who purge from those who do not. These two alternatives will be presented in the DSM-IV Options Book in order to elicit comment and additional data.

Although the Work Group was not entirely satisfied with the somewhat arbitrary criterion for binge frequency of twice a week for 3 months, the review by Wilson[4] did not uncover sufficient data on which to base a change in this criterion. The Work Group did recommend that "rapid" be removed from criterion A for bulimia nervosa, and recommended rewording the definition of a binge provided in the diagnostic criteria. The proposed definition of a binge in DSM-IV includes what in DSM-III-R was separated into two criteria:

1. Excessive eating, which is now defined as "eating, in a discrete period of time (e.g., in any 2-hour period), an amount of food that is definitely larger than most people would eat in a similar period of time."

2. A sense of lack of control over eating during the episode (e.g., a feeling that one cannot stop eating or control what or how much one is eating).

The Work Group believed that, although quantitative guidelines could not be provided regarding a minimum number of calories to be considered "large," a binge could be described in more operational terms. In doing so, the Work Group has used terminology initially developed by Cooper and Fairburn in the Eating Disorder Examination and modified slightly by a consortium of investigators studying binge eating disorder.[5]

Finally, the literature review conducted by Devlin and colleagues[6] suggested that there are a significant number of individuals who do not meet criteria for bulimia nervosa but who do have a significant problem with binge eating. Among patients seeking treatment for obesity, for example, approximately one quarter to one half report significant problems with binge eating. However, the characteristics of such a "binge eating disorder" remain unclear, and the Work Group felt that a recommendation for the inclusion of a new diagnostic category in the DSM-IV could not be made on the basis of the currently available literature. It is possible that, in the time before final decisions regarding the DSM-IV are made, sufficient data will become available to merit the addition of this disorder.

SUMMARY

The major changes proposed in the diagnostic criteria for eating disorders in the DSM-IV are the subtyping of anorexia nervosa into bulimic and nonbulimic groups, the restriction or subtyping of bulimia nervosa on the basis of purging behavior, and the possible inclusion of a new diagnostic category for binge eating disorder. It should be emphasized that the recommendations outlined here are not final, but are currently under consideration for the DSM-IV and will be presented in the DSM-IV Options Book.

ACKNOWLEDGMENTS

The members of the Eating Disorder Work Group of the American Psychiatric Association's Task Force for DSM-IV are: Paul E. Garfinkel, M.D., Katherine A. Halmi, M.D., James E. Mitchell, M.D., B. Timothy Walsh, M.D. (chair), and G. Terence Wilson, Ph.D.

REFERENCES

1. DaCosta M, Halmi KA: Classifications of anorexia nervosa; question of subtypes. Int J Eating Disord (in press).

2. Garfinkel PE: Evidence in support of attitudes to shape and weight as a diagnostic criterion of bulimia nervosa. Int J Eating Disord (in press).
3. Mitchell JE: Subtyping of bulimia nervosa. Int J Eating Disord (in press).
4. Wilson GT: Diagnostic criteria for bulimia nervosa. Int J Eating Disord (in press).
5. Spitzer RL, Devlin MJ, Walsh BT, et al: Binge eating disorder: A multisite field trial of the diagnostic criteria. Int J Eating Disord (in press).
6. Devlin MJ, Walsh BT, Spitzer RL, et al: Is there another binge eating disorder?: A review of the literature on overeating in the absence of bulimia nervosa. Int J Eating Disord (in press).

BULIMIA NERVOSA

MARTINA DE ZWAAN, M.D. and JAMES E. MITCHELL, M.D.

DIAGNOSIS AND CLINICAL FEATURES

While bulimia nervosa was first described as a distinct disorder over 10 years ago by Russell,[1] binge eating and purging had long been associated with obesity and anorexia nervosa. The diagnostic system for bulimia nervosa is still in the process of evolution. The diagnostic criteria usually applied today are those described in the DSM-III-R[2]:

A. Recurrent episodes of binge eating (rapid consumption of a large amount of food in a discrete period of time.

B. A feeling of lack of control over eating behavior during the eating binges.

C. The person regularly engages in either self-induced vomiting, use of laxatives or diuretics, strict dieting or fasting, or vigorous exercise in order to prevent weight gain.

D. A minimum average of two binge eating episodes a week for at least three months.

E. Persistent overconcern with body shape and weight.

Binge Eating

Binge eating is difficult to define, and at some point merges with overeating, but the amount consumed during eating binges is usually far in excess of the amount most people would consider simply overeating (up to 11,500 kcal or more). During binge eating, patients typically experience loss of control over eating, and most describe being unable to stop eating once they have commenced. There is often an all-or-none pattern to the sequence of eating.

The behavior often starts during a period of restrictive dieting associated with a period of increased concern about body weight, when the individual loses control and overeats. The onset sometimes can be associated with stressful life events, most commonly family or relationship problems, leaving home, failure at school or work, or work transition. A binge eating episode usually lasts less than 2 hours but can last as long as 8 hours. During binge eating episodes, people consume foods that are considered primarily snack or dessert foods and in general consume foods they usually avoid at other times because they consider them fattening. They tend to consume high-calorie, easily ingested foods rich in fat, with a texture that facilitates rapid eating (e.g., ice cream). During an episode most individuals eat very rapidly, and many report that they do not really taste the food or do not remember what they have eaten.

Binge eating is a secretive habit. For most individuals the episodes become institutionalized parts of their daily routine and are often planned in advance. Sometimes they are precipitated by unpleasant events, or by feelings of depression, anxiety, boredom, and loneliness. The episodes often follow what the individual perceives as breaking of a rigid, restrictive dietary rule, such as eating a forbidden food. Frequency data indicate that most patients with bulimia nervosa binge eat once a day or more often. Bulimic episodes are usually terminated by some form of purging behavior. After each binge eating episode most patients feel distressed because of the prospect of gaining weight from ingested food.

Methods of Weight Control

Self-induced vomiting is the method most commonly employed by bulimic individuals (70 to 95 per cent). Self-induced vomiting is performed as soon as possible after eating in order to minimize the absorption of food. Relative to the course of the illness for most individuals, self-induced vomiting either begins at about the same time as binge eating, or follows the development of binge eating. Early in the illness, many individuals insert their fingers into the throat to induce the gag reflex. However, the vomiting becomes progressively easier over time and may eventually require only drinking a quantity of water toward the end of the binge-eating episode, or bending over the toilet and applying pressure to the abdomen. Some individuals abuse the over-the-counter drug Ipecac syrup, which contains the alkaloid emetine, as a way of promoting vomiting, a particularly dangerous procedure.

Abuse of laxatives is another method to counteract the effects of ingested food. Some individuals take laxatives only after episodes of overeating; others take them as a routine weight-control method. Laxative abuse is a relatively ineffective method of avoiding calorie absorption, because such drugs primarily affect the large intestine, where primarily fluid absorption takes place. Consequently, laxatives, which act directly on the colon, produce a temporary fluid loss caused by watery diarrhea that gives patients a sense of weight loss. Reflex fluid retention and weight gain leads to further usage, and over time tolerance to the laxatives develops and the dosage must be increased. Some individuals ingest up to 60 or more tablets daily. Patients misuse primarily stimulant-type laxatives containing phenolphthalein, examples being Ex-Lax and Correctol.

A variety of other less frequent abnormal eating-related behaviors have been described in patients with bulimia nervosa, such as diuretic abuse, abuse of appetite suppressants, vigorous exercise, excessive use of enemas, chewing and spitting out food without swallowing it, rumination (the regurgitation, chewing, and reswallowing of food), and the misuse of saunas as a weight loss technique. Patients with diabetes mellitus may utilize an effective and very dangerous way of achieving weight loss by neglecting their insulin requirements: they intentionally underdose as a way to purge calories by means of glucosuria.

Attitudes to Shape and Weight

Bulimic individuals are deeply concerned about their shape and weight and are in persistent fear of weight gain. These concerns have been characterized as a "morbid fear of fatness" or as "weight phobia." Even small weight changes may result in marked alterations in mood and behavior. Concerns about body shape usually focus on the appearance of the patient's stomach, hips, buttock, and thighs. It is interesting that these are the body areas about which most women in western societies are most concerned.

EPIDEMIOLOGY

The prevalence of the syndrome of bulimia nervosa as described in the DSM-III-R is about 1 to 2 per cent in female high school or college students, but we still know little about the true prevalence in the general population.[3] Markedly lower rates have been found among nonwhites than whites. There is evidence that eating disorders might be more common among female athletes. An association between bulimia nervosa and diabetes mellitus has been reported, although the data are conflicting. Bulimia nervosa occurs almost exclusively in developed "western" societies that have an excess of food and in which a high emphasis is placed on slimness as a model of attractiveness. Very little is known about the changes in prevalence over time, and about the longitudinal course of bulimia nervosa. Results so far suggest that bulimia nervosa many times does not remit spontaneously, but instead waxes and wanes in severity over time.

DEMOGRAPHIC CHARACTERISTICS

Bulimia nervosa is almost exclusively confined to young women, with less than 10 per cent of the total cases reported in the literature being male.[4] The usual age of onset is between 16 and 19 years, and the average age of first treatment contact is about 24. The delay in presentation is most likely due to the guilt and shame that accompany the disorder and the assumption that it is not treatable; therefore, most do not seek help until they have developed secondary impairment from the disorder, such as depression and school or work problems. Approximately 70 per cent of all cases are within a normal weight range at the time of assessment. It seems that there is a greater heterogeneity of socioeconomic status in bulimia nervosa than is typically cited for individuals with anorexia nervosa.

ASSOCIATED PROBLEMS

Affective Disorder

Depression scores are usually significantly higher among bulimic patients than normal control subjects, and clinically significant depressive disorders occur far more frequently in bulimic patients than in the general population.[5] The point prevalence of major affective disorder—usually of the depressive type—in patients with bulimia nervosa is between 21 and 45 per cent (average 37 per cent); lifetime prevalence ranges between 36 and 92 per cent (average 61 per cent). The rates are surprisingly high given our knowledge of the base prevalence of affective disorders. The nature of the relationship between depression and bulimia nervosa is unclear, but regardless of the causal direction (what is causing what), the comorbidity problem is significant.

Anorexia Nervosa

Some patients with bulimia nervosa have a history of weight loss sufficient to qualify for a prior diagnosis of anorexia nervosa. Furthermore, binge eating is relatively common in patients with anorexia nervosa, and characterizes a subgroup of anorectics.

Personality Disorders and Personality Traits

Different authors have found markedly different rates for personality disorders in patients with bulimia nervosa. The most common types of personality disorders described have been histrionic and borderline, followed by compulsive and avoidant. Clinical experience reveals that some patients with bulimia nervosa tend to be industrious, perfectionistic, and achievement oriented. These individuals are usually very critical, and punitive in their evaluation of themselves. Certain styles of thinking are common, such as black-or-white thinking and overgeneralization. Finally, bulimia nervosa is often characterized by low self-esteem, negativity, and a sense of personal ineffectiveness. Interestingly, self-esteem seems to be an important predictor of success in treatment.

Alcohol/Drug Abuse

As with depression, there is clearly a problem of comorbidity. Research has shown that the rate of alcohol and drug abuse problems is significantly higher among bulimic women compared to age- and sex-matched controls. In addition, studies have suggested a familial relationship between alcohol/drug abuse problems and bulimia nervosa.

Other Associated Problems

Several problems are reported at high frequencies by this patient group, including a history of self-injurious behavior such as self-cutting, and stealing behavior.[6]

MEDICAL COMPLICATIONS

Fortunately, most disturbances common in bulimia nervosa are not severe, and most resolve quickly after symptom remission.

Signs and Symptoms

Complaints are frequently nonspecific: weakness, amenorrhea, abdominal fullness, feeling bloated, constipation, fatigue, puffy cheeks, headache, dental problems, nausea, and lethargy. There are signs observable on examination that should alert the clinician to the possible diagnosis of bulimia nervosa:

1. Lesions on the skin over the dorsum of the dominant hand, resulting from the use of the hand to stimulate the gag reflex (Russell's sign).

2. Hypertrophy of the salivary glands, particularly the parotid glands, which is usually bilateral and painless. The patient's serum amylase level may be modestly elevated.

3. Dental complications, which are frequent in these patients and are caused by the highly acid gastric contents producing erosion of the enamel and, secondarily, decalcification. The erosion is often particularly marked on the lingual surface of the upper teeth.

4. A flushed appearance and petechial hemorrhages on the cornea, soft palate, or face seen shortly after a binge-and-vomiting episode.

Dehydration and Electrolyte Abnormalities

Nearly 50 per cent of bulimic patients demonstrate fluid or electrolyte abnormalities due to vomiting, laxative, or diuretic abuse as well as low salt intake. The most common abnormalities are metabolic alkalosis, hypochloremia, hypokalemia, and hyponatremia. Dehydration may result in volume depletion, which leads to a secondary hyperaldosteronism, and reflex peripheral edema. Vomiting tends to generate metabolic alkalosis (high serum bicarbonate) through loss of gastric hydrochloric acid and volume contraction. Metabolic acidosis (low serum bicarbonate) may be present in patients who have recently abused laxatives as a result of loss of alkaline fluid from the bowel. Clinical manifestations of hypokalemia, such as cardiac conduction defects and a variety of arrhythmias, have been observed in eating disorder patients. Hypomagnesemia is an important and often overlooked electrolyte abnormality in eating disorder patients. Other rare but potentially dangerous electrolyte abnormalities are hypocalcemia and hypophosphatemia.

Gastrointestinal

Laxative abuse can cause constipation, especially during withdrawal, and in rare cases permanent impairment of colonic functioning. Other medical complications of bulimic behavior include delayed gastric emptying, gastrointestinal bleeding, gastric and duodenal ulcer, malabsorption syndromes, steatorrhea and protein-losing gastroenteropathy, pancreatic dysfunction, osteomalacia, and pseudofractures. Rare but very serious side effects are esophageal tearing with bleeding or perforation due to repeated vomiting, and gastric dilatation and perforation due to the ingestion of large amounts of food during an eating binge. Pancreatitis may result from abrupt pancreatic stimulation during frequent binge eating.

Cardiovascular

Electrolyte disturbances may cause electrocardiographic changes and heart failure. Peripheral edema can develop from rebound fluid retention after purging. The alkaloid emetine, which is included in Ipecac syrup, is apparently responsible for the serious myopathy that can develop, including fatal cardiomyopathy.

Renal

High blood urea nitrogen and decreased glomerular filtration may be suggestive of renal function impairment due to hypokalemic nephropathy in patients with chronic dehydration and chronic hypokalemia.

Endocrine

While amenorrhea is an infrequent symptom in bulimia nervosa as compared to anorexia nervosa, irregular menses is quite common. Some patients, probably as a result of dieting and semistarvation, may develop low levels of estradiol, progesterone, luteinizing hormone, and particularly follicle-stimulating hormone, hyperprolactinemia, or both.

TREATMENT

Published treatment studies show quite clearly that most individuals with this disorder improve dramatically with therapy, and many apparently recover from the condition. While controlled studies suggest that both pharmacotherapy and psychotherapy can have a significant impact on bulimia nervosa in the short run, the long-term outcome for bulimia nervosa is less encouraging, and patients are still at substantial risk of relapse.[7,8] Unfortunately, there are no predictors to date indicating which treatment fits best for which patient.

Most patients with bulimia nervosa can be treated effectively out of hospital. It probably is wise to attempt to avoid inpatient admission, since it is better for patients to gain control of their eating out of hospital, where they are dealing with the same internal and external cues that they will have to face after treatment. Furthermore, outpatient treatment is cost effective, less socially disruptive, and less stigmatizing.

Medical Management

Careful physical examination and laboratory assessment are indicated for each patient. Of particular importance are screening determinations of serum electrolytes.[9] An electrocardiogram with a rhythm strip may be indicated.

In extreme cases of hypokalemia, intravenous potassium supplementation may be necessary, since laxative abuse, diuretic abuse, and vomiting may result in a severe contraction alkalosis that makes correction of potassium levels difficult. Hydrogen ion shifts into the extracellular fluid to compensate, and potassium shifts into the cells. Furthermore, renal excretion of potassium is increased as a result of the secondary hyperaldosteronism resulting from the hypovolemia. Sodium is reabsorbed instead of potassium in order to retain water, since the body's highest priority is the maintenance of an adequate blood volume. However, in most cases supplemental oral potassium will be sufficient.

All stimulant-type laxatives must be discontinued immediately. Patients should drink a minimum of 6 to 10 cups of water or decaffeinated beverage a day. No salt should be added to food. Exercise is a way to stimulate bowel function. Bulk may be added to the diet. Patients should monitor their stools, and if they do not have bowel movements every 3 to 4 days, they should consult an expert. Bulimic patients withdrawing from laxatives or diuretics need to be told that they may temporarily gain as much as 2 to 5 kg through temporary fluid retention.

Pharmacotherapy

Many different drugs have been used in the treatment of bulimia nervosa. They include tricyclic antidepressants (amitriptyline, imipramine, desipramine), nontricyclic antidepressants (mianserin, fluoxetine, phenelzine, trazodone, bupropion, tryptophan), and appetite suppressants (fenfluramine, methylamphetamine), as well as anticonvulsants (carbamazepine, phenytoin), lithium, and naltrexone.[10]

Antidepressants

Antidepressant drugs were first used because of the association of bulimia with depressive illness. The results of the controlled trials so far (Table 6–1) indicate that antidepressants are more effective than placebo in reducing the frequency of bulimic episodes and the intensity of some of the other symptoms of the disorder. Interestingly, antidepressants are apparently equally effective whether or not the patient is depressed. Thus, the effectiveness of antidepressants may result from a direct activation of neurotransmitter systems known to control food intake, rather than from their antidepressive action per se. Although many patients are improved in terms of the percentage reduction in bulimic symptoms, in most studies only a minority of patients are free of the behavior. No study has systematically examined the maintenance of change, nor have the effects of drug discontinuation been investigated. There is, however, a strong impression in the literature that many patients relapse, suggesting that many patients did not learn more adaptive behavior patterns. Furthermore, there is a marked difference in placebo response rates across these studies, suggesting po-

TABLE 61–1. RESULTS OF CONTROLLED TREATMENT STUDIES USING
ANTIDEPRESSANTS

	Daily Dosage (mg)	Outcome
Drug vs. Placebo		
Imipramine	200–300	Imipramine > placebo
Desipramine	150–200	Desipramine > placebo
Fluoxetine	60	Fluoxetine > placebo
Phenelzine	60–90	Phenelzine > placebo
Buproprion	450	Buproprion > placebo
Mianserin	60	Mianserin = placebo
Amitriptyline	150	Amitriptyline = placebo
L-Tryptophan	3000	L-Tryptophan = placebo
Drug vs. Psychotherapy		
Desipramine vs. CBT	200–300	CBT > desipramine
Imipramine vs. CBT	200–300	CBT > imipramine
Drug vs. Drug		
Desipramine vs. Fenfluramine	150 vs 60	Fenfluramine > desipramine

tential differences in the supportive psychotherapy component inherent in the medication management in these studies.

Imipramine and desipramine are the best studied tricyclic drugs. The dosage levels reported in the literature appear to be similar to those used in the treatment of major depression. The time course of action of the medication appears to be similar to that for the treatment of depression, with improvement occurring after 2 or 3 weeks of treatment.

In clinical practice, monoamine oxidase (MAO) inhibitors are used less frequently because of the dietary restrictions required of patients taking them. Foods containing a high concentration of tyramine or dopamine may cause rapid and excessive rises in blood pressure that may be life threatening.

Bupropion, an antidepressant chemically unrelated to tricyclics and MAO inhibitors, cannot be recommended in the treatment of patients with bulimia nervosa, despite its significant superiority to placebo. In a multicenter controlled trial, 5.8 per cent of the subjects experienced grand mal seizures during treatment with 450 mg bupropion, leading to an early termination of the study. This is the only published study to date reporting an increased seizure frequency in bulimic subjects during treatment with an antidepressant, but it does suggest that this drug should be avoided in individuals with eating disorders.

Recent research has focused on the use of serotonergic drugs, since they are able to enhance satiety. There is some evidence that underactivation of serotonergic transmission may be involved in the pathogenesis of bulimia nervosa. Fluoxetine hydrochloride has been shown to have a considerable effectiveness in the treatment of bulimia nervosa at high dosages (60 mg/day). This drug also has a very favorable side effect profile compared to traditional tricyclic compounds, and is generally well tolerated, with the major side effects being anxiety, nausea, sleeplessness, and rash. In a large, unpublished, multicenter placebo-controlled trial, 60 mg of fluoxetine was significantly superior to 20 mg fluoxetine and placebo. Subjects usually tolerate 60 mg well even when therapy is initiated at this dosage.

Given the relatively low cost of medication therapy, a trial with antidepressants might be the first step in the treatment of some bulimic patients; however, one must be aware that only a few bulimic patients completely cease binge eating and purging on antidepressants, and many patients will require further treatment such as cognitive behavior therapy (CBT). We suggest, therefore, that antidepressants be prescribed when there is a clear history of an affective disorder, in particular if there is evidence that the affective disorder preceded the onset of the eating disorder, but that CBT is currently the treatment of choice. Furthermore, antidepressants may be helpful for patients who remain depressed despite improvement in their eating symptoms, and for those patients who show only a partial response or a lack of response to a psychotherapy intervention, whether or not they are depressed.

One long-term study with antidepressants indicated that many patients needed to take the medication for long periods of time, at minimum 6 months to 1 year. It is then reasonable to try to taper antidepressant responders off the drug, to see if the drug is still necessary.

Two recent studies examined the relative effectiveness of psychological (CBT) and pharmacological (desipramine and imipramine) treatments. The results suggest superiority for CBT, with or without the antidepressant, over drug therapy alone. These studies raise the question of whether or not antidepressant treatment should be employed as the sole treatment, since CBT may be superior.

Anticonvulsants

According to the hypothesis that bulimia nervosa might represent a seizure equivalent, antiepileptic drugs were used experimentally. There is no convincing evidence to date for a correlation between seizure disorders, or eletroencephalographic abnormalities, and bulimia nervosa, or for the efficacy of phenytoin or carbamazepine in most of these patients.

Lithium Carbonate

In the one double-blind trial to date, the utility of lithium was not established. Also, lithium should be used cautiously in eating disorder patients, given the fluid and electrolyte abnormalities to which they are prone.

Opiate Antagonists

Like the serotonergic system, the endogenous opioid peptide system appears to be quite important in the control of feeding behavior, and there is evidence that, in particular, stress-induced feeding is linked to this system. To date there is only one long-acting, orally active narcotic antagonist available in the United State: naltrexone. Controlled studies suggest that naltrexone at high dosages may be useful in the treatment of some patients with bulimia nervosa, but it carries the risk of hepatotoxicity at this dosage and therefore cannot be recommended for clinical practice.

Psychotherapy

Many psychotherapeutic approaches have been developed for the treatment of bulimia nervosa: cognitive, behavioral, and psychodynamic approaches, as well as family therapy and even hypnosis have been suggested.[11-13] Some are highly structured and can be recognizably reproduced by a variety of therapists. Structured behaviorally and cognitively oriented programs that use specific techniques to alter distorted eating behavior (problem oriented) have been studied most extensively in numerous controlled studies, and have proven to be reasonably effective. They have consistently been found to benefit most patients with changes in eating habits, attitudes, and associated psychopathology. Therefore, the CBT approach employing both performance-based behavioral techniques and verbal cognitive elements may be considered as the treatment of choice for bulimia nervosa to date, and is explained here in more detail.

The treatment may be provided in group, individual, or mixed group/individual formats. Most of these programs are time limited, lasting from a minimum of 6 weeks to a maximum of 18 weeks. A few provide more than weekly sessions early in the course of treatment. Central to all CB treatments for bulimia nervosa are techniques such as education; self-monitoring of relevant behavior, feelings, and cognitions; the instruction to eat three regular meals a day; exposure to feared foods at some time in treat-

ment; and cognitive restructuring, designed to change attitudes toward shape and weight. However, there is evidence that psychological treatment methods that do not directly address eating patterns and exclude behavioral techniques, but instead focus on interpersonal issues, may be equally effective. Central to these treatments is the notion that eating problems constitute a maladaptive solution for other "underlying difficulties." Once identified, such problems then become the focus of treatment.

The Cognitive-Behavioral Approach

EDUCATIONAL TECHNIQUES

Lectures may provide general information about the physical and emotional consequences of bulimia. Patients receive information about food intake, metabolism, the effect of binge eating, vomiting, and laxative abuse on physiological functioning, electrolyte balance, and caloric intake. General information on depressive symptomatology in bulimia is also provided. The relationship between bulimia, drug abuse, stealing, and lying is reviewed. Some behaviors are obviously pathological to most patients; most know that binge eating and self-induced vomiting or laxative abuse are problems. However, patients might not label other practices, such as using over-the-counter diuretics, drinking large amount of caffeine-containing liquids, restrictive eating and dieting, fasting, and excessive, inappropriate exercise for weight loss, as problem behaviors.

SELF-MONITORING

To better understand the role of food and eating in her life, it is important for the patient to keep records of her deviant eating behaviors, and to link these eating behaviors to specific thoughts or feelings, which may occur before, during, or after the eating behaviors. Self-monitoring techniques are used to increase awareness of bulimic behavior in particular and eating patterns in general. It brings the problem into better focus. In addition, a food diary is used to record meal plans and food intake. Most important, it is well known that self-monitoring per se may have a significant effect upon the observed behavior. It is of utmost importance for the therapist to review these records carefully.

NUTRITIONAL COUNSELING

Nutritional education should be implemented early as a component in the treatment of this disorder. It is important for the patient to understand that the goal of treatment is not just to eliminate the binge eating and other associated bulimic behaviors such as vomiting, but also to institute a plan of eating regular, balanced meals. Most patients are initially quite resistant to this suggestion, since they are convinced that eating regular meals will lead to weight gain. It is most important for the therapist to assume a firm and directive position. A good way to reach the goal of three balanced meals a day is to instruct patients in meal planning techniques. Patients should be instructed to try to eat these meals at fairly standard times regardless of their appetite, and regardless of binge-purge episodes that might occur. Patients should set aside 10 to 30 minutes each day to make the meal plan for the next day.

Early in the course of treatment patients may be asked to avoid foods that are associated with binge eating episodes in order to facilitate the interruption of the eating pathology. Patients are encouraged to weigh themselves only once a week to interrupt the unhealthy weighing behaviors often associated with fear of weight gain. This part of a CBT program can be conducted either by a dietitian (team approach) or by the mental health practitioner if his or her knowledge of nutrition is adequate.

CUES, RESPONSES, AND CONSEQUENCES

Many sorts of cues may be involved in triggering bulimic behavior (social, situational, physiological, and mental). There are three types of responses: thoughts, behaviors, and feelings. The thoughts a person has regarding a situation or cue will influence how she feels and how she subsequently behaves. Many people with eating problems have certain styles of thinking that are problematic, including overgeneralization, catastrophizing, dichotomous thinking, self-fulfilling ideas, and overreliance on the opinion of others. Thoughts derived from these styles of thinking may eventually become automatic, and patients may be unaware of them.

Both negative and positive consequences may result from bulimic behaviors. Although the positive consequences (e.g., relief of anger, thoughts about avoiding weight gain) are more immediate than the negative consequences, it is very important for the patient to understand that, in the long run, the negative consequences will dominate. One way to improve eating habits is to identify and learn to control the cues that lead to bulimic symptoms by breaking the relationship between the cue and the response (stimulus control). This includes the avoidance of stimulus cues, the delay of binge eating response to a cue, and the use of competing alternative behaviors to binge eating as a way of responding to certain cues. Formal exposure and vomiting prevention sessions may be employed, wherein patients are asked to overeat (= cue), but are then prevented from the vomiting response. It is also helpful to rearrange the consequences of behavior, so that appropriate behaviors will be rewarded and inappropriate behaviors not rewarded. The reward should follow the behavior, should be contingent on the occurrence of the behavior, and should follow the behavior as quickly as possible. Patients are taught to reward themselves cognitively and materially for abstinent behavior.

Occurrence of behavior often cannot be explained using only one sequence of cues-response-consequences. Much of the time, behavior consists of a series of components, with responses that can become cues themselves for another set of responses, and so on. The focus then becomes an investigation of the ways that such a chain can be broken early in the cycle.

RESTRUCTURING THOUGHTS

Although behavioral procedures are the most effective means of producing changes in cognitive processes, and adherence to behavioral instructions usually reduces the strength of irrational beliefs, it is also helpful to address the irrational beliefs in treatment directly, since they may support resistance to behavioral change. After becoming aware of the thoughts, feelings, and behaviors that are triggered by particular cues and that result in specific consequences, and after the attempt to trace connections between an affective reaction and specific cognitions, patients need to evaluate their thoughts in order to determine whether or not those thoughts are accurate and reasonable. One technique is to challenge irrational thoughts by questioning their content. A second method is to test erroneous assumptions prospectively.

RELAPSE PREVENTION

Relapse prevention is a particularly important area, since there is a significant potential for relapse. Patients should practice exposure to high-risk situations and high-risk foods. If these remain "feared," this may preordain a relapse upon exposure. Avoided foods are gradually incorporated into patients' diet at times when they feel they are in good control. This practice is broadened to include feared social situations.

It is important to teach patients the differences between lapses or slips and relapse. The former are common minor recurrences of symptoms that provide an opportunity to learn and are not evidence of failure. Patients must be aware that they may experience future episodes of poor control, especially during times of stress. Participation in self-help groups should be emphasized, and plans for crisis situations should be prepared.

BODY IMAGE

Many individuals with bulimia nervosa have a distorted body image, and their ideas about their own body size and shape are often inaccurate. This might be attributable to problematic cultural expectations of women's bodies and social roles. Mainly cognitive techniques are used to challenge specific negative thoughts about body size and shape.

In roleplaying exercises and different types of homework, *social skills* and *assertiveness*, *stress management*, and *problem-solving* techniques can be learned by practical examples. *Relaxation* and *exercise* can be used as stress management techniques.

FAMILY ISSUES

The need for family involvement varies depending primarily on the age of the patient. If family involvement is desirable, interviews are conducted to promote the development of an open, honest relationship between the patient and family or friends, and to enlist support for the treatment program. Patients are also helped to identify family roles that may be influencing their eating behavior.

Psychodynamic Approaches

Two highly structured, brief psychodynamic approaches that have been adapted for the treatment of bulimia nervosa have been shown to be equally effective as CBT in controlled studies.

STRUCTURED BRIEF PSYCHOTHERAPY

The underlying theoretical approach is based on the understanding of behavior using psychodynamic principles. An attempt is made to uncover feelings, make meaning out of behavior, and explore the development of current attitudes. A problem or focus of treatment is selected, which is not the disturbed eating behavior per se, but difficulties in relationships, for example.

INTERPERSONAL PSYCHOTHERAPY

This approach focuses on the patients' current social adjustment and interpersonal relations and attachments. Social relationships are systematically reviewed, and social problems are identified and then related to the pathological behavior.

REFERENCES

1. Russell G: Bulimia nervosa: An ominous variant of anorexia nervosa. Psychol Med 9:429–448, 1979.
2. American Psychiatric Association: Diagnostic and Statistical Manual of Mental Disorders. 3rd ed, rev. Washington, DC: American Psychiatric Association, 1985.
3. Fairburn CG, Beglin SJ: Studies of the epidemiology of bulimia nervosa. Am J Psychiatry 147:401–408, 1990.
4. Pyle RL, Mitchell JE, Eckert ED, Halvorson PA, Neuman PA, Goff GM: The incidence of bulimia in freshman college students. Int J Eating Disord 2:75–85, 1983.
5. Hatsukami DK, Mitchell JE, Eckert ED: Eating disorders: A variant of mood disorders? Psychiatr Clin North Am 7:349–365, 1984.
6. Mitchell JE, Hatsukami D, Pyle RL, Eckert ED: The bulimia syndrome: Course of the illness and associated problems. Compr Psychiatry 27:165–170, 1986.
7. Freeman CPL, Munro JKM: Drug and group treatment for bulimia/bulimia nervosa. J Psychosom Res 32:647–660, 1988.
8. Mitchell JE, Hoberman H, Pyle RL: An overview of the treatment of the bulimia nervosa. Psychiatr Med 7:317–332, 1989.
9. Mitchell JE, Pyle RL, Eckert ED, Hatsukami D, Lentz R: Electrolyte and other physiological abnormalities in patients with bulimia. Psychol Med 13:273–278, 1983.
10. Mitchell JE: Psychopharmacology of eating disorders. The psychobiology of human eating disorders: Preclinical and clinical perspectives. Ann NY Acad Sci 575:41–49, 1989.
11. Cox GL, Merkel WT: A qualitative review of psychosocial treatments for bulimia. J Nerv Ment Dis 177:77–84, 1990.
12. Fairburn CG: The current status of the psychological treatments for bulimia nervosa. J Psychosom Res 32:635–645, 1988.
13. Fairburn CG: A cognitive behavioral approach to the management of bulimia. Psychol Med 11:707–711, 1981.

62

TREATMENT OF ANOREXIA NERVOSA

LYNNE HOFFMAN, M.D. and KATHERINE A. HALMI, M.D.

ANOREXIA NERVOSA: GENERAL DESCRIPTION

Anorexia nervosa is a psychiatric disorder whose diagnosis is based on both psychological and physiological criteria. Psychological criteria include an intense fear of becoming fat and disturbance in body image. Physiological requisites for the diagnosis are amenorrhea of at least 3 months' duration and a persistent low body weight at least 15 per cent below that expected for height and age. All these conditions must be fulfilled for the diagnosis of anorexia

nervosa to be given. Although it is not a common illness, anorexia nervosa is often a chronic disorder associated with considerable morbidity and may have a devastating impact on the developing adolescent and young adult.

Anorexia nervosa primarily affects adolescent and young adult women, with approximately 85 per cent of the cases developing between the ages of 13 and 20. There appears to be a bimodal distribution of age onset, with peaks at 14.5 and 18 years.[1] Both of these ages are associated with times when adolescents are usually becoming more independent from their family. The earlier peak also occurs at the same time that many physical changes secondary to puberty are taking place. Anorexia nervosa is quite rare in males, who account for approximately 5 per cent of the patients.

There is considerable evidence that the incidence of anorexia nervosa has been increasing in the past two decades, especially in western industrialized countries, and in the age group between 15 and 24. Most of the evidence comes from reports that more patients with the disorder are being diagnosed and treated in clinics and hospitals. In Monroe county, New York, the annual incidence of anorexia nervosa rose from 0.35:100,000 through the 1960s to 0.64:100,000 in the 1970s.[2] The best estimate of prevalence rate came from a large-scale English study that revealed one severe case of anorexia nervosa per 200 girls aged 12 to 18.[3]

The etiology of anorexia nervosa remains obscure. Although the illness invariably follows a period of food restriction, dieting is certainly not uncommon in the vulnerable population and clearly does not solely account for the development of anorexia nervosa. In the past, most investigators focused on a specific causative factor such as psychodynamic issues, cognitive defects, developmental concerns, phobic mechanisms, or particular endocrine disturbances. More recently, a broader etiological perspective has been adopted that attempts to integrate a variety of biological, psychological, and sociological factors.

The course of anorexia nervosa varies from a single episode with weight and psychological recovery, to nutritional rehabilitation with relapses, to an unremitting course resulting in death. Most studies show a mortality rate of about 5 per cent, although the few very long-term studies available (i.e., 20 years or more) suggest the ultimate mortality rate may be as high as 15 to 20 per cent.[4] Many anorectic patients have considerable improvement in their medical and nutritional status; however, the majority still suffer from the characteristic psychological aspects of the illness for many years, including a distorted body image and an obsessive preoccupation with food. Poor outcome has been associated with longer duration of illness, older age of onset, multiple hospitalizations, premorbid personality difficulties, and poor social adjustment in childhood.

Reports indicating an increased familial occurrence of anorexia have existed in the literature for over two decades. In a study of 30 female twin pairs in London, 9 out of 16 of the monozygotic pairs and 1 out of 14 of the dizygotic pairs were concordant for anorexia nervosa.[5] Several investigators have focused on the first-degree relatives of anorectic probands. In a recent large-scale family study (539 relatives of anorectics and 833 relatives of controls), a fivefold increased risk of an eating disorder (anorexia, bulimia, or atypical) was noted for the relatives of anorectics compared to the relatives of the controls. The authors believed these findings "indicated quite clearly that familially mediated variables play a crucial role in the etiology and pathogenesis of anorexia nervosa."[6]

Although there are no laboratory tests that are pathognomonic for anorexia nervosa, there are many endocrine and physiological abnormalities, primarily induced by the starvation state, that are commonly found in anorectics. Anorectics are notoriously resistant to therapy, and thus the diagnosis is often first made by an internist or pediatrician. In addition to the state of malnutrition and emaciation, physical signs associated with anorexia include the following:

1.   Skin changes such as dryness and scaliness reflect the state of nutrition and hydration. Lanugo, or fine soft hair, may cover body surfaces. Scalp hair may be thinning or even falling out in clumps.

2.   In anorectics who also vomit, the serum amylase level is often elevated and serial measurements may be useful in following the patient's progress in treatment. Enlarged salivary glands and lesions on the knuckles of patients' fingers (from inducing vomiting) are also associated with purging behavior. Both vomiting and laxative abuse can produce clinically significant dehydration and electrolyte imbalances. The latter include potentially fatal hypokalemia.

3.   Changes in cardiovascular status are also commonly present. Most frequently observed are bradycardia and hypotension. Electrocardiograms, which should be taken in all patients, are frequently abnormal on initial evaluation.

4.   Emaciated anorectics usually present with a moderately severe leukopenia with a relative lymphocytosis. The erythrocyte sedimentation rate is often low. Nutritional anemias (usually iron or vitamin B_{12} deficient) are frequent.

All of these physiological changes are readily reversible with nutritional rehabilitation.

Many endocrine abnormalities characteristically accompany anorexia nervosa. Amenorrhea is a major diagnostic criterion of the disorder. The loss of menses may actually precede significant weight loss and often persists for many months after weight restoration. Low levels of urinary and plasma gonadotropins have been documented in anorectics. The circadian pattern of luteinizing hormone and follicle-stimulating hormone secretion, which changes with maturation, shows a regression to prepubertal levels in adult women with anorexia. Although the precise cause of amenorrhea is still to be clarified, it is believed to be due to a disturbance at the level of the hypothalamus.

Anorexia nervosa is associated with a state of hypercortisolism due to increased production of cortisol. Recent studies provide strong evidence that the increase in cortisol results from an increase in the hypothalamic production of corticotropin-releasing factor (CRF). This is of particular interest because CRF has been shown in animal studies to cause decreased feeding, increased activity, and hypothalamic hypogonadism, all of which are common manifestations of anorexia nervosa. Although the mechanism underlying the increase in CRF remains obscure, the elevated CRF may be involved in perpetuating some of the psychological disturbances characteristic of anorectics.

Anorectics frequently have abnormalities of thyroid function. Thyroxine (T_4) is usually within normal range but triiodothyronine (T_3) levels are generally below normal. Thyroid-stimulating hormone is generally not elevated. The disturbances in thyroid function found in anorexia nervosa appear to be primarily a consequence of malnutrition.

Elevated levels of serum growth hormone are found in approximately half of emaciated anorectic patients and generally return to normal with treatment and weight gain. However, while nutritional status clearly plays a role in the disturbance of growth hormone secretion in anorexia nervosa, there may be differences in the mechanism underlying growth hormone hypersection in simple malnutrition compared to anorexia. Evidence for this comes from reports showing an absence of a correlation between the extent of weight loss and the degree of growth hormone elevation in anorectics. For reviews of the characteristic physiological and endocrine changes in anorexia, see Owen and Halmi[7] and Newman and Halmi.[8]

The diagnosis of anorexia nervosa is not difficult to make in patients who are motivated for treatment and honest about their symptomatology, two relatively rare events in this population. The differential diagnosis requires careful consideration of other conditions that can produce weight loss. Medical illness such as Crohn's disease can produce significant weight loss, and an organic basis for the malnutrition needs to be excluded. Patients who are medically ill do not present with the characteristic fear of fatness or peculiarities in handling food seen in anorectics. Interviewing family members and friends may be necessary to obtain this information.

Other psychiatric illnesses may also present with weight loss. Many depressed patients have decreased appetite and significant weight loss. Depressed patients do not, however, exhibit the characteristic fear of weight gain seen in anorexia, nor are they preoccupied with the caloric content of food and food preparation. Anorexia nervosa and depression are closely associated; care must be taken to make the appropriate diagnosis, and both conditions should be treated when they coexist. Schizophrenic patients may present with food refusal as a result of their delusions, but they are rarely preoccupied with the fear of becoming obese and they do not usually have the hyperactivity characteristic of anorectic patients. Weight loss and vomiting can occur in somatization disorder as well. However, anorectics are far more preoccupied with weight, body size, and dieting than individuals with somatization disorder.

TREATMENT OF ANOREXIA NERVOSA

General Considerations

Unlike most psychiatric illnesses, anorexia nervosa has both powerful physiological and psychological components. The first step in treating the anorectic patient must include nutritional rehabilitation and weight restoration. It is exceedingly difficult to accomplish change with psychotherapy in a patient who is suffering the psychological effects of emaciation. The states of emaciation and starvation produce dramatic effects on mood and behavior. These were well documented over 40 years ago in the Minnesota Experiment, in which healthy male conscientious objectors voluntarily participated in a semistarvation experiment.[9] All reported lethargy, poor concentration, loss of sexual interest, moodiness, and insomnia and many developed bizarre eating habits and unusual food preoccupations. These effects did not resolve for many weeks after nutritional rehabilitation was completed.

There is some disagreement as to the preferred initial treatment setting for patients. However, most would agree that severe emaciation, the presence of vomiting, failed outpatient treatment, severe depression or suicidal feelings, or physical complications indicate the need for hospitalization. Treatment goals should include weight restoration, normalization of eating behavior, change in the pursuit of thinness and prevention of relapse (which may be as high as 50 per cent the first year after hospital treatment).

Anorectic patients are notoriously disinterested in treatment. Gaining the patients' trust and cooperation can be very difficult. This is often best accomplished by acknowledging their desire for thinness and control but emphasizing the negative and dangerous consequences of their behavior, including medical risk, depression, interfering preoccupation with food and exercise, social isolation, and damaged peer relationships.

The remainder of this chapter reviews the use of pharmacotherapy and psychotherapy in the treatment of anorexia and describes an inpatient treatment program.

Medication

Although many medications have been used to treat anorectics, there are surprisingly few large-scale, controlled studies demonstrating the efficacy of pharmacology in the treatment of anorexia. To date, several drugs have proven useful in aiding weight gain. No medication has been shown at this time to be effective in maintaining weight gain, changing anorectic attitudes, or preventing relapse over the long term.

Neuroleptics

The first medication used in the treatment of anorexia nervosa, over 30 years ago, was chlorpromazine. This medication is still frequently used in low doses and is generally considered to be especially effective in severely obsessive or agitated anorectics. Surprisingly, however, there are no controlled, double-blind studies definitively demonstrating the efficacy of chlorpromazine in inducing weight gain. There have been controlled studies of two other neuroleptics, the selective dopamine antagonists pimozide and sulpiride. In a study of 18 patients, pimozide, at doses of 4 to 6 mg, showed some beneficial effects on weight gain (in a behavioral modification program), especially initially, and some minor attitudinal improvements, including less weight phobia and better motivation.[10] However, in a double-blind crossover study by the same group using 300 to 400 mg of sulpiride, there was no significant drug effect on weight gain, weight phobia, or body distortion.[11] Given the relative lack of proven drug efficacy, the paucity of well-controlled, large-scale studies, and the considerable side effects associated with neuroleptics, this class of medication should be used sparingly and with caution in this patient population.

Following several case reports suggesting that lithium carbonate might prove useful in the treatment of anorexia, a single double-blind trial of lithium was conducted.[12] Lithium carbonate had a minimal effect on facilitating weight gain in anorectics. However, the marginal results combined with the high risk of lithium toxicity in patients who restrict fluids or purge make it difficult to justify the use of lithium in this population.

Antidepressants

Considering the strong association between anorexia nervosa and depression, it is surprising that antidepressants have not been studied more extensively in the treatment of anorexia nervosa. Following several case reports showing good results with the tricyclic antidepressant amitriptyline, two controlled studies with this medication have appeared. In the first study 25 patients received either active medication or placebo for a period of 5 weeks; another group of 18 patients receiving a pure psychosocial intervention provided another control group.[13] In this study there was no statistically significant benefit on any measure for the medication group compared to the placebo group. Significant side effects were reported by the medicated patients. No correlation between plasma levels of amitriptyline and degree of improvement was found. However, in a recent large-scale multicenter study comparing amitriptyline, cyproheptadine (an antihistamine and a serotonin antagonist), and placebo, amitriptyline did show a marginal effect compared to placebo, decreasing the time it took for patients to reach their target weight and increasing the rate of weight gain.[14] Again, amitriptyline was associated with significant side effects. Interestingly, in that study, cyproheptadine was as effective as amitriptyline in inducing weight gain in the anorectic restrictors (but not in the bulimic subgroup) and also had an unexpected effect on depression as demonstrated by a significant decrease in Hamilton depression ratings. Cyproheptadine was used in large doses ranging from 12 to 28 mg/day. Cyproheptadine has the advantage of not having the tricyclic antidepressant side effects of reducing blood pressure and increasing heart rate. This makes it especially attractive for use in emaciated anorectics.

Some promising results have been reported for two structurally different medications, both of which are relatively selective inhibitors of serotonin reuptake. Clomipramine has a tricyclic structure and is currently available for the treatment of obsessive-compulsive disorder. In a recent controlled study in England, anorectics were treated with either 50 mg of clomipramine (a relatively low dose) or placebo.[15] The medication group showed initial improvement in appetite, hunger, and caloric consumption, although there was no impact on ultimate outcome. The group was followed for 4 years. At 1 year the medication group had maintained their weight better than the control group (although not to a statistically significant extent). By 4 years the groups were identical in weight and sexual and social adjustment. Although these results are far from dramatic, it must be remembered that only 50 mg of active drug was used; up to 250 mg is recommended in the treatment of obsessive-compulsive disorder. Moreover, the sample size (a total of 16 patients) was very small. Clearly a large-scale study with higher doses of clomipramine is indicated to properly assess the potential efficacy of this medication in the treatment of anorexia nervosa, especially after nutritional rehabilitation, and in preventing relapse.

Fluoxetine, a nontricyclic antidepressant, was recently reported to be beneficial in the treatment of six anorectics who were also suffering from depression.[16] In general, depressed patients treated with fluoxetine lose a small amount of weight (1 to 2 kg). However, the patients in this study not only had improvements in their depression but all gained significant amounts of weight. Fluoxetine has also been useful in ameliorating the frequency and intensity of obsessive-compulsive symptomatology. Several, but not all, of these six patients reported a diminution in their preoccupation with food and weight. These preliminary reports clearly indicate the need for a large-scale, controlled trial of fluoxetine in the treatment of anorexia nervosa.

General Comments

Many medications appear to facilitate weight gain in anorexia nervosa and may be helpful in conjunction with other treatment strategies. These medications have many side effects, and the decision to use them must always involve careful consideration of the associated risks. Controlled studies are needed to evaluate the role of medication in preventing relapse after a healthy weight has been obtained.

Psychotherapy

Behavioral Therapy

Over two and a half decades ago, single case studies demonstrating the effectiveness of behavioral therapy in the treatment of anorexia began appearing in the literature. Although there are few controlled comparison studies demonstrating the superiority of behavioral therapy to other treatment strategies, it is clear from the literature that behavioral therapy is effective at inducing short-term weight gain in anorectics, and this approach is now incorporated, in some form, into most structured treatment programs for anorexia.

Behavioral management is most easily accomplished in the context of a hospital treatment program. Using an operant conditioning paradigm, weight gain is the reinforced variable. An individual behavioral assessment should be made on all patients to determine and implement individualized reinforcers. These will usually include increased physical and social activities and increased privileges within the hospital. Whenever possible, negative reinforcers should be avoided. A combination of daily reinforcements with more delayed reinforcements will provide the most effective behavior therapy program. Information feedback is also important; thus patients are weighed daily (at the same time and under the same conditions) to keep track of their progress. Once a healthy weight has been obtained, behavior modification can continue, but in a different form. Now weight maintenance, and increasingly normal eating behavior, become the reinforced parameters. On days when weight drops too low (i.e., outside of a 5-pound range with the target weight in the middle), patients lose privileges. As they show they are able to maintain their weight appropriately, they may be reinforced with more opportunity to choose their own meals in the hospital and out on passes with family and friends. Behavioral contracts for weight maintenance should continue on an individualized basis once the patient has been discharged.

Another behavioral approach, the response prevention technique, can be used to stop vomiting and laxative abuse. Patients all sit in a common living area for at least 1 hour after each meal to prevent vomiting. Moreover, open access to toilets is initially prevented, and patients exclusively use a commode in their rooms. These measures effectively stop vomiting in most patients. (For a comprehensive review of the use of behavioral therapy in anorexia nervosa, see Halmi.[17])

There are several case studies in the literature suggesting that systematic desensitization may be effective in treating a subgroup of anorectics. The approach assumes that anorexia nervosa can be conceptualized as a weight phobia or fear of eating. Other treatment modalities were used as well in most of these cases. The techniques might be useful in combating the fear of fatness in weight-restored anorectics. Unfortunately there has been no recent research on the use of systematic desensitization in anorexia nervosa.

Cognitive Therapy

Cognitive therapy techniques have also been developed for use in anorexia nervosa. The goal is to help the patient challenge the validity of the overvalued and distorted beliefs and perceptions that are perpetuating their illness. The assessment of cognitions is the first step, and patients can be asked to write down thoughts on an assessment form that can then be examined for systematic distortions in the processing and interpretation of events. Garner and Bemis[18] have clearly described the modification of cognitive techniques for the treatment of anorexia nervosa, including decentering, operationalizing beliefs, examination of underlying assumptions, modifications of basic assumptions, reinterpretation of body image misperceptions, and the "what if" technique. Patients are gradually taught to recognize the connection between some of their ideas and maladaptive behaviors and to gradually exchange their beliefs for more realistic ones.[18]

Family Therapy

Most treatment protocols now incorporate some form of family therapy in their approach. The initial goal is to support the family and alleviate their anxiety, provide education, and evaluate family interactions and experiences. Interactions within the family that may contribute to perpetuating the illness in patients are identified and attempts are made to provide strategies to change the harmful patterns of communication. In the families of anorectics, difficulties typically include enmeshment, rigidity, and failure to resolve conflict. Few working in the field believe that family therapy alone is likely to be sufficient in treating anorexia, and clearly the approach is both more feasible and more essential for the young patient still living at home.

Like most forms of psychotherapy popular in the treatment of anorexia nervosa, family therapy has not been adequately investigated in controlled studies. In the one study that compared family therapy to individual supportive therapy, 57 anorectics were divided into three subgroups depending on age and duration of illness.[19] Treatment lasted for a year (generally weekly) and outcome was conducted at 1 year follow-up. In all groups the outcome was discouraging, with a majority of the patients (60 per cent) having a poor outcome. Family therapy was found to be more effective than the individual approach in the subgroup of anorectics that had an early age of onset (less than 18 years) and relatively brief duration of illness (less than 3 years). This provides some evidence for the routine inclusion of family therapy, particularly in younger patients.

Individual Psychotherapy

Almost all therapists working in the field have advocated some form of individual psychotherapy, although again there are no controlled comparison studies to show the superiority of any particular approach. Most of those who have worked extensively in the field believe that the traditional psychoanalytical approach is rather ineffective. Themes that are commonly encountered in treating anorectics include low self-esteem, self-hatred, perfectionistic striving, inner emptiness, and a profound sense of ineffectiveness. Although no one approach is universally effective, it is believed that successful psychotherapy requires a highly interactive therapist who is able to explore, educate, negotiate, challenge, and encourage the patient directly and openly. (For a comprehensive summary of therapeutic approaches to anorexia nervosa, see Hsu.[20])

An Inpatient Treatment Program

Severe anorexia nervosa is most easily and safely treated in a hospital setting. A typical program is described here. Although the cornerstone of the program is behavioral, various therapeutic modalities are employed.

Initial Phase

The initial phase includes a full medical, psychiatric, and family evaluation, followed by weight restoration. Laboratory data are collected on all patients in the first 24 hours and include complete blood count, electrolytes, liver and thyroid function tests, serum amylase levels, and an electrocardiogram. Weekly complete blood counts, serum electrolytes, and amylase levels are obtained throughout the hospital stay.

A target weight is set within 48 hours of admission, although the patients may not be informed initially of their endpoint. One specific approach to weight gain involves using a liquid formula, Sustacal, which is easily adjusted calorically, well tolerated, and devoid of the symbolic value anorectics impose on many solid foods. Weight gain proceeds at 2 to 3 pounds a week. If necessary (and this is a rare event), Sustacal is fed via a nasogastric tube—patients will rarely refuse to drink the formula once aware of this outcome. Patients remain in a central living area for 1 hour after all meals to prevent vomiting. Inputs and outputs are strictly measured, and patients use a commode during their initial weeks on the unit. Activities are highly limited initially, and

privileges are clearly correlated with weight gain initially, then weight maintenance and appropriate eating behavior. Patients are weighed daily each morning after their first void and told their weights to provide them with feedback on their progress and a sense of control.

Phase Two

Once their target weight has been attained, patients are fed off of prearranged trays for at least 2 weeks to help them visualize the amount of food needed to maintain their weight in a healthy manner. They are slowly allowed to choose their own food, one meal at a time, and eventually to eat in the hospital cafeteria and on passes with family and friends. If their weight drops too far (outside a range of which they are aware), they lose all privileges and are unit restricted. If this occurs frequently, a patient must be placed back on trays or even Sustacal if necessary. Decisions such as these are made at weekly "team" meetings and are presented as team decisions. This strategy minimizes struggles between patients and individual staff members.

While the focus is on weight gain, weight maintenance, and eating behavior, a wide variety of therapeutic techniques are employed from the start of the hospital stay. All patients receive individual psychotherapy, which usually has both cognitive and insight-oriented aspects. There are several groups run on the unit, including an adult and adolescent group that focuses on age-appropriate interpersonal issues; an eating disorders group that examines ongoing difficulties with eating behavior, body perception, and specific foods; and a discharge group that looks at aftercare planning. Family counseling and therapy occur weekly. Most patients receive a vocational assessment during their hospital stay. Finally, milieu therapy and peer interactions are central to the success of the program and are fostered through community meetings and patient government.

Medications are used as required. If depression exists following weight gain, a tricyclic antidepressant is often prescribed. In the nonbulimic anorectic group, cyproheptadine will often be advised for the highly anxious or mildly depressed patient. Neuroleptics, especially chlorpromazine, may be recommended for the severely agitated or extremely obsessional patient, and are usually used briefly.

Particular concern and attention is paid to appropriate discharge planning. Relapse is estimated to occur in up to 50 per cent of patients in the first year following hospitalization, and many patients follow a chronic course for many years.[21] Unfortunately, little research has been conducted into the prevention of relapse. There is no good evidence suggesting any treatment is effective in preventing relapse. Individual psychotherapy is always recommended. Often a structured living situation, day hospital program, or both are arranged to ease the transition from the hospital. Weekly weigh-ins are always arranged as part of outpatient treatment, and the recommendations for allowable weight loss before re-hospitalization are clearly outlined.

SUMMARY

Anorexia nervosa remains an enigmatic disorder whose multifaceted etiology is only beginning to be understood. Perhaps because so many questions regarding the pathophysiology of the illness remain unanswered, there have been few treatment breakthroughs in the last decade. Behavior modification remains the cornerstone of most treatment centers. Family and cognitive therapy also play important roles in treatment, and medications are helpful in some patients in facilitating weight gain and dealing with the intense anxiety and obsessive behavior that anorexia often generates. It is hoped that as research clarifies the biological and psychological bases of anorexia nervosa, more specific and efficacious treatment strategies will evolve.

REFERENCES

1. Halmi KA, Casper R, Eckert E, et al: Unique features associated with age onset of anorexia nervosa. Psychol Res 3:209, 1979.
2. Jones D, Fox MM, Babigian HM, et al: Epidemiology of anorexia nervosa in Monroe County N.Y. 1960–1976. Psychosom Med 42:551, 1980.
3. Crisp AH, Palmer RL, Kalucy RS. How common is anorexia nervosa? A prevalence study. Br J Psych 128:549, 1976.
4. Theander S: Outcome and prognosis in anorexia nervosa and bulimia: Some results of previous investigations compared with those of a Swedish long term study. J Psychiatric Res 19:493, 1985.
5. Holland AJ, Crisp A, Russell GFM, et al: Anorexia nervosa: A study of 34 twin pairs and one set of triplets. Br J Psych 145:414, 1984.
6. Strober M, Lampert C, Morrell W, et al: A controlled family study of anorexia nervosa: Evidence of familial aggrega-

tion and lack of shared transmission with affective disorders. Int J Eating Disord 9(3):239, 1990.
7. Owen WP, Halmi KA: The medical management of anorexia nervosa. *In* APA Taskforce on Psychiatric Treatments; Eating Disorders, vol 1, book 1. Washington, DC: American Psychiatric Association, 1989:451.
8. Newman MM, Halmi KA: The endocrinology of anorexia nervosa and bulimia nervosa. Neurol Clin 6(1):195, 1988.
9. Keys A, Brozek J, Henschel A, et al: The Biology of Human Starvation, Minneapolis: University of Minnesota Press, 1950.
10. Vandereycken W, Pierloot R: Pimozide combined with behavior therapy in the short term treatment of anorexia nervosa: A double-blind, placebo controlled crossover study. Acta Psychiatr Scand 66:445, 1982.
11. Vandereycken W: Neuroleptics in the short term treatment of anorexia nervosa: A double-blind placebo controlled study with sulpiride. Br J Psychiatry 144:288, 1984.
12. Gross HA, Ebert MH, Faden VB, et al: A double-blind controlled trial of lithium carbonate in primary anorexia nervosa. J Clin Psychopharmacol 1(6):378, 1981.
13. Biederman J, Herzog DB, Rivinus TM et al: Amitriptyline in the treatment of anorexia nervosa: A double-blind, placebo controlled study. J Clin Psychopharmacol 5(1):10, 1985.
14. Halmi KA, Eckert E, LaDau TJ, et al: Anorexia nervosa: Treatment efficacy of cyproheptadine and amitriptyline. Arch Gen Psychiatry 43:117, 1986.
15. Crisp AH, Lacey JH, Crutchfield M: Clomipramine and "drive" in people with anorexia nervosa. Br J Psychiatry 150:355, 1987.
16. Gwirtsman HE, Guze BH, Yager J, et al: Fluoxetine treatment of anorexia nervosa: An open trial. J Clin Psychiatry 51:378, 1990.
17. Halmi KA: Behavioral management for anorexia nervosa. *In* Garner DM, Garfinkel PE, eds. Handbook of Psychotherapy for Anorexia Nervosa and Bulimia. New York: Guilford Press, 1985:147–159.
18. Garner DM, Bemis KM: Cognitive therapy for anorexia nervosa. *In* Garner DM, Garfinkel PE, eds. Handbook of Psychotherapy for Anorexia Nervosa and Bulimia. New York: Guilford Press, 1985:107–146.
19. Russell GFM, Szmukler GJ, Dare C et al: An evaluation of family therapy in anorexia nervosa and bulimia nervosa. Arch Gen Psychiatry 44:1047, 1987.
20. Hsu LKG: Eating Disorders. New York: Guilford Press, 1990:124–186.
21. Hsu LKG: Outcome of anorexia nervosa—a review of the literature (1954–1978). Arch Gen Psychiatry 37:1041, 1980.

Section J

PERSONALITY DISORDERS

63

PROPOSED DSM-IV CRITERIA FOR PERSONALITY DISORDERS

BRUCE PFOHL, M.D.

Proposed changes for the DSM-IV are outlined in the *DSM-IV Options Book.*[1] These proposals grow out of several problems that have become apparent from empirical studies using the DSM-III and -III-R personality criteria. First, when Axis II criteria are systematically assessed, it is more common for patients to meet criteria for several personality disorders than to meet criteria for one. It is not clear whether this is due to overlap at the conceptual level or lack of specificity of individual criteria. In either case, high levels of overlap make it difficult to demonstrate differential etiological and treatment implications for the various personality disorders.

A second problem is the fact that several personality disorders appear to be related to Axis I disorders in ways that are not fully addressed by the structure and content of the DSM-III-R. For example, family studies link schizotypal personality disorder with schizophrenia. If schizotypal personality disorder represents one end of the spectrum of schizophrenic illnesses, is it wrong to classify it as a personality disorder? Borderline personality disorder is associated with affective instability, and most cases have a past or present diagnosis of major depression. Is this really an atypical affective disorder? The criteria for avoidant personality disorder share much in common with the criteria for social phobia. Is it possible that different researchers have been studying the same disorder using different names?

A third problem is that the DSM-III-R ignores the large body of research that suggests that many personality traits are normally distributed in the general population. In applying Axis II criteria, it is clear that patients vary greatly in level of severity of symptoms. Patients who are below threshold for a given personality diagnosis may still experience difficulties related to personality traits. Would a rating system based on a series of continuous dimensions better represent the true state of nature?

The proposals for the DSM-IV attempt to address these problems while recognizing that major changes in diagnostic criteria disrupt research progress. The changes between the DSM-III and DSM-III-R were major for many of the personality disorders, making it hard to compare studies across the time periods covered by these two manuals. For the most part, the proposed changes for the DSM-IV are more modest. In order to reduce overlap between personality diagnoses, changes in wording or replacement criteria have been suggested when data from several studies indicated that a given criterion lacked specificity. In a few cases, major changes are being considered.

The discussion of proposals for specific personality disorders in this chapter is organized around the three personality clusters described in the DSM-III-R. It should be noted that this cluster structure was originally adopted for heuristic purposes. Since empirical studies provide only weak support for this system of clustering, the DSM-IV may adopt a different organization.

PROPOSED CHANGES FOR CLUSTER A PERSONALITY DISORDERS

The DSM-III-R describes cluster A as the odd/eccentric cluster and includes paranoid, schizoid and schizotypal personality disorders. Minor changes in wording have been suggested for these disorders to clarify meaning and reduce overlap with other personality disorders. Schizotypal and borderline personality disorders present the most problematic overlap because the former is theoretically and empirically related to schizophrenia and the latter is more often associated with affective syndromes. There is a proposal that the criteria for schizotypal personality disorder specify that the odd behavior and perceptual experiences not be counted if they are limited to periods of mood disturbances and affective instability. Field trials are being conducted to determine whether this change decreases overlap with borderline personality disorder.

Because of family history findings, there has been some discussion of a proposal to move schizotypal personality disorder out of Axis II and place it in the schizophrenia section as a milder form of the schizophrenia spectrum. Alternatively, it has been argued that, regardless of any association with Axis I, this syndrome is a personality disorder since it manifests as a lifelong pattern of maladaptive behavior involving "a wide range of important social and personal contexts." The latter point of view does not rule out the possibility that some schizotypal personality disorder symptoms might improve in response to medications normally used for schizophrenia.

PROPOSED CHANGES FOR CLUSTER B PERSONALITY DISORDERS

Cluster B, the dramatic/emotional/erratic cluster, includes antisocial, borderline, histrionic, and narcissistic personality disorders. Ironically, antisocial personality disorder is the most well studied of the criteria sets and also the one with the most radical proposals for change. There is concern that the DSM-III-R criteria for this disorder are too cumbersome and that the criteria are overoperationalized to the extent that patients who manifest disregard for the rights of others in more subtle and sophisticated ways fail to get the diagnosis. Proposed alternative criteria include such items as deceitful and manipulative, glib or superficial, callous unconcern for the feelings of others, and incapacity to maintain enduring relationships. Field trials are currently being conducted to determine if these criteria can be rated reliably and how this criteria set relates to external validators and other personality disorders.

Relatively minor changes are proposed for narcissistic, histrionic, and borderline personality disorder. For borderline personality disorder, a new criterion is proposed that refers to the potential for stress-related "psychotic-like" experiences.

PROPOSED CHANGES FOR CLUSTER C PERSONALITY DISORDERS

Cluster C, the anxious/fearful cluster, includes a more diverse group of disorders—avoidant, dependent, obsessive-compulsive, and passive-aggressive personality disorders.

The criteria for avoidant personality disorder and social phobia are semantically similar, and preliminary reports suggest high rates of comorbidity for these two disorders. One proposal is to combine the two concepts under one set of criteria and cross-list the diagnosis in both the anxiety disorder and personality disorder sections of the DSM-IV. Another proposal is to develop a consensus about theoretical distinctions that might be used to separate the two disorders. Future research studies would then determine whether the two syndromes are truly distinct. In the mean time, a more practical question is whether patients diagnosed as having avoidant personality disorder might respond to antianxiety medications.

Passive-aggressive personality disorder appears to define a behavior style common to several other personality disorders. The DSM-III-R criteria for this disorder have been criticized for being too narrow in scope to be considered a complete personality style. Proposals range from eliminating the diagnosis to developing additional criteria to broaden the concept. Proposals for obsessive-compulsive personality disorder and dependent personality disorder are limited to fine tuning the criteria to reduce overlap with other disorders.

OTHER PROPOSED CATEGORIES

Sadistic personality disorder and self-defeating personality disorder are listed in an appendix of the DSM-III-R as "proposed diagnostic categories needing further study." Given that the data supporting these categories are still very limited, there is little likelihood that they will be promoted to the body of the DSM-IV and a possibility that they may be dropped altogether. This will hinge in part on a decision about whether it is desirable for the DSM-IV to have an appendix for diagnoses needing further study.

The category of depressive personality disorder has been proposed and is currently the subject of field trials. Criteria include such traits as mood dominated by dejection and gloominess; critical, blaming, and punitive toward oneself; judgmental toward others; and prone to feeling guilt. The field trials will examine how this diagnosis relates to the affective disorders, especially dysthymia.

PERSONALITY RATINGS AS CONTINUOUS DIMENSIONS

While there is little enthusiasm for completely replacing the current personality categories with a series of continuous trait measures, there are several proposals to supplement the categories with dimensional ratings. This could be accomplished by using the number of criteria present for a given Axis II disorder as a continuous dimensional rating. Another proposal is to base supplemental dimensional ratings on traits derived from research using psychological tests. For example, there is considerable research supporting the validity of such trait dimensions as neuroticism, extraversion, openness to experience, agreeableness, and constraint.

SUMMARY

The DSM-IV will generally feature the same personality disorder categories as the DSM-III-R. In most cases the criteria are similar except for occasional modifications and substitutions aimed at reducing overlap between personality disorders. Depending on the outcome of field trails, the criteria for antisocial personality disorder may be simplified and altered in ways that broaden the scope of this diagnosis. It is likely that the DSM-IV will more clearly acknowledge the associations between Axis I and Axis II disorders. It has not been resolved whether this will involve clarification in the text of the manual or some system of cross-listing certain personality disorders in different sections. Finally, the system of categorical personality diagnosis may be supplemented by some method of coding severity of individual personality disorders or traits.

REFERENCES

1. American Psychiatric Association: The DSM-IV Options Book. Washington, DC: American Psychiatric Association, 1991.

64

CLUSTER A PERSONALITY DISORDERS

MADELEINE M. O'BRIEN, M.D., ROBERT L. TRESTMAN, PH.D., M.D., and
LARRY J. SIEVER, M.D.

The cluster A personality disorders include schizoid, schizotypal, and paranoid personality disorders in the DSM-III-R.[1] Cluster A is often referred to as the "odd" or "eccentric" cluster. For each of these three personality disorders, we present in this chapter a clinical description including epidemiological factors, course of illness, any pertinent family history or genetic data, any pertinent laboratory or testing findings, differential diagnosis, and treatment approaches. The treatment section is divided into three parts: psychopharmacological treatments, psychological treatments, and combined approaches.

SCHIZOID PERSONALITY DISORDER

The defining clinical feature of schizoid personality disorder is pervasive indifference to social and familial relationships and a constricted range of affect. The diagnosis arose from the work of German descriptive psychiatrists who sought to describe the premorbid personality structure of schizophrenic patients and their functioning between psychotic episodes as well as the functioning of their relatives.

There are seven diagnostic criteria for schizoid personality disorder, and four are required for the diagnosis. People with schizoid personality disorder do not want, seek, or enjoy close relationships. They prefer solitary activities, have a decreased interest in sexual activity, seem incapable of experiencing or expressing strong emotions, and are indifferent to praise or criticism or the feelings of others. Some clinicians believe that this cold and aloof behavior is not simply related to a disinterest but may be the outcome of a tension created from vacillating between wanting and not wanting social contact[2] or from familially determined predispositions to schizophrenic illnesses.[3]

Epidemiology

There are few epidemiological data available for schizoid personality disorder. The prevalence of schizoid personality disorder is presumably very low in the general population, but is specifically unknown. In clinical studies using DSM-III-R criteria, the prevalence rate ranged from 1 to 16 per cent, with a median of 8.5 per cent.[4] Clinical observations of outpatient populations have suggested that it may occur in males more than females. During DSM-III-R Advisory Committee meetings, there was consideration of eliminating the category schizoid personality disorder. Interestingly, revised criteria that allowed for the concomitant diagnosis of schizoid and schizotypal personality disorders resulted in an increase in the clinical diagnosis of schizoid personality disorder.[5]

Etiology

While the etiology of schizoid personality disorder remains unclear, various formulations have been proposed. These include a genetic basis, a psychological basis, and the impact of both of these operating simultaneously. For example, there has been an association made between social isolation and eye movement dysfunction (EMD). A neurointegrative deficit reflected in EMD might hamper the development of the relationship between parent and child, creating a dysynchrony in attachment with subsequent psychological sequelae.[6] Psychologically, theories of schizoid personality development involve the failure to achieve developmental milestones of object relations, which depend upon adequate mothering.

Differential Diagnosis/Comorbidity

The diagnosis of schizoid personality disorder rests upon the identification of a long-term pattern of social isolation. The differential diagnosis may include avoidant personality disorder, and a clear distinction must be made between the indifference to people and the chosen social withdrawal of the schizoid personality versus fear of rejection by people and the social withdrawal of the avoidant personality. Schizophrenic disorders and delusional disorders must be eliminated from the differential diagnosis. It is also very important to identify any coexisting diagnoses such as major depressive disorders. Finally, other personality disorders, particularly schizotypal personality disorder, may coexist.

Treatment

There have been very few systematic treatment studies on patients with schizoid personality disorder. These patients rarely seek treatment, and most often do so in the context of a precipitating crisis, during which they seek relief from the acute symptomatology but not from the long-lasting patterns of social isolation. Treatment is multifaceted and must be individually tailored to the needs of the given patient. Psychoanalytical concepts have been employed to help the clinician understand the developmental deficits and the defenses the patient has developed to provide adequate intrapsychic protection and to preserve a sense of self. Traditional psychoanalysis per se, however, is relatively contraindicated with most schizoid patients. The schizoid patient will not be able to tolerate the frequency of the contact, and the overall neutrality of the analyst would not be corrective for a patient with such severe difficulties with relatedness.

It is the use of the real relationship between patient and therapist and secondarily that of the transference relationship that will allow the patient to develop trust and subsequently improve relatedness.[7] The psychotherapy of schizoid patients is usually overall a supportive psychotherapy, with less emphasis on insight-oriented work and with particular sensitivity to the patient's ability to tolerate interpretations and confrontations.[8] To optimize treatment, the clinician may employ various cognitive or behavioral techniques, particularly geared at reducing socially isolative behaviors, reinforcing socially outgoing behaviors, and facilitating adjustments to shifts in life circumstances. Some clinicians believe that, despite improvements in group psychotherapy and psychopharmacology, individual verbal psychotherapy remains the mainstay of treatment.

In the beginning of the individual treatment with the schizoid patient, it is important to allow the patient to determine the necessary distance, to respect the patient's need to be distant or isolative, to express tolerance of this distance, and to remain flexible in meeting the patient's needs. Since some of the treatment entails social reeducative measures, some therapists will refer a schizoid patient to a social skills group or to a psychotherapy group. In a psychotherapy group, some of the difficulties in forming, sustaining, and appreciating relationships with others can be explored effectively. Group psychotherapy can be a very productive treatment modality provided that the individual needs of each patient in the group are adequately assessed and met.[9]

The use of medication in schizoid personality disorder can play an important role in the overall treatment of schizoid personality disorder. Since a patient with schizoid personality disorder usually presents for treatment following a crisis that has exacerbated symptoms, it is important to take a full and detailed history of both chronic and acute symptoms. The clinician should also evaluate the patient for comorbid psychiatric syndromes or diagnoses. It may be useful to conceptualize symptoms as falling into dimensions of cognitive organization, affective regulation, impulse control, and anxiety modulation. It has been shown that patients diagnosed with cluster A personality disorders, when under stress, are especially vulnerable to cognitive distortion.[10]

Depending on a patient's symptoms, there may be a role for chronic medication in the schizoid personality, but more often than not, medication would be of short-term use for the control of acute symptomatology. Antipsychotic medications, antidepressants, and anxiolytics may be useful in treatment; but there is, as of yet, no compelling evidence that specific medications are especially helpful for the enduring patterns of thinking, feeling, and behaving of the schizoid patient. A trial of low-dose antipsychotic medication may relieve several symptoms: anger, hostility, suspiciousness, illusions, ideas of reference, paranoid ideation, anxiety, and obsessive and compulsive symptoms.[10] The judicious use of medication at times when symptoms become more intense can be extremely helpful in the overall treatment and in the patient's continued participation in psychotherapy.

Clinical Course

Regarding the course of the patient with schizoid personality disorder, many of the symptoms seem chronic and not particularly amenable to treatment; however, by virtue of targeted psychorehabilitative and social reeducative strategies in individual and group psychotherapies, other people may begin to respond to the patient more affirmatively, thereby affording the patient with more opportunities for personal growth. This cycle can become positively self-perpetuating. If, through therapy, the patient can begin to relate more effectively by using the relationship with the primary therapist as the springboard for relationships outside therapy, some of the more fixed character traits may be modified. There are no definitive data that suggest that patients with schizoid personality disorder are at greater risk for the development of schizophrenic illnesses, but if schizoid personality disorder is present before schizophrenia develops, it is associated with a poorer outcome.[11]

SCHIZOTYPAL PERSONALITY DISORDER

The defining clinical features of schizotypal personality disorder are pervasive deficits in interpersonal relatedness and peculiarities of ideation, appearance, and behavior. Historically, "schizotype" was a term applied to those individuals identified as predisposed to the development of schizophrenia.[12,13] Schizotypal personality disorder was first introduced in the DSM-III when it seemed necessary to delineate between the loss of reality testing seen transiently in borderline personality disorder from so-called borderline schizophrenia, in which a phenomenological and genetic relatedness to schizophrenia was proposed. The criteria for schizotypal personality disorder were developed from a review of records of "borderline schizophrenic" relatives of

probands with schizophrenia in the Danish Adoption studies of schizophrenia.[14]

There has been considerable interest in research with schizotypal personality disorder because of the possibility that it may be another phenotypic expression of the genotype predisposing to schizophrenia. Furthermore, schizotypal personality disorder was the only personality disorder in the DSM-III derived partially from empirical studies and not solely from clinical consensus. Its inclusion set the tone for a more scientific approach to the delineation of personality disorders and their relationship to Axis I disorders.[15]

There are nine diagnostic criteria in the DSM-III-R for schizotypal personality disorder, and five are required for the diagnosis. The diagnostic criteria of schizotypal personality disorder are the nonpsychotic, albeit bizarre, symptoms that are amplified to their florid psychotic counterparts in schizophrenia. People with schizotypal personality disorder experience ideas of reference, magical thinking, extreme anxiety in certain social situations, recurrent illusions, and paranoid ideation. There may be odd speech patterns and eccentric appearance or mannerisms. People with schizotypal personality disorder are usually poorly related and tend to have only one or two friends outside of the immediate family. Of the nine diagnostic criteria, the first four are akin to the "positive" or psychotic symptoms of schizophrenia and the remaining five are akin to the "negative" or deficit symptoms of schizophrenia. The psychotic-like symptoms of schizotypal personality disorder are less intense and pervasive than those of major Axis I psychotic disorders and are more amenable to reality testing.

Epidemiology

There has been no published study reporting the prevalence of schizotypal personality disorder in a sample of adults that is representative of the general population.[15] The prevalence of this personality disorder in the general population is very low; however, it is one of the more frequently diagnosed personality disorders because the symptoms can be very severe and disabling. Patients are more likely to seek treatment and clinicians are more likely to identify this disorder. As with schizoid personality disorder, there are relatively few epidemiological data. There seems to be no gender difference in distribution.

Etiology

In understanding the etiology of schizotypal personality disorder, researchers have focused on identifying psychobiological markers, and particularly on testing whether markers seen in schizophrenia occur in increased frequency in schizotypal personality disorder. It has been shown that there is an increased prevalence of schizotypal relatives in the biological relatives of schizophrenics as compared with relatives of controls and that these schizotypal relatives had decreased activity of plasma amine oxidase.[16] Eye movement dysfunction was associated with schizotypal personality disorder in a group of college students identified to be at high risk for the development of schizophrenia.[17] Inferior backward masking performance has also been demonstrated in patients with schizotypal personality disorder, as in patients with schizophrenia.

Evidence has continued to accumulate more recently that corroborates that there are strong psychophysiological similarities between schizotypal personality disorder and schizophrenia. In a recently published study, eye tracking accuracy in patients with schizotypal personality disorder was compared with controls with non–schizophrenia-related personality disorders and with normal controls. Both schizotypal and schizophrenic subjects demonstrated significantly more impaired tracking than did the other personality disordered control group and the normal control group.[18] These parallels between schizotypal personality disorder and schizophrenia suggest not only genetic and biological similarity but also raise the possibility of similarity in treatment responses.

Differential Diagnosis/Comorbidity

There are no extensive data on the overlap between schizotypal personality disorder and Axis I disorders, but evidence suggests that there is a substantial overlap with major depressive disorders.[15] Schizotypal personality disorder also showed the highest rate of overlap with schizophrenia; however, the diagnosis of schizotypal personality disorder cannot be made concomitantly with the diagnosis of schizophrenia according to the exclusionary criteria as set forth in the DSM-III-R. Premorbid diagnosis of schizotypal personality disorder has been shown to be a significant predictor of positive outcome in schizophrenia. Schizotypal personality disorder often coexists with other personality disorders, particularly with other odd cluster disorders but also with borderline personality and avoidant personality disorders. Finally, it is important to distinguish schizotypal personality disorder from the Axis I diagnoses of schizophrenia and delusional disorders.

Treatment

The treatment of schizotypal personality disorder resembles that of schizoid personality disorder in that individual and skills-oriented psychotherapy may be of value. Again, the benefits that can be gained in psychotherapy will depend upon the therapist's skill in respecting the social isolativeness and suspiciousness of these patients while concomitantly encouraging the very gradual development of a therapeutic relationship. Cognitive and behavioral measures may be valuable in, for example, helping the patient learn how to establish and maintain eye contact or how to determine appropriateness of certain behaviors for specific social situations. There is a body of research, however, that suggests that when there is a comorbid diagnosis of obsessive personality disorder, those patients with schizotypal personality disorder are less amenable to behavioral interventions.[19] Another useful strategy is to help the patients accept and adapt to their solitary lifestyle.[8] Clinically, it has also been observed that the more schizophrenic-like the patient with regard especially to paranoid ideation and suspiciousness, the more resistant he or she is to change.

There seems to be an increasing number of clinical studies paralleling those of psychophysiological and psychobiological testing demonstrating statistically significant efficacy of low-dose antipsychotic medication. Treatment with low-dose haloperidol (2 to 12 mg/day) in a single-blind trial of 17 schizotypal patients resulted in significant improvement of schizotypal symptoms, particularly with regard to ideas of reference, odd communication, and social isolation.[20] Unfortunately, these patients exhibited a high sensitivity to side effects that led to problems with medication compliance and dropout. In another study, the efficacy of thiothixene versus placebo in the treatment of borderline and schizotypal patients was examined. Although clinically some of the patients obviously improved, there was not a statistically significant drug effect by psychological instrument measures. Upon further clinical assessment of results, it seemed that the patients who benefited the most from treatment with low-dose antipsychotics were the most impaired patients with high degrees of psychoticism.[21] A study of patients with both schizotypal personality disorder and obsessive-compulsive disorder treated with low-dose thiothixene showed significant reduction in several schizotypal symptoms.[22]

Since the use of an antipsychotic medication in schizotypal personality disorder may be on an ongoing basis, it is essential to assess overall effectiveness very carefully and thoroughly. One way to approach the use of antipsychotic medication with the patient is to inform the patient that the medication may be helpful with certain specified symptoms and to encourage a clinical trial for an agreed upon length of time and at a specific dosage. The extent of clinical effectiveness can then be assessed. It is very important to be extremely thoughtful and careful in the use of even low-dose antipsychotic medication because of the risk of tardive dyskinesia. Each patient needs to be informed fully about this potential side effect. In order for an antipsychotic medication to be continued at a low dose in a maintenance fashion, the benefits should unequivocally outweigh the risks. As previously discussed with regard to the pharmacologic treatment of schizoid personality disorder, the clinician should always be aware of symptoms that may arise in the context of acute stressors or that may represent comorbid diagnoses; appropriate medication should be started.

Clinical Course

The clinical course of schizotypal personality disorder is fairly stable. The gains from psychotherapy and psychopharmacology are usually modest at best, but to a patient who suffers from serious symptoms that can be very disabling and at times require hospitalization, even modest gains can be significant. The percentage of patients with schizotypal personality disorder who will develop schizophrenia is unclear. One study found that as many as 25 per cent of patients diagnosed with schizotypal personality disorder met criteria for schizophrenia at a 2-year follow-up.[22]

PARANOID PERSONALITY DISORDER

The prominent clinical feature of paranoid personality disorder is lifelong suspiciousness, mistrust, hypervigilance, and hypersensitivity to praise and criticism, and a pervasive tendency to ascribe malicious intent to the actions of others and events. Paranoid personality disorder first entered the official psychiatric nomenclature in 1942.

There are seven diagnostic criteria for paranoid personality disorder in the DSM-III-R, and four are required for the diagnosis. People with paranoid personality disorder are easily slighted and swiftly become extremely defensive. They demonstrate a pervasive and unwarranted mistrust of others. They have an extraordinarily difficult time letting go of grudges. Fearing that they might be betrayed or demeaned, they tend not to confide in others and appear cold and aloof. They question without justification and read hidden meaning into the intentions or activities of others. They have been described as pathologically jealous, constantly questioning the fidelity of their partners. They read hidden meaning into the actions or statements of others.

Epidemiology

There has been no study employing the DSM-III-R criteria that has established the prevalence of paranoid personality disorder in the general population. Its incidence is very low, and a range of 1 to 3 per cent seems a reasonable estimate.[23] Certain groups with a proclivity for paranoid ideation, such as prisoners, refugees, the elderly, and the hearing impaired, have been identified as at risk for paranoid personality disorder, but the results of such studies are difficult to evaluate. Therefore, there are no known specific epidemiological risk factors, but clinical observation suggests that paranoid personality disorder may be more common in men.

Etiology

The etiology of paranoid personality disorder remains unclear. Familial and adoption studies of the biological relatives of schizophrenics have suggested that genetic factors may play an etiological role in this disorder. Moreover, it has been shown that the risk for paranoid personality disorder was highest in relatives of patients with paranoid delusional disorder.[24] It is thought that paranoid personality disorder and delusional disorder may share a genetic basis with each other, which is perhaps stronger and distinct from that which may be shared with schizophrenia.[23]

Psychologically, an understanding of paranoid personality disorder would entail a grasp of hypotheses and explanations of paranoid ideation and suspiciousness. Many theories have been proposed to explain and understand paranoid ideation, most of which involve homosexual feelings, hostile feelings, and feelings of shame and humiliation.

Differential Diagnosis/Comorbidity

The differential diagnosis of paranoid personality disorder must exclude those individuals who become mildly paranoid under stress and who remit swiftly and spontaneously with no interepisodic suspiciousness. Furthermore, individuals with paranoid personality disorder often meet criteria for other personality disorders, particularly schizotypal personality disorder (with which it shares the diagnostic criterion of paranoid ideation), schizoid, and other personality disorders. In most clinically based samples, fewer than 25 per cent of patients diagnosed with paranoid personality disorder are free of other personality disorder diagnoses.[23] It is important to distinguish between the diagnosis of paranoid personality disorder and that of paranoid delusional disorder. The clinical distinction can be made by differentiating between paranoid ideation and paranoid delusions. People with paranoid delusional disorder tend to have more fixed and intense beliefs, whereas people with paranoid personality disorder tend to have muted and less organized ideas that are more amenable to reality testing. Finally, and as with all cluster A personality disorders, to make the diagnosis of paranoid personality disorder, the symptoms must not solely occur during the course of a schizophrenic illness.

Treatment

There have been no systematic treatment studies of paranoid personality disorder. Patients with paranoid personality disorder are very difficult to treat because it is so difficult to develop a working, trusting relationship with these patients. Paranoid individuals will tend to mistrust their therapists' motives and avoid disclosing personal information. Although patients with paranoid personality disorder tend to deny their difficulties, they can become very disturbed by their symptoms and will sometimes seek treatment. In individual psychotherapy, these patients are often intimidated by the threat of intimacy. Initially, it is advisable for the therapist to maintain a somewhat distant stance with a predictably professional and impersonal attitude. Such consistency and perserverance may allow a modicum of trust to be established. If the therapist listens to their difficulties nonjudgmentally over time and is empathically supportive, a holding environment may eventually be created in which trust may be experienced, learned, and fostered. Once a therapeutic alliance is established, the therapist may encourage the patient to test out paranoid ideas during sessions. Eventually, it may be possible to introduce some cognitive and behavioral techniques that will encourage the patient to interface with his or her environment more and to reevaluate paranoid ideas. People with paranoid personality disorder often do poorly in group psychotherapies.

Regarding the use of medication in paranoid personality disorder, is it again useful to identify acute and chronic symptoms and to target symptoms accordingly. Since patients with paranoid personality disorder are especially vulnerable to cognitive distortion, the use of low-dose antipsychotic medication may be of some help. Again, under stress certain symptoms may worsen, and other medications may be indicated for short-term use.

There have to date been no controlled medication trials in patients with paranoid personality disorder.

Clinical Course

Modest improvements may be made in psychotherapy or with the use of medication.[23]

REFERENCES

1. American Psychiatric Association: Diagnostic and Statistical Manual of Mental Disorders. 3rd ed. Revised. Washington, DC: American Psychiatric Association, 1987.
2. Lively WJ, West M, Tanney A: Historical comment on DSMIII schizoid and avoidant personality disorders. Am J Psychiatry 142:1344–1347, 1985.
3. Frances A: The DSMIII personality disorders section: A commentary. Am J Psychiatry 137:1050–1054, 1980.
4. Kalus O, Bernstein DP, Siever LJ: Schizoid personality disorder: A review of current status and implications for DSM-IV. J Pers Disord (in press).
5. Morey LC: Personality disorders in DSMIII and DSMIII-R: Convergence, coverage and internal consistency. Am J Psychiatry 145:573–577, 1988.
6. Siever LJ, Coursey RD, Alterman IS, et al: Clinical, psychophysiological, and neurological characteristics of volunteers with impaired smooth pursuit eye movements. Biol Psychiatry 26:35–51, 1989.
7. Robbins A: The interface of the real and transference relationships in the treatment of schizoid phenomena. Psychoanal Rev 75(3):393–417, 1988.
8. Stone M: Psychotherapy with schizotypal borderline patients. J Am Acad Psychoanal 11:87–111, 1983.
9. Leszcz M: Group psychotherapy of the characterologically difficult patient. Int J Group Psychother 39(3):311–335, 1989.
10. Siever LJ, Davis KL: A psychobiologic perspective on the personality disorders. Am J Psychiatry (in press).
11. Soloff PH: What's new in personality disorders: An update in psychopharmacologic treatment. J Pers Disord 4(3):233–243, 1990.
12. Rado S: Theory and therapy: The theory of schizotypal organization and its application to the treatment of decompensated schizotypal behavior. In Rado S, ed. Psychoanalysis of Behavior, Vol 2. New York, Grune & Stratton, 1962:127–140.
13. Meehl PE: Schizotaxia, schizotypy, schizophrenia. Am Psychologist 17:827–838, 1962.
14. Spitzer RL, Endicott J, Giggon M: Crossing the border into borderline personality and borderline schizophrenia: The development of criteria. Arch Gen Psychiatry 36:17–24, 1979.
15. Siever LJ, Bernstein DP, Silverman JM: Schizotypal personality disorder: A review of its current status. J Pers Disord 5:193–208, 1991.
16. Baron M, Asnis L, Gruen R, et al: Plasma amine oxidase and genetic vulnerability to schizophrenia. Arch Gen Psychiatry 40:275–282, 1983.
17. Siever LJ: Biological markers in schizotypal personality disorder. Schizophr Bull 11(4):564–575, 1985.
18. Siever LJ, Keffe R, Bernstein D, Coccaro EF: Eye tracking impairment in clinically identified patients with schizotypal personality disorder. Am J Psychiatry 147(6):740–745, 1990.
19. Minichiello WE, Baer L, Jenike MA: Schizotypal personality disorder: A poor prognostic indicator for behavior therapy in the treatment of obsessive-compulsive disorder. J Anxiety Disord 1(3):273–276, 1987.
20. Hymowitz P, Frances A, Jacobsberg L, et al: Neuroleptic treatment of schizotypal personality disorder. Compr Psychiatry 27:267–271, 1986.
21. Goldberg SC: Borderline and schizotypal personality disorders treated with low dose thiothixene versus placebo. Arch Gen Psychiatry 43(7):680–686, 1986.
22. Schulz SC: The use of low dose neuroleptics in the treatment of "schizo-obsessive" patients. Am J Psychiatry 143(10):1318–1319, 1986.
23. Bernstein DP, Useda D, Siever LJ: DSM-IV sourcebook: Paranoid personality disorder. J Pers Disord (in press).
24. Kendler KS, Masterson CL, Davis KL: Psychiatric illness in first-degree relatives of patients with paranoid psychosis, schizophrenia, and medical illness. Br J Psychiatry 147:524–531, 1985.

CLUSTER B PERSONALITY DISORDERS

REBECCA A. DULIT, M.D., DEBORAH B. MARIN, M.D., and
ALLEN J. FRANCES, M.D.

The DSM-III-R contains 11 personality disorder diagnoses that are grouped into three clusters. This chapter discusses the treatment of the four disorders in the dramatic cluster, which include borderline personality, antisocial personality, narcissistic personality, and histrionic personality disorders. These personality disorders differ substantially in the degree of empirical support available to inform their treatment. This review focuses primarily on systematically researched treatment approaches and briefly reports on less systematically studied, but widely conducted techniques.

The reader is cautioned to keep the following considerations in mind. There is no treatment of choice for any of the dramatic cluster disorders. Some treatments do result in favorable short-term outcomes for some patients, but nothing is known about long-term treatment outcome. The treatment techniques described must be viewed only as recommendations that may or may not be effective for individual patients. A combined pharmacological and psychotherapeutic approach may be necessary for some patients who meet cluster B diagnostic criteria, and efforts should be made to assess and prioritize target symptoms for clinical intervention.

BORDERLINE PERSONALITY DISORDER

Clinical Description

Borderline personality disorder (BPD) is characterized by a pervasive pattern of stormy interpersonal relationships, unstable affect, and behavioral dyscontrol. While the syndrome can be identified with reasonable reliability, the concept of the disorder has been evolving for a number of decades. Prevalence rates for BPD vary substantially across studies because of differences in diagnostic criteria and setting, but it appears that BPD is one of the more common psychiatric diagnoses. Prevalence rate estimates based on available studies are 1 to 2 per cent of the general population, 11 per cent of psychiatric outpatients, 19 per cent of psychiatric inpatients, 33 per cent of psychiatric outpatients with a personality disorder, and 63 per cent of psychiatric inpatients with a personality disorder.[1]

Borderline personality disorder appears to be more prevalent among women than among men. The average percentage of females in 38 studies was 74,[2] but the ratio might be lower if studies were conducted in military or correctional settings. Some investigators have also raised the possibility of gender bias in the application of diagnostic criteria.[3] Empirical data on socioeconomic variables in BPD are insufficiently and inconsistently reported across studies, and the disorder may be overdiagnosed in some cultural and ethnic groups and underdiagnosed in others.

Comorbidity of BPD with Axis I and other Axis II disorders is substantial. Borderline personality disorder typically obtains the most overlap with histrionic, antisocial, schizotypal, narcissistic, and dependent personality disorders, and overlaps to a lesser but still common degree with passive-aggressive, avoidant, and paranoid personality disorders.[2] Affective disorder is particularly common in BPD, with rates ranging from 24 to 74 per cent for major depression, 4 to 20 per cent for bipolar disorder, and 3 to 14 per cent for dysthymia.[1] BPD has been reported to occur in as many as 25 per cent of bulimics,[4] and up to 67 per cent of BPD patients may meet criteria for at least one substance use disorder diagnosis.[5]

Several long-term follow-up studies of hospitalized BPD patients have been conducted during the past decade[6] and have shed fascinating light on the natural course of the disorder. Most BPD patients show persistent morbidity with multiple hospitalizations, severe symptomatology, unstable relationships, and poor work performance during their teens and twenties, and cannot be distinguished functionally from schizophrenic controls on 2- to 5-year follow-up. The rate of completed suicide is significant (3 to 10 per cent), and self-mutilation and suicide attempts are common. On longer term follow-up, however, it appears that as many as two thirds of BPD patients who survive gradually achieve reasonably stable employment and interpersonal lives during their thirties.

In the past decade, there have been about ten family studies of the prevalence of psychiatric disorders in relatives of BPD patients.[2] No study has identified a linkage between BPD and schizophrenia. Some studies have shown an increased prevalence of affective disorder in the relatives of BPD subjects, but the linkage is neither uniform nor strong. Some family prevalence studies have suggested that BPD breeds true and may be linked to other types of impulse disorders, such as antisocial personality disorder.

Neurobiological studies of BPD are rapidly proliferating.[7] Several investigations have consistently found that dysregulation of the central serotonergic system correlates with impulsivity, physical aggression, and suicidality. Abnormal dexamethasone suppression test and thyrotropin releasing hormone test results have been found in up to 61 per cent and 46 per cent, respectively, of BPD patients and lend support to the hypothesis that BPD may be a type of mood disorder. Borderline personality disorder patients demonstrate a significantly higher percentage of abnormal electroencephalograms (EEGs) than depressed, nonborderline subjects and normal controls, and EEG abnormalities have included generalized slow wave activity, localized slow wave activity, and spike phenomena.

Treatment Approaches

Ninety-seven per cent of BPD outpatients presenting for treatment have been in previous outpatient treatment and 63 per cent have significant histories of psychotropic medication use.[8] Although there is an extensive literature on the treatment of borderline personality disorder, there have been few systematic studies of treatment efficacy, and it is clear that there is no treatment of choice for the entire group of patients who meet BPD criteria.

Pharmacotherapy of BPD

NEUROLEPTICS

Historically, there has been much interest in the use of neuroleptics for BPD. Goldberg and colleagues[9] conducted a 12-week, double-blind, placebo-controlled study of low-dose thiothixene in 50 high-functioning outpatients with DSM-III criteria–defined BPD and/or schizotypal personality disorder (SPD). The neuroleptic was superior to placebo for all patient groups, but was less strikingly so for the pure BPD subjects than for the SPD and mixed subjects. Thiothixene resulted in improvements in psychotic symptoms, obsessive-compulsive symptoms, and phobic anxiety. Interestingly, the placebo response was also strong, with decreased ratings of anger, hostility, sensitivity, BPD criteria, and schizotypal symptoms.

Soloff and colleagues[10] conducted a 5-week, randomized, double-blind, placebo-controlled study comparing the efficacy of haloperidol and amitriptyline in 90 inpatients with DSM-III criteria–defined BPD, SPD, or both. Haloperidol was significantly superior to amitriptyline and placebo in decreasing depression, paranoia, impulsivity, hostility, and schizotypal symptoms. Patients reported greater improvements than trained raters, and improvements began during the drug washout period.

Most recently, Cowdry and Gardner[11] conducted a crossover study of trifluoperazine, tranylcypromine, carbamazepine, alprazolam, and placebo in 16 criteria-defined BPD outpatients with a history of severe behavioral dyscontrol. Each trial was designed to last 6 weeks, but only five of ten patients completed the full neuroleptic trial; 50 per cent discontinued during the first 3 weeks because of clinical deterioration or medical complications. Subjects who completed the neuroleptic trial had a somewhat favorable outcome, with significant improvement relative to placebo in physician-rated anxiety and suicidality and patient-rated depression, anxiety, and rejection sensitivity. No patients, however, responded to neuroleptic better than to other active medication.

In summary, low-dose neuroleptic treatment may be effective for certain target symptoms in BPD, including psychotic-like, impulsive, and depressive symptoms. There is, however, a high incidence of side effects, and the placebo response appears substantial.

ANTIDEPRESSANTS

The high prevalence of affective symptomatology in BPD has led to considerable interest in the efficacy of antidepressant treatment for BPD. Emerging empirical evidence suggests that tricyclic antidepressants are of limited value and may be counterproductive in some patients. The study by Soloff et al.[10] is the only one that evaluated a tricyclic medication in a double-blind, placebo-controlled trial in criteria-defined BPD patients. Amitriptyline was minimally effective for depressive symptoms compared to placebo and was not superior to the antidepressant effects of haloperidol. The presence of a concurrent major depression did not predict response to amitriptyline. Furthermore, many subjects who did not respond to amitriptyline did worse than subjects on placebo. These amitriptyline nonresponders developed increased paranoid ideation, behavioral dyscontrol, suicidal threats, and assaultive behavior.

The high prevalence of atypical depressive symptoms in BPD has led other investigators to conduct systematic trials of monoamine oxidase inhibitor (MAOI) antidepressants. Liebowitz and Klein have studied the efficacy of phenelzine in patients with hysteroid dysphoria, many of whom meet criteria for borderline personality disorder. In a randomized placebo-controlled, crossover design study of MAOIs in combination with intensive psychotherapy,[12] improvement was noted in chronic emptiness, loneliness, and impulsivity. Another placebo-controlled study of atypical depressive subjects by Liebowitz et al.[13] used phenelzine and imipramine. Subjects with panic attacks or hysteroid dysphoria or both responded more consistently to an MAOI than to imipramine or placebo.

Cowdry and Gardner[11] reported that tranylcypromine was the only medication that both subjects and clinicians rated as having significant positive effect. Improvements were noted in a variety of symptoms, including anxiety, rage, depression, rejection sensitivity, impulsivity, and suicidality. The authors noted that the MAOI had its primary effect on mood, with behavioral changes being a secondary effect, but this study also found no correlation between medication effect and a concurrent diagnosis of major depression.

Preliminary trials of fluoxetine for BPD[14] suggest that some patients may respond well to fluoxetine. Target symptoms that may be most responsive include rejection sensitivity, anger, depressed mood, mood lability, and impulsivity. However, some patients may develop an acute onset of dysphoria and suicidal behavior from fluoxetine.[15]

In summary, tricyclic antidepressants may have limited positive effects in some BPD patients, but significant behavioral toxicity and dyscontrol may also occur. Monoamine oxidase inhibitor antidepressants may be more effective for certain target symptoms, including mood lability, self-image, and impulsivity, but the potential for serious side effects and dietary noncompliance must be considered.

Minor Tranquilizers

There are few systematic treatment studies using minor tranquilizers in criteria-defined BPD patients. Clinical improvement on alprazolam was initially suggested by a case report of three DSM-III criteria–defined BPD patients.[16] Cowdry and Gardner,[11] however, found no significant improvements in physician or patient ratings during a double-blind alprazolam trial. Of note, this study did find a statistically significant worsening of suicidality and behavioral dyscontrol, including suicide attempts and assaultive behavior, in 7 of 12 patients. Interestingly, two other patients responded more favorably to alprazolam than to any other medication trials, and some patients who developed impulsivity reported feeling less anxious and depressed prior to behavioral dyscontrol.

Carbamazepine

Cowdry and Gardner[11] included this anticonvulsant in their multidrug crossover study and found that the frequency and severity of episodes of behavioral dyscontrol were significantly reduced for 10 of 11 subjects during the carbamazepine trial. Physician raters also noted a modest but significant improvement in subjects' mood. Patients, however, did not report feeling significantly improved in mood ratings, and three subjects developed melancholia during treatment with carbamazepine.

Lithium Carbonate

No systematic study has assessed the efficacy of lithium carbonate in BPD patients defined by modern criteria, but Rifkin and colleagues[17] conducted a double-blind, placebo-controlled study of lithium carbonate in patients with emotionally unstable character disorder. They found a decrease in mood lability in 67 per cent of subjects on active medication and in 19 per cent on placebo.

Psychotherapy of BPD

Individual psychotherapy is probably the most common type of treatment conducted with BPD patients, and the literature on the psychotherapeutic approaches to BPD is extensive. Unfortunately, little is known about the efficacy of specific forms of psychotherapy for BPD. Long-term follow-up studies of hospitalized BPD patients have not shed light on this issue and, to our knowledge, only the behavioral treatment of BPD has even begun to be systematically studied.

Despite theoretical differences among the major contributors on intensive psychodynamic psychotherapy of borderline personality, there is much agreement about basic treatment principles. Waldinger and Gunderson[18] summarized these principles as follows:

1. A stable treatment framework must be defined and deviations from the framework should be actively addressed.
2. The therapist should be verbally active in identifying, confronting, and directing patient behavior during sessions in order to diminish transference distortions.
3. The therapist must be able to tolerate and explore negative transference without retaliating or withdrawing.
4. The therapist must help the patient to be aware that he or she communicates affect through behavior.
5. The therapist must make the BPD patient's self-destructive behaviors ungratifying and set limits on behaviors that endanger the patient or the therapy.
6. The therapist should focus on clarifications and interpretations of the transference in the here and now, since genetic reconstructions early in therapy are likely to be counterproductive.
7. The therapist must pay careful attention to countertransference feelings.

In this brief review of the psychodynamic therapeutic approaches to BPD, it is not possible to describe the work of many important contributors. We briefly discuss two major treatment models and highlight their differences. Kernberg et al.'s[19] approach to intensive psychotherapy of the borderline patient is based on their conceptualization of BPD as a disorder of internalized object relations. They regard the BPD patient's inability to tolerate primitive aggression as the primary source of pathology and recommend that psychotherapy be organized around early interpretation of negative transference and primitive defenses, such as splitting and projective identification. They also emphasize the importance of the therapist setting limits to prevent the patient from acting out negative transference and to maintain the technical neutrality of the therapist.

In contrast to Kernberg's model of primitive defenses mobilized in the service of conflict resolution, Buie and Adler[20] emphasize the core difficulty with these patients as being an inability to maintain evocative soothing memories of significant others at times of separation or stress. They maintain that the central therapeutic task is the creation of an empathic relationship in which the patient can experience and eventually internalize real memories of being sustained and soothed by the therapist. The therapist may have to utilize certain holding actions (extra appointments, phone calls, postcards during vacations) early in treatment to protect patients from destructive enactments of abandonment fears. Later in treatment, emphasis is placed on patients exploring their idealization of the therapist and accepting the therapist as he or she is.

Despite the theoretical differences among those who have written about psychodynamic psychotherapy with BPD patients, there is agreement that basic personality change is the goal. Thus far, such treatments have not been subjected to systematic study, although a detailed review[18] of five successfully completed intensive psychotherapies suggests the potential for treatment efficacy.

Despite the fact that BPD patients present a multitude of problem behaviors, little attention has been focused on the behavioral treatment of these patients. Linehan and Wasson[21] have developed an outpatient behavioral psychotherapy for chronically suicidal BPD patients that combines weekly individual and group sessions. Behavioral targets are hierarchically arranged as follows: (1) suicidal behaviors, (2) therapy-interfering behaviors, (3) quality of life–interfering behaviors, and (4) skill acquisition. Their approach emphasizes problem solving and empathic validation of patients. Linehan recently conducted a 1-year prospective outcome study of 46 subjects, randomly assigned to behavioral treatment or treatment as usual in the community, and found that patients in behavioral treatment had a significant reduction in the frequency and severity of parasuicidal behavior, were less likely to drop out of treatment, and had fewer days of inpatient psychiatric care.[22] No outcome differences were found between groups in suicidal ideation, depression, or hopelessness.

ANTISOCIAL PERSONALITY DISORDER

Clinical Description

The DSM-III-R criteria for antisocial personality disorder (ASPD) include behaviors from both childhood and adulthood. Childhood behaviors include aspects of conduct disorder, such as truancy, frequent fights, cruelty to people and animals, and theft. Adolescent and adult behaviors are characterized by impulsivity, lack of remorse and empathy, and a sense of moral, vocational, and social irresponsibility. The antisocial patient typically engages in behaviors that defy conventional societal limitations, although disregard for others may be masked by charming and seductive behavior. Impulsivity may be manifested by engagement in physical fights, criminal behavior, and substance abuse.

Antisocial personality disorder is the only Axis II diagnosis that has been well studied in several large-scale epidemiological studies. Prevalence rates range from 0.2 to 9.4 per cent in the general population, from 3 to 37 per cent in psychiatric inpatients, and up to 75 per cent in prison populations.[1,23] Antisocial personality disorder is more common in males, and the sex ratio ranges from 2 : 1 to 7 : 1.[24] Antisocial personality disorder has been most commonly observed in young adults, in urban settings, and in lower socioeconomic classes. The disorder typically begins in late childhood and peaks in adolescence. Importantly, studies suggest that there is a significant risk of suicide in ASPD patients.[25]

Antisocial personality disorder often coexists with Axis I and other Axis II disorders. Borderline, histrionic, and passive-aggressive personality disorders are the most common comorbid Axis II diagnoses.[1] Affective, anxiety, and substance use disorders are also observed in antisocial patients.[1] Substance abuse has been identified in over 83 per cent of antisocial patients in the general population, and 18 per cent of substance abusers exhibit ASPD.[23] While some have suggested that substance abuse may lead to antisocial behavior, it has also been observed that conduct disorder in adolescence is a strong predictor of subsequent antisocial behavior.

Twin and adoption studies suggest a strong genetic component for both ASPD and criminal behavior.[26] Concordance for antisocial behavior among monozygotic and dizygotic twins is as high as 51 per cent and 22 per cent, respectively. Offspring of adult criminals have rates of ASPD ranging from 6 to 36 per cent. Environmental factors also play a role in the development of ASPD. Family discord, lack of affection, multiple temporary placements, and institutional care contribute to subsequent antisocial behavior.[26]

Biological and psychophysiological studies have focused on the sensation-seeking, impulsive, and criminal behaviors exhibited by ASPD patients. Diminished functioning of both the serotonergic and noradrenergic systems has been associated with impulsivity and violence.[7] Electroencephalographic abnormalities, especially in the frontal and temporal lobes, have been correlated with antisocial and criminal behavior.[27]

Treatment Approaches

Unfortunately, most clinicians agree that the prognosis for treatment of ASPD is extremely bleak. The choice of treatment should be based in part on the predominant symptomatology and the clinical setting. There is little research on the pharmacotherapy of ASPD, but the literature on the treatment of impulsive and aggressive behavior may be applicable to these patients. There are suggestions that lithium carbonate and β-adrenergic antagonists can control violent behavior and explosive rage in prison settings.[28,29] Fluoxetine has also been shown to lessen the aggression displayed by patients with ASPD.[30] Carbamazepine may be useful for the antisocial patient who has evidence of EEG abnormalities, particularly temporal lobe dysrhythmias. It is also essential to systematically assess and treat coexisting Axis I conditions, since ASPD itself is generally so difficult to treat. Antidepressant medication may effectively treat not only depressive symptomatology, but also alcohol and cocaine abuse.

The goal of a therapeutic environment for the antisocial patient is to alter maladaptive behavior patterns and to enhance the patient's sense of responsibility for self and others. A general inpatient psychiatric facility is not the optimal environment for treatment of ASPD. Antisocial patients are often manipulative and disruptive in such environments and elect to leave when faced with limits. Specialty units to which patients are mandated by the court are more likely to provide successful treatment.[31] Once external controls limit the ability to flee, an environment that provides consistent responses to patients' behaviors and a strictly enforced hierarchical structure for determining progress is essential throughout the treatment program. Outpatient programs that adopt a similar approach have also been shown to be effective milieus for treatment.[31]

Early intervention for children with conduct disorders has been utilized to prevent the development of antisocial behavior later in life.[31] Treatment of such children focuses in part on altering dysfunctional patterns in the family environment by teaching parents to more effectively manage the child and to feel less guilt. Specialized milieu programs are often useful for the antisocial adolescent to attenuate an adult antisocial syndrome.[31]

NARCISSISTIC PERSONALITY DISORDER

Clinical Description

Narcissistic personality disorder (NPD) was established as a diagnostic category in the DSM-III. Diagnostic criteria were derived from a review of the psychodynamic literature and focus on the narcissist's grandiosity in fantasy and behavior, hypersensitivity to evaluation by others, feelings of entitlement, and lack of empathy. A recent exploratory effort to empirically identify criteria for NPD found that the following characteristics were significantly more common in NPD subjects than in those with other Axis I

and II diagnoses: a sense of superiority and uniqueness, exaggeration of talents, boastful and pretentious behavior, grandiose fantasies, self-centered and self-referential behavior, need for attention and admiration, arrogant and haughty behavior, and high achievement.[32]

Prevalence rates of NPD in clinical populations vary substantially across studies and range from 2 to 16 per cent.[1] Little is known about the demographic features and family history of patients with NPD, although the disorder may be more common in men.[32] Narcissistic personality disorder patients frequently meet criteria for other Axis II diagnoses, and the highest comorbidity rates occur with antisocial, histrionic, dependent, and borderline personality disorders.[1] Little is known about comorbidity with Axis I disorders and, to our knowledge, no information is available regarding the neurobiology of NPD.

Treatment Approaches

Individual psychotherapy or psychoanalysis is the recommended treatment for patients with NPD, but empirical studies do not exist to support the efficacy of any particular treatment approach. The treatment of NPD is precarious because of the patient's tendency to initially idealize and later devalue the therapist. The risk is high that patients will abruptly terminate treatment in response to an everyday failure on the part of the therapist.

Debate exists in the clinical literature regarding the use of confrontative techniques. Kernberg[33] argued that the NPD patient's grandiosity and need for self-sufficiency are defenses against primary feelings of helplessness, rage, and envy. He viewed the NPD patient's idealization of the therapist as a projection of his or her grandiosity onto the therapist and recommended active confrontation and interpretation of idealization and grandiosity.

Kohut,[34] in contrast, defined the core feature of NPD patients as an intense need for others to help them in regulating self-esteem and to make up for deficiencies in internal structure. He viewed the NPD patient's idealization of the therapist as a reactivation in the transference of previously unsuccessful idealizations of parents in childhood. He recommended that an idealizing transference be allowed to unfold in order for the patient to understand the parental failures of childhood, and emphasized the importance of empathic listening and vicarious introspection.

To our knowledge, there are no pharmacological treatments that have been studied for NPD. Since many NPD patients develop depressive symptoms, especially in response to perceived rejection, antidepressant trials with MAOIs or tricyclic agents may be useful in this population. We would recommend systematic assessment of comorbid diagnoses and target symptoms since these may respond well to pharmacological intervention.

HISTRIONIC PERSONALITY DISORDER

Clinical Description

The DSM-III criteria–defined histrionic personality disorder (HPD) is a revision of the DSM-II criteria–defined hysterical personality, and its core features include self-dramatization, self-centeredness, seductiveness, excessive demands for approval, and shallow and labile expressions of affect. The psychoanalytical literature often subdivides HPD patients into two groups: one that is fairly high functioning and another that is more regressed, impulsive, and disturbed.

Estimates of the prevalence of HPD in clinical populations range from 6 to 45 per cent.[1] Although the disorder does occur in men, it is predominantly diagnosed in women, and the possibility of gender bias has been raised.[35] Many patients with HPD meet criteria for other personality disorders, including borderline, narcissistic, passive-aggressive, antisocial, dependent, avoidant, and schizotypal personality disorders.[1] The area of comorbidity with Axis I disorders has not been well researched, and there are no empirical data on the family history or neurobiology of HPD.

Treatment Approaches

Little empirical research is available to inform the treatment of patients with HPD. There is an extensive literature on psychotherapeutic approaches to HPD, and these depend in part on the psychopathology of the patient. There is general agreement that a central dynamic in treatment is the extreme dependency of these patients and their tendency to use flirtation, idealization, and self-destructive behaviors to obtain gratification of dependency needs.[36] The goal in psychotherapy is to help patients become consciously aware of their infantile and often unrealistic dependency fantasies through transference interpretation. The risk of the classical psychoanalytical approach leading to patient disillusionment and either serious acting out or termination must be considered, especially with more severely disturbed patients. Some[36] recommended maintaining a flexible balance between fulfilling and withholding gratification of dependency needs in order to help the patient understand the limits of gratification they can expect from others.

Psychopharmacotherapy may be effective for some patients with HPD. Liebowitz and Klein[12] have reported on the favorable effects of MAOIs for a condition called hysteroid dysphoria. These patients have much in common with DSM-III criteria–defined HPD patients and are highly rejection sensitive, crave attention and admiration, and are vulnerable to acute atypical depressive reactions to disappointment. Careful assessment of comorbid Axis I and II disorders in HPD patients may be useful in identifying and prioritizing target symptoms that might respond to pharmacotherapy.

CONCLUSION

The research on treatment outcome for the dramatic cluster of personality disorders has been directed primarily toward BPD. Even for this diagnosis, however, the available research is remarkably thin. This results from the fact that research on treatment outcome for personality disorders is beset with methodological difficulties—for example, the lack of well-established outcome measures, the overlap among personality disorders and Axis I conditions, and the lack of standardized treatments for comparison. In the absence of empirical data, the clinician must base treatment decisions on clinical judgments.

A few general guidelines about each of the dramatic cluster diagnoses may be useful. Because of the heterogeneity of the presentation of BPD patients, it is unlikely that any one treatment will ever be the treatment of choice. It is therefore crucial to assess comorbidity and to select target symptoms that are likely to be most amenable to intervention. A combination of psychotherapy and medication is often necessary. There is no effective treatment for ASPD, but the syndromes that accompany it may be amenable to treatment. Although HPD and NPD have not received systematic research attention, an extensive clinical literature suggests a wide range of treatment techniques. The treatment of personality disorders is a difficult area for research, but the extensive research now available on the descriptive features of personality disorders should soon help us to develop a more comprehensive research literature to inform clinical practice.

REFERENCES

1. Widiger TA, Rogers JH: Prevalence and comorbidity of personality disorders. Psychiatr Ann 19:132, 1989.
2. Widiger TA, Frances AJ: Epidemiology, diagnosis, and comorbidity of borderline personality disorder. In Tasman A, Hales RE, Frances AJ, eds. Review of Psychiatry, Vol 8. Washington, DC: American Psychiatric Press, Inc, 1989:8.
3. Pollack WS: Psychotherapy. In Bellack AS, Hersen M, eds. Handbook of Comparative Treatments for Adult Disorders. New York: John Wiley & Sons, 1990:393.
4. Levin A, Hyler S: DSM-III personality diagnosis in bulimia. Compr Psychiatry 27:47, 1986.
5. Dulit RA, Fyer MR, Haas GL, et al: Substance use in borderline personality disorder. Am J Psychiatry 147:1002, 1990.
6. Stone MH: The course of borderline personality disorder. In Tasman A, Hales RE, Frances AJ, eds. Annual Review of Psychiatry. Vol 8. Washington, DC: American Psychiatric Press, Inc., 1989:103.
7. Marin DB, De Meo M, Frances AJ, et al: Biological models and treatments for personality disorders. Psychiatr Ann 19:143, 1989.
8. Skodel AE, Buckley P, Charles E: Is there a characteristic pattern to the treatment history of clinical outpatients with borderline personality? J Nerv Ment Dis 171:405, 1983.
9. Goldberg SC, Schulz SC, Schulz PM, et al: Borderline and schizotypal personality disorders treated with low-dose thiothixene vs placebo. Arch Gen Psychiatry 43:680, 1986.
10. Soloff PH, George A, Nathan S, et al: Progress in pharmacotherapy of borderline disorders. Arch Gen Psychiatry 43:691, 1986.

11. Cowdry RW, Gardner DL: Pharmacotherapy of borderline personality disorder. Arch Gen Psychiatry 45:111, 1988.

12. Liebowitz MR, Klein DF: Interrelationship of hysteroid dysphoria and borderline personality disorder. Psychiatr Clin North Am 4:67, 1981.

13. Liebowitz MR, Quitkin FM, Stewart JW, et al: Antidepressant specificity in atypical depression. Arch Gen Psychiatry 45:129, 1988.

14. Norden MJ: Fluoxetine in borderline personality disorder. Prog Neuropsychopharmacol Biol Psychiatry 13:885, 1989.

15. Teicher MH, Glod CA, Cole JO: Emergence of intense violent suicidal ideation in patients treated with fluoxetine. Am J Psychiatry 147:207, 1990.

16. Faltus FJ: The positive effect of alprazolam in the treatment of three patients with borderline personality disorder. Am J Psychiatry 141:802, 1984.

17. Rifkin A, Quitkin F, Carrillo C, et al: Lithium carbonate in emotionally unstable character disorder. Arch Gen Psychiatry 27:519, 1972.

18. Waldinger RJ, Gunderson JG: Effective Psychotherapy with Borderline Patients. Washington, DC: American Psychiatric Press, Inc., 1987.

19. Kernberg OF, Selzer MA, Koenighsberg HW, et al: Psychodynamic Psychotherapy of Borderline Patients. New York: Basic Books, Inc., 1989.

20. Buie DH, Adler G: The definitive treatment of the borderline personality. Int J Psychoanal Psychother 9:51, 1982.

21. Linehan MM, Wasson EJ: Behavior therapy. In Bellack AS, Hersen M, eds. Handbook of Comparative Treatments for Adult Disorders. New York: John Wiley & Sons, 1990:420.

22. Linehan MM, Armstrong HE, Suarez A, et al: Cognitive-behavioral treatment of chronically parasuicidal borderline patients. Arch Gen Psychiatry 48:1060, 1991.

23. Regier DA, Farmer ME, Rae DS, et al: Comorbidity of mental disorders with alcohol and other drug abuse. Results from the epidemiologic catchment area (ECA) study. JAMA 264:2511, 1990.

24. Merikangas KR, Weissman MM: Epidemiology of DSM-III Axis II personality disorders. In Frances AJ, Hales RE, eds. Annual Review. Vol 5. Washington, DC: American Psychiatric Press, Inc., 1986:258.

25. Martin RL, Cloninger R, Guze SB, et al: Mortality in a follow up of 500 psychiatric outpatients II. Cause-specific mortality. Arch Gen Psychiatry 42:58, 1985.

26. Rutter M, Macdonald H, Couteur AL, et al: Genetic factors in child psychiatric disorders—II. Empirical findings. J Child Psychol Psychiatry 31:39, 1990.

27. Kandel E, Freed A: Frontal-lobe dysfunction and antisocial behavior: A review. J Clin Psychology 45:404, 1989.

28. Yudofsky S, Williams K, Gorman J: Propranolol in the treatment of rage and violent behavior in patients with chronic brain syndromes. Am J Psychiatry 138:218, 1981.

29. Wickham EA, Reed JV: Lithium for the control of aggressive and self-mutilating behavior. Int Clin Psychopharmacol 2:181, 1987.

30. Coccaro EF, Still JL, Herbert JL, et al: Fluoxetine treatment of impulsive aggression in DSM-III-R personality disorder patients. J Clin Psychopharmacol 10:373, 1990.

31. Reid WH: The antisocial personality: A review. Hosp Community Psychiatry 36:831, 1985.

32. Ronningstam E, Gunderson J: Identifying criteria for narcissistic personality disorder. Am J Psychiatry 147:918, 1990.

33. Kernberg O: Borderline Conditions and Pathological Narcissism. New York: Jason Aronson, 1975.

34. Kohut H: The Restoration of the Self. New York: International Universities Press, 1977.

35. Chodoff P: Hysteria and women. Am J Psychiatry 139:545, 1982.

36. Chodoff P: Histrionic personality disorder. In Treatment of Psychiatric Disorders: A Task Force Report of the American Psychiatric Association. Washington, DC: American Psychiatric Association, 1990:2727.

66

CLUSTER C PERSONALITY DISORDERS

MICHAEL H. STONE, M.D.

The personality disorders described in the DSM-III-R[1] have been grouped into three "clusters." Cluster C includes four personality types whose common property is the tendency to experience anxiety and to show outward signs of fear. The four types—dependent, obsessive-compulsive, avoidant, and passive-aggressive—share in another feature: inhibition in the assertion of socially acceptable impulses. Customarily, these include inhibitions in the sexual sphere, but also a fearful reluctance to express irritation or anger, even when the interpersonal circumstances (an unfair coworker, an unreasonably demanding family member) would justify such emotion. This inhibitedness is encountered commonly in histrionic personality disorder (currently classified within the "dramatic"cluster), the as yet nonofficial "self-defeating" personality disorder, and in dysthymic persons, who, although presently classified in Axis I, can usually be said to show a "depressive" personality disorder.[2]

These inhibited personality types are precisely the ones that Freud and the psychoanalytic pioneers first encountered and sought to treat. Psychoanalysis and the related psychotherapies have their greatest efficacy in this domain: in the alleviation of inappropriate inhibition.[3] Whereas we are taught to regard *personality* attributes as ego *syntonic*, inhibition inevitably carries with it a measure of suffering, and therefore of ego *dystonicity*. It is this suffering that constitutes the internal motor impelling the patient to seek help, and, having done so, to endure the discomforts that accompany the steps toward recovery: self-revelation and the gradual entry into the territory of fear.

Inhibited patients typically *internalize* blame for the frustrations in their life, even in situations in which observers (including the therapist) would hold the patient blameless. This quality, too, facilitates treatment, in the sense that the patient shows a willingness to accept some responsibility for contributing to the unhappiness in his or her personal life. This puts therapist and patient on the same wavelength and fosters the cooperative dialogue we now refer to as the therapeutic alliance. Those who blame others (externalizers, such as antisocial, paranoid, and sadistic patients) pose far greater challenges to the therapeutic process; their prognosis is correspondingly more guarded.

DEPENDENT PERSONALITY DISORDER

Clinical Description and Etiology

The traits that most readily call to clinicians' attention the likelihood that they are dealing with a dependent personality are submissiveness, passivity, timidity, and clinginess. The psychodynamic wellspring from which these traits develop in early life is fear of being abandoned. This fear does not always originate from the same source: in some persons, death of a parent during one's childhood seems the most important causative agent, but in others, repeated experiences of neglect or outright rejection by caretakers is the primary noxious influence.

At least three of the defining items in the DSM-III-R for dependent personality disorder (DPD) may be viewed as reparative tactics designed to maintain a hold on the important other(s) in one's life: pressuring others for reassurance, mindlessly agreeing with others lest disagreement lead to rejection, and doing favors and tasks one would rather not do simply to ingratiate oneself with these "vital" others. These are true "dependency" attributes.[4] The remaining six items may be seen more as characterological symptoms of the failure of these defensive maneuvers. Being inordinately hurt by criticism or mild disapproval, for example, represents an adaptive failure. The dependent person may try, at the same time, to turn such failure into a victory, as when breaking into tears at some slight criticism elicits volumes of reassurance, and perhaps a hug from a lover or spouse one was afraid of "losing." Letting others make all the decisions is both a failure and a defense: here the defensive aspect takes the form of

overcompliance (submissiveness). Submission reduces the probability of offending the other person, hence "ensuring" loyalty or steadfastness. Clinginess—never letting the other out of one's sight—is one of the most common manifestations of the dependent personality, and is a sign of "pathological attachment."[4] This tendency often backfires, in the sense that it alienates most people and threatens to drive away the very person(s) to whom one clings the most tightly.

Dependent personality will often be found in conjunction with the features of avoidant personality,[5] or with the characterological attributes of depressive persons (low self-esteem, pessimism, constant worrying). In the older classification of borderline conditions[6] the "healthiest" type of borderline was the "anaclitic depressed type": the patient who was simultaneously depressed and clingy. Many patients with DSM-III-R criteria–defined borderline personality disorder are also markedly dependent. At the extremes of DPD one may encounter erotomania (including erotomanic preoccupation with the therapist).

Although patients with DPD have a higher than expected proportion of first-degree relatives with dependent and other anxious cluster personality disorders,[7] especially avoidant personality disorder, much of the psychopathology stems from "cultural transmission" via a similarly dependent parent, who inculcates in the future patient a propensity to fearfulness and clinging.

Treatment

The treatment of dependent personality, unless the disorder is found in conjunction with distinctive symptoms (belonging, e.g., to Axis I disorders) amenable to various pharmacological or other biological measures, relies upon verbal therapies. Currently, these might include any of the following: psychoanalysis, psychoanalytically oriented psychotherapy, supportive therapy, cognitive therapy, behavioral therapy, or group therapy. Apart from "classical" psychoanalysis (which cannot be admixed with any other of the modalities without ceasing to be "classical"), the other forms of psychotherapy will often need to be combined in different ways during the course of treatment. How many modalities are used depends on the breadth of training of the therapist as well as on the nature and severity of the problems presented by the patient. The best approach is pragmatic, not parochial.

The length of therapy likewise cannot be determined on theoretical or doctrinal grounds, but rather only on the basis of the patient's motivation, the intensity and urgency of the problems, and the realistic goals of the patient. A dependent patient who, for example, is young, single, highly motivated, and possessed of some inner resources (e.g., hobbies, skills) may wish to overcome the pathological dependency in a thorough way, with the goals of living autonomously, relying less on parents, becoming self-reliant at work, and forming a sexual partnership. These goals might be realized in an intensive therapy (two or more visits per week) spanning 2 to 5 years, or even longer. With a more seriously handicapped patient, one might use the same forms of psychotherapy, but with the more modest goals of substituting dependency upon the original family with a less severe dependency upon a marital partner—bypassing what might be the unrealizable ambition of "complete" autonomy.

Dependent patients are usually exquisitely sensitive to being alone and, worse yet, to being jilted. Many will have devoted years to "perfecting" the techniques of clinging to others, to the utter neglect of outside interests, casual reading, the cultivation of friends, or any other potentially sustaining activities. To be alone for an evening or a weekend, for such a patient, is like being parachuted into the desert. In this situation, supportive interventions are of critical importance. Therapists must encourage dependent patients of this sort to expand upon whatever activities (if any) they may have found enjoyable and diverting in the past, or (and what is substantially more difficult) to develop such interests for the first time. Joining church groups, political organizations, lecture series, and the like may go a long ways toward conquering the fear of being alone, while also helping to expand the patient's social network. In the meantime, psychotherapy (of whichever mode is most congenial with the therapist) can assist in helping the patient overcome fears connected with meeting new people at social gatherings, expressing opinions in public, and the like. Group therapy may be useful in helping such patients see that other people can continue to like and to accept them even if they should give vent to an opinion discordant with views of the others (a step dependent persons experience as extremely risky).

Patients who are particularly clingy will need to be taught (via a supportive or cognitive intervention) about the terrible "Catch 22" inherent in this tendency: that excessive demands upon the attentions of others will (almost invariably) drive away—and provoke abandonment by—the very persons upon whom they have so tenaciously clung. The lesson (that if someone loves you, he or she will stay if given breathing space but flee if confined), although absolutely crucial to the amelioration of dependent personality disorder, goes contrary to a lifetime of thought on the part of the patient. The therapist's task here will be no brief skirmish, but will have more the characteristics of a fight to the finish. Inevitably, the therapist will be caught up in the clinginess (e.g., demands for extra time, nighttime calls, symptom outbreaks before vacations). This will elicit countertransference annoyance, riddance wishes, and the like, all of which must be controlled and dealt with reflectively and compassionately, so that the resulting emotional material can be used rewardingly for the patient's benefit. Otherwise,

such feelings may lead to a redramatization of the patient's original plight (of getting rejected), intensifying the dependency and clinginess.

When under the stress of personal loss or rejection, patients with DPD often become anxious— in a way that will warrant the employment of the milder anxiolytic drugs, such as the benzodiazepines. These medications reduce the "crisis" atmosphere and help restore the patient's equilibrium, permitting the strengthening effects of therapy to solidify.

OBSESSIVE-COMPULSIVE PERSONALITY DISORDER

Clinical Description and Etiology

The traits of obsessive-compulsive personality disorder (OCPD), as enumerated in the DSM-III-R, reflect abnormalities in all three "compartments" of mental life: behavior, thought and mood. "Compulsive" refers to the behavioral aspects: preoccupation with lists, rules, schedules, and the like; indecisiveness; hoarding; overemphasis of work, to the exclusion of pleasurable activities; and stinginess with money or time (unless there is "something in it" for oneself). The cognitive component usually takes the form of overconscientiousness, moral rigidity, or repetitive worries and self-reproaches that one cannot obliterate from one's mind. These "obsessions" are often dystonic, just as the preoccupation with "doing the right thing" can pass over into truly symptomatic ritualistic compulsive behavior (making sure the door is locked, the stove turned off . . .). Some patients with OCPD, in other words, also show the Axis I obsessive-compulsive disorder (OCD). Although each disorder figures in the differential diagnosis of the other, one must keep in mind that OCD patients may show any of a number of personality disorders (e.g., avoidant, histrionic, dependent) besides OCPD.[8]

Regarding the sex ratio in OCPD, it is usual to find a male excess in the range of 6:4. Men and women tend to have similar dynamics and personality traits, but gender gives rise to different caricature types within the culture: women with OCPD often appearing as fussbudget housewives for whom every ashtray and curio must be in exactly the same place, and who beg off from sex because the laundry isn't yet finished; men appear as "uptight" professionals who check their watch every 5 minutes to make sure they're "on schedule," and who feel unnerved by the understructured time of holidays and weekends, to which they bring no spontaneity.

The abnormality of mood associated with OCPD is in the characteristic restriction in the expression of emotion (the situation opposite, in effect, to that of the histrionic person).

As can be seen, many of the traits upon which the contemporary diagnosis of OCPD rests reflect the original notions of Freud, who believed that obsessionality derived from abnormalities in the "anal" stage of development and showed itself via the triad of "orderliness, obstinacy and parsimony." From a dynamic standpoint, OCPD patients are overwhelmed with concern about loss of control (being too messy, or sexy, or naughty . . .), hence their over-controllingness, their urge to dominate others rather than submit, and their striving for "machine-like" perfection and for the stifling of the "messiness" of emotional life. Loss of control also of *angry* feelings looms as a major issue in most patients with OCPD. Their fear of retaliation is often so great as to lead to "magical thinking," wherein they fear if they were to reveal (say, to a therapist) an angry thought about a parent, the parent, although living miles away, would somehow "know" what they had said and would exact punishment.

The ritualistic behavior may also be understood as having a propitiatory quality—as though the anger of the parent (or other authority figure) over one's "badness" can be warded off by double-checking that one's tie is straight, that one hasn't stepped on any cracks in the sidewalk, and so forth.

Other important defensive maneuvers encountered in OCPD patients are intellectualization, rationalization, and reaction-formation.[9] All these represent attempts to deal with fears and other disturbing emotions via *logic*. As a result, speech in OCPD patients becomes arid, peppered with irrelevant detail, such that one never quite gets to what should have been the emotional "point" of any discussion. The patient talks *around* the central issues, not directly about them.[10]

Since reason and logic are part of the normal mechanisms of survival, it is a matter of clinical judgment as to when these mechanisms have "spun out of control" enough to warrant a diagnosis of OCPD. Reliance on these mechanisms will differ from one culture to another, so one must also take into consideration the patient's cultural background. In general it may be said that, whereas the *histrionic* "style" represents exaggerations having to do with the ability to *love*, the *compulsive* style concerns the domain of *work*.

From the standpoint of etiology, some data suggest a measure of heritability in OCPD, but the evidence is not strong and is partly indirect. The genetic contribution to the emergence of the personality traits of "neuroticism" (roughly similar to the set of anxious cluster disorders) has been assessed as 50 per cent,[11] but what breeds true is not so much the whole disorder as certain specific traits. The concordance rate for compulsive personality in monozygotic twins is greater than that in dizygotic twins, yet in a family study of OCPD, despite the higher incidence of mental illness in the close relatives of the patients (as compared with those of the controls), those illnesses were more apt to be either depressive or other types of cluster C disorders than OCPD itself.[12] OCPD may thus gets its impetus from a genetic factor (predisposing, perhaps, to a predilection for structure; e.g.,

lining objects up in neat rows), but is given final shape by rearing patterns that overemphasize conformity, neatness, and punitiveness.

Although psychological test findings show characteristic abnormalities in OCPD (spikes in the "2-7-8" scales of the Minnesota Multiphasic Personality Inventory[13]; overattention to fine details on the Rorschach test), the diagnosis can usually be made readily enough simply on the basis of the clinical presentation.

Treatment

The treatment of OCPD tends at best to be time consuming and tedious, owing to the patient's adroitness at evading the significant emotional issues. The therapist is apt to hear endless monologues of self-justification, of lofty goals and ambitions, and of "reasons" why the patient's family members and intimates need to be rigidly controlled ("the wife'd buy out the dress-shop if I let her have a credit card"), browbeaten ("my daughter'd go to bed with any guy that'd look at her, unless I got a private investigator to check out his family"), or neglected ("work comes first: I don't have time for all this romantic stuff when there's a job to be done"). The loneliness that underlies possessiveness, or the fear (of love's "chaoticness") that pushes the compulsive person to frenzies of unnecessary work or trivial pursuits, remains buried underneath the patient's verbiage and diversionary concerns. Obsessive-compulsive personality disorder is often found in conjunction with passive-aggressive, paranoid, or avoidant personality disorders, or at least with some of their traits. The prognosis, and the optimal strategy the therapist must employ, will depend on these factors. When OCPD is characterized mainly by inhibition of enjoyment—with little in the way of meanness, pettiness, hostility, or controllingness—the response to treatment will be better (although not necessarily briefer) than when those qualities dominate the clinical picture.

Whichever form of psychotherapy is used, therapists working with compulsive patients must develop ways to parry the thrust of the patient's indecisiveness, ruminative thinking, and suppression of emotion. When using short-term therapy or cognitive therapy,[14] the therapist will have to establish priorities as to which problems deserve the most urgent attention (lest the patient set up endless "decoy" problems to throw the therapist off the scent). Problem-solving methods will be useful. As an antidote to perfectionism, it is useful to point out that (1) the fastest way to conquer certain problems is to acquire skills gradually, and to be willing to make mistakes without undue embarrassment, whereas (2) the patient's hope to succeed even quicker by being "perfect" the first time around is illusory. When time is not a pressing consideration, a psychoanalytically oriented approach may be especially useful; the use of dreams and free association are helpful in piercing the compulsive patient's intellectual armor, and in getting through to the painful feelings underneath.

Obsessive-compulsive personality disorder patients, particularly those with the passive-aggressive trait of procrastination, often evoke countertransference irritation, boredom, and fatigue. These problems, and the stalemated treatment that might result, can usually be circumvented by forthrightness and honesty—in letting the patient know that, "yes, you have gotten me a bit tired or cranky with all this talk about unimportant things, so perhaps you're doing this to avoid something uncomfortable. Let's see if we can't discover what that may be."

Despite the obstacles that confront the therapist who works with OCPD patients, their dogged persistence and task orientedness are positive traits that often help create a good therapeutic alliance and lead eventually to a favorable outcome. In the long-term follow-up of borderline patients, for example, those whose next most prominent personality traits were obsessive-compulsive outperformed those with all other accompanying personality features.[15]

AVOIDANT PERSONALITY DISORDER

Clinical Description and Etiology

The description in the DSM-III-R of avoidant personality disorder (APD) is composed of several key traits (e.g., reticence in social situations, avoidance of activities that demand interpersonal contact) and mild symptoms (e.g., easily hurt by criticism, fear of showing visible signs of anxiety in public). The latter are at the crossroads between trait and symptom proper: a pronounced *fear* of blushing or crying is still one step removed from the actual outbreak of these symptomatic behaviors. There appears to be a dynamic equilibrium between APD and certain symptom disorders of Axis I,[16] most notably social phobia but also agoraphobia and OCD. Patients with these conditions often show an underlying APD. Some patients with social phobia create for themselves an environmental niche in which social contacts are reduced to a bare minimum of superficial encounters, such that they are "left with" only the APD. If unanticipated circumstances suddenly pushed them into the social arena, signs of severe anxiety (e.g., crying in public, marked blushing, or sweating) will quickly reappear.

It is common for persons with APD to manifest traits of DPD or OCPD—enough to justify diagnosis of either or both of these disorders by DSM-III-R criteria. This situation is called comorbidity, although it does not imply two distinct illnesses; rather, it signifies a pervasive personality abnormality that happens to satisfy criteria for two arbitrarily defined disorders in the category-based manual.

Patients with APD often have close relatives with cluster C conditions, including APD itself.[7] In a twin study, however, concordance was noted in monozygotic pairs in which the proband was agoraphobic but not in which the proband had social phobia.[17] It may be that genetic loading for mild depressive illness predisposes to APD (and to social phobia), since patients with major (including recurrent) depression or with dysthymia often have concomitant avoidant traits, along with a family history of affective illness and cluster C disorders.[18] Environmental influences are important, and in many instances probably sufficient, in the etiological background of APD. Children "programmed" to fear and to avoid many kinds of persons and situations most people consider harmless will tend to develop APD, and often have a parent who is as fearful and avoidant as the future patient. This tendency may carry down the generations.

Certain traumatic patterns in early development seem sufficient by themselves as causative of APD. Parental brutalization, incest, and sexual molestation in childhood have been implicated not only in post-traumatic stress disorder, but in a lasting pattern of social avoidance and fearfulness toward those who even remotely resemble the victimizers of the past.[19] Early sexual exploitation often leads to pain-dependent, self-defeating (i.e., "masochistic") personality traits, alongside those of avoidance[20]; in this setting, APD may be accompanied by gaze avoidance and intense shame.

Treatment

Fashioning a suitable program of treatment for the patient with APD will depend in part upon whether the personality traits themselves are admixed with symptomatic phobia or with such anxiety symptoms as palpitations, blushing, and trembling. The psychodynamic underpinnings of each case also enter into the equation: patients who have been "taught" the language of fearfulness and withdrawal by a similarly avoidant parent will require a different therapeutic strategy than would be appropriate for an avoidant patient who had been an incest victim. Fortunately, there is a wider array of potentially useful modalities to choose from than is so for most of the other personality disorders. As for psychopharmacological measures, the social anxiety that often accompanies APD may respond to a monoamine oxidase inhibitor such as phenelzine. For patients with blushing, stage fright, and the like, β-blockers such as atenolol may interrupt the autonomically mediated anxiety symptoms.[21] Benzodiazepine anxiolytics may curtail the brief panic episodes to which APD patients are prone. Favorable response to medication often converts a highly symptomatic, hence highly fearful, avoidant person into someone far less afraid of the once anxiety-engendering life situations. This, in turn, helps psychotherapy make a more convincing case that these stressors (meeting people, going on a date) need not be so frightening. The patient can then respond more enthusiastically to whatever form of psychotherapy seems most useful.

Because of the conjunction of APD, in so many instances, with social phobia, various forms of treatment that focus on the latter will often prove useful.[21] These include social skills training, desensitization, cognitive therapy, and other methods under the umbrella of behavioral treatment. One technique involves the selection of social tasks graded hierarchically as to their difficulty: once a level of comfort is achieved in talking with salesclerks in a store, a harder task could be tried, such as making small talk with strangers in a "singles" bar. As for social phobia, in vivo exposure techniques of this sort are considered more effective than desensitization; cognitive, group, and dyadic therapies seem the most effective.[22] Group therapy, even though forced exposure to strangers in an atmosphere of acceptance would seem particularly advantageous, has thus far proven neither more nor less effective than one-on-one supportive or exploratory psychotherapies.[22] When APD has been a sequel to incest or other interpersonal traumata, however, special groups composed of patients with similar backgrounds are considered especially helpful.

PASSIVE-AGGRESSIVE PERSONALITY DISORDER

Clinical Description and Etiology

Although, in actual practice, many persons with OCPD show varying degrees of anger, irritability, resentment, and hostility, these traits are not part of the definition of OCPD, nor are they for the other two cluster C disorders thus far discussed. In contrast, passive-aggressive personality disorder (PAPD) implies at least some measure of hostility; three of the nine DSM-III-R criteria ("becomes sulky, irritable, or argumentative . . . ," "resents useful suggestions . . . ," "scorns people in positions of authority") speak of hostility directly. The remaining items center around obstructionism and procrastination. This is not to say that many such persons are not also anxious—especially when confronting authority—but manifest anxiety is seldom as prominent as would be observed in DPD or APD. Obsessive-compulsive personality disorder covers a broad spectrum, some of whose members are as openly anxious as those with DPD or APD while others are as customarily free of anxiety as are most PAPD patients. In this regard PAPD shares some common ground with the (admittedly much more severe and openly aggressive) sadistic personality disorder, in that persons of either sort typically *externalize* and cannot accept blame for any of their shortcomings. Even those who do accept some responsibility for their plight (e.g., for alienating superiors or for causing unhappiness to their intimates) will set up counterarguments to nullify any positive suggestion, such

that no beneficial change occurs. This tendency asserts itself just as strongly, of course, in the therapeutic milieu, and constitutes a major impediment to treatment.

The captiousness, verbal nitpicking, contrariness, and sulkiness that characterize PAPD are not known to be the latter-day phenotype of any genetic influence; rather, the condition would seem to have its origin in a pattern of unending power struggles with one's parents. The comparative helplessness of youth made it impossible to "win" these battles at the time, certainly not in any directly confrontative way. Instead, the future PAPD patient developed face-saving techniques of passive resistance. One such technique has been brilliantly pictorialized in the children's cartoon in which the mother asks her youngster, "Where did you go?" (Answer: "Out!"); "What did you do?" ("Nothing!"). Parental overcontrol is arguably the most common and most important psychodynamic factor in PAPD, but it is not the only underlying mechanism. In some cases parental neglect or blatant favoring of another sibling can alienate a child, and conduce to the formation of the silent protest and grudging obedience we associate with this condition.

Within the realm of PAPD, several subtypes have been described: (1) those with anxiety or depression (about one patient in three); (2) a self-defeating type, locked in a frustrating relationship with a "punishing partner"; (3) those who are primarily vindictive; and (4) those who voluntarily, but begrudgingly, keep their lives on hold by caring for aging parents.[23] Those with a "punishing partner" will occasionally erupt into outbursts of not so passive aggression.

Treatment

Problems in treatment usually center on extreme indecisiveness and on the undermining of one's own ambitions, alienating others via uncooperative or argumentative interactions. Medications have not been found beneficial, except in patients who are prone to episodes of depression or anxiety. Because of their externalization and argumentativeness, these patients do not do well in group therapy, usually quitting or being extruded by the other members. Cognitive therapy may be helpful, if one can get the patient to understand, and to modify, the entrenched pattern of expecting the worst from others—and then of creating a self-fulfilling prophecy by bringing out the worst in others. Supportive and analytically oriented psychotherapy may also succeed in selected patients, although the task is long and arduous.[24] The analysis of dreams is potentially helpful in getting to the heart of the central conflicts, especially since passive-aggressive patients are so adroit at trivializing the therapist's interpretive remarks. Dreams may provide the "smoking gun," demonstrating the patient's anger, fear, and the like in an undeniable fashion. First, however, the therapist must make a convincing case that this therapeutic approach is not (as the patient will artfully contend) so much hocus-pocus. This may consume many months of "resistance analysis." If successful, the therapist will arrive at the underlying feelings of littleness, of unworthiness, of having received only conditional love (i.e., "if you get straight As . . . "). Optimally, the therapist will also enable the patient to see that an authority figure can actually be benign and genuinely concerned about his or her welfare, whereas in the patient's view the therapist's only motives were to emerge "superior" and to "keep the patient down."

The recommendations offered here should not be construed as an indication that treatment can succeed with any regularity in PAPD. The battle is not even. On the therapist's side (it is to be hoped) are wisdom, skill, compassion, and nearly infinite patience. However, these may be no match for the passive-aggressive patient's skipping appointments, paying late, coming in a few minutes before the session was to end, saving the emotionally crucial material until 2 minutes before the session is over, and then announcing a few weeks later that "not much is happening here, so I'm quitting." In the absence of adequate follow-up data on this disorder, it is unclear what are the proportions of favorable and unfavorable outcomes, but in the opinion of most seasoned clinicians, good outcomes are the exception.

REFERENCES

1. Diagnostic and Statistical Manual of Mental Disorders. 3rd ed. Revised. Washington, DC: American Pschiatric Association Press, 1987.
2. Phillips KA, Gunderson JG, Hirschfeld RMA, Smith LE: A review of the depressive personality. Am J Psychiatry 147:830–837, 1990.
3. Stone MH: Treatment of borderline patients: A pragmatic approach. Psychiatr Clin North Am 13:265–285, 1990.
4. Livesley WJ, Schroeder ML, Jackson DN: Dependent personality disorder and attachment problems. J Pers Disord 4:131–140, 1990.
5. Trull TJ, Widiger TA, Frances A: Covariation of criteria sets for avoidant, schizoid and dependent personality disorders. Am J Psychiatry 144:767–771, 1987.
6. Grinker RR Sr, Werble B, Drye RC: The Borderline Syndrome. New York: Basic Books, 1968.
7. Reich JH: Familiality of DSM III dramatic and anxious personality clusters. J Nerv Ment Dis 177:96–100, 1989.
8. Mavissakalian M, Hamann MS, Jones B: DSM III personality disorders in obsessive-compulsive disorder: Changes with treatment. Compr Psychiatry 31:432–437, 1990.
9. Freud A: The Ego and the Mechanisms of Defense. New York: International Universities Press, 1966.
10. Horowitz M, Marmar C, Krupnick J et al: Personality Styles and Brief Psychotherapy. New York: Basic Books, 1984.
11. Andrews G, Stewart G, Allen R, Henderson AS: The genetics of six neurotic disorders: A twin study. J Affective Disord 19:23–29, 1990.
12. McKeon P, Murray R: Familial aspects of obsessive-compulsive neuroses. Br J Psychiatry 151:528–534, 1987.
13. Greene RL: The Minnesota Multiphasic Personality Inventory: An Interpretive Manual. New York: Grune & Stratton, 1980.
14. Beck AT, Freeman A: Cognitive Therapy of Personality Disorders. New York: Guilford Press, 1990.
15. Stone MH: The Fate of Borderline Patients. New York: Guilford Press, 1990.
16. Tyrer P, Casey P, Gall J: Relationship between neurosis and personality disorder. Br J Psychiatry 142:404–408, 1983.
17. Torgersen S: Genetic factors in anxiety disorders. Arch Gen Psychiatry 40:1085–1089, 1983.
18. Akiskal HS, Bitar AH, Puzantian VR et al: The nosological status of neurotic depression. Arch Gen Psychiatry 35:756–766, 1978.
19. Stone MH: Individual psychotherapy with victims of incest. Psychiatr Clin North Am 12:237–255, 1989.
20. van der Kolk BA: Compulsion to repeat the trauma: reenactment, revictimization and masochism. Psychiatr Clin North Am 12:389–412, 1989.
21. Liebowitz MR, Stone MH, Turkat ID: Treatment of personality disorders. In Annual Review of Psychiatry, vol 5. Washington, DC: American Psychiatric Press, Inc. 1986:356–393.
22. Emmelkamp PMG, Scholing A: Behavior treatment for simple and social phobics. In Noyes R Jr, Roth M, Burrows GD, eds. Handbook of Anxiety, vol IV. Amsterdam: Elsevier, 1990:327–361.
23. Perry JC: Passive aggressive personality disorder. In Treatment of Psychiatric Disorders, vol III. Washington, DC: American Psychiatric Press, Inc., 1989: 2783–2789.

Section K

CHILD AND ADOLESCENT DISORDERS

67

PROPOSED CHANGES IN THE DSM-IV CRITERIA FOR CHILD PSYCHIATRY

MAGDA CAMPBELL, M.D., MONIQUE ERNST, M.D., Ph.D,
STEPHEN R. SETTERBERG, M.D., and DAVID SHAFFER, M.D.

Certainly the DSM-III[1] represented a major improvement over the DSM-II[2], particularly in the area of disorders of childhood and adolescence. This was clearly reflected in the quality of psychopharmacological studies, especially those involving autistic children[3,4] and conduct disorders.[5] However, the DSM-III-R included major changes, and autism received a much broader definition.[6–9] Under the subclass of disruptive behavior disorders, the categories of attention-deficit hyperactivity disorder (ADHD), conduct disorder, and oppositional deficit disorder were reorganized in the DSM-III-R. Conduct disorder was (now) typed into group type, solitary aggressive type, and undifferentiated type. Furthermore, conduct disorder now had a long list of symptoms, and was biased toward an older age group.

The changes in the DSM-IV, if any, will be based on a critical review of the literature in regard to issues identified in the DSM-III-R, secondary data analyses, and field trials. The field trials, funded by the National Institute of Mental Health will involve two major categories: pervasive developmental disorders (PDDs) and disruptive behavior disorders.

PERVASIVE DEVELOPMENTAL DISORDERS

The issues regarding PDDs in the DSM-III-R were as follows: (1) age of onset in autism, (2) removal from Axis II to Axis I, (3) the overinclusiveness of autistic disorder and the cumbersomeness of the criteria, and (4) that the category pervasive developmental disorders not otherwise specified (PDDNOS) was used for syndromes that had achieved diagnostic status in the tenth revision of the International Classification of Diseases (ICD-10).[10] Specifically, Rett's syndrome, Asperger's syndrome, childhood disintegrative disorder, and atypical autism were defined in the ICD-10 as discrete entities within the pervasive developmental disorders.[11]

On the whole, the secondary analyses of data collected on subjects with autism confirmed the findings from the literature review, indicating that autism diagnosed by DSM-III-R criteria is significantly broader than when diagnosed by other, including DSM-III, criteria.

The international field trial will involve a large number of autistic subjects and appropriate controls; ICD-10, DSM-III, and DSM-III-R criteria will be employed, as well as criteria developed by the DSM-IV Work Group.[9]

In order to render the DSM more compatible with the ICD-10, it has been proposed that in addition to

The views expressed in this paper are those of the authors and do not represent the official positions of the American Psychiatric Association or its DSM-IV Task Force.

autism, Rett's syndrome, Asperger's syndrome, childhood disintegrative disorder, and atypical autism should be included in the category of PDDs. Furthermore, autistic disorder has a long list of criteria that makes it difficult to use. The objective is to attempt to reduce the number of criteria, which should perhaps render greater simplicity to the system and make diagnosis more accurate. The inclusion of operationally defined criteria for additional disorders may help to distinguish responders from nonresponders in clinical drug trials and studies of psychosocial interventions involving PDD populations.

DISRUPTIVE BEHAVIOR DISORDERS

With regard to disruptive behavior disorders, the revisions made for the DSM-III-R involved major changes in criteria format: "polythetic" lists of specific criteria replaced the more conceptually organized criterion subsets of the DSM-III. However, a polythetic format requires specifying precise thresholds for a diagnosis (e.g., requiring that 8 of a possible 14 criteria be present for ADHD). The thresholds used in the DSM-III-R for these disorders were not based upon systematic empirical research. There have now been several reports that the DSM-III-R revisions resulted in significant prevalence changes, with conduct disorder (CD) becoming less prevalent. This change in prevalence is likely to be clinically significant, because there is evidence that the new criteria fail to identify a significant number of impaired children and adolescents.[12] The DSM-IV field trials have been designed to examine, and if necessary revise, these thresholds. This should result in a better alignment between diagnosis and the characteristics of young people who are in a treatment situation because of a disruptive disorder.

The absence of subgroupings of ADHD criteria in the DSM-III-R have been held to obscure the essence of the hyperactivity and inattention constructs. This will be rectified in the DSM-IV by regrouping the ADHD criteria into a hyperactivity-impulsivity (the distinction between impulsivity and hyperactivity has not been supported by several factor-analytic studies) subset and an inattention subset. It is not clear that this will have any significant impact on treatment or clinical issues.

As conceived in the DSM-III, oppositional defiant disorder (ODD) was a mild condition that featured contrary, defiant, and stubborn behavior that fell short of clearly antisocial conduct. In the DSM-III-R, the criteria for ODD involved a shift toward more clearly antisocial behavior, with ODD being seen as a milder or early form of CD. One of the options being considered for the DSM-IV would formalize this and would class ODD as a less severe form of CD.

The DSM-III's category attention deficit disorder without hyperactivity was relegated to a not otherwise specified category in the DSM-III-R. However, there is increasing evidence that supports the existence of that clinical picture, and the disorder will be reinstated in the DSM-IV.

ANXIETY DISORDERS

Children with various anxiety disorders (e.g., separation anxiety disorder) may also meet DSM-III-R criteria for overanxious disorder of childhood (OAD-C). This is at least partly because several of the criteria for those disorders overlap. Thus a patient who meets criteria for one of those disorders may, with few additional symptoms, also meet criteria for OAD-C. It has been held that this is a spurious comorbidity. The DSM-IV proposes to both eliminate the structural overlap and re-describe OAD-C in a way that better fits empirical descriptions of anxiety symptoms in the child and teen population. Overanxious disorder of childhood will be characterized by symptoms of anticipatory and performance anxiety that are unrelated to social fears or fears of separation.

The symptoms of avoidant disorder of childhood are similar to those of social phobia. Although there is as yet no evidence to show that the one condition is continuous with the other, as a matter of principle, it is desirable to avoid categories that duplicate one another symptomatically, and that can be distinguished only by the age of the patient. One option proposed in the DSM-IV will eliminate the separate category for children and include text and criteria in the category social anxiety disorder, generalized type (formerly social phobia, generalized type), that will make it applicable to children.

Finally, it has been proposed to delete the category of identity disorder. The reasons for this are that, despite its wide use, its separate existence has never been illustrated by satisfactory case histories, it incorporates many normal concerns, and its criteria include psychological mechanisms that can only be inferred.

DISORDERS OF INFANCY

In the DSM-IV, the category reactive attachment disorder of childhood will include two subtypes: (1) socially withdrawn or inhibited, and (2) socially indiscriminate. These subtypes are consistent with research and the ICD-10 nomenclature.

ADJUSTMENT DISORDERS

A new subtype, adjustment disorder with suicidal behavior, has been proposed in which the predominant stress-related manifestation is suicidal behavior (ideation, threats, or attempts) in the absence of evidence of major depression or other Axis I diagnoses.

It was believed that the introduction of this category would help regularize a commonly occurring presentation among adolescents who may now get a potentially misleading diagnosis of adjustment disorder with depressive features.

TREATMENT IMPLICATIONS

Increases in the precision of diagnostic categories allow for research and practice more specifically tailored to a patient's needs. This is true to the extent that clinicians actually use carefully applied diagnostic criteria to guide their treatment planning. There is evidence that many clinicians often employ DSM categories merely as conceptual guides.[13] Subtle criterion changes are unlikely to influence practice in such cases. However, basic differential diagnostic choices may significantly alter treatment planning. For example, choosing between diagnosing mild major depression or adjustment disorder with depressed mood may influence psychopharmacological planning.

The specific changes proposed for the DSM-IV will make more accurate diagnoses available for several groups of children. The changes will:

1. Enable diagnosis of milder forms of conduct disorder.

2. Include a diagnosis for attention deficit disorder without hyperactivity.

3. Increase the specificity of autism and of ADHD.

4. More clearly differentiate between childhood anxiety disorders.

5. Include a diagnostic category for suicidal children who are not accurately represented by the other adjustment disorders.

6. Differentiate between clinically meaningful subtypes of reactive attachment disorder and of PDDNOS (Rett's syndrome, Asperger's syndrome disintegrative disorder, and atypical autism).

It is hoped that the DSM-IV changes for conduct disorder will be simpler and thus facilitate its use. Unless this work results in a subgroup of children[14] and adolescents[15] with conduct disorder characterized by bullying, physical fight, destroying property, and explosiveness (and verbal aggression), a rational treatment will be difficult to prescribe. The cluster of aggressiveness is certainly responsive to treatment with certain psychoactive agents.[14] Stealing, cruelty, truanting, and forcing someone into sexual activity are usually observed at an older age, and for these symptoms pharmacotherapy is not indicated. These types of antisocial behaviors may be responsive to psychosocial interventions.[16]

No major change is planned for the remaining diagnostic categories in children and adolescents, although there will be revisions in the text.

ACKNOWLEDGMENT

This work was supported in part by U.S. Public Health Service Grants MH-40177, MH-32212, and MH-18915 (Dr. Campbell) and MH-18915 (Dr. Ernst) from the National Institute of Mental Health.

REFERENCES

1. American Psychiatric Association: Diagnostic and Statistical Manual of Mental Disorders. 3rd ed. Washington, DC: American Psychiatric Association, 1980.
2. American Psychiatric Association: Diagnostic and Statistical Manual of Mental Disorders. 2nd ed. Washington, DC: American Psychiatric Association, 1968.
3. Campbell M: The use of drug treatment in infantile autism and childhood schizophrenia: A review. In Lipton MA, DiMascio A, Killam KF, eds. Psychopharmacology—A Generation of Progress. New York: Raven Press, 1978:1451.
4. Campbell M: Drug treatment of infantile autism: The past decade. In Meltzer HY, ed. Psychopharmacology: The Third Generation of Progress. New York: Raven Press, 1987:1225.
5. Campbell M, Spencer EK: Psychopharmacology in child and adolescent psychiatry: A review of the past five years. J Am Acad Child Adolesc Psychiatry 27:269, 1988.
6. American Psychiatric Association: Diagnostic and Statistical Manual of Mental Disorders. 3rd ed. Revised. Washington, DC: American Psychiatric Association, 1987.
7. Frances A, Pincus HA, Widiger TA, et al: DSM-IV: Work in progress. Am J Psychiatry 147:1439, 1990.
8. Hertzig M, Snow M, New E, et al: DSM-III and DSM-III-R diagnosis of autism and PDD in nursery school children. J Am Acad Child Adolesc Psychiatry 29:123, 1990.
9. Volkmar FR, Bregman J, Cohen DJ, et al: DSM-III and DSM-III-R diagnoses of autism. Am J Psychiatry 145:1404, 1988.
10. Shaffer D, Campbell M, Cantwell D, et al: Child and adolescent psychiatric disorders in DSM-IV: Issues facing the work group. J Am Acad Child Adolesc Psychiatry 28:830, 1989.
11. World Health Organization: Mental and behavioral disorders. In International Classification of Diseases, 10th rev. Geneva: World Health Organization, 1989: chap V (F).
12. Lahey BB, Loeber R, Stouthamer-Loeber M, et al: Comparison of DSM-III and DSM-III-R diagnoses for prepubertal children: Changes in prevalence and validity. J Am Acad Child Adolesc Psychiatry 29:620, 1990.
13. Setterberg SR, Ernst M, Rao U, et al: Child psychiatrists' views of DSM-III-R: A survey of usage and opinions. J Am Acad Child Adolesc Psychiatry 30:652–658, 1991.
14. Campbell M, Small AM, Green WH, et al: Behavioral efficacy of haloperidol and lithium carbonate: A comparison in hospitalized aggressive children with conduct disorder. Arch Gen Psychiatry 41:650, 1984.
15. Rifkin A, Karajgi B, Perl E, et al: Lithium treatment of conduct disorders in adolescents. Presented at the 29th Annual Meeting of NIMH-NCDEU, Key Biscayne, FL, 1989.
16. Werry JS, Wollersheim JP: Behavior therapy with children and adolescents: A twenty-year overview. J Am Acad Child Adolesc Psychiatry 28:1, 1989.

DISORDERS IN CHILDREN:
Autistic Disorder, Psychosis, Attention-Deficit Hyperactivity Disorder, Anxiety Disorders, and Depression

CARRIE SYLVESTER, M.D., M.P.H. and CATHERINE A. NAGEOTTE, M.D.

AUTISTIC DISORDER

Clinical Description

Autistic disorder (AD) is the well-defined pervasive developmental disorder (PDD) characterized by qualitative impairment in social interaction, communication, and imaginative activity, as well as markedly constricted interests. Associated features include uneven cognitive functioning, abnormal motor behavior such as stereotypies, odd responses to sensory stimulation, self-injurious behavior, atypical mood, and abnormalities in eating, sleeping, and drinking. Most children with PDD are mentally retarded, but some have normal intelligence and a few have special (savant) abilities. They are at increased risk for seizures in childhood, and may develop seizures during adolescence.[1]

Prevalence of AD is about 4:10,000, and of all PDD is about 10:10,000 to 15:10,000 children.[2] The sex ratio is about three boys for every girl. There is higher concordance for monozygotic twins, and siblings have a prevalence 50 times that of the general population. Fragile X syndrome is found in up to 16 per cent of autistic males. There is an increased prevalence of PDD in children with perinatal and postnatal central nervous system infections, congenital neurocutaneous disorders, and metabolic disorders. The most problematic area of differential diagnosis is that of mental retardation, but impaired socialization characterizes PDD. Other differential diagnoses that may overlap with PDD are attention-deficit hyperactivity disorder, psychomotor seizures, Tourette's syndrome, and developmental disorders of language, motor, or visuospatial skills. Usually distinct diagnoses are Rett's syndrome, progressive disintegrative psychosis, elective mutism, and psychosocial deprivation.[2]

Onset is typically noted early with lack of social smiling and cuddling, and the core impairments are usually obvious between 18 and 36 months of age. Children with higher intelligence, developed speech by 5 years, and later onset do best. Residual aloof-ness, rigidity, and oddness persist in the best outcomes. Autistic disorder does not deteriorate to schizophrenia. There is no characteristic physical or laboratory finding specific to AD or PDD. Evaluation should focus on detecting remediable abnormalities, including tests for sensory impairments, metabolic disorders, seizures, language disorders, and mental retardation.

Treatment

Haloperidol, in dosage ranges of 0.5 to 4.0 mg/day, can reduce irritability, uncooperative behavior, anger, and labile affect. Dose reduction or discontinuation leads to rapid return of pretreatment symptoms.[3] Pharmacological management of mood disorders, attention-deficit hyperactivity disorder, and seizures with special attention to subtle partial seizures is beneficial. Propranolol may be tried to reduce rage outbursts, aggression, and severe anxiety.[2,4] Narcotic antagonists may be useful adjuncts in managing self-injurious behavior, but data are preliminary and hepatotoxicity in immature individuals is a concern.[5,6] Fenfluramine may positively affect motor behavior and reduce hyperactivity. Its utility is restricted because it may retard discriminate function learning and causes bowel dysfunction, insomnia, weight loss, and possibly neurotoxicity.[6]

The first issue in comprehensive treatment is to explain carefully to parents that their child suffers from a neurodevelopmental disorder through no fault of their own in order to begin to support and guide them in the demanding task of parenting a chronically impaired child. Therapeutic attention to the developmental needs of the family unit is crucial for an optimal outcome. The most effective intervention has been highly structured behavior modification in an educational setting and teaching parents to use that approach.[2,7] Recurrent evaluation to determine management in a least restrictive setting consistent with the Education for Handicapped Children Act of 1978 (federal law PL 94-142) is essential.

CHILDHOOD PSYCHOSES

Clinical Description

As in adults, childhood psychosis may be an element of various disorders, and children who would have formerly been diagnosed as schizophrenic are now viewed as having PDD, affective disorders, or atypical psychosis. Hallucinations in children may particularly occur in a number of nonpsychotic conditions.[8] The phenomenology of childhood-onset schizophrenia separate from other disorders has been only recently subjected to careful scrutiny largely because it is an extremely rare disorder. It is believed to be more common in boys, which is consistent with the later onset of schizophrenia in women. In carefully studied 4- to 13-year-old children with DSM-III-R criteria–defined schizophrenia, onset of psychotic symptoms was at about 7 years.[9] Twin and adoption studies of adult schizophrenics support a strong genetic contribution to risk for the disorder. Other risk factors that have been of interest are subtle neonatal central nervous system injuries, including viral infection. Burke et al.[8] found a high rate of psychosis in relatives of nonpsychotic and psychotic children with hallucinations, suggesting familial factors for psychotic symptoms regardless of diagnosis.

Because childhood psychosis is relatively rare, the initial evaluation should focus on exclusion of organic etiologies such as brain tumor (second only to leukemia in childhood malignancies), toxicity due to heavy metals or poisoning, seizures, occult brain trauma, and nutritional deficiency. Schizophrenia should be considered in individuals with AD or PDD only when there are prominent delusions or hallucinations.[2] Stress-related states, especially after catastrophe, can mimic psychosis.[10] Also, children with affective disorders may have psychotic symptoms.

Treatment

Although there is no double-blind, placebo-controlled study of any treatment for childhood schizophrenia, neuroleptics are of use in the treatment of acute psychotic or agitated states and for acute exacerbations of chronic psychotic disorders. Long-term (greater than 6 months') use of neuroleptics has been of only modest benefit in childhood schizophrenia, but sufficient to warrant their carefully monitored use.[11] Non-neuroleptic management of associated disorders is important because reduced use of neuroleptic medication is a goal. Neuroleptics disrupt learning, including that dependent on attendance to social cues, and cause tardive dyskinesia even in young patients. Their long-term use is strongly discouraged in any childhood situation where a specific

medication (e.g., antidepressant, anxiolytic, or lithium carbonate) can be used.

The low-potency, sedating neuroleptics, such as thioridazine, have the advantage of long use in child psychiatry and reduced risk of frightening dystonic reactions. Nevertheless, the additional burden of sedation is unwarranted because learning, including social learning as a basis for behavioral modification, is the main work of children. High-potency neuroleptics such as haloperidol and thiothixene are less sedating and interfere less with learning.[6] They have less anticholinergic activity, which minimizes the risk for delirium, which could be mistaken for medication nonresponse and lead to erroneous increase in neuroleptic dose. Thiothixene may cause less akathisia in children than haloperidol.[11] A complete blood count and liver function studies should be obtained before beginning these medications.

Haloperidol, for example, is initiated at 0.01 to 0.05 mg/kg/day in two divided doses. Dosage can be titrated upward by 0.25 to 0.5 mg every 3 to 4 days. The usual therapeutic range is 0.5 to 4 mg/day in divided doses because, although children metabolize and clear neuroleptics rapidly, they are more sensitive to the main effects. Larger, nearly adolescent children may require slightly higher doses. For schizophrenia, a trial of 4 weeks should be adequate to determine efficacy. After 4 to 6 months, medication should be discontinued and need for further medication reassessed.[6]

The issues of family and school described for autistic disorder apply to childhood schizophrenia. There are no treatment outcome studies of DSM-III-R criteria–defined childhood schizophrenia. Although it has been believed that residential placement is usually required, that may be based on mixed populations. Treatment in the home is dependent on supports available to the family, and day hospitalization may be considered.

ATTENTION-DEFICIT HYPERACTIVITY DISORDER

Clinical Description

Attention-deficit hyperactivity disorder (ADHD) is characterized by age-inappropriate impulsivity, distractibility, and motoric activity with associated emotionality and apparent intrusiveness, aggressiveness, and destructiveness due to impulsivity. Impaired academic and social learning is probably due to constantly shifting cognitive focus and inability to modulate behavior in response to social cues. Prevalence rates in community samples range from 2.2 to 9.9 per cent.[12] Comorbidity with conduct disorder and specific learning disabilities and an approximately eightfold male predominance are well known. Girls have a substantially greater (40:1) risk for comorbid conduct disorder, but outcome for these dually affected girls is unknown.[13] While the outcome for ADHD may be regarded optimistically, symptoms persist to adulthood in about 50 per cent of cases.[14]

The family-genetic risk for this disorder has been confirmed, but no clinically applicable biological marker has been described. Positron emission tomography has revealed reduced cerebral glucose metabolism in hyperactive adults who are also biological parents of children with ADHD.[14] Physical examination provides baseline height, weight, blood pressure, and complete blood count. It may reveal limitations in vision or hearing, but specialized examinations may be required. A neurology consultation is useful in selected cases. A speech pathologist, who may be available in the school, may find subtle receptive language difficulties that are causing the behavior or aggravating ADHD. Psychological testing with individually administered intelligence testing and achievement testing is necessary for comprehensive treatment planning. The Connors rating forms, which are completed by parents and teachers, are accepted, specialized instruments for evaluation at baseline and in the course of treatment for ADHD.[15]

The differential diagnosis of ADHD includes situational intolerance of developmentally appropriate overactivity as an exclusionary diagnosis. Conduct disorder with calculated aggressiveness and lying, oppositional disorder, an anxiety disorder including post-traumatic stress disorder, affective disorder with predominant irritability, neuropsychiatric difficulties including receptive language deficits, Tourette's syndrome, sensory impairments, and partial seizures may be responsible for the symptoms or may be comorbid conditions. Other differential diagnoses include any painful or pruritic condition and Sydenham's chorea.

Treatment

There is a relative wealth of data based on adequately controlled studies of the short-term pharmacological management of ADHD. The stimulants have been studied for over half a century and improve motor behavior, attention, distractibility, impulsiveness, and short-term memory in about 75 per cent of hyperactive children.[16] There is also mounting evidence of short-term improvements in relationships with adults, especially mothers and teachers, in stimulant-treated children with ADHD.[17] Poor short-term improvements in achievement in the context of a good behavioral response to the stimulants has been a troublesome outcome. There may be a kind of therapeutic window at which adequate behavioral control and superior academic, or cognitive, response are found at lower doses. Thus, it has been suggested that routinely advancing beyond 0.6 mg/kg/dose of methylphenidate in the interest of further behavioral control may degrade cognitive performance.[17] There are, unfortunately, no controlled studies of long-term effects of treatment on achieve-

ment, interpersonal relationships, or legal difficulties in essentially pure ADHD patients.

The stimulants used in the treatment of ADHD are methylphenidate, dextroamphetamine, and magnesium pemoline. Methylphenidate is the most commonly prescribed medication for ADHD, in part because its central site of action is associated with less marked cardiac effects than dextroamphetamine.[18] The usual starting dose for children is 5 mg in the morning, with an option to begin a noon dose then or to add the second dose at noon 3 to 5 days later. This can be advanced by 5 mg/dose or every other dose every 3 to 14 days depending upon the sense of urgency and comfort with reliability of observer data. The target is 0.3 to 0.6 mg/kg/dose, with no single dose more than 20 mg and a maximum total daily dosage of 60 mg. The amount of distractibility during after-school activities should be considered in deciding whether to prescribe a 4:00 P.M. dose, which may be lower than the earlier doses. There is sufficient variability in reported duration of effect that close communication with parents and teachers is necessary to determine whether the dosing frequency should be shortened to 3 hours or lengthened to as much as 6 hours.[16,18] The dosage for dextroamphetamine is one half that for methylphenidate, except that the total daily dose may be as much as 40 mg with no single dose to exceed 10 mg. Dextroamphetamine sulfate is available in elixir. Both are available in sustained release preparations, which may have psychosocial advantages in school but are expensive and controversial in terms of effects comparable to the standard preparations. The effects of these stimulants can be noted in a few days and should be apparent within 2 weeks of reaching maximum dose. If tolerance develops after months of successful treatment, it is reasonable to switch to another stimulant. Magnesium pemoline has the advantages of single daily dosing, chewable tablets, and no abuse potential coupled with the disadvantage of effectiveness taking up to 3 weeks. (Stimulants are not abused by individuals affected by ADHD, but have "street value" to any antisocial individual who may be affiliated with a patient.) The starting dose is 18.75 mg in the morning, with weekly increases of 18.75 mg to a maximum of 112.5 mg or 0.5 to 3 mg/kg/day.

The common, transient short-term side effects of stimulants are headaches, abdominal pain, irritability, moodiness, and anorexia. Growth reduction may occur despite return of appetite. Height should be monitored at least every 4 months so that drug holidays to allow for rebound growth can be planned for school vacations. The potential for a brief but dramatic increase in symptoms upon sudden cessation of medication is an important issue in patient education. Tachycardia and hypertension, especially in blacks, are of particular concern with dextroamphetamine. There is a strongly suspected risk for exacerbation of tics and other movement disorders, but not for significantly lowering seizure threshold.[16] Psychotic symptoms may be a side effect, but are also a toxic effect. Methylphenidate may reduce white blood cell count and magnesium pemoline may cause elevation in liver function tests, so those should be monitored at least every 6 months.

Other useful medications are tricyclic antidepressants and clonidine. The use of neuroleptics in this population has the clear risk of tardive dyskinesia and little to recommend it for this long-term indication. Desipramine has been the most carefully studied antidepressant for this indication. Dosages above 3.5 mg/kg/day with the concomitant requirement for careful monitoring described here may be necessary for adequate control.[19] Clonidine is not as effective as the stimulants in managing distractibility and attention, but is a particular consideration when there is a family history of tics suggestive of Tourette's disorder or when aggressiveness, oppositionality, or hyperarousal secondary to early stress or abuse are complicating features.[20] The usual dosage of clonidine for school-age children with ADHD is 0.15 to 0.3 mg/day in three to four divided doses. Because sedative effects peak about 30 to 90 minutes after each dose, clonidine is started at night, with dosage increments of 0.05 mg/day every third day. Mild hypotension, orthostatic hypotension, and lowered pulse have not been clinically significant in carefully monitored patients. Rebound hypertension is a potentially serious side effect if the medication is abruptly discontinued. Another concern is the induction of depression in children at risk for comorbid depression.[20]

Current consensus is that, in the absence of compelling evidence for efficacy of medications alone, multimodal treatment is indicated. Close work with the school with respect to appropriate placement, remediation services, and behavioral modification techniques is a generally agreed upon strategy. Psychotherapies include cognitive-behavioral with an emphasis on self-verbalization and planning of activities, social skills groups, family therapy, parent training in behavioral techniques, and individual therapy focused on self-esteem issues. There are few studies of these techniques, but it is clear that no single therapy or one combination thereof will serve for all, or perhaps most, ADHD patients.[7,21]

ANXIETY

Clinical Description

The anxiety syndromes of childhood are separation anxiety disorder, avoidant disorder, and overanxious disorder. Children may develop any of the so-called adult anxiety disorders and may be especially at risk for prolonged post-traumatic stress disorder (PTSD).[10,22] Anxious children may have a predominance of somatic complaints, social withdrawal, or hyperarousal with impulsivity. Their symptoms may be situationally exacerbated or essentially nonspecific. Anxiety, fears, and simple phobias are common symptoms in childhood, but rare presenting complaints. School refusal, abdominal or chest pain, refusal to sleep alone due to either separation anxiety or PTSD, prominent symptoms of intercurrent major depression, or particularly troublesome phobias may prompt parents to bring an anxious child to psychiatric attention.

The prevalence rates for separation anxiety disorder, overanxious disorder, and simple phobia each are about 5 per cent.[12] Sex differences in rates of anxiety symptoms are not impressive in younger children.[23] The familial nature of the anxiety disorders has been a topic of much study over the past decade. While the contribution of inborn factors undoubtedly varies for specific syndromes, the likelihood of an anxious child being parented by an anxious and/or depressed parent(s) or subjected to controlling, anxious behavior by an anxious sibling is an important consideration in treatment planning. There has been much speculation as to the relationship of separation anxiety disorder to panic disorder, and anxious adults report having been fearful or anxious children, but specific relationships between child and adult syndromes have not been established. There are no pathognomonic laboratory or psychometric tests for the anxiety disorders. In addition to determining the specific anxiety disorder, the differential diagnosis includes affective disorders, somatization disorder, psychotic withdrawal, ADHD, adjustment disorder with anxiety, and real worries in a dangerous environment.

Treatment

Medical management of childhood anxiety has been tricyclic antidepressants, benzodiazepines, antihistamines, β-adrenergic blockers, or clonidine.[4,24] Buspirone has been used in young adolescents, and information may be forthcoming on its use in prepubertal children. There are no positive double-blind controlled studies of management of childhood anxiety using medication alone. All medication recommendations should therefore be made in the context of a comprehensive treatment plan.

Behavioral management of separation anxiety disorder or school refusal may be enhanced, especially with reference to the child's discomfort, by the use of a tricyclic antidepressant in antidepressant dosages (see later) or alprazolam beginning at 0.25 mg/day and advanced 0.25 mg. every 3 to 4 days to a total daily dosage of 3 mg/day in three divided doses.[24] The usual pediatric dosage for alprazolam is 0.25 to 2 mg/day with a maximum of 4 mg/day. The starting dosage of diazepam is 0.25 mg/day, advancing 0.5 mg every 3 to 4 days to the usual pediatric dosage of 1 to 10 mg/day in three to four divided doses. The maximum recommended dosage of diazepam for anxiety or sleep disorders in prepubertal children is 15 mg/day.

Antihistamines such as diphenhydramine and hydroxyzine have long been used for management of anxiety and insomnia in children. There is therefore a conspicuous lack of data on child pharmacokinetics or from controlled clinical trials. Sedation and anticholinergic effects are common, and lowered seizure threshold, delirium, and worsening of tic disorders are serious, less common side effects.[4] The maximum pediatric dosage for diphenhydramine or hydroxyzine is 5 mg/kg/day, with a maximum of 300 mg/day in three to four divided doses. Although one half the maximum total daily dose may be used as a hypnotic, as little as 1 mg/kg at bedtime may be effective. Similarly, pediatric clinical experience has been that a starting dose of one quarter of the maximum dose may be sufficient for anxiety without causing undue side effects.

The theoretical efficacies of β-blockers, such as propranolol, and of clonidine in regulating hyperarousal and consequent irritability and behavioral difficulties in children with PTSD are showing promise in preliminary studies.[4,20] β-Blockers are contraindicated in asthma and diabetes. Because they can cause bradycardia and peripheral vasoconstriction, careful monitoring of peripheral circulation and cardiovascular function to maintain blood pressure above 90/60 mm Hg and pulse above 60/min is necessary. Fatigue and depression are troublesome side effects in children at risk for depression. The usual pediatric dosage of propranolol is 2 to 4 mg/kg/day in two divided doses up to no more than 16 mg/kg/day, with a maximum of 300 mg recommended for psychiatric indications in older children. Advancement of dosage is guided by cardiovascular as well as psychiatric response. β-Blockade should not be stopped abruptly; tapering over 7 to 14 days is recommended. (See section on ADHD for clonidine recommendations.)

Despite evidence that a majority of anxious adults can achieve symptomatic relief from psychosocial treatments, there are no systematic data on individual or family therapies of these disorders in children.[21,25] Behavioral therapies, including desensitization and cognitive strategies, have been studied, but mostly in less severe anxiety disorders.[7] They are prone to failure if the family is not sufficiently engaged and supported or if the child is too uncomfortable and becomes resistant or explosive. For children whose anxiety is a response to specific stressors, play therapy focused on reenactment and mastery is probably beneficial, but requires advanced skills.[10]

DEPRESSION

Clinical Description

Major depression or dysthymic disorder meeting DSM-III-R criteria occurs in prepubertal children. Children may also develop seasonal affective disorder, but diagnosis is especially problematic because of synchrony of onset of symptoms and school. Although depressive symptoms are not uncommon in childhood, major depression has a prevalence estimated at less than 3 per cent without a notable sex difference in prepubertal children.[26] This rate is much less if comorbidity with anxiety disorders and disruptive disorders is considered. These children are, unfortunately, usually not brought to clinical attention unless disruptive behaviors, school failure or refusal, insomnia or refusal to sleep alone, or appetite change become seriously apparent. Furthermore, the well-known familial nature of major affective disorders contributes additional risk for parental inattention to subtle symptoms. Although outcome data are limited, childhood onset confers obvious additional risks resulting from cognitive interference with acquisition of academic skills and the impact of depressive symptoms on development of interpersonal skills. There is a growing consensus that early onset of major depression is associated with increased genetic loading.[27] Depressed children are therefore at a significant disadvantage in terms of family context for evaluation and treatment.

There have been downward extensions of many of the biological studies of adult depression with similar results, but clinical applications are not established. Similarly, psychological testing usually contributes little to the clinical diagnosis of depression, and use of specific instruments in monitoring treatment response remains primarily of research interest. A physical examination is important to rule out organic etiologies such as those mentioned for psychosis as well as thyroid and adrenal endocrinopathies. In addition to determining the relative weight of symptoms of anxiety disorders, disruptive disorders, and psychosis, the possibility of substance abuse in preadolescent children must be considered.

Treatment

Psychopharmacological treatment of major depression in children has not been substantially supported by double-blind, placebo-controlled studies. Children have a very high placebo response rate, and a placebo washout period has not been incorporated into most child psychopharmacology studies. Small numbers of subjects have also limited conclusions from available studies. It has been suggested that careful monitoring of adequacy of plasma levels and the use of state markers such as the dexamethasone suppression test may better define depressed children who respond to antidepressants.[28] The dose of dexamethasone for prepubertal children is 0.5 mg and for pubertal children is 1.0 mg, or 20 μg/kg.[27]

Desipramine, imipramine, and amitriptyline are used at dosages up to 5 mg/kg/day and nortriptyline in dosages of 0.5 to 2.0 mg/kg/day, all in two to three divided doses.[28] A tricyclic starting dosage of 1.5 mg/kg/day has been recommended, with advances of 1.0 to 1.5 mg/kg/day every 3 days.[27] A maximum starting and advancing dosage of 25 mg/day may be consistent with less toxicity and greater patient comfort.[29] Children also rapidly, but very variably, metabolize heterocyclic antidepressants. Monitoring of plasma levels is important to ensure adequate plasma levels—probably above 150 ng/ml for imipramine or amitriptyline and between 75 and 150 ng/ml for nortriptyline.[28] It is also important to attempt to stabilize treatment at the lowest potentially therapeutic level to reduce risk in the face of inadequate data to support therapeutic efficacy of these medications in children.

Children are at risk for worsening of or developing cardiac conduction problems with tricyclic antidepressants, but the clinical risk in carefully monitored cases is uncertain.[29] An electrocardiogram (ECG), blood pressure measurement, and resting pulse at baseline and careful monitoring of ECG at least twice during dosage adjustment coupled with parent training in monitoring pulse, are advisable.[30] Other toxic symptoms and side effects are similar to those found in adults. A particular concern is that children may develop nausea, abdominal pain, and tiredness upon abrupt withdrawal of antidepressants, which may be confused with continuing depression.[27]

Lithium augmentation may be of use in tricyclic-resistant childhood depression. Monoamine oxidase inhibitors have received recent attention in adolescents and older children, but the need for dietary supervision is a limiting factor. Fluoxetine may be a useful addition, but its use should be limited until experience with several million adults over a few years has been compiled.

As for the other disorders of childhood, there are few data to guide specific selection of psychotherapeutic approach for depression. Ideally, young children should be treated in a family context with support for parents and child. However, if a child is suicidal and the family is not able to adequately supervise the child, hospitalization may be required. Thus far, studies of family therapy have focused on depressed mothers and on suicidal adolescents, so the particular approach to family therapy that might be most helpful is unclear.[25] School consultation is essential if academic deterioration or difficulties with teachers and peers are significant. Structured evaluation of those features of a child's presentation as well as formulation of recommendations to the school system may also require inpatient assessment where a variety of staff, including a teacher, can interact with the child.

REFERENCES

1. Volkmar FR, Nelson DS: Seizure disorder in autism. J Am Acad Child Adolesc Psychiatry 29:127–129, 1990.
2. Pomeroy JC: Infanitle autism and childhood psychosis. In Garfinkel BD, Carlson GA, Weller EB, eds. Psychiatric Disorders in Children and Adolescents. Philadelphia: WB Saunders, 1990:271–290.
3. Perry R, Campbell M, Adams P, et al: Long-term efficacy of haloperidol in autistic children: Continuous versus discontinuous drug administration. J Am Acad Child Adolesc Psychiatry 28:87–92, 1989.
4. Coffey BJ: Anxiolytics for children and adolescents: Traditional and new drugs. J Child Adolesc Psychopharmacol 1:57–83, 1990.
5. Bernstein GA, Hughes JR, Mitchell JE, Thompson T: Effects of narcotic antagonists on self-injurious behavior: A single case study. J Am Acad Child Adolesc Psychiatry 26:886–889, 1987.
6. Campbell M, Spencer E: Psychopharmacology in child and adolescent psychiatry: A review of the past five years. J Am Acad Child Adolesc Psychiatry 27:269–279, 1988.
7. Werry JS, Wollersheim JP: Behavior therapy with children and adolescents: A twenty year overview. J Am Acad Child Adolesc Psychiatry 28:1–18, 1989.
8. Burke P, DelBeccaro M, McCauley E, Clark C: Hallucinations in children. J Am Acad Child Adolesc Psychiatry 24:71–75, 1985.
9. Russell AT, Bott L, Sammons C: The phenomenology of schizophrenia occurring in childhood. J Am Acad Child Adolesc Psychiatry 28:399–407, 1989.
10. Terr L: Too Scared to Cry: Psychic Trauma in Childhood. New York: Harper & Row, 1990.
11. Teicher MH, Glod CA: Neuroleptic drugs: Indications and rational use in children and adolescents. J Child Adolesc Psychopharmacol 1:33–56, 1990.
12. Costello EJ: Developments in child psychiatry epidemiology. J Am Acad Child Adolesc Psychiatry 28:836–841, 1989.
13. Szatmari P, Boyle M, Offord D: ADDH and conduct disorder: Degree of diagnostic overlap and differences among correlates. J Am Acad Child Adolesc Psychiatry 28:865–872, 1989.
14. Zametkin AJ, Nordahl TE, Gross M, et al: Cerebral glucose metabolism in adults with hyperactivity of childhood onset. N Engl J Med 323:1361–1366, 1990.
15. Connors CK, Barkley RA: Rating scales and checklists for psychopharmacology. Psychopharmacol Bull 21:809–815, 1985.
16. Dulcan MK: Using psychostimulants to treat behavioral disorders of children and adolescents. J Child Adolesc Psychopharmacol 1:7–20, 1990.
17. Jacobvitz D: Treatment of attentional and hyperactivity problems in children with sympathomimetic drugs: A comprehensive review. J Am Acad Child Adolesc Psychiatry 29:677–688, 1990.
18. Greenhill L: Attention-deficit hyperactivity disorder in children. In Garfinkel BD, Carlson GA, Weller EB, eds. Psychiatric Disorders in Children and Adolescents. Philadelphia: WB Saunders, 1990:149–192.
19. Biederman J, Baldessarini RJ, Wright V, et al: A double-blind controlled study of desipramine in the treatment of ADD: II. Serum drug levels and cardiovascular findings. J Am Acad Child Adolesc Psychiatry 28:903–911, 1989.
20. Hunt RD, Capper L, O'Connell P: Clonidine in child and adolescent psychiatry. J Child Adolesc Psychopharmacol 1:87–102, 1990.
21. Barrnett RJ, Docherty JP, Frommelt GM: A review of child psychotherapy research since 1963. J Am Acad Child Adolesc Psychiatry 30:1–14, 1991.
22. Kinzie JD, Sack W, Angell R, et al: A three-year follow-up of Cambodian young people traumatized as children. J Am Acad Child Adolesc Psychiatry 28:501–504, 1989.
23. Orvaschel H, Weissman MM: Epidemiology of anxiety disorders in children: A review. In Gittelman R, ed. Anxiety Disorders of Childhood. New York: Guilford Press, 1986:58–72.
24. Bernstein GA, Garfinkel BD, Borchart CM: Comparative studies of pharmacotherapy for school refusal. J Am Acad Child Adolesc Psychiatry 29:773–781, 1990.
25. Combrink-Graham L: Family systems research. J Am Acad Child Adolesc Psychiatry 29:501–512, 1990.
26. Fleming JE, Offord DR: Epidemiology of childhood depressive disorders: A critical review. J Am Acad Child Adolesc Psychiatry 29:571–580, 1990.

27. Weller EB, Weller RA: Depressive disorders in children and adolescents. In Garfinkel BD, Carlson GA, Weller EB, eds. Psychiatric Disorders in Children and Adolescents. Philadelphia: WB Saunders, 1990:3–36.

28. Ryan ND: Heterocyclic antidepressants in children and adolescents. J Child Adolesc Psychopharmacol 1:21–31, 1990.

29. Bartels MG, Varley CK, Mitchell JC, Stamm SJ: Pediatric cardiovascular effects of imipramine and desipramine. J Am Acad Child Adolesc Psychiatry 30:100–103, 1991.

30. Popper CW, Elliot GR: Sudden death and tricyclic antidepressants: Clinical considerations for children. J Child Adolesc Psychopharmacol 1:125–132, 1990.

69

PSYCHOSIS AND MANIA IN ADOLESCENTS

GABRIELLE A. CARLSON, M.D.

The subject of adolescent psychosis is deserving of a separate section not so much because the treatment is different but because diagnostic issues require separate consideration. Basically, as is expanded upon in this chapter, our ability to diagnose accurately and predict outcome in adolescents presenting with psychotic symptoms has been only slightly better than 50–50. With that sobering observation in mind, it seems important both to find ways of increasing predictive ability and to avoid being too dogmatic about initial diagnosis, thus the decision to discuss adolescent psychosis generically. Furthermore, the emphasis of this chapter is on ways in which adolescent psychoses—predominantly psychotic depression, mania, schizophrenia, schizoaffective disorder, and atypical psychosis—differ from the psychoses presenting in adults. Similarly, since the psychopharmacological treatment of the psychoses is similar regardless of age at onset, only areas in which treatment considerations are different are covered here.

It is important to note at the outset that the definition, occurrence, and treatment of major psychiatric disorders in the adolescent years are woefully understudied. First, until recently, childhood "psychosis" studies lumped autism and a number of other uncommon developmental disorders with more classically defined schizophrenia beginning in childhood, making their data impossible to interpret. Second, child psychiatry studies, when they include adolescents, rarely go past age 14 and only recently have tried to define puberty rather than age as a relevant feature. Conversely, most investigators of adult populations of affective or schizophrenic disorder have lower age cutoffs, between 16 and 18, and virtually never examine the subjects at those ages separately. Finally, young people from ages 13 through 19 are not developmentally homogeneous; thus it may be unwise to generalize to the whole population of adolescents. While these considerations are true for all psychiatric disorders in this age group, the relative rarity of "functional" psychosis in adolescents means that even greater effort and time must be spent in accruing significant sample sizes than is spent for adults, where not only are the disorders more common but also the age availability is greater.

DEFINITION, PREVALENCE, AND DIAGNOSTIC ISSUES

Gillberg and colleagues[1] defined adolescent psychosis as follows: the presence of hallucinations, formal thought disorder of the schizophrenic kind, delusions, disorientation, and mania or major depression with mood congruent features. In systematically reviewing clinical records of 401 13- to 19-year-olds, they found that 0.5 per cent of all youngsters developed "clear cut psychotic symptoms" sometime during their teenage years. Of the 61 cases (32 boys, 29 girls) meeting the above criteria, the mean yearly prevalence for hospitalized psychosis ranged from 0.9 : 10,000 at age 13 to a peak of 17.6 : 10,000 at age 18, for a cumulative prevalence of 53.8 : 10,000.

Using DSM-III[2] criteria to diagnose from records, these authors found 41 per cent of psychoses could be diagnosed as schizophrenia, 27.9 per cent as major affective disorder (of the 17 cases in question, 8 had a psychotic depression, 4 had a bipolar disorder,

3 were manic, and 2 had a cycloid psychosis), 21.3 per cent as substance-induced disorder, and 9.8 per cent as atypical psychosis. However, this means only that the *symptoms presented at the time of hospitalization* best fit these diagnostic categories.

A number of studies have emphasized the fact that bipolar disorder is frequently misdiagnosed in adolescence.[3,4] Most pointedly, Joyce[5] observed that 38 per cent of adolescent-onset depressives were called schizophrenic (this did not occur with patients over age 30) and 72 per cent of adolescent manics versus 24 per cent of older manics were misdiagnosed. Werry et al.[6] reported on 61 young people admitted to an inpatient unit in New Zealand over a 16-year period with "psychosis" and found that 79 per cent met schizophrenia or schizophreniform disorders criteria (DSM-III), and 21 per cent were bipolar, had a psychotic depression, or were schizoaffective. A follow-up study of 59 of these subjects was completed 1 to 16 years (average 5) after admission. Rediagnosis was accomplished using information from personal interview, medical and coroner records, parents, and the like. They found that only 49 per cent of the subjects could still be classified as schizophrenic, and 37 per cent had followed a bipolar course and 10 per cent a schizoaffective course. In other words, only 57 per cent of the bipolar patients and 63 per cent of the schizophrenics were originally identified accurately. This is only slightly worse than studies of adults with psychosis, however, in which about 70 per cent of the schizophrenia and bipolar diagnoses remained stable over time.[7]

Does adolescence additionally complicate diagnostic accuracy? As I have pointed out elsewhere,[3] there are several unavoidable reasons why it might. Kraepelin originally distinguished the two basic functional psychoses by course. The DSM-III, DSM-III-R, and probably DSM-IV continue to build a number of course variables into their diagnostic criteria. For instance, to diagnose schizophrenia, one must have a continuous disturbance for 6 months and a clear deterioration in function. By definition, then, it is impossible to diagnose the first episode of an acute disorder in an adolescent as schizophrenia. Even though it is possible to diagnose bipolar disorder with only one manic episode, it helps if the patient has had an episodic course. If the first and only episode is of depression, one cannot diagnose bipolar disorder. Furthermore, two of the melancholia criteria require a prior episode of depression. These problems are true of any first episode of illness, however. At the outset, one will not have had the luxury of time to enhance diagnostic accuracy. The major reason adolescence makes the situation more complicated is that there has been less time in the young person's life to have established a history of stable premorbid function against which to contrast a clear behavioral change.

Other reasons for erroneous diagnosis of adolescent psychosis include a combination of phenomenological reality and clinical bias. Mild episodes of depression or mania can often be dismissed as results of the vicissitudes of adolescence. In young people with histories of stable premorbid functioning, careful delineation of how the presenting problems differ from previous function is critical.[3] In characterologically stormy children and adolescents, distinguishing clinical episodes from severe emotional lability is extremely difficult.[4] Even in these cases, however, the presence of unequivocal psychotic symptoms that are not drug induced cannot be dismissed as "adolescent turmoil."

While it has not been established definitively because of the absence of data, it appears that the "formes fruste" of many psychiatric (and medical, for that matter) disorders are somewhat atypical. Several studies suggest that bipolar disorder in adolescence is characterized by more intense psychotic symptoms than it is when onset is later.[3] It is unclear if the same observation can be made for acute psychoses that follow a schizophrenic course, again because data are lacking.

WHAT ARE THE BEST DIAGNOSTIC PREDICTORS?

The predictors of a deteriorating course after a psychotic episode appear to be the same in children and adolescents[6,8,9] as they are in adults.[10] Poor premorbid adjustment, including such personality variables as introversion, extreme shyness, schizoidal temperament, emotional instability, aggression, lack of affective contact, and obsessiveness, occur more often in youngsters with nonremitting courses. Other important contributors include insidious onset of psychosis, attentional and information processing abnormalities, and other developmental problems such as neuromuscular problems and low IQ.[11,12] Family history of schizophrenia may be higher in younger onset schizophrenics as well.[13]

Conversely, the best predictors of a bipolar outcome are good premorbid functioning, normal or better IQ,[6] and clear diagnosis of mania at first episode.[14] Bipolar disorder and major depression in first- and second-degree relatives occur with significantly greater frequency in adolescent- and prepubertal-onset bipolar patients than in their adult counterparts.[15] The symptoms presented during the acute psychotic episode, with the exception of prominent affective symptoms, have virtually no predictive validity. These are also virtually the same predictors reported in the adult literature.[10] Finally, if the first episode of severe depression in an adolescent is characterized by acute onset, psychotic symptoms, psychomotor retardation, and family history of major depression and bipolar disorder, there is substantial likelihood that a bipolar course will occur.[16]

It is interesting that even with a disorder characterized by its episodic nature, premorbid functioning may predict course to some extent. In adolescent bipolar patients with prepubertal histories of behavior disorder, lithium response is unimpressive and intermorbid function is poor.[15,17] Thus, serious psychopathology in prepubertal youngsters appears to be a marker for continued disturbance regardless of the nature of the subsequent psychosis.

TREATMENT

There are embarrassingly few systematic studies of psychopharmacological treatment of acute psychosis specifically in an adolescent population. Those drugs whose efficacy has been specifically studied include haloperidol and loxapine[18] and thioridazine and thiothixine.[19] Strober et al.[20] examined the prophylactic use of lithium in adolescent bipolar subjects. In general, there is nothing to suggest that the strategies for treating an acute psychosis, whether it is classified as schizophrenic, schizophreniform, manic, psychotic depressive, or atypical, are any different in adolescents than in adults.

Psychopharmacological Treatment

Neuroleptics

Since most adolescents are still in school, it is necessary to be particularly sensitive to the cognitive impairment conferred by many neuroleptics. This does not mean undermedicating the person or withdrawing medication in an injudicious way. It is likely that the more sedating neuroleptics and higher dose account for much of the observed adverse effect.[21] In an individual child, therefore, it is important to track school performance and compare it to best levels of prior function. It is also unclear if children and adolescents are any more vulnerable to movement disorders and tardive dyskinesia than adults. Most studies of neuroleptics in this age group have been done in autistic and mentally retarded youngsters, for whom abnormal motor movements may represent baseline problem or unusual vulnerability.[21] Given the potential extended use of these drugs starting at an early age, low-dose strategies should be adopted wherever possible. In addition, if one is dealing with a first episode of psychosis in a youngster with good premorbid functioning, it is worth considering a "drug holiday" sooner rather than later. This should take place after the child has been without psychotic symptoms for 6 to 12 months, preferably when the child is not in school, and with the consent and education of everyone who has contact with the child.

Medication compliance is a problem in all psychiatric disorders at all ages. It may be worse in adolescents, in whom perceived invulnerability to adversity is part of the gestalt and may not necessarily represent illness denial. Under these circumstances, if maintenance drug is needed, depot neuroleptics should be considered.

Lithium Carbonate

Interest in using this medication has increased dramatically in recent years with the hope that it will solve many adolescent behavior problems reformulated as bipolar disorder to lend credence to its use. A diagnostic rationale for the use of lithium is summarized in Table 69–1.

Adolescents are usually healthy and tolerate lithium fairly well. In fact, given the young person's rapid renal clearance, it may take higher doses of lithium to maintain therapeutic levels (0.7 to 1.2 mEq/liter in blood drawn 12 hours after the last dose).[3] In prepubertal children there is a significant positive correlation between total daily lithium dose and weight,[22] but it is not clear that the same is true for adolescents, especially manic adolescents. Finally, the only systematic report of side effects was also in prepubertal children treated for conduct disorder. Campbell et al.[23] reported that weight gain, decreased motor activity, excessive sedation, gastrointestinal complaints, pallor, headache, and polyuria were complaints noted in decreasing order of frequency. Less than half the sample experienced these problems, however. Among the more serious concerns in children are the accumulation of lithium in bones and the known effects on thyroid function and on kidney function.[24] Although Platt et al.[25] reported some cognitive impairment in prepubertal children treated with lithium, other studies of the subject are more equivocal in their results.[26]

The most pressing management questions revolve around how long to continue and when to stop lithium. How long to continue lithium depends in part on the certainty of the patient's diagnosis and where he or she is in life. Common sense is the best guide here. In a young person who had had a destructive manic or depressive episode largely treated by medication, who is still young and facing several years of school, the longer a period of stability he or she has, the better. Relapse is most likely to occur within the first 4 to 6 months after episode remission[20] and may occur within the first year and a half of first episode

---

TABLE 69–1. REASONS FOR INITIATING LITHIUM TREATMENT IN JUVENILE BIPOLAR DISORDER[a]

1. Presence or history of disabling episodes of mania and depression
2. Episode(s) of severe depression with a possible history of hypomania
3. Presence of an acute, severe depression characterized by psychomotor retardation, hypersomnia and psychosis, positive family history of major depression or bipolar disorder
4. An acute psychotic disorder with affective features
5. Behavior disorders characterized by severe emotional lability and aggression where there is a positive family history of major affective or bipolar disorder or lithium responsiveness

[a] Reprinted with permission from Carlson GA: Bipolar disorders in children and adolescents. In Garfinkel B, Carlson GA, Weller E, eds. Psychiatric Disorders in Children and Adolescents. Philadelphia, WB Saunders, 1990:21–36.

in treatment-compliant youngsters. It makes some sense, therefore, not to consider a drug holiday in such cases for at least 2 years unless there is some very compelling reason. In contrast, in an emotionally labile adolescent for whom clear treatment effect has not been demonstrated after 6 to 9 months, a drug holiday may be helpful in discerning whether change has taken place.

Treatment of lithium-refractory bipolar disorder is likely to be the same in adolescents as it is in adults. There are only anecdotal reports of carbamazepine use in adolescents.[27,28] Treatment of concurrent personality disorder, conduct disorder, and substance and alcohol abuse poses the same dilemmas in adolescents as it does in adults. The question of subsyndromal disorder versus comorbidity is difficult to resolve prior to treatment. Although there are as yet no data to substantiate this contention, it is my impression that a clear history of good function prior to adolescence suggests that other psychopathology occurring concurrent with the mood disorder is part of the mood disorder and not another Axis II problem.

Antidepressants

There are two observations that may be unique to adolescents with mood disorder. First, it has been very difficult to demonstrate treatment efficacy for those antidepressants that have been studied.[29] Most clinicians use these medications in their practice and have anecdotal support for their utility, but demonstrating this with adequate sample size with the rigors of double-blind, placebo-controlled trials has so far been unsuccessful. Second, the question of antidepressant use in an adolescent who may have a manic episode precipitated by antidepressant use needs to be addressed in discussing treatment with patient and family. Development of hypomania sometimes occurs in an at-risk population[16] and usually subsides with the withdrawal of the antidepressant. This occurrence also provides an important predictor of bipolar course. The question of whether or not a rapid cycling course ultimately can occur, or if it can be prevented by "covering" the patient with lithium before instituting antidepressants, has not been resolved. In making a decision about how to proceed if one believes a bipolar course is a possibility, it is necessary to review especially carefully risks versus benefits with the family.

Psychosocial Interventions

Treating adolescents with any serious disorder involves understanding the patient, his or her family, and the other needs both of them have. At the onset of the illness, one is dealing with the admitted diagnostic ambiguity inherent in our predictive ability. Seeing one's child severely psychotic, regardless of the diagnostic label assigned, is an unimaginably frightening and painful experience. Psychoeducational approaches that appear to be valuable in the treatment of schizophrenics[30] are likely to be helpful with psychotic adolescents and their families. Basically, one is providing as much manageable information as possible to enhance the family members' understanding and observations so they can help the clinician make informed decisions with them. Initially, this includes a collaborative effort to establish a diagnosis more reliably. One of the reasons diagnoses change over time is that more information is obtained (e.g., it is revealed that a hypomanic episode had occurred some months earlier or that, in fact, the teenager had been delusional for longer than he or she had admitted).

Ultimately, decisions must be made as to whether a mood stabilizer should be added to the neuroleptic, whether a special education placement will be needed on follow-up, what kinds of additional structure might be needed, and for how long and how to help the adolescent and family manage symptoms that do not remit in spite of optimal psychopharmacological treatment. In the simplest cases, an obvious manic episode will respond well to lithium and the young person can return to high school or college having, at worst, missed a semester of school. Although there is initial and realistic anxiety about recurrence, education and supportive management may be all that is needed. In a less compliant youngster or family, or one in whom symptoms have not completely remitted, ongoing psychotherapy will be important to maintain close observation and a trusting relationship to enhance compliance with treatment recommendations. Where postpsychotic impairment (and in this case it probably does not matter if the affective symptoms or residual "schizophrenic" symptoms are causing the impairment) is a continuing problem, a more structured school environment must be sought regardless of whether there is documented academic impairment. Maintaining a therapeutic posture between optimism and informed realism is important. Accomplishing these goals in families often beset by the same psychopathology afflicting the adolescent is daunting.

CONCLUSION

It is important to try to clarify the nature of psychotic symptoms when they occur for the first time in an adolescent. However, it is particularly important to ascertain information on the adolescent's emotional, behavioral, intellectual, interpersonal, and social functioning prior to the onset of acute psychosis, because these factors appear to have more predictive validity than the nature of the psychotic symptoms themselves. This information is relevant not only for the psychopharmacological treatment implemented but also for the kind of treatment planned subsequently.

REFERENCES

1. Gillberg C, Wahlstrom J, Forsman A, Hellgren L, Gillberg IC: Teenage psychoses—epidemiology, classification and reduced optimality in the pre-, peri-, and neonatal periods. J Child Psychol Psychiatry 27:87–98, 1986.
2. American Psychiatric Association: Diagnostic and Statistical Manual of Mental Disorders. 3rd ed. Washington, DC: American Psychiatric Association, 1980.
3. Carlson GA: Bipolar disorders in children and adolescents. In Garfinkel B, Carlson GA, Weller E, eds. Psychiatric Disorders in Children and Adolescents. Philadelphia: WB Saunders Company, 1990:21–36.
4. Carlson GA: Annotation: Child and adolescent mania—diagnostic considerations. J Child Psychol Psychiatry 31:331–341, 1990.
5. Joyce PR: Age of onset in bipolar affective disorder and misdiagnosis as schizophrenia. Psychol Med 14:145–149, 1984.
6. Werry JS, McClellan JH, Chard L: Childhood and adolescent schizophrenic, bipolar and schizo-affective disorders: A clinical and outcome study. J Am Acad Child Adolesc Psychiatry 30:457–465, 1991.
7. Beiser M, Iacono WG, Erikson D: The temporal stability in major mental disorders. In Robins LN, Barrett JE, eds. The Validity of Psychiatric Diagnosis. New York: Raven Press, 1989:77–98.
8. Eggers C: Course and prognosis of childhood schizophrenia. J Autism Child Schizophr 8:21–36, 1978.
9. Eggers C: Schizo-affective psychoses in childhood: A follow-up study. J Autism Dev Disord 19:327–342, 1989.
10. McGlashan TH: A selective review of recent North American long-term follow-up studies of schizophrenia. Schizophr Bull 14:515–542, 1988.
11. Nuechterlein K: Childhood precursors of adult schizophrenia. J Child Psychol Psychiatry 27:133–144, 1986.
12. Hellgren L, Gillberg C, Enerskog I: Antecedents of adolescent psychoses: A population-based study of school health problems in children who develop psychosis in adolescence. J Am Acad Child Adolesc Psychiatry 26:351–355, 1987.
13. Gottesman II, Shields J: A critical review of recent adoption, twin and family studies of schizophrenia: Behavior genetics perspectives. Schizophr Bull 2:360–401, 1976.
14. Tohen M, Waternaux CM, Tsuang MT, Hunt AT: Four-year follow up of twenty-four first episode manic patients. J Affective Disord 19:79–86, 1990.
15. Strober M, Morrell W, Burroughs J, et al: A family study of bipolar I in adolescence: Early onset of symptoms linked to increased familial loading and lithium resistance. J Affective Disord 15:255–268, 1988.
16. Strober M, Carlson GA: Bipolar illness in adolescents with major depression: Clinical, genetic and psychopharmacologic predictors. Arch Gen Psychiatry 39:549–555, 1982.
17. Kutcher SP, Marton P, Korenblum M: Adolescent bipolar illness and personality disorder. J Am Acad Child Adolesc Psychiatry 29:355–358, 1990.
18. Pool D, Bloom W, Mielke DH, et al: A controlled evaluation of Loxitane in seventy-five adolescent schizophrenic patients. Curr Ther Res 19:99–104, 1976.
19. Realmuto GM, Erikson WD, Yellin AM, et al: Clinical comparison of thiothixene and thioridazine in schizophrenic adolescents. Am J Psychiatry 141:440–442, 1984.
20. Strober M, Morrell W, Lampert C, Burroughs J: Lithium carbonate in prophylactic treatment of bipolar illness in adolescents: A naturalistic study. Am J Psychiatry 147:457–461, 1990.
21. Campbell M, Green WH, Deutsch SI: Child and Adolescent Psychopharmacology. Beverly Hills, CA: Sage Publications, 1985.
22. Weller EB, Weller RA, Fristad MA: Lithium dosage guide for prepubertal children: A preliminary report. J Am Acad Child Adolesc Psychiatry 25:92–96, 1986.
23. Campbell M, Perry R, Green WH: Use of lithium in children and adolescents. Psychosomatics 25:95–105, 1984.
24. Jefferson JW: The use of lithium in childhood and adolescence—an overview. J Clin Psychiatry 43:174–177, 1982.
25. Platt JE, Campbell M, Green WH, Grega DM: Cognitive effects of lithium carbonate and halperidol in treatment-resistant aggressive children. Arch Gen Psychiatry 41:657–662, 1984.
26. Carlson GA, Rapport MD, Pataki CS, Kelly KL: Lithium in hospitalized children at 4 and 8 weeks: Mood, behavior and cognitive effects. J Child Psychol Psychiatry (in press).
27. Hsu LKG: Lithium-resistant adolescent mania. J Am Acad Child Adolesc Psychiatry 25:280–283, 1986.
28. Reiss AL, O'Donnell DJ: Carbamazepine-induced mania in two children: Case report. J Clin Psychiatry 45:272–274, 1984.
29. Ryan N: Heterocyclic antidepressants in children and adolescents. J Child Adolesc Psychopharmacol 1:21–32, 1990.
30. Larson J: Something old and something new: Integrating pharmacologic and psychosocial approached in schizophrenia treatment. Psychiatr Ann 20:645–654, 1990.

70

TREATMENT OF DEPRESSIVE
DISORDERS IN ADOLESCENTS

ELIZABETH McCAULEY, Ph.D. and KATHLEEN MYERS, M.D., M.S., M.P.H.

Considerable progress has been made in the characterization of depression in young people, while identification and investigation of treatment strategies are in a more formative stage. This chapter provides a brief overview of adolescent depression and then focuses on treatment considerations, with a critical review of the intervention literature.

OVERVIEW OF DEPRESSION IN ADOLESCENCE

Clinical Features

Depression appears to occur in 0.4 to 6.4 per cent of adolescents from the general population,[1] and rates among clinical samples vary from 13 to 34 per cent.[2–4] Major depression has been described in young children,[5] but most studies[6] report a marked increase in incidence in the pre- to early adolescent years, with increased frequency among adolescents. Girls are overrepresented in clinical samples of major depressive disorders, as compared to other childhood disorders, and during adolescence increasingly outnumber boys.[7] Differences in social and cultural pressures that may account for the pattern of female versus male presentation have yet to be investigated.

Depression in young people is currently diagnosed using the same criteria as for adults; however, some differences in presentation have been identified. Young people are more likely to present with increased somatic complaints and irritability[8,9] than are adults. This has clinical importance since, when either of these symptoms predominates, families and clinicians may overlook other signs of depression. Somatic complaints may be more acceptable within a family, and many depressed young people first present in adolescent medicine clinics with diffuse somatic complaints.[10] Irritability is equally important because it quickly leads to intensified parent-child conflict, and the child's depression can be overlooked while parents and teachers focus on issues of compliance and attitude. Guilt feelings, low self-esteem, and suicide gestures are also more frequent in young people, whereas adults display more of the vegetative signs of depression.[8,9,11]

Frequently, psychiatrically disturbed young people present with a complex clinical picture and meet diagnostic criteria for more than one disorder. Many depressed young people present with concurrent disorders, with reports of 33 to 59 per cent of samples of children and adolescents having coexisting separation anxiety, 7 to 37 per cent having coexisting conduct disorders, and 17 to 38 per cent having a predisposing or coexisting dysthymic disorder.[6,8,9] The data suggest that many young people become depressed after a prodromal period of dysthymia, and others have had an early history of separation anxiety that precedes, but may co-occur with, clinical depression.[6,8] The co-occurrence of conduct disorder is seen most frequently with boys, and with increasing age in boys, depressive and externalizing symptoms show great overlap.[12] Significant anxiety symptoms are also associated with depression, particularly as severity increases.[13,14] It has also been suggested that young people with prolonged difficulties with anxiety are at significant risk for eventually becoming clinically depressed as well.[15]

Clinical Course

Prospective data on the clinical course of depression suggest that depression in young people has the same episodic course as found in adults. Kovacs et al.'s[6,16] longitudinal study of prepubertal depressed children found a mean length of episode of 32 weeks and a relapse rate of 72 per cent within a 5-year follow-up period. Strober and Carlson[17] conducted 3- to 4-year follow-up evaluations on 60 young people who had been hospitalized for major depression at 13 to 16 years of age. Of these juveniles, 31 per cent went on to have subsequent depressive episodes and 20 per cent developed mania. In a 3-year prospective study of depressed youths, McCauley and colleagues[18] found a mean length of episode of 36 weeks, with 54 per cent relapsing during the follow-up period. Duration of initial episode and relapse were associated with factors reflecting severity of the young person's initial episode rather than environmental or family background variables. Finally, follow-up studies of depressed children and adolescents seen again as young adults indicate ongoing difficulties with depression[19] and residual impairments in psychosocial functioning.[20]

Family History

Parental history of depression is associated with increased risk of psychopathology, as has been substantiated in studies of the offspring of affectively disturbed adults[21-24] as well as in investigations of parents of depressed youth.[25-27] However, specificity of transmission is less clear. Parental history of depression alone does not distinguish depressed from nondepressed psychiatric controls,[25,26] whereas parental history of affective pathology and alcoholism or anxiety[25,27] shows a more clear-cut relation with affective disturbance in offspring.

Laboratory Studies

Few investigations have included adolescents in attempts to replicate the findings of hypothalmic abnormalities identified in depressed adults. Dexamethasone suppression tests, as a measure of dyscontrol cortisol output, have, however, been included in many studies of depressed youths with highly variable results.[28-31]

Abnormalities in growth hormone production in response to laboratory challenge tests have been found in both adults and prepubertal depressed subjects.[32] Two studies with adolescents yielded more equivocal results. Kutcher and colleagues[33] studied the nocturnal secretion pattern of growth hormone in adolescent males with and without major depression. The depressed youths showed a variable output pattern with greater secretion during the first half of the sleep period, whereas normal controls had a steady output throughout the night. Jensen and Garfinkel,[32] however, did not find differences in a small sample (eight) of adolescent boys whose growth hormone response to oral clonidine and L-dopa was assessed. Finally, initial attempts have been made to document changes in sleep patterns, such as shortened rapid eye movement (REM) latency, found in adult populations. The data, thus far, suggest that polysomnographic irregularities may be documented in depressed adolescents but are more likely to be present in older versus younger adolescents.[34-36]

In sum, the laboratory findings are limited and inconsistent, making conclusions difficult at this time. Biochemical profiles as well as familial risk factors might be somewhat different for prepubertal versus adolescent depressed youths, with biological loading being more evident in earlier onset cases. These findings, if borne out with further research, could have significant implications for both diagnosis and treatment.

Differential Diagnosis

As described earlier, the differential diagnosis of depression in young people can be complicated by the presentation of unique symptom clusters and the presence of coexisting disorders. Differential diagnosis must also take into account the various presentations of mood disorder, with consideration of unipolar depression, bipolar disorder, and dysthymia, as well as adjustment reactions with depressed mood. Depression with psychotic features may appear more like a schizophreniform disorder at this age, and some depressed adolescents are at the very early stages of an evolving bipolar disorder. Depressive symptoms alone, including suicidality, are very common during adolescence, such that it may be difficult to distinguish adolescent depressive adjustment reactions from dysthymia or major depression.

The possibility of personality disorders in relation to adolescent depression has not been addressed. Given the complexity of these issues, adolescent depression may best be conceptualized within the framework of atypical depression.[37]

THERAPEUTIC INTERVENTIONS

General Considerations

Intervention with depressed adolescents presents a complex set of challenges and, as yet, there is not a "proven" approach to guide clinicians. Any approach must take into account not only the clinical presentation of the adolescent, but the broader context in which his or her depression occurs. Assessment of home environment and parent functioning is essential because many adolescents become depressed in response to overwhelming environmental demands, and, in some cases, the youth's depression is related to parental psychopathology or negligence. The parents' own histories of depression and response to treatments should be reviewed, and, in some cases, consideration of treatment for parents may be an essential part of the adolescent's therapeutic intervention. Input from parents is critical in obtaining an accurate sense of the course of the child's difficulties, preexisting functioning, and response to prior interventions. It is equally important to assess how the parents view the adolescent and his or her depression, and how ready and able they are to facilitate therapeutic interventions that might include increased social contact, autonomy, and activity on the part of the adolescent.

Adjunct therapeutic involvement with school and community resources is also necessary. Many depressed adolescents find large-scale, traditional high schools too overwhelming to handle and present with significant histories of school avoidance. The therapist must be prepared to work with the youth, parents, and the school system to identify an appropriate alternative educational plan or setting. Educators, parents, and the youths themselves will need guidance regarding the impact of depression on social and academic functioning. Input to school officials is especially required in cases in which suicidality, significant anxiety symptoms, or both are predominant, because these symptoms will undoubtedly challenge the school's ability to manage the student. Furthermore, since it appears that adolescent depression is episodic, with residual impairment, long-term case management may be necessary to track these adolescents over time, making sure that necessary services are available to them with the hope of minimizing the negative consequences of repeated, debilitating depressive episodes.

Pharmacotherapy

Pharmacotherapy has become increasingly accepted as an early intervention in the treatment of adolescent depression. The reasons are not clear, since there are very few data to support its efficacy. The trend may reflect the conceptualization of childhood and adolescent depression as the same disorder that occurs in adulthood. Alternatively, the increasing use of briefer therapies and managed care systems may influence physicians' treatment decisions. Until scientific studies clarify the role of pharmacotherapy, current practices must be considered empirical.

Efficacy of Antidepressant Therapy

Clinical reports in the 1960s and 1970s reported success with tricyclic antidepressants in the treatment of childhood depression. More recent studies in the 1980s using an "open-label" design also suggested a response to imipramine[38–40] and to amitriptyline or its metabolite nortriptyline.[41–44] These earlier studies suffered from many methodological flaws, including difficulties in inclusion criteria, diagnostic specificity, outcome measures, and non-blinded or noncontrolled design. In the later 1980s, two studies addressed these issues by using double-blind, placebo-controlled designs with adequate sample sizes.[45,46] Geller and colleagues[46] failed to find superiority for nortriptyline over placebo despite adequate plasma levels. Puig-Antich and colleagues[45] found no difference between imipramine- and placebo-treated groups. However, a maintenance plasma level of 150 ng/ml discriminated responders from nonresponders. Higher levels were associated with an 85 per cent response rate, whereas lower levels produced 30 per cent response. Earlier studies[38–40] also suggested that plasma levels of imipramine over 125 ng/ml were associated with a better response. Recently, Preskorn and colleagues[47] reported that a small sample of depressed children who responded preferentially to imipramine demonstrated nonsuppression on the dexamethasone suppression test.

Overall, the possible occurrence of a response threshold may suggest specificity of antidepressant action in children. However, paucity of studies and the lack of replication, as well as the relatively small sample sizes, severely limit interpretations.

Adolescent studies are even more rare. Most studies have been conducted with tricyclics. Using a double-blind, placebo-controlled design, two studies failed to demonstrate a beneficial response to amitriptyline[48] or its metabolite nortriptyline.[49] With a less rigorous open-label design, Ryan and colleagues[50] did not find a relationship between imipramine serum levels and clinical response for depressed outpatients. Strober and colleagues did find such a trend with inpatients.[51]

There is only one study reported of the serotonergic antidepressant fluoxetine. Using a double-blind, placebo-controlled design, Simeon and colleagues[52,53] found that about two thirds of adolescents responded with marked or moderate improvement in both the fluoxetine and placebo groups. However, there was a statistical trend suggesting better subjective response in those adolescents taking fluoxetine.

Systematic studies of other antidepressants are lacking. Using a chart review methodology, Ryan and colleagues[54] reported "good or fair response" in 74 per cent of 23 outpatients treated with monoamine oxidase inhibitors (MAOIs) following failure to respond to tricyclic antidepressants. Some of these teens were treated with both a tricyclic and a MAOI concurrently. These authors hypothesized that developmental factors may predispose adolescents to respond differentially to nontricyclic medications. In another chart review study of nonbipolar depressed adolescents who responded partially to imipramine, Ryan and colleagues found that lithium augmentation produced a "good" response in 6 of 14 youths.[55] Lithium levels were maintained in the therapeutic range of 0.5 to 1.2 mEq/liter. Improvement occurred gradually over the first month of treatment, consistent with most recent reports of adult responsivity.

Overall, these studies do not suggest general benefits of antidepressant medications in depressed adolescents. It is possible that some subset of depressed adolescents do respond. Well-designed studies are now needed to determine whether adolescent major depression is generally responsive to pharmacotherapy, whether adolescents respond differently from adults, or whether only subgroups of adolescents benefit.

Pharmacokinetics, Plasma Levels, and Dosing Schedules

The lack of established efficacy precludes formal recommendations for the use of antidepressants in adolescents. Guidelines discussed here have been established empirically. The use of antidepressants in adolescents requires additional considerations over those recommended for adults. The tricyclics are the most commonly used antidepressants with adolescents. Their elimination appears to follow first-order kinetics, with a logarithmically linear rate of disappearance similar to that in adults and children.[56] Steady state plasma levels appear to be achieved by day 7,[57] also consistent with adult studies. Wide variability in plasma levels occurs[39,58–60] that does not appear to be determined by age, weight, height, or body surface area.[39]

The tricyclics are metabolized more quickly in adolescents than in adults, but less quickly than in children,[56,61] as a result of increased first-pass hepatic metabolism and decreased protein binding. The rapid metabolism may require twice-daily or three-times-daily dosing for younger adolescents in order to maintain constant plasma levels and prevent withdrawal reactions. However, this more frequent dosing schedule may also lead to greater noncompliance, especially with adolescents who are self-conscious about taking medications.

The Food and Drug Administration (FDA) has provided dosing guidelines only for the use of imipramine, desipramine, amitriptyline, and nortriptyline in adolescents. No age limits are given by the FDA for the use of fluoxetine. Monoamine oxidase inhibitors are not recommended for use with youths under 16 years of age.

Younger and smaller adolescents are prescribed imipramine, desipramine, and amitriptyline in dosages of 1.0 mg/kg/day up to 5.0 mg/kg/day, with the dose titrated up from the lower dosages to attain serum levels of 150 to 300 ng/ml. Higher plasma levels have been reported in some studies, but are not recommended even in the absence of adverse effects. Nortriptyline generally requires 0.5 to 2.0 mg/kg/day to achieve a plasma level of 75 to 150 ng/ml. Older adolescents may be prescribed tricyclics according to adult schedules, rather than on a weight basis. In clinical practice fluoxetine has generally been used in dosages recommended for adult depression. Monoamine oxidase inhibitors are also prescribed in adolescents over 16 years according to adult schedules.

Frequent plasma level determinations and electrocardiograms (ECG) are required early in the course of establishing medication regimens for all tricyclic antidepressants and MAOIs. The younger the adolescent, the more frequently monitoring may be required, especially in the higher dosage ranges (above 150 mg for imipramine, desipramine, and amitriptyline). Some authors state that plasma levels are not needed, if ECG findings are normal.[60,62] However, some youths are slow hydroxylators, which could increase plasma levels beyond expected ranges.[60]

Side Effects and Complications

Systematic studies of adverse effects in adolescents are lacking. Most of the adverse effects noted in adults also occur with adolescents, particularly anticholinergic effects, although these are usually mild and do not interfere with ongoing treatment.[61,62] The most common anticholinergic effects are probably dry mouth and constipation, and less commonly blurred vision and urinary retention.[61]

Cardiovascular effects occur frequently, although again they rarely limit treatment.[61,62] The most common is mild tachycardia. Mild cardiac conduction delays may also be observed, including increase in P-R interval and QRS complex and nonspecific intraventricular conduction delays. Tricyclics may increase youths' blood pressure,[63] but serious hypertension is uncommon. Also uncommon is orthostatic hypotension. A preexisting sinus arrhythmia does not preclude treatment with a tricyclic, which may in fact regulate the sinus arrhythmia, similar to the effect noted in geriatric patients.

Potentially serious complications occur less commonly, but may be fatal. These include heart blocks and arrhythmias with conduction slowing, leading to seriously impaired cardiac function. The immature cardiac system appears to be susceptible to the cardiotoxic effects of the tricyclic antidepressants.[60,61] Younger adolescents may have risks similar to those of children. However, the spontaneous sudden deaths observed in a small cluster of 8- to 9-year-olds treated with desipramine[64,65] have not been reported with adolescents. Large increases in the P-R interval (to greater than 0.21 second) or in the QRS complex (to greater than 0.12 second) should be considered potentially lethal. Pulses up to 120 beats/minute are common, but values above this need to be closely followed and may require discontinuation of the medication.[59–62]

Central nervous system (CNS) effects that should be considered serious include confusional states[59,61] and the induction of mania or psychoses. There has been concern that the early treatment of child and adolescent depressions with medications may accelerate an underlying bipolar disorder. Seizures may be more common in youths than in adults, resulting from a reduced seizure threshold due to CNS immaturity.[59]

Discontinuing a tricyclic antidepressant may lead to withdrawal effects, especially in younger adolescents, because of the greater rate of metabolism of these medications.[66] These effects have been attributed to the withdrawal of anticholinergic effects. Some youths may even demonstrate withdrawal effects daily, if receiving once-daily dosing. These withdrawal symptoms include a flu-like syndrome, sleep disturbances, and psychic or motoric activation.[61,66] For youths experiencing these effects, gradual decreases and more frequent dosing schedules are indicated.

Ryan and colleagues[54] reported that adolescents tolerated MAOIs and the dietary guidelines well, with mo major adverse effects. Reports of the use of fluoxetine 10 to 40 mg/day in nondepressive adolescent disorders note that the major side effects included behavioral activation in both verbal and motoric functions and mild gastrointestinal distress.[67–69] These symptoms were evident within the first few days of therapy. No adverse cardiovascular effects were noted on ECGs, blood pressure, or pulse.

Monitoring Medications and Somatic Response

Before starting an antidepressant each adolescent should receive a physical examination.[61] Height and weight should be followed twice yearly. Baseline laboratory assessment should include a urinalysis, complete blood count (CBC), and ECG. Many clinicians also advise a chemistry panel to assess hepatic and renal functions, and thyroid studies. The ECG is crucial before starting a tricyclic antidepressant. An ECG or rhythm strip should also be obtained at each dose increase. The ECG guidelines for continuing the tricyclic antidepressants are as follows[61]: P-R interval less than or equal to 0.21 seconds, QRS complex widening to no more than 30 per cent over baseline complex width, heart rate no greater than 130 beats/minute, systolic blood pressure no greater than 130 mm Hg, and diastolic blood pressure no greater than 85 mm Hg. Since adolescence is a time of rapid growth and endocrine change, plasma monitoring is recommended to assure maintenance of therapeutic levels.

Psychotherapy

Psychotherapy is an umbrella term covering a vast array of individual, family, and group therapy approaches. Although many papers devote themselves to issues related to the treatment of depressed youths or case reports, few actual treatment outcome studies are available. The following review focuses on treatment outcome studies only.

Efficacy of Psychotherapy

FAMILY AND INDIVIDUAL PSYCHOTHERAPY

The literature on systematic, controlled studies of family approaches to the treatment of depression in adolescents is very limited.[70] Furthermore, recent reviews of both behavioral and nonbehavioral psychotherapy with children and adolescents indicate that no well-controlled studies of individual approaches to mood disorders have been reported.[71,72] Barnett and colleagues[71] reviewed the nonbehavioral individual psychotherapy studies from the last 27 years (43 studies) and found that most studies "lack clear specification of the nature of the problems of the group included for study."

Werry and Wollersheim's[72] review of the behavior therapy literature from the last 20 years also found no studies directed specifically toward the depressive syndrome or symptom complex. They did, however, find many reports of successful behavioral interventions with anxiety symptoms, particularly separation anxiety and simple fears, suggesting that at least some of the symptomology that occurs concomitantly with depression can be successfully addressed. It should be noted, however, that separation anxiety seen in younger children has been the major focus of study. Werry and Wollersheim[72] cautioned that separation anxiety seen in adolescence has not been carefully investigated and may constitute a more treatment-resistant problem.

GROUP THERAPY

In contrast to the scarcity of studies of individual or family approaches, there is a small but very encouraging literature on group approaches to treatment of depression in late childhood and adolescence. All of these studies explored the use of strategies adapted from interventions effective with adults. Most build on cognitive and behavioral theoretical models of depression. Elements of three models are particularly represented: Beck et al.'s[73] model of the negative view of self, world, future, and importance of underlying negative cognitions; Rehm's[74] self-control model, in which depression is perpetuated by the establishment of excessive standards, inaccurate monitoring of performance, and little self-reinforcement; and Lewinson's[75] model, which posits inadequate social skills and overall loss of positive reinforcement as central features that maintain depression.

In one of the earliest reports, Butler and colleagues[76] described the use of two group intervention techniques with 10- to 12-year-olds identified as "withdrawn, self-deprecating, and underachieving." The groups included a roleplay group with focus on problem solving and social skills; a cognitive restructuring group that taught skills related to negative thinking; a placebo attention group; and a no-treatment group. Child and teacher reports were used to assess change, and both active interventions were associated with greater improvement in index symptoms than the control groups, with the roleplay group showing greatest gains.

Reynolds and Coats,[77] using a multistage process to screen a high school population for depressed students, investigated the relative efficacy of two brief interventions: cognitive-behavioral versus relaxation training therapy. A wait-list control was also included. Both treatment groups were associated with greater improvement in measures of depression at the end of the treatment program and also at the 5-week follow-up evaluation, but no significant differences between treatment groups were found.

Stark and colleagues[78] conducted a similar study with 9- to 12-year-olds using self-control and behavioral problem solving therapeutic approaches, again with a wait-list control group. Subjects were also identified via a multilevel screening of a school-based population, and in both studies the therapy was conducted at the school. Again the therapeutic interventions proved to be associated with greater reduction in depressive symptomology at the completion of therapy and at follow-up than did the wait-list control condition. There were no consistent findings of differences between the two therapeutic approaches.

A fourth school-based study has been reported by Kahn and colleagues[79] utilizing the same multistage screening process to identify depressed students from a middle school sample. They included a cognitive-behavioral treatment cell that was modeled on Clarke and Lewinsohn's[80] Coping with Depression Course for adolescents, a relaxation therapy cell, a self-modeling treatment cell, and a wait-list control group. Interventions were brief—12 sessions over a 6- to 8-week period—and follow-up evaluations were completed at the end of treatment and then at 1 month after treatment. Post-treatment evaluations revealed improvement in depression for all three treatment groups in contrast to the wait-list controls. More students in the cognitive-behavioral and relaxation groups showed clinical improvement that persisted through the 1-month follow-up period.

These studies provide support for the use of structured, time-limited, school-based interventions in the treatment of depression in young people. The implications of this work are limited because all four studies drew from school-based rather than clinical samples and none used the DSM-III or Research Diagnostic Criteria for identification of major depression. Therefore, the results may apply only to those youths with mild to moderate depressive disorders that have not required clinical attention. Further drawbacks are the small sample sizes reflected in each study (9 to 17 per treatment group), the limited time of follow-up evaluations (4 to 5 weeks), and the fact that not all follow-up evaluators were blind to the experimental conditions.[79]

Two recently published studies have employed group techniques with clinical populations of depressed youths.[81,82] Both have used structured diagnostic interviews to establish depression and have identified groups of youths with major depression, minor or intermittent depression, or, in a minority of cases, dysthymia. Fine and colleagues[81] compared a social skills training group intervention with a therapeutic support group but did not include a wait-list control group. The interventions each consisted of weekly meetings for 12 weeks with follow-up evaluations at the conclusion of treatment and again 9 months after treatment. The results indicated greater initial improvement in the subjects who participated in the less structured therapeutic support group, although those in the social skills group appeared to have made equal gains by the 9-month follow-up. The investigators hypothesized that, for those in the social skills group, there was a latency period before their depressed mood remitted and their new skills jelled. It is not clear what role the social skills training was thought to play in the actual remission of the depressed mood.

In the most carefully designed study to date, Lewinsohn and colleagues[82,83] compared two versions of their Coping with Depression Course for Adolescents (CDCA) and a wait-list control. The CDCA is a psychoeducational approach that teaches skills in the areas of relaxation, pleasant event scheduling, constructive thinking, social skills, communication negotiation, and problem solving. The two treatment cells differed in that one included a parent intervention component and the other involved direct intervention with the adolescents only. The outcome indicated improvement in both treatment conditions in contrast to the wait-list control, with a trend toward greater gains in the group with parent involvement. Positive treatment effect was retained at the 2-year follow-up. The study was carefully designed and executed; however, implications for clinical efficacy are limited given the small samples involved, especially in the follow-up, and the inclusion of only depressed young people with no co-occurring diagnoses.

Clinical Implications

Although these studies have not yet isolated treatment components key to alleviating depression, they do provide important information that can be applied to clinical work with adolescents. The studies suggest that certain techniques are effective, at least in group work with moderately depressed adolescents. Application of similar approaches in individual work seems feasible and allows the clinician to draw upon intervention strategies in which initial efficacy has been shown. These techniques include the use of relaxation training. The training utilized in these studies follows a straightforward format beginning with the introduction of information regarding the relation between anxiety, stress, and depression, then teaching progressive relaxation skills, including practice of new skills as homework. Training in muscle relaxation, use of mental imagery in relaxation, and generalization of relaxation skills is incorporated.

In the self-control[77,78,79] framework, young people are taught, in a psychoeducational approach, how to monitor mood, pleasant events, and positive self-statements as well as how to increase self-reinforcement and decrease self-punishment. Similarly, problem-solving and social skills training are presented using a didactic, skill-building approach. Finally, Lewinsohn and colleagues[82,83] have incorporated many of these elements into one course that also includes communication and problem-solving skills. This model suggests an avenue for addressing some of the relevant family issues by teaching communication and problem-solving skills to both parents and adolescents.

While most of the studies utilized specific skills that can be adapted for individual work, Fine et al.[81] found a less structured, more traditional process group to be more effective than social skills training. This suggests that the group process itself, rather than specific skill building, may be the important element that is effective with adolescents. However, not all group approaches were equally effective. The combination of skills that teach young people how to handle their depression per se, as well as the related social problems, that was utilized in some of these studies may be central to an enduring, effective intervention.

Finally, some preliminary thoughts regarding age and therapy strategy may also be drawn from these initial studies. The more strictly cognitive interventions (e.g., identification of automatic thoughts) did not appear as effective with young adolescents as those that incorporated more concrete social and problem-solving skills training.[76] This may reflect the more concrete thinking of the younger adolescent.

CONCLUSIONS AND RECOMMENDATIONS

The available data do not suggest a clear protocol for the treatment of depression during adolescence. Efficacy of pharmacotherapy has not been established and, although more promising, the group psychotherapy data are still preliminary. Moreover, while there is an abundant adult literature on the relative and combined benefits of medications and psychotherapy, such studies are not yet available on adolescents. Meanwhile, the clinician is faced with severely depressed adolescents, many of whom have coexisting disorders and multiple psychosocial stressors. The studies to date represent an important beginning but do not address the treatment complexities of the clinical population. They do, however, offer some guidelines.

It appears at this time that medication should not be considered as the primary therapy or first form of intervention offered. The practicing clinician needs to use medication interventions judiciously, not resorting to medication too early in treatment but not denying an individual adolescent the possible benefits of a medication trial. In most cases primary intervention with introduction of relaxation, cognitive, social and problem-solving skills allows the clinician to introduce effective coping tools. Parallel family assessment/intervention is indicated. Individuals or families with more complex diagnostic makeup, more dysfunctional systems, or inadequate response to these initial interventions might then require ongoing individual or family treatment or the addition of a medication trial.

More immediate use of medications would be considered in those cases in which the adolescent has significant, pervasive vegetative or psychotic features, or both. Use of medication as a conjoint treatment modality appears more indicated when the adolescent presents with persistent depressive symptoms that do not suggest an acute reaction to stress or an underlying longstanding dysthymia. Adolescents in stable, well-functioning families with positive family histories of affective disorder and responsivity to medication may be mostly likely to benefit from the addition of a medication.

Finally, special consideration must be given to those adolescents with suicidal ideation and behaviors. There is no proven treatment approach for dealing with the suicidal youths. In all cases careful assessment of risk factors and intent, coupled with repeated follow-ups to assess ongoing risk, are indicated. Initial intervention focus is typically on the need to hospitalize, and only after the youth is more stable are long-term treatment decisions made. Strategies regarding longer term treatment differ with the individual case. Suicide in adolescents is frequently associated with significant depression, but many suicidal young people have other primary diagnoses, including conduct disorders and substance abuse. Impulsivity is more highly associated with suicidal behavior in young people than in adults. Thus for each case the type of therapy, pharmacological and psychological, depends in great part on the primary psychiatric problem presented. The treatment of the depressed, suicidal adolescent would follow the same guidelines and suffer the same limitations as outlined above. Special consideration must be given to choice and management if medication is considered in light of the risk for overdose and the lethality of some antidepressant medications.

REFERENCES

1. Fleming JE, Offord DR: Epidemiology of childhood depressive disorder. J Am Acad Child Adolesc Psychiatry 29:571, 1990.
2. Kashani J, Simonds JF: The incidence of depression in children. Am J Psychiatry 136:1203, 1979.
3. Klerman GL: The current age of youthful melancholia: Evidence for increase in depression among adolescents and young adults. Br J Psychiatry 152:4, 1988.
4. Strober M, Green J, Carlson G: Phenomenology and subtypes of major depressive disorder in adolescence. J Affective Disord 5:37, 1981.
5. Kashani JH, Carlson GA: Seriously depressed preschoolers. Am J Psychiatry 144:348, 1987.
6. Kovacs M, Feinberg TL, Crouse-Novak MA, et al: Depressive disorders in childhood: I. A longitudinal prospective study of characteristics and recovery. Arch Gen Psychiatry 41:229, 1984.
7. Rutter M: The developmental psychopathology of depression: Issues and perspectives. In Rutter M, Izard CE, Read PB, eds. Depression in Young People: Developmental and Clinical Perspectives. New York: Guilford Press, 1986:38.
8. Mitchell J, McCauley E, Burke PM, et al: Phenomenology of depression in children and adolescents. J Am Acad Child Adolesc Psychiatry 27:12, 1988.
9. Ryan ND, Puig-Antich J, Ambrosini P, et al: The clinical picture of major depression in children and adolescents. Arch Gen Psychiatry 44:854, 1987.
10. Smith M, Mitchell J, Corey L, et al: Chronic fatigue in adolescents. Pediatrics 88:195, 1991.
11. Baker M, Dorzab J, Winokur G, et al: Depressive disease: Classification and clinical characteristics. Compr Psychiatry 12:354, 1971.
12. McGee R, Williams S: A longitudinal study of depression in nine-year-old children. J Am Acad Child Adolesc Psychiatry 27:342, 1988.
13. Bernstein GA: Comorbidity and severity of anxiety and depressive disorders in a clinic sample. J Am Acad Child Adolesc Psychiatry 30:43, 1991.
14. Strauss CC: Anxiety disorders of childhood and adolescence. School Psychol Rev 19:143, 1990.
15. Puig-Antich J, Rabinovich H: Relationship between affective and anxiety disorders in childhood. In Gittelman R, ed.

Anxiety Disorders of Childhood. New York: Guilford Press, 1986:136.

16. Kovacs M, Feinberg TL, Crouse-Novak M, et al: Depressive disorders in childhood: II. A longitudinal study of the risk for subsequent major depression. Arch Gen Psychiatry 41:643, 1984.

17. Strober M, Carlson G: Bipolar illness in adolescents with major depression. Arch Gen Psychiatry 39:549, 1982.

18. McCauley E, Myers K, Calderon R, et al: Three year follow-up of depressed youth. Paper presented at the Society for Research in Child and Adolescent Psychopathology, Costa Mesa, CA, January 1990.

19. Harrington R, Fudge H, Rutter M, et al: Adult outcomes of childhood and adolescent depression. Arch Gen Psychiatry 47:465, 1990.

20. Kandel DB, Davies M: Adult sequelae of adolescent depressive symptoms. Arch Gen Psychiatry 43:255, 1986.

21. Kashani JH, Burk BA, Reid JC: Depressed children of depressed parents. Can J Psychiatry 30:265, 1984.

22. Kashani JH, Burk BA, Horwitz B, et al: Differential effect of subtype of major affective disorder on children. Psychiatry Res 15:195, 1985.

23. Keller MB, Beardslee WR, Dorer DJ, et al: Impact of severity and chronicity of parental affective illness on adaptive functioning and psychopathology in children. Arch Gen Psychiatry 43:930, 1986.

24. Gammon GD, John K, et al: Children of depressed parents: Increased psychopathology and early onset of major depression. Arch Gen Psychiatry 44:487, 1987.

25. Mitchell J, McCauley E, Burke P, et al: Psychopathology in parents of depressed children and adolescents. J Am Acad Child Adolesc Psychiatry 28:352, 1989.

26. Puig-Antich J, Goetz D, Davies M, et al: A controlled family history study of prepubertal major depressive disorder. Arch Gen Psychiatry 46:406, 1989.

27. Strober M: Familial aspects of depressive disorder in early adolescence. In Weller EB, Weller RA, eds. An Update of Childhood Depression. Washington, DC: American Psychiatric Press, Inc., 1984:38.

28. Crumley FE, Clenenger J, Steinfink D: Preliminary report on the dexamethasone suppression test for psychiatrically disturbed adolescents. Am J Psychiatry 139:942, 1982.

29. Robbins DR: Preliminary report on the dexamethasone suppression test in adolescents. Am J Psychiatry 139:942, 1983.

30. Hsu GLK, Molcan K, Cashman MA, et al: The dexamethasone suppression test in adolescent depression. J Am Acad Child Adolesc Psychiatry 22:470, 1983.

31. Targum SD, Capadanno AE: The dexamethasone suppression test in adolescent psychiatric inpatients. Am J Psychiatry 140:589, 1983.

32. Jensen JB, Garfinkel BD: Growth hormone dysregulation in children with major depressive disorder. J Am Acad Child Adolesc Psychiatry 29:295, 1990.

33. Kutcher SP, Williamson P, Silverberg J, et al. Nocturnal growth hormone secretion in depressed older adolescents. J Am Acad Child Adolesc Psychiatry 27:751, 1988.

34. Emslie GJ, Roffwarg HP, Rush AJ, et al: Sleep EEG findings in depressed children and adolescents. Am J Psychiatry 144:668, 1987.

35. Goetz RR, Puig-Antich J, Ryan N, et al: Electroencephalographic sleep of adolescents with major depression and normal controls. Arch Gen Psychiatry 44:61, 1987.

36. Lahmeyer JW, Poznanski EO, Bellur SN: Sleep in depressed adolescents. Am J Psychiatry 140:1150, 1983.

37. Liebowitz MR, Quitkin FM, Stewart JW, et al. Phenelzine v. imipramine in atypical depression. Arch Gen Psychiatry 41:669, 1984.

38. Preskorn SH, Weller EB, Weller RA: Depression in children: Relationship between plasma imipramine levels and response. J Clin Psychiatry 43:450, 1982.

39. Weller EB, Weller RA, Preskorn SH, et al: Steady-state plasma imipramine levels in prepubertal depressed children. Am J Psychiatry 139:506, 1982.

40. Conners CK, Petti T: Imipramine therapy of depressed children: Methodologic considerations. Psychopharmacol Bull 19:65, 1983.

41. Brumback RA, Stanton RD: Neuropsychological study of children during and after remission of endogenous depressive episodes. Percept Mot Skills 50:1163, 1980.

42. Stanton RD, Wilson H, Brumback RA: Cognitive improvement associated with tricyclic antidepressant treatment of childhood major depressive illness. Percept Mot Skills 53:219, 1981.

43. Geller B, Perel JM, Knitter EF, et al: Nortriptyline in major depressive disorder in children: Response, steady-state plasma levels, predictive kinetics, and pharmacokinetics. Psychopharmacol Bull 19:62, 1983.

44. Kashani JH, Shekim WO, Reid JC: Amitriptyline in children with major depressive disorder: A double blind cross-over pilot study. J Am Acad Child Adolesc Psychiatry 23:348, 1984.

45. Puig-Antich J, Perel JM, Lupatkin W, et al: Imipramine in prepubertal major depressive disorders. Arch Gen Psychiatry 44:81, 1987.

46. Geller B, Cooper TB, McCombs HG, et al: Double blind, placebo-controlled study of nortriptyline in depressed children using a "fixed plasma level" design. Psychopharmacol Bull 25:101, 1989.

47. Preskorn SH, Weller EB, Hughes CW, et al: Depression in prepubertal children: Dexamethasone nonsuppression predicts differential response to imipramine vs. placebo. Psychopharmacol Bull 23:128, 1987.

48. Kramer AD, Feiguine RJ: Clinical effects of amitriptyline in adolescent depression. A pilot study. J Am Acad Child Adolesc Psychiatry 20:636, 1981.

49. Geller B: A double-blind placebo-controlled study of nortriptyline in adolescents with major depression. New Clinical Drug Evaluation Unit (NCDEU) Annual Meeting Abstracts. Washington, DC: National Institute of Mental Health, 1989.

50. Ryan ND, Puig-Antich J, Cooper TB, et al: Imipramine in adolescent major depression: Plasma level and clinical response. Acta Psychiatr Scand 73:275, 1986.

51. Strober M: Effects of imipramine, lithium, and fluoxetine in the treatment of adolescent major depression. New Drug Evaluation Unit (NCDEU) Annual Meeting Abstracts. Washington, DC: National Institute of Mental Health, 1989.

52. Simeon JG: Pediatric psychopharmacology. Can J Psychiatry 34:115, 1989.

53. Lapierre YD, Ravel KJ: Pharmacotherapy of affective disorders in children and adolescents. Psychiatry Clin North Am 12:951, 1989.

54. Ryan ND, Puig-Antich J, Rabinovich H, et al: MAOIs in adolescent major depression unresponsive to tricyclic antidepressants. J Am Acad Child Adolesc Psychiatry 27:755, 1988.

55. Ryan ND, Meyer V, Dachille S, et al: Lithium antidepressant augmentation in TCA-refractory depression in adolescents. J Am Acad Child Adolesc Psychiatry 27:371, 1988.

56. Geller B, Cooper TB, Chestnut E, et al: Nortriptyline pharmacokinetic parameters in depressed children and adolescents: Preliminary data. J Clin Psychopharmacol 4:265, 1984.

57. Geller B, Cooper TB, Chestnut EC: Serial monitoring and achievement of steady state nortriptyline plasma levels in depressed children and adolescents: Preliminary data. J Clin Psychopharmacol 5:213, 1985.

58. Geller B, Cooper TB, Chestnut EC, et al: Child and adolescent nortriptyline single dose kinetics predict steady state plasma levels and suggested dose: Preliminary data. J Clin Psychopharmacol 5:154, 1985.

59. Preskorn SH, Weller EB, Weller RA, et al: Plasma levels of imipramine and adverse effects in children. Am J Psychiatry 140:1332, 1983.

60. Preskorn SH, Bupp SJ, Weller EB, et al: Plasma levels of

imipramine and metabolites in 68 hospitalized children. J Am Acad Child Adolesc Psychiatry 28:373, 1989.

61. Ryan ND: Heterocyclic antidepressants in children and adolescents. J Child Adolesc Psychopharmacol 1:21, 1990.

62. Campbell M, Spencer EK: Psychopharmacology in child and adolescent psychiatry: A review of the past five years. J Am Acad Child Adolesc Psychiatry 27:269, 1988.

63. Lake CR, Mikkelsen EJ, Rapoport JL, et al: Effect of imipramine on norepinephrine and blood pressure in enuretic boys. Clin Pharmacol Ther 39:647, 1979.

64. Riddle MA, Nelson JC, Kleinman CS, et al: Sudden death in children receiving Norpramin: A review of three reported cases and commentary. J Am Acad Sci Adolesc Psychiatry 30:104, 1991.

65. Biederman J: Sudden death in children treated with a tricyclic antidepressant: A commentary. Biol Ther Psychiatry 14:1, 1991.

66. Dilsaver SC, Greden JF: Antidepressant withdrawal phenomena. Biol Psychiatry 19:237, 1984.

67. Riddle MA, Hardin MT, King R, et al: Fluoxetine treatment of children and adolescents with Tourette's and obsessive compulsive disorders: Preliminary clinical experience. J Am Acad Child Adolesc Psychiatry 29:45, 1990.

68. Gwirtzman HE, Guze BH, Yager J, et al: Treatment of anorexia nervosa with fluoxetine: An open clinical trial. J Clin Psychiatry 51:378, 1990.

69. Riddle MA, Brown N, Dzubinski D, et al: Fluoxetine overdose in an adolescent. J Am Acad Child Adolesc Psychiatry 28:587, 1989.

70. Shaw JA: Childhood depression. Med Clin North Am 72:831, 1988.

71. Barnett RJ, Docherty JP, Frommelt GM: A review of child psychotherapy research since 1963. J Am Acad Child Adolesc Psychiatry 30:1, 1991.

72. Werry JS, Wollersheim JP: Behavior therapy with children and adolescents: A twenty-year overview. J Am Acad Child Adolesc Psychiatry 28:1, 1989.

73. Beck At, Rush AJ, Shaw BF, et al: Cognitive Theory of Depression. New York: Guilford Press, 1979.

74. Rehm LP: A self-control model of depression. Behav Ther 8:787–804, 1977.

75. Lewinsohn PM: A behavioral approach to depression. In Friedman RJ, Katz MM, eds. The Psychology of Depression: Contemporary Theory and Research. Washington, DC: Winston-Wiley, 1974:157.

76. Butler L, Miezitis S, Friedman R, et al: The effect of two school-based intervention programs on depressive symptoms in preadolescents. Am Educ Res J 17:110, 1980.

77. Reynolds WM, Coats KI: A comparison of cognitive-behavioral therapy and relaxation training for the treatment of depression in adolescents. J Consult Clin Psychol 54:653, 1986.

78. Stark KD, Reynolds WM, Kaslow NJ: A comparison of the relative efficacy of self-control therapy and a behavioral problem-solving therapy for depression in children. J Abnorm Child Psychol 15:91, 1987.

79. Kahn JS, Kehle TJ, Jenson WR, et al: Comparison of cognitive-behavioral, relaxation, and self-modeling interventions for depression among middle-school students. School Psychol Rev 19:196, 1990.

80. Clarke GN, Lewinsohn PM: The Coping with Depression Course—Adolescent Version: A psychoeducational intervention for unipolar depression in high school students. Unpublished manuscript, Oregon Research Institute, Eugene, 1986.

81. Fine S, Forth A, Gilbert M, et al: Group therapy for adolescent depressive disorder: A comparison of social skills and therapeutic support. J Am Acad Child Adolesc Psychiatry 30:79, 1991.

82. Lewinsohn PM, Clarke GN, Hops H, et al: Cognitive-behavioral treatment for depressed adolescents. Behav Ther 21:385, 1990.

83. Clarke G, Lewinsohn P, Hops H: Leader's Manual, Adolescent Coping with Depression Course. Eugene, OR: Castalia Publishing Company, 1990.

71

SAFETY OF PSYCHOTROPIC AGENTS IN THE TREATMENT OF CHILD AND ADOLESCENT DISORDERS

ALAN S. UNIS, M.D.

By conservative estimates, 10 to 15 per cent of the child and adolescent population of the United States is afflicted with psychiatric disorders. This chapter provides a framework for evaluating the safety of psychotropic agents for children and adolescents. By examining the components of safety, it is possible to obtain a preliminary sense of the risks that the physician assumes when administering psychotropic agents to young patients. Some practical methods to minimize the most common risks associated with drug treatment, as well as some suggestions for case management, are included.

COMPREHENSIVE ASSESSMENT OF DISORDER

The DSM-III-R describes and summarizes the American Psychiatric Association's system for classifying psychiatric disorders. The DSM-III-R utilizes specific criteria for diagnosing a psychiatric disorder. Such criteria (in the absence of a specific underlying pathophysiological process) are, furthermore, the sole means for monitoring the course of the disorder and its response to treatment with psychotropic agents. A comprehensive DSM-III-R diagnosis entails the collection of clinical data using clinical interviews, psychometric testing, and the physical examination.

Comprehensive assessment of the young patient requires the development of a clinical data base from multiple information sources. The historical information obtained from the primary caregiving parent (usually the mother) is generally reliable and correlates well with direct observations of the child.[1,2] However, the presence of psychiatric disorder in the parent must also be determined during the clinical assessment. A number of adult disorders (e.g., depression) introduce predictable biases in reporting that result in a decrease in the specificity of clinical problems and an exaggeration of clinical severity.

Information obtained from teachers can be uniquely useful in describing a child or adolescent's response to demanding situations. Other family members (e.g., grandparents) and involved social agency professionals can likewise provide valuable clinical information. Standardized clinical questionnaires have become an indispensable component of the evaluation of child and adolescent psychopathology. Questionnaires can be subdivided into those that assay specific episodes of a clinical phenomenon (e.g., those that count behaviors) and those that more globally describe clinical symptoms or behaviors. The Child Behavior Checklist (CBCL) is an example of a globally oriented questionnaire that can be completed by parents, teachers, and the patient (if 11 years or older) and that assays a broad range of symptomatic behavior.[3] Intellectual and academic achievement testing are indispensable components of the psychiatric evaluation when a history of school maladjustment is elicited, even in the absence of poor grades.

The physical examination is as important as the mental status examination in children and adolescents with psychiatric symptoms and warrants completion prior to the initiation of any medication trial. Clinical history and physical examination are still the best predictors of abnormal laboratory test results. Thus, laboratory tests should be obtained only when clinical judgment dictates rather than in a "screening" fashion.[4] Obviously, some psychotropic agents require baseline laboratory studies, such as an electrocardiogram, prior to treatment with a tricyclic antidepressant. Such testing falls more into the realm of management than diagnosis in that normal values are expected.

TARGET AND BASELINE AGENT-RESPONSIVE SYMPTOMS

Targeting is the identification of specific clinical symptoms or behaviors that are the focus of (drug) treatment. The clinician should select a means of following symptoms across settings and take advantage of the unique strengths of the various historians who contributed to the initial evaluation of the patient. Whenever possible, a consistent review of the patient's concurrent clinical status in comparison to that obtained in the initial history can be supplemented using a list of standard questions developed from the clinical history. Standardized questionnaires (which tend to be developed for evaluating symptom severity in selected disorders) may not be relevant to the specific clinical presentation of a patient. Some psychiatric symptoms (and their drug responsiveness) are common to a number of child and adolescent disorders. Psychotic symptoms are the best example of this phenomenon. Standardized questionnaires can never the less be extremely useful in targeting if such questionnaires are relevant to the clinical presentation of the patient (Table 71–1). It should be remembered, however, that standardized questionnaires are developed to supplement clinical assessment and assay only a narrow aspect of the patient's presentation.

Baselining requires the repeated measurement, using some of the procedures or instruments noted above, of the untreated symptoms or behaviors over a period of time that is considered clinically sufficient to establish the stability and severity of the disorder. A number of clinical realities curtail the acquisition of adequate baseline data. Life-threatening behaviors or symptoms, the incipient expulsion from or refusal to attend school, or even the approach of a camping trip in the young patient with enuresis or separation anxiety, for example, are all familiar events that force premature closure on therapeutic decision making. The length of the baseline period clearly will vary from case to case and situation to situation.

CHOOSING THE APPROPRIATE AGENT

Clinicians who prescribe psychotropic medications for young patients frequently choose agents based upon unsubstantiated beliefs that one drug is safer than another. For example, pemoline or the tricyclics are frequently used for attention-deficit hyperactivity disorder (ADHD) instead of the more efficacious psychostimulants, *d*-amphetamine and methylphenidate, because of the reported abuse potential of the latter. Likewise, trazodone or fluoxetine are preferred over the classical tricyclics, imip-

TABLE 71–1. EXAMPLES OF STANDARDIZED QUESTIONNAIRES AND RATING SCALES FOR ASSESSING CHILD AND ADOLESCENT PSYCHIATRIC DISORDERS[a]

	Standardized Questionnaires	
Assessment of	*Global Assessments*	*Direct Observational Assessments*
General psychopathology	Child Behavior Checklist[3]	Rutter-Graham Psychiatric Interview Children's Psychiatric Rating Scale
Disruptive behavior disorders	Connors Parent and Teacher Symptom Questionnaire	Continuous Performance Testing Classroom Observation Code
Tics and Tourette's syndrome	Yale Global Tic Severity Scale[8]	
Autism and pervasive developmental disorders	Child Autism Rating Scale	Timed Stereotypies Rating Scale
Mental retardation syndromes	Aberrant Behavior Checklist	
Anxiety disorders	Children's Manifest Anxiety Scale: Parent and Child forms	
Obsessive-compulsive disorder		Yale-Brown Obsessive Compulsive Scale[9,10]
Anorexia nervosa	Anorectic Attitude Questionnaire	Anorexic Behavior Scale
Depressive disorders	Bellevue Index of Depression Child Depression Inventory	School-age Depression Listed Inventory Depression Rating Scale, Revised

[a] Explanations of the instruments can be found in Rapoport and Conners[7] unless otherwise referenced.

ramine or desipramine, for major depressive episode because the potential for fatal overdosage is markedly diminished in the former even though efficacy of the latter in the child and adolescent disorder is somewhat better determined. Although understandable in its intent, this practice overlooks the fact that patients may not be optimally helped by choosing an agent based primarily upon hearsay rather than upon demonstrated therapeutic effects and side effects. A comprehensive working knowledge of a half-dozen or so effective agents is preferable to embarking upon a treatment with a newer, less characterized agent.

Once symptomatic behavior in a young patient is characterized, the clinician might consider listing the agents that have been reported as effective in treating such behaviors (Table 71–2). The potential agents, listed in order of the most characterized and effective to the least characterized and possibly effective, can then be systematically administered to the patient until an effective agent is found.

TABLE 71–2. EXAMPLE OF A POTENTIAL LIST OF PSYCHOTROPIC AGENTS BASED ON REPORTED EFFECTIVENESS FOR DISRUPTIVE BEHAVIOR DISORDERS[a]

Psychostimulants	d-Amphetamine Methylphenidate Pemoline
Tricyclic antidepressants	Imipramine Desipramine
Antihypertensives	Clonidine Propranolol
Anticonvulsants	Carbamazepine Valproic acid

[a] The agents are listed in order of more commonly to less commonly prescribed.

TABLE 71–3. FACTORS THAT MAY ASSIST THE CLINICIAN IN ASSESSING DESIRABLE AND UNDESIRABLE EFFECTS OF A GIVEN PSYCHOTROPIC AGENT[a]

Reports of effectiveness.
Reports clarifying therapeutic doses from toxic doses.
Reports of common as well as uncommon side effects during acute and chronic treatment.
Reports of carcinogenesis or growth retardation.
Reports of impaired school performance or diminished scores on formal cognitive testing.
Reports of teratogenesis or diminished fertility.

[a] Literature searches using any number of medical data bases (e.g., Medline, Teris, and Toxnet) will quickly identify useful articles.

By answering the following questions (see also Table 71–3), the clinician can determine the relative desirability of typical and atypical agents for the various child and adolescent psychiatric disorders.

1. Are there clinical studies to predict an average amount of improvement in relation to the baseline symptoms?

2. Is there a published therapeutic index (therapeutic dose/toxic dose) in children or adolescents?

3. Is there adequate clinical experience with the agent to predict the nature and incidence of acute and chronic side effects of the agent during a typical therapeutic trial?

4. Are there known developmental effects in terms of somatic maturation or cognitive functioning?

5. Are there any known reproductive risks that occur concurrent with treatment or that extend beyond the therapeutic trial?

6. What are the risks, based upon past behavior

or based upon what is known about the disorder, of *not* treating the patient with medications?

If these questions cannot be answered with any certainty, then medication treatment might be the more risky course in comparison to more traditional psychosocial interventions. This is not to say that medications should not be tried, but patients and their families should be able to embark upon a therapeutic drug trial after being informed as much as possible as to the nature of the risks involved. In fact, most patients and their families are not daunted by the risks if there is some hope of some symptomatic change.

EDUCATION OF THE PATIENT AND FAMILY

The ethical practice of medicine (and especially psychiatry) requires the clinician to educate the patient and the responsible caregivers regarding the nature of the disorder and the treatments being offered. The social and psychological sequelae of diagnostic labeling, the relative lack of complete information regarding the risks of treatment, and the relative inability to predict the specific effectiveness of the agent should be addressed before proceeding with a drug treatment. Handouts regarding the expected effects, side effects, and potential hazards of a particular drug are commonly available and should be used. An explanation to the child, in age-appropriate or developmentally appropriate terms, that a medicine is expected to help with a particular behavior or problem, goes a long way toward ensuring compliance.

BASELINE PHYSICAL PARAMETERS, LABORATORY STUDIES, AND SIDE EFFECTS REVIEW

Height, weight, and vital signs are generally obtained during the initial physical examination and are repeated during follow-up visits as indicated or no less than twice annually. Changes in clinical status or the emergence of new symptoms warrant reexamination of the patient.

There is not uniform agreement on which laboratory studies are absolutely indicated with the various agents. Serial monitoring of white cell counts tends to be unreliable in predicting carbamazepine-induced leukopenia. Nevertheless, the usual practice in the United States includes baseline and follow-up complete blood counts (CBCs). Serial electrocardiographic (ECG) monitoring during a trial of a tricyclic antidepressant, until recently, was probably less regularly obtained by most clinicians because of limited access to testing facilities. Most recent studies of the tricyclic antidepressants sug-

gest that such monitoring is indicated even though clinically relevant cardiotoxicity is unusual. Because the cardiac effects of the tricyclics correlate with serum concentration, the ECG is most likely to identify cardiac conduction anomalies when it is obtained during peak serum concentrations. Most clinicians, however, obtain trough serum samples to determine the adequacy of the daily dose and, while the patient is in the clinic, perform the ECG. This practice may not be adequate for identifying potentially life-threatening arrhythmias.

The review of systems obtained during the initial assessment permits the clinician to document those symptoms that might be substantially mistaken for side effects of a particular drug. The administration of the Subjective Treatment Emergent Side-Effects Scale (STESS) prior to initiating drug treatment likewise ensures that baseline physical complaints are not mistaken for treatment side effects.

DOSING STRATEGIES IN CHILDREN AND ADOLESCENTS

The most common preventable error in medicating a young patient is in failing to appreciate the individual and developmental differences in the absorption, distribution, and metabolism of the various psychotropic agents.[5] A number of factors are responsible for this variability in drug metabolism in children. Children tend to have a brisker absorption of almost any orally administered agent in comparison to infants and adults. Thus, orally administered agents frequently result in higher peak plasma concentrations that occur sooner than is seen after the same unit dose is given to an adult. In addition, a child's hepatic mass per kilogram of body weight is larger than an adult's. Thus, serum half-lives (the time from peak serum concentration to half-maximal serum concentration) of hepatically metabolized agents tend to be shorter. This increased efficiency in the absorption and metabolism of drugs together diminishes the overall steady state concentration of many psychotropic agents and supports the use of smaller multiple doses throughout the day over larger doses given in once- or twice-daily schedules.

In choosing a titration strategy, it is important to remember that the best predictor of subsequent compliance is the severity of acute side effects. Titration strategies that utilize low initial dosages and increase daily dosages based upon the patient's tolerance of side effects will be more likely to be successful. The completion of a review of systems or a STESS will permit the clinician to discriminate pre-existing physical symptoms from treatment-associated side effects. The reader is referred to Popper and Frazier[6] for detailed dosing protocols for many of the more commonly prescribed psychotropic agents for child and adolescent psychiatric disorders.

FOLLOW-UP

How soon or how often to see a patient back for follow-up is determined by a number of clinical and pharmacological factors. The obviously distressed patient or parent might be seen back more frequently (weekly or even semiweekly) even though a therapeutic response to a particular agent is not expected. During the titration with a tricyclic antidepressant for treatment of a mood disorder, more frequent visits might be warranted initially, perhaps in the context of obtaining appropriate laboratory studies, even though the clinical response would not be expected for as long as a month after a therapeutic serum concentration is achieved.

Clinical response, rather than patient distress, also might determine follow-up frequency. The child with ADHD will likely show a dramatic and quick response to psychostimulant treatment, and a follow-up appointment every other week during the titration phase of treatment should provide the clinician with adequate clinical data to determine whether to increase, maintain, or decrease the daily dose or adjust the daily schedule. Although a specific recommendation for follow-up cannot be uniformly made, the clinician should convey accessibility by providing an avenue for interim contact by telephone or by notifying the patient or parent of services available during evenings and weekends should questions arise before the next appointment.

Maintenance phase follow-up generally can be managed on a monthly basis or less, depending upon the degree of symptomatic relief and the expected length of treatment. Six months of continuous symptomatic remission for a major depressive episode is suggested before an attempt is made to wean the antidepressant. A monthly review of symptomatic relief is warranted in such a case. The child with ADHD may require monthly prescription refills, but generally a quarterly review of behavioral symptoms, potential chronic side effects, growth and vital signs, and social and academic adjustment is sufficient.

Other therapeutic interventions are likely indicated in the majority of disorders that afflict children and adolescents. Individual, group, and family therapies, social skills training, behavioral parenting education, and educational supplementation all require a degree of follow-up over and above that which is provided for medication management.

UNSUCCESSFUL TRIALS

Establishing criteria for an unsuccessful trial, either by virtue of unacceptable side effects or by virtue of drug nonresponsiveness, will create some a priori expectations about when a new agent is warranted. A failure to obtain partial or complete symptomatic relief after the administration of an adequate dose for a sufficient period of time, or the development of intolerable side effects on doses that are inadequate to provide any symptomatic relief, is not unusual. Assuring the patient of such is important before a new agent is tried.

Invariably, clinicians will encounter the patient with some symptomatic relief and some troublesome side effects on perfectly acceptable doses of a drug. The belief that the next agent will be better than the present one is best pursued after reviewing the initial assessment and the course of treatment.

Specific protocols for weaning a drug are not always explicitly discussed as part of most overall drug treatment protocols. A number of psychotropic agents are associated with specific withdrawal syndromes. Sudden withdrawal of imipramine after therapeutic doses can result in a flu-like syndrome attributed to cholinergic rebound. Antipsychotic withdrawal can be associated with orofacial dyskinesia or acute dystonic reactions. Carbamazepine withdrawal may precipitate a seizure even in the patient with no previous history or epilepsy. By gradually decreasing the daily dose by some convenient fraction of the maximal dose, such withdrawal-emergent symptoms can be attenuated.

SOCIAL AND PROFESSIONAL RESPONSIBILITIES

Clinicians who prescribe psychotropic agents to children and adolescents have a unique responsibility to these patients and to the practice of medicine to report unusual effects of the various agents to the Food and Drug Administration or to an appropriate journal for professional review. This is especially true in the case of agents that have come to market without specific testing in children and adolescents. The apprehension that one may have wrongly prescribed an agent must be countered by the need to educate colleagues and share clinical experiences. Under the current system of approving and marketing psychotropic agents, only physicians who prescribe such agents are in a position to actually describe and report the effects of their use.

REFERENCES

1. Rutter M, Graham P: The reliability and validity of the psychiatric assessment of the child. I: Interview with the child. Br J Psychiatry 114:563–579, 1968.
2. Graham P, Rutter M: The reliability and validity of the psychiatric assessment of the child. II: Interview with the parent. Br J Psychiatry 14:581–592, 1968.
3. Achenbach TM, Edelbrock C: Manual for the Child Behavior Checklist, and Revised Child Behavior Profile. Queen City Printers, Inc., 1983.
4. Ricciuti A, Morton R, Behar D, Delaney MA: Medical findings in child psychiatric inpatients. J Am Acad Child Adolesc Psychiatry 26:554–559, 1987.
5. Biederman J, Ross J, et al: A double-blind placebo controlled

study of desipramine in the treatment of ADD: II. Serum drug levels and cardiovascular findings. J Am Acad Child Adolesc Psychiatry 28:903–911, 1989.

6. Popper CW, Frazier SH, eds: J Child Adolesc Psychopharmacol 1(1):1–103, 1990.

7. Rapoport J, Conners CK, eds: Rating scales and assessment instruments for use in pediatric psychopharmacology research. Psychopharmacol Bull 21(4):1113–1125, 1985.

8. Leckman JF, Riddle MA, et al: The Yale Global Tic Severity Scale: Initial testing of a clinician-rated scale of tic severity. J Am Acad Child Adolesc Psychiatry 28:566–573, 1989.

9. Goodman WK, Price LH, et al: The Yale-Brown Obsessive Compulsive Scale. I. Development, use and reliability. Arch Gen Psychiatry 46:1006–1011, 1989.

10. Goodman WK, Price LH, et al: The Yale-Brown Obsessive Compulsive Scale. II. Validity. Arch Gen Psychiatry 46:1012–1016, 1989.

Section L

TREATMENT IN THE MEDICAL SETTING

72

PSYCHIATRIC EMERGENCIES

CHRISTOS S. DAGADAKIS, M.D., M.P.H.

Effective management of psychiatric disorders requires a systematic assessment and treatment approach. Overlearned, practiced approaches maximize the likelihood that essential elements will be completed accurately even in high-stress and time-pressured situations. A sequential format can help structure the efforts for care. A sequence of evaluation that is particularly useful in psychiatric emergencies involves first making a screening for level of urgency and safety, followed by screening for medical problems and etiology for the mental disorder, psychosis, substance abuse, and nonpsychotic disorder. Based on the above sequential evaluation, the patient's history and interest in care, and available care options, a treatment plan can be developed and put into operation.

SCREENING FOR URGENCY AND SAFETY

Maximizing safety for the caregiver and the patient is a primary element for emergent care. The risk that the individual may harm himself or herself or others needs to be rapidly assessed. Once safety is addressed, a determination can be made of how soon the individual needs to be seen and the appropriate requirements for assessment.

Risk to Self

Immediate risk to self can be determined by assessing the following elements: (1) presentation or history of a recent attempt at self-harm or behavior resulting in risk to self, (2) statements about suicidal ideation and/or intent to harm himself or herself, (3) command hallucinations for self-harm, (4) inability to care for basic human needs and/or confusion, (5) sense of hopelessness, and (6) recent use of and/or impairment from alcohol or other substances of abuse, usually in addition to one of the five previous elements. An individual with immediate risk for self-harm needs to be placed in a secure environment. This may involve frequent direct observation, a locked door, and physical restraints, as well as attempts to lower the risk by detoxification, psychotherapeutic efforts, medication intervention, or some combination of these.

An individual who has a history of a recent suicide attempt or suicidal ideation and who denies it or minimizes the problems warrants more data gathering. Family and friends or roommates can frequently give a history of elements of risk for self-harm. It is not unusual for an individual to express suicidal thoughts and plans to family and not to caregivers, especially if the caregivers might prevent that effort. A history of self-harm in the more distant past, impulsivity, affective disorder, psychosis (especially with delusions that support hopelessness or imply invulnerability), recent losses of important people or valued elements, and family history of suicide are elements that increase risk. An individual who has continuing active suicidal or self-harm ideation and intent needs to be hospitalized, whether voluntarily or involuntarily. Suicidality and self-harm are frequently on a continuum from absolute intent to no real intent. Therapeutic interventions help to move the individual to the lower risk end. It is important to clarify how suicide or self-harm solves a problem for the individual and develop other alternatives. Frequently, distorted thoughts or perceptions result in conclusions that suicide is the only way out. The patients may have a thought that no one cares about them, therefore they might as well die. In a careful interview, caring individuals in their environment may be identified, in effect decreasing some of that person's logic for suicide. Statements about suicidality may cease once a significant other appears and realizes how upset the individual was.

Prior to any release to outpatient care, it is important that the suicide risk again be assessed. If the individual now denies suicidal ideation, questions must be asked and answered about what is different and what caused the change. A follow-up plan that is appropriate to the individual's situation is necessary. If a person has a substance abuse problem that was related to the suicidality, this also must be addressed. The more concrete and lethal the suicide attempt (either because of means or low likelihood of discovery), the more convincing the change must be before the person is released. With a very lethal attempt a hospitalization may still be useful to help ensure that the change is real and that all elements have been examined and addressed.

Risk to Others

Immediate risk to others can be determined by assessing the following elements: (1) violence toward others or property in the recent past by history; (2) threats toward others in the recent past; (3) overt anger (e.g., loud voice, clenching fists, angry verbal content, and facial expression of anger); (4) signs of recent physical conflict (e.g., facial scars, stitches, wounded knuckles, and ecchymoses); (5) past history of violence or explosiveness; (6) impairment from alcohol or other substance of abuse; (7) confusion; (8) antisocial personality disorder; and (9) psychosis, especially mania or involving paranoia. The risk to others includes the public, family or friends, caregivers, and other patients in the care environment. Individuals at risk require placement in a secure environment that may include physical restraints, seclusion in a preferably locked room or an unlocked room if in more control, and immediate stabilization through anger-reducing strategies such as listening to the patient, sitting the patient down, decreasing stimulation, and/or use of medication.

SCREENING FOR MEDICAL PROBLEMS AND ETIOLOGY FOR THE MENTAL DISORDER

Multiple studies have shown that what appear to be psychiatric symptoms are frequently caused by medical problems.[1] As many as 10 per cent of psychiatric admissions are primarily caused by a medical problem, between 20 and 25 per cent of psychiatric admissions have a medical problem that contributed to or exacerbated an underlying psychiatric problem, and 50 per cent of people admitted to psychiatric services have a medical problem that needs to be addressed.[2,3] In assessing an apparently psychiatrically emergent patient, the patient's medical history should be determined, including current medications, current illnesses and treatments, and past significant illnesses. Rapid onset of totally new psychiatric symptoms or visual or olfactory hallucinations, or both, suggests medical causes. Cardiovascular, endocrine, infectious, pulmonary, gastrointestinal, hematological, central nervous system, and cancerous conditions are frequent causes of psychiatry symptoms.[3] Table 72–1 lists many frequently encountered medical problems with psychiatric presentations.

Screening laboratory tests can also be helpful in clarifying a medical or toxic etiology for the symptoms (Table 72–2). A metabolic derangement such as low sodium, infection with elevated white blood cell count, or brain damage with a history of head injury are examples of disturbances that can be identified by these tests. Psychiatric symptoms are also frequently related to medications the individual is taking (Table 72–3). Steroids are a particularly frequent cause for depression, mania, psychosis, or a combination of these. People who have psychiatric disorders may have their underlying disorder made worse with concomitant medical illness or medication reactions. A physical examination, including vital signs and screening neurological evaluation, can help detect underlying medical illness and help in assessing the individual's level of self-care. When the problem is still primarily psychiatric, that individual may have neglected his or her health care because of the psychiatric illness, and the physical exam can help in directing the patient to treatment for these problems. It is important not to attribute automatically exacerbations to the underlying condition. For many individuals treatment of the medical condition or stopping the exacerbating medication alone resolves or improves the psychiatric symptoms. With some conditions, especially psychoses such as those caused by steroids, neuroleptic medications may be helpful or necessary.

Individuals who have such symptoms as disorganized thinking, incoherence, concentration deficits with fluctuating levels of consciousness, perceptual disturbances, disorientation, disturbances in sleep, memory difficulties, or changes in psychomotor activity have delirium and require a full medical assessment to identify the organic etiology. The onset is usually rapid. Dementia is usually characterized by short- and long-term memory problems along with judgment impairment, personality changes, disturbances in higher cortical function, and impaired abstract thinking.[4] Dementias usually de-

TABLE 72–1. MEDICAL PROBLEMS WITH PSYCHIATRIC SYMPTOMS[a]

Medical Problem	Psychiatric Symptoms
Adrenal cortical insufficiency (Addison's disease)	Thought disorder, depression, suspiciousness, anxiety, confusion, markedly fluctuating affect and behavior
Brain damage (from trauma, circulatory abnormalities, and/or anoxia)	Confusion, disorientation, irritability, affective lability, memory disturbance, hallucinations, delusions
Hyperadrenalism (Cushing's disease)	Somatic delusions, anxiety, agitation, irritability, hallucinations, emotional lability, hypervigilance, referential thinking
Hyperthyroidism	Anxiety, clouded sensorium, paranoia, agitation, delusions
Hyperparathyroidism and hypoparathyroidism	Hyperactivity, anxiety, irritability, confusion, disorientation, clouded sensorium
Hepatolenticular degeneration (Wilson's disease)	Rapid mood swings, hallucinations, irritability, memory problems
Hypoglycemia	Agitation, confusion, anxiety
Hypothyroidism	Anxiety, depression, fatigue, paranoid delusions
Hypoxia	Visual hallucinations, depression, disorientation, confusion, memory problems
Infections (especially of the CNS)	Confusion, irritability, disorientation, hallucinations, agitation
Intracranial tumors	Clouding of consciousness, hallucinations (especially visual, gustatory, and olfactory), rapid shifts in mental state
Porphyria (acute intermittent type)	Mood swings, depression, confusion
Postpartum psychosis	Confusion, mood lability, irritability, delusions, hallucinations
Seizures	Affective lability, paranoia, confusion, disorientation, visual, gustatory, olfactory, and/or auditory hallucinations, automatic behaviors, anger outbursts; note: patients in postictal states may have confusion, combativeness, and affective lability
Systemic lupus erythematosus	Thought disorder, confusion, anxiety, elation, affective lability, hallucinations, delusions, paranoia, confusion, disorientation

[a] Modified with permission from Dagadakis CS: The emergent psychotic patient. In Schwartz G, et al, eds. Principles and Practice of Emergency Medicine. 3rd ed. Philadelphia: Lea & Febiger (in press).

velop gradually; thus history of deterioration and functioning are particularly important, along with prior history of prior medical assessments. If there is insufficient history, a probable dementia must have a thorough medical screening as above. The current situation may be acute and not be a dementia or may involve a rapid deterioration of an individual with dementia from another medical problem.

SCREENING FOR PSYCHOSIS

Whenever an individual presents with psychiatric symptoms, that person should be evaluated for psychotic symptoms. Psychosis is defined as a "major mental disorder of organic or emotional origin in which a person's ability to think, respond emotionally, remember, communicate, interpret reality, and behave appropriately is sufficiently impaired so as to interfere grossly with the capacity to meet the ordinary demands of life."[5] The above features will usually be obvious or elicited in the history of the present problem and the general interview or in formal and informal mental status examinations. Unusual uses of words, ideas, behavior, and intensity of focus suggest further exploration. When the affect and content of behavior are not concordant, psychosis is a greater possibility. A regression or major change in activities of daily living may be a clue to psychosis. Fixed or unmodifiable beliefs (delusions) that are out touch with reality and that are not a usual part of the individual's cultural background are an indication of psychosis. Hallucinations, usually auditory, are frequently present in psychosis. It is important to distinguish whether voices are heard inside an individual's head or are distinct voices heard outside. The latter may be hallucinations, but the former may represent that person's own thoughts and internal dialogue, and no psychosis may be present. An occasional sound or hearing of a name being called may be an illusion (a stimulus in the environment that is misinterpreted) and may not indicate psychosis. The individual's comfort with the presence of psychotic symptoms such as hallucinations or delusions usually indicates that the symptoms are chronic. For most people new psychotic symptoms are a cause for alarm or concern. The longitudinal history of the symptoms and disorder are frequently as useful diagnostically as the mental status examination. A history of overall functioning can also help to clarify onset. The more acute the onset, the more likely a medical or toxic cause contributes or that the disorder is the manic phase of bipolar disorder. The latter disorder can have a change from normal affect and function to mania in hours.

The treatment of emergent psychosis requires structure to minimize ambiguity, avoidance of excess stimulation, understanding and acknowledgment of the individual's concerns, setting clear limits, and a safe setting. At times only removing an individual from a stressing environment can help

TABLE 72–2. SCREENING LABORATORY TESTS FOR EMERGENT PSYCHOSIS AND OTHER PSYCHIATRIC DISORDERS[a]

Laboratory Test	Indications	Pitfalls
Complete blood count	Elevated temperature History or appearance of poor self-care Possible trauma Substance abuse history Question of hypoxia	White counts are elevated in high stress states
Electrolytes, glucose, and blood urea nitrogen	Rule out hypoglycemia Assess dehydration and metabolic abnormality Possible delirium	Abnormalities may not be causative of psychosis but a result of poor self-care
CT scan	Focal neurological signs History or recent head injury Unexplained delirium	Paranoid patients may be agitated by CT scan apparatus
EEG	Loss or alteration of consciousness prior to confusion or psychosis Signs of encephalopathy	Agitated or uncooperative patients preclude an EEG since the head must be held relatively still to connect electrodes and attempts at sedation may mask abnormality
Blood alcohol level	Apparent alcohol use Alcohol on breath, staggering, and/or slurred speech History of recent alcohol use	Negative alcohol level does not preclude psychosis secondary to withdrawal
Toxicology screen	History of drug ingestion Apparent signs and symptoms of drug use	Presence of drugs may be in addition to underlying psychosis and not causative Negative screen does not preclude psychosis secondary to past drug use or current withdrawal
Skull x-ray	Suspected skull fracture or penetration wound	Rarely useful except in head trauma and then the utility is for medical-legal reasons
Pregnancy test (hCG in serum or urine)	Prior to use of psychotropic emergent medications, especially benzodiazepines, in women at risk for pregnancy	If urine is too dilute (less than 10 specific gravity), test unreliable Inaccurate histories in psychotic individuals
T_3, T_4, TSH	Depression, anxiety	If obtained while agitation is prominent, values may be temporarily elevated

[a] Modified with permission from Dagadakis CS: The emergent psychotic patient. *In* Schwartz G, et al, eds. Principles and Practice of Emergency Medicine. 3rd ed. Philadelphia: Lea & Febiger (in press).

decrease the psychotic symptoms. Once elements that may have contributed to the stress, such as a family conflict or loss of housing, are clarified, potential solutions can be crafted. If the agitation and/or psychotic symptoms are severe and are not improved by environmental and support efforts, or both, medications may be helpful. In emergent psychosis, generally there are three pharmacological options: a benzodiazepine, a neuroleptic, or a combination. Both benzodiazepines and neuroleptics have similar short-term effectiveness for agitation and psychosis in most patients. Neuroleptics are generally more effective in decreasing psychotic symptoms.[6]

The advantages to using benzodiazepines are that, if psychotic symptoms cease during their brief use,

longer term preventive use of neuroleptics can be avoided with avoidance of risk for tardive dyskinesia, other side effects of neuroleptics can be avoided, and anxiety symptoms can be helped. The disadvantages of the use of benzodiazepines are oversedation with possible respiratory arrest if the patient already has taken other sedative hypnotics or alcohol; potential physical and/or psychological addiction, especially in substance abusers; delay in starting a neuroleptic that may be more effective for longer term use in a chronic psychosis; and disinhibition and increased agitation in a small number of individuals. Neuroleptics are generally the most useful for individuals who have responded to them effectively in the past, have a likelihood of a longer term psychotic illness, have particularly marked level of psychosis

TABLE 72-3. PSYCHOSIS AND OTHER PSYCHIATRIC DISORDERS FROM PRESCRIPTIVE DRUGS[a]

Prescription Drug	Psychiatric Symptoms
Antidepressants (mainly tricyclics and tetracyclics)	Disorientation, anxiety, confusion, paranoia, hallucinations
Atropinic action medications	Anticholinergic psychosis ("dry as a bone, red as a beet"), disoriented, confused, visual hallucinations, agitation
Barbiturates	Agitation, confusion, hallucinations, depression, somnolence
Benzodiazepines	Depression, and rarely agitation and disinhibition
Bromides	Emotional lability, delusions, hallucinations, confusion, disorientation, irritability
Cimetidine	Psychosis, paranoia, agitation, depression, delirium
Digoxin	Psychosis with visual hallucinations and/or apathy
Disulfiram	Delirium with manic, depressive, and paranoid states, psychotic depression, schizophreniform psychosis
L-Dopa	Hypomania, hallucinations, dementia, paranoid delusions, delirium, depression, agitation
Lidocaine	Psychosis with visual hallucinations
Penicillin (intravenous)	Agitation, hallucinations, anxiety, convulsions
Phenylbutazone (in large doses)	Delirium, hallucinations
Podophyllin (oral and cutaneous)	Visual hallucinations, sedation, paranoia, nausea
Propranolol	Psychosis with visual hallucinations, delirium, depression with or without psychosis
Quinidine	Psychosis with visual hallucinations, depression, excitement
Ranitidine	Depression, agitation, hallucinations, confusion
Reserpine	Depression with or without psychosis, nondepressed psychosis, catatonia
Salicylates (high doses)	Confusion, agitation, delirium, hallucinations
Steroids (prednisone)	Affective instability, depressions, manic-like state, schizophreniform state, confusion, disorientation

[a] Modified by permission from Dagadakis CS: The emergent psychotic patient. In Schwartz G, et al, eds. Principles and Practice of Emergency Medicine. 3rd ed. Philadelphia: Lea & Febiger (in press).

and/or agitation that may only respond to neuroleptics, and have a clinical state in which respiratory depression is likely or particularly risky (minimized with low-sedation neuroleptics such as haloperidol). Neuroleptics have a higher incidence of tardive dyskinesia in people with bipolar disorder.[7] Since for many people in manic states lithium and carbamazepine can help treat the psychosis in brief periods (5 days to weeks), initial management with a benzodiazepine may be sufficient. In mania, a neuroleptic can be used for psychosis that is particularly prominent and upsetting for the patient.

The evidence is equivocal and not convincing that adjunctive use of benzodiazepines and neuroleptics is more effective for psychosis. Some individuals may have benefit from both.[8] The use of the combination can decrease the amount of neuroleptic used and thus potentially decrease the risk for both side effects and tardive dyskinesia. There is usually little more antipsychotic effect beyond the 400- to 600-mg chlorpromazine equivalent level.[9] Doses above this generally are helpful by giving sedation to help in decreasing agitation. Adding a benzodiazepine at that point may help with sedation.

Among the benzodiazepines, lorazepam is preferred for intramuscular use, since it is well absorbed in 1 to 1.5 hours and has an intermediate half-life of 10 to 18 hours. The usual dose for both IM and oral modes is 1 to 2 mg, with a frequent daily maximum of 10 mg. Intramuscular diazepam and chlordiazepoxide have much more erratic absorption. If these latter two are given, absorption is the best from the deltoid muscle, assuming there is enough muscle mass to give an injection safely. Orally, diazepam is absorbed the most rapidly, in 0.5 to 2 hours, with a half-life of 20 to 50 hours; chlordiazepoxide is absorbed in 0.5 to 4 hours, with a half life of 5 to 30 hours. The usual dose for diazepam is 5 to 10 mg p.o. or IM, and the dose for chlordiazepoxide is 5 to 25 mg p.o. or IM. Clonazepam is generally more sedating and is given in dosages of 1.5 to 10 mg/day initially, with a half-life of 18 to 50 hours.

There is little evidence that any neuroleptic except clozapine in selected individuals is more effective with psychosis than others. The difference is side effect profile and sedation.[10] In emergent settings, haloperidol, loxapine, fluphenazine, and thiothixene are frequently used since these can be given both p.o. and IM. Chlorpromazine IM is used infrequently since it has a higher frequency of orthostatic hypotension, sedation, and other adverse side effects.[11] When compared to the IM form, the frequency of cardiac and respiratory arrest was much higher than with haloperidol. Haloperidol has been extensively studied in emergent settings and is frequently used.[12] The advantages of using haloperidol are relatively less sedation than most neuroleptics; availability of small volume injectable version (1 ml for 5 mg), a clear, tasteless concentrate, and a pill form; and the availability of a long-acting depot injectable form. Its major disadvantage is a higher frequency of extrapyramidal symptoms, especially dystonias in young males. In an average-size person, a frequent dose would be 5 mg p.o. or IM repeated every hour up to about 20 to 30 mg/day. Little further antipsychotic effect is obtained from higher doses. In an elderly or small person doses range from 0.5 to 1 mg. Fluphenazine also has a long-acting depot version. Generally the long-acting versions are usually preceded by trials of shorter acting versions to minimize duration of particularly adverse side effects. In addition, there is a delay of effective blood levels being reached, and frequently other forms must be given. These properties of the long-acting versions limit their utility in emergent settings. Thiothixene and loxapine are more sedating.

Extrapyramidal symptoms (EPS), including dystonias and akathisia, are frequent with neuroleptics and in emergent settings. Dystonias that frequently involve rigidity of muscles and cramping in the neck, tongue, and back can be effectively treated with anticholinergic agents such as benztropine or diphenhydramine. Benztropine can be given IM or p.o. in a dose of 1 to 2 mg. It has the advantage of having a longer half-life (12 to 15 hours) than most anti-EPS agents. Diphenhydramine (dose 25 to 50 mg IM or p.o.) is more sedating and has a half-life of 4 to 6 hours. Its main advantage is that it is available over the counter in the 25-mg size. For most acute EPS the IM form is preferable and is effective within one-half hour. Since the frequency of EPS is high, ambivalence about medications is frequent and enhanced by EPS, and agitation can increase with EPS, giving regular anti-EPS agents when starting a neuroleptic is an option. The disadvantages of some decrease in neuroleptic blood level, increased anticholinergic symptoms, and occasional anticholinergic psychosis are frequently outweighed by the advantages in the acute situations. In acute settings, it makes sense to develop familiarity with a few medications in the benzodiazepine, neuroleptic, antimanic, and anti-EPS classes. This limiting of options results in fewer errors by staff who are under frequent stress and need to make rapid decisions.

SCREENING FOR SUBSTANCE ABUSE

Substances of abuse can cause and exacerbate a wide range of psychiatric disorders and behavioral problems. Many individuals who complete suicide or attempt it have alcohol present in their blood.[12] The frequency of polydrug abuse is high. Many users of drugs also abuse alcohol. Individuals with psychiatric illness who have been stabilized on medications frequently stop these medications when drinking or using drugs and then deteriorate. Every individual who is evaluated psychiatrically must be asked about alcohol and drug use. It needs to be recognized that the history may not be accurate and tends to be understated, since alcohol and drug abuse have some social stigma. The more vague the history, the more likely there is abuse. Statements such as "I can take it or leave it," "I can stop any time," or "I stopped for one year" frequently indicate abuse. It is important in the history to determine when and what was the last use and the use in the last week. This gives some measure of the current physiological effect in the individual and the risk for withdrawal and immediate impairment. A longer term history is important to assess the cumulative potential effect on brain function, social relations, compliance with treatment, and correlation with psychiatric symptoms. It is helpful to identify the pattern of use, such as binge drinking versus steady and frequent use. An attempt should be made to identify the number of ounces of alcohol ingested per day. A statement that a person drinks two glasses of whiskey per night could mean two 8-ounce glasses. It is also helpful to identify if the individual attempts to treat his or her mental disorder and symptoms with substances of abuse. Some drink only when they are manic in an attempt to slow down. Others drink to try to prevent panic attacks. The use pattern may help in identifying the psychiatric disorder, and the treatment of that disorder can help decrease or stop the abuse. Effective treatment and support of abstinence have been facilitated by support groups such as Alcoholics Anonymous and Narcotics Anonymous. Changing life-style and patterns that result in cues to drink or use are also helpful and can be developed in formal substance abuse treatment settings.

Alcohol

Alcohol is the most pervasive drug of abuse. In emergency situations it is frequently related to suicidal behavior and violence. Alcohol disinhibits higher levels of cognitive control. In addition, both in acute use and chronic use, it can decrease mood and add to affective instability. Individuals who drink frequently may significantly neglect self-care and have additional alcohol-related physical problems that may also affect their mental state. Alcohol can cause hypoglycemia and thus can result in a confusional state in some individuals. Some individuals with chronic alcohol use can develop delusional syndromes, especially with paranoia. Dementing syndromes are frequent with chronic users, both from the alcohol and from the frequent head injuries they acquire. Alcohol blood levels are helpful in assessing the level of intoxication and level of abuse. An individual who has a 200-mg/dl level and who talks and appears to think clearly is very likely to have a severe and chronic problem. A rough estimate of blood level decrease is 50 mg/dl/hr, although it often is much slower depending on the individual's liver function.

Alcohol withdrawal symptoms can occur within 24 hours of stopping. About 5 per cent of individuals who withdraw develop delirium tremens within 2 to 10 days of cessation if untreated. Withdrawal is characterized by tremor, anxiety, increases in blood pressure and pulse, and diaphoresis. Early signs of delirium tremens are hallucinations or illusions; anxiety or panic feelings or both, especially when trying to fall asleep; and insomnia. As the condition progresses, delirium, psychosis, disorientation, and/or agitation become prominent. Delirium tremens is a medical emergency and requires sedation, hydration, and correction of electrolyte imbalances. Auditory hallucinations with no vital sign changes and normal electrolytes usually represent not withdrawal or delirium tremens, but an alcohol hallucinosis that can be treated with neuroleptics, benzodiazepines, or both. Similarly, delusions with a chronic history of alcohol abuse, no other indications of withdrawal, and no other psychiatric or organic disorder can be considered an organic delusional disorder and treated with neuroleptics. If these delusions are longstanding, they may not resolve with neuroleptics or may require an extended treatment course. People with chronic alcohol abuse are frequently vitamin deficient and should be treated with thiamine 50 to 200 mg IM initially and 100 mg p.o./day for 3 days. In addition, other multivitamin supplements may help.

Sympathomimetics: Cocaine and Amphetamines

Cocaine users, whether they employ an intravenous, nasal, or smoking (crack) route, can present with anxiety, irritability, depression, psychosis, affective lability, paranoia, visual and/or auditory hallucinations, and sensations of insects or worms underneath the skin. Amphetamine use can present with all of the above symptoms except skin sensations. Some individuals may have a manic presentation. Intravenous users have a particular risk for human immunodeficiency virus (HIV) infections, since needles are shared in the expansive state after use and the frequency of use is higher than with heroin. Neuroleptics, benzodiazepines, or both can help the psychotic symptoms. Frequently the symptoms improve in a few days in cases of cocaine use but tend to be longer in duration in cases of amphetamine use. The depression may be more longstanding. The use of desipramine has been shown to decrease relapse to cocaine use and also to minimize depressive symptoms after stopping the use.[13]

Sedative-Hypnotics

The two classes of sedative-hypnotics most frequently encountered in emergent settings are benzodiazepines and barbiturates. Withdrawal syndromes are possible with both classes. Barbiturate withdrawal, especially when the drug has been taken in large dosage for a long period (months), is a medical emergency with a high risk for delirium, seizures, and death. The short-acting barbiturates (amobarbital, secobarbital, and pentobarbital) are the most fre-

quently abused. There is little abuse of phenobarbital. Frequently, barbiturates given in combination compounds for pain problems are abused. Benzodiazepine withdrawal is most frequent in shorter acting compounds such as alprazolam, lorazepam, and oxazepam. Longer acting compounds such as diazepam and chlordiazepoxide can cause withdrawal, but it is less frequent and severe, since there is built-in detoxification. For these long-acting compounds, higher doses for longer periods are required to result in withdrawal on cessation (e.g., diazepam daily doses in the 30- to 40-mg range for many months). The withdrawal syndrome is similar to that described earlier for alcohol. Preventive management of barbiturate withdrawal, which frequently develops as long as 1 week after barbiturate cessation, involves first finding the point of barbiturate tolerance with either pentobarbital or phenobarbital and then decreasing the dose 10 per cent per day. Benzodiazepine detoxification can use a similar method, with phenobarbital or other benzodiazepines given to the point at which symptoms of withdrawal stop and then gradually decreased. Recently, carbamazepine has been used effectively in benzodiazepine withdrawal, especially with alprazolam.[14] If an individual has been using sedative-hypnotics or alcohol in the immediate past, caution must be used in giving another sedative-hypnotic to help with agitation or psychosis since the individual can become overly sedated and respirations can be inhibited. Toxicology testing for benzodiazepines and barbiturates is useful in identifying their use, but quantification is not generally available.

Narcotics

Drug seeking and withdrawal phenomena are the most frequent issues involving narcotics in emergent settings. Specific requests for narcotics, especially oxycodone and meperidine, often come from drug abusers. Elaborate histories and symptom complexes are presented. At times psychiatric symptoms are presented in attempts to get drug treatment and detoxification that would not otherwise be available. Narcotic withdrawal does not have serious and longstanding consequences other than discomfort for a few days. Symptoms of withdrawal include nausea, vomiting, piloerection, diaphoresis, tremor, and increased blood pressure and pulse. Individuals who are addicted often have little tolerance for physical and emotional discomfort. Detoxification usually is done with either benzodiazepines or hydroxyzine to help with the agitation and anxiety in the first few days. Longer term use of benzodiazepines should be avoided because of these individuals' abuse potential. Other symptom-related medications can be used, such as antiemetic agents or propranolol for tremor and blood pressure changes. Unless an individual is going to and is accepted in or already in a methadone treatment program, usually methadone is not used. One exception in which methadone is used is in detoxification through the use of pain cocktails, generally in pain clinics, where the methadone and an amount of phenobarbital, if sedatives are also abused, is given in a flavored liquid mixture and decreased by 10 per cent per day.

Drug abusers have the same increased risk for suicide and organic affective syndromes as alcohol abusers. Intravenous narcotic users have an increased risk for HIV and other infections that may produce organic brain syndromes. In addition, intravenous use has a higher likelihood of other toxic substance introduction through cutting or adulterating the heroin or other narcotic. In narcotic overdoses, naloxone can be given to reverse the narcotic depressive effect.

Hallucinogens

The most frequently encountered hallucinogens include lysergic acid diethylamide (LSD), marijuana, hashish, phencyclidine (PCP or angel dust), mescaline, and psylocybin. A frequent presentation is hallucinosis and distortion of visual stimuli and body image. In addition, frequently there are confusion, vivid colors, mood changes and lability, depersonalization, paranoia, time distortion, expansiveness and sense of special experiences, violent behavior (especially with PCP), and anxiety. It is frequently difficult to identify what the substance was. History from the patient or others sometimes helps, but compounds are frequently mixed or sold as other drugs. Individuals with mental disorders and psychoses can also take such substances and have their condition exacerbated. Toxicology testing can help identify the substance. In all the above compounds except PCP, decreasing the stimulation may help calm the symptoms. The disordered person using PCP does not necessarily respond to low stimulation. Benzodiazepines can be used as sedation. If the psychotic symptoms are particularly prevalent or benzodiazepines have not been helpful, haloperidol can be given. Phencyclidine is released from fat stores, which can result in a return of all of the symptoms even after the individual appears stabilized, especially after medications have worn off. Other hallucinogens, especially LSD, can result in brief flashbacks or return of some of the original symptoms of anxiety, illusions, depersonalization, vivid colors, and depression. Usually, lowered stimulation and social support for minutes to hours or a benzodiazepine, or both, helps to control the flashback.

Inhalants

Inhalants are generally hydrocarbons or solvents that evaporate easily. Some individuals inhale the vapors from glue or gasoline, which are both readily available, in an attempt to achieve an altered mental state. This frequently results in an organic brain syndrome with confusion, decreased concentration, memory problems, lability, and apathy. Individuals who have long term, (even at low levels), exposure to solvents and hydrocarbons may have depressive mood, decreased energy, and some cognitive changes. Individuals who abuse inhalants tend to be people with few social skills and resources. Prolonged use of inhalants can result in dementia-like clinical states.

SCREENING FOR NONPSYCHOTIC DISORDERS

Once medical problems have been assessed, organic etiologies have been considered, the possibility of psychosis has been explored, and substance abuse has been assessed, then nonpsychotic disorders can be considered. Only disorders that have a higher frequency in emergent settings or circumstances are discussed here. Short term management is discussed.

Anxiety Disorders

Panic disorder, generalized anxiety disorder, and post-traumatic stress disorder are the most frequently encountered anxiety disorders in emergent settings. Panic disorder usually presents with somatic concerns, especially of impending doom, concern about heart problems (especially palpitations or accelerated heart rate), shortness of breath, shaking, dizziness, sweating, choking, flushing or chills, numbness or tingling, and depersonalization. Lowered stimuli, support, assessment of physical problems and explanation of the findings, and a benzodiazepine if the symptoms persist can be helpful. If the individual meets the DSM-III-R[4] criteria for panic disorder, imipramine, phenelzine, or alprazolam with or without behavioral therapy may be indicated. It usually is not wise to start these medications in an emergent setting unless the starting individual is going to be following the patient or the individual who will be following the patient recommends one of these. A patient needs to establish an ongoing relationship for monitoring and assessment to effectively use these medications. The improvement may not be immediate, and there is some risk of abuse and addiction with alprazolam. Depression is frequent with panic disorder, and suicide is a risk. A few weeks' supply of imipramine or phenelzine can be fatal.

The individual with generalized anxiety disorder frequently has motor tension, autonomic hyperactivity, vigilance, and scanning lasting for at least 6 months, with concerns about at least two life circumstances. These individuals often present in emergent settings when a life stressor either highlights their concerns or increases their baseline anxiety. Assessment of their medical concerns and explanations of the findings, exploration of stressors, and development of a structure and a strategy to deal with concerns until they can see someone in follow-up can help decrease the baseline tension. An intermediate half-life benzodiazepine like lorazepam or diazepam can be helpful emergently; buspirone may be useful for longer term use, but it may require weeks to be fully effective. The use of buspirone and longer term benzodiazepine use requires ongoing care and should not be started in an emergent setting unless a definite follow-up option is available. In post-traumatic stress disorder an individual who experienced an event outside of the usual human experience can have recurrent intrusive thoughts, recurrent distressing dreams related to the event, or re-experience of the event. Re-experiencing the event may involve illusions, hallucinations, or dissociative episodes or distress when exposed to a somewhat parallel situation. The individual with such symptoms needs structure, support, and symptomatic treatment in the emergent setting. A benzodiazepine may help with anxiety and agitation. If the hallucinations and agitation do not respond to the benzodiazepine, addition of a neuroleptic may help. More ongoing care may involve therapy, especially group therapy, and possibly an antidepressant or ongoing benzodiazepine, again from a follow-up source.

Affective Disorders

Individuals who have depression present in emergent settings with somatic complaints usually related to depression and a somatic focus. Suicidality is often present in depression, especially with a sense of hopelessness. Usually it is not appropriate to start depressed people with antidepressants in emergent settings unless a clear-cut follow-up option exists and the treating source agrees with the treatment choice. No antidepressants are quickly effective in treating depression, and all require from 1 week at the earliest to 8 weeks for full effect. During this treatment period many adjustments need to be made, and a therapeutic relationship is frequently necessary to maximize compliance through support and modification of treatment regimens. Many antidepressants have significant side effects and can provide a lethal means for suicide. The risk for suicide occasionally increases when an individual is improving and has the energy to carry out suicidal impulses. Two antidepressants are relatively safe if taken in overdose alone: trazodone and fluoxetine. There is some controversy currently whether fluoxetine increases suicidal risk in some individuals; thus careful monitoring is necessary until the risk is clarified by research. Approximately 1500 mg of tricyclic antidepressants is a lethal dose. This lethal dose may be lower if alcohol or other drugs are also ingested. This should be considered when medications are started or refilled in at-risk individuals.

For individuals who have depression and are agitated, occasionally benzodiazepines are helpful. Sedative-hypnotics tend to add to individuals' depression; thus this needs to be monitored in their

use. Where an individual meets the criteria for major depression and has significant psychosis, generally the use of both antidepressants and neuroleptics is more effective than either alone. Generally only depressed individuals who are actively suicidal or at particular risk for suicide, are not able to provide self-care or have care provided, and/or whose medication management is complicated require hospitalization.

Individuals who are in a manic state usually require hospitalization, since their likelihood of engaging in high-risk behaviors is quite high. In addition, their moods are quite variable. They can move from what appears to be quite rational and appropriate behavior to high levels of irritability and expansive behavior. In addition, judgment is impaired in mania. In the emergent setting, manic individuals can benefit from sedation with benzodiazepines such as lorazepam, diazepam, or clonazepam. Lithium carbonate or carbamazepine, the usual treatment and preventive medications for bipolar disorder, take in the range of 5 to 7 days or more to ameliorate symptoms and should be started on admission if there are no contraindications. If psychosis is prominent, neuroleptics can be used, but frequently benzodiazepines are sufficient for management until the antimanic agent becomes fully effective. It is useful to lower the stimulation in helping to manage a manic person.

Somatoform Disorders

The frequent somatoform disorders encountered in emergent settings are conversion disorder, hypochondriasis, somatoform pain disorder, and somatization disorder. Most of these individuals present with medical complaints, and when no etiology is determined, they are referred for psychiatric evaluation. It is important to acknowledge the individual's somatic complaints and attempt to understand the individual's concerns about them. It is often helpful to describe the psychiatric evaluation as an attempt to address their symptoms from a different angle. It helps to note that having such symptoms can be quite upsetting and stressful and that this can add to the severity of the symptoms. If a way can be discovered to decrease this stress and anxiety, the symptoms may be helped. Usually the most that can be done in an emergent setting is to make a diagnostic assessment and set the stage for further care, generally on an outpatient basis. Some individuals with a conversion disorder have symptoms of such severity, such as paralysis or blindness, that acute intervention or inpatient psychiatric hospitalization is required. Occasionally empathy and understanding and developing an approach to deal with an individual's conflicts can help to resolve or decrease the conversion, especially if a plausible avenue can be given for the individual to give up the symptoms. Often such intervention is beyond the scope of emergent outpatient settings. Appropriate referral to individuals and agencies who have experience and are relatively effective in dealing with somatoform disorders is important, as is the framework for which that referral is given. Usually the approach described above, focusing on the patient's response to his or her symptoms, is fruitful.

Personality Disorders

Usually people with personality disorders present in emergent settings when their disorder results in interpersonal difficulties, internal states become unacceptable, their behavior becomes alarming to others (e.g., suicidal behavior or violence), they seek support from others, or they attempt to use the encounter to avoid negative consequences. It is useful to first understand why the individual is in the setting, and then to make hypotheses about how the disorder contributed. A diagnostic formulation is based on obtaining a longitudinal history that includes social and occupational functioning and legal history. This formulation can also help in directing the form of approaching the patient.

With a paranoid personality disorder, an interviewer would need to be unambiguous, business-like, and not overly warm. With a narcissistic individual, it would be important to avoid criticism and recognize how important that individual's appearance and role are to him or her. Specific personality disorders have frequent comorbidity with other disorders, and knowing the personality disorder can direct the search for another disorder. Substance abuse is very frequent in people with antisocial personality disorder. Similarly, depression is frequent in individuals with borderline and obsessive-compulsive personality disorders. The personality disorders frequently encountered in emergent settings are borderline, antisocial, and dependent disorders. The impulsivity, self-mutilation, depressive features, interpersonal difficulties, and suicidality of borderline disorders result in many encounters. The staff need to be firm and consistent and to maintain good communication, since borderline individuals may see, and attempt to place, some staff in roles as "good" caregivers and others as "bad" caregivers. Development of treatment approaches for individuals may help provide consistency to the multiple episodes. Brief hospitalizations can help get the behavior and the affect under control, and rapid return to the community helps minimize a high risk for dependency and regression.

Individuals with antisocial personality disorders, especially when intoxicated, have a higher frequency of violence to staff and others. Histories may be given in an attempt to obtain a hidden agenda, often involving drug seeking, helping in avoiding legal consequence, or help in obtaining a place to stay. Substance-abusing individuals with antisocial personality disorders have a higher risk for suicide than do persons with many mental disorders. Firm, nonpunitive, and clear limits, and a business-like demeanor are helpful in dealing with antisocial individuals. Dependent personality disorders may seek care and provide symptoms to maximize caregiving. It is important to encourage as much individual action as the patient can tolerate and to avoid situations that foster regression. Attempts can be made to match the personality-disordered individual's perceived needs to options that are available and are the most likely to succeed.

Adjustment Disorder

Individuals with adjustment disorder are frequently seen in emergent settings. These individuals have not adjusted effectively to identifiable psychosocial stressors and may have symptoms in excess of what would normally be expected for the stressor. If the disturbance is one instance in a pattern of overreaction to stress, the individual may have a personality disorder or another mental disorder. Individuals with adjustment disorder are frequently helped by an empathic interview that helps to clarify the concerns, resources, and options. Developing a plan of action may lower the individual's stress sufficiently to move on to the next task or work with another caregiver. Identification of providers who are able to deliver short-term pragmatic crisis intervention and therapy is important. They can continue the stabilization that begins with the first interview, if more is needed. Occasionally benzodiazepines can help in temporarily decreasing anxiety and with sleep. These are not a substitute for problem-solving efforts, support, and development of other external support.

PATIENT DISPOSITION

The disposition of the patient usually involves deciding whether to recommend inpatient or outpatient treatment. Individuals who have an immediate risk, by actions or stated intent, to harm themselves or others require inpatient hospitalization unless this risk can be significantly reduced in the emergent setting. The more overt the action, the more likely that an inpatient stay may be warranted, even if the risk is decreased, since the improvement may be transient. An individual who was suicidal when drunk and who ordinarily does not abuse alcohol may be less at risk when detoxified. A person who had homicidal thoughts in the belief that his or her partner had been unfaithful and later changed that idea may be less at risk. Short-term no-harm contracts have been used by mental health practitioners for many years. These are primarily useful in cases in which a person cannot make such a contract, which usually indicates a hospitalization is warranted. If an individual agrees to the contract, other factors of risk need to be taken into account. The contracts are most meaningful when the contracting parties have a positive, trusting, longer term therapeutic relationship. Individuals who cannot take care of their basic human needs or who, because of their behavior, are likely to significantly harm relationships, employment, resources, or others usually need to be admitted. Familiarity with the local civil commitment system is essential, and it can be used when an individual in one of the categories described here is not willing to be hospitalized, if the law applies. Inpatient treatment may also be indicated for individuals who have very complex medication regimens or who have other complicating medical or social problems that require more monitoring and structure. Individuals who are noncompliant with outpatient treatment may also warrant hospitalization.

Outpatient treatment is appropriate for those who are not at immediate risk, whose problems are less severe, and whose resources on an outpatient basis are adequate. A broad support structure of family and friends could provide the monitoring and help in the treatment compliance of an individual who otherwise would need an inpatient stay. These resources and options need to be explored before a plan is made. In developing a plan, accessibility and acceptability of options need to be considered. The person's preferences, impediments to care, and past history of compliance need to be considered. It makes little sense to give an individual a referral that he or she cannot afford or for which transportation would be extremely difficult. Compliance is enhanced by making the referral very concrete and written out for the patient. A specific name, place, address, telephone number, and time for an appointment maximize the likelihood of successful referral. Asking patients to call the emergent caregiver when they have made the connection, or calling them, also helps and gives them the message that the follow-up treatment is important and the provider cares. Patients are more likely to follow instructions from those they perceive as caring. It is often helpful to ask the patient to repeat the instructions and to ask if there are any questions about them. Clinicians may spend a great deal of time in making as assessment and diagnosis, but most of it may go for naught if not enough effort and time are spent on the disposition.

REFERENCES

1. Hall RC: Medically induced psychiatric disease—an overview. *In* Hall R, ed. Psychiatric Presentation of Medical Illness. New York: Medical & Scientific Books, 1980:6–9.
2. Herride CF: Physical disorders in psychotic illness: A study of 209 consecutive admissions. Lancet 2:949, 1960.
3. Hall RC, Popkin MK, DeVaul R, et al. Physical illness presenting as psychiatric disease. Arch Gen Psychiatry 35:1315, 1978.
4. American Psychiatric Association: Diagnostic and Statistical Manual of Mental Disorders. 3d ed. Revised. Washington, DC: American Psychiatric Association, 1987.
5. American Psychiatric Association: The American Psychiatric Association Psychiatric Glossary. Washington DC: American Psychiatric Press, Inc., 1984:114.
6. Greenblatt DJ, Raskin A: Benzodiazepines: New indications. Psychopharmacol Bull 22:79, 1986.
7. Sachs GS: Adjuncts and alternatives to lithium therapy in bipolar affective disorder. J Clin Psychiatry 50(12, suppl):31, 1989.
8. Easton MS, Janicak PG: The use of benzodiazepines in psychiatric disorders: A review of the literature. Psychiatr Ann 20(9):525, 1990.
9. Baldessarini RJ, Cohen BM, Teicher, MH: Significance of neuroleptic dose and plasma level in pharmacological treatment of psychosis. Arch Gen Psychiatry 45:79, 1988.
10. Kane JM: The current status of neuroleptic therapy. J Clin Psychiatry 50:9:322, 1989.
11. Pang LM, Chen CH: Rapid tranquilization of acutely psychotic patients with intramuscular haloperidol and chlorpromazine. Psychosomatics 14:59, 1973.
12. Hirschfield MI, Davidson L: Clinical risk factors for suicide. Psychiatr Ann 15(11):428, 1988.
13. Gawin FH, Kleber HD: Cocaine abuse treatment: Open pilot trial with desipramine and lithium carbonate. Arch Gen Psychiatry 41:903, 1984.
14. Ries RK, Roy-Byrne PP, Ward NG, et al: Carbamazepine treatment for benzodiazepine withdrawal. Am J Psychiatry 146:536, 1989.

SUGGESTED READINGS

Treatment of Psychiatric Disorders: A Task Force Report of the American Psychiatric Association. Washington, DC: American Psychiatric Association, 1989.

Hall RCW, ed: Psychiatric Presentations of Medical Illness: Somatopsychic Disorders. New York: SP Medical & Scientific Books, 1980.

Hyman SE: Manual of Psychiatric Emergencies. Boston: Little, Brown & Company, 1988.

Hyman SE, Arana GW: Handbook of Psychiatric Drug Therapy. Boston: Little, Brown & Company, 1987.

Slaby AE, Lieb J, Trancredi LR: The Handbook of Psychiatric Emergencies. 3rd ed. New York: Medical Examination Publishing Company, 1986.

73

CONSULTATION-LIAISON PSYCHIATRY

LAWRENCE G. WILSON, M.D.

This chapter describes the place of consultation-liaison psychiatry in the field of psychiatry as a whole and focuses on some of its most frequent clinical, teaching, and research activities. Activities that are of most importance to the practicing physician as well as the student and resident are highlighted.

Consultation-liaison psychiatry is a relatively young subspecialty, having been present in an embryonic form for many decades but as a defined area for only about 40 years. Psychosomatic medicine, as an academic enterprise as well as a clinical discipline, has been active since the 1930s and has gradually merged in some respects with the activities of consultation-liaison psychiatry. Psychosomatic medicine, under the influence of several psychoanalysts and physiologists, came to focus on seven diseases originally theorized to develop rather directly from specific emotional influences: ulcerative colitis, peptic ulcer, rheumatoid arthritis, hyperthyroidism, essential hypertension, neurodermatitis, and bronchial asthma. These diseases were thought to be psychophysiological responses to strong emotions, such as fear, anger, rage, disgust, resentment, and grief. The initial hypotheses were rather simplistic and have since been largely disproved, but early investigators led by Franz Alexander were pioneers in beginning to investigate affects and their physiological consequences. Other investigators followed who expanded beyond the original "Holy Seven" diseases to study the role of stress, emotions, and other psychosocial influences in all illnesses. This opening up of virtually every medical condition as meriting psychosomatic interest and study has led to the current challenge to medicine to deal with every illness as a biopsychosocial event deserving of analysis, study, and treatment from biological, psychological, and sociocultural angles.[1] Consultation-liaison psychiatry can be considered the practical or action-oriented branch of of psychosomatic medicine. It is a specialized field of psychiatry focusing on evaluation and treatment of the whole person in a hospital setting, with recently expanded interest in the outpatient clinical environment. Consultation-liaison psychiatry is involved with bringing psychiatric principles of evaluation, diagnosis, and treatment to the nonpsychiatric health care system.

THE HOSPITAL SETTING

The concerns of consultation-liaison psychiatry have traditionally been with medical, surgical, or rehabilitation patients in the hospital. The hospital environment is one rich with clinical situations recognized by many caregivers as needing or benefitting from psychiatric assistance. Frequently, however, the request for consultation will be framed in the most vague way: "Could you come help us with this guy who's going crazy down here," or "We've got a woman here tearing up the place," or "We need a consult on a guy whose behavior is real strange." Anxiety or frustration on the part of the referring doctor may be the most obvious fact gleaned from the initial request. The first goal will frequently be clarification of the perceived problem and helping the consultee formulate a question.

The consultant arriving on the scene will need the skills of any good clinician: the ability to listen to staff, to efficiently review any existing records, and to conduct an interview appropriate to the situation. The interview by a consultation-liaison psychiatrist may need to be conducted in a semiprivate or noisy public setting, with a patient frequently uncomfortable from pain or lethargic from sedatives. It will likely be more focused than other interviews, since the referring clinician will have given some idea of the problem, and a true "open-ended" style would not be appropriate or effective. The need is even greater than in other settings for a thorough mental status examination, with a particular focus on tests for cognitive functioning.

Requests for hospital consultation largely result from what some have tagged "the three Ds"—delirium, depression, and dementia. Since the clinical presentations of these syndromes overlap to a large degree and sometimes are suffused with anxiety or agitation as the most obvious clinical characteristic, this seems like accurate clinical lore.

Delirium

Delirium has been reviewed in detail in Chapter 10, and its historical, theoretical, and physiological bases thoroughly discussed. In a busy hospital, delirium can truly be a "great initiator," a modern institutional equivalent of syphilis. Delirium can be described as the acute or subacute onset of diffuse cognitive dysfunction, with prominent features of an altered state of consciousness and alertness, failure to attend, and anxiety and agitation. It can also be accompanied by irritability, illusions, delusions, hallucinations, and bizarre behavior. Sometimes these last elements are the most obvious to hospital ward staff, and there is an immediate assumption of a schizophrenic or other psychotic breakdown while the cognitive dysfunction or confusional state with its many possible metabolic or toxic causes is totally overlooked. The list of causes of delirium is long but can be approached in the usual manner of possible categories of etiology (Table 73–1): metabolic, endocrine, drug withdrawal, toxic, cardiovascular, infectious, neurological, or the less common causes outlined in Chapter 10.

Initially, the main focus should be on finding a treatable or changeable cause for the delirious state. Management of the agitation or anxiety that is a result may also be a collateral focus, with neuroleptics or benzodiazepines possible alternative choices. Haloperidol (Haldol and others) is probably the safest choice in delirium of unknown cause. It can be started in doses of 1 to 2 mg orally or 0.5 mg IM every 30 to 60 minutes, with intravenous administration (0.5 mg) in cases of severe symptomatology. Doses are repeated or titrated upward as needed until the patient is calm, then an estimated daily dosage is given in three or four divided doses. The medication should be continued for 2 to 3 days, then tapered over 2 to 3 days. A benzodiazepine such as lorazepam is a possible choice, but is less predictable because of its sedating quality, and in older people or patients with pulmonary problems, respiratory de-

TABLE 73–1. POSSIBLE CAUSES OF DELIRIUM (ABBREVIATED LIST)

Category	Posible Etiology
Metabolic disorders	Electrolyte imbalance, hypoxia, hypercarbia, hepatic encephalopathy, uremia, thiamine deficiency
Endocrine disorders	Thyroid, parathyroid, adrenal
Drug withdrawal states	Alcohol, sedative-hypnotics, anxiolytics
Intoxications	Alcohol, sedative-hypnotics, opiates, anticholinergics, stimulants, exogenous steroids, cardiac medications, heavy metals
Cardiovascular disorders	Congestive heart failure, arrhythmias, myocardial infarction
Infections	Meningitis, encephalitis, pneumonia, sepsis
Neurological disorders	Seizures, head injury, space-occupying lesion, hypertensive encephalopathy

pression remains a concern. Protection of the delirious patient by physical restraints is frequently a coequal necessary part of the management.

Many drugs cause the onset of new abnormal mental states or exaggerate existing ones. Some classes of drugs are fully predictable causes of confusion in older people or medically compromised patients if taken in overdose or higher dose form (e.g., those with anticholinegic effects). Common causes of anticholinergic delirium are tricyclic antidepressants, over-the-counter sedative-hypnotics, and the low-potency phenothiazine antipsychotics. Some new or exotic drugs have unpredictable effects, and a few can cause delirium, depression, excitability, and other negative states. The number of drugs used particularly in the many acquired immunodeficiency syndrome (AIDS)-related problems is rapidly changing and expanding, and each new year brings more drugs of which the consultant must be aware.

Depression

Depression in all its many ramifications can be seen in many medical or surgical patients. Some patients express their psychological distress through various somatic manifestations (the "somatic idiom") rather than experiencing or expressing the distress in mood-related words or affect. These manifestations may be particularly prevalent in some inpatient medical settings. Studies utilizing explicit criteria have diagnosed mood disorders in as many as 22 to 33 per cent of medically ill patients in the hospital.[2] However, it may be much more difficult to diagnose depression in the hospital than in other settings because of the symptoms of medical illness present. Vegetative signs of depression, so important in the DSM-III-R scheme of diagnosis, may be severely disrupted by the medical illness or condition and be nearly useless in diagnosis. For example, symptoms such as decreased energy, loss of concentration, anorexia, and sleep disturbance in a medically ill patient may not be indicative of depression. Some researchers have found that the presence of mood and cognitive symptoms as well as persistent anhedonia is far more important in separating those medically ill patients who have major depression from those who have adjustment disorder with depressed mood related to the medical illness.[3] Deciding whom to treat with antidepressant medications, some of which have side effects potentially problematic for the medical illness, is a consistent concern in this situation. The development of agents with few or no cardiac effects or anticholinergic actions has been helpful to the psychiatrist doing consultations. Fluoxetine (Prozac) starting at a 10- to 20-mg/day dosage (given in the morning to prevent nighttime restlessness) has been helpful in many medically ill patients with major depression, as have tricyclics with less anticholinergic activity (desipramine) or newer agents with virtually none (trazodone).

One of the most vexing problems for a consultant is the obviously depressed patient who has severe multiple medical problems, is withdrawn and apathetic, may have marginal cardiac status, and is very fragile even at baseline. Older or newer antidepressants need to be started at low doses and increased slowly to limit side effects that may be dangerous as well as uncomfortable. An increasingly utilized safe and rapid way to brighten the mood and stimulate activity and more interest in surroundings is the use of an agent from the stimulant category, such as dextroamphetamine (Dexedrine) or methylphenidate (Ritalin). Both anecdotal and semicontrolled studies have pointed to the safety and usefulness of stimulants in depressed patients, who may represent a large percentage of the patients evaluated in some hospitals or nursing homes. Methylphenidate has been used more frequently in medically ill patients, since it is slightly less potent. Ironically, improvement in appetite frequently occurs, although concern about the opposite effect is reasonable. The suggested dose is 5 mg at 8:00 A.M. and 12:00 noon (with none later in the day that might disrupt sleep) as a start. If no improvement occurs in 2 days, this dose can be advanced to 10 mg at 8:00 A.M. and noon. Particularly fragile or weak patients should be started at 2.5 mg at 8:00 A.M. and noon and advanced if the drug is tolerated. It is rare that more than 20 mg/day is required to get the desired effect. Improvement is usually evident in 2 to 3 days, and the duration of use is several days to several weeks. This regimen has been used safely and successfully in cardiac patients (after surgery and after myocardial infarction), neurology patients (those with seizure disorders, or after surgery or stroke), and cancer patients. Some will need to be switched to usual antidepressants for maintenance after improvement in mood, activity, and general interest in life.[4]

Acute reactive mood disturbances are common in hospitals. Many of these episodes are brief, are obviously related to the stress of the medical illness, and clearly need only supportive therapy. Medical illness or injury can be a provocative stressor to nearly everybody, and persons with preexisting life issues can temporarily decompensate into dependency, withdrawal, rage, self-blaming, or any number of other states. Many of these persons will be receptive to verbal approaches, and brief, focused, problem-centered psychotherapy is quite feasible to undertake in the hospitalized patient.

Dementia

Dementia, with its slow onset of cognitive dysfunction in a patient with a clear sensorium, can manifest in many different ways. Particularly in the early or mild type of dementia with only minor memory disturbance, the diagnostic challenge can be great. With the insult of medical illness or trauma, patients with mild preexisting cognitive dysfunction can develop major states of anxiety or agitation, necessitating restraints and need for pharmacotherapy. In addition, patients with dementia seem particularly sensitive to metabolic changes or mild central nervous system toxic insults from medications or anoxia leading to mild states of delirium, which, superimposed on the baseline condition, can appear as serious psychotic reactions. Misperceptions, illusions, hallucinations, gross delusions, and resultant agitation may require both benzodiazepine sedation and brief neuroleptic treatment to suppress the intensity of the psychotic phenomena. The combination of delirium superimposed on preexisting dementia is particularly common in hospitals serving large numbers of elderly patients. Another variant is the dramatic increase in the severity of cognitive dysfunction seen in many patients with Alzheimer's disease who become depressed. Accurate diagnosis and appropriate treatment of the associated depressive component can frequently reverse some of the most alarming cognitive deterioration, and forestall pessimistic plans by the patient's family to embark on permanent institutionalization.[5]

Patient Evaluation

When seeing a patient who is delirious or has recent onset of signs of dementia, the psychiatrist will frequently be in a position of suggesting additional tests or procedures to elucidate possible treatable or correctable causes or precipitants of the delirium or dementia. Sometimes it will be evident that a computed tomography scan or spinal fluid exam will be necessary to investigate possible medical causes of diffuse cognitive dysfunction; some have called this the search for "coarse brain disease."[6] Similarly, in other situations there will be indicators that metabolic, infectious, toxic, or other factors are possible causes for the symptoms of depression or acute psychosis that are manifested. Medical or surgical colleagues will usually be grateful for suggestions of new or additional avenues to pursue these possible causes.

Sometimes the ward physicians and nurses will need help with patients who do not have a clear psychiatric diagnosis but have very problematic behavior such as demandingness or abusiveness to the staff. In fact, these patients still need very careful diagnostic interviewing and consideration of the possibility of delirium, since many times irritability and abusiveness will result from the diffuse and subtle cognitive dysfunction of delirium. For those who do not have delirium, there are several principles that have been helpful in the management of ward behavioral problems. The general outlines of behavioral modification have been helpful, with the following points kept in mind: (1) one consistent nurse or contact person per shift to deal with the patient to ensure clear communication regarding procedures, treatment plans, and the like; (2) consistent and simple behavioral requirements to attain a reward (such as a scheduled talk with a nurse if there is decreased yelling, no talk with a nurse if the yelling continues); and (3) reinforcement of good behavior with praise, or time out of the room on the ward for socially appropriate behavior. Nursing and medical staff will sometimes appreciate help with these kinds of situations as much as with situations involving more florid manifestation of psychiatric symptoms.

SPECIFIC MEDICAL CONDITIONS: PSYCHIATRIC ASPECTS

Some specific medical or traumatic problems have a high rate of psychiatric complication. Investigations into several of these have revealed unexpectedly high rates of manifestation of organic mental syndromes and disorders. Research over the past 15 years has delineated the high rate of mood disorders associated with brain injury after *cerebral vascular infarcts or hemorrhages (stroke)*. Left-sided lesions are associated with a higher rate of mood disorder, and the more anterior lesions seemingly increase vulnerability to symptoms. Depressive disorders may occur in up to 47 per cent of acute stroke patients, with about half of these having the full major depressive episode. These patients represent a group in which aggressive pharmacotherapy can be extremely helpful in preventing or limiting the poor rehabilitation that might result when depression is a concomitant of the neurological damage. Many antidepressant medications have been found to work well in this group, but some work has indicated that nortriptyline is particularly well tolerated and efficacious.[7] Avoidance of orthostatic hypotension is particularly important after stroke, and nortriptyline has an excellent record in this regard. Methylphenidate (Ritalin), as described previously, is another generally safe and effective possibility.

Many patients suffering industrial accidents, vehicular injury, or violent assault suffer *closed head injury* and have varying degrees of damage and dysfunction of the brain. Although such injury is generally the province of the neurologist or the rehabilitative medicine specialist, many of these patients become quite aggressive and sometimes violent during the stage of cognitive dysfunction and delirium. As described earlier, haloperidol can be safely used in initial doses of 1 to 2 mg orally or 0.5 mg IV every 30 to 60 minutes until the patient is calm. A daily dose can be selected based on initial requirements, then tapered down after the patient is stable for a day or two. It should be the objective to discontinue neuroleptics as soon as possible when using them in this manner, particularly when the aggressiveness has become more chronic and is not related to delirium. Many patients could then be classified as having organic personality syndrome, explosive type, although some researchers have preferred the term

organic aggressive syndrome.[8] Some excellent work has been done utilizing β-blocking agents for patients with longer lasting symptoms. Propranolol (Inderal) and several other β-blockers have been studied. High levels of propanolol will be required for some patients (up to 800 mg), and there will usually be a lag time of 4 to 8 weeks after reaching therapeutic levels before clinical response. Titration to higher doses needs to be carefully monitored, with a close watch on pulse and blood pressure. Patients with a number of medical conditions (asthma, chronic obstructive pulmonary disease, congestive heart failure, persistent angina, and others) must be excluded from this treatment because of possible aggravation of coronary and systemic vasoconstriction.[8] A β-blocker with a more benign profile of side effects, pindolol, has been used recently with good success in aggressiveness and other behavioral problems related to brain injury. It seems to have intrinsic sympathomimetic effects that prevent some of the possibly dangerous cardiac or hypotensive effects.[9] Aggression in the elderly that seems related to diffuse or focal brain damage also is increasingly being managed by the use of β-blockers, as is the case when the condition manifests anxiety as the predominant symptom (i.e., organic anxiety syndrome). Specific directions for monitoring and carefully titrating up to effective levels of these β-blocking agents can be found in the neuropsychiatric references to this topic and should be reviewed before initiating this therapy.

Patients with *temporal lobe epilepsy (complex partial seizures)* have a high incidence of psychotic symptoms. Sometimes these symptoms are not adequately managed by the treatment for the seizure disorder itself, and psychiatric opinion will be sought. Although carbamazepine (Tegretol) has been helpful in stabilizing this particular group, at times these patients will demonstrate such severe mood disorder or psychotic symptomatology that aggressive treatment with antidepressants, lithium, or antipsychotic medications will be needed. Patients with *Parkinson's disease* and *multiple sclerosis* (MS) will also frequently manifest symptoms of mood disorder. Treatment with antidepressants will frequently be useful for some, particularly with the labile mood of MS.[10]

Systemic lupus erythematosus (SLE) patients are another group representing frequent consultation requests. The basic lupus process, including cerebritis, may produce such problems as psychosis and cognitive impairment as well as seizures, but it also may produce depression, insomnia, and high levels of anxiety. Many of these patients will be on moderate to high-dose steroid treatment, and possible toxicity to that class of drugs may be hard to tease out from the basic disease process. A close working relationship with the primary physician in working out the role of disease versus treatment effects is important in all the diseases discussed here.

MANIFESTATIONS OF SUBSTANCE ABUSE PROBLEMS IN CONSULTATION-LIAISON WORK

In many hospital settings, the manifestation of substance abuse is pervasive. In one recent study, all new medical-surgical admissions to a major hospital were screened and a rate of diagnosed alcohol dependence of 25 per cent was found.[11] There was significant underdiagnosis of the patients' alcohol problems: surgeons identified it in only one fourth of cases and obstetrician-gynecologists in less than one tenth. In some settings, the rate is undoubtedly much higher than 25 per cent. Mental disorders coexisting with substance abuse disorders ("dual diagnosis") have been studied more carefully in the last few years, and in some hospitals the rates are similarly high. The consultant will frequently be called initially to help manage a patient in alcohol withdrawal, and the primary physician will need some suggestions on the amount and scheduling of benzodiazepine administration to suppress the autonomic signs as well as the tremulousness and agitation of withdrawal. Aggressive and early treatment will usually prevent the development of the hypertension, fever, and delirium of delirium tremens. Opiate, sedative-hypnotic, or anxiolytic withdrawal present other challenges to appropriate treatment. After withdrawal from any addicting substance is complete, many patients will manifest dysphoria of an extreme degree, but unless suicidality is associated with it, the dysphoric mood will generally improve as the patient gets further away from the acute withdrawal. This mood disturbance, however, can be quite prominent, and if it lasts more than several weeks after withdrawal and the symptoms are not subsiding, most clinicians would initiate treatment with antidepressant medication. If followed for a number of months, however, a high percentage of patients with depression secondary to alcohol abuse (organic mood syndrome) will slowly clear without specific drug treatment.

Many hospitals are developing aggressive on-site identification and counseling programs for hospitalized substance abusers. These programs are particularly aimed at patients hospitalized for longer periods of time, such as on rehabilitation units, spinal injury centers, orthopedic units, and trauma centers. Dual diagnosis problems are prevalent in postinjury patients, and ample opportunities exist to observe the psychiatric aspect of this combined problem and to attempt both psychotherapeutic and drug therapy. Obviously, for the opiate and cocaine abuser with psychiatric problems, specific programs available for referral after discharge are less abundant than for alcohol abusers. However, in all groups a brief intervention or instructing of the patient about arranging follow-up treatment may be crucial. The specific instructions to the patient will often be translated into a strong motivational element to seek posthospital care.

ASSESSMENT OF SUICIDE ATTEMPTS

Depending on the hospital in which one works, assessing people who have attempted, threatened, or alluded to possible suicide can be a major activity of the consulting psychiatrist. In some central city hospitals, a large percentage of requests for consultation will be to assess people who have poisoned themselves, cut themselves, or in some way purposely inflicted a wound or a burn upon themselves. As in other consultation-liaison areas, a careful diagnostic assessment with a particular focus on the mental status exam as well as on past history and the social support system is unquestionably the initial need. Another requirement is for the consultant to clearly know the appropriate state laws pertaining to involuntary detention of persons who have attempted to harm themselves. The person who has attempted or threatened suicide may have a great range of needs, but those who require only outpatient follow-up will be relatively easily handled. The patient needing inpatient evaluation and possible treatment because of the severity of the attempt or ongoing suicidality will be more difficult. Restraints to protect the person from self-injury or elopement while on the medical or surgical unit will be a sensitive topic for many patients, ward staff, and family. The specific hospital regulations and the appropriate laws regarding detaining persons until they can be officially evaluated for involuntary treatment will all need to be known with clarity. A sizeable proportion of lawsuits against psychiatrists arise from this setting, where it may be asserted that there has been negligence by not properly protecting a person who has attempted or has verbally threatened suicide.[12]

THE CHALLENGE OF AIDS

Our health care system is being confronted in nearly every respect by the multiple needs of those persons with human immunodeficiency virus (HIV)-related problems. For the consultation-liaison psychiatrist, HIV seropositivity, ARC (AIDS-related complex), and AIDS are challenges to the ideal of the "biopsychosocial approach" that seems best for these illnesses, since they represent real or potential disturbances in the biological, psychological, and social realms. Not only are the three Ds of delirium, depression, and dementia (AIDS dementia complex) seen, but the D of demoralization is frequently another stark manifestation. This predictably fatal disease, striking largely a very young population, can result in severe dislocation of life, and the widespread social reaction to persons with HIV illness adds yet another dimension for the patient to experience.

The psychiatrist needs to become familiar with the toxicities of the drugs used for all the various problems that AIDS patients experience. The common side effects and toxic phenomena of the anti-HIV agent Zidovudine (AZT), as well as the usual anti-bacterials, antifungals, and antineoplastic agents used in treating AIDS, should be familiar to psychiatrists consulting to AIDS patients. The neuropsychiatric aspects of AIDS are becoming more familiar, and some studies have shown as many as 50 to 70 per cent will have cognitive impairment at some point in their illness, usually evidence of chronic organic brain dysfunction with occasional associated features of delirium or mood disorder.[13] Sometimes it will be very difficult to distinguish between demoralization and depression that is of sufficient severity to necessitate specific medical treatment. As with the association of depression in other medical illnesses, sometimes the zone of difference will be so gray as to lead the consultant to think "Why not treat them all?" Antidepressants can be helpful, but those with minimal anticholinergic side effects (such as desipramine, trazodone, or fluoxetine) should be chosen because of the extreme sensitivity of many ill AIDS patients to this side effect. Again, in this particular group, the use of methylphenidate (Ritalin) to lift mood and correct lethargy and withdrawal can sometimes be strikingly helpful. In some patients nearing the final stages, maintenance methylphenidate may be justified to ensure as high a quality of life as possible.

MEDICAL-LEGAL AND ETHICAL ISSUES

The psychiatrist working in consultation and liaison will frequently be involved in clinical situations tinged with medical-legal issues. In addition to the post–suicide attempt patient who may need involuntary treatment, other patients may be seen on medical or surgical services who are quite psychotic and unable to care for their medical condition. Perhaps the level of psychosis by itself would not be severe enough to justify involuntary psychiatric care, but with the chronic medical condition not being attended to, severe deterioration and danger to life may be a possibility. Again, a clear understanding of the applicable state laws is a necessity. Very frequently the psychiatrist will be asked by the attending physician to help decide whether a person is competent to consent to surgery or highly technical diagnostic procedures that require a considerable level of understanding.[14] Older persons who need amputation for a gangrenous extremity or severe injury may show limited ability to discuss and weigh the risks and benefits of such a procedure. The psychiatrist will frequently need a legal consultant such as the hospital attorney to go over both the clinical and legal issues to be able to guide the attending physician.

The consultation-liaison service has become an arena for many ethical concerns and issues to be expressed, discussed and considered with medical colleagues. In situations that are considered medically futile, sometimes the consultation-liaison psy-

chiatrist becomes another person to include in the discussion regarding decisions about "do not resuscitate" (DNR) orders. Quality of life in the future and treatable or untreatable past and current psychiatric problems will all become possible elements to this discussion. In a time of scarce resources, medical teams will often fervently search out help from the consultation-liaison service, particularly if a patient has a "psych history." This element may actually be totally inappropriate to the decision at hand, but will sometimes get brought into the discussion regardless and will need help in resolution.

LIAISON

While many psychiatrists do hospital consultations in the midst of doing other kinds of work in general psychiatry both in and outside the hospital, a lesser number do liaison psychiatry. This term is used to describe a close collaborative relationship between psychiatry and another medical department, either inpatient or outpatient. The focus in liaison work is more on general issues related to clinical syndromes and patient care, rather than on specific cases. It is concerned more with common clinical situations faced, rather than a particular situation. The setting is usually in teaching or staff conferences rather than at the bedside with the patient. For example, the focus might be working with a burn service staff on the early recognition of delirium in the acutely burned patient and the various approaches, both medical and nonmedical, to managing the delirious patient. The burn service is frequently an excellent area for collaborative clinical and teaching work, and also a good area for joint research (e.g., the use of antidepressants in the pain and dysphoria of burn patients). Renal dialysis units present many challenges in the area of psychiatric and psychological management of patients and are excellent places for liaison collaboration. A high prevalence of mood disorders and sexual dysfunction and a high suicide rate exist among patients on chronic dialysis, and strong psychiatric involvement can lead to early identification and intervention.[15] Rehabilitation medicine units, with their high proportion of patients with very long recovery periods, are also excellent places for liaison work. High rates of depression exist because of the severe trauma that brings many patients to these units, and also because of the relatively high percentage of poststroke and post–closed head injury cases that result in significant levels of mood disorder, delirium, and organically derived aggressiveness and assaultiveness. Close liaison work with the nursing and medical staff of these units can help them become better at recognition and appropriate early management and referral for specific psychiatric evaluation. On geriatric units, the identification and treatment of organic mental disorders, especially the syndrome of delirium superimposed on dementia, is a common liaison focus. This calls for the liaison psychiatrist to be very familiar with the effects of drugs on the elderly and how they are absorbed, distributed, metabolized, and excreted differently than in younger individuals, and the need to use reduced and individualized dosing schedules. The staff will usually be very appreciative of specific teaching about psychosocial intervention techniques to decrease the behavioral disruption that is common on geriatric units.

Outpatient primary care medical clinics have become a more frequent locale for liaison activity. Studies have pointed to outpatient units as having a high prevalence of mixed substance abuse and mental disorder. Early identification and treatment can be a main focus of liaison activities in this area. The techniques of behavioral medicine will be particularly important in liaison work with outpatient medical clinics. Since nicotine dependence, adherence to medical regimens, and poor stress coping represent major problems among many medically ill persons, approaches arising from behavioral medicine may be particularly helpful for patients in this setting.[16] Special techniques, such as behavior modification, progressive relaxation, and hypnosis, have all become utilized more frequently by liaison psychiatrists in these clinics. Couples and group therapy as well as specific educational programs have also been initiated by psychiatrists working here. Focused, time-limited psychotherapy is another excellent skill to know and to teach others as a liaison or consultant psychiatrist, particularly in the outpatient setting.

CONCLUSION

Consulting to the various areas of the modern hospital brings the consultation-liaison psychiatrist into intimate contact with the whole range of modern medicine, from high-tech imaging methods of the brain to the medically futile sustaining of life of the person in a terminal state. It is challenging to bring meaningful, up-to-date, and effective psychiatric expertise to bear on the care of the medically or surgically ill patient, whether that be knowledge of an appropriate pharmacological approach or what outpatient program would be best for an alcoholic after going through withdrawal. The whole range of applicable treatment, from new technology to brief psychotherapy to community referral, is the realm of the consultation-liaison psychiatrist.[17]

The modern medical center of the 1990s is a meeting place for many current controversies in diagnosis and biopsychosocially oriented patient care of a humane kind. It is also a focal point for many of society's present problems with health care, including ensuring equitable access to care, determining how to allocate costs, and deciding how to ethically determine when to let life end. It is a challenge for consultation-liaison psychiatry to continue to play a critical, helpful, and decisive role in this crucial meeting ground of professional and societal need.

REFERENCES

1. Engel GL: The clinical application of the biopsychosocial model. Am J Psychiatry 137:535–544, 1980.
2. Katon W, Sullivan M: Depression and chronic medical illness. J Clin Psychiatry 51(6, suppl):3–11, 1990.
3. Rodin G, Voshart K: Depression in the medically ill: An overview. Am J Psychiatry 143:696–705, 1986.
4. Satel S, Nelson JC: Stimulants in the treatment of depression. J Clin Psychiatry 50:241–249, 1989.
5. Rovner BW, Broadhead J, Spencer M, et al: Depression and Alzheimer's disease. Am J Psychiatry 146:350–353, 1989.
6. Taylor MA, Sierles FS, Abrams R: General Hospital Psychiatry. New York: The Free Press, 1985:194.
7. Robinson RG, Forrester AW: Neuropsychiatric aspects of cerebrovascular disease. In Hales RE, Yodofsky SC, eds. Textbook of Neuropsychiatry. Washington, DC: American Psychiatric Press, Inc., 1987:191–208.
8. Silver JM, Yudofsky SC, Hales RE: Neuropsychiatric aspects of traumatic brain injury. In Hales RE, Yudofsky SC, eds. Textbook of Neuropsychiatry. Washington, DC: American Psychiatric Press, Inc., 1987:179–190.
9. Greendyck RM, Berkner JP, Webster JC, et al: Treatment of behavioral problems with pindolol. Psychosomatics 30:161–165, 1989.
10. Silver JM, Hales RE, Yudofsky SC: Psychopharmacology of depression in neurologic disorders. J Clin Psychiatry 51(1, suppl):33–39, 1990.
11. Moore RD, Bone LR, Geller G, et al: Prevalence, detection, and treatment of alcoholism in hospitalized patients. JAMA 261:403–407, 1989.
12. Soloff PH, Gutheil TG, Wexler DB: Seclusion and restraint: A review and update. Hosp Community Psychiatry 38:882–886, 1987.
13. Perry SW: Organic mental disorders caused by HIV: Update on early diagnosis and treatment. Am J Psychiatry 147:696–710, 1990.
14. Applebaum PS, Grisso T: Assessing patients' capacities to consent to treatment. N Engl J Med 319:1635–1638, 1988.
15. Levy NB: Current issues in psychonephrology (special section). Gen Hosp Psychiatry 10:255–279, 1988.
16. Garrick T, Lowenstein R: Behavioral medicine in the general hospital. Psychosomatics 30:123–134, 1989.
17. Brody EB: New horizons for liaison psychiatry: Biomedical technologies and human rights (editorial). Am J Psychiatry 146:293–295, 1989.

74

PSYCHIATRIC EFFECTS OF NONPSYCHIATRIC MEDICATIONS

ROBERT H. GERNER, M.D.

When we consider the possibility of central nervous system (CNS) psychiatric effects of nonpsychiatric medication, we must bear in mind that we commonly are not expecting such a side effect, usually because attention is focused on some other disorder or because the agent in question is not considered a psychotropic. In some instances the nonpsychotropic designation is related purely to an arbitrary assignment when the agent is approved by the Food and Drug Administration (FDA). For example, carbamazepine and valproic acid are not considered psychotropics, but have been discovered to be equipotent to lithium in treating mania, and clonazepam is considered an anticonvulsant even though it has all of the properties of other long–half-life benzodiazepines.

Some reasons that "medical drugs" may cause CNS effects are because they: (1) cross the blood-brain barrier routinely, (2) affect susceptible individuals who have an idiosyncratic sensitivity to them, (3) produce secondary effects that then have CNS consequences, and (4) have effects that are dose related and occur in many individuals. Some pharmacological effects are relatively predictable with regard to CNS functioning. For example, depleting norepinephrine by any means is likely to be associated with depression. With many drugs, however, the level of understanding of CNS physiology and pharmacology is not precise enough to explain, much less predict, the CNS effects that are occasionally observed. This is especially true when the incidence of such effects is rare. The differential diagnosis can rarely be made with investigative tests since both psychological and physiological tests will show the same patterns as a true "idiopathic" psychiatric illness. Electroencephalograms (EEGs) are useful only when a delerium (as opposed to a depressive, manic, psychotic, or anxious syndrome) is present and abnormalities on the EEG are present. A negative EEG is not meaningful in "ruling out" a pharmacologically induced CNS syndrome.

This issue has direct clinical significance, since it means that the presentation of CNS effects may vary considerably from one individual to another. Thus, on the same dose or at the same serum level, one patient may experience sedation, another confusion, and another psychosis. Attempts to directly link a specific drug to a specific psychiatric syndrome are therefore to be eschewed. Empiricism is the rule with these relatively unpredictable phenomena.

The ability to attribute an etiology to these reactions may lead the primary care physician and the family to err in undertreatment. Patients will often not realize they are affected mentally and usually will not make the connection to a medication that they, and their physician, view as a nonpsychotropic. Yet, even though the syndrome is exogenously caused, the patient's thoughts and mood are disordered, and he or she may act out their depressed, manic, or other symptoms with grave consequences. Insight may not be preserved, and simply telling the patient that this is a drug side effect will not necessarily obviate behaviors seen in pure psychiatric disorders. Furthermore, in some cases a primary psychiatric disorder has been induced, and it is incorrect to think of the clinical situation as a drug side effect. Hence, in most cases in which a CNS-psychiatric syndrome occurs, a psychiatric consultation is indicated and a defined intervention needs to be carefully thought out.

Treatment of CNS effects that are intolerable can be chosen based on the prevalent symptoms or postulated action of the drug. In most cases the best course of action is to consider changing to another primary therapeutic agent. Even another drug in the same class may relieve symptoms, since the exact mechanism of CNS action is rarely understood. If this is not feasible, or the symptoms are severe or persistent, the traditional course is to treat the patient as if he or she were presenting with the primary psychiatric disorder most similar to the symptoms, using a relatively simplistic treatment plan (e.g., use antipsychotics if the major symptoms are confusion or psychosis). However, extreme care should be taken not to choose psychotropic agents that will increase the likelihood of CNS complications (i.e., low-potency neuroleptics with marked anticholinergic and hypotensive effects are usually contraindicated).

The opinions expressed here do not necessarily reflect the official position of the Department for Veterans Affairs.

The groups of patients most susceptible to CNS side effects are: (1) the elderly; (2) those with organic impairment from disease or trauma; (3) those on multiple drug regimens; (4) those who are under physiological stressors such as sleep deprivation; (5) those with stimulation deprivation (i.e., in an intensive care unit); and (6) those with a concomitant psychiatric illness, or personal or first-degree family history of a major psychiatric disorder. When considering the pharmacological agent, the physician should consider the range of action of the medication (not merely "what is the current indicated use") and to what degree this individual is likely to fall in a higher risk group for CNS side effects.

This chapter discusses general categories of common nonpsychiatric pharmacological agents and psychiatric sequelae that are known from the literature or from extensive clinical experience. Understandably, replication of any specific patient's reaction always contains some element of conjecture, since rechallenge is rarely ethical or possible. Furthermore, even with many case reports, neither the numerator nor the denominator is accurately known and a valid incidence usually cannot be calculated.

CARDIOVASCULAR AGENTS

Cardiac Glycosides

While perhaps the best known historical CNS reaction from a cardiovascular agent was originally reported by William Withering, who described the CNS effects of foxglove, others have described a combination of visual illusions/hallucinations and delerium with digitalis. The incidence of this effect with all of the cardiac glycosides is not rare[1] and, taken in total, such CNS effects may be expected in approximately 20 per cent of patients prescribed normal doses.

Hypotensive Agents

More commonly, CNS effects are found to be associated with hypotensive agents of various types. Classically, the agents that deplete presynaptic stores of catecholamines are notoriously associated with depressive syndromes, which may be minor, major, or psychotic and present with agitated or retarded features. These agents are α-methyl-dopa, reserpine, and, although it is not very permeable across the blood-brain barrier, guanethidine.[2] All of the β-blockers can cause the depressive syndromes described above, although atenolol and nadolol appear to have the least incidence because of their low lipophilic affinity and, hence, low CNS concentrations at usual therapeutic doses.[3–7] Psychiatric effects such as hallucinations and nightmares are more common with longer duration of treatment with the β-blockers. However, it is accepted clinical lore that propranolol (or equivalent doses of other lipophilic

β-blockers) rarely produces CNS-depressive states at dosages below 80 mg/day. For this reason it can be used to effectively treat tricyclic antidepressant– and lithium-induced tremors without difficulty. However, many patients will not tolerate it at the high doses used for cardiovascular conditions (hypertension, angina pectoris, arrhythmias, and myocardial infarction) or migraine prophylaxis. Clonidine is a presynaptic α2-agonist that reduces the release of norepinephrine. It is active centrally and has been used as an antimanic agent. Not surprisingly, it can produce marked depressive syndromes.

It is reasonable practice to always change from one of these agents in any patient with a psychiatric syndrome since the presentation cannot reliably be predicted in an individual patient. We have never found that an acceptable alternative was not available for cardiovascular control.

Other Cardiac Drugs

The angiotensin-converting enzyme inhibitors (captopril, enalapril, lysinopril) may have an antidepressant effect and rarely have been reported to induce depressive symptoms.[8] Lidocaine and related compounds (mexiletine, tocainide) may cause dose-dependent CNS effects of confusion and agitation. Procainamide may cause symptoms similar to lidocaine, but less frequently. Idiosyncratic CNS reactions of anxiety, depression, agitation, and psychosis/confusion have occurred with quinidine, prazosin, and disopyramide (Norpace) via their anticholinergic effects, which are one tenth that of atropine.

Diuretics

Diuretics have very rarely been associated with psychiatric syndromes. Some cases that may be due to hypokalemic states, with weakness and fatigue mimicking depression or anxiety, have been reported, but these agents are not considered to be a common etiology of psychiatric syndromes.

GASTROINTESTINAL AGENTS

Metoclopramide

Metoclopramide (Reglan) is a potent dopamine receptor blocker and readily crosses the blood-brain barrier. Because of this, it will act as do most traditional neuroleptics in reducing psychotic symptoms and producing extrapyramidal syndromes (EPS).[9,10] In a nonpsychiatrically ill person the EPS of akinesia may mimic depression since this syndrome will include flat facies, blunt affect, loss of interests, and psychomotor retardation. More acutely disturbing to the patient is akathisia or the EPS of motor restlessness that presents as anxiety, agitation, extreme worry, and difficulty sitting still. Other concomitant parkinsonian symptoms of tremor, cogwheeling, rigidity, and impaired gait may be present.

Prochlorperazine

Prochlorperazine (Compazine) is a neuroleptic and may produce the same EPS as described for metoclopramide.

Histamine-2 Receptor Blockers

Cimetidine (Tagamet) is the oldest specific histamine-2 receptor blocker, and other, newer agents may also have similar CNS side effects, although not yet appreciated. Depression and confusional syndromes are not uncommon and may not be dose dependent.[11] The mechanism of action for this is not understood. We have observed patients who have had this effect from cimetidine and who have been subsequently treated without ill effects with ranitidine (Zantac) (which also can cause depression),[12] suggesting that histamine-2 blockade per se is not the etiology.

Anticholinergic Agents

Anticholinergic agents are present in many formulations and occur as side effects in many other drugs that have a very wide range of indications [atropine, scopolamine, propantheline (Banthine), dicyclomine (Bentyl), many over-the-counter hypnotics, trihexyphenidyl (Artane), benztropine (Cogentin), etc.] The full presentation of the anticholinergic syndrome ("hot as a hare, red as a beet, dry as a bone, blind as a bat, and mad as a wet hen")[13] is not usually present and, if so, is a medical emergency. More commonly, the initial symptoms are impairment in memory recall that may be initially subtle, followed by either a euphoric and confused state or, more commonly, a depressive syndrome. If treatment is continued, patients may develop hallucinosis (usually visual) and delerium. It is a general consensus that the susceptibility to such effects is highly correlated to the age of the patient.

Antihistamines

Antihistamines of the histamine-1 receptor, such as diphenhydramine (Benadryl), dimenhydrinate (Dramamine), chlorpheniramine (Chlortrimeton), brompheniramine (Dimetane), hydroxyzine (Atarax, Vistaril), meclizine (Antivert), and promethazine (Phenergan), commonly cause sedation in "normal doses" that may be dysphoric and may be interpreted by some patients as depression. In high doses or mild overdosage they cause hallucinations (usually visual) and agitation/confusion. The syndrome is quite similar in presentation to that of anticholinergics.

Disulfiram

Disulfiram (Antabuse) is typically given to patients who are at relatively high risk of CNS side effects. Approximately one third of alcoholics have a concomitant psychiatric disorder, usually in the affective spectrum. In addition to its intended use (blocking oxidative metabolism of acetaldehyde), it also inhibits dopamine-β-hydroxylase, the enzyme that converts dopamine to norepinephrine. One may reasonably conclude that it will increase central dopamine and decrease central norepinephrine. Not surprisingly, the increased dopamine can exacerbate or precipitate psychoses in manic-depressive or schizophrenic patients, or in normal patients. The CNS depletion of norepinephrine may also appear as a delerium or a depression.[14,15]

Antibiotics

Antibiotics are among the most commonly prescribed agents, and therefore many patients may be taking them and may develop nonrelated psychiatric symptoms. However, the correlation of acute symptoms during and ending following an antibiotic trial would lend credence to an association. Since most antibiotic treatments are short, mild CNS reactions are usually tolerated. We have observed unsystematically that the potent gram-negative agents are reported by patients to sometimes produce a syndrome of fatigue, malaise, poor concentration, and depression that was not present while they were ill before treatment with antibiotics. Since this ended when the antibiotics were discontinued, linkage is tentatively assumed. Although case series are lacking, we have observed this with doxycycline, erythromycin, and cefadroxil. Panic and hallucinations can occur after injection of procaine penicillin, but are due to the procaine moiety.[16]

Cycloserine (Seromycin) is both a broad-spectrum and antitubercular antibiotic and has been reported to produce psychosis, depression, paranoia, and hallucinations.

Isoniazid CNS reactions are much more common. Patients may develop depression or manic or schizophrenic-like syndromes. Usually the treatment must be stopped, although, like the peripheral neuropathy, some CNS syndrome cases may respond to treatment with vitamin B_6.[17]

Cyclosporine

The immunosuppressive agent cyclosporine has a relatively high incidence of CNS effects (e.g., a 30 per cent rate of tremors). Numerous case reports document a variety of CNS syndromes, usually of a psychotic nature—paranoia, hallucinations (visual), anxiety, and depression. The mechanism of CNS action is unknown, but cyclosporine is very lipophilic, and most reports indicate a dose-dependent effect.[18]

CENTRAL NERVOUS SYSTEM AGENTS

Baclofen

Baclofen (Lioresal) is a gamma-aminobutyric acid (GABA) agonist used for muscle spasms. It has been found to rarely produce or exacerbate depression,[19,20] and may exacerbate schizophrenia.[21] Certainly in overdosage baclofen may produce a delirium.[22] Because it is a GABA agonist, a withdrawal syndrome like that with alcohol or benzodiazepines can occur, with anxiety and insomnia being the initial manifestations.

Antiparkinsonian Agents

Antiparkinsonian agents that increase central dopamine tone consequently may be expected to exacerbate or precipitate schizophrenic or manic syndromes or episodes. Naturally, treatment of such secondary psychiatric syndromes should not include use of neuroleptics, which will worsen the primary parkinsonian disorder.

L-*Dopa* increases dopamine and norepinephrine and was noted in initial trials to produce mania or other activated psychiatric syndromes in 20 to 50 per cent of patients.[23] These reactions have been considered to be much more likely in individuals who have a previous or concomitant psychiatric history.

Bromocriptine (Parlodel) is a dopamine agonist and has been used as an effective antidepressant. At lower doses it may act to turn off presynaptic release of dopamine and cause depression,[24] whereas at higher doses it clearly can cause hallucinations and paranoid ideation in up to 10 per cent of patients.[25]

Amantadine (Symmetryl) is a dopamine agonist used both as an antiparkinsonian and an antiviral agent. Ironically, it is often used to treat EPS secondary to neuroleptics in schizophrenia. It can aggravate schizophrenic and manic symptoms, and can cause hallucinations and confusion in normal patients.[26,27]

L-*Deprenyl* (Eldepryl) is a monoamine oxidase (MAO) inhibitor specific for MAO-A at low doses and is used to treat parkinsonian syndromes. However, at higher doses that often would be encountered clinically (e.g., 30 mg/day) it is nonspecific and inhibits both MAO-A and MAO-B. It has the same CNS effects as the other MAO inhibitors that are usually used to treat depression. Thus, while it may have an antidepressant effect, it also may provoke a hypomanic episode in some individuals. Currently, it appears that this is most likely in patients who have a history of manic depressive illness in themselves or close relatives.

Tetrabenazine is similar in action to reserpine, depleting presynaptic catecholamine stores. It may produce lethargy, depression, insomnia, and confusion.[28]

Antinociceptive Agents

Antinociceptive agents are usually without serious CNS effects. This is particularly true for the opiates when used at usual prescribed doses.

Pentazocine (Talwin) is an opiate agonist that has a high incidence of CNS side effects, producing acute hallucinations (usually visual), confusion, nightmares, and depression in up to 10 per cent of patients.[29,30] Since patients in such states may act out their delusional fears, and the incidence is frequent, measures to prevent untoward consequences should be taken when patients are given pentazocine.

Acetylsalicylic acid (aspirin) does not cause CNS side effects at normal doses. Chronic salicylate intoxication can produce a mild delirium with confusion, agitation, and behavior that is bizarre and may imitate a personality disorder.[31] In contrast, actual poisoning from overdosage is usually associated with CNS symptoms ending in coma.

Nonsteroidal anti-inflammatory agents (NSAIDs) may produce a dose-dependent depressive syndrome of lethargy, reduced concentration, anhedonia, and apathy. Cases related to indomethacin, ibuprofen, and naproxen have been reported.[32] The mechanism of such a reaction is unknown, as is the frequency, as well as the extent the plethora of similar agents that might produce such a phenomena. The NSAIDs also increase the concentration of lithium by reducing excretion in the renal tubule that is of clinical consequence.[33]

Anticonvulsants

Anticonvulsants have a wide range of mechanism of action and so need to be considered individually.

Barbiturates (e.g., *phenobarbital, mysoline*) produce a dose/blood level–dependent intellectual dulling but have not been found to specifically precipitate other psychiatric states. Porphyria attacks are usually associated with CNS symptoms of depression or manic-like states and can be precipitated by barbiturates. The differential diagnosis of patients (especially of European heritage) who are mentally disturbed following barbiturate ingestion must include porphyria.

Phenytoin (Dilantin) has been considered at various times to relieve many psychiatric disorders, to have no psychiatric effects, and to produce nonspecific cognitive dysfunction. As with any consideration with this class of agents, the literature is confounded by the wide range of patient pathology. Furthermore, phenytoin can produce folate deficiency, which is a cause of depression. Attention and psychomotor performance appear to be inversely correlated to phenytoin levels.[34,35] Psychomotor performance is generally improved when the anticonvulsant regimen is changed to *carbamazepine* or *valproic acid*.[36]

HORMONES

Corticosteroids

Corticosteroids, but not mineralocorticoids, have the most notoriety of medical agents causing CNS syndromes. The differential diagnosis is often complicated, however, because the underlying disease may cause CNS symptoms that may remit if the steroids are increased. The mechanism of action for steroid psychoses is not clear.

It is interesting that in both mania and depression cortisol is very significantly increased in the cerebrospinal fluid.[37] Corticosteroids do affect the sodium-potassium ion pump and alter norepinephrine and serotonin metabolism. The incidence of frank steroid psychosis ranges from less than 10 per cent to greater than 50 per cent, with a consensus that about 25 per cent of patients will exhibit some CNS syndrome of at least a mild degree.[38-40] These milder syndromes should be evaluated for treatment (see later in this section), since the dysphoria endured by patients may significantly interfere with activities of daily living or compliance with treatment. Severe syndromes probably occur in only about 5 per cent of patients. While at one time it was thought that females were at greater risk for steroid psychoses, this appears to be an artifact of the higher incidence of illnesses treated by steroids in females.

Most patients who have a CNS side effect from corticosteroids have an affective syndrome—approximately 50 per cent are depressed, 25 per cent are manic/euphoric, and the rest have schizophreniform symptoms or delirium. It is now established that these symptoms are relatively dose dependent, with a low incidence at doses below 30 to 40 mg/day prednisone equivalents. At higher doses the CNS symptoms are likely to start within the first week of treatment. It is also noteworthy that steroid withdrawal psychosis can occur.[41,42] Adrenocorticotropic hormone also can precipitate the same clinical CNS phenomena[43] as direct steroid administration.

The risk of developing such a reaction to steroids is notably not predicted by past response to steroids or by past psychiatric history. When a full-blown case presents, the treatment of choice is a neuroleptic. It is our opinion that treatment should usually be given, since the behavior of the patient is unpredictable and may worsen suddenly. Virtually all patients will remit after the steroid is withdrawn. Lithium has been reported to abort the CNS side effects if given early,[43] and tricyclic antidepressants are relatively contraindicated because they may worsen the symptoms.[44] The mechanism of action of this is not known, but if it is due to anticholinergic side effects from the tricyclics, then the newer nonanticholinergic antidepressant agents may be useful.

Anabolic Steroids

Anabolic steroids include a wide range and increasing number of agents. Regardless of the reason for use (impotence, body building), they have a relatively high incidence of CNS side effects. Pope and Katz[45,46] have reported both depression or manic states in 22 per cent and psychotic symptoms in 12 per cent of a series of 41 subjects who used a variety of agents, including *methandrostenolone, testosterone, nandrolone, methenolone, boldenone,* and *oxandrolone.* While such reactions are much more likely to occur at high doses, case reports abound where "normal" doses were used in patients with no previous psychiatric history[47] and who remitted with symptomatic treatment and time.

Hormone Affecting Sexual/Reproductive Function

Female hormones given as *oral contraceptives* or as replacement therapy may have an antidepressant effect or induce depression. The field is controversial as to whether women who develop depression on oral contraceptives are usually predisposed by a past history of affective illness.[48] This area is confused by the use of such agents to successfully treat some affective disorders in women. The incidence of depression on oral contraceptives is not insignificant (5 to 7 per cent),[49,50] and the syndrome of depression is usually characterized by nonendogenous features such as rejection sensitivity that are associated with "atypical depressions."[51] However, the consequences of depression in this group are very real: social disruption, suicidality, and the like. There is a general consensus that the risk of depression is correlated with the amount of progesterone in the preparation, with the possible mechanism of action being an increase in MAO and a decrease in biogenic amines.[48] The depression usually responds to discontinuation. Women with a history of depression should be systematically evaluated in a prospective manner if placed on oral contraceptives, and depressed women who are on such agents should usually have them discontinued as part of a treatment plan.

Leuprolide (Lupron) is an injectable gonadotropin-releasing hormone agonist that reduces follicle-stimulating hormone and luteinizing hormone levels and is used in women for severe premenstrual syndromes. We have seen several women who developed an exacerbation of their mild depression when placed on it. The incidence of de novo depression/anxiety is greater than 20 per cent.

Danazol (Danocrine) is an androgenic steroid that has antiestrogenic effects and is used to treat endometriosis. We have collected scores of cases of severe depressive syndromes in women treated with normal doses of this agent (R. H. Gerner, unpublished observations). The general incidence of depressive/anxious symptoms is greater than 20 per cent. Treatment with antidepressants may be necessary in addition to discontinuing the danazol.

Yohimbine (Yocon) is an α_2-antagonist and consequently increases the release of norepinephrine. It is used to enhance erectile competence. While normal patients may experience mild anxiety at usual therapeutic doses of 5 to 10 mg, individuals with a predisposition to panic attacks (past panic attacks or family history) are likely to have a panic episode after ingesting yohimbine. The panic episode is seen as typical for that individual patient and is not merely a misinterpretation of mild sympathomimetic arousal. The incidence is very high in vulnerable individuals, with panic occurring in five of seven panic patients given oral yohimbine,[52] confirming earlier parenteral placebo-controlled studied demonstrating significant differences between normal and panic patients.[53]

Bariatric Agents

Bariatric agents (appetite suppressants) all act via the release of presynaptic norepinephrine or dopamine [*diethylpropion* (Tenuate), *benzphetamine* (Didrex), *phenmetrazine* (Preludin), *dextroamphetamine, methamphetamine*] or serotonin [*fenfluramine* (Pondimin)]. Anxiety from sympathomimetic effects is dose dependent. More marked psychiatric syndromes appear to be uncommon when the agents are used at "normal" doses, and the more publicized psychotomimetic effects are almost always due to acute or chronic excessive dosage in patients with a history of drug abuse or personality disorder. In such cases, the presence of paranoia accompanied by agitation is the common feature, with (visual) hallucinations being common. These effects are thought to be due to dopamine and respond well to neuroleptics. Withdrawal depression is similarly associated with high dosages and can be treated with antidepressants, albeit it usually remits quickly without specific treatment.

Ketamine

Ketamine (Ketalar) is a dissociative anesthetic agent that is no longer widely used in adults because of the frequency of hallucinatory phenomena lasting hours to days following induction. Treatment concomitantly with benzodiazepines (diazepam) may reduce this phenomenon, and symptomatic neuroleptic can be given if symptoms persist.

Bronchodilator Sympathomimetics

Bronchodilator sympathomimetics may produce anxiety syndromes via two mechanisms. First, the peripheral activation that occurs is often perceived as anxiety by the patient even if no drug entered the CNS. Second, many of these agents freely cross the blood-brain barrier, especially the nonselective agents such as *ephedrine, phenylephrine*, and the over-the-counter dilators and decongestants. Similarly, *theophylline* has a dose/blood level–dependent anxiogenic effect. Although psychotic symptoms can occur, this is very rare. The treatment of sympathomimetic-induced anxiety is complicated, since the most simple treatment (β-blockers) is contraindicated. *Atenolol* has been advocated as a β-blocker that has minimal effect on the pulmonary system but will reduce tachycardia and tremors. Benzodiazepines may be useful if chronic obstructive pulmonary disease (COPD) is not severe, and buspirone can be used with apparent impunity in COPD since it does not depress respiration at any dose. If anxiety symptoms persist, the selective β2-agonists (*albuterol, isoetharine, metaproterenol*, and *terbutaline*) and *terfenadine* (Seldane) and similar new histamine-1 blockers (*azelastine*) do not cause anxiety and should be tried.

CONCLUSION

It is apparent that the psychiatric effects of many of these nonpsychiatric medications are unpredictable with regard to frequency and presentation. New medications may have such effects that were not detected in initial clinical trials because of size or exclusion criteria of vulnerable patients. All patients who develop psychiatric symptoms should be carefully questioned for possible temporal relationships to changes in pharmacotherapy, and consideration should be given for referral for psychiatric consultation. Patients and their families may not make appropriate cause-effect relationships and may seek nonmedical psychotherapists who themselves are unaware of potential etiologies from these treatments.

REFERENCES

1. Learoyd BM: Psychotropic drugs in the elderly patient. Med J Aust 1:1131–1133, 1972.
2. Goodwin FK, Ebert MH, Bunney WH: Mental effects of reserpine in man: a review. In Shader RI, ed. Psychiatric Complications of Medical Drugs. Raven Press, New York: 1972:73–102.
3. Betts T, Alford C: β-Blocking drugs and sleep. Drugs 25(suppl 2):268–272, 1983.
4. Greminger P, Vetter H, Boerlin HJ, et al: A comparative study between 100 mg atenolol and 20 mg pindolol slow-release in essential hypertension. Drugs 25(suppl 2):37–41, 1983.
5. Cove-Smith R, Kirk CA: Letter to Editor. Postgrad Med J 59(suppl 3):161–163, 1983.
6. Westerlund A: Central nervous system side-effects with hydrophilic and lipophilic β-blockers. Eur J Clin Pharmacol 28(suppl):73–76, 1985.
7. Gengo FM, Gabos C: Central nervous system considerations in the use of β-blockers, angiotensin-converting enzyme inhibitors, and thiazide diuretics in managing essential hypertension. Am Heart J 116:305–310, 1988.
8. Williams GH: Angiotensin converting enzyme inhibitors in the treatment of hypertension. N Engl J Med 319:1517–1525, 1988.
9. Breitbart W: Tardive dyskinesia associated with high-dose intravenous metoclopramide. N Engl J Med 315:518–519, 1986.
10. Lazzara RR, Stoudemire A, Manning D, et al: Metoclopramide-induced tardive dyskinesia. Gen Hosp Psychiatry 8:107–108, 1986.

11. Flind AC, Jones DR: Mental confusion with cimetidine. Lancet 1:379, 1979.

12. Silverstone PH: Ranitidine and confusion. Lancet 1:1071, 1984.

13. Hollender MH, Jamieson RC, McKee EA, et al: Anticholinergic delirium in a case of Munchausen syndrome. Am J Psychiatry 135:1407–1409, 1978.

14. Liddon SC, Satran R: Disulfiram (Antabuse) psychosis. Am J Psychiatry 123:1284, 1967.

15. Reisberg B: Catatonia associated with disulfiram therapy. J Nerv Ment Dis 166:607–609, 1978.

16. Green RL, Lewis JE, Kraus J, Frederickson EL: Elevated plasma procaine concentrations after administration of procaine penicillin G. N Engl J Med 291:223–226, 1974.

17. Jackson SLO: Psychosis with isoniazid. Br Med J 2:743–746, 1957.

18. Craven JL: Cyclosporine-associated organic mental disorders in liver transplant recipients. Psychosomatics 32:94–102, 1991.

19. Pinto OS, Polikar M, DeBono G: Results of international clinical trial of Lioresal. Postgrad Med J 48(suppl, Oct):18–23, 1972.

20. Brogden RH, Speight TN, Avery GS: Baclofen: A preliminary report on pharmacological properties and therapeutic efficacy in spasticity. Drugs 8:1–14, 1974.

21. Davis KL, Hollister LE, Berger PA: Baclofen in schizophrenia. Lancet 1:1245, 1976.

22. Goldstein ET, Murray KB, Preskorn SH: Baclofen-induced delirium. Ann Clin Psychiatry 3:223–224, 1991.

23. Goodwin FK: Behavioural effects of L-dopa in man. In Shader RI, ed. Psychiatric Complications of Medical Drugs. New York: Raven Press, 1972:149–174.

24. Boyd AE, Reichlin S, Turksoy N: Galactorrhoea-amenorrhea syndrome: Diagnosis and therapy. Ann Intern Med 87:165–175, 1977.

25. Calne DB, Plotkin C, Williams AC, Nutt JG: Neophytides A, Teychenne PF: Long-term treatment of parkinsonism with bromocriptine. Lancet 1:735–738, 1978.

26. Borison RL: Amantadine-induced psychosis in a geriatric patient with renal disease. Am J Psychiatry 136:111–112, 1979.

27. Hausner RS: Amantadine-associated recurrence of psychosis. Am J Psychiatry 137:240–241, 1980.

28. McClellan DL, Chalmers RJ, Johnson AH: A double-blind trial of tetrabenazine, thiopropazate and placebo in patients with chorea. Lancet 1:104–107, 1974.

29. Byrd GJ, Kane FJ: Persistent psychotic phenomena following one dose of pentazocine. Texas Med 72:68–69, 1976.

30. Taylor M, Galloway DB, Petrie JC, et al: Psychomimetic effects of pentazocine. Br Med J 2:1198, 1978.

31. Anderson RJ, Potts DE, Gabow PA, et al: Unrecognized adult salicylate intoxication. Arch Intern Med 138:481, 1978.

32. Griffith JD, Smith CH, Smith RC: Paranoid psychosis in a patient receiving ibuprofen, a prostaglandin synthesis inhibitor: Case report. J Clin Psychiatry 43:499–500, 1982.

33. Ragheb M: Ibuprofen can increase serum lithium level in lithium-treated patients. J Clin Psychiatry 48:161–163, 1987.

34. Reynolds EH: Chronic antiepileptic toxicity: A review. Epilepsia 16:319–352, 1975.

35. Smith MC, Bleck TP: Convulsive disorders: Toxicity of anticonvulsants. Clin Neuropharmacol 14:97–115, 1991.

36. Thompson PJ, Trimble MR: Anticonvulsant drugs and cognitive functions. Epilepsia 23:531–544, 1982.

37. Gerner RH, Wilkins J: CSF cortisol in affective illness. Psychiatric Med 3:33–40, 1985.

38. Mitchell DM, Collins JV: Do corticosteroids really alter mood? Postgrad Med J 60:467–470, 1984.

39. Lewis DA, Smith RE: Steroid-induced psychiatric syndromes: A report of 14 cases and a review of the literature. J Affective Disord 5:319–332, 1983.

40. Hall RCW, Beresford TP: Psychiatric manifestations of physical illness. In Michels R, Cavenar JO, Brodie HKH, eds. Psychiatry, vol 2. Philadelphia: JB Lippincott, 1989:9.

41. Gupta VP, Ehrlich GE: Organic brain syndromes in rheumatoid arthritis following corticosteroid withdrawal. Arthritis Rheum 19:1333–1338, 1976.

42. Gifford S, Murawski BJ, Kline NS, Sachar RE: An unusual adverse reaction to self-medication with prednisone. Int J Psychiatry Med 7:97–122, 1976.

43. Falk WE, Mahnke MW, Poskanzer C: Lithium prophylaxis of corticotropin-induced psychosis. JAMA 241:1011–1012, 1979.

44. Hall RCW, Popkin MS, Kirkpatrick B: Tricyclic exacerbation of steroid psychosis. J Nerv Ment Dis 166:738–742, 1978.

45. Pope HG, Katz DL: Affective and psychotic symptoms associated with anabolic steroid use. Am J Psychiatry 145:487–490, 1988.

46. Pope HG, Katz DL: Psychiatric effects of anabolic steroids. Psychiatr Ann 22:24–29, 1992.

47. Pope HG, Katz DL: Body builders psychosis. Lancet 1:863, 1987.

48. Parry BL, Rush J: Oral contraceptives and depressive symptomatology. Compr Psychiatry 20:347–358, 1979.

49. Malek-Ahmdi P, Behrman PJ: Depressive syndrome induced by oral contraceptives. Dis Nerv Sys 37:406–408, 1976.

50. Herzberg BN, Johnson AL, Brown S: Depressive symptoms and oral contraceptives. Br Med J 4:142–145, 1970.

51. Herzberg BN, Draper KC, Johnson AL, Nichol GC: Oral contraceptives, depression and libido. Br Med J 3:495–500, 1971.

52. Uhde TW, Ballenger JP, Vittone B, et al: Human anxiety and noradrenergic function: Preliminary studies with caffeine, clonidine and yohimbine. In Proceedings of the Seventh World Congress of Psychiatry. New York: Plenum Press, 1985.

53. Charney DS, Heninger GR, Breier A: Noradrenergic function in panic attacks. Arch Gen Psychiatry 41:751–763, 1984.

Section M

OTHER SPECIFIC DISORDERS AND CONDITIONS

75

PREMENSTRUAL SYNDROME

JEFFREY L. RAUSCH, M.D.

Premenstrual syndrome (PMS) is a clinical disorder that represents a cyclical complex of behavioral and emotional symptoms occurring in the latter half of the menstrual cycle. Although over 150 different symptoms have been described to vary with the menstrual cycle, the most common symptoms include mood changes, irritability, swelling, and breast pain. Premenstrual syndrome is distinguished from the syndrome of painful menstruation (dysmenorrhea), although PMS and dysmenorrhea may coexist in some patients.

Premenstrual syndrome appears to be a prevalent disorder, comprising a significant proportion of depressive symptoms in the community. Blazer and colleagues[1] studied PMS prevalence using a multivariate classification procedure that examined patterns of depressive symptoms in the Piedmont region of the Epidemiological Catchment Area. Their method was free of a priori assumptions about the existence of any diagnoses. They found that premenstrual dysphoric symptoms clustered into a relatively pure type of syndrome, comprising 15 to 16 per cent of the population sample with depressive symptoms in that region of the country.

Although precise estimates about the prevalence of PMS in the U.S. population at large are not yet available, one study of 1852 women from a county in Sweden found a 73 per cent prevalence of mild premenstrual symptoms.[2] Only 7.5 per cent of women felt they needed to see a physician for their complaints. In another study, approximately 5 per cent of college women met symptomatic criteria for a 30 per cent increase in premenstrual symptoms, using proposed DSM-III-R criteria.[3]

Although most women may report at least some physical or emotional changes associated with specific phases of the menstrual cycle, for most these changes are not severe. In the study of Hallman,[2] 28 per cent of the women who reported premenstrual symptoms noted that their social functioning was negatively affected by their symptoms; 2.1 per cent had been absent from work as a result of premenstrual symptoms.

The onset of PMS may be at any time after menarche; complaints tend to be more frequent in women over 30.[2,4] Although precise information about the natural history of the disorder is not available, many women seeking treatment for the condition indicate that symptoms tend to worsen with age[2] or with the number of pregnancies. Premenstrual syndrome tends to abate after age 45,[1] or after menopause. It is not known whether there is a familial pattern to PMS, which would indicate a genetic or constitutional vulnerability to develop the disorder, although some evidence suggests that familial patterns may be present.

No specific laboratory tests are available. Although several findings have supported the possibility of low luteal progesterone, high estrogen, or low progesterone/estrogen ratios, other studies have not been supportive of such a pattern.[5,6] Some studies support the possibility of an asynchrony between progesterone and estrogen, or early ovulation, or decrease in progesterone over time relative to estrogen.

TREATMENT

Over 50 different treatment methods have been proposed for PMS. This chapter reviews the newer, more widely recognized, and better studied treatments. These treatments can be generally divided into three categories: (1) conservative measures, (2) pharmacological therapies in menstruating women, and (3) treatments that suppress the menstrual cycle itself.

Conservative Measures

Many women may not require specific medical treatment for mild premenstrual symptoms. For those who do, a conservative approach may be initially indicated. A number of studies have shown that the rate of placebo response often exceeds 40 per cent, and others have observed that symptoms may diminish with longitudinal monitoring.

In one study, only 20 per cent of women seeking treatment for PMS had their symptoms prospectively confirmed; of those, 81 per cent felt their symptoms no longer interfered with functioning after a 2-month observation period. Therefore, a 2-month period of prospective monitoring is indicated before establishing a diagnosis. In women diagnosed with PMS, conservative measures may include counseling on effective coping strategies, exercise, and diet.[7-9]

It has been postulated that a subgroup of women may benefit from a diet low in refined sugar, with frequent meals and avoidance of caffeine. Differences between follicular- and luteal-phase plasma glucose levels have not been found. Hypoglycemic symptoms induced with a glucose tolerance test are not specific to the luteal phase, and do not resemble the PMS symptoms. Some data suggest a potential dose-dependent association between caffeine consumption and the appearance of premenstrual symptoms, however.

Vitamin therapy with B_6 has been found to be more effective than placebo in dosages of 50 to 500 mg daily in four studies. Improvements in symptoms of depression, irritability, tiredness, dizziness, and nausea have been cited. However, four other studies do not find B_6 better than placebo at similar dosages (50 to 300 mg daily). High or prolonged dosages of pyridoxine may be associated with neurological toxicity in PMS sufferers.[10,11]

Vitamins E and A and magnesium have also been suggested for use in the treatment of PMS, although there are currently no convincing placebo-controlled data demonstrating their efficacy. Levels of vitamins A and E and magnesium have not been found to be lower in PMS sufferers. One well-conducted study indicated that 1000 mg daily of calcium carbonate was more effective than placebo for negative affect, water retention, and pain in premenstrual sufferers.[12]

Medical Treatments in Cycling Patients

Pharmacological Treatment

PROGESTERONE

Progesterone treatment is commonly used to relieve PMS, and there are many PMS sufferers who attest to its benefit. However, there is no weight of scientific proof for its effectiveness over placebo. Although good results have been occasionally reported with open progesterone administration, nearly all controlled studies have not found progesterone to be superior to placebo.[13] The same pattern was evident for synthetic progestogens, including ethisterone, norethisterone, and medroxyprogesterone acetate, although one study found norethisterone to be more effective than placebo for breast tenderness.[14]

ORAL CONTRACEPTIVES

Studies using oral contraceptives have yielded inconsistent results. Surveys have differed as to whether PMS symptoms are more commonly found in oral contraceptive users versus nonusers.[2,15] Oral contraceptives have their own psychological side effects that vary between subjects and between different available formulations. It is difficult to predict an individual's response to these agents.

DIURETIC/ANTIMINERALOCORTICOID TREATMENTS

One older theory of PMS held that PMS symptoms were analogous to a subclinical form of cerebral edema. Women with PMS have been found to have higher body water/potassium ratios in the luteal phase compared to controls. Also, fluctuations in capillary filtration rate and permeability to plasma proteins have been observed premenstrually. These observations have supported a rationale for the diuretic treatment of PMS.

The diuretic effects of metolazone 1 to 5 mg daily were more effective for irritability, tension, depression, headache, and water retention symptoms in a placebo-controlled study of women with premenstrual weight gain. A triamterene and benzthiazide combination was also found to be more effective than placebo for depressed mood and irritability. Spironolactone has been found to be better than placebo for bloatedness. In other double-blind placebo-controlled studies, however, neither chlorothalidone nor potassium chloride were better than placebo. We found atenolol, a drug that inhibits plasma renin activity, to reduce self-reports of irritability, although most other symptoms were not significantly improved over placebo. Diuretic therapy is effective for symptoms of water retention, but indications for the use of diuretics in the treatment of other mood symptoms appear less robust.

BROMOCRIPTINE

Bromocriptine has been tried for treatment of premenstrual symptoms because of the observed increases in prolactin levels during the luteal phases, and because breast pain (mastodynia) is a common symptom of PMS. Most studies indicate that bromocriptine is effective for the treatment of mastodynia, although a few other studies have found significant improvements in mood, including depressive symptoms, and irritability.[14]

PROSTAGLANDIN TREATMENTS

Mefenamic acid, a prostaglandin synthesis inhibitor, has had mixed results, with efficacy shown for mood symptoms in some, but not all, controlled studies. Efamol (evening primrose oil), a prostaglandin synthesis precursor, has also had different effects. Naproxen sodium is effective for pain. Prostaglandins are known to mediate dysmenorrheic somatic complaints, and the results of some previous treatment studies are confounded by the inclusion of dysmenorrheic women into the study samples.

Psychopharmacological Treatments

CLONIDINE

Multiple neurotransmitter systems interact with ovarian steroids through complex mechanisms. Consequently, several investigators have attempted to treat premenstrual mood symptoms directly with various psychopharmacological strategies. The central α_2-adrenergic presynaptic autoreceptor agonist properties of clonidine have been theorized to compensate for a putative excess of central noradrenergic activity via presynaptic noradrenergic inhibition. One study of clonidine indicated efficacy over placebo in reducing premenstrual psychiatric (Brief Psychiatric Rating Scale) ratings. Clonidine can reduce plasma renin activity and aldosterone excretion, and these results suggest that further study would be worthwhile.

ALPRAZOLAM

Alprazolam has been found to be more effective for premenstrual mood symptoms than placebo in at least two published reports.[16,17] This treatment appears to be useful when alprazolam is used 8 to 12 days prior to menses.[16] Doses have ranged from 0.25 to 4 mg daily; Smith et al.[17] found 0.25 mg t.i.d. to be effective. Therefore, it appears that potentiating gamma-aminobutyric acid inhibition of neuronal cell firing may be effective for the mood lability and irritability found during the late luteal phase.

NALTREXONE

There is evidence that an increased late luteal opioid receptor sensitivity, or a blockade of midcycle opioid agonist activity may be therapeutic for premenstrual dysphoria. One study examined naltrexone given on days 9 through 18 of the cycle, prior to the expected midcycle rise and fall of β-endorphin. The active treatment group did better than those on placebo for concentration difficulties, behavioral changes, and negative affect. The gastrointestinal effects of naltrexone may be limiting in some patients, however.

ANTIDEPRESSANTS

Recently, premenstrual mood symptoms have been studied in connection with response to antidepressant drug treatment. Two open studies have indicated encouraging results with nortriptyline and clomipramine, and several groups have also reported promising anecdotes of responses to fluoxetine, including one controlled study. Further studies are presently underway to confirm these initial positive impressions, but so far, the antidepressants appear promising for the treatment of premenstrual mood changes.

SEROTONIN AGONISTS

Fenfluramine, a drug that promotes serotonin release, has been found to relieve appetite changes, depression, and anxiety in PMS sufferers compared to placebo.[18] Also, the 5-hydroxytryptamine$_{1A}$ partial agonist buspirone was found to be effective in the treatment of premenstrual irritability, fatigue, pain, and social functioning in 34 patients treated with a mean daily dose of 25 mg of buspirone 12 days prior to menstruation. These studies are supportive of the hypothesis that raphe serotonin neuron functioning may be etiologically relevant in the expression of premenstrual mood symptoms.

Sleep Deprivation

One interesting report has suggested that eight of ten women with premenstrual depression responded to one night's total sleep deprivation.[19] These findings are interesting in comparison with the recent evidence suggesting a seasonal variation in PMS, with approximately 70 per cent of women experiencing fewer symptoms during the summer.[3]

Menstrual Cycle Suppression

The most effective methods for treating PMS derive from the suppression of ovulation. Premenstrual symptoms appear to be associated with hypothalamic-pituitary-gonadotropic cyclicity, since symptoms do not occur before puberty, during pregnancy, or after menopause. Premenstrual symptoms persist in hysterectomized women with ovariectomy, whereas ovariectomy appears to be effective.

Surgery

Surgical hysterectomy and bilateral oophorectomy with estrogen replacement appears to attenuate premenstrual mood symptoms. In one study, 14 women with severe debilitating PMS were treated with hysterectomy, oophorectomy, and continuous estrogen replacement. Psychological measures 6 months after the operation showed clear improvement in mood as indicated by ratings on the Overall Life Satisfaction (OLS) and the Profile of Mood States (POMS).[20] Currently there is no general consensus that PMS is an appropriate indication for ovariectomy, although this treatment may offer a potential alternative for the severely refractory patient.

Induction of Anovulation

Medical approaches to inducing anovulation include gonadotropin-releasing hormone (GnRH) agonist, a peptide capable of attenuating the menstrual cycle with chronic administration through a down-regulation of pituitary gonadotropin secretion. Muse and colleagues found that GnRH effectively and reversibly interrupted the menstrual cycle during a 3-month administration.[21] Concomitant with the abolishment of the menstrual cycle, there were improvements in both behavioral and physical symptoms over the 3 months during which the women were studied. Two subsequent reports substantiated improvements in bloating and breast tenderness, with perhaps less clear effects on mood. Both studies have noted, however, that certain women may suffer adverse effects, including worsened symptoms. Hypoestrogenemia induced by GnRH may be remedied by estrogen supplementation, without a loss of the therapeutic response.

Another medical anovulatory approach is danazol, a synthetic androgen that can suppress the hypothalamic-pituitary-gonadal (HPG) axis. Danazol has been shown to significantly attenuate premenstrual symptoms such as lethargy, irritability, and anxiety at doses of 200 to 400 mg, in comparison to placebo. The androgenic properties of danazol may limit its utility in women of childbearing age, and hirsutism may be problematic in some patients.

Ovulation may also be suppressed with estradiol treatment. Subcutaneous estradiol implants or percutaneous estradiol patches have been found more effective than placebo in anovulatory doses. In such patients, progestogen therapy is necessary during the last week of the cycle to prevent endometrial hyperplasia. The progestogen treatment may induce intolerable cyclical symptoms in some patients, and skin irritation and pigmentation may be associated with percutaneous patches.

SUMMARY

Premenstrual symptoms are prevalent in the population, and constitute a significant proportion of depressive symptoms in the community at large. Most women do not experience significant impairment from premenstrual symptoms, although perhaps 5 to 8 per cent do experience symptoms severe enough to legitimately warrant medical attention at some time.

Among women seeking attention, many may not meet strict criteria for the syndrome, and many will meet criteria for other psychiatric diagnoses. Among confirmed premenstrual sufferers, many will demonstrate an improvement with time, short of any specific medical intervention. However, for the remainder, several approaches are available for treatment of the core syndrome.

Conservative treatments and prospective monitoring may select placebo nonresponders as candidates for more interventive treatments. Fluid retention and complaints of bloating may be relieved with diuretics, and breast pain may respond to bromocriptine or norethisterone. Mood symptoms appear to respond to alprazolam, clonidine, antidepressants, fenfluramine, buspirone, atenolol, naltrexone, or calcium, although more research is necessary before the relative usefulness of each of these agents is known.

For the patient whose severe premenstrual symptoms cannot be ameliorated short of menstrual cycle suppression, GnRH, estradiol, and danazol are available as treatments to suppress the HPG axis itself and improve menstrual symptoms concomitant with the induction of amenorrhea.

More research is clearly necessary. What is evident is that the symptoms are common and represent a significant proportion of depressive symptoms in the community. Women benefit from attention to these symptoms. Recognizing that treatment responses may vary, a hierarchy of interventions can be advanced until satisfactory relief is achieved at the minimum level of intervention necessary to achieve a response.

ACKNOWLEDGMENT

This work was supported by the Department for Veterans Affairs.

REFERENCES

1. Blazer D, Swartz M, Woodbury M, et al: Depressive symptoms and depressive diagnoses in a community population. Use of a new procedure for analysis of psychiatric classification. Arch Gen Psychiatry 45:1078–1084, 1988.
2. Hallman J: The premenstrual syndrome—an equivalent of depression? Acta Psychiatr Scand 73:403–411, 1986.
3. Rivera-Tovar AD, Frank E: Late luteal phase dysphoric disorder in young women. Am J Psychiatry 147:1634–1636, 1990.
4. Gise LH, Lebovits AH, Paddison PL, et al: Issues in the identification of premenstrual syndromes. J Nerv Ment Dis 178:228–234, 1990.
5. Dennerstein L, Spencer-Gardener C, Burrows GD: Mood and the menstrual cycle. J Psychiatr Res 18:1–12, 1984.
6. Bäckström T, Sanders D, Leask R, et al: Mood, sexuality, hormones, and the menstrual cycle. Hormone levels and

their relationship to the premenstrual syndrome. Psycho-som Med 45(6):503–507, 1983.

7. Asso D: Levels of arousal in the premenstrual phase. Br J Soc Clin Psychol 17:47–55, 1978.

8. Canty AP: Can aerobic exercise relieve the symptoms of premenstrual syndrome (PMS)? J School Health 54:410–411, 1984.

9. Abraham GE: Nutritional factors in the etiology of premenstrual tension syndromes. J Reprod Med 28:446–464, 1983.

10. Dalton K: Progesterone, fluid and electrolytes in the premenstrual syndrome. Br Med J 281:61, 1980.

11. Dalton K, Dalton MJ: Characteristics of pyridoxine overdose neuropathy syndrome. Acta Neurol Scand 76:8–11, 1987.

12. Thys-Jacobs S, Ceccarelli S, Bierman A, et al: Calcium supplementation in premenstrual syndrome: A randomized crossover trial. J Gen Intern Med 4:183–189, 1989.

13. Maddocks S, Hahn P, Moller F, et al: A double-blind placebo-controlled trial of progesterone vaginal suppositories in the treatment of premenstrual syndrome. Am J Obstet Gynecol 154:573–581, 1986.

14. Ylostalo P, Kauppila A, Puolakka J, et al: Bromocriptine and norethisterone in the treatment of premenstrual syndrome. Obstet Gynecol 59(3):292–298, 1982.

15. Graham CA, Sherwin BB: The relationship between retrospective premenstrual symptom reporting and present oral contraceptive use. J Psychosom Res 31:45–53, 1987.

16. Harrison WM, Endicott J, Rabkin JG, et al: Treatment of premenstrual dysphoria with alprazolam and placebo. Psychopharmacol Bull 23:150–153, 1987.

17. Smith S, Rinehart JS, Ruddock VE, et al: Treatment of premenstrual syndrome with alprazolam: Results of a double-blind, placebo-controlled, randomized crossover clinical trial. Obstet Gynecol 70:37–43, 1987.

18. Brzezinski AA, Wurtman JJ, Wurtman RJ, et al: d-Fenfluramine suppresses the increased calorie and carbohydrate intakes and improves the mood of women with premenstrual depression. Obstet Gynecol 76:296–301, 1990.

19. Parry BL, Wehr TA: Therapeutic effect of sleep deprivation in patients with premenstrual syndrome. Am J Psychiatry 144:808–810, 1987.

20. Casper RF, Hearn MT: The effect of hysterectomy and bilateral oophorectomy in women with severe premenstrual syndrome. Am J Obstet Gynecol 162:105–109, 1990.

21. Muse KN, Cetel NS, Futterman LA, Yen SCC: The premenstrual syndrome: Effects of the "medical ovariectomy". N Eng J Med 311:1345–1349, 1984

76

PSYCHIATRIC TREATMENT OF ADULTS WITH HUMAN IMMUNODEFICIENCY VIRUS INFECTION

SAMUEL PERRY, M.D.

For over a decade psychiatrists have been treating the emotional, behavioral, and neuropsychological problems associated with infection by human immunodeficiency virus-1 (HIV), the etiological agent of acquired immunodeficiency syndrome (AIDS). Ironically, the main thing we have learned is that we knew a lot already. We brought to this new epidemic a vast clinical and research experience regarding the psychopathology associated with medical illness—depression, anxiety, delirium, dementia, adjustment disorders, and the like. The concern that we would have to start from scratch has not been realized. Those psychotherapeutic and psychopharmacological treatments that have proven effective for other patients are similarly effective for adults with HIV infection. Psychiatrists need not feel that they need

to acquire special expertise before they can help these patients.

As with any physical illness, however, the psychiatrist familiar with some basic information about HIV infection and its medical management will feel more comfortable treating such patients and helping them deal with the inevitable uncertainty associated with a chronic and ultimately fatal disease. This chapter therefore begins with a medical overview about the course of the illness, its various stages and physical manifestations, and the side effects of common treatments that may be confused with psychiatric problems. Against this backdrop, the chapter then presents some special considerations for pharmacotherapy, psychotherapy, and psychiatric inpatient management.

MEDICAL OVERVIEW

Epidemiology

HIV is a retrovirus that has been around for a long time, certainly decades and probably much longer. The best hunch is that HIV had been smoldering at low prevalence within isolated cultures in central Africa; then with migration into the cities, transportation of blood products, and international travel, HIV spread around the globe. Because HIV can be transmitted parenterally, it at first primarily infected those who received contaminated blood (e.g., hemophiliacs given factor VIII from pooled donations) or who shared contaminated drug paraphernalia (e.g., intravenous drug users); and because HIV can be transmitted sexually, it also at first primarily infected those most likely to be exposed by intercourse with many different partners (e.g., gay men within sexually active urban communities).

As a result, when the disease was first described in the early 1980s, those at risk in the United States were clustered into three "H" groups: hemophiliacs, heroin addicts, and homosexuals. With the spread of HIV, this early clustering into risk groups is less and less true: the development in 1985 of sensitive and specific serological assays (enzyme-linked immunosorbent assay with Western blot confirmation) has helped protect the blood supply, with the result that very few current transfusion recipients are now at risk. Conversely, heterosexual partners of infected parenteral drug users and bisexuals are now relatively more at risk as the epidemic has spread. Accordingly, although the public still may be influenced by the early spread of the illness among stigmatized individuals, the estimated 1 million persons infected in the United States comprise a heterogeneous population of males and females. A focus on "risk behaviors" rather than "risk groups" is a more accurate way of considering the likelihood of infection.

Pathogenicity

Although HIV has a simple structure—a strand of RNA encased within a protein capsule—its effects on the entire immune system are complex and devastating. Exquisitely targeted for a surface antigen on CD4 "helper" lymphocytes, HIV invades these cells, uses reverse transcriptase to reverse the usual DNA to RNA process, and encodes its own genetic message within the nucleus of the host cell. When the lymphocyte is then stimulated to reproduce, millions of HIV are made, destroying the CD4 cell as they exit and invading other CD4 cells. The diminution of total CD4 lymphocytes ("T cells") is therefore a rough clinical indication of how suppressed the immune system has become and how vulnerable the individual is to infections and tumors that opportunistically take advantage of this situation.

Of particular note for psychiatrists, HIV also directly affects the central nervous system (CNS). Soon after infection has occurred, and usually years before opportunistic infections and tumors appear, the spinal fluid will show evidence of HIV's presence. In most infected individuals, no clinically significant mental changes result from the leukoencephalopathy in predominantly subcortical areas, but a few physically asymptomatic adults will show a subtle "subcortical dementia" characterized by apathy, social withdrawal, avoidance of complex tasks, and complaints of "mental slowing" despite adequate function on the usual mental status questions that test memory, attention, concentration, and simple calculations. More sophisticated neuropsychological tests may detect a subtle impairment.

Unfortunately, with disease progression into frank AIDS (see "Staging"), a more significant dementia does develop in at least half the individuals before death. At this point it may be difficult to discern to what degree the notable cognitive decline is due to the direct effects of HIV on the CNS and how much it is due to systemic illness, to wasting, to opportunistic infections and tumors within the CNS, or to the iatrogenic effects of various medications.

Staging

Efforts to characterize the variable course of HIV infection are continually being revised as we learn more about the disease. The "four-stage" classification prepared by the Centers for Disease Control (CDC) is the most commonly used.

Stage I represents acute infection in which some patients may develop flu, a rash, a transient mononucleosis-like syndrome, or, more rarely, an acute meningoencephalitis, but most cannot identify the exact time when HIV infection occurred. Psychiatrists do not often see patients in stage I.

Stage II represents the period in which individuals are infectious but do not have any AIDS-related physical symptoms or signs. This latency phase lasts on average about 10 years, but the range is wide.

Stage III is similar to stage II except for the development of persistent and palpable lymphadenopathy at two or more extrainguinal sites. This chronic lymphadenopathy is due to antibody-ridden debris floating through the lymphatic system and is not in itself prognostic. At this point in the epidemic, most HIV-infected patients are in either stage II or III and are not physically symptomatic, but may be living with the fear of an ultimately fatal infection.

Stage IV-A represents the development of constitutional symptoms, such as persistent fever, diarrhea, fatigue, and at least 10 per cent of body weight. This stage has replaced the less precise term "AIDS-related complex" (ARC), but still encompasses a range of disability, with some patients being only mildly symptomatic and others being severely impaired even though they do not meet criteria for "frank AIDS" (Stages IV-B, -C, -D, and/or -E).

Stage IV-B indicates HIV-related neurological disease, including dementia, peripheral neuropathy, and myelopathy (effects of the virus on the spinal cord). *Stage IV-C* designates the wide array of opportunistic infections secondary to immunosuppression, including relatively milder infections such as oral candidiasis (thrush). *Stage IV-D* lists cancers indicative of a defect in cell-mediated immunity, such as Kaposi's sarcoma (KS), non-Hodgkin's lymphoma, or primary lymphomas of the brain. *Stage IV-E* is reserved for diseases that are not listed in other categories, but could be attributed to or complicated by HIV infection, such as anemia or chronic lymphoid interstitial pneumonitis.

This CDC staging is not intended to convey prognosis or severity of illness. Patients in earlier stages (I through IV-A) may die abruptly, whereas patients with frank AIDS may have relatively mild KS or may have recovered from an effectively treated opportunistic infection and live for several years with only minor physical problems, especially if complying with maintenance medications (see later in the chapter). Furthermore, patients with AIDS commonly have more than one disease within a given category (e.g., different opportunistic infections concurrently or sequentially) as well as diseases in different categories (e.g., neuropathy and KS).

PSYCHIATRIC ASPECTS OF MEDICAL TREATMENTS

Psychiatrists treating patients with HIV infection do not have to become experts about the medical aspects of the disease, but three attributes are helpful. First, because the course of the illness is so variable from one individual to another, because the physical complications are so unpredictable, because it is often so hard to tease apart which symptoms are psychological and which physical, and because the understanding of the infection and its treatment are changing so rapidly, the psychiatrist should have a tolerance for uncertainty and ambiguity. However, not knowing everything is not the same as not knowing anything. Psychiatrists can help patients appreciate this distinction and thereby convey a sense of control despite understandable concerns about the unknown and unknowable.

Second, because the physical complications and their treatments can be so complex, the psychiatrists must establish and maintain an alliance with medical colleagues involved in the patient's care. The psychiatrist does not need to know every esoteric detail about the medical management, just as the internist need not be told about more confidential psychosocial issues, but the nature of HIV infection usually requires that the psychiatrist step outside the isolated magic circle and work collaboratively with other physicians.

Third, the psychiatrist should have a basic knowledge about the psychological aspects of the more common physical illnesses and their treatments as well as an updated manual on the bookshelf for quick and easy reference (e.g., *Confronting AIDS: Update 1988*[1]). For starters, the following summary is provided.

Maintenance Medications

Zidovudine (AZT), which partially interferes with reverse transcriptase, has been found effective in controlled studies for reducing the mortality during the first year or so after HIV-infected adults develop *Pneumocystis carinii* pneumonia (PCP) or have total CD4 cells less than 500. Since not all patients can tolerate AZT (e.g., some develop severe anemia) and since many become refractory to the benefits after a couple of years, other related antiviral drugs are being tested; but these also are associated with adverse effects, such as the pancreatitis and neuropathy associated with dideoxyinosine (DDI). Maintenance antibiotics have also been shown to be beneficial in reducing PCP, such as trimethoprim-sulfamethoxazole (Bactrim), diaminodiphenylsulfone (Dapsone), and aerosolized pentamidine, which can be self-administered at home.

The efficacy of these and other treatments has been a reason to encourage HIV testing and determine who may benefit from early medical care, but psychiatrists must recognize that the initiation of these treatments in previously physically asymptomatic adults has emotional consequences. It is a benchmark in their illness; denial and minimization are much more difficult to sustain when one is taking a medication frequently throughout the day. Furthermore, the drugs can induce mental changes. AZT, for example, can cause not only headaches and nausea but severe insomnia and even agitation and mania, which may require more gradual induction or temporarily stopping the drug and administering inderal, benzodiazepines, or even lithium and neuroleptics. Even if serious side effects do not occur, the psychiatrist may need to help with the patient's long-term compliance, a problem because no immediate physical benefits are experienced.

Pneumocystis carinii Pneumonia

Caused by an organism that ordinarily colonizes human alveoli without consequence, PCP is the most common severe opportunistic infection. The initial symptoms are easy enough to ignore, just a mild and unproductive cough with maybe a little dyspnea on exertion, and several weeks may pass before the fever and respiratory distress require hospitalization. Even then chest radiographs may be normal, but usually they show a diffuse infiltrate radiating symmetrically from the hilum. Bronchoscopic washings or biopsy confirms the diagnosis.

From a psychiatric view, two points about PCP should be kept in mind. First, the early symptoms are easy to dismiss or, conversely, patients aware of how subtle these symptoms can be may become hypochondriacally preoccupied with each little cough. Generally, in the absence of fever and dyspnea, there is little cause for alarm. Second, although PCP was often rapidly fatal early in the epidemic, acute treatments and prophylaxis have improved considerably. It is no longer an imminent death sentence. Most patients recover after a brief hospitalization from their first or even second and third bouts and return to relatively active and productive lives for at least a couple of years.

Candida

When this fungus infects the esophagus and lungs, the effects can be devastating, but usually it just causes a white blanketing of the tongue and mouth (thrush), which may be uncomfortable but is not dangerous and responds promptly to topical nystatin or chlortrimazole troches. The psychiatrist who helps provide early effective treatment can help tighten the doctor-patient bond and reduce anxiety by indicating concretely that many manifestations of HIV infection can be treated if not cured.

Other Pathogens and Tumors

Psychiatrists may live with the fear that they will miss some opportunistic infection or tumor within the CNS and attribute the associated symptoms to some functional disorder, but the chances are quite slim. True, cryptococcal encephalitis can cause subtle changes in thinking and mood without diagnostic meningeal signs or focal findings, but by this time patients are usually quite sick with fulminant multisystemic infections caused by the fungus. Similarly, when *Toxoplasma gondii* infects the CNS, the encephalitis is characterized by headaches, fever, delirium, and coma and the mass brain lesions are characterized by seizures, focal neurological findings, and brain abnormalities detected by computed tomography (CT) scan or magnetic resonance imaging (MRI). Psychiatrists are not likely to be fooled by this protozoan. The CNS lymphomas, although more rare, are a bit more tricky in that mental changes can occur before headache and neurological signs and before CT scan or MRI confirms the diagnosis, but it is not as if other specialists would have necessarily made the diagnosis sooner, nor is there evidence that a few weeks' delay in diagnosis affects the prognosis.

However, there are two medical problems that might fool psychiatrists. First, complaints of blurry or diminished vision should not automatically be attributed to anxiety or to the side effect of a psychotropic medication. The complaint may be due to retinitis caused by cytomegalovirus (CMV) and therefore warrants prompt referral for evaluation since the potential blindness can be prevented, or at least delayed for months, by dihydroxypropoxymethylguanine (DHPG), provided the drug's effects on the

bone marrow can be tolerated. Second, the psychiatrist should be wary about attributing weight loss, apathy, sleep disturbance, and fatigue solely to depression. These symptoms can be caused by HIV itself or, potentially more treatable, by *Mycobacterium tuberculosis* (MTb), by *Mycobacterium avium-intracellulare* (MAI), herpes simplex virus (HSV), tertiary lues, coccidiomycosis, and histoplasmosis. An expert in infectious diseases may miss rare pathogens as well but, when confronted with the dilemma about what is physical and what is emotional, the psychiatrist will make a more informed decision after consulting with other members of the treatment team.

Finally, in regard to the psychiatric aspects of HIV illnesses, it must be emphasized that most often the psychiatrist is *not* struggling with the possibility of some unrecognized disease within the CNS or worried that depressive symptoms are due to some undiagnosed systemic infection. Instead, the psychiatrist is primarily focused on two other areas: first, helping the patient cope with physical problems that are apparent, such as the severe chronic pain of postherpetic neuralgia, the cosmetic and radiotherapeutic needs of KS, or the discouragement, pain, and fatigue of chronic diarrhea; and second, helping with the HIV-related psychiatric and psychosocial problems that are discussed next.

PSYCHOPHARMACOTHERAPY FOR HIV-INFECTED ADULTS

Antidepressants

In general, standard antidepressants are effective, are well tolerated at usual dosages, and do not increase immunosuppression. There is no reason to withhold antidepressants for an HIV-infected patient with a major mood disorder or with a dysthymia that has not responded to a brief trial of psychotherapy. There are, however, six things psychiatrists may want to keep in mind when considering antidepressants for this population.

First, there is a temptation to recommend antidepressants prematurely to these patients. Many are suffering an understandable normal grief over loss of loved ones and over their own incurable and ultimately fatal infection, but they do not have a loss of self-esteem, irrational guilt, or other psychological symptoms of depression. Often clinicians, feeling helpless themselves and wanting to do something, prescribe antidepressants without first noting if empathic support and the assurance of follow-up care will be enough.

Second, and paradoxically, many HIV-infected patients who are depressed and have a good chance of responding to medication are reluctant to take an antidepressant for fear that it will adversely affect their immune system or interact with other drugs.

Offering reassurance or even having them read scientific articles[2] will often be to no avail, and the psychiatrist is left with recommending psychotherapy alone (see later in the chapter).

Third, if and when antidepressants are recommended and accepted, their side effect profile should be tailored to the individual. Those patients with persistent severe diarrhea or with agitation and insomnia may respond better to a heterocyclic that is relatively more anticholinergic and sedating, such as amitriptyline; however, in general, HIV-infected depressed patients do better with a more activating antidepressant, such as imipramine, desipramine, or fluoxetine, because of increased sensitivity to anticholinergic side effects, because depressive symptoms more often include fatigue and lethargy, or both.

Fourth, for depressed patients with problems with intestinal absorption, there is an advantage in choosing agents with known therapeutic blood levels so that the appropriate dose can be determined (e.g., desipramine, imipramine, nortriptyline).

Fifth, some preliminary studies have suggested that individuals at risk for AIDS have high lifetime prevalence of affective disorders.[3] The psychiatrists should recognize this constitutional and perhaps biological predisposition to depression, not view symptoms as only reactive in nature, and consider that prolonged maintenance or intermittent pharmacotherapy may be necessary.

Sixth, if antidepressants are not well tolerated or the depression is severe, with marked suicidal ideation and vegetative decline, electroconvulsive therapy (ECT) should be considered. It has been safely and effectively administered to depressed patients with AIDS.[4]

Anxiolytics and Hypnotics

Unusually high levels of emotional distress have been found among some HIV-infected populations who are currently physically asymptomatic (CDC stages II/III) or have relatively mild prodromal symptoms (CDC stage IV-A). Some such patients describe feeling "like a walking time bomb." Chronic anxiety may also be associated with frequent medical monitoring (e.g., number of "T cells"), with real or feared experiences of stigmatization and discrimination, and with the need to modify sexual behaviors. The psychiatrist should therefore not assume that this distress is unwarranted because the patient does not yet have AIDS.

Because this anxiety can cause undue hopelessness, impede daily functioning and compliance with medical care, and disrupt the doctor-patient relationship, it must be addressed; however, many patients and some clinicians are tempted to overuse anxiolytics and hypnotics (e.g., lorazepam, diazepam, alprazolam). Benzodiazepines should be reserved for situational anxiety and transient insomnia. Daily maintenance over the years of HIV infection can lead to rebound insomnia, tolerance, and physical and psychological dependence. It is therefore preferable to use psychotherapeutic techniques for the chronic and mild to moderate distress associated with HIV infection. If the patient insists upon medication rather than "talk therapy," busipirone might be helpful as long as there is an understanding that a week or two may be necessary before the dysphoria improves.

Neuroleptics

Unless the HIV-infected patient has an underlying psychotic illness, such as bipolar disorder or schizophrenia, neuroleptics are rarely indicated. The exception is a psychotic delirium related to an organic mental disorder caused by HIV itself or secondary to CNS or systemic infections and tumors. Some reports have suggested that such patients are especially prone to severe dystonic reactions or neuroleptic malignant syndromes when high-potency neuroleptics are administered.[5] The psychiatrist may therefore prefer to prescribe lower potency neuroleptics in combination with shorter acting benzodiazepines for sedation and reduction of the agitation and combative behavior accompanying delirium.

Psychostimulants

Some studies have suggested that mild HIV-induced mental changes may precede the development of physical symptoms in an unknown, but small percentage of patients.[6] This milder impairment may be detected by a battery of neuropsychological tests that emphasize timed and subcortical tasks; however, since baseline testing is usually not available for comparison and since the tests are burdensome and not often easily available, psychiatrists more often make the diagnosis of "subcortical dementia" or "AIDS dementia complex" on the basis of a careful history that focuses on daily functioning and its deterioration over time. Especially suspect is the complaint of "slowed thinking" even in the presence of a normal mental status exam. For such patients, a trial of psychostimulants might be helpful (e.g., methylphenidate 5 to 10 mg at 8:00 A.M. and 12:00 noon).

PSYCHOTHERAPY FOR HIV-INFECTED ADULTS

Given the heterogeneity of HIV-infected populations, no single therapeutic strategy is universally applicable. As always, therapy must be tailored to the needs and capacities of the individual patient. There are, however, four components that tend to be shared by all HIV-related psychotherapies: psychosocial support, psychoeducation, behavioral modification, and distress reduction.

Psychosocial Support

The stigmatization often accompanying HIV infection may cut off the usual sources of support, a void the psychiatrist is left to fill by providing empathy, problem solving, and rather straightforward advice about whom to tell and whom not to tell about the infection as well as when to tell and how. Although stated briefly here, support in the context of a confidential setting is the scaffolding on which all other psychotherapeutic strategies are built.

Psychoeducation

Generally, three areas must be covered. First, the patient needs to be informed about the reasons medical monitoring is advisable. The role of "matchmaker" may fall upon the psychiatrist, who will need to consider the personality of the patient and make a referral to an appropriate internist, who in turn will follow the patient, provide HIV testing with counseling if not yet conducted, prescribe maintenance medication if and when necessary, and be available for prompt treatment of opportunistic infections and tumors. The first few weeks of psychotherapy are often focused on overcoming the patient's denial and resistance, reducing undue concerns about confidentiality, and increasing awareness about the medical benefits of early interventions.

Second, HIV-infected patients should be informed about the possibility of neuropsychological impairment. This discussion is best conducted in the context of an ongoing relationship and before an organic mental disorder has developed, thereby proving sufficient notice for the patient to make informed personal and financial arrangements while still having the time, capacity, and judgment to do so and decreasing the chance of contested wills. This information need not be alarming. The psychiatrist can honestly state that HIV-related mental changes are not inevitable, may not be severe, and differ in both cause and course from Alzheimer's dementia, which may be the patient's association. Many patients will have already heard of this possibility, so an open discussion is often experienced as relieving: "The devil that you see is less frightening than the devil you don't."

If permission is granted by the patient, family members and loved ones should participate in some of these psychoeducational sessions, preferably before but certainly soon after the onset of organic mental changes. Otherwise, along with the patient, they are likely to view more subtle changes in behavior and mood as purely volitional or psychological. Although cure is not yet available, the organic changes should not be described as untreatable, a description that conveys therapeutic nihilism and reduces hope. Instead, the psychiatrist can point out the value of medications; for example, AZT may delay or even temporarily reverse HIV-induced organic changes, and psychotropic medication can provide symptomatic treatment for associated agitation, irritability, and misperceptions. Furthermore, the provision of a familiar and structured environment with titration of stimuli can reduce the associated confusion.

The third psychoeducational task is discussing modes of HIV transmission. Most patients will know that the virus is definitely transmitted through semen, cervical secretions, and blood (including transplacentally and via shared drug paraphernalia), and most will have heard—even if they are unconvinced—that although HIV has been isolated in low concentrations from tears and perspiration, infectivity by this route has not been documented and "casual contact" is safe. Family members of patients with AIDS living in confined apartments and sharing meals, bathrooms, and other essentials of daily living have not acquired the infection.

More time is required to go over areas of relative and not absolute risks, areas in which little is known other than that there is wide variability.[7] Current estimates are that the chance of infection for a single sexual exposure using a condom with a low-risk partner who has recently tested seronegative is 1 in 5 billion, whereas the estimated risk for 5 years of regular unprotected sex with a known seropositive partner is 2 in 3. The risk of infection increases with the number of partners, with receptive anal intercourse, and with practices that lead to rectal trauma. More efficient sexual transmission has also been related to coexisting genital ulcers, to greater immunosuppression in the infected partner, and to a history of sexually transmitted diseases, such as syphilis and genital herpes. Male-to-male and male-to-female transmission is probably more efficient than female-to-male; but in the United States, as an increasing number of females become infected, relatively more males will become infected by heterosexual spread. A few case reports have indicated possible female-to-male and female-to-female orogenital transmission.[8]

The risk of a mother with HIV infection giving birth to an infected child is between 20 and 50 per cent for a first child and somewhat higher if a previously born child was infected. Because the infant will have maternal antibodies to HIV for about 15 months, the presence of infection during this period is often established by culture of the virus.

In regard to parenteral transmission, the risk of infection from a single exposure through shared "works" is not known, but it is known that once HIV-infected blood is given for transfusion, at least 89 per cent of recipients become infected. The risk of occupational exposure among medical professionals is also unknown, but after an accidental needle stick is estimated at 1 in 250 if the patient was infected with HIV, although the risk no doubt depends on the depth of the stick and the amount of fresh blood transmitted. The hurried pace during cardiac resuscitation or for surgical procedures for acute trauma may make medical staff more vulnerable. Although HIV cannot pass through intact epidermis, infection has been reported among health care workers who were splashed on mucous membranes and broken skin with the blood of patients with AIDS.

The information about relative risks cannot be presented dogmatically. The "facts" are changing every day as epidemiologists take aim at a moving target. Instead, the discussion should be considered a process that teaches the patient how to deal with certain ambiguities, weigh available and future data, and, within limits, make a reasonable personal decision along the spectrum of behaviors that are definitely safe (e.g., sexual abstinence and cessation of intravenous drug use) to behaviors that are somewhat safe (e.g., using latex condoms with nonoxynol-9 spermicidal jelly and chlorine bleaching of intravenous "works") to behaviors that are unsafe (e.g., douching, penile withdrawal, and reducing the number of sexual partners).

Behavioral Modification

For some patients, psychoeducation will not be sufficient to sustain a reduction in risk behaviors. This situation is not surprising. Education alone has failed to eliminate other life-threatening habitual behaviors, such as cigarette smoking, alcohol and drug abuse, noncompliance with medication, and seat belt recommendations. Furthermore, behaviors that are chronic, biologically driven, pleasurably reinforced, ego syntonic, linked to mental states of high arousal, and associated with a distant rather than immediate threat tend to be more refractory to change.

Based on paradigms developed and tested before the AIDS epidemic (e.g., the Health Belief Model, Social Learning Theory, Theory of Reasoned Action), investigators are examining therapeutic strategies to reduce risk behaviors, including cognitive reframing to increase personal effectiveness, roleplaying to increase skills at refusing unsafe sex, modeling to increase the perception that safer sex is the social norm, and, more often, an admixture of different theories and techniques.[9] As with most psychotherapies, we still do not know which approach is best for whom in decreasing HIV transmission, with one exception: it is already clear that drug rehabilitation programs are effective in reducing needle use and sharing and, to a lesser extent, in reducing unsafe sexual practices. Furthermore, since nonintravenous drug and alcohol use during sex is associated with increased rates of unsafe sex, the psychiatrist faced with the challenge of patients who are placing themselves or others at risk for HIV infection should always assess drug abuse or dependence and target interventions at these disorders if present.

The courts have not yet made a definitive decision about the psychiatrist's obligations if an HIV-infected patient is known to be placing others at risk, but the American Psychiatric Association has recommended that the physician has the ethical right but not the obligation to breech confidentiality and notify identified third parties at risk if attempts at counseling the patient have failed.[10]

Distress Reduction

One study has found that a six-session stress prevention training, which is based on the general principles of cognitive-behavioral therapy and on the specific techniques of stress inoculation, is more effective than psychoeducation alone in reducing anxiety and depression among physically asymptomatic HIV-seropositive patients.[11] Accumulating clinical experience suggests that other approaches are effective as well, including interpersonal psychotherapy to resolve role disputes and aberrant grief responses, psychodynamic psychotherapy to help provide a psychological meaning to and an intellectual mastery over distress, and client-oriented psychotherapy to help convey an unqualified positive regard to buffer the acidic reactions from self and others. These techniques may be implemented in all formats—individual, couple, family, and group.

PSYCHIATRIC HOSPITALIZATION OF HIV-INFECTED ADULTS

To the extent possible, patients with HIV infection should be admitted and treated for their mental illnesses similarly to other patients. They need not be excluded from recommended ward activities, and their infection need not be disclosed to other patients. Staff should practice the universal precautions recommended by the CDC for *all* patients, including disposal of needles without recapping, use of gloves when handling potentially hazardous material, and accessible biohazard bags for disposing equipment and waste. Patients infected with HIV do not require nursing in a single room unless there is bleeding, blood-stained fluids, or secretions, or the patient is so immunocompromised that he or she is likely to acquire infections from other patients, or the patient has tuberculosis or some other organism in addition to HIV that poses a risk to others.

Exceptions to these general guidelines do exist. Some wards are not equipped to handle serious medical problems, necessitating transfer either to a medical unit or to a facility more closely allied with a general hospital. HIV-infected patients who are potentially violent evoke rational and irrational fears among staff members and other patients. Appropriate tranquilization, restraint, and seclusion should be implemented sooner rather than later to reduce these fears and in turn make the patient more accessible to treatment. The staff has an ethical and legal responsibility to protect others from sexual transmission. Manic, antisocial, regressed, or disinhibited patients should be placed in wards that are sufficiently well staffed to prevent such an occurrence, and other patients should be encouraged to report any sexual advances so that staff can promptly intervene. Condoms should be readily available for HIV-infected patients on pass and at discharge, and unescorted activities should only be granted after reasonable assurance that unsafe sexual practices will not occur.

CONCLUSIONS

Although AIDS has only been around a short time, we already know that it is similar to many other severe illnesses that affect emotions, behavior, and brain function and that have meaning both to the individual and to society. True, the epidemic has highlighted ethical and legal problems and national deficiencies in delivery of health care, but it has also provided psychiatrists an opportunity to tighten our alliance with medical colleagues, to advance our understanding about the relationship between the mind and body, and to apply past knowledge and current advances to treat this population. Psychiatry has responded and will continue to respond to this challenge.

REFERENCES

1. Institute of Medicine/National Academy of Sciences: Confronting AIDS: Update 1988. Washington, DC: National Academy Press, 1988.
2. Rabkin JG, Harrison WM: Effect of imipramine on depression and immune status in a sample of men with HIV infection. Am J Psychiatry 147:495–497, 1990.
3. Perry S, Jacobsberg L, Fishman B, et al: Psychiatric diagnosis before serological testing for human immunodeficiency virus. Am J Psychiatry 147:89–93, 1990.
4. Schaerf FW, Miller RR, Lipsey JR, et al: ECT for major depression in four patients infected with human immunodeficiency virus. Am J Psychiatry 146:782–784, 1989.
5. Breitbart W, Marotta RF, Call P: AIDS and neuroleptic malignant syndrome. Lancet 2:1488–1489, 1988.
6. Perry S: Organic mental disorders caused by HIV: Update on early diagnosis and treatment. Am J Psychiatry 147:696–710, 1990.
7. Curran JW, Jaffe HW, Hardy AM, et al: Epidemiology of HIV infection and AIDS in the United States. Science 239:610–616, 1988.
8. Perry S, Jacobsberg L, Fogel K: Orogenital transmission of human immunodeficiency virus. Ann Intern Med 111:951–952, 1989.
9. Kelly JA, St. Lawrence JS, Hood HV, et al: Behavioral interventions to reduce AIDS risk activities. J Consult Clin Psychol 57:60–67, 1989.
10. Perry S: Warning third parties at risk of AIDS. Hosp Community Psychiatry 39:731–739, 1989.
11. Perry S, Fishman B, Jacobsberg L, et al: Effectiveness of psychoeducational interventions after HIV antibody testing. Arch Gen Psychiatry 48:143–147, 1991.

77

INTERMITTENT EXPLOSIVE DISORDER

ROLAND D. MAIURO, Ph.D.

CLINICAL DESCRIPTION

As defined in the DSM-III-R, intermittent explosive disorder consists of dyscontrol episodes of impulsive aggression characterized by serious assaultive behavior or property damage. The quality and magnitude of the aggressive response are "explosive" in that it appears to be grossly out of proportion to identifiable precipitating events or psychosocial stressors. Moreover, the pattern is "intermittent" or episodic, without signs of generalized impulsivity or aggressiveness between the episodes.

The type of aggression exhibited in intermittent explosive disorder is distinct from other acts of aggression in that it appears to be impulsively driven by poorly controlled affect or "rage." Socially damaging acts thus appear as "crimes of passion" as opposed to instrumental acts (e.g., gang or underworld assault, terrorism, hate crimes) or predatory aggression of a primary psychopathic nature (e.g., vandalism, serial murder, or rape). The individual exhibiting this behavior pattern may, in fact, describe the violent behavior in an ego-dystonic fashion as "something that came over" them in the form of a "spell" or "attack," and express subsequent guilt or regret.

Diagnostic classification of intermittent explosive disorder requires that the practitioner rule out other DSM-III-R disorders associated with aggression. These include psychotic disorders, organic personality syndrome, antisocial or borderline personality disorder, and conduct disorder. The behavior must also occur, at least at times, independently of intoxication with a psychoactive substance.

Prevalence and Course

In a 2-year study of a general psychiatric inpatient population at the University of Maryland, Monopolis and Lion[1] reported that 2.4 per cent of the 830 patients met criteria for explosive disorder, a figure similar to those reported in early DSM-III field trials (1.8 to 2.8 per cent). The age and sex distribution in their sample also conformed to DSM-III field trial data in that a large percentage (80 per cent) of patients were young males, with many in their 20s and 30s. The observed gender difference in favor of men is congruent with cross-cultural findings of greater aggressivity in men, particularly when indices of physical aggression are employed.

Clinical researchers specializing in violent behavior have suggested that explosive disorders are, in fact, quite prevalent, but are rarely seen or appropriately identified by practitioners in general psychiatric or health care settings.[2] Studies that have described the victim as well as the perpetrator have reported that commonly the violence is directed toward spouses or family members.[3] Recent reviews of diagnostic protocols used in hospital emergency room and psychiatric settings indicate that domestic violence is a major public health concern that is grossly underreported and inadequately treated by health care practitioners.[4] These reports, together with the knowledge that violent and assaultive behavior problems often come to the attention of criminal justice systems rather than mental health systems, seriously limit our ability to develop reliable prevalence rates. Enough data exist, however, to suggest that existing prevalence figures are probably a low estimate of the actual frequency with which such problems occur in the general community.

Limited data exist regarding the long-term course for cases identified as intermittent explosive disorder. Longitudinal studies of aggressive personality traits indicate that aggressive behavior is quite stable developmentally and often resistant to traditional, nonspecialized psychotherapeutic interventions.[5] In a controlled treatment study of domestically violent men, many of whom would easily meet the criteria for explosive disorder, there was little change in aggression for a group that received minimal treatment and monitoring over a 6-month period.[6]

Family History

Studies of violent and aggressive individuals indicate that many have a history of violence in their family of origin. In fact, when all developmental risk variables are examined, this is probably the strongest predictive factor associated with violence toward strangers as well as intimates. In national surveys of

domestic and nondomestic assault, Straus and Gelles[7] found the risk for violence in men to be eight- to tenfold if a violent parent was present in their family of origin.

While some researchers have suggested that some diagnosable conditions associated with temper problems (e.g., antisocial personality disorder, attention-deficit hyperactivity disorder) may have a degree of genetic heritability, others have doubted whether this actually occurs. In a small but well-controlled study of familial history, Mattes and Fink[8] found evidence that a personality trait or disposition to temper outbursts was more strongly transmitted than were specific diagnoses such as intermittent explosive disorder or antisocial personality disorder. Approximately 14 per cent of the explosive disorder sample had first-degree relatives with temper problems, compared to 4 per cent of a general psychiatric control sample. However, sociological and psychological researchers have noted that intergenerational transmission occurs through a variety of nongenetic mechanisms, making the exact role of genetics difficult to determine. These factors include direct parental modeling of aggression as a response to conflict, instilling attitudes that condone or facilitate aggression, and emotional desensitization regarding the consequences of such behavior for self and others.

Differential Diagnosis

In evaluating well over 1000 cases of anger dyscontrol and assaultive behavior, Maiuro and his colleagues identified a broad spectrum of diagnosable profiles in addition to intermittent explosive disorder.[6] In accord with the findings of other investigators, many cases met criteria for personality disorders, various types of depression, impulse control disorder, unresolved learning disabilities or attention deficit disorder, alcohol abuse, cyclic mood or arousal disorders, adjustment reactions, organic personality syndromes, and, to a lesser extent, formal thought disorder. Table 77–1 provides a description of the different patterns of violent and aggressive behavior commonly reported for various diagnostic categories in the clinical research literature.

Differential diagnosis requires that many of the diagnoses listed be ruled out before a diagnosis of intermittent explosive disorder is applied. Exceptions include nonpsychotic depressions and secondary, intermittent alcohol and substance abuse problems, which may coexist in many cases and require treatment as related but separate problems.

Despite the presence of diagnosable psychological conditions in many cases, it should be emphasized that violent behavior can be found in a broad cross section of the population. Moreover, with the exception of intermittent explosive disorder, which includes violent behavior by definition, many diagnostic categories list aggressive behavior as one of many possible manifestations of affective instability and

TABLE 77–1. PSYCHIATRIC DIAGNOSIS AND COMMON PATTERNS OF VIOLENCE
REPORTED IN THE CLINICAL LITERATURE

Diagnostic Label	Common Pattern of Violence
Schizophrenia (paranoid)	Interpersonal; directed toward others who are delusionally perceived as persecuting or depriving; methodic; use of weapons; high risk due to severity and lethality
Schizophrenia (undifferentiated)	Trespassing, property damage; interpersonal in context of need for avoidance and escape; early or acute phases of disorder
Antisocial personality impulse control disorder	Multiple forms of aggressive behavior; intimate and non-intimate victims; early onset; repetitive; sometimes instrumental nature
Intermittent explosive disorder	Interpersonal violence toward intimates and/or nonintimates; property damage; episodic in otherwise controlled or overcontrolled individual; ego dystonic
Organic brain syndrome	Unfocused; disorganized; confused; destructive attempts at self-protection; generalized irritability and pathologically low frustration tolerance
Manic-depressive	Short fused; quickly subsiding; high ratio of verbal and physical posturing with actual interpersonal violence less likely; high-frequency but low-severity displays
Grief reaction, dysthymic disorder, adjustment disorder, dependent personality, mixed personality disorder with paranoid features	Spouse abuse; exit blocking in response to threatened loss of mate; destructive and maladaptive attempts to restore power, predictability, and control

impulse dyscontrol. In those cases in which diagnosable psychopathology exists, it is most profitably viewed as a vulnerability factor that makes the angry and assaultive behavior more likely, rather than a causal entity. Most researchers now agree that violent behavior is a complex, multidetermined phenomenon that occurs in the context of a variety of situational, interpersonal, psychological, and sociocultural variables.

CLINICAL ASSESSMENT AND TREATMENT

Comprehensive treatment of aggressive behavior requires that the clinician consider multiple avenues of intervention, including crisis management,[9] psychopharmacological methods, cognitive-behavioral methods, and, if needed, a coordinated public health response with referring agencies. Increasingly, health care providers are held accountable by the public to recognize cases at risk for assault and to make reasonable efforts to intervene.[10] Therefore, a carefully conducted assessment is essential to adequately evaluate and manage the risk and to develop an appropriate treatment plan.

Clinical Assessment

Effective intervention with explosive or violent behavior is often a difficult and time-consuming process. Angry emotions may be covered and distorted by a variety of defense mechanisms, including denial, minimization, suppression, repression, and isolation. Given the social undesirability of interpersonal violence and the legal duress that many clients face, care must be taken to ensure satisfactory levels of trust and predictability in the therapeutic relationship as part of the assessment process. Sufficient time must be allowed for the patient to overcome the discomfort associated with the sharing of socially undesirable acts and attitudes. It may take a number of visits before sufficient trust is established between the intake worker and the patient, and a multiple-stage assessment process should be considered.

Checks should be conducted on test-taking attitude if psychometric or self-report indices are employed, and multiple sources of information should be gathered to help ensure a reliable and comprehensive evaluation. The multiple sources of information may include: all relevant offense history (police and victim reports on both current and prior infractions of all types), comprehensive mental health data through psychiatric interviewing, extended interviewing with respect to anger control and violence history, a battery of psychometric indices, and reports from the spouse, friends, or relatives.

It is not uncommon for angry and violent patients to feel distressed and ambivalent about their need for help. It is important for the clinician to know about the individual's source of motivation for seeking help (e.g., court, family, personal dissatisfaction), potential stressors or impending losses, and the consequences associated with the violent and abusive behavior (e.g., divorce, separation, reconciliation, access to children, fines, legal proceedings, conditions of probation). While some therapists may use such information to help determine the patient's amenability to their particular approach or program, there are currently few data to suggest that these variables have predictive power regarding outcome in the individual case. They do, however, appear to be useful in alerting the clinician to areas that may require further assessment, case management, clarification regarding client expectations, and strategies to overcome treatment resistance, compliance issues, and dropout problems.

Whether or not the spouse or mate is to be actively involved in the treatment process, it is important to involve them in the assessment stage. The spouse may be a more reliable source for describing the violence since he or she is on the receiving end of the punches, pushes, and blows. Some clinicians believe that the memory of perpetrators may be impaired or limited during periods of extreme rage, and that this adds to the risk of underreporting already present as a result of psychological defensiveness and social undesirability.[3] It is also essential to establish contact with the spouse for purposes of assessing and monitoring dangerousness. The clinician who treats intermittent explosive disorder cases should be prepared to assume case management responsibility for family safety issues and be aware of community shelter and advocacy resources for potential victims.

Clinical protocols should be used to identify risk factors for serious forms of injury. It is important to ask questions focused on the frequency and severity of previous violent episodes, injuries, specific intent to harm, and the availability of weapons. A number of investigators have also found similarities in emotional state between suicidal and homicidal men,[3,11] indicating the need to ask about history of suicide in the family, personal attempts, threats, and ideation. Intermittent explosive disorder may also be complicated by depression, which may not be apparent until a comprehensive assessment is performed.[12,13] Alcohol or substance abuse has been associated with violent episodes of greater frequency, longer duration, and greater severity of injury and should be assessed.

Laboratory Studies

Clinical researchers appear to differ on the importance of neurological signs in the diagnosis and treatment of intermittent explosive disorders. This is reflected in the changes in the DSM-III-R compared to the DSM-III, which previously listed a number of essential and associated features of neurological significance. These signs include prodromal affective or autonomic symptoms in the form of an "aura," subtle changes in sensorium during an episode, hypersensitivity to sensory stimuli, and partial amnesia.

Some investigators have suggested that intermittent explosive behavior may be due to limbic system dysfunction[3] or seizure disorder.[14] However, when tests are conducted, actual findings generally fall

into the category of "soft" neurological signs. When an electroencephalogram (EEG) is performed, nonspecific rhythm abnormalities have been documented in many cases along with some theta activity. Importantly, no consistent relationships between history, symptoms, or response to treatment have emerged in association with EEG findings. Currently, neither hard nor soft neurological signs are required to diagnose intermittent explosive disorder according to the DSM-III-R. Clear organic symptoms may be helpful in differentially identifying organic mood syndrome, organic personality syndrome, or organic personality disorder.

Toxic screening for abuse of drugs such as cocaine, lysergic acid diethylamide (LSD), amphetamines, and phencyclidine (PCP) is indicated in some cases, particularly in young males with a history of conduct disorder. Such drugs increase the risk for violence secondary to increasing arousal and irritability, as well as the possible induction of psychosis and paranoia. PCP has a track record of inducing out-of-control behavior of particularly high intensity. It can also return to circulation from fat stores in the body and precipitate a toxic state after the patient has been stabilized.

Psychological Testing

In cases of explosive and assaultive behavior, the patient is best assessed with a comprehensive battery of measures. Such measures might include: a general psychopathology inventory [e.g., Minnesota Multiphasic Personality Inventory (MMPI), Millon Clinical Multiaxial Inventory]; a depression measure (e.g., Beck Depression Inventory); a measure of assertiveness or coping strategies (e.g., Assertiveness-Aggressiveness Inventory, Revised Ways of Coping Checklist); an index of drug or alcohol abuse (e.g., Michigan Alcohol Screening Test); and specific measures of angry, violent, and abusive behavior (e.g., Index of Spouse Abuse, Spielberger State-Trait Anger Expression Inventory).

Despite its length, the MMPI has a number of advantages, including subscales focused on various subtypes of anger and hostility (e.g., Overcontrolled Hostility) and validity scales to measure the subject's test-taking attitudes and response style (e.g., lying, minimization, defensiveness). These issues are very important when assessing anger and hostility because of the social undesirability commonly associated with the anger and abusive behaviors. The MMPI also allows anger dyscontrol issues to be examined in the context of other emotional tendencies (e.g., paranoia, anxiety, and depression) as well as the subject's general personality features.

Practitioners in busy, time-limited clinical settings might consider the Brief Anger-Aggression Questionnaire (BAAQ) as a more limited screening measure.[15] The BAAQ is a six-item measure derived from the Buss-Durkee Hostility Inventory (BDHI) specifically developed for the rapid assessment and identification of violence-prone men (Table 77–2). Factor-analytic studies indicate that the BAAQ is a measure of overtly expressed anger characterized by generalized irritability and a tendency to act in an aggressive and violent fashion. It has been useful in distinguishing domestically violent men from nonviolent control subjects. The BAAQ also correlates highly with the full BDHI ($r = .78$) and is sensitive to psychological and behavioral changes associated with treatment. Advantages of the BAAQ include the fact that it usually takes about a minute to administer, it has normative data for both domestically violent and generally assaultive men, and there are two forms of the instrument that allow for direct assessment of the patient and an independent rating of the patient by the spouse, a friend, or a relative (BAAQ-O).

Pharmacological Treatment

Eichelman[16] has proposed a "rational pharmacotherapy" approach based upon four biological systems implicated in the genesis of aggressive behavior. Three are neurotransmitter systems. These include: the gamma-aminobutyric acidergic (GABA-ergic) system, the noradrenergic system, and, of more recent interest, the serotonergic system. The fourth system is a neurophysiological system associated generally with electrical activity in the brain and specifically with seizure activity in the form of "kindling" patterns and epilepsy.

Animal studies have demonstrated that the GABA system inhibits various types of aggression. Psychopharmacological intervention enhances GABA activity through activation of the benzodiazepine receptor system. The human clinical literature suggests that benzodiazepines (diazepam, chlordiazepoxide) can be useful in the management of agitated, aggressive patients. Intramuscular doses of lorazepam have been used in emergent situations to attenuate aggressive behavior in out-of-control patients. It should be noted, however, that paradoxical rage reactions have been observed in a minority of patients, suggesting the need for careful monitoring of response. Some writers indicate that more cases of increased aggressiveness have been reported for diazepam and chlordiazepoxide than oxazepam.

The noradrenergic system has long been recognized for its activating influence upon aggression in animals. Elevated levels of norepinephine metabolites have been found in human studies of aggressive behavior. Cerebral spinal fluid (CSF) assays have shown elevated levels of 3-methoxy-4-hydroxylphenylglycol, and blood tests have yielded elevated levels of phenylethylamine, in some aggressive patients.

Early studies have demonstrated lithium carbonate to be associated with decreased aggressive acts in violent patients who had been institutionalized.[17] Like lithium, β-adrenergic antagonists also act to decrease the functional availability of norepinephine. Based upon case studies, various clinical researchers have reported that β-blockers such as propranolol, metoprolol, pindolol, and nadolol may decrease aggressive behavior, even when used with chronically disturbed patients.

Animal studies have demonstrated that manipulation of brain concentrations of serotonin upward and downward can predictably increase and decrease aggressive behavior in rats. Diagnostic studies of chronically aggressive inpatients have yielded parallel data suggesting a link between low CSF levels of 5-hydroxyindoleacetic acid and chronic aggressivity. Serotonin-enhancing compounds (tryptophan, fluoxetine) are now being tested for antiaggressive effects.

Neurophysiological studies in animals have demonstrated that affective aggression episodes can be elicited through brain stimulation. Moreover, subictal levels of electrical activity can potentiate "kindling" patterns in which fearful and aggressive behaviors occur in the absence of clearly identifiable seizures.

TABLE 77–2.   BRIEF ANGER-AGGRESSION QUESTIONNAIRE[a]

Directions: Read the statements listed below. Rate each one so that it describes your current way of feeling or behaving.

1. When I really lose my temper, I am capable of hitting or slapping someone.

0	1	2	3	4
Extremely Unlikely	Unlikely	Possible	Likely	Very likely

2. I get mad enough to hit, throw, or kick things.

0	1	2	3	4
Not at all	Rarely	Sometimes	Frequently	Very frequently

3. I easily lose my patience with people.

0	1	2	3	4
Not at all	Rarely	Sometimes	Frequently	Very frequently

4. If someone doesn't ask me to do something in the right way, I will avoid, delay doing it, or not do it at all.

0	1	2	3	4
Not at all	Rarely	Sometimes	Frequently	Very frequently

5. At times I feel I get a raw deal out of life.

0	1	2	3	4
Not at all	Rarely	Sometimes	Frequently	Very frequently

6. When I get mad I say threatening or nasty things.

0	1	2	3	4
Not at all	Rarely	Sometimes	Frequently	Very frequently

[a] Reprinted with permission from Maiuro RD, Vitaliano PP, Cahn TC: A brief measure for the assessment of anger and aggression. J Interpersonal Violence 2:166–178, 1987.

Diagnostic studies of aggressive patients frequently yield histories of head injury, soft neurological signs, and abnormal EEG results. Such findings have led to trials of anticonvulsants in some cases of intermittent aggression. Early work with phenytoin has been supplanted by carbamazepine, which numerous investigators have found effective. It should be noted, however, that some clinicians believe other medications should be tried before carbamazepine because of potential side effects of bone marrow suppression in some cases.

Eichelman[16] offered the following suggestions to clinicians considering psychopharmacological approaches: (1) use the most benign intervention when beginning treatment; (2) select the medication that most closely addresses the primary illness, because the dyscontrol episodes may be a by-product of this problem; (3) have some quantifiable means of assessing efficacy and side effects (repeated structured interviews or psychometrics); and (4) institute drug trials systematically by applying one intervention at a time, assessing its impact, and monitoring therapeutic levels through routine lab work.

Cognitive-Behavioral Approaches

Many practitioners believe that psychoeducational and cognitive-behavioral approaches are particularly well suited for patients with anger, violence, and impulse control problems. These approaches tend to be highly structured and directive and are generally offered as an opportunity for "self-improvement" (educational classes, personal growth workshops) rather than as treatment of illness or pathology. As a result, this type of programming can facilitate the entry of patients who might otherwise be reluctant to seek services.

Recent programming efforts have focused upon specific populations defined by the setting or victim of the abusive behavior (e.g., domestic violence, spouse abuse). A variety of methods are employed to: (1) increase the patient's awareness, appreciation, and accountability for their acts; (2) enhance the patient's ability to identify and manage the attitudes and emotions that are associated with violent behavior; (3) decrease social isolation and provide a supportive milieu for change; (4) decrease hostile-dependent relationships, in those cases in which they exist; and (5) develop nonviolent and constructive conflict resolution skills.

Anger management training has become a core component of cognitive-behavioral treatment programs for assaultive individuals. The seemingly uncontrollable and unanticipated episodes of violence perpetrated by many patients can be explained by the patients' poor sense of their own irritability and anger. To increase patients' awareness of anger cues and dynamics, we have developed a psychoeducational videotape that portrays a variety of vignettes related to anger and assaultive behavior. Patients view the videotape in a group setting and are encouraged to compare their own experiences to those illustrated in the vignettes. Patients are also taught cognitive, behavioral, and physiological signals related to anger and impending loss of control to help them recognize and short circuit an aggressive response in the early stages of arousal. Discrimination training can be employed to help the patients differentiate their emotional response (anger, frustration, threat), which is appropriate and acceptable, from their behavioral response or expression (verbal abuse, violent tirade), which is inappropriate and damaging.

Anger reactions in assaultive individuals often appear to be deeply ingrained traits[7] and are often experienced as "automatic" or reflexive reactions. Cognitive restructuring techniques such as Ellis' ABC model of emotional response can be useful in pinpointing the self-generated components of an anger response. Having the client repeatedly record and examine the antecedent events and the mediating appraisals or beliefs that are associated with his or her emotional response can help foster the development of self-control strategies.

In some cases, anger may be used to mask a variety of other feelings related to threat and vulnerability. As a result, the emotion of anger tends to be overly used and abused. Moreover, the powerful surge of adrenaline experienced during an angry and violent tirade can dissipate feelings of hurt and helplessness and create a vicious and addictive cycle of aggressiveness. Some programs[6,18] employ a variety of structured exercises (feeling journals, videotaped scenarios, and discussion) to help spouse abusers recognize and label a more flexible range of emotions and feelings. These exercises are designed to develop alternative responses to anger and to desensitize the patient to emotions that may have been socially or developmentally counter-conditioned (e.g., hurt, sadness) or anxiety provoking (e.g., fear, jealousy, insecurity).

Intense arousal can interfere with higher cortical functioning and interpersonal problem solving during stressful encounters. Clients can be taught a variety of arousal reduction strategies such as progressive muscle relaxation, imagery, and deep breathing exercises. Other clients may employ more naturalistic techniques such as going for a walk or listening to soothing music. Such "self-control" techniques can help increase the probability that the client will maintain a state of body and mind that is conducive to good communication and rational problem solving.

Individuals who commit acts of violence often lack appropriate conflict resolution skills and resort to more primitive and physical ways of acting and responding. A number of clinicians have identified a lack of assertive or problem-solving skills as an area of dysfunction for violent men. The assertiveness deficits fall into two general domains: skill deficits and discrimination problems in which the individual confuses assertiveness with aggressiveness.[19]

These deficits can be addressed with a variety of techniques, including bibliotherapy (providing reading assignments that define, describe, and legitimize assertive behavior), therapist modeling, roleplay methods, and videotaped feedback focused on discrimination training regarding noncoercive and nonabusive communication styles.

Training patients to use "time out" techniques can be useful. The use of such techniques is particularly important in those phases of treatment when other self-control skills are not well developed, or in the inevitable situation when conflict resolution skills may be tested and overwhelmed. The purpose of the technique is to provide a behavioral safety valve to decrease the likelihood of continued abuse and an opportunity for de-arousal to promote rational problem solving.

Sonkin and Durphy[18] have summarized the time out procedure as the systematic application of the following steps:

1. The violence-prone man recognizes cues that signal the presence of intense anger.
2. He assertively states that he "needs to take a time-out" or simply makes a "T" sign with his hands without speaking.
3. He leaves the house for a period of time (up to 1 hour) to "cool off" and collect his thoughts. Some practitioners suggest seeking the social support of a friend or group member at these times. Drinking, driving, or going to a bar or tavern are all discouraged.
4. He returns home in 1 hour as agreed, to reestablish contact, rebuild trust, and discourage avoidance as a coping strategy.
5. He returns to "check in" and calmly states and discusses the issue related to his anger.

Many practitioners cite advantages to group treatment: it permits the anger and aggression to be addressed as an interpersonal process, provides multiple models for social learning, and provides a source of support to overcome problems. Good practice requires that anger be dealt with in the context of a variety of factors such as permissive attitudes toward violence, devaluation of potential victims, power and control issues, interrelated emotional problems, problem solving, and social skill deficits, as well as the specific behaviors that constitute the violence and abuse.

CONCLUDING REMARKS

Individuals prone to anger and assaultive behavior have been increasingly recognized as a public health concern. A wealth of case studies and a few controlled investigations now exist that indicate that many individuals with intermittent explosive disorder are treatable if specialized assessment and intervention protocols are employed. Although much work remains to delineate the exact mechanisms and outcomes of drug treatments and the long-term efficacy of cognitive-behavioral treatments, initial reports appear promising. Sophisticated models of aggressive behavior suggest the need to attend to multiple issues during intervention. Psychopharmacological interventions may be most useful in emergent situations, when complicating depression and arousal disorders are present, and when modification of biological substrates otherwise associated with irritability and impulsivity is required to make the patient amenable to additional therapy. Cognitive-behavioral methods may have a greater likelihood of changing attitudes and imparting new coping strategies and interpersonal skills. In any case, intervention should be empirically guided by a comprehensive assessment; be oriented toward patient, family, and community health concerns; and be evaluated to determine the actual impact of the treatment employed.

REFERENCES

1. Monopolis S, Lion JR: Problems in the diagnosis of intermittent explosive disorder. Am J Psychiatry 140:1200–1202, 1983.
2. Elliott FA: Neurology of aggression and episodic dyscontrol. Semin Neurol 10:303–312, 1990.
3. Maletzky BM: The episodic dyscontrol syndrome. Dis Nerv Syst 36:178–185, 1973.
4. Domestic violence intervention calls for more than treating injuries. JAMA 264:939–944, 1990.
5. Huesmann LR, Eron LD, Lefkowitz MM, Walder LO: Stability of aggression over time and generations. Dev Psychol 20:1120–1134, 1984.
6. Helping angry and violent people manage their emotions and behavior. Hosp Community Psychiatry 38:1207–1210, 1987.
7. Straus MA, Gelles RJ: Physical Violence in American Families: Risk Factors and Adaptations to Violence in 8,145 Families. New Brunswick, NJ: Transactional Publishers, 1990.
8. Mattes JA, Fink M: A family study of patients with temper outbursts. J Psychiatr Res 21:249–255, 1987.
9. Dagadakis CS, Maiuro RD: The assaultive patient. In Schwartz GR, Caten CJ, Mangelsen MA, Mayer TA, eds. Principles and Practice of Emergency Medicine. 3rd ed. Philadelphia: Lea & Febiger (in press).
10. Gross BH, Southard MJ, Lamb HR, Weinberger LE: Assessing dangerousness and responding appropriately: Hedlund expands the clinician's liability established by Tarasoff. J Clin Psychiatry 48:9–12, 1987.
11. Maiuro RD, O'Sullivan MJ, Michael MC, Vitaliano PP: Anger, hostility, and depression in assaultive versus suicide attempting males. J Clin Psychol 45:531–541, 1989.
12. Fava M, Anderson K, Rosenbaum JF: "Anger Attacks": Possible variants of panic and major depressive disorders. Am J Psychiatry 147:867–870, 1990.
13. Maiuro RD, Cahn TS, Vitaliano PP, et al: Anger, hostility, and depression in domestically violent versus generally assaultive men and nonviolent control subjects. J Consult Clin Psychol 56:17–23, 1988.
14. Monroe RR: Dyscontrol syndrome: Long-term follow-up. Compr Psychiatry 30:489–497, 1989.

15. Maiuro RD, Vitaliano PP, Cahn TC: A brief measure for the assessment of anger and aggression. J Interpersonal Violence 2:166–178, 1987.
16. Eichelman B: Toward a rational pharmacotherapy for aggressive and violent behavior. Hosp Community Psychiatry 39:31–39, 1988.
17. Sheard MN: Clinical pharmacology of aggressive behavior. Clin Neuropharmacol 7:173–183, 1984.
18. Sonkin DJ, Durphy M: Learning to Live without Violence: A Handbook for Men. San Francisco: Volcano Press, 1982.
19. Maiuro RD, Cahn TS, Vitaliano PP: Assertiveness deficits and hostility in domestically violent men. Violence and Victims 1:279–289, 1986.

ACKNOWLEDGMENTS

The author would like to thank Meg Crager, John Brinkley, M.D., and Jane Eberle for their assistance in the preparation of this manuscript.

Requests for reprints should be addressed to Roland D. Maiuro, Ph.D., Associate Professor & Director, Harborview Anger Management and Domestic Violence Program, Department of Psychiatry & Behavioral Sciences, University of Washington School of Medicine, ZA-31, Seattle, Washington 98104, USA.

78

THE DIAGNOSIS AND TREATMENT OF ATTENTION-DEFICIT HYPERACTIVITY DISORDER IN ADULTS

PAUL H. WENDER, M.D.

The major point to make in discussing attention-deficit hyperactivity disorder (ADHD) in adults is that it is a common and usually undiagnosed condition of adult life. That it is common is not surprising because ADHD occurs in 5 to 10 per cent of preadolescent children and the symptoms of ADHD persist into adult life in one to two thirds of those cases.

DIAGNOSIS

Suitable diagnostic criteria for ADHD in adults are not provided by the DSM-III criteria or the DSM-III-R criteria because both focus on age-specific symptoms (e.g., "has difficulty sticking to a play activity" or "has difficulty waiting turn in games or group situations"). Persisting ADHD is referred to as attention deficit disorder, residual type by the DSM-III criteria. The criteria are: "signs of hyperactivity are no longer present, but other signs of the illness have persisted to the present without periods of remission, as evidenced by signs of both attentional deficits and impulsivity (e.g., difficulty organizing work and completing tasks, difficulty concentrating, being easily distracted, making sudden decisions without thought of the consequences)." The DSM-III-R notes that associated features may change with age and that some adults may continue to show some signs of the disorder.

Since neither the DSM-III or the DSM-III-R provides specific diagnostic criteria for ADHD in adults, our research group constructed operational diagnostic criteria—the "Utah Criteria." The first prerequisite is that the adult must have merited the diagnosis of ADHD in childhood with both hyperactivity and inattentiveness. DSM-III-R criteria permit ADHD to be diagnosed in the absence of motor hyperactivity, but we wished to focus on the more typical instances in which hyperactivity was present. Since most adult psychiatric patients were not evaluated in childhood and because the symptoms DSM-III-R uses are too specific, we make the retrospective diagnosis of ADHD on the basis of the following criteria.

Childhood Criteria

As a child the subject had both symptoms and signs of #1 and #2 and at least one of #3 through #6 (below): (1) more active than other children, unable to sit still, fidgety, restless, always on the go, talking excessively; (2) attention deficits, sometimes described as a "short attention span," characterized by inattentiveness, distractibility, inability to finish school work; (3) behavior problems in school; (4)

impulsivity; (5) overexcitability; (6) temper outbursts.

As an additional aid in retrospective diagnosis, we employ the Parents' Rating Scale (see Table 78–1), which is the Conners Abbreviated Teachers' Rating Scale filled out by the patient's mother (or father or older sibling if the mother is not available) describing the adult subject's behavior when he or she was between the ages of 6 and 10. The Parents' Rating Scale has been normed and a cutoff point of 12 or greater places an individual within the 95th percentile of childhood "hyperactivity." All putative ADHD adults must meet these retrospective diagnostic criteria.

Adult Criteria

The adult criteria were also designed to focus on the more typical instances in which inattentiveness and restlessness existed in childhood and persist to the time of diagnosis. The following are the adult symptoms required by the Utah Criteria (childhood ADHD having been diagnosed by the previous methods).

The presence in adulthood of both characteristics #1 and #2—which the patient observes or says other observe about him—together with two of the characteristics #2 through #7 (below).

1. **Persistent motor hyperactivity:** manifested by restlessness, inability to relax, "nervousness" (i.e., inability to settle down—not anticipatory anxiety), inability to persist in sedentary activities (e.g., watching movies, TV, reading newspaper), being always on the go, dysphoric when inactive.

2. **Attention deficits:** manifested by the inability to keep mind on conversations, distractibility (being aware of other stimuli when attempts are made to filter them out), inability to keep mind on reading materials, difficulty keeping mind on tasks, frequent "forgetfulness"—often losing or misplacing things, forgetting plans, "mind frequently somewhere else."

3. **Affective lability:** usually described as antedating adolescence and in some instances beginning as far back as the patient can remember; manifested by definite shifts from a normal mood to depression or mild euphoria or excitement; the depression described as being "down," "bored," or "discontented"; mood shifts usually last

TABLE 78–1. PARENTS' RATING SCALE

Patient's name _____ # _____ Date _____ Physician _____

To be filled out by the *mother* of the subject (or father only if mother is unavailable).

Instructions: Listed below are items concerning children's behavior and the problems they sometimes have. Read each item carefully and decide how much you think your child was bothered by these problems when he/she was between *six* and *ten* years old. Rate the amount of the problem by putting a check in the column that describes your child at that time.

		NOT AT ALL	JUST A LITTLE	PRETTY MUCH	VERY MUCH
1.	RESTLESS (OVERACTIVE)				
2.	EXCITABLE, IMPULSIVE				
3.	DISTURBS OTHER CHILDREN				
4.	FAILS TO FINISH THINGS STARTED (SHORT ATTENTION SPAN)				
5.	FIDGETING				
6.	INATTENTIVE, DISTRACTIBLE				
7.	DEMANDS MUST BE MET IMMEDIATELY; GETS FRUSTRATED				
8.	CRIES				
9.	MOOD CHANGES QUICKLY				
10.	TEMPER OUTBURSTS (EXPLOSIVE AND UNPREDICTABLE BEHAVIOR)				

Scoring: Not at all, 0; Just a little, 1; Pretty much, 2; Very much, 3.

hours, at most a few days, and are present without significant physiological concomitants; mood shifts may occur spontaneously or be reactive.

4. **Inability to complete tasks:** lack of organization in job, running household or performing school work; tasks frequently not completed; switches from one task to another in haphazard fashion; disorganization in activities, problem solving, organizing time.

5. **Hot temper:** experiences explosive short-lived outbursts; may have transient loss of control and be frightened by his own behavior; easily provoked or shows constant irritability.

6. **Impulsivity:** makes decisions quickly and easily without reflection, often on the basis of insufficient information and to his own disadvantage; inability to delay acting without experiencing discomfort; manifestations include poor occupational performance; abrupt initiation or termination of relationships (e.g., multiple marriages, separations, divorces); antisocial behavior, such as joy-riding, shop-lifting; excessive involvement in pleasurable activities without recognizing risks of painful consequences (e.g., buying sprees, reckless driving).

7. **Stress intolerance:** cannot take ordinary stresses in stride and reacts excessively or inappropriately with depression, confusion, uncertainty, anxiety or anger; emotional responses interfere with appropriate problem solving; experiences repeated crises in dealing with routine life stresses.

The Utah Criteria exclude patients with current major depression, antisocial personality disorder, or schizotypal or borderline traits. These exclusionary criteria were chosen in order to study samples that would be as pure as possible. There is no doubt that some patients have mixtures of ADHD and these other disorders, but we elected to perform our research on a sample with no apparent psychiatric comorbidity.

Features suggesting the diagnosis of ADHD in patients are certain symptoms and diagnoses in siblings and parents: hot temper and lability of mood; disorders that appear to be genetically related to adult ADHD, such as antisocial personality disorder (or traits of antisocial personality disorder), alcoholism, and drug abuse; and ADHD ("hyperactivity") in the patients' children. Associated features—consequences of ADHD—are histories of academic or vocational underachievement and instability of relationships.

A further aid in diagnosis is the Parents' Rating Scale, a questionnaire that has been discussed previously.

PHARMACOLOGICAL MANAGEMENT OF ADHD IN ADULTS

When effective, medication relieves symptoms in all of the seven target areas described above (the adult criteria) and allows patients to function at a better level than they ever have previously: hyperactivity and feelings of restlessness decrease or disappear; attentiveness is increased; distractibility and forgetfulness disappear; lability of mood diminishes and patients experience neither "highs" nor "lows"; explosive temper, impatience, and irritability all tend to decrease; and resilience to stress improves and disorganization diminishes, as does impulsivity.

Stimulants

Amphetamine was first used in 1937 in the treatment of children whom we would now diagnose as afflicted with ADHD. Methylphenidate began to be widely used in the 1960s and is now (of the two drugs) the more frequently employed. In both children and adults there appears to be no difference between the amphetamines (D-amphetamine and methamphetamine) and methylphenidate in efficacy. Both types of stimulants are useful in approximately three quarters of ADHD cases. Currently, the use of the amphetamines has decreased relative to that of methylphenidate. However, the preferential use of methylphenidate is not based on scientific findings; rather, it seems to be based on fashion and perhaps on the belief that the amphetamines are more abusable than methylphenidate. Although the therapeutic effects of methylphenidate and D-amphetamine appear to be similar, some patients find that excessive doses of methylphenidate make them groggy (the "zombie" effect in children), whereas excessive doses of the amphetamines may make them feel edgy. Any patient may do better on any one of the three drugs than on the others, and the most effective treatment may have to be determined by trials of all three agents. One major difference between the amphetamines and methylphenidate is that the duration of action of the former is considerably longer than that of methylphenidate. Euphoria is not produced by amphetamine or methylphenidate in the therapeutic dosage ranges. Tolerance occurs uncommonly, only to a slight degree, and usually the effective dose retains its efficacy indefinitely. Whether ADHD adults will manifest a euphoriant response to very large oral doses or to intravenous administration of the stimulants is not known.

Amphetamines

The dosing regimen for D-amphetamine and methamphetamine is as follows. The drugs are administered three times a day, generally starting with 2.5 mg at 8:00 A.M., noon, and 3:00 or 4:00 P.M., and the dose is gradually increased to a maximum of 15 mg t.i.d. The duration of action of the amphetamines is approximately 3 to 4 hours, and a fourth daily dose is rarely required. While the differences between amphetamine and methamphetamine have not been studied, some patients have reported that methamphetamine is more sedating (and sometimes undesirably so), as compared with D-amphetamine. Both D-amphetamine and methamphetamine are available in long-acting preparations (Dexedrine Spansules and Desoxyn Gradumets, respectively). The two preparations do not seem to function equally effectively. Patients' responses to the Dexedrine Spansules have been variable: some patients have reported them to be satisfactory, some have noted that too much of the medication is released immediately, producing irritability and edginess, while still others report that the onset of action is delayed for a few hours. Our experience with Desoxyn Gradumets is less extensive than that with Dexedrine Spansules; in most instances the Gradumets' action appears to persist for 10 to 12 hours. Finally, the therapist should remember that the practical value of these timed-release preparations is limited by their considerable cost.

Methylphenidate[1,2]

Methylphenidate is currently the drug most frequently used in the treatment of ADHD in children, although it and the amphetamines appear to be effective in the same fraction of children. We have used methylphenidate in our controlled trials, not because of any superiority to D-amphetamine but because its widespread use has made it the "gold standard." Again, as noted, methylphenidate has a shorter duration of action than do the amphetamines and, therefore, requires a greater number of doses per day. In controlled trials we are currently conducting, patients who are maintained on methylphenidate report that its duration of action is somewhere between 2 and 3 hours. Our standard practice is to begin our patients with doses of 5 mg t.i.d. and to increase the dose—and particularly its frequency—gradually thereafter. Most patients appear to require four to seven doses per day. A typical dose schedule might be: 10 mg q 2 h, six to seven times per day; 15 mg q 2.5 h, five times per day; 20 mg q 3 h, three to four times per day. Because of the frequent dosing necessary—as reported by adults, and which can only be guessed at in children—these total daily doses may exceed those recommended in the *Physicians' Desk Reference*. Our maximum daily dosage is 90 mg/day. Absolute adherence to the dose schedule is essential, and we have our patients purchase digital watches that have a "countdown alarm" (i.e., the watch is set to go off, for example, at 2.5-hour intervals).

Methylphenidate is available in an ostensibly long-acting preparation, Ritalin-SR. Most of our patients report that it lasts only 3 to 4 hours and that a 20-mg dose of Ritalin-SR is actually less efficacious than a 20-mg tablet. Since allergic reactions have been reported to occur with Ritalin-SR (and rarely occur with the standard preparation), the use of the slow-release form will probably decrease.

Pemoline[3]

We have employed pemoline (Cylert) in controlled trials and have found it to produce moderate to marked improvement in approximately 45 per cent of patients. This response rate is lower than that seen with the amphetamines or methylphenidate. Unlike those drugs, pemoline should be administered on a once-daily dose schedule (e.g., 18.75 mg or one half of that size tablet) in the morning and gradually increased to the point at which symptoms are controlled or the side effects (particularly headache and insomnia) prevent further increase. In our placebo-controlled study, the average maintenance dosage was approximately 75 mg/day. Some patients may require a divided dose, morning and early afternoon, but this is uncommon. Approximately 2 to 3 per cent of patients receiving pemoline develop abnormalities of their liver enzymes; therefore, liver function tests must be run periodically (at what intervals is uncertain). There may be a few patients who respond to pemoline who do not respond to the amphetamines or methylphenidate. Pemoline's major advantage is not related to its therapeutic efficacy but to the fact that it is a Schedule IV drug and has little "street value," and so may be dispensed to patients with histories of alcohol or substance abuse; however, no controlled trials of its usefulness in such populations have been reported. Nevertheless, in individuals with histories of alcohol or substance abuse, pemoline should still be employed with caution.

Other Medications

Because the stimulant drugs can be abused by others, if not the patient, and because their duration of action is short, we have conducted open trials of the monoamine oxidase inhibitors pargyline and selegiline and of bupropion.[4–6] All appear to warrant further study, but the documented efficacy of the stimulant drugs, together with their safety in the prescribed dose range, make them the treatment of choice.

Because of their affective lability, many ADHD patients have been diagnosed as cyclothymic, and because of their frequent dysphoria, as suffering from dysthymic disorder. Based on these misdiagnoses, they are frequently treated with tricyclic antidepressants and lithium. In general, ADHD adults do not manifest a therapeutic response to the tricyclic antidepressants or lithium. Our experience with fluoxetine is limited, but it, too, seems to be ineffective in treating ADHD symptoms. Systematic studies of these agents have not been conducted.

Some patients respond satisfactorily to stimulants but have problems with insomnia. This is because the duration of the arousing effect is longer than that of the "anti-ADHD" effect, and if doses are taken later in the day, to provide psychological and behavioral control during the evening, patients may have difficulty falling asleep. This insomnia can generally be reversed by the use of a modest dose of a low-potency neuroleptic (e.g., 5 to 20 mg thioridazine 1 hour before bedtime). Patients do not become tolerant to the effects of the antipsychotic, but frequent use (and presumed retention in the brain) *may* require the use of larger doses of stimulants. In such instances, the time of stimulant dosing and the amount of neuroleptic must be carefully titrated.

PSYCHOLOGICAL MANAGEMENT OF THE ADULT WITH ADHD

Treatment of the ADHD adult without the help of a spouse or significant other is very difficult. ADHD adults, like ADHD children, have had the syndrome all their lives and have little awareness of their differences or the effect of their behavior on others. They likewise are frequently unaware of even substantial improvements in their functioning; it is not infrequent for a patient to report a slight diminution in symptoms and describe himself or herself as only minimally improved, while a spouse or other will rate the patient as very much improved. During the course of pharmacological management, the therapist should monitor the patient's symptoms within each of the seven target areas. We have found it useful to list target symptoms in the seven areas and rate them as: none, slight, moderate, and marked. In each area we query specifically about those problem symptoms identified in the diagnosis, such as inattentiveness, affective lability, and temper.

It is important to emphasize that medication constitutes only one aspect of the treatment of adult ADHD. Other facets of treatment include education of the patient about ADHD and psychotherapy. After many years of teaching parents and adult sufferers, I summarized my teaching program in a book, *The Hyperactive Child, Adolescent, and Adult.*[7] I have found that its use expedites patients' understanding of ADHD, the meaning of the diagnosis, and the rationale of treatment and is more convincing to that subgroup of patients who are more believing of the written than the spoken word.

Finally, it should be emphasized that having ADHD does not prevent the patient from having comorbid disorders or maladaptive patterns that remain even when medication has eliminated the target symptoms. Frequent areas of difficulty that remain are those in the patient's marital relationship and relationships with his or her children. With the ADHD symptoms controlled by medication, it is our impression that patients who were previously refractory to psychotherapy are now able to benefit from individual, marital, and family therapies.

REFERENCES

1. Wood DR, Reimherr FW, Wender PH: Diagnosis and treatment of minimal brain dysfunction in adults. Arch Gen Psychiatry 33:1453–1461, 1976.
2. Wender PH, Reimherr FW, Wood DR, et al: A controlled study of methylphenidate in the treatment of attention deficit disorder, residual type. Am J Psychiatry 142:547–552, 1985.
3. Wender PH, Reimherr FW, Wood DR: Attention deficit disorder ("minimal brain dysfunction") in adults. Arch Gen Psychiatry 38:449–456, 1981.
4. Wender PH, Wood DR, Reimherr FW, et al: An open trial of pargyline in the treatment of attention deficit disorder, residual type. Psychiatr Res 9:329–336, 1983.
5. Wood DR, Reimherr FW, Wender PH: The use of L-deprenyl in the treatment of attention deficit disorder, residual type. Psychopharmacol Bull 19:627–629, 1983.
6. Wender PH, Reimherr FW: Bupropion treatment of attention deficit hyperactivity disorder in adults. Am J Psychiatry 147:1018–1020, 1990.
7. Wender PH: The Hyperactive Child, Adolescent, and Adult: Attention Deficit Disorder through the Lifespan. New York: Oxford University Press, 1987.

THE SUICIDAL PATIENT:
Assessment, Crisis Management, and Treatment

JOHN A. CHILES, M.D. and KIRK STROSAHL, PH.D.

DIMENSIONS OF SUICIDAL BEHAVIOR

The term "suicidal behavior" indicates a variety of thoughts and actions, including completed suicide (the least common), attempted suicide or parasuicide, and suicidal ideation (the most common). National or regional studies about suicidal behavior tend to focus on completed suicides because the data kept, generally by medical examiner offices, report only this condition. Studies of completers are generally retrospective, and there are clear ethical problems with prospective designs for completed suicide.

The term "attempted suicide" defines individuals who have committed some form of deliberate self-injury with some degree of suicidal intent. Noting that many patients who "attempt suicide" are not attempting to kill themselves, Kreitman[1] introduced the phrase "parasuicide" to define a condition distinct from that of suicide. Kreitman (and others) have shown the epidemiology of parasuicide to be quite distinct from that of suicide and have made a convincing case that the clinical issues involved in managing the parasuicidal patient are different.

The term "parasuicide" causes some confusion, so in this chapter we use "attempted suicide," as defined previously. While most suicide attempters will not ultimately die by suicide, as a group they remain significantly more at risk than the general population. Follow-up studies report a rate of suicide of approximately 1 per cent per year continuing over at least 10 years following a suicide attempt.[2] Attempted suicide is a major public health problem in the United States, with a lifetime incidence of 7 to 12 per cent and a repetition rate around 50 per cent.[3] Suicidal ideation in some form is a common phenomenon, occurring in perhaps as high as 20 per cent of the general population,[3] and many would agree with the anonymous statement "Thoughts of suicide have gotten me through many a bad night." References to the frequency of suicidal ideation are scant, because most studies focus on behavior. Suicidal ideation is a common reason for psychiatric inpatient admission.

Suicidal behavior occurs across the spectrum of mental illnesses. For example, about the same percentage of schizophrenic patients commit suicide as do patients with major depressive disorder.

DEMOGRAPHIC FEATURES

Suicide is more common in the elderly, and the rates are higher for males. In addition to age and sex, other important demographic factors are race, marital status, religion, employment, and seasonal variation.[4] In the United States, Caucasians are more suicidal than non-Caucasians (13.7 : 100,000 versus 6.9 : 100,000). Suicide is more common among the single, separated, divorced, or widowed. Loss of a spouse increases suicide risk for at least 4 years following the spousal death. Suicide rates are higher among Protestants than Catholics and Jews, and suicide rates and unemployment correlate positively in many countries.

PERSONALITY AND ENVIRONMENTAL CHARACTERISTICS

Most personality studies of suicidal patients have been conducted with attempted suicides or suicidal ideators. These studies focus on four areas of functioning: cognition, emotional distress, interpersonal functioning, and environmental stress. Each of these factors is known to play a role in the genesis of suicidal behavior, and they probably interact in an interdependent fashion. Studies of cognitive functioning generally show that suicidal individuals are poor problem solvers. They often engage in dichotomous thinking, and have difficulty performing flexible cognitive operations.[5]

Suicidal patients have troubled emotional lives characterized by depression, anxiety, anger, guilt, and boredom. Many suicidal individuals have a *low threshold for emotional pain*. They engage in extreme solutions earlier than non–suicide-prone individuals because of their trouble accepting and working with the way they feel.

The interpersonal environment of suicidal patients has limited social networks marked by frequent conflict. Personal loss or the threat of rejection are common precipitating events for suicidal behavior. Suicidal patients often lack *competent* social support, that is, individuals who can provide emotional support without routinely cajoling or lecturing.

Life stress, either negative or positive, is a major precipitant of the suicidal behavior. Suicidal patients have a higher rate of negative life stress. These stresses include physical illness, financial uncertainty, and life phase changes. Attempts at marshalling support and reassurance from the social network usually fail, increasing the sense of stress and emotional distress.[6]

GENETIC AND BIOLOGICAL CHARACTERISTICS

Family history is pertinent to suicidal behavior, and more information is available about completed suicides than about suicide attempts or ideation. Suicide does cluster in families, suggesting that genetic factors may have a role to play. Recent data from work with monozygotic and dizygotic twins indicate that this clustering may really represent a genetic disposition to the psychiatric disorders associated with suicide.[7] The question remains open whether there is an independent genetic component for suicide.

Laboratory work in the last decade and a half has focused attention on serotonin as it relates to suicidal behavior. Asberg et al.[8] reported a bimodal distribution of the serotonin metabolite 5-hydroxyindoleacetic acid (5-HIAA) in the cerebral spinal fluid (CSF) of 68 depressed patients. Those depressed patients with low CSF 5-HIAA were more likely to have attempted suicide than those in the high group. The clinical implications of an association between serotonin metabolism and suicidal behavior are unclear.

A CLINICAL MODEL OF SUICIDAL BEHAVIOR

The basic tenet of our inpatient and outpatient approach is that suicidal behavior is a *learned* problem-solving behavior.[9] It arises when individuals feel they have no other meaningful problem-solving options available to them. Any individual can become suicidal. Reinforcements, both prior to the act and following it, are essential in developing and stabilizing a person's behavior pattern. Two types of reinforcements, internal and external, are heavily implicated in shaping and maintaining suicidal behavior. The internal reinforcement for suicidal behavior is its *expressive* function. The behavior itself serves to alleviate anxiety.

The external reinforcements for suicidal behavior follow the act. Frequently, the immediate consequence is for the individual to be removed from the stressful environment and freed from the daily hassles that accompany it. Persons in the social support network who have been critical or rejecting may now have second thoughts. In the short term, suicidal behavior is a very potent problem-solving behavior: it works.

There are three basic conditions that predispose an individual to suicidal behavior. First, the person must be experiencing some emotional and/or physical pain that is viewed as *intolerable*. Second, the pain must be viewed as *inescapable*. The person believes that he or she has little power to effectively change the situation at hand. Third, this pain must be viewed as *interminable*: it is unlikely to end. When these "three Is" are in effect, the task of coping with pain appears to be a never-ending one. Suicidal behavior can be viewed as a viable problem-solving option by nearly everyone if the problem is perceived as intolerable, inescapable, and interminable.

INPATIENT HOSPITAL TREATMENT OF SUICIDAL BEHAVIOR

It has not been established that hospitalization is an effective treatment for suicidal behavior, and, indeed, the majority of suicidal patients referred to an emergency service are not psychiatrically hospitalized. The indications for psychiatric inpatient care for those patients with suicidal behavior who require it are:

1. Serious psychiatric disorders, disorders that in their own right require hospitalization for diagnosis and treatment. This can include psychotic depression, schizophrenia, organic states, and substance abuse.

2. Patients who need a "time out" period, a brief respite from significant current stress. In this sense, the hospital is being used as a sanctuary and, if there were less intense alternatives, they would be more appropriate. These hospitalizations should be brief, and efforts should be made to increase effective social support.

3. If the admission is planned as part of a treatment strategy.

OUTPATIENT THERAPY WITH THE SUICIDAL PATIENT

The most difficult aspects of working with the suicidal patient are reactions elicited from the therapist. These reactions generally center around affective, ethical, and legal issues. Affective issues refer to personal reactions to the act of self-destructive behavior, suicidal ideation, and/or suicidal verbalizations to others. Ethical issues entail the responsibility of each therapist to adhere to ethical standards within his or her discipline. Often, one of these ethics is to administer no harmful treatment and to use only effective treatment approaches. Legal concerns arise mainly around the dictates of state statutes, which almost invariably require involuntary hospitalization of a patient who is an "imminent threat" to commit suicide. If such steps are not followed, the therapist is potentially liable for any damages that could accrue from such a failure. This can be a legal double bind for the therapist. On the one hand, a lawsuit is possible if there is a failure to hospitalize given the presence of certain key suicide risk indicators. On the other hand, there is a growing body of civil rights lawsuits arising from authorizing such detentions for patients who later claim that they were never suicidal in the first place.

THE INITIAL TREATMENT PHASE: REFRAMING SUICIDAL BEHAVIOR

The initial session with a patient often takes the form of describing the problem-solving model and then integrating the patient's experiences into that model. It does not help to lecture the patient about the negative consequences of suicide or suicide attempting. The key therapeutic intervention is to teach the patient alternative strategies to use at the same time that they would have used suicidal behavior. Thus, the initial session has a *positive overtone* rather than a "problem-seeking" focus.

The second objective in the initial phase of therapy is to teach the concept of situational specificity: recognition that discrete events in the patient's daily life trigger suicidal behavior. At times, suicidal ideation is *functional*; attempting or completing suicide is seen as an effective way to solve the problem. At other times, the suicidal ideation is expressive in form; the individual expresses anxiety relief at the thought of committing suicide. To teach effective problem-solving and tolerance for emotional distress, patients need to look at individual situations and to start thinking about their life difficulties as an accumulation of events over which they can exercise some control.

An immediate goal of therapy is to help the patient discover what she or he is already doing that works. It is rare to find someone who is malfunctioning in every phase of life. The overall objective of this "what works and what doesn't" approach is to get the patient to increase coping behaviors that are reasonably effective, and to begin to substitute those for ones that are not working.

Another initial strategy in therapy is to teach the personal scientist approach to suicidal behavior.[10] The patient collects information in between therapy sessions that helps to answer important questions that are generated by clinician-patient discussions. New responses to old situations are viewed as "experiments," rather than absolute truth. The empha-

sis is on what *really* works rather than what ought to work. This personal science model also underscores a very important point of our therapy process: the recurrence of suicidal behavior in therapy is not evidence that the treatment has failed. It simply means that suicidal behavior is being used to address an intrapsychic or environmental crisis because other potential options have not been sufficiently experientially validated.

Self-monitoring is the technical term used to describe the collection of data about key target behaviors in between therapy sessions. While it is important not to overfocus on suicidal behavior, it is still necessary to make some links between day-to-day situations the patient encounters and the appearance of suicidal problem-solving behavior. Assignments that have the patient record key events, cognitions, feelings, and problem-solving responses are a good way to develop this linkage. The objective in reviewing these forms is to allow the issue of suicidal ideation, verbalization, and even attempts to be talked about openly and matter-of-factly in an objectified way. This allows the patient and therapist to discuss problem-solving options that worked well and those that did not. As this therapy proceeds, its effect is to systematically attack the "three Is" through experience. The patient is discovering that there are coping behaviors that work, that pain seldom maintains itself at the same level of intensity over a 24-hour period, and that situations that appear to be hopeless can, in fact, be managed through a step-by-step problem-solving procedure.

THE INTERMEDIATE TREATMENT PHASE

During the intermediate phase of therapy, the therapist and patient begin to recontextualize the relationship between thoughts, feelings, and behavior. This intervention begins to target the patient's understanding of tolerance for emotional distress. The clinician can give a homework instruction that encourages the patient to allow suicidal ideation to be present while observing its different contours and connotations. Patients perform this assignment with the instruction to come back prepared to discuss the topography of the suicidal ideation. Our tack is to encourage acceptance and, in fact, anticipation of distressing thoughts or feelings while doing what needs to be done in the real world.

THE TERMINATION PHASE

The final stages of therapy are marked by a focus on improved problem solving and development of an intermediate-term life plan. The goal is to bolster the patient with problem-solving strategies that have already worked, and to practice applying these responses to situations that previously have generated suicidal ideation. The emphasis is not to prevent the occurrence of suicidal ideation as much as it is to strengthen alternative problem-solving responses. The patient needs to repetitively practice the alternatives in a solution-focused way.

Even termination from therapy is described as a field experiment. The patient is praised for coming far enough in therapy to warrant a field trial with a planned follow-up visit. There is ample encouragement to see this 1-, 3-, or 6-month period as an experiment in the application of new behaviors to old situations. Although the recurrence of suicidal ideation or verbalizations is addressed, it is certainly not the focus of the interventions at this point. It is acknowledged as a potential event that can actually be used as a "signal" to re-initiate effective problem solving. A written plan for handling these recurrences is generated between the clinician and the patient. This plan describes "at risk" situations, the effective alternative coping responses to be used, obstacles to implementation of those alternatives, and a method for systematic evaluation and follow-up. Experiential learning is more potent than therapy, and therefore patients should be moved quickly into the field trial stage. With repetitiously suicidal patients, this has the effect of undercutting their reliance upon therapy and the therapist as a substitute for generating effective real-life problem-solving strategies.

CRISIS MANAGEMENT: A LEARNING APPROACH

One of the challenges of every clinician's professional life is addressing the suicidal crisis, a situation that tends to elicit both the most positive and most negative aspects of affective, ethical, and legal issues. The key therapeutic plan for effective crisis management is to form a clear and mutually agreed upon contract from the onset of therapy. This means that the therapist must understand his or her own affective, ethical, and legal stance with respect to suicidal behavior, and this has to be communicated effectively to the patient. We also encourage following a behaviorally based protocol, so that the clinician does not inadvertently reinforce the occurrence of suicidal behavior if it occurs during the course of therapy.

We also make use of a crisis card strategy, completed in the first therapy session. The crisis card lists instructions that the patient is required to follow in the event of a suicidal crisis. The card is stored in a wallet or purse. We often spend a good deal of time generating the specific steps to be followed. The goal in this procedure is to encourage the patient to first contact natural community supports that are capable of providing competent social support. A second tier is to contact a local crisis clinic or crisis agency if there is one available. Finally, after all other options have actually been tried and have failed, the patient is encouraged to contact the therapist.

When hospitalization is employed, it is advisable to adopt a short-term acute care approach. This means that the patient is seeking a short "time out" from the environment in order to marshall an effective problem-solving plan. This type of admission is generally well received by inpatient staff, as compared to the very mixed reaction often given to suicide attempters after the fact.

There is an intangible element about crisis management that is probably more important than the specific technical steps that have just been described—that is, the clinician's capacity to provide a caring, emotionally validating therapeutic environment while remaining consistent and true to the therapeutic model. The suicidal patient often looks to the therapist to provide a sense of balance and calm, and this is best done through direct modeling. The degree to which a therapist's own anxiety is projected into this situation will affect the patient's sense of self-control and sense of personal balance.

CLOSING COMMENTS

Recently, a consortium of 300 national organizations and state health departments[11] formulated 14 objectives for mental health to be reached by the year 2000. Included in this was the task of reducing the suicide rate in the United States to no more than 10.5 : 100,000 people, down from the recent figure of 11.7 : 100,000. To reach this goal, as well as to reduce the troubling and costly problem of suicide attempting, much work needs to be done. We need to increase our understanding of all aspects of suicidal behavior, and effective intervention strategies need to be developed and thoroughly investigated.

REFERENCES

1. Kreitman N: The clinical assessment and management of the suicidal patient. In Roy A, ed. Suicide. Baltimore: Williams & Wilkins, 1986.
2. Paerregaard G: Suicide among attempted suicides: A 10-year follow up. Suicide 5:140–144, 1975.
3. Strosahl K, Linehan M, Chiles J: Will the real social desirability and the prediction of suicidal behavior. J Consult Clin Psychol 52:449–457, 1984.
4. Buda M, Tsuang MT: The Epidemiology of Suicide. Implications for Clinical Practice. Blumenthal SJ, Kupfer DJ, eds. Washington, DC: American Psychiatric Press, Inc., 1990.
5. Rotheram-Borus M, Trautman P, Dopkins S, Shrout P: Cognitive style and pleasant activities among female adolescent suicide attempters. J Consult Clin Psychol 58:554–561, 1990.
6. Chiles J, Strosahl K, Cowden L, et al: The 24 hours before hospitalization: Factors related to suicide attempting. Suicide Life Threat Behav 16:335–342, 1986.

7. Roy A, Segal N, Centerwall B, et al: Suicide in twins. Arch Gen Psychiatry 48:29–32, 1991.

8. Asberg M, Thoren P, Traskman L, et al: Serotonin depression: A biochemical subgroup within the affective disorders? Science 191:478–480, 1976.

9. Chiles JA, Strosahl KD, Yanping Z, et al: Depression, hope-lessness, and suicidal behavior in Chinese and American psychiatric patients. Am J Psychiatry 146:339–344, 1989.

10. Beck A, Rush A, Shaw B, Emery G: Cognitive Therapy of Depression. New York: Guilford Press, 1979.

11. Ment Health Report 14(9):145–152, 1990. (Business Publishers, Inc., Silver Spring, MD.)

Section N

TREATMENTS NOT SPECIFIC FOR DISORDER

80

BRIEF PSYCHOTHERAPIES

MICHAEL E. ADDIS, B.A. and KELLY KOERNER, B.A.

This chapter provides a framework for thinking about brief psychotherapy treatments. It is not a "how to" manual, although there are a number of brief therapy treatment manuals readily available.[1-3] Instead, we consider such questions as: What exactly is brief psychotherapy?, What are the similarities and differences between brief psychotherapy treatments?, and When is brief psychotherapy indicated or not indicated?

WHAT IS BRIEF PSYCHOTHERAPY?

The terms "brief," "time-limited," or "short-term" psychotherapy are commonly used to describe a subset of psychosocial treatment interventions. The communalities among all brief therapies include a limited number of sessions, a well-defined therapeutic focus, greater clinician involvement, prompt intervention, and a focus on the "here and now."[4] Brief treatments stand in historical contrast to the more open-ended, time-unlimited approaches typified by psychoanalysis.

A number of trends within the mental health field over the past 30 years have provided impetus for the increase in brief psychotherapy approaches. First, there has been a growing recognition that not all people seeking psychological help need long-term treatment. For many patients short-term, limited treatment goals may be more desirable.[5] For example, Gelso and Johnson[6] have suggested that the public's

heightened awareness of the importance of psychological factors in functioning has led more people to seek help for issues other than total personality reconstruction. Second, the number of available treatments other than psychoanalysis has increased concurrent with a greater specificity in the classification of emotional disorders.[5] Both of these trends have helped to develop brief standardized interventions for specific problems. Finally, the availability of various alternative treatment formats such as crisis intervention, free clinics, and "rap" groups has normalized the process of seeking help on a short-term basis.[4]

Economic considerations have also led to wider spread use of brief treatment formats. Outside the mental health field, policy makers and third-party reimbursement agencies have exerted pressure for clinicians and researchers to provide shorter term treatments with empirically demonstrated efficacy.[7] Moreover, many third-party reimbursement agencies will pay only for a limited number of psychotherapy sessions, thus placing a practical limit on the feasibility of long-term treatment.

Many of the available brief treatments have evolved from the behavior therapy tradition, which has always strived for empirical validation of treatment.[8] Behavior therapists, however, are not the only ones seeking evidence for the efficacy of psychotherapy. Since Eysenck[9] drew serious doubt on the efficacy of traditional psychotherapy approaches, a surge of studies have attempted both to

499

demonstrate the efficacy of psychotherapy in general and to evaluate the relative merit of different treatments.[10] Thus, research studies and corresponding trends in clinical practice seem to reflect a growing consensus that empirically validated treatments should be brief (averaging 20 sessions), and should produce replicable results with respect to treatment outcome.

OVERVIEW OF THE BRIEF PSYCHOTHERAPIES

Ten years ago it was estimated that there were upwards of 240 different therapeutic orientations in existence.[11] No doubt many of these schools are still influential, and many utilize brief interventions whereas others are generally practiced on a long-term basis. Moreover, a given orientation may give rise to a large number of therapies. There are, for example, many different dynamic psychotherapies, although all are of a psychodynamic orientation. Even assuming only a percentage of available therapies are standardly brief, the sheer multitude of approaches makes any general discussion of "brief therapy" a difficult prospect. This section addresses the questions, What qualifies as brief therapy? and What are the major brief therapy approaches available? To help in summarizing this information, distinctions can be drawn between the stances, the styles, and the structures of brief psychotherapy. A stance refers to common goals or values held by brief therapists. Style refers to such variables as the content of treatment interventions as well as the clinician's theoretical orientation. Structure applies to formal aspects of an approach, such as the number of sessions.

The Brief Therapy Stance

Despite the variety of brief therapies, there are common goals and values across approaches. By definition, clinicians who practice brief psychotherapy place limits on time. The need to produce change in a limited amount of time forces the clinician to establish a therapeutic relationship, to develop a focus, and to become more active in the therapeutic process in a relatively short period of time.[4,12] Consequently, it is not surprising that many clinicians find it difficult to do brief therapy.[6,12] Clinicians who standardly do brief as opposed to long-term therapy also tend to maintain different views about the definition of health and the absolute value of psychotherapy. Psychological health is viewed as synonymous not with total personality reconstruction but rather with an ongoing process of adaptation to current life circumstances. Moreover, many clinicians who practice brief therapy do not view psychotherapy as unconditionally beneficial. At times psychotherapy may do more to prevent change than to promote it.[12]

Styles of Brief Psychotherapy

Brief psychotherapy styles can be broadly classified into psychodynamic, crisis-oriented, and cognitive-behavioral approaches. There are numerous entire books discussing the specifics of each approach, and space limits us from providing detailed discussions of specific approaches in this chapter. A comprehensive list of brief therapies is available in Koss and Butcher.[4] Our comments are largely drawn from their overview and are intended to provide a general flavor for each of the three main styles.

Brief psychodynamic therapies utilize insight as a means to change through short-term treatment. Techniques common to long-term psychodynamic therapies are utilized in brief approaches but toward a different end. As opposed to total personality reconstruction, the focus remains more on the patient's current life circumstances. The clinician strives to develop a single focus by isolating a central conflict currently operating in the patient's life. Various brief psychodynamic approaches offer a set of interpretive principles, or lenses through which the clinician can organize core issues. Representative core issues include interpersonal conflicts,[3] oedipal issues such as grief and loss,[13] or the very nature of limited time.[14] Having developed a focus, the clinician may then use any number of traditional psychodynamic techniques (e.g., transference interpretation) to elucidate the core issue and to produce change primarily through insight or some form of corrective emotional experience.[15]

All crisis-oriented therapies are intended to help a patient with a particularly stressful life event (e.g. a "crisis"). Interventions in crisis-oriented approaches can take place in a number of ways. The clinician may simply intervene in the patient's environment by, for example, arranging to hospitalize a suicidal patient. Alternatively, clinicians may help patients tolerate a period of intense emotional distress through supportive listening. There are also crisis-oriented approaches designed for work on specific crises such as grief due to loss, or debriefing from an acute traumatic event.[16]

Behavioral and cognitive therapies are generally brief by nature. Almost without exception, brief behavioral and cognitive therapies are intended for use with specific problems. A maladaptive set of cognitive or overt behaviors related to the presenting problem is isolated and then standardized interventions are introduced to bring about change. Examples of overt behavioral techniques include systematic desensitization[17] and exposure-based therapy for obsessive-compulsive disorder.[18] Cognitive behavioral treatments include cognitive therapy for depression,[1] rational-emotive therapy,[19] and self-instructional therapy.[20]

Structure of Brief Psychotherapies

Some notion of abbreviated time is obviously a defining structural feature of brief therapies. Short-term approaches seek to produce the most change possible with the least amount of time investment and cost to the patient.[12] This brief therapy stance means that the total number of sessions may or may not reflect a brief or long-term approach. Still, some[4] have suggested that 25 sessions or fewer best characterizes brief psychotherapies. Others[12] have argued that the gross number of sessions is not a meaningful index of short-term intervention. Twenty-five sessions can be divided into five sessions a week for 5 weeks or five sessions a year for 5 years. The problems addressed, the types of interventions utilized, and the nature of the therapeutic relationship will certainly vary between these two formats. We would argue that, as a structural variable, the absolute number of sessions cannot adequately define brief therapy. Behavior therapists, for example, often considered the prototypic brief therapists, have been known to see patients for 100 or more sessions.[21] However, it is difficult to think of calling a 100-session treatment a brief therapy. What is probably true is that most, but not all, brief therapies occur in 25 sessions or fewer. Many highly structured, empirically validated brief interventions[1,2,22] are structured for a 20-session limit. However, in addition to the number of sessions, and perhaps more importantly, brief therapy is characterized by the clinician's attitudes and goals going into treatment.

The structure of brief therapies also varies according to the function of time-limiting in a given approach. Brief approaches can be divided into: (1) those that are intended to be brief and are conducted according to a strict treatment protocol, (2) those that are intended to be brief and in which therapy is more loosely structured, and (3) specific cases in which brevity is unintentional.

In planned and manualized brief treatments, therapy proceeds through a specific, predetermined process in order to alleviate a specific set of problems. A treatment manual guides the clinician through the course of treatment by prescribing specific interventions at roughly standard points in therapy. Moreover, these treatments are usually designed to alleviate problems associated with specific psychiatric diagnoses. In cognitive therapy for depression,[1] for example, the clinician begins by helping the patient to schedule and structure pleasant activities. As therapy progresses, the clinician moves to more cognitive interventions, focusing on the patients' beliefs and assumptions about themselves and their life circumstances. Therapy almost invariably follows this progression, and the manual details specific interventions for each phase of treatment.

In contrast to planned manualized treatments are brief therapy approaches, which are intended to be brief but are not so highly structured. Although non-manualized brief therapy may still be planned and well conceptualized, it is probably true that many treatments of this form rely on abbreviated long-term interventions.[4] Many short-term dynamic psychotherapies, for example, do not provided the clinician with a step-by-step manual of interventions for a specific problem. Rather, they offer a set of guidelines or interpretive principles from which the brief therapy clinician can conceptualize an array of problems and select a therapeutic focus for a given patient.[14,23] Although these therapies may require the clinician to be more active than their long-term counterparts, the clinician is still responding to a general set of principles rather than to specific guidelines set forth by a treatment manual.

Brief treatment can also take place unintentionally. If a patient terminates therapy prematurely, or a clinician sees a patient for a few sessions and then makes a referral, it is possible to describe the treatment as brief therapy. Alternatively, one could describe the process as unsuccessful long-term therapy due to either the patient's or the therapist's actions. As Koss and Butcher[4] noted, "It is inappropriate to conclude that a patient has received brief psychotherapy when actually he or she received three history taking sessions prior to long-term psychotherapy and then dropped out." We would agree with Koss and Butcher that the above scenario does not represent brief therapy. Short-term approaches are not defined by the absolute amount of time spent in therapy, but rather by the intentional structuring of time limits and the designation of specific therapeutic goals.

WHEN IS BRIEF THERAPY APPROPRIATE?

A great deal has been written on the selection of patients for brief psychotherapy. The strict selection criteria probably reflect an implicit assumption that brief treatments are fundamentally different than long-term interventions and should be undertaken only under certain conditions. However, if one turns to the research literature on the efficacy of long-term versus brief treatments, there is little if any support for the superiority of long-term approaches.[4,6] It would seem more logical, then, to reverse the question from, What select group of patients is appropriate for brief therapy? to What group, if any, is inappropriate for short-term treatment?[12] Here the clinical literature demonstrates some consistency regarding patient selection criteria.

Extreme problems such as psychosis or chronic suicidal behavior are almost always contraindications for brief treatment. Otherwise, brief therapies vary on how explicit and how broad or narrow are their criteria for patient selection. In general, psychodynamic brief therapies tend to be more explicit and narrow in their selection criteria. Sifneos,[13] for example, has suggested that suitable patients should have a circumscribed chief complaint, a history of "meaningful" relationships, a flexible interaction style, a high motivation to change, and an above-average psychological sophistication and intelligence. In contrast, Mann[14] has suggested that a wide difficulty range of problems can be addressed in short-term treatment provided that the patient possesses basic ego functions such as the ability to form quick attachments and to tolerate loss. It is questionable, however, whether these criteria are actually less stringent than those cited by other brief psychodynamic approaches.[3]

Behavioral and crisis-oriented therapies have, for the most part, not stated explicit patient selection criteria. There are conceptual and pragmatic reasons why this is so. Because most overt-behavioral and cognitive-behavioral treatments are brief by nature, historically there have not been longer term treatments as possible alternatives for patients unsuitable for briefer therapy. Moreover, most behavioral therapies are geared toward intervention for a specific disorder (e.g., anxiety, depression). These disorders can be conceptualized as occurring across individuals varying greatly in their intelligence, ability to relate to a clinician, and motivation to change. Although these factors may have important implications for the therapy process, they are not stated as specific selection criteria. The same is true for crisis-oriented therapies. It is simply not practical to select patients for crisis intervention based on the above dimensions. A highly intelligent, psychologically sophisticated person may have a crisis and need brief intervention as much as a less intelligent, angry person who finds it difficult to relate to mental health professionals. A crisis is a crisis, and crisis-oriented therapy would not be useful if it always ruled out those people who might be more difficult to work with.

What, then, is the value of selection criteria for brief psychotherapy? Koss and Butcher[4] reported that only 6 to 20 per cent of patients meet criteria for inclusion in specific brief dynamic therapies. Moreover, the majority of people in need of mental health services cannot afford long-term therapy, not to mention the fact that there is no research attesting to the superiority of long-term interventions.[4,6,12] We would argue that, for practical, ethical, and empirical reasons, we are not in a position to exclude from brief treatment a majority of people seeking help because of variables such as level of intelligence, psychological sophistication, or even motivation to change.

Failing to exclude people based on these dimensions does not, however, prevent clinicians from considering how these and other relevant variables may be related to individual outcome in brief therapy. We review research linking specific variables to therapeutic outcome and then suggest some clinical implications for practicing brief psychotherapy across a variety of styles.

There is a wide body of literature examining client variables in relation to therapeutic outcome (see Garfield[24] for a thorough review). We highlight dimensions that have been shown to be consistently related to outcome and are clinically relevant across styles of brief therapy. For example, social class rank is positively related to continuation in psychother-

apy.[24] Although there is little a clinician can do about a patient's social class, he or she can be aware that lower class patients may be more likely to terminate prematurely and take steps to keep them engaged in therapy (e.g., role initiation procedures).

The ability of clinician and patient to develop some form of collaborative relationship is an integral part of any therapeutic venture. In brief therapy the process is necessarily accelerated. Whether the clinician is active, passive, assigns homework, or makes interpretations, the nature of the therapy relationship is for one person to help another. In brief therapy, if a patient does not feel he or she is being helped, if a clinician does not like a patient, or if clinician and patient cannot agree on what the problem is, that relationship may be jeopardized and outcome may be negatively affected. In support of this, some researchers have found relationships between variables such as the quality of the "helping alliance,"[25,26] patient involvement,[27] and outcome in brief therapy, with high-quality helping alliance and high patient involvement positively correlated with better outcomes. However, at least two points are still unclear from this research. First, what exactly is a good helping alliance or high patient involvement? Is it more than how difficult the patient is and whether the clinician and patient like each other?[28] Second, it is possible that patients who improve in therapy rate themselves as more involved and like their clinicians more. If this is the case, then the relationship between therapeutic alliance and outcome is reversed. Although research demonstrates an association between the therapeutic relationship and outcome, the exact nature of that relationship remains unclear.

What is clear is that, in brief psychotherapy, the clinician must quickly engage both himself or herself and the patient in therapy so that each stays involved throughout the course of treatment. This would suggest that the clinician should pay close attention to the initial few sessions of brief therapy. In many brief therapies the quality of the therapeutic relationship begins to evolve through an initial orientation process. In brief dynamic therapies the beginning phase of therapy is dedicated to developing a focus.[3] Through this process clinician and patient come to isolate a particular problem and establish an agenda for working on it. In many behavioral therapies the orientation process is very explicit. The clinician tells the patient what his or her impression of the problem is, what the patient can expect from therapy, and how change will occur. Regardless of the style of brief therapy, careful attention to the initial orientation process is important.

In addition to developing a mutually agreed upon focus and providing any necessary role induction, the initial orientation process should probably include a clear statement of the treatment rationale that accommodates the patient's understanding of the problem. Some research has found that patients who respond positively to an initial treatment rationale have better long-term outcomes.[29] Others have found that varying the rationale associated with time limits predicts patient expectancies for change.[6] Patients may be especially sensitive to time limits and, although some[14] would consider this a central therapeutic issue, in other approaches excessive attention to time may undermine the credibility and effectiveness of brief therapy. Whichever approach is taken, clinicians should monitor the patient's response to time limits. The treatment rationale and therapy goals can then be modified in such a way that limited time is viewed not as a shortcoming buy rather an integral part of therapy.

Flexibility on the part of the clinician has been described as a defining characteristic of brief therapy.[4] This flexibility is best seen in the resourcefulness with which the clinician who does brief therapy makes use of what he or she has. The clinician finds ways to engage the patient in therapy by taking advantage of natural changes outside of therapy. For example, if a patient is seeking short-term treatment as an adjunct to a 12-step program, the therapy rationale can be modified accordingly. In brief therapy the clinician is likely to select interventions that use and complement the strengths the patient brings to treatment. For example, the clinician might recruit a supportive family member as a "co-therapist" to assist in an in vivo exposure-based treatment. A patient who is psychologically minded might be encouraged to read about the process of treatment and change from a prepared bibliography.

SUMMARY AND CONCLUSION

The terms "brief," "time-limited," and "short-term" therapy refer to psychosocial interventions that place limits on the amount time in therapy. The absolute number of therapeutic sessions, however, is not a defining characteristic of a brief psychotherapy approach. Brief interventions are best characterized by the clinician's goals and attitudes going into therapy. Brief therapists try to produce significant change with the smallest investment of time and money. They tend to set limited therapeutic goals and expect to be more active in the therapeutic process than their long-term counterparts. This stance gives rise to a number of styles, including psychodynamic, behavioral, and crisis-oriented approaches. Each style can be implemented in any of three ways. First, time limits can be planned and therapy conducted according to a specific treatment protocol. Second, time limits can be planned while therapy is conducted in a more loosely structured format. Third, time limits can be unplanned, as in a premature termination. Of the three, only the first two can realistically be called brief therapy. While there is considerable clinical lore regarding the selection of patients for brief therapy, there is very little empirical evidence consistently demonstrating superior outcome for specific types of patients.

Moreover, the demands on mental health professionals to provide services to an increasing number of people make rigid selection of brief therapy patients impractical. The question, "Who is appropriate for brief psychotherapy, should be restated, Who is *inappropriate* for brief psychotherapy?

REFERENCES

1. Beck AT, Rush AJ, Shaw BF, Emery G: Cognitive Therapy of Depression. New York: Guilford Press, 1979.
2. Klerman GL, Weissman MM, Rounsaville BJ, Chevron ES: Interpersonal Psychotherapy of Depression. New York: Basic Books, 1984.
3. Strupp HH, Binder JL: Psychotherapy in a New Key: A Guide to Time-Limited Dynamic Psychotherapy. New York: Basic Books, 1984.
4. Koss MP, Butcher JN: Research on brief psychotherapy. In Garfield SL, Bergin AE, eds. Handbook of Psychotherapy and Behavior Change. New York: John Wiley & Sons, 1986:627–670.
5. Pardes H, Pincus HA: Brief therapy in the context of national mental health issues. In Budman SH, ed. Forms of Brief Therapy. New York: Guilford Press, 1981:7–21.
6. Gelso CJ, Johnson DH: Explorations in Time-Limited Counseling and Psychotherapy. New York: Teachers College Press, 1983.
7. Strupp HH: Psychotherapy: Research, practice, and public policy (how to avoid dead ends). Am Psychol 41:120–130, 1986.
8. Masters JC, Burish TG, Hollon SD, Rimm DC: Behavior Therapy. San Diego: Harcourt Brace Jovanovich, 1987.
9. Eysenck HJ: The effects of psychotherapy: An evaluation. J Consult Psychol 16:319–324, 1952.
10. Jacobson NS: The efficacy of psychotherapy: Fact or fiction. Unpublished manuscript, University of Washington, Center for Clinical Research, Seattle, 1991.
11. Corsini RJ, ed. Handbook of Innovative Psychotherapies. New York: John Wiley & Sons, 1981.
12. Budman SH, Gurman AS: The practice of brief therapy. Professional Psychol Res Pract 14:277–292, 1983.
13. Sifneos PE: Short-term anxiety-provoking psychotherapy: Its history, technique, outcome, and instruction. In Budman SH, ed. Forms of Brief Therapy. New York: Guilford Press, 1981:45–80.
14. Mann J: Time-Limited Psychotherapy. Cambridge, MA: Harvard University Press, 1973.
15. Alexander F, French TM: Psychoanalytic Therapy: Principles and Applications. New York: Ronald Press, 1946.
16. Mitchell J, Bray G: Emergency Services Stress: Guidelines for Preserving the Health and Lives of Emergency Personnel. Englewood Cliffs, NJ: Prentice-Hall, 1990.
17. Wolpe J, Lazarus AA: Behavior Therapy Techniques. Oxford, England: Pergamon Press, 1966.
18. Steketee G, Foa EB: Obsessive-compulsive disorder. In Barlow DH, ed. Clinical Handbook of Psychological Disorders. New York: Guilford Press, 1985:69–144.
19. Ellis A, Grieger R: Handbook of Rational Emotive Therapy. New York: Springer-Verlag, 1977.
20. Meichenbaum D: Cognitive Behavioral Modification. New York: Plenum Press, 1977.
21. Wilson GT: Behavior therapy as a short-term therapeutic approach. In Budman SH, ed. Forms of Brief Therapy. New York: Guilford Press, 1981:131–161.
22. Jacobson NS, Margolin G: Marital Therapy: Strategies Based on Social Learning and Behavior Exchange Principles. New York: Brunner/Mazel, 1979.
23. Malan DH: The Frontier of Brief Psychotherapy. New York: Plenum Press, 1976.
24. Garfield SL: Research on client variables in psychotherapy.

In Garfield SL, Bergin AE, eds. Handbook of Psychotherapy and Behavior Change. New York: John Wiley & Sons, 1986:213–256.

25. Luborsky L, Crits-Christoph P, Alexander L, et al: Two helping alliance methods of predicting outcomes of psychotherapy. J Nerv Ment Dis 171:480–491, 1983.

26. O'Malley SS, Suh CS, Strupp HH: The Vanderbilt Psychotherapy Process Scale: A report on the scale development and a process-outcome study. J Consult Clin Psychol 51:581–586, 1983.

27. Gomes-Schwartz B: Effective ingredients in psychotherapy: Predictions of outcome from process variables. J Consult Clin Psychol 46:1023–1035, 1978.

28. Jacobson NS, discussant. Three perspectives on the therapeutic alliance. Panel presented at the 24th annual meeting of the Association for the Advancement of Behavior Therapy, San Francisco, 1990.

29. Fennel JV, Teasdale JD: Cognitive therapy for depression: Individual differences and the process of change. Cognitive Ther Res 11:253–271, 1987.

81

BRIEF DYNAMIC THERAPY

PETER E. MAXIM, M.D., Ph.D.

As he or she engages in discussion on different topics with a patient, the therapist develops a model of the patient's difficulties. This model will serve as the basis for developing a set of treatment goals and methods for achieving them. To develop the model, the therapist attends to four connected areas of patient experience: (1) the way the patient processes current relationships and comprehends and reasons about goals he or she wants to achieve; (2) the expectations and perceptions that the patient brings to this way of processing as they have been influenced by his or her prior experience with these people or similar others; (3) the memory content, meanings, and organization from his or her previous life development that resonate with issues on the current topics under discussion; and (4) the schematic organization and content of the self that will be affirmed or put in conflict with different outcomes from current life events. To help in tracking these areas one can condense them into four metaphors. The first is the equations of conflict. These equations contain the elements and relevant content about which the patient is seeking help. The second is the triangles of conflict that relate these equations and their elements to significant past and present relationships. The third metaphor is the epigenetic principle of life stage development. The elements of both the equations of conflict and triangles of conflict are connected to a time line of residual life stage issues. The fourth metaphor in our model connects these first three to sets of schemata, and to the structures and processing apparatus that represent the self.

AREAS OF PATIENT EXPERIENCE

Equations of Conflict

On first entering a session, patients are often anxious to tell the therapist about a series of personal episodes that convey their problems. Patient and therapist listen to each unfolding story from the assumption that it contains a script made up of a set of intentions or needs, a goal that will achieve them, a set of expectations on the method of reasoning to be used and a behavioral result that is predictably unsatisfactory. The dissatisfaction comes either from the goal not being achieved, unsatisfactory feelings or meanings that result when the goal is achieved, or the fact that achieving one equation stops the achievement of another desired one. Often such equations come in pairs in which the equation elements of needs, goals, or the outcome of affects or beliefs in one pair member contradict those of the other. An example might be where a husband says: "If I say what I want to do on the weekend, I get to do what I want, but she gets angry, tells me I'm selfish, and I feel guilty. But, if I keep quiet and get her to say what she wants and we do that, I feel resentful and trapped and can't enjoy it."

Triangles of Conflict

The triangles of conflict separate the elements of the belief equation into three parts. There are mismatches between expected incoming information resulting in a maladaptive explanation of perceived causes. The patient struggles to appraise and cope as well with the information mismatch. To the extent that he or she fails, he or she experiences symptoms, affects, beliefs, and maladaptive behavior. A second triangle, of people, highlights the patient's memories of his or her relationships with significant people in the past and in the present, and the importance that the therapist will take on for him or her. The conflict triad of need information agenda; failed appraisal and coping; and resulting symptoms, affects, beliefs, and behaviors that the patient experiences with significant others presently can be superimposed at all three points of the triangle of people. Those that occur at present have occurred with significant others in the past, and will develop in the relationship with the therapist.

Life Stage Development

The developmental metaphor[1] presumes that the individual's personality develops by an epigenetic principle similar to biologic growth:

1. Personality growth occurs in a ground plan and differentiated structures in the self arise from that plan.
2. Formation of the personality is mostly a unidirectional process, and movement in the opposite direction is seen as regressive and maladaptive, as is stagnation.
3. At each stage in differentiation the unfolding of the ground plan carries its requirements that the individual solve new types of interactions with the world.
4. Features of the personality that develop later will be determined by the way earlier features are resolved.
5. Plasticity inherent in correcting defects in early phases of the ground plan decreases as the person differentiates.
6. There are appropriate sequences and rates of interaction that the individual should go through for proper differentiated development. Changes in sequences and rates will produce maladaptive identity formation. This maladaption will be most severe with early stage sequence and timing defects.

An individual's memory is normally seen as a mosaic of more or less successful experiences. The therapist thus assumes the patient's memory organization is strongly influenced by his or her experiences and varying success in resolving life stage issues.

To further comprehend the significance of a patient's narration of current conflict episodes, the therapist links the issues under discussion to knowledge of relevant levels of life stage development: specific stages in childhood that resonate with the conflict issue, aspects of adolescent identity formation that also may be tied in, and later adulthood-stage tasks and experiences that are relevant (Table 81–1). One asks oneself to what degree the people, types of

relationships, beliefs, perceptual distortions, appraisal, coping, and needs under discussion can be tied to particular life stages. Having identified the stages, one can then broaden the enquiry to seek more information about why the patient is operating as if still in these earlier stages. More pointedly, one can ask oneself what the next developmental stage task was and what parts of that task were not resolved then that are now similar to the current conflict episodes elements.

Schematic Organization and Content of the Self

Nunn[2] proposed a model of the self on three axes: memory (conscious, unconscious, preconscious), perceived reality and the three Freudian components of structural theory (ego, id, superego), and schemata or representation of prior experience. There are five characteristics of the self that one experiences in the operation of the self-processing apparatus: intentionality, causal construction, affective reactions, time sense, and imagination. Their effects are briefly summarized here. *Intentionality* heavily influences one's constructed memories as they are abstracted from different experiences.[3–5] The maturation of *causal reasoning*[6,7] is partly determined by childhood completion of myelination of corpus callosum fibers. During childhood, right hemisphere dominance thus changes to adult left hemisphere experiential construction.[8] Experientially, the gestaltic, affect-laden focus on similarities in right hemisphere–dominated reasoning moves to a discriminative, propositional, and logical focus coming from the left hemisphere. From a clinical standpoint, causality constructed on the basis of negative reinforcement contingencies dominates the generation of operating rules stored in schemata more than does causality based on positive reinforcement. In assessing maladaptive behavior, it is much more important to ask "What would be worse for the patient than doing this?" than "What does the patient get out of doing this?"

Like causal reasoning, one's *affective reactions* mature from predominantly experiencing affective feelings that can "take one over" to expressed emotion in which the affect is fused with speech and under more control. One's affective reactions are a major bias in the processing of elements in the equations of belief conflict.[9–12]

Time perception, perspective, orientation, and dominance are particular aspects in our overall *sense of time* that importantly bias how we construe our current experiences.[13–15] In normal functioning one perceives events as not coming too fast to process, one has the perspective that events are occurring about as quickly as expected, one's internal orientation to time matches apparent time passing, and one easily ties thoughts of the past to those of the present and projects them into the future.

In using *imagination*, one is capable of synthesiz-

TABLE 81–1. THE DEVELOPMENTAL LIFE STAGES METAPHOR

Stage	Age	Issues	Normal Outcomes	Maladaptive Outcomes
I	0–2	Separation/individuation: a) differentiation b) practice c) rapprochement d) physiological needs	Development of grandiose and idealizing roles; advanced sensorimotor reasoning; ideational and speech. Pragmatic speech functions. Myths of efficacy and belonging. Assumption of trust.	Prolonged need for mirroring or idealizing self-objects; early sensorimotor reasoning; private or restricted myths of being nobody or being destroyed. Distrust.
II	2–4	Categorical view of self: e) individual object constancy; emergence of variation in temperament; safety needs	Differentiation of subjective "I" from social "me's," gender identity formation. Concrete operational reasoning. Public speech development. Myths of invulnerability. Trust leads to faith. Collaborative and creative relational processing.	Failed differentiation of "I" from social me's." Confused gender identity. Reliance on sensorimotor reasoning. Poor public speech. Myths of defectiveness or perfection. Doubts about autonomy. Power assertion or love manipulation types of relational processing.
III	4–5	Mastery and autonomy Belonging and love needs	Concrete operational reasoning onset. Moral development issues. Sex role identity begins. Myth of multipotentiality; autonomy.	Cycles of avoidant or aggressive behavior. Affective lability. Failed integration of self across contexts. Loss of sense of subjective "I"; guilt.
IV	5–8	Initiative Esteem needs	Formal operational reasoning onset. Roles broaden. "Warrior/maiden" aspects of the subjective "I" begin; chum relationship onset (alter-ego self objects. Apprenticeship.	Black/white, concrete operational reasoning continues; decreased school performance. Few hobbies or interests; peer isolation, stealing, lying, cruelty. Attempts to rework idealizing relationships. Inferiority.
V	8–10	Competence	Formal operational reasoning; perceptual empathy; self-reflective capability; myth of integration of needs.	Compartmental, variable reasoning; projective self-object searches; self-reflective futility; myth of defective character; work paralysis, runaway, drug abuse onset
VI	10–early adolescence	Youth	Sex-role behavior onset. Social obedience based on reciprocity. Self-reflective articulation. Peer group broadens. Achievement is pursued.	Sex-role confusion. Role identity lability. Affective and behavioral lability. Drug abuse, sociopathic behavior.
VII	Early adolescence–young adult	Identity formation: a) differentiation b) practice c) rapprochment d) consolidation	Distinguishable self-identity roles. Jobs/career directions. Intimate relationships. Resolution of ambivalence.	Identity confusion. Role diffusion; job expediency; impulse disorder problems; variable psychopathology; persistent ambivalence.
VIII	Young–to middle adulthood (18–30)	Trying out the identity	Flexibility in subjective "I"; investment in many social "Me's." Try out different job/career, geographic moves. Marriage, couples identity; children, parenting	Lack of "I" investment in social roles, social isolation; job expediency or welfare. Problems with intimacy, couples identity, sex-role interactions.
IX	Middle age (30–70)	Making the most of it	High energy in creativity, job/career, family, social goals. Flexibility in crises. Reassessment of identity and life goals every 10 years, Managing cross-generational roles.	Lack of energy to generate, achieve; lack of pleasure in success; loss of function in crises. Boredom with work. Repeated divorce; integrational conflict.
X	Mature age (65–death)	Summing it up	Energy conservation with selected expenditure; interest in a legacy, identity review, articulation of ideology, granting rights. Adjust to grieving, loss, ill health	Difficulty with continued energy demands; passivity with ill health. Chronic depression and hostility; social isolation.

ing new forms with invented meanings and locating them at any time in any space. This capacity is thought to have evolved from "open" genetic programming, in which the structuring and acquisition of content of the self have not been genetically predetermined but left to be shaped by one's experience.[16] The phases of creative or imaginative construction—preparation, incubation, illumination, and verification—have been well described by Wallas.[17]

These five characteristics bias the operating rules used by the processing apparatus to construct as well as remember "relevant" schemata. Many of these biases are summarized in current attribution theory.[18–20] The framework of a schemata comes from Quillian's[21] description of the principles that establish a semantic network. These principles are used first to construct an "episode" schemata. Here are recorded the goals, expectations, appraisals, and coping elements as well as the sequential interaction, outcome beliefs, and future operating rules from an experience. Content and structure of elements of similar "episode" schemata are then used by the self-processing apparatus to build three versions of an "abstract" schemata. These have the same internal structures but have varying content depending on whether they are "me as I am," "ought," or "ideal" schemata. In "ought" schemata the apparatus modifies the content to emphasize what others think one ought to need, feel, and value. In "ideal" schemata, the self-processing apparatus modifies the content to emphasize awareness of the self's own needs, interactions, affects, time sense, and imagination. These two versions may be stored in superego and id parts of the state-space and be arrayed along grandiose and idealizing poles. Contradictory schemata may be stored at preconscious and unconscious levels.

In therapy sessions one observes patients making context associations from one episode scheme to another where there are salient similarities. Some similarities are also directly linked to particular levels in relevant abstract schemata through indexing registers, as mentioned previously.

DEVELOPMENT OF THE BRIEF DYNAMIC THERAPY METHOD

Marmor[22] has nicely traced the development of brief dynamic therapy methods out of the psychoanalytic method. There are at least six components to this methodological shift: (1) the emphasis on developmental stage IV or later was seen to be often preceded by difficulties at earlier stages; (2) the narrated myth that formed a closed-system, linear, causal model of self-dynamics became an open-system, interactive, modular model; (3) the data to be discussed in therapy sifted from products and states to relationships and processes; (4) the explicit goal of the relationship between patient and therapist shifted from guided attempts to resolve internal, structural, and content conflicts, so as to achieve life's meaning, to interactive attempts to resolve conflicts in one's current world so as to facilitate evolution of meaning; (5) the implicit goals of interactional processing between patient and therapist shifted from collaborative dependency to collaborative emancipation; and (6) the language employed in therapy broadened from descriptive, linear reasoning accompanied by constrained interpersonal messages to an interactive experiencing of the parallel, conflicting determinants of reasoning discussed through mutual use of performatives, imperatives, and other pragmatics. Clare[23] saw this shift as moving the method from a focus on flaw, failure, symptom, and disease to a focus on growth, self-esteem, and achievement of potential.

As these shifts have occurred, all four of the previously described metaphors have come to be integrated as the general model for a range of brief dynamic therapy methods. Anxiety-provoking psychotherapy methods with an oedipal focus,[24] brief therapy methods with both oedipal and loss foci,[25] time-limited loss focus,[26] and multiple-foci, short-term dynamic therapy methods[27] formed a clinical core for therapeutic practice in the 1970s that utilized the first three metaphors. One effect of this core development has been to move to identifying combinations of affects with cognitions as the determinant of specific behaviors, in particular relationships. The theoretical differences in dynamic and cognitive-behavior therapy (CBT) methods are thus coming together. In the CBT method, Beck[28] saw emotions following meanings (automatic thoughts) attributed to events, thereby emphasizing a progression from cognition to affective reaction and then to behavioral reaction. However, Meichenbaum[29] started with affect and progressed to cognition. He first set up the affective bias in the "stress innoculation" experience so as to be able to bring out the resulting distorted cognitions of inner speech and try to override them with propositional, logical reasoning. This affective-to-cognitive process is also what one observes in much of the dialogue of psychoanalytical and brief dynamic therapy sessions.

Recent additions to the brief dynamic method have expanded its focus to new areas of the self's structures. The contribution of crisis-oriented therapy methods[30] distinguished between (1) one's need to alter defenses in the self-processing apparatus, or the dynamic self-concept, and heuristic integrational links during one's schematic construction of new experiences; and (2) the range of coping strategies one could promote at the interactional processing link. Environmental and specific hazard manipulation techniques were described that were distinct from patient-directed interactions. The client-centered therapy method[31] brought renewed emphasis on the quality of the patient-therapist relationship as a necessary condition for change accompanied by an expanded use of the therapist's interpersonal messages. Havens[32] has further contributed new ideas on the use of pragmatic speech to collaborate with patients whose malfunctioning involves the top schemata levels of the self "as being." Understanding the importance of the idealizing pole to self-organization, as well as the grandiose pole,[33] has led to new techniques to correct relational processing problems in one's current abstract schemata. Interpersonal therapy techniques for depression[34] focused on intervening at the connections between relational processing, plans and strategies, and the metabelief link to role transitions. These techniques also emphasized the linking of issues to developmental stages VIII to X. Cashdan[35] more recently has developed techniques for addressing relational processing malfunctioning in patients with cluster B personality disorders.

These new techniques are part of a trend to relate types of patient-induced countertransferance responses to high-level defects in self-organization. In Cashdan's[35] object relations therapy technique, the therapist experiences the patient's particular type of projective identification: power, dependency, sexuality, or ingratiation. He or she then uses a range of self-expressions to openly identify and counter this type of relational processing. The trend to expand the rational use of therapist self-expression in this way in brief dynamic therapy best distinguishes this method from trends in CBT method development. In the latter, new prescriptive cognitive and behavioral techniques are evolving in an attempt to address problems of patients with cluster B personality disorders.[36,37] The method's emphasis remains, however, on the therapist using clinical knowledge of opposing plans, strategies, belief elements, and interactional processing, the "working" and "behaving" levels of himself or herself, to effect patient change. In contrast, technical developments in the dynamic method continue to explore new applications of the "corrective emotional experience"[38] as it can be induced in genuine patient-therapist experiencing[31] under the guidance of elements and content at levels I and II in therapists' clinical schemata, the therapists' "self as being." The therapist uses his or her knowledge of structure and content at these levels to identify maladaptive patient myths and rituals and reorganize their inherent assumptions into counter-myths. Through dialogue about these counter-myths, the therapist corrects information about how he or she appears to be experienced by the patient, and how he or she experiences the patient.[39]

A rationale for greater use of the therapist's self in promoting change in patient state-space organization, self-processing apparatus, and upper levels of constructed schemata comes from Weiss'[40] studies on the unconscious control hypothesis. The original analytical dynamic hypothesis assumed that one could not exert control over unconscious content in one's self-organizational processing. The opposing unconscious control hypothesis assumes that one originally kept some ideas or impulses unconscious because experiencing or expressing them would be too dangerous. This hypothesis predicts that active collaboration that lifts into consciousness one's old unexamined intentions and affects will now be reacted to not with tension and anxiety, but with an increased sense of recall and broadened patient experiencing. Weiss' affirmative results provide theoretical underpinnings to the therapists' intervening by actively identifying and discussing with the patient elements from his or her unconscious constructions that are biasing his or her interactions. Epstein[41] and Gabbard[42,43] thus describe active "containment" techniques for aggression or fear in paranoid and schizoid patients. The treatment of Axis II, cluster B patients similarly benefits from active focusing techniques[44] that correct poor heuristic integration due to affective dissociation and defensive denial. The therapist uses a sequence of instructions to contain and direct affect, leading the patient to experience ideas and feelings in the context of a "holding" patient-therapist relationship. Such active containment techniques are also part of the method to unify the personas of multiple personality disorder.[45]

This trend in the brief dynamic therapy method to develop specific techniques for correcting the malfunctioning of specific self-structures is accompanied by a change in our conceptualization of patient pathology. Adopting an open-ended, modular, process-oriented model of individual functioning means that the patient and therapist meet in each new session not with an expectation of picking up on the threads of a single, unwinding, predetermined script of one's life, but for a recurring fresh review of "where are we" in the patient's "states of mind,"[46] "self-identities,"[35] or "working self" schematas. Future shifts in this model may lead to a greater specification of both the necessary patient-therapist relationship variables and the sufficient explicit dialogue needed to correct particular malfunctions in the self.

REFERENCES

1. Erickson EH: Identity: Youth and Crisis, New York: Norton, 1968.
2. Nunn R: On the ego and the id. Unpublished manuscript, Department of Psychiatry and Behavioral Sciences, University of Washington, Seattle, 1989.
3. Whitehead AN: Process and Reality. New York: Macmillan Co, 1929.
4. Atkinson RL, Shiffrin RM: Human memory: a proposed system and its control processes. In Spence KW, Spence JT, eds. The Psychology of Learning and Motivation: Advances in Research and Theory, vol 2. New York: Academic Press, 1968:90–191.
5. Dennett DC: Brainstems: Philosophical Essays on Mind and Psychology. Cambridge, MA: MIT/Bradford Books, 1978.
6. Lane RD, Schwartz GE: Levels of emotional awareness: A cognitive-developmental theory and its application to psychopathology. Am J Psychiatry 144:133–143, 1987.
7. Baker HS, Baker MN: Heinz Kohut's self psychology: An overview. Am J Psychiatry 144:1–9, 1987.

8. Dimond SJ: Neuropsychology: A Textbook of Systems and Psychological Functions of the Human Brain. London: Butterworth, 1980.
9. Werner H: Comparative Psychology of Mental Development. New York: Science Editions, 1961.
10. Koestler A: The Logic of the Moist Eye, The Act of Creation. London: Hutchinson, 1964, chap. 12.
11. Frijida NH: The laws of emotion. Am Psychol 43:349–358, 1988.
12. Kippax S, Crawford J, Benton P, Gault U: Constructing emotions: Weaving meaning from memories. Br J Social Psychol 27:19–33, 1988.
13. Fraisse P: Perception and estimation of time. Annu Rev Psychol 35:1–36, 1984.
14. Tismer KG: Psychological aspects of temporal dominance during adolescence. Psychol Rep 61:647–654, 1987.
15. Munzel K, Gendner G, Steinberg R, Raith L: Time estimation of depressive patients: The influence of internal content. Eur Arch Psychiatr Neurol Sci 237:171–178, 1988.
16. Mayr E: Behavior programs and evolution strategies. Am Sci 62:650–659, 1974.
17. Wallas G: Stages of control. In Rothenberg H, Hansman C, eds. The Creativity Question. Durham, NC: Duke University Press, 1976:69–73.
18. Rhodewatt F, Agustdottir S: The effects of self-presentation on the phenomenal self. J Personal Social Psychol 50:47–55, 1986.
19. Dawes RM: Statistical criteria for establishing a truly false consensus effect. J Exp Social Psychol 25:1–17, 1989
20. Ginosaur Z, Trope Y: Problem solving in judgment under uncertainty. J Pers Social Psychol 52:464–474, 1987.
21. Quillian MR: Semantic memory. Unpublished doctoral dissertation, Carnegie Institute of Technology, Pittsburgh, PA, 1966.
22. Marmor J: Historical aspects of short-term dynamic therapy. Psychiatr Clin North Am 2:3–11, 1979.
23. Clare AW: Brief psychotherapy: New approaches. Psychiatric Clin NA 2:93–109, 1979.
24. Sifneos P: Short-Term Psychotherapy and Emotional Crisis. Cambridge, MA: Harvard University Press, 1972.
25. Malan DH: A Study of Brief Psychotherapy. London: Tavistock Publications, 1963.
26. Mann J: Time Limited Psychotherapy. Cambridge, MA: Harvard University Press, 1973.
27. Davanloo H: Techniques of short-term dynamic therapy. Psychiatr Clin North Am 1:11–22, 1979.
28. Beck AD, Thinking and depression: II. Theory and Therapy. Arch Gen Psychiatry 10:561–571, 1964.
29. Meichenbaum M: Cognitive Behavior Modification: An Integrative Approach. New York: Plenum Press, 1977.
30. Jacobson GF: Crisis oriented therapy. Psychiatric Clin NA 2:39–54, 1979.
31. Rogers C: Carl Rogers on Personal Power. London: Constable, 1978.
32. Havens L: Making Contact. Cambridge, MA: Harvard University Press, 1986.
33. Kohut H: The Analysis of the Self. New York: International University Press, 1971.
34. Klerman GL, Weissman MM, Rounsaville BJ, et al: Interpersonal Psychotherapy of Depression. New York: Basic Books, 1984.
35. Cashdan S: Object Relations Therapy. New York: WW Norton and Co, 1988.
36. Linehan M: Dialectical behavior therapy: A cognitive behavioral approach to parasuicide. J Personal Disord 1:328–333, 1987.
37. Glantz K, Goisman RM: Relaxation and merging in the treatment of personality disorders. Am J Psychother 4:405–413, 1990.
38. Alexander F, French T, et al: Psychoanalytic Therapy. New York, Ronald Press, 1946.
39. Frayn DH: Regressive transference—a manifestation of primitive personality organization. Am J Psychother 44:50–60, 1990.
40. Weiss J: Unconscious mental functioning. Sci Am 262:103–109, 1990.
41. Epstein L: An interpersonal-object relations perspective on working with destructive aggression. Contemp Psychoanal 20:651–662, 1984.
42. Gabbard G: On "doing nothing" in the psychoanalytic treatment of the refractory borderline patient. Int J Psychoanal 70:527–534, 1989.
43. Gabbard G: Psychodynamic Psychiatry in Clinical Practice. Washington, DC: American Psychiatric Press, Inc., 1990.
44. Gendlin ET: Focusing. New York: Bantam, 1981.
45. Braun BG, ed: Treatment of Multiple Personality Disorder. Washington, DC: American Psychiatric Press, Inc., 1986.
46. Horowitz MJ: Formulation of states of mind. Psychiatr Clin North Am 2:39–54, 1979.

82

GROUP THERAPY AND MARITAL/FAMILY TREATMENT

ELSA O'CONNOR, Ed.D. and JAMES W. CROAKE, Ph.D.

GROUP PSYCHOTHERAPY

There is a broad spectrum of group psychotherapy that occurs in a vast array of settings. Groups may be held in an inpatient unit, an outpatient clinic, a community mental health center, a health maintenance organization, or a variety of other public and private facilities. The theoretical foundations for the group may be cognitive-behavioral, interpersonal, object relations, or some other modality utilized in individual psychotherapy.

Preparation

A pregroup interview with each prospective member can address erroneous beliefs. During this time, patient fears and apprehensions are solicited, as well as expectations for change. The leader can clarify the goals and objectives of the group, create accurate expectations about desirable patient behavior, describe leadership roles, and discuss realistic outcomes of therapy.[1]

Exclusion Criteria

In discussing criteria for exclusion, it is important to note that the frame of reference utilized is heterogeneous, intensive, outpatient group treatment. The patients described may therapeutically benefit from a specialized form of group psychotherapy with a homogeneous population (i.e., those who have poor impulse control due to organicity or sociopathy and would be disruptive to the group process), as would patients who are paranoid, hypochondriacal, addicted to alcohol or other drugs, or actively psychotic. These patients soon develop a role in the group that inhibits group process and becomes injurious both to the participant and other members.

Patients undergoing recent traumatic life crises may do better in individual therapy because they are able to have the undivided attention they require. The same holds true for the deeply depressed and suicidal patient. The criteria for exclusion are not precise and provide only a rough guideline for the practitioner to follow in maximizing the efficacy of group psychotherapy. Practitioner skill and specific areas of expertise may alter these recommendations.[2]

Inclusion Criteria

Individuals who are socially and psychologically isolated, shy, and inhibited can derive benefits from supportive and empathic interactions with others. Those who are experiencing conflict with interpersonal relationships may learn alternative behaviors and test new understandings within the safety of the group environment.

Group therapy can also be useful for working on issues of intimacy and individuation, through the mechanism of relatedness experienced within the group setting. The limited criteria for inclusion indicate that group psychotherapy is the treatment of choice for a multitude of people. It is the therapist's task to determine which form of therapy will bring about the desired change based on the patient's psychological resources, the skills of the group leaders, and the types of groups available.[2,3]

Group Stages

The initial stage of group therapy can be thought of as a time for orientation and exploration. Safety and trust are major concerns for participants as they determine how actively they will participate and whether they can identify with this setting. As the group establishes norms, and members gradually begin to reveal their thoughts and feelings, the group will enter the second stage, which is characterized by increased anxiety and defensiveness. The anxiety is an outgrowth of the fear and vulnerability resulting from being known by other group members on a deeper level. Concerns about being judged and misunderstood are bound to surface, followed by demands for an increase in structure. This stage may be perceived as a struggle related to power and dominance among the members, including the leader. Before these issues can be resolved, conflict must be recognized as an inevitable part of all relationships. If disagreement can be brought forward with the integrity and acceptance of members remaining intact, a foundation of trust will have been established. This will enable further movement to the third stage of development, distinguished by cohesiveness and productivity.

Group cohesiveness refers to the members' experience of belonging to the group, being accepted by the group, and feeling a sense of solidarity with the group. At this stage, participants take risks and work on painful conflictual material. They have learned to take responsibility for their actions and are willing to practice behavioral changes both inside and outside the group environment. They have also begun to accept personal responsibility for group progress, and will speak up with increased frequency if they are dissatisfied.

The final stage is termination. It is essential that group members be given the opportunity to consolidate their learning and grieve the loss of the group. They discover that the group has meant something unique to each member. Integrating and interpreting this significance for one another becomes a critical component in weaving loose ends together. Participants are able to assess their progress and decide how they will continue to effect change in their lives.[3,4]

Leadership

In reviewing leadership variables, researchers have frequently stated that the therapist-patient relationship is more important for group process and therapeutic success. Numerous research efforts have focused on leader genuineness, empathy, and warmth. Yet, with psychologically impaired populations, it appears that relationship variables are not as significant in mediating therapeutic outcome as are the technical aspects of leadership that involve structuring activity within the group, clarity of instructions, and concrete behaviors that are reinforcing to the members. In addition, there are therapeutic factors that emphasize interpersonal processes unique to group treatment, and these factors do not directly involve the therapist-patient relationship. Thus, while the therapist plays a significant role in shaping group development, particularly in its early stages, once the dynamics of group process take hold, the group becomes the medium for change.[3,5]

Caution is advised regarding the introduction of confrontation before sufficient trust has been established. As for therapist self-disclosure, it has not been sufficiently researched to provide conclusive guidelines. The role of the leader is complex and requires sensitivity, flexibility, and a willingness to both engage and withdraw from the group process as needed.

Co-therapy

Since the mid-1960s co-therapy has received growing attention and acceptance. There are several advantages to this approach: (1) two viewpoints offer increased understanding of group process and patient perspective; (2) transferences can be split among two therapists and will usually emerge with greater clarity; (3) treatment will be continuous, since one therapist can lead the group in the absence of the other; (4) the co-therapy team can provide information to members about a collaborative relationship by modeling behaviors that are beneficial to interpersonal functioning, (5) each therapist can offer the other balance when one therapist is being confronted by group members, and the other can assist the process by elucidating the issues; and (6) if a leader is overly idealized by the group, the other therapist can provide perspective and discuss errors that may have been overlooked. The co-therapy team allocates time to process their interactions before and after group sessions. The major disadvantage of co-therapy arises when competitiveness and divisiveness interfere with group process.[6]

Problematic Patients and Interventions

Pretherapy interviews can only go so far in preventing problematic patients from entering an outpatient long-term psychotherapy group. Each participant brings to therapy a unique constellation of issues. They enter a group in the hope of learning how to remove obstacles that impede effective interpersonal functioning. Consequently, the question arises as to what constitutes problematic behavior, since most participants are troubled individuals trying their utmost to cope with difficult situations. When members display behaviors that obstruct the group's progress and prevent other participants from learning, they have become problematic. Therapists respond to these situations with a step-by-step assessment that takes into consideration their own reactions and then allows decision making to occur by examining when, why, and how to intervene.

After self-assessments have assured therapists that they can intervene without significant interference from personal issues, the next question is when to intervene. Two approaches to intervention may be useful. It has been recommended that leaders share their feelings and thoughts about the disruptive behavior. Alternatively, it is suggested that leaders involve the group in probing its own intentions by asking why it allows this behavior to continue. An example would be, "I'm wondering why the group allows Gerry more time to speak than any other member?" Helping members learn how to offer and accept feedback is a further dimension of therapist effectiveness in dealing with problematic behavior. As a last resort, should the disruption of the group not be resolvable through leader or member interventions, the participant is asked to leave during an individual conference outside the group. The focus is on the member's needs not being reconcilable to the purpose of the group. If there are co-therapists, both are present for the conference.[7]

Concurrent Individual and Group Therapy

Combined therapy refers to individual and group therapy with the same practitioner. Conjoint therapy is the circumstance in which a group member sees another therapist for individual work. Rutan and Alonso suggested that group therapy be added to individual work when the patient does not have sufficient associational material to maintain energy in individual sessions.[8] Individual therapy may be added to group work for patients unable to express themselves in a group format.

Concurrent therapy has several pitfalls, the most prominent being the opportunity for splitting to occur. It is essential that the therapist keep communication channels open and gain an agreement from the patient that secrets will not be kept between the individual and group therapy. Each therapy needs to be viewed as adjunctive to the other, and even though the patient may feel that one is more important at times, an overall perspective of cooperation is required.

Short-Term Group Psychotherapy

Short-term, brief, or time-limited group psychotherapy has become a widely known and practiced modality. These groups are marked by setting a specific time frame, which may range from a minimum of eight to ten sessions to a maximum of 20 to 25 sessions. The process includes establishing limited treatment goals, rapid assessment of group inclusion, an active therapist who manages each session, promptness of intervention, and ventilation (patient expression) as a critical element in short-term group psychiatry.

The goals for short-term group therapy should be explicit and agreed upon by the patient and the therapist. They include reduction of symptom distress, reestablishment of the patient's former sense of equilibrium, efficient use of patient resources, developing the patient's understanding of the current disturbance, and increasing coping skills for the future.[9,10]

MARITAL THERAPY

According to behavioral theory, distressed couples tend to have more rigid structural patterns of interactions and display more negative affect and greater reciprocity of negative effect.[11] Assisting couples to see that their behavior is reciprocal and mutually controlled is perceived as one of the most important concepts in treatment.[12] Before therapy the couples use aversive maneuvers in attempting to change each others' behavior. Showing them how to switch to a system of rewards such as the *quid pro quo* contract allows couples to learn more mutually satisfying ways of addressing wants.[13] Behavioral marital therapists use contracts to further positive reinforcers within the relationship. Helen may wish to have Thursday evenings with friends. She makes a contract with Fred that if he cares for the children on Thursday evenings, she will take care of the children on Saturday, which will free him to play handball.

Psychiatric Disorders

In the case of a depressed patient complaining of marital distress, marital therapy has been shown to be at least as effective as cognitive-behavioral therapy conducted only with the depressed spouse.[14] In agoraphobia, the spouse is primarily engaged as a supporter of the patient and not as a partner in marital therapy. This form of education, although not marital therapy, enhances treatment results. Depression and agoraphobia severely disrupts the equilibrium of a partnership. Marital therapy provides an effective treatment option. This is also the case if marital problems have precipitated panic attacks, phobia, or depressive episodes.

The functions of alcohol on the marital system are varied and may include regulation of emotional disturbance, stabilizing a chaotic system, and an expression of stress within the family. More frequently, alcohol precipitates marital dysfunction just as it can mimic signs and symptoms of most psychiatric disorders. Studies have shown that marital therapy can assist outpatient treatment for alcohol dependence.[14]

Treatment Approaches

Psychoanalytic Theory

Psychoanalytically oriented therapy emphasizes the need for insight into unconscious childhood experiences that are the source of current maladaptive behavior in the relationship. The nature of the marital system is affected by shared fantasies and the defenses used by each partner. Couples are offered either individual or conjoint sessions to understand both themselves and each other. The therapist may address transferential material that will shed light on sources of difficulty.

Partners may be asked to recall situations or experiences with parental figures that resemble current difficulties with a spouse. Separating the past from the present can assist the partners in releasing feelings that generate discomfort and lead to destructive projections in the present relationship. Critics of this approach contend that insight does not necessarily lead to behavioral change, and that the time of change, if it occurs, may involve months or years of therapy. The analytical approach has provided creative ways of viewing relationships, but lacks empirical validation.[15]

Systems Theory

With the emergence of the systems perspective, the intrapersonal structure of the individual is deemphasized. The focus of attention is on each person as part of a system that shapes a specific context. Spouses act and react to one another based upon their biased apperceptions. Communication within the interactional system is a key determinant of a successful relationship. Role expectations are focal in communication. Verbal and nonverbal exchanges, body movements, and voice inflections are all part of the system that transmits information both within the partnership and to outside institutions.

Unspoken ideas of what makes a "good" marriage or a "wonderful" partner affect the duties and rights designated to each person as well as the activities generated by the couple. The therapist serves as an observer and a teacher while maintaining a neutral stance to the couple. By making systems interventions (e.g., "How do you decide who will drive the car?"), the therapist brings to the surface areas of unspoken role behaviors or expectations that are a source of conflict. Expectations can be redefined so that conscious choices are made that will increase the stability and adaptability of the partnership.[16]

Behavioral Marital Therapy

Behavioral marital therapy (BMT) stresses intensive short-term treatment. It draws on the social learning hypothesis of marital distress, which correlates the subjective quality of a relationship to the rates of pleasant and unpleasant interactions. Couples are taught communication and problem-solving skills and are given opportunities to expand their repertoire of pleasing behavior. Therapy averages 12 to 16 sessions, which are usually 60 to 90 minutes in length. Meetings are structured with the therapist setting the agenda.

The therapist plays many roles that include teacher, director, model, and evaluator, and actively participates in sharing perceptions and insights. Relationship strengths are highlighted, as are strategies that promote feelings of competency in conflict resolution. Self-report questionnaires provide structure for the interviews. Homework assignments are a regular part of each session—for example, recording daily satisfactions on a five-point Likert-type scale (always to never)—and serve as a catalyst for discussions within the session.[17]

Emotionally-Based Therapy

Emotionally focused therapy (EFT) rests on the theoretical framework that an individual's emotional and experiential state will lead to construction of conscious meaning, perceptions, and organization, which in turn will determine the person's behavior. Thus, if one of the partners organizes experience in terms of feelings of anger and rejection, this person will attribute these expressions to the partner. If the organization of experience is one of feeling valued, the same behavior of the partner is taken to have positive connotations. EFT tries to understand each person's emotionally based self-organization and the variables that have an impact on this organization. EFT is an integration of experiential and systematic perspectives. Therapists help the couple access and communicate emotional experiences such as anger, fear, and vulnerability, which generates dialogues that lead to interpretation of the interactive process between the partners. The style of the quarrel takes precedence over why they quarrel. By bringing forth the emotional experiences that underlie their interaction, the couple is able to restructure intrapsychic and interpersonal processes.[18]

Patient Selection

A primary consideration in recommending marital therapy is the investment of both partners in improving the relationship. A thorough assessment to determine the degree of involvement is important. Evidence suggests that difficulties in communication, mutual responsiveness, and conflict resolution are major contributors to marital distress. The therapist not only addresses the process consideration of these factors but also determines the psychological foundations that are the underpinnings for the distress.

Criteria for elimination of patients for marital therapy may include couples whose patterns of interaction would not allow a display of vulnerability to be respected, as in physically violent and abusive relationships, or couples who exhibit rigid attack-attack interactional processes. These couples may benefit from strategic systems approaches, or they may require individual psychotherapy before couple work can be effective.[19] Commitment to change by both partners is critical in marital therapy. If improvement of the relationship is not desired by one member, then separation or divorce may be realistic options to be explored.

Combination with Other Treatments

Sex Therapy

Marital therapy is frequently integrated into sexual dysfunction therapy. Sexual behavior of the couple is viewed as a microcosm of the overall dynamics within the partnership.

Pharmacotherapy

There are also times when psychopharmacological interventions are useful. Physicians may choose to have a colleague administer medication to one of the partners, thus enabling the therapeutic alliance to remain balanced.

Individual and Group Therapy

It is not unusual for one or both members of the relationship to be engaged in individual or group work during the time of marital therapy. The essential ingredient in this process is the flow of information and energy into the couples' work. It is hoped that the other modalities will assist the development of the individual as well as the system. When simultaneous therapy is in progress, guidelines are established for determining boundaries of confidentiality and consultation.

Course of Treatment

Couples arriving for marital therapy will typically bring a presenting problem. The individual who conducts therapy will strive to create an atmosphere of neutrality and impartiality so that each partner's perception of the difficulty may be safely aired. During these presentations the therapist will be listening for conflictual material that has polarized the couple (e.g., "I am outgoing and enjoy being with people all the time, while my wife would much rather be alone and shop through catalogues.") Neither statement is totally accurate, but in a distressed relationship the couples are so distanced from one another that they are at opposite ends of the continuum. Hence, they see polarities and view one another with antithetical, biased modes of apperception.

In addition to the presenting problem, the couple will also bring along past family experiences, personal values, role expectations about men and women, and varying desires for independence and interdependence. As therapy proceeds, each partner will learn to define his or her family heritage. They will also learn how to conceptualize in terms of "the relationship," as well as "Jeff and Anne."

Gradually they will understand their interactional dances that promote closeness or extend distance. They will practice modifying behaviors and learn to gauge marital interactions in a more sensitive manner. The goals of marital therapy will vary from couple to couple.

Strategies and Interventions

Pinpointing behaviors that lead to marital satisfaction is a way of addressing the question "What constitutes health?" Interventions are treatment strategies based upon a defined paradigm of marriage. Couples may do their homework assignment by going out to dinner with increased frequency. However, if they do not grasp the connection between behavior and the overall functioning of the partnership, attachment and communication will not develop further. Instead, they may go out to dinner with each reading the evening newspaper.

Goals

The therapist may encounter conflicts about organization, structure, and rules within the marriage. Exploring relationship goals and identifying collusional patterns are part of the process that enables each partner to assume greater responsibility for the system. At any time the therapist may reinterpret a symptom or sign from a negative to a positive. A wife may feel ashamed that her husband wept out of frustration in front of their son. She sees this as a sign of her husband's weakness. Reframing this scenario so that the son was able to witness his father's vulnerability and courage to be imperfect allows each partner and their son freer expression of affect.

Communication training may involve teaching skills that include empathic response and active listening (as well as modeling the communication of personal feelings, both negative and positive). Training in problem solving teaches the couple to define issues, specify behaviors that are to be changed, address one problem at a time, paraphrase partner responses before speaking, learn negotiating skills, and not overgeneralize one negative interaction as the sum of the marriage or one behavior as the sum of the spouse's being. Helping each partner change the locus of control from the other (e.g., "She is making me feel guilty") to themselves (e.g., I feel frustrated when I'm asked a question, and a particular response is required") increases self-determination and leads to feelings of inclusion and investment in the marriage.

FAMILY THERAPY

In family therapy, the family system is treated as a unit. The diagnostic features of the individuals are an ongoing consideration of the therapist, but the attention is given to the family's dynamics.[20] In the case of family conflict, the systems approach attends to the family interaction. Applicable individual diagnoses are kept in mind by the therapist as potential limitations to technique; however, the diagnoses are secondary to the attention given to the family coalition.

Therapists working with psychopathology know that the identified patient is the frequent object of complaint by the other family members. The "healthy" members wish to focus upon the signs and symptoms of the identified patient. This focus shunts other interpersonal problems and permits the members to deny the family and subfamily interactions as contributory to the identified patient's diagnoses, as well as permitting individual self-delusions of salubrious functioning apart from the identified patient. It is not uncommon for everyone to believe that, if it were not for the interpersonal and intrapersonal dynamics of the identified patient, there would be no dysfunction in the family.[21]

Formulation

It is often quite surprising to the beginning therapist to have an entirely different view of each of the family members once they are all seen together. Talking with each of the family members separately or together about the identified patient's problems allows for each of them (including the patient) to present themselves in a healthy, rational manner.

Theoretical Structures

There have been many attempts to determine patterns of interaction that support specific diagnoses. To date, only general familial patterns are noted in functional and dysfunctional families.[22] The enmeshed family[23] contains alliances and divisions that keep the dysfunction in place. Assisting each family member to become more independent and to change the alignments is the therapeutic goal.

The "double bind" as viewed by Bateson[24] is an interaction within the family that does not allow for a satisfactory communication. None of the parties involved seem to be able to extract themselves from the no-win transaction. Double bind communication places impossible limits on those for whom the interactions is intended. For example, a mother may say to her child, "Stop being so obedient and listen to me." If the child is obedient by listening to the mother, she is angry because the child doesn't think for himself. If the child disobeys the mother, he isn't listening to her. Any response by the child reinforces the mother's idea that the child is impossible. She may also be thinking that she is a failure or the child would be able to respond effectively. The child usually cannot pinpoint the source of the frustration and anger, but nonetheless may feel totally inept. The feeling of ineptness may well carry over to relationships outside of the family. Certainly this type of communication reinforces the dysfunctional familial pattern and precludes a positive family dynamic.

Communication schools of family therapy attempt to disrupt the no-win transactions with interventions that preclude double binds. The use of "antisuggestion,"[25] also termed "paradoxical intention," is a direction by the therapist to do more of that which has been labeled as irrational. Sending the family home to reenact the exact fight about which they came into the therapeutic session complaining would be an example of antisuggestion. The family is given the assignment to return home and carry out the very behaviors that formerly felt out of control and unpleasant. Purposive reenactment interferes with the maladaptive patterns of communication and may even result in a humorous outcome.

The late Murray Bowen coined the term "fusion," which indicates pathological families who seemingly cannot act independently and are glued together in an indefinable, dysfunctional mass.[26] Bowen further made note of the multigenerational transmission of pathology. Without interruption of the fusion, the next generation reengages in impairment.

Melanie Klein,[27] who is generally credited with moving psychoanalytical theory toward an emphasis on the ego rather than instinctual drives, opened the door for the possibility of psychoanalytical theory to be modified (object relations theory) to accommodate family therapy. She believed that interaction with others in the family was aimed not at drive reduction but rather at the development of the self. She emphasized a movement toward satisfying objects. This changed the function of the libido away from the pleasure principle as Freud conceived it.

Henry Dicks[28] made use of projective identification, wherein unacceptable aspects of one's personality are projected onto another member of the family. As an example, a mother's unconscious promiscuous desires are projected onto the teenage daughter, with resultant accusation and arguments. The use of the concept of projective identification is seen as an extension of Klein's ideas and becomes the foundation for family therapy from an object relations point of view.

Patient Selection

Family treatment is seen by systems theory as the therapy of choice when family members are available. If one accepts the principles that undergird the therapy, working with individuals is generally less effective. There are, however, situations that are not conducive to family therapy. A patient in an acute psychotic state is not able to function within any social situation. Once medications, seclusion, and other standard techniques have stabilized the patient, family therapy can begin. It is best to begin working with the family in the hospital if the identified patient is in the hospital, so that from nearly the beginning of the acute situation the family becomes accustomed to being seen as the patient, even if only one of the members is hospitalized.

Combination with Other Treatment

Family therapy can readily be used in combination with other forms of treatment. Biological interventions would be the most obvious. Medications or electroconvulsive therapy may be necessary for the patient to attend during the family sessions. Many physicians prefer to have a colleague administer the biological intervention in order to avoid a compromised position when attempting to make the family the patient.

It is often desirable to see a couple separately from the rest of the family. Some issues are specific to the primary coalition, the marital unit. Sexual problems would be a case in point. The couple's diagnosis, assessment, goals of treatment, and therapy can be worked with freely apart from other family members. Not only is the couple's sex life none of the rest of the family's business, but allowing other family members to be privy to such information can be confusing at best and would enhance pathology at worst. Certainly it weakens the marital coalition and strengthens intergenerational ties. The latter is deleterious to salubrious family functioning.

Individual family members can also be seen for skills training. This training would take many forms depending upon the problem. Occupational training and physical therapy are obvious. Parent training is appropriate. Classes in how to make small talk and groups for learning how to make friends might be other examples.

Individual psychotherapy with the identified patient is not a good idea. This only furthers the misconception that one of the family members is the problem. Additionally, when there is individual therapy, important issues affecting the family are discussed more easily in individual treatment and never are mentioned or resolved in the family context.

Group therapy on a limited basis can be simultaneously used with family therapy. A single parent, for example, may be in a group for sexual dysfunction. Again, the important point is that material properly discussed and resolved within the family should not be discussed in another therapy context because this increases the possibility of sabotaging the family therapy.

Course of Treatment

Family therapy is generally more time limited than individual treatment. Family therapy focuses on here-and-now problem solving. Individual personalities are secondary to the family style and therefore rarely discussed in any depth. A family member's pattern of movement is clarified only to the extent that it facilitates immediate communication, alters transactions, or assists in solving the problem at hand.

The family rules—particularly those that are tacit, not privy to all members, or impossible—receive attention. Patterns of interaction that regularly exclude some members and inappropriately coalesce others are addressed. Patterns of communicating through one member to another rather than addressing those involved are discouraged by the therapist. The goal of the therapist is to open and clarify communication, correct negative interactions, eliminate scapegoating, and promote independence within the greater concern for the family group.

Strategies and Techniques

Attending to the family rather than the individual gives rise to questions such as: "What do each of you wish to have accomplished in this session?" "What can each of you do to bring this expressed desire to an equitable solution?" "What have each of you done to improve the situation?" "What have each of you done to solve the problem about which you are complaining?" "What can each of you do that will ensure that the problem continues?" "What can each of you do that will sabotage agreed upon plans?" In response to the latter two questions, it is frequently another family member who will point out what each of the other members is likely to do to ensure that the problems continue and treatment plans will be sabotaged.

The family will fight any suggestion that they, not the identified patient, are the problem. The interventions by the therapist to alter the family's perception will be met by intensified signs and symptoms that provide the necessary evidence to the other family members that they are fine, and only the identified patient is sick.

Attempts to weaken intergenerational ties will be met with a host of reasons as to why the attention must be directed to a particular child by one of the parents for the child's or grandchild's benefit. The role of the therapist consists of giving assurance to the parent that their concerns are understood, and the welfare of the child, parent, or whomever is the motivation. Since these previously expressed concerns have not been useful, would the family consider an alternative approach?

Whatever the strategy and technique employed, each of the family members must feel that they are a part of the problem solving and decision making, that their ideas are considered, and that their personal welfare is clearly evident in each stage of the therapy. Each member needs to become aware of the contribution he or she can make to the betterment of the family. A simple question offered any time during the therapy will clarify this point: "Will what you're suggesting or planning to do work out well for each member of the family six months from now?"

REFERENCES

1. Piper WE, Perrault EL: Pretherapy preparation for group members. Int J Group Psychother 39:17–33, 1989.
2. Tosselane RW, Siporin M: When to recommend group treatment: A review of the clinical and the research literature. Int J Group Psychother 36:171–201, 1986.
3. Yalom ID: The Theory and Practice of Group Psychotherapy. 3rd ed. New York: Basic Books, 1985:252.
4. Corey G: Theory and Practice of Group Counseling. Belmont, CA: Brooks/Cole Publishing Co, 1990:85–93.
5. Dies RR: Practical, theoretical and empirical foundations for group psychotherapy. In Frances AJ, Hales RE, eds. Psychiatry Update: Annual Review, vol 5. Washington, DC: American Psychiatric Press, Inc, 1987:669.
6. Shaffer J, Galinsky MD: Models of Group Psychotherapy. 2nd ed. Englewood Cliffs, NJ: Prentice-Hall, 1989:59–60.
7. Corey MS, Corey G: Process and Practice. 3rd ed. Monterey, CA: Brooks/Cole Publishing Co, 1987:111–112.
8. Rutan JS, Alonso A: Group therapy, individual therapy, or both? Int J Group Psychother 32:267–282, 1982.
9. Poey K: Guidelines for the practice of brief dynamic group therapy. Int J Group Psychother 35:331–354, 1985.
10. Klein RH: Some principles of short-term group therapy. Int J Group Psychother 35:309–329, 1985.
11. Gottman JM, Levenson RW: Assessing the role of emotion on marriage. Behav Assessment 8:48, 1986.
12. Jacobson NS, Margolin G: Marital Therapy: Strategies Based on Social Learning and Behavior Exchange Principle. New York: Brunner Mazel, 1979:40.
13. Fish RC, Fish LS: Quid pro quo revisited: The basis of marital therapy. Am J Orthopsychiatry 56:371, 1986.
14. Jacobson NS, Holtzworth-Munroe A, Schmaling KB: Marital therapy and spouse involvement in the treatment of depression, agoraphobia, and alcoholism. J Consult Clin Psychiatry 1:9, 1989.
15. Crowe M, Ridley J: Therapy with Couples: A Behavioral Systems Approach to Marital and Sexual Problems. London: Blackwell Scientific Publications, 1990:29–32.
16. Morofka V: Marital therapy from a systems approach. Perspect Psychiatr Care 22:146, 1984.
17. Jacobson NS, Holtsworth-Munroe A: Marital therapy: A social learning-cognitive perspective. In Jacobson NS, Gurman AS, eds. Clinical Handbook of Marital Therapy. New York: Guilford Press, 1986:29–71.
18. Greenberg LS, Johnson SM: Emotionally Focused Therapy for Couples. New York: Guilford Press, 1988:36–38.

19. Johnson SM: Marital therapy: Issues and directions. Int J Family Psychiatry 8:67, 1987.
20. Sperry L, Carlson J: Case formulation in family psychology: Systemic or integrative? Fam Psychologist 7:14, 1991.
21. Croake JW: The use of the mental status exam in family therapy. Fam Psychologist 6:25, 1990.
22. Croake JW, Myer KM: Holistic medicine and chronic illness in children. Individual Psych 40:463, 1984.
23. Hirschorn H: Structural therapy. In Sherman R, Dinkmeyer D, eds. Systems of Family Therapy. New York: Brunner/Mazel, 1987:200.
24. Bateson G: Mind and Nature. New York: Daulton, 1979:83.
25. Croake JW: Ellis' rational emotive therapy. In Sherman R, Dinkmeyer D, eds. Systems of Family Therapy. New York: Brunner/Mazel, 1987:254.
26. Bowen M: Family Therapy in Clinical Practice. New York: Aronson, 1978:221.
27. Klein M: Feminist concepts of therapy outcome. Psych Theory Res Pract 13:91, 1976.
28. Dicks HV: Marital Tensions. London: Routledge & Kegan Paul, 1976:31.

83

HYPNOSIS FOR PSYCHIATRIC DISORDERS

DAVID SPIEGEL, M.D. and JAMES SPIRA, Ph.D., M.P.H.

DEFINITION

Hypnosis is a state of attentive, receptive concentration, with a relative suspension of peripheral awareness. This intense concentration, or absorption, is accompanied by an experience of dissociation, separating normally related experiences into discrete units. Because of their intense absorption in the trance experience, hypnotized individuals usually accept instructions relatively uncritically; hence the term "suggestibility." Hypnotic phenomena occur spontaneously, and the alteration of consciousness that hypnotized individuals experience has a variety of therapeutic applications. Hypnotic experience involves three factors: absorption, dissociation, and suggestibility.

Absorption

Hypnotized individuals are intensely absorbed in their trance experience. Research has shown a correlation between hypnotizability and a tendency for people to undergo spontaneous absorbing experiences.[1] Relative to normal daily activity, what a person in a hypnotic trance concentrates on is attended to completely.

Dissociation

This intense absorption means that many routine experiences that would ordinarily be consciously reflected upon occur out of ordinary conscious awareness. Even rather complex emotional states or sensory experiences may be dissociated. These experiences may range from the simple, such as a hand feeling not as much a part of the body as usual, to the complex, such as a fugue episode in which, for a period of hours to months, an individual functions as though he or she had a different identity. Such experiences can be both induced and reversed with the structured use of hypnosis.

Suggestibility

While hypnotized individuals are not deprived of their will, they do have a tendency to uncritically accept instructions in trance, suspending the usual conscious editing function that raises the question, "Why?" when an instruction is given. Thus, hypnotized individuals are more prone to accept instructions, no matter how irrational. They are also less prone to distinguish an instruction as coming from another rather than themselves (hypnotic source amnesia), and so will tend to act on another person's ideas as though those ideas were their own. This aspect of hypnosis implies that a hypnotized individual is especially vulnerable to the nature of the therapeutic intervention, meaning that the trance state can enhance responsiveness, either for good or for ill.

MYTHS

There are a variety of common "mythunderstandings" about hypnosis, the most prevalent deriving from the name itself: the Greek root *hypnos* means "sleep." The hypnotized individual is not asleep but, rather, awake and alert. Hypnosis is not something done *to* a subject or patient. It is a capacity in an individual, which varies from individual to individual, is highest in late childhood, and declines gradually throughout adulthood. About one out of four adults is not hypnotizable, and one out of ten is highly hypnotizable. There are no apparent gender differences in hypnotizability—men and women are equally hypnotizable. There is nothing intrinsically dangerous about hypnosis. It is a benign procedure, tolerated well by patients. However, there is nothing intrinsically therapeutic about hypnosis, and it is not in and of itself a therapy. Many patients find it a relaxing and comfortable state and may be reassured by the fact that they can produce in a formal state of hypnosis some or all of the symptoms they have experienced spontaneously, such as conversion symptoms, hysterical seizures, or fugue episodes. It is the use to which the trance state is put, however, that is the crucial issue in determining treatment outcome. Hypnotizability is not a susceptibility, or a sign of weak mindedness. It is rather a capacity for focused concentration that is associated, if anything, with the absence of serious psychiatric and neurological disorder.[2]

MEASURING HYPNOTIZABILITY

Because hypnotizability is a stable and measurable trait, a clinical assessment of hypnotizability can become a useful starting point for the use of hypnosis in treatment.[3] This approach combines a hypnotic induction with a procedure that provides the psychiatrist with a deduction of the patient's hypnotic ability. Hypnotizability scales have existed since the early part of the century and have been widely used in research. They involve a structured hypnotic induction and an assessment of the subject's response to a variety of instructions, including alterations in involuntary movement, sensation, temporal orientation, and perception (e.g., hallucinatory experiences). One such scale, the Hypnotic Induction Profile (HIP),[3] calls for rapid induction commencing with upward gaze and lowering of the eyelids, followed by a series of instructions to the subject to elevate the left hand and keep it in the air, even if the examiner pulls the hand down. Subjects are rated on (1) their ability to experience a sense of dissociation of the left hand from the body; (2) evidence of the hand floating back up in the air after being pulled down, accompanied by (3) a sense of involuntariness while elevating the hand; (4) response to the cutoff signal ending the hypnotic experience; and (5) a physical sensation of floating during the trance experience. The entire procedure can be administered and scored in less than 10 minutes. It predicts responsiveness to a variety of treatments and facilitates differential diagnosis. About three out of four psychiatric outpatients are hypnotizable; one in ten is highly hypnotizable.[3]

Hypnotizability also varies according to psychiatric diagnosis. For any disorder, there may be patients who are more or less hypnotizable. Yet, in general, it appears that patients with dissociative disorders such as multiple personality disorder and post-traumatic stress disorder are more frequently found to be highly hypnotizable, whereas those experiencing affective disorders, generalized anxiety, and schizophrenic thought disorders are relatively less hypnotizable.[2,4] Research also indicates that, even among a seriously disturbed psychiatric population, the use of appropriate psychoactive medication does not hamper hypnotizability.

METHODS OF SELF-HYPNOSIS

There are several different approaches to hypnosis, most notably therapist-facilitated or self-hypnosis. Essentially, all hypnosis is self-hypnosis in that a patient must be willing to enter into a state of focused attention that involves abandonment of monitoring extraneous information. For this to occur, the patient must be able to trust the therapist and the surroundings.

Presented in this section are methods we have found to be most beneficial for a large variety of psychiatric problems. They are simple to learn and to apply, and can be varied according to the patients and their problems. Since hypnosis is a simple shift in the focus of attention, a simple induction is sufficient, followed by the appropriate utilization exercise. Patients who are relatively less hypnotizable might benefit from slightly longer inductions. This can be accomplished in group therapy by offering options or being general in the use of suggestions during the induction ("The utilization can begin whenever you have reached the appropriate level of relaxation/trance that is appropriate for you at this time," or "You may experience a sense of floating, or perhaps another very comfortable, pleasant sensation").

For those patients who are low in hypnotizability, the trance induction can act to help them relax, while the utilization of this state can help them to examine various issues while remaining in that state of calmness and relaxation. The hypnotic induction can be talked through at first by the therapist. After several sessions of being guided through the self-hypnosis, the patients can begin to utilize the method on their own whenever it is most useful for them. Nonetheless, it can be beneficial for the therapist to lead the patient or group during each session through different hypnotic exercises as appropriate to the particular circumstances. Different ways to utilize the hypnotic state are described later in the chapter. Although longer sessions are beneficial, it is also useful to employ a simple 5-minute exercise at the close of each session, so that patients can leave with a sense of restfulness and completion.

Simple Self-Hypnosis

Patients can be told the following:

The way to go into a state of self-hypnosis is simply to count to yourself from 1 to 3. On "1," do one thing: look up. On "2," do two things: slowly close your eyes, and take a deep breath. On "3," do three things: let the breath out, let your eyes relax but keep them closed, and let your body float. Then allow one hand to float up in the air like a balloon, and this will be the signal to me that you are ready to concentrate.

Once these instructions have been given and responded to, the first of the series of metaphors can be selected on the basis of the patient's hypnotizability (see "Utilizations," later in this section).

More Involved Self-Hypnosis

For those who find it difficult to go into trance from the simple induction above, several modifications are suggested. These suggestions are simple elaborations of each stage of the trance induction.

First Time

Hypnosis is nothing unusual. It is simply an increased state of relaxation that helps you to focus more effortlessly on things that can help you, or issues that you are interested in.

Beginning

Get as comfortable as possible with your arms resting on the arm of the chair. Take a moment to quiet yourself as you begin to rest into the chair.

Induction (Added to the Suggestion of Floating)

Imagine a feeling of floating, floating right down through the chair . . . . There will be something pleasant and welcome about this sensation of floating. And no matter what else might be going on, you can continue to concentrate on this pleasant feeling. You might feel this comfortable sensation in your body, or you might picture yourself floating effortlessly in a safe and comfortable environment . . . whatever is most comforting for you.

INDUCTION VARIATION 1

As you sit there, you can concentrate on the floating, floating, floating. Sometimes you can make it more vivid by imagining that you're floating in water. Or, if it's more helpful, imagine you're an astronaut floating above the field of gravity, or a bird soaring effortlessly in the clouds. The focus on floating leads to an inevitable sense of muscle relaxation; with the muscles more relaxed, anxiety itself is reduced. It is very difficult to instruct the muscles to relax through intellectual means, but to feel yourself floating is a direct communication with the muscle to shift into a state of buoyant repose. A pleasant consequence of this buoyant repose is that thinking and feeling can actually occur with greater ease.

This is a multimodality induction, useful for those with various cognitive styles, merging visual with kinesthetic.

INDUCTION VARIATION 2

As you allow yourself to float effortlessly, you might notice a part of you that remains tense or resistant, as if you are fighting yourself for some reason. There is really no need to fight yourself. You can help yourself even more by letting that floating feeling spread throughout your entire body and mind, into every nook and cranny, until as much of you as possible feels comfortable, safe, and secure in this pleasant and freeing experience. The more comfortable your body, the freer your thoughts and feelings, and the more creative solutions you can find to your questions.

This induction emphasizes the fact that the hypnotized individual remains in control.

Utilization for Anxiety Control and Problem Solving

The specific way one wishes to utilize this trance state depends upon the therapeutic issues. However, a general utilization can begin as follows:

As you continue to float, you can continue to concentrate effortlessly on that pleasant floating feeling. At the same time, while you imagine yourself floating, in your mind's eye visualize a huge screen. It can be a movie screen, a TV screen, or, if you wish, a piece of clear blue sky that acts like a screen. On that screen you project your thoughts, ideas, feelings, memories, fantasies, plans, while you float here. You establish this clear sense of your body floating here, while you relate to your thoughts and ideas out there. First picture a pleasant scene—somewhere you enjoy being. [*Pause 30 to 60 seconds, then add:*] Notice how you can use your store of memories and fantasies to help yourself and your body feel more comfortable. It is a place to become more aware of your own thoughts, feelings, and wishes.

SCREEN VARIATION 1

Now on that screen you can place anything you need to, and you might find that some images appear their automatically for you. It could be some difficulty that you have not previously had the time to consider. Or it could be some unfinished issues from the meeting that you want to more deeply explore. No matter what happens on the screen, maintain this pleasant floating sensation in your body. Whatever appears on the screen, it's nice to be able to remain in this comfortable feeling here in the chair, while your mind effortlessly explores different possibilities up there on the screen. And whenever you need to, you can let the screen fade and come even more back into this comfortable feeling. Then, if you like, you can go back to that screen some more, all the time keeping that comfortable feeling here in the chair.

Screen Variation 2

Insert a summary theme from the meeting for group members to work on in an individual and imaginative way. For example, if the group was working on lost abilities due to cancer, the themes on the imaginary screen might be structured in this manner:

> Now divide the screen in half, and on the left half picture something you have lost—an ability such as hiking, a role such as teaching, the completion of a project. At the same time as you face this loss, picture on the other side of the screen a new goal or role that you have, something you want to, can, and will accomplish.

Screen Variation 3

This approach is a good counseling method for helping patients to appreciate their current situation, realistic goals that would improve their quality of life, and ways to make this transition within the context of their lives. It takes approximately 5 to 8 minutes.

Induction Into Trance.   This can be simpler for highly hypnotizable patients, or more elaborate for those who are more highly vigilant and self-monitoring. Build a safe and comfortable resource state (sitting here, floating comfortably, feeling safe and secure; finding some place that is very pleasant, relaxed, untroubled).

Imagining Two Screens Off in the Distance.

> Imagine that off in the distance are two large screens, side by side.

Left Screen Is Problem State.

> Look up to the screen on the left. Imagine up on that screen a film being shown where you are in a difficult situation, a situation that you are not currently handling very well. It could be a problem with a family member, friends, work, your doctor, some pain or sadness, or whatever is a major concern to you. [*pause*] Imagine what you look like in that situation. [*pause*] How do you feel there? What sounds are there around you, or thoughts you might be having? [*pause*]

Return to Control State.

> Now you can let that image go, and return to this simple, comfortable, safe and relaxed state (back

here) where your mind is calm and untroubled. [*pause*]

This can be accessed more strongly for beginners; experienced practitioners can access/return to this state more readily.

Right Screen Is Goal State.

> Now imagine that you are watching a movie playing up on the right screen. Since this is the realm of imagination, anything is possible. And you can watch what it would be like to go through this difficult situation, but this time go through it more successfully. [*pause*] What would it be like to be able to handle this situation even better? [*pause*] What would you look like in this situation? [*pause*] How would you feel? [*pause*] How would others hear the sound of your voice; how would you hear their voices; what thoughts might you be having? [*pause*]

Return to Comfort State.
Look at Screens Again.

Look at both screens off there in the distance. See them side by side.

Access Resources.

> What would you need to get from the situation in the left screen to the situation in the right screen? What would help you make this transition?

Transition.

> Imagine very gradually going from the situation on the left to the situation on the right, with whatever resources help you. You might open a door or go through a corridor between the two screens. Or you might find some other way to flow over to the right screen. These resources that assist you to make this change could be feelings or ideas, people or places; they might be conscious or unconscious. [*pause*] Notice how you change as you move from the left screen to the right screen. [*pause*] How do you look different as you make this transition? [*pause*] What feelings change? [*pause*] How do you or others sound? [*pause*]

Suggestions for Future Use.

> This exercise can help you face and deal with problems by putting them into a new perspective and discovering new ways of coping with them. Try this exercise on your own several times a day, and any time you feel anxious or that your problems are weighing on you.

Ending the Trance Session

Variation 1

The exercise can be concluded by instructing the patient to practice producing the sense of comfort every time they wish to explore some problem, reduce their anxiety, or control the pain. For example

> It's nice to know that you can always return to this state whenever you want, just by counting backward: 3, 2, 1. You can use this exercise to help you with [*pain, stress, anxiety, etc.*] several times

throughout the day . . . . And now you can come back by simply counting from 3 to 1. On 3, get ready. On 2, with your eyelids closed, roll up your eyes. On 1, open your eyes, let your hand float back down, make a fist, open it, and that will be the end of the exercise.

VARIATION 2

Occasionally, patients are somewhat reluctant to exit from the trance state. In such cases, the following can be utilized:

It's nice to know that you can return to this comfortable place any time in the future that you like. And now, wherever you are, whatever you are doing, you can begin to follow my voice back to this room. And you can bring back all of the beneficial energy you have now to this room, as you begin to reorient to my voice. In the next couple of breaths, you can allow the inhale to come in even more fully, helping to lift up your chest, eyes, and eyelids.

In a group setting it is important to ensure that all patients have formally ended their trance experience. Watch each person to be sure his or her eyes are open, and chat casually for a few moments to ascertain that everyone is out of trance. Ask for any comments or questions about the experience.

Applications

This technique can be used individually or with a group. The therapists can lead the groups through the exercises, encouraging patients to try these exercises at home whenever they like. It is best to use simpler techniques first with patients until they begin practicing on their own. After a few months, it is very easy for most patients to practice more advanced self-hypnosis methods.

USES OF HYPNOSIS IN PSYCHOTHERAPY

Dissociative Disorders

Hypnosis has been used in intensive psychotherapy as a means of gaining access to repressed memories that have not emerged using other techniques—for example, when both the patient and the psychotherapist have worked on resistance issues and feel that some additional leverage is necessary. Such a use of hypnosis comes up particularly in regard to traumatic events that may have occurred during childhood and have been dissociated.

Hypnosis can be a helpful tool in the psychotherapy of dissociative disorders. These patients experience their fugue states, multiple personalities, and conversion symptoms as occurring suddenly and being beyond their control. The formal use of hypnosis can serve therapeutic as well as diagnostic purposes. The controlled access to the hypnotic state often spontaneously triggers the dissociative symptom (e.g., hysterical pseudoseizures). If not, it is possible

to induce the symptom, for example, by using age regression and having the patient reexperience the last time the dissociative symptom was present. In this structured manner, the patient can be taught to practice bringing on the symptom and thereby learn to control it.

The use of hypnosis in the psychotherapy of trauma was initially thought to be limited to abreaction, based on Freud's cathartic method. The idea was that some intense affect associated with the traumatic event needed to be released, and that simply repeating the event with its associated emotion in the trance state would suffice to resolve the symptoms. However, it became clear to Freud that conscious, cognitive work must be done on the material.[5] For therapy to be effective, the patient must reexperience the traumatic events with an enhanced sense of control over the experience. This may take the form of a symbolic restructuring of the traumatic experiences in hypnosis[3] along with the use of a grief work model.[6] Hypnosis can be used to provide controlled access to the dissociated or repressed memories of the traumatic experience and then to help patients restructure their memories of the events.

Post-Traumatic Stress Disorder

One of the most beneficial uses of hypnosis is found in the treatment of post-traumatic stress disorder. Since there is growing evidence that many people enter a dissociated state during physical trauma,[7,8] it makes sense that enabling them to enter a structured dissociated state in therapy would facilitate their access to memories of the traumatic experience, memories that must be worked through in order to resolve the post-traumatic symptomatology. Hypnosis can be helpful in allowing the victim to review aspects of the trauma in a controlled manner. The memories can be experienced for a time with the assurance that they can be put aside afterward. In a trance, patients can be quickly taught how to produce a state of physical relaxation despite whatever psychological stress they experience. They can then find a condensation image that symbolizes some aspect of the trauma. It is often helpful to have them do this on an imaginary screen, giving them some sense of distance from the event. It is also useful to divide the screen in half, having them picture on one side some aspect of the event (e.g., a rape victim's image of the assailant) and on the other side something they did to protect themselves (e.g., struggling with the assailant, talking with him, running away). This enables patients to restructure their view of the assault, facing it but not only in terms of the humiliation, pain, and fear with which it was initially associated. Victims can better acknowledge their helplessness when they also recognize their efforts to protect themselves.

Bereaved individuals can picture themselves at the graveside on one side of the screen and in an earlier moment of joy with the deceased on the other side. They can then be taught to use this exercise as a kind of self-hypnosis in which they grieve and work through the loss. It is crucial that this be conducted in such a way that patients feel in control of the process. The most distressing thing about a traumatic event is a sense of absolute helplessness. This takes the form in a post-traumatic stress disorder of a loss of control over the state of mind, with spontaneous dissociative states, startle reactions, or intrusive recollections of the event. Furthermore, such patients may tend to identify the therapist with the assailant and feel that the therapy amounts to a reinflicting of the trauma. It is crucial that the process of the therapy, especially using a technique such as hypnosis, be structured so that it enhances patients' sense of control. This approach can allow them to integrate the image of themselves as victims with the ongoing, more global image of themselves as persons, making the repressed material conscious and therefore less powerful, and enabling them to establish a new, more congruent self-image, absorbing the loss into the ongoing flow of their lives.

Treatment of Victims of Sexual Abuse

The therapeutic challenge in treating victims of sexual abuse is one of forging a new sense of unity after an experience that produces profound fragmentation. Victims of rape and incest have undergone one or more sudden and radical discontinuities in their personal experience. The very extremity of the assault and the violation of physical boundaries leaves victims with polarized and incompatible views of the self. One is the view of the self prior to the assault: a relatively intact person who controls his or her physical and personal boundaries and feels able to provide protection and continuity of experience. The other view is of the self that experienced the assault: helpless, unable to control physical experience, soiled by becoming the victim of someone else's rage.

Victims of sexual abuse can be taught either to relive the memories by hypnotic age regression or to picture them on an imaginary screen. It is important to teach such subjects to dissociate their mental experience of going through the traumatic event from the physical one, both to remind them that it is not again physically recurring and to prevent the snowball effect of mental and physical tension that can lead to many of the symptoms of anxiety or panic states. Thus, they can be taught first to "float" physically, affiliating with a metaphor that connotes physical relaxation, such as being in a pool or bath, even while they picture traumatic events on an imaginary screen.

It is then helpful to have victims divide the screen in half, putting some condensation of the traumatic experience on one side and picturing on the other side something they did to protect themselves. Some rape victims talk to their assailant to try to humanize themselves and decrease the likelihood that they

will be murdered. Others fight back physically, warning the assailant that they will not surrender without an all-out battle. Many incest victims go so far as to consciously provoke attack as a way of protecting younger siblings from the same fate. In any event, their memory of the assault can be made more bearable when they can see the part of themselves that attempted to provide protection, maintain dignity, or protect others during the attack. Thus, the image on the right side of the screen is meant to balance that on the left, to help them show that while they were indeed being victimized, they were also attempting to master the situation, that they displayed courage or compassion, and that the humiliation of the attack is only one component of the experience.

Psychosomatic Disorders

Since highly hypnotizable individuals show an unusual capacity for psychological control over somatic function, it makes sense that hypnotic phenomena may be involved in both the etiology of some psychosomatic symptoms and their control. For example, Andreychuk and Skriver[9] found that hypnotizability not only was a predictor of treatment response for migraine headaches, but also was a correlate of pretreatment symptom severity: that is, more highly hypnotizable individuals complained of more severe migraine symptoms prior to treatment but responded better to intervention. Highly hypnotizable individuals have been shown to have the capacity to control peripheral skin temperature and blood flow and to be able to suppress cortical evoked response to a perceptual stimulus while hallucinating an obstruction to the stimulus.[10] It makes sense that certain classical conversion disorders such as hysterical paralyses may well represent dissociative phenomena, since profound alterations in sensation and experience of control over motor function are standard hypnotic phenomena. Nonetheless, these have been documented rather rarely.

In general, hypnosis is useful in two senses, one diagnostic, the other therapeutic. Patients who are highly hypnotizable are more likely to have conversion symptoms, such as hysterical pseudoseizures, than those who are not, especially if hypnotic induction tends to bring on, worsen, or ameliorate the symptom. Even among highly hypnotizable patients, it is rare for a conversion symptom to simply disappear; indeed, pushing patients to relinquish it too quickly may humiliate them, since it conveys the message that the problem was "all in their head." Hypnosis can be quite appropriately used as part of a rehabilitation strategy, particularly insofar as it can help patients master the reactive anxiety that is associated with real physical dysfunction as well as conversion symptoms. A patient can be taught to use a state of self-hypnosis to develop the sense of floating relaxation while picturing problems that bother him or her on an imaginary screen. The patient can then work on improving function, in a dysfunctional hand, for example, by developing tremors that gradually build up strength and circulation.

Hypnosis has been quite effective in helping asthmatics. They can learn to use it as a first resort rather than medication when they begin to feel an attack coming on, thereby interrupting the vicious cycle of anxiety and bronchoconstriction. Hypnotizability is correlated with treatment response.[11] Relaxation instructions have been similarly helpful for some patients with stress-related bowel disease such as ulcerative colitis and regional enteritis. Patients have found it helpful to imagine in trance something soothing in their gut, which gives them a sense of control over a syndrome that renders them feeling especially helpless, thereby diminishing the cycle of reactive anxiety. Similarly, warts have been treated with hypnosis, and one carefully controlled study demonstrated that simple hypnotic instructions to the effect that the warts would tingle and disappear resulted in a rate of improvement that was significantly better than the spontaneous rate of remission of warts.[12] Thus, hypnosis can be quite helpful in controlling the psychosomatic interaction, which can lead to either deterioration or improvement of somatically related symptoms.

CONCLUSION

Hypnosis as an adjunct to psychotherapy can be of great value. This is especially true for those patients who are hypnotizable and for psychiatric disorders such as dissociation, trauma, phobias, addictions, and somatic-related disorders. It has been used to further enhance treatment in a number of different ways. Hypnosis can be utilized at the beginning of the therapeutic session with a brief hypnotic exercise in order to elicit material that can be the focus of the remainder of the session. It can be used to enhance the recall of old information or the consideration of new ways to restructure information by having the patient in a trance during a major portion of the treatment. Also, hypnosis can be helpful in finishing the treatment as a way of relaxing the patient, integrating issues raised in the session, and providing self-help methods that will increase patient compliance with therapist recommendations.

Hypnosis can be used in individual, couple, or group therapy.[13] Given the low cost of utilizing hypnosis, the minimal danger of complications, and the high efficacy across so many patients and psychiatric problems, hypnosis should definitely be considered a standard part of every therapist's repertoire.

REFERENCES

1. Tellegen A, Atkinson G: Openness to absorbing and self-altering experiences ("absorption"), a trait related to hypnotic susceptibility. J Abnorm Psychol 83:268–277, 1974.
2. Spiegel D, Detrick D, Frischholz E: Hypnotizability and psychopathology. Am J Psychiatry 139:431–437, 1982.
3. Spiegel H, Spiegel D: Trance and Treatment: Clinical Uses of Hypnosis. Washington DC: American Psychiatric Press, 1987.
4. Spiegel D: Uses and abuses of hypnosis. Integr Psychiatry 6:211–222, 1989.
5. Freud S: Remembering, repeating, and working-through (further recommendations of the technique of psycho-analysis). In Strahey J, Freud A, eds, transl. The Standard Edition of the Complete Psychological Works of Sigmund Freud, vol XII. London, Hogarth Press, 1958:145–156.
6. Spiegel D: Vietnam grief work using hypnosis. Am J Clin Hypn 24:33–40, 1981.
7. Spiegel D: Hypnosis in the treatment of victims of sexual abuse. Psychiatr Clin North Am 12:295–305, 1989.
8. Spiegel D, Cardena E: New uses of hypnosis in the treatment of posttraumatic stress disorder. J Clin Psychiatry 51:39–43, 1990.
9. Andreychuk T, Skriver C: Hypnosis and biofeedback in the treatment of migraine headache. Int J Clin Exp Hypn 23:172–183, 1975.
10. Spiegel D, Cutcomb S, Ren C, et al: Hypnotic hallucination alters evoked potentials. J Abnorm Psychol 94:249–255, 1985.
11. Collison DR: Which asthmatic patients should be treated by hypnotherapy? Med J Aust 1:676–681, 1975.
12. Surman OS: Hypnosis in the treatment of warts. Arch Gen Psychiatry 23:439–441, 1973.
13. Spiegel D, Spira J: Supportive-expressive group therapy: A treatment manual of psychosocial intervention for women with recurrent breast cancer. Unpublished manuscript, Department of Psychiatry and Behavioral Sciences, Stanford University, Stanford, CA, 1991.

84

ELECTROCONVULSIVE THERAPY

DAVID H. AVERY, M.D.

Electroconvulsive therapy (ECT) continues to be one of the most effective treatments in psychiatry since its introduction over 50 years ago. Early clinicians recognized that psychotic patients who had spontaneous seizures often experienced a remission of symptoms. During the 1930s several attempts to induce seizures in psychiatric patients were made. Von Meduna in 1935 used camphor and subsequently metrazol to induce seizures. Cerletti and Bini in 1938 introduced ECT, which, because of its simplicity and ease of application, became the most common method of inducing seizure activity. Since then, research has clarified a great deal about the efficacy, side effects, optimal mode of administration, and mechanism of action of ECT.

EFFICACY OF ECT

Depression is by far the most common indication for ECT. It should be emphasized that depression is not simply sadness, but is a syndrome in which a persistent low mood is associated with altered sleep, altered appetite, weight change, agitation or retardation, poor concentration, decreased sex drive, low self-esteem, hopelessness, and suicidal ideation. Prior to the advent of ECT, depressive illness was associated with high death rates—10 to 15 per cent 1-year mortality rates in some studies. With the introduction of ECT, death rates decreased, both from suicide and nonsuicidal causes. Subsequent controlled studies of patients from the same era have confirmed the life-saving effect of ECT in depression. Several studies using sham ECT controls have demonstrated the efficacy of ECT.

With the introduction of antidepressant medication in the 1960s, numerous studies compared medication, both tricyclic antidepressants and monoamine oxidase inhibitors, with ECT. Most studies have shown ECT to be superior to antidepressant medication, some have shown the two treatments equal, but none have shown medication to be superior to ECT. Typically, these studies show 80 to 90 per cent response rates of hospitalized depressed patients to ECT compared to 60 to 80 per cent response rates with tricyclic antidepressants (even when given in dosages of 200 to 250 mg/day). Comparisons with monoamine oxidase inhibitors and tryptophan

also support the superiority of ECT. The antidepressant effect of ECT may be faster than medication: the duration of hospitalization is shorter for patients treated with ECT. The response to ECT may also be more complete than with medication.

Depressive illness is associated with high suicide rates, with most suicides occurring within 8 months of hospitalization, and a person with a partially treated depression may be at increased risk. Suicide attempts in depressed patients are seen less frequently following treatment with ECT than with antidepressant medication. Treatment with ECT is associated with decreased suicide rates compared with depressed patients treated with neither ECT nor antidepressant medication. Because of the more complete, faster response seen with ECT compared with medication, ECT may be the treatment of choice in the suicidal depressed patient.

Psychotic depression often responds poorly to antidepressant medication alone, but has an 80 to 90 per cent response rate to ECT. Some recent data suggest that adding an antipsychotic to an antidepressant may improve the response to the ECT response rate, but replication is needed. Several investigators have found that the presence of psychosis in depressed patients is neither a good nor a poor prognostic sign for ECT response.

Many prognostic factors for ECT response have been studied. In general, endogenous depression has been found to have a better ECT response compared to neurotic or reactive depression. Bipolar and unipolar patients appear to respond equally well. Primary depressions respond better than depressions that are secondary to other psychiatric or medical problems. The presence of an Axis II personality disorder diagnosis in addition to the major depression diagnosis worsens the prognosis. Individual signs and symptoms of depression in general are poor predictors of response. Psychomotor agitation and a pyknic habitus are good prognostic factors. Guilt and a previous episode of depression may be good prognostic factors. Possible poor prognostic factors include a duration greater than 1 year, a fluctuating course in the episode, emotional lability, paranoia, and anxiety.

Electroconvulsive therapy continues to be an important treatment for depression in the elderly. Recently elderly patients referred for ECT were noted to have a leukoencephalopathy when studied with magnetic resonance imaging: subcortical hyperintensity was more common compared to control group of normal elderly subjects. These patients responded well to ECT, and ECT caused no changes in the magnetic resonance image.

The natural history of depression is often associated with frequent relapses following recovery from an episode. Electroconvulsive therapy is clearly effective in treating the depressive episode, but does not decrease (or increase) the likelihood of a clinical relapse. Therefore, antidepressants, which are effective maintenance medications, are usually prescribed for 6 to 9 months after an ECT response. Some recent data indicate that relapse is much more likely following ECT in patients who had failed adequate antidepressant trials prior to the ECT than in patients who had not been determined to be medication resistant. For some patients with recurrent depression, maintenance ECT—single ECT sessions given every few weeks on an outpatient basis—may be helpful in preventing relapse.

Electroconvulsive therapy is also an effective treatment for mania. One recent naturalistic study found a 78 per cent response rate to ECT, significantly better than the 62 per cent response rate in those receiving lithium. Bilateral electrode placement is superior to unilateral in treating mania. Even those patients who had had a poor response to lithium had a high response rate to ECT. Electroconvulsive therapy has stopped the rapid cycling in some bipolar patients, but ECT should not be considered the first line of treatment for this problem.

The possible role of ECT in the treatment of schizophrenia is obscured by diagnostic problems. "Schizophreniform" psychoses, although associated with hallucinations and delusions, will frequently respond well to ECT. Good prognostic signs for ECT response in atypical psychoses include the presence of symptoms of endogenous depression or mania, a relatively acute onset, a good premorbid personality, and a family history of affective disorder. Patients with catatonia often respond well. If the duration of illness is less than 1 year, the prognosis is favorable. Thus, patients with "acute schizophrenia" often respond well, whereas schizophrenics with chronic symptoms usually do not. In a well-controlled study of schizophrenics who were neither acutely ill nor extremely chronic, ECT was found to be equal to phenothiazines and superior to psychotherapy. The possible effectiveness of ECT in some schizophrenics takes on special significance in view of the concern over phenothiazine-induced tardive dyskinesia.

Electroconvulsive therapy has been used with some success in other disorders. Patients with neuroleptic malignant syndrome frequently respond to ECT. However, some of these patients may have been in the process of developing lethal catatonia and happened to have received neuroleptics. Electroconvulsive therapy is effective in some patients with Parkinson's disease, but the effect may be only temporary. Patients with chronic pain and patients with tardive dyskinesia have responded to ECT. Depressed patients with coexisting medical problems such as brain tumors, positive human immunodeficiency virus status, Down's syndrome, and mental retardation have responded well to ECT. While not routine, ECT has been effective in some depressed adolescents. There is no evidence that ECT is effective in treating personality disorders or autism.

ADMINISTRATION OF ECT

Before a patient is given ECT, a careful history, physical and neurological exam should be completed. Liver function tests, measures of creatinine, and electrolytes, a complete blood count, urinalysis, electrocardiogram, and radiographs of the chest and the thoracic and lumbar spine should be obtained. Any physical problems must be considered and evaluated appropriately. There are several relative contraindications for ECT: intracranial neoplasm, a recent cerebral vascular accident, subdural hematoma, a recent myocardial infarction, congestive heart failure, angina pectoris, and acute or chronic respiratory disease. As with any therapy, the risks of withholding treatment must be weighed against the risks of the treatment itself. For example, in a depressed patient who has postural hypotension, the possible hypotensive effects of tricyclic antidepressants might be avoided by giving ECT and carefully monitoring the electrocardiogram during treatment. Electroconvulsive therapy has been used successfully during pregnancy and can be an alternative to the possible teratogenic effects of antidepressant medication.

The patient should be informed of the risks and benefits of the treatment and a consent form should be signed. The patient should take no water or food by mouth for at least 8 hours prior to the treatment. The patient's temperature is taken in the morning before each treatment to rule out a febrile process. Some centers give atropine 1 mg IM 30 minutes prior to treatment to prevent the bradycardia that sometimes accompanies ECT. However, atropine has not been shown to be critical to successful ECT. The patient voids completely, and is placed on the treatment table in a supine position. Then the patient is given an anesthetic. In the past, thiopental or methohexital IV has been used, but in recent years etomidate has been used by some because it does not have significant anticonvulsant effects like the barbiturates.

Succinylcholine is injected to induce muscle relaxation and the patient is ventilated with oxygen. A rubber mouthpiece is inserted to prevent possible damage to the teeth. The electrodes are applied to the head. When relaxation is complete, the current is delivered. Depending on the degree of muscle relaxation induced, the tonic-clonic activity of the seizure may be seen, with the tonic phase lasting approximately 10 to 20 seconds and the clonic phase 30 to 60 seconds. An adequate seizure should have a duration of at least 25 seconds. Rarely, a seizure may continue for 120 seconds or more. Under these circumstances, the seizure may be stopped by administering IV diazepam. The patient is ventilated with oxygen and usually begins breathing spontaneously within a few minutes after the seizure ends. The patient is usually awake after 10 to 15 minutes. Most patients experience a transient postictal confusion and memory disturbance.

The seizure duration is monitored by using the blood pressure cuff technique. Inflating a blood pressure cuff on one arm to above systolic pressure prevents the muscle relaxant from reaching the muscles of that arm and allows the seizure activity to be observed. However, this technique underestimates the actual electroencephalographic (EEG) seizure duration. Many ECT machines now have the capability of EEG monitoring. Some preliminary data suggest that the effectiveness of the treatment may correlate with the total seizure duration up to 750 seconds of seizure activity.

For most patients, an adequate course of ECT consists of 6 to 12 treatments; usually three treatments are given per week. The number of treatments is determined by the clinical improvement of the patient. Many clinicians believe that one or two additional treatments are necessary after clinical remission has occurred to prevent early relapse. Some have advocated the use of multiple monitored ECT, giving several seizures in a single session, and have claimed that fewer sessions are necessary. However, controlled studies have not yet supported this claim.

The administration of lithium to patients undergoing ECT is associated with a clear increase in cognitive dysfunction and is contraindicated. The administration of antidepressant medication during ECT treatment offers no increased efficacy and may be associated with increased memory disturbance. Concomitant benzodiazepine use may interfere with the induction of the seizure or shorten the seizure. One study has even demonstrated reduced ECT efficacy associated with concomitant benzodiazepine use. Sometimes it is difficult to induce seizures, or the seizures are short even in patients not taking benzodiazepines or barbiturates. Recently, intravenous administration of caffeine has been successfully used in such patients.

Very rarely, the patient may have prolonged apnea because of decreased metabolism of the succinylcholine. Succinylcholine is metabolized by plasma pseudocholinesterase. Decreased pseudocholinesterase activity may be associated with decreased liver function and severe anemia, as well as certain medications, including amitriptyline and some antibiotics.

Succinylcholine, a depolarizing muscle relaxant, has been shown to release large amounts of potassium from skeletal muscle in patients with burns, muscle trauma, central nervous system trauma, peripheral nerve injury, spinal cord injury, and muscle changes due to prolonged inactivity. Since a rapid rise in potassium may cause ventricular arrhythmia and cardiac arrest, patients with these conditions may require the use of a nondepolarizing muscle relaxant such as atracurium.

A low dose of succinylcholine (about 0.7 mg/kg) has been associated with post-ECT agitation; no agitation was noted in these patients after increasing the succinylcholine dose to a mean of about 1.0 mg/kg. It has been hypothesized that a low dose of succinylcholine might allow enough muscle activity to produce high lactate levels and thus create a situation analogous to a lactate infusion–induced panic attack.

The use of brief-pulse ECT can reduce the postictal memory disturbance relative to the traditional sinusoidal wave form.

Some investigators have advocated titrating the dose of electricity to assess the seizure threshold. For example, one might begin with pulse frequency of 20 Hz, a pulse width of 1.5 msec, and a duration of 1 second. If there is no seizure elicited, the next stimulus might be given after a 40-second waiting period with a higher dose (e.g., 40 Hz, 1.5-msec pulse width, and 1 second duration). Subsequent doses might be 70 Hz, 1.5 msec, and 1.0 second, and 70 Hz, 1.5 msec, and 2.0 seconds. Using the lowest threshold that elicits a seizure might decrease the memory disturbance. The seizure thresholds may vary as much as 12-fold among patients with higher thresholds, which are seen among men and older patients and with bilateral placement. As patients recover with ECT, the seizure threshold increases.

Unilateral (both electrodes over the same hemisphere) and bifrontal ECT clearly cause less of the transient memory disturbance than the traditional bilateral (bitemporal) treatments. When unilateral treatments are used, right unilateral placement is usually used since its effects on verbal memory are less than with left unilateral treatment. However, controversy continues over whether unilateral treatments are as efficacious as bilateral treatments. Some studies show the two treatments to be equal; others show bilateral treatments to be superior. Unilateral ECT failures will usually respond to bilateral treatments. Unilateral treatments often yield shorter seizures. Even when seizure duration is controlled, bilateral treatments appear to have a greater physiological effect, as measured by prolactin secretion and heart rate increase, compared to unilateral treatments. Some clinicians begin with bilateral treatments and, if the patient experiences significant memory disturbance, switch to right unilateral treatments.

ADVERSE EFFECTS OF ECT

The risk of death during ECT is estimated at about 1:10,000 patients treated. The most common cause of death is cardiovascular problems. Since the modification of the ECT technique with muscle relaxants, anesthesia, and hyperoxygenation, there have been no reports of structural neurological damage in patients given ECT. Magnetic resonance imaging and cerebral computed tomography performed before and after ECT show no changes. Furthermore, studies of animals given ECT have revealed no neuropathological changes, even with electron microscopic tissue examination.

Memory disturbance has long been associated with ECT use. Both retrograde memory (memory of past events) and anterograde memory (capacity to remember newly acquired material) are impaired during the days following ECT. Within 6 to 9 months after a course of ECT, the capacity to learn new material returns to normal. In addition, the ability to remember past events returns except for the days prior to and during the course of treatment.

As with other antidepressant treatments, ECT can precipitate mania. Those who experience ECT-induced mania have an earlier age of onset and a longer duration of illness compared to those who do not experience this. Mania should be distinguished from organic euphoric states, which are more brief and usually associated with more severe cognitive impairment and silly, inappropriate laughter.

MECHANISM OF ACTION OF ECT

Theories of ECT's mechanism of action have changed as the theories of the etiology of depression have changed. Some have believed that depression represents "introjected anger" and that ECT worked by satisfying the persons's needs for self-punishment. However, the effectiveness of the modified technique, during which the patient is unconscious, speaks against this theory. It has also been hypothesized that ECT works by interfering with the memory of stressful events. However, there is no association between clinical effectiveness and memory disturbance.

The *sine qua non* for an effective treatment appears to be seizure activity. Chemically-induced seizures are efficacious. When electrically-induced seizures are prevented with lidocaine, the electrical stimuli are not effective in relieving the depression.

Some evidence suggests that deficiencies of neurotransmitters are associated with the depressed state; some animal studies show increased release of serotonin and norepinephrine during seizures. Like many antidepressant medications, repeated seizures may decrease postsynaptic β-adrenergic sensitivity.

Affective disorders may be associated with desynchronization of circadian rhythms; ECT has been hypothesized as a *Zeitgeber* that resynchronizes these rhythms. Electroconvulsive therapy may work in a way analogous to cardiac defibrillation, resetting desynchronous clocks back to time zero. One catatonic patient who responded to ECT was noted to have a high temperature (38.3°C) and no 24-hour rhythm prior to ECT. With the ECT treatments, a circadian rhythm developed and the 24-hour temperature amplitude and mean gradually returned to normal. During the second week of treatment, the timing of the minimum of the temperature rhythm corresponded with the time of ECT administration even on non-ECT days.

Electroconvulsive therapy has also been hypothesized to work as an anticonvulsant in a manner analogous to carbamazepine. Electroconvulsive therapy has been proposed to work by restoration of the equilibrium between the cerebral hemispheres. The "nonphysiological" depolarizations may be important for the restoration of aberrant intravesicular transmitter ratios.

Response to ECT is associated with normalization of a variety of physiological functions that have been found to be abnormal in depression: dexamethasone nonsuppression, short rapid eye movement sleep latency, reduced slow wave sleep, and high nocturnal temperature.

Electrophysiological evidence indicates that centrocephalic structures are implicated in the mechanism of the ECT process. As with antidepressant medication, it is too early to formulate a definite model for the mechanism of action of ECT. However, the lack of a theoretical construct does not diminish the empirical evidence for its efficacy and relative safety.

LEGISLATION OF ECT

Controversy concerning ECT has led to legislative changes restricting its use, particularly in the United States. After passage of such legislation in California, the rate of ECT use was approximately 6:100,000 persons per year; in Great Britain, Denmark, and Sweden, the rate is approximately seven to 15 times greater. The use and availability of ECT is particularly low in public hospitals in the United States. In California, minorities are probably untreated, with whites accounting for 92 per cent of the ECT use.

In spite of the controversy, ECT remains the most effective treatment for severe endogenous depressions, especially psychotic depressions.

ACKNOWLEDGMENT

This work was supported in part by Research Scientist Development Award 5 KO MH00493-04.

SUGGESTED READINGS

Abrams R: Electroconvulsive Therapy. New York: Oxford University Press, 1988.
American Psychiatric Association Task Force Report on Electroconvulsive Therapy. Report no. 14. Washington, DC: American Psychiatric Association Press, 1978.

American Psychiatric Association Task Force Report on Electroconvulsive Therapy. "The Practice of Electroconvulsive Therapy: Recommendations for Treatment, Training, and Privileging." Washington, DC: American Psychiatric Association Press, 1990.

Avery DH, Mills M: Electroconvulsive therapy and antidepressants in the treatment of depression. *In* Ayd F, Taylor IJ, eds. Mood Disorders: The World's Major Public Health Problem. Baltimore: Ayd Medical Communications, 1978:138–153.

Avery DH, Winokur G: Mortality in depressed patients treated with electroconvulsive therapy and antidepressants. Arch Gen Psychiatry 33:1029–1037, 1976.

Coffey CE, Figiel GS, Weiner RD, Saunders WB: Caffeine augmentation of ECT. Am J Psychiatry 147(5):579–585, 1990.

Fink M: Convulsive Therapy: Theory and Practice. New York: Raven Press, 1979.

King BH, Liston EH: Proposals for the mechanism of action of convulsive therapy: A synthesis. Biol Psychiatry 27:76–94, 1990.

Sackeim HA, Decina P, Portnoy S, Neeley P, Malitz S: Studies of dosage, seizure threshold, and seizure duration in ECT. Biol Psychiatry 22:249–268, 1987.

Squire LR: ECT and memory loss. Am J Psychiatry 134(9):997–1001, 1977.

Squire LR, Zouzounis JA: ECT and memory: Brief pulse versus sine wave. Am J Psychiatry 143(5):596–601, 1986.

Section O

FUTURE PSYCHOPHARMACOLOGY

85

THERAPEUTIC DRUG MONITORING

GARY A. FAST, M.D. and SHELDON H. PRESKORN, M.D.

Therapeutic drug monitoring (TDM) is an important tool when using certain psychotropic drugs. Therapeutic drug monitoring enhances the clinician's ability to rationally adjust the dose of selected medications (e.g., tricyclic antidepressants, lithium, carbamazepine) to increase therapeutic efficacy and reduce adverse side effects. Patients have substantial interindividual differences in the metabolism and elimination rates (up to 40-fold) of such drugs (e.g., tricyclic antidepressants) and, therefore, may obtain vastly different plasma concentrations while receiving standard doses of the same medication. Therapeutic drug monitoring allows the clinician to identify subtherapeutic plasma concentrations as well as potentially toxic plasma concentrations. Certain general features of various psychotropic drugs make TDM advantageous (Table 85–1), but not all psychotropic drugs (e.g., benzodiazepines) share these features.

THERAPEUTIC DRUG MONITORING GOALS

Assess Compliance

Approximately 40 per cent of patients receiving psychotropic medications are noncompliant with their regimen.[1] Noncompliance can lead to subtherapeutic plasma concentrations and therefore prolong the duration of the illness, or lead to supratherapeutic plasma concentrations and serious toxicity. Checking compliance is also an important issue with

regard to maintenance treatment, especially with psychiatric patients, whose concentration, motivation, and thought processes may be impaired.

Enhance Therapeutic Response

Well-defined plasma concentration–efficacy relationships exist for some psychiatric medications (e.g., nortriptyline, desipramine, amitriptyline, imipramine, and lithium carbonate). Knowing the plasma level can allow the clinician to adjust the drug dose more rationally to enhance therapeutic effect. Such relationships for other medications, such as the psychiatric use of anticonvulsants (e.g., carbamazepine and valproic acid), have not been as precisely defined.

Avoid Toxicity

Because of a narrow therapeutic index and substantial interindividual pharmacokinetic variability, toxicity can result from the administration of standard doses of drugs such as lithium carbonate and the tricyclic antidepressants. Factors that contribute to wide interindividual variability in the elimination rates may predispose to toxicity.

Minimize Cost

Noncompliance and subtherapeutic plasma concentrations of some psychotropic drugs can delay

529

TABLE 85–1. PSYCHOTROPIC MEDICATIONS: SUMMARY OF FEATURES THAT MAKE MONITORING PLASMA DRUG LEVELS USEFUL

Feature	Mood Stabilizers			Antidepressants				Antipsychotics		
	Lithium Carbonate	Carbamazepine	Valproate	Tricyclic Antidepressants[a]	Bupropion	Fluoxetine	Trazodone	Haloperidol	Thiothixene	Chlorpromazine[b]
Multitude of actions	+	+	−	+	−	−	−	−	−	+
Small therapeutic index	+	−	−	+	+	−	±	+	−	+
Large interindividual variability in metabolism	±	+	−	+	+	+	±	+	+	+
Difficult early detection of toxicity	±	±	−	+	+	−	−	+	+	+
Long delay in onset of action	+	+	+	+	+	+	±	+	+	+
Well-defined concentration-response relationships										
Beneficial effects	+	−	−	+	?	−	−	±	±	?
Nuisance effects	±	±	−	±	?	−	−	?	?	?
Toxic effects	+	+	±	+		−	−	±	±	?

[a] General statements apply to all TCAs, but empirical data bases are best for nortriptyline, desipramine, amitriptyline, and imipramine.
[b] Same general statements would hold for thioridazine and mesoridazine.

the remission of a psychiatric illness, leading to additional outpatient office visits or prolonged hospital stay. Identifying supratherapeutic plasma concentrations can help to avoid toxicity and hence unnecessary or prolonged hospitalization. Such hospitalizations will typically require a myriad of laboratory tests and procedures to work up and then treat toxicity.

Avoid Medicolegal Problems

Therapeutic drug monitoring is important in this era of malpractice suits. The lack of TDM in the case of sudden death and substantially elevated postmortem plasma concentrations may be seen as negligence. Therapeutic drug monitoring can also provide objective evidence to substantiate the need for and safety of unusually high doses of medications in certain patients.

THERAPEUTIC DRUG MONITORING OF TRICYCLIC ANTIDEPRESSANTS

The antidepressants that have been most extensively studied with regard to TDM are the tricyclic antidepressants (TCAs). These medications have been the first-line pharmacotherapy in the treatment of depression for the last 30 years. While a comprehensive review of the TCA plasma concentration–antidepressant response relationship studies is beyond the scope of this chapter, Perry et al.,[2] in a meta-analysis, summarized the TCA efficacy literature using logistic regression analysis. Their results follow.

Nortriptyline

Studies on nortriptyline are generally consistent in demonstrating a curvilinear concentration–antidepressant response relationship, with an optimum range of 50 to 150 ng/ml. Within this range, 70 per cent of patients with primary major depressive disorder experience complete remission (e.g., a final Hamilton Depression Rating Scale score equal to or less than 6) versus 29 per cent of patients who develop TCA plasma concentrations outside this range. Of note, the response rate is generally higher in the lower end of this range than at the upper limit. This observation may be relevant to the often-asked question: "If my patient has gotten somewhat better but is in the middle of nortriptyline's range, should I push the dose up?" We would recommend augmenting the drug with lithium carbonate or thyroid supplement rather than adjusting the dose. If the clinician wants to adjust the dose, a modest reduction would seem most prudent.

Desipramine

Desipramine studies demonstrate a curvilinear concentration–antidepressant response relationship similar to the one observed with nortriptyline. The "therapeutic window" for desipramine according to the meta-analysis was 100 to 160 ng/ml. In this range, there is a remission rate of 59 per cent versus 20 per cent outside the range.

Amitriptyline

The results for this tertiary amine tricyclic are less robust in terms of its concentration–antidepressant response relationship. However, its optimal range is based on both efficacy data and data demonstrating that the central nervous system (CNS) cardiovascular system (CVS) toxicity and dropout rates for adverse effects are a function of TCA plasma levels. The optimum plasma level range for this medication is 75 to 175 ng/ml. Within this range, the remission rate is 48 per cent versus 29 per cent outside the range.

Imipramine

Imipramine is the only TCA reviewed that does not show a curvilinear relationship between concentration and antidepressant response in adult patients. A linear relationship appears to best fit the data with this drug in adults. However, a curvilinear relationship has been described for imipramine when used to treat depressed children.

Basd on the meta-analysis, the threshold for optimum antidepressant response to imipramine was close to the threshold for CNS and CVS toxicity. Thus, the upper limit to the therapeutic range is a function of toxicity rather than reduced efficacy, as it is with the other TCAs. At present, the threshold proposed from the meta-analysis is 265 ng/ml, with a remission rate of 42 per cent above this threshold versus 15 per cent below it.

Comments

A summary of the concentration-efficacy data for these four TCAs supports the use of TDM at least once as a routine aspect of TCA therapy for major depressive disorder. The data are consistent across all four TCAs in indicating that optimum TCA plasma levels are associated with a greater likelihood of achieving a full remission of the depressive episode after 4 weeks of TCA treatment. Translated into clinical terms, there is a 1.7- to 3.0-fold increase in clinical response to TCAs if the depressed patient obtains an optimal TCA plasma level.[2] Studies have also focused on issues of TDM and enhanced safety (e.g., using TDM to avoid CNS toxicity, CVS toxicity, and catastrophic outcomes). Preskorn and Jerkovich,[3] in a meta-analysis, demonstrated that

TCA-induced CNS toxicity is concentration dependent. Based on the meta-analysis, the risk of CNS toxicity is 13 times higher when the TCA plasma levels exceed 300 ng/ml and 37 times higher when the TCA plasma levels exceeds 450 ng/ml. Interestingly, peripheral anticholinergic side effects (e.g., blurry vision, dry mouth, and constipation) were reported as being more than routinely expected in only 8 per cent of patients with TCA-induced CNS toxicity. In otherwise neurologically uncompromised patients, plasma concentrations of less than 250 ng/ml rarely present with manifestations of CNS toxicity. However, as the threshold concentration of 250 ng/ml is exceeded, patients develop asymptomatic nonspecific electroencephalographic (EEG) abnormalities.[4] As the TCA plasma concentration increases beyond 450 ng/ml, the risk of seizures in addition to delirium increases.[5]

The role of TDM with TCAs is also important to avoid iatrogenic cardiotoxicity. The cardiac effects of TCAs are concentration dependent, with the possible exception of orthostatic hypotension and tachycardia. While all TCA-induced cardiac conduction disturbances are more likely to occur with someone who is predisposed to cardiac disease, data demonstrate these effects will occur routinely in healthy individuals if the appropriate threshold concentration is exceeded. In healthy middle-aged subjects with TCA plasma concentrations of less than 200 ng/ml, intracardiac conduction defects are unusual. However, at a TCA plasma threshold of 200 ng/ml, slowing of the His bundle–ventricular system was found to routinely occur in otherwise healthy individuals.[6] At TCA plasma concentrations above 350 ng/ml, first-degree atrioventricular block occurred in 70 per cent of physically healthy patients treated with desipramine or imipramine.[7] Although there have been no published studies on the incidence of cardiac arrhythmia or sudden death in physically healthy subjects during routine TCA therapy, based on overdose studies, cardiac arrhythmias occur at a mean ($\pm$SD) plasma concentration of 1275 ± 290 ng/ml and cardiac arrests occur at a mean ($\pm$SD) plasma concentration of 1700 ± 150 ng/ml.[8]

Technique

Generally, the physician starts the patient on a standard TCA dose—for example, 50 to 75 mg/day of nortriptyline in a physically healthy adult. After 1 week, the vast majority of patients will be at steady state. A blood sample is then drawn 10 to 12 hours after the last dose. The reason for this interval is to ensure that absorption and distribution of the drug are complete. Virtually all the data on optimal concentration ranges are based on 10 to 12-hour postdose samples. If the sample cannot be drawn at 10 to 12 hours after the last dose, drawing it later is better than drawing it earlier. These drugs have half-lives on the order of 24 hours or more.

THERAPEUTIC DRUG MONITORING OF OTHER ANTIDEPRESSANTS

Monoamine Oxidase Inhibitors (e.g., Phenelzine)

Antidepressant efficacy of phenelzine has been correlated with an 80 to 85 per cent inhibition of monoamine oxidase (MAO) enzyme inhibition. Studies indicate that 60 mg of phenelzine daily is needed to inhibit MAO by at least 80 per cent.[9] Monitoring of platelet MAO inhibition levels at baseline and during treatment can permit more optimal phenelzine dosing. This approach is more cumbersome than the more conventional method of TDM, which involves making a single measurement of the plasma drug concentration. That fact, coupled with the infrequent use of monoamine oxidase inhibitors (MAOIs), has kept this approach from gaining more widespread acceptance.

Bupropion

Bupropion, an aminoketone structurally distinct from other antidepressants, shows considerable interindividual variability in plasma levels among even physically healthy patients. Studies indicate there is a relationship between trough steady state plasma bupropion levels between 50 and 100 ng/ml and optimal antidepressant response; high plasma levels of bupropion and its metabolites are associated with a poor response.[10]

Fluoxetine

Plasma concentration–antidepressant response studies have not demonstrated a positive correlation for fluoxetine. The inability to use TDM may actually be a substantial disadvantage for fluoxetine given its long half-life coupled with the failure to demonstrate a minimally effective dose of the drug.[11]

Trazodone

Trazodone, a triazolopyridine, is used for the treatment of depression at doses between 200 and 600 mg/day and at lower doses as a hypnotic. This drug does not meet the criteria for utility of TDM and TDM would not be predicted to be critical when prescribing this agent. Consistent with this prediction, most plasma concentration–antidepressant response studies have not demonstrated a critical relationship.

THERAPEUTIC DRUG MONITORING OF MOOD STABILIZERS

Lithium

Therapeutic drug monitoring is important with lithium because of its narrow therapeutic index. To induce remission in acute manic episodes, the serum lithium concentration needs to be in a range between 0.8 and 1.2 mEq/liter. The range for maintenance therapy is between 0.6 and 0.8 mEq/liter. The risk of toxicity begins to outweigh efficacy at concentrations exceeding 1.5 mEq/liter.

Technique

Generally, the physician starts a patient on lithium with a divided dosage schedule, 300 mg either b.i.d. or t.i.d., and measures a trough serum level 4 to 5 days after initiation of therapy and 10 to 12 hours after the last dose. At this time a steady state plasma level has been achieved. Because lithium generally follows first-order kinetics, dose adjustment can be rationally performed based on a serum lithium concentration. If the lithium level is obtained too early, prior to reaching steady state levels, the clinician may increase the dose inappropriately, causing potentially toxic concentrations.

Single dose–plasma concentration nomograms for lithium have also been used to more efficiently reach therapeutic lithium plasma concentrations.[12] Twelve hours after a nightly dose of 450 to 600 mg of lithium, a blood sample is obtained for plasma concentration determination. Based on established nomograms, a prospective dosing regimen can then be determined.

Carbamazepine

While plasma concentrations of carbamazepine correlate well with its anticonvulsant activity and toxicity, the plasma concentration–antimanic efficacy relationship has yet to be adequately determined. Typical anticonvulsant therapeutic ranges for carbamazepine are 4 to 12 μg/ml. Until adequate plasma concentration–antimanic efficacy studies are performed, plasma carbamazepine levels much above 12 μg/ml should be avoided, especially from a medicolegal standpoint. Additional psychiatric uses of carbamazepine may involve the treatment of depression, schizoaffective illness, impulse control disorder, organic affective disorders, and agitated schizophrenia. Again, there are minimal concentration-efficacy data for these uses.

Technique

Carbamazepine chemotherapy is initiated with a 200-mg b.i.d. dosing schedule with meals. As with the previous medications mentioned, there is substantial interindividual variability in the metabolism and elimination rates of carbamazepine. An initial steady state trough serum level is checked in 5 to 7 days. Because of the hepatic autoinduction, initial plasma carbamazepine levels will typically not predict chronic plasma levels. Therefore, multiple blood draws may be necessary to adequately adjust the dose to obtain concentrations that fall within the

therapeutic range for anticonvulsant activity. In this regard, carbamazepine is anomalous relative to other psychiatric medications, for which repeated drug level monitoring to adjust the dose is generally not needed.

Valproic Acid

While the plasma concentration–antimania efficacy relationship for valproate has not been adequately assessed, the anticonvulsant range for valproate is 50 to 100 μg/ml. The response threshold of between 50 and 80 μg/ml is approximately the concentration at which plasma albumin sites saturate.[13] Some studies indicate that a threshold plasma level of 75 μg/ml is needed in the treatment of schizoaffective disorder patients.[14] At levels greater than 100 μg/ml, increased efficacy is not usually seen and the risk of cognitive impairment is increased.[15]

THERAPEUTIC DRUG MONITORING OF ANTIPSYCHOTICS

Haloperidol has received considerable attention recently in the debate over the concept of a "therapeutic window." An inverted U relationship between concentration and response has been demonstrated by some studies, indicating the presence of a therapeutic window for optimal antipsychotic response.[16] The therapeutic range for haloperidol is between 5 and 20 ng/ml, with toxicity occurring above 50 ng/ml. Empirically, it appears that patients with different diagnostic profiles may show decreases in Brief Psychiatric Rating Scale scores at varying haloperidol concentrations. For example, patients who have been diagnosed as having schizophreniform disorder may respond to concentrations that would typically be subtherapeutic for chronic schizophrenia, whereas patients with subchronic schizophrenia may respond to haloperidol concentrations that are at the lower end of the therapeutic range for chronic schizophrenic patients.[17]

Wolkin et al.[18] reported a well-defined curvilinear relationship between plasma level and dopamine receptor occupancy and response, suggesting the utility of TDM with neuroleptics. Schulz et al.[19] proposed that the extent to which a neuroleptic blocks D_2 dopamine receptors determines the degree to which psychotic symptoms are manifested. At low plasma haloperidol concentrations (e.g., less than 5 ng/ml), minimal D_2 dopamine receptor blockade occurs; thus the result is an excessive amount of dopamine and the presence of psychotic symptoms. At therapeutic plasma concentrations (e.g., 5 to 20 ng/ml), sufficient D_2 dopamine receptor blockade occurs and the result is a remission of psychotic symptoms. At concentrations greater than 20 ng/ml little additional receptor blockade occurs. Seeman[20] suggested that excessive plasma haloperidol concentrations could enhance the presynaptic release of dopamine, leading to an overabundance of neuro-transmitter in the synaptic cleft, and hence cause a return of symptomatology. While the aforementioned ideas are consistent with the "dopamine hypothesis" of psychosis, clinically, patient presentation is often not as clear cut as these theories might suggest.

CONCLUSION

Therapeutic drug monitoring in psychiatry is useful with a number of psychotropic medications in which a positive relationship between plasma drug concentration and efficacy can be demonstrated. These drugs include lithium carbonate, four tricyclic antidepressants (nortriptyline, desipramine, imipramine, and amitriptyline), some antipsychotics (haloperidol and thiothixene), and monoamine oxidase inhibitors. Psychotropic medications that have not been adequately studied but are good candidates for having a meaningful relationship between plasma concentration and efficacy include bupropion and mood-stabilizing anticonvulsants (carbamazepine and valproate). Therapeutic drug monitoring allows for the rational dose adjustment of these aforementioned medications, identifies potentially toxic drug levels, and is a cost-effective tool in the management of certain psychiatric illness.

ACKNOWLEDGMENTS

Parts of this paper first appeared in "NPL Facts," a newsletter written by Dr. Preskorn and supported by the National Psychopharmacology Laboratory, Inc. Additional parts of this paper appeared in Preskorn, SH, Fast, GA: Therapeutic drug monitoring for antidepressants: Efficacy, safety, and cost effectiveness. J Clin Psychiatry, 52(6, suppl): 23–33, 1991.

The authors thank Ms. Marianne Eyles for manuscript preparation.

REFERENCES

1. Ley P: Satisfaction, compliance and communication. Br J Clin Psychol 21:241–244, 1981.

2. Perry PJ, Pfohl BM, Holstad SG: The relationship between antidepressant response and tricyclic antidepressant plasma concentrations. Clin Pharmacokinet 13:381–392, 1987.

3. Preskorn SH, Jerkovich GS: Central nervous system toxicity of tricyclic antidepressants: Phenomenology, course, risk factors, and role of therapeutic drug monitoring. J Clin Psychopharmacol 10:88–94, 1990.

4. Preskorn SH, Othmer S, Lai C, et al: Tricyclic antidepressants and delirium. J Clin Psychiatry 139:822–823, 1982.

5. Preskorn SH, Fast GA: Tricyclic antidepressant-induced seizures and plasma drug concentration. J Clin Psychiatry (in press).

6. Vohra J, Burrows G, Hunt D, et al: The effects of toxic and therapeutic doses of tricyclic antidepressant drugs on intracardiac conduction. Eur J Cardiol 3:219–227, 1975.

7. Veith RC, Friedel RO, Bloom B, et al: Electrocardiogram changes and plasma desipramine levels during treatment. Clin Pharmacol Ther 27:796–802, 1980.

8. Petit JM, Spiker DG, Ruwitch JF, et al: Tricyclic antidepressant plasma levels and adverse effects after overdose. Clin Pharmacol Ther 21:47–51, 1977.

9. Ravaris CL, Nies A, Robinson DS, et al: A multiple-dose, controlled study of phenelzine in depression-anxiety states. Arch Gen Psychiatry 33:347–350, 1976.

10. Preskorn SH: Antidepressant response and plasma concentrations of bupropion. J Clin Psychiatry 44(5, sec 2):137–139, 1983.

11. Preskorn SH, Silkey B, Beber, et al: Antidepressant response and plasma concentrations of fluoxetine. Ann Clin Psychiatry 3:147–151, 1991.

12. Cooper TB, Bergner PE, Simpson GM: The 24-hour serum lithium as a prognosticator of dosage requirements. Am J Psychiatry 130:601–603, 1973.

13. Penry KJ, Dean JC: The scope and use of valproate in epilepsy. J Clin Psychiatry 50(3, suppl):17–22, 1989.

14. McElroy SL, Keck PE Jr, Pope HG: Sodium valproate: Its use in primary psychiatric disorders. J Clin Psychopharmacol 7:16–24, 1987.

15. Brown R: US experience with valproate in manic depressive illness: A multi-center trial. J Clin Psychiatry 50(3, suppl):13–16, 1989.

16. Smith RC, Baumgartner R, Misra CH, et al: Haloperidol: Plasma levels and prolactin response as predictors of clinical improvement in schizophrenia: Chemical v radioreceptor plasma level assays. Arch Gen Psychiatry 41:1044–1049, 1984.

17. Santos JL, Cabrones JA, Vazquaez C, et al: Clinical response and plasma haloperidol in chronic and subchronic schizophrenia. Biol Psychiatry 26:381–388, 1989.

18. Wolkin A, Brodie JD, Barouch F, et al: Dopamine receptor occupancy and plasma haloperidol levels. Arch Gen Psychiatry 46:482–484, 1989.

19. Schulz SC, Butterfield L, Garicano M, et al: Beyond the therapeutic window: A case presentation. J Clin Psychiatry 45:223–225, 1984.

20. Seeman P: Antischizophrenic drugs—membrane receptor sites of action. Biochem Pharmacol 26:1741–1748, 1977.

86

FUTURE ANTIDEPRESSANTS

WILLIAM F. BOYER, M.D. and JOHN P. FEIGHNER, M.D.

No one can doubt that antidepressant pharmacotherapy has made tremendous strides since the accidental discovery of the mood-elevating effect of imipramine. Despite these gains, several significant problems remain. These include nonresponse, delay in onset, toxicity in overdose, and side effects. Side effects, in turn, may lead to medical and psychiatric morbidity (including induction of mania), treatment with an inadequate dose, complete inability to take the medication, a poor *quality* of response, or premature termination of maintenance therapy. Relapse after discontinuing treatment is another important issue in pharmacotherapy, although it is not, strictly speaking, a problem with medication. Future antidepressants, if they are to be valuable, will improve in several of these areas.

Several general factors will affect antidepressant use in the future. One of these is the development of antidepressant drugs that are considerably better tolerated than first- and second-generation agents. This shifts the risk-benefit ratio in favor of continuing maintenance treatment for most patients. Another factor is the continuing modification and improvement of the diagnostic criteria as shown in the DSM-III, DSM-III-R, and DSM-IV and the tenth revision of the International Classification of Diseases (ICD-10). Prior to the development of operationalized diagnostic criteria, such as the Feighner and the Research Diagnostic Criteria, it was difficult to reliably show the superiority of antidepressants to placebo. As diagnoses become more reliable and scientifically based, it may be possible to show the superiority of some antidepressants over others in specific populations. This will be especially important as the number of antidepressant drugs continue to multiply. Some suggestion of this trend can already be seen in the findings that (1) monoamine oxidase inhibitors (MAOIs) are superior to tricyclic antidepressants (TCAs) in atypical depression and (2) strongly serotonergic antidepressants are superior in obsessive-compulsive and perhaps panic disorders.

Most of the recent antidepressants were discovered by their effects in animal models of depression. These include prevention of tetrabenzine-induced sedation, inhibition of behavioral despair, and potentiation of L-dopa after pargyline pretreatment. Pharmaceutical companies are devoting considerable time and resources to using and developing these and newer models. This aggressive and sophisticated preclinical work should not discourage clinicians from making and reporting observations of the antidepressant properties of other substances. The pharmaceutical screening process inevitably produces a certain uniformity among the drugs. It should be remembered that the phenothiazines were discovered by chance in the investigation of antihistamines, TCAs were discovered by chance in the investigation of phenothiazines, and MAOIs were discovered by chance in the investigation of antitubercular drugs. Therefore there is still a need for astute clinical observations.

The broad spectrum of action of many antidepressants will also affect the use of these drugs. In some ways the development of antidepressants parallels that of the β-blockers or calcium channel blockers. Although these agents were introduced for the treatment of specific disorders, such as hypertension and angina, they have found use in many other conditions. However, instead of being narrowly labeled as "antihypertensives" or "antianginal" drugs, they retained names that referred to their presumptive modes of action. Antidepressants have found a similar broad range of psychiatric and nonpsychiatric uses, including migraine prophylaxis and enuresis, chronic pain, and antiarrhythmic therapy, plus several in psychiatry, but are still referred to by the inappropriately narrow name of "antidepressants." This can be a practical clinical problem in explaining the rationale for treatment selection to patients. It may be appropriate in the future to refer to these medications with names such as "amine uptake inhibitors" or "amine receptor regulators."

Another important development may be a broadening of the concept of "antidepressant" to include nonpharmacological treatments. The efficacy of bright light therapy is reasonably well established for seasonal affective disorder. There is some evidence that it may also be helpful for nonseasonal depression. The mechanism of action of light therapy is not established, but interest centers on its effects on altered circadian rhythms and serotonin function. Similarly, sleep deprivation has significant but temporary beneficial effects on 50 per cent or more of patients with major depression. The mechanism of sleep deprivation is also not established, but may likewise involve alterations in circadian rhythms or suppression of a depressogenic substance produced during sleep.[1,2]

SPECIFIC ANTIDEPRESSANTS

Drugs Acting on Serotonin Uptake

The major antidepressants in this class selectively inhibit serotonin reuptake. The selection serotonin reuptake inhibitors (SSRIs) include fluoxetine, sertraline, paroxetine, fluvoxamine, and citalopram (Table 86–1; Fig. 86–1). The SSRIs are selective in that their physiological effects in normal doses are limited to inhibition of serotonin reuptake. They do not directly affect any receptor function. This contrasts markedly to the original generation of antidepressants, which inhibit reuptake of several neurotransmitters and interact with a variety of neuroreceptors. The SSRIs are a very important new class of medications for at least two reasons. First, the narrow scope of biological activity translates to fewer side effects and lower toxicity in overdose. Second, the SSRIs may also have a broader scope of clinical indications than TCAs. For example, drugs with potent serotonin reuptake inhibition are significantly superior to those that selectively inhibit norepinephrine reuptake in the treatment of obsessive-compulsive disorder and perhaps panic disorder. There is also some suggestion that SSRIs are more effective in reducing suicidal ideation than noradrenergic antidepressants. However, comparative trials for this indication have not been done.

Other possible relative indications include eating disorders (obesity, bulimia, and anorexia nervosa), substance abuse (alcohol as well as possibly stimulant and nicotine dependence), aggressive impulsivity, headaches, and chronic pain. This breadth of indications is exciting for theoretical as well as clinical reasons. The efficacy of selective serotonergic drugs for these disorders provides some insight into the central role of serotonin in these conditions.

Over the next few years several SSRIs will be approved for marketing in the United States. The avail-

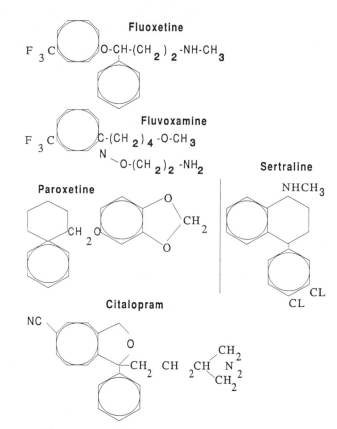

Figure 86–1. Selective serotonin reuptake inhibitors.

ability of a number of drugs in this class will be important for clinicians. The newer SSRIs will have much shorter half-lives than fluoxetine. One of these, paroxetine, has no known active metabolites. These features will be important in minimizing side effects and avoiding drug interactions. An important example of the latter is the need to discontinue fluoxetine for a month or more before initiating treatment with a MAOI.

The side effect profile of the different SSRIs will vary in important ways. Paroxetine, for example, appears to have a lower risk of anxiety, nervousness,

TABLE 86–1.   SOME DIFFERENCES BETWEEN THE SSRIs

SSRI	Potency at 5-HT Receptors	Dosage Range (mg)	Half-Life (Hours)	Active Metabolites	Weight Loss	Common Side Effects
Fluoxetine	25.0	20–80	48–72	Yes	Yes	Nausea, restlessness, diarrhea, agitation
Sertraline	7.3	50–200	25	Yes	Yes	Nausea, diarrhea, restlessness, insomnia
Paroxetine	1.1	20–50	24	No	No	Nausea, diarrhea, mild drowsiness
Fluvoxamine	6.2	100–300	15	No	No	Nausea, diarrhea, insomnia, restlessness
Citalopram	2.6	10–80	35	No	No	Nausea, dry mouth, diarrhea

and weight loss than fluoxetine. In contrast, fluvoxamine may have a higher incidence of nausea than fluoxetine.[3]

Another new class of serotonergic antidepressants has so far received relatively little attention in the United States. Tianeptine is a prototype of this group. It is an atypical TCA that appears to act as a selective serotonin reuptake *agonist*. Clinical trials have shown it also effectively relieves symptoms of anxiety and depression.[4] Drugs of this type are important not only because they may offer important new clinical alternatives, but because they also pose a significant issue in our understanding of how antidepressants work.

5-Hydroxytryptamine$_{1a}$ Partial Agonists

This category includes the azaspirodecanedione derivatives buspirone, ipsapirone, gepirone, and tandosiprone. These drugs are relatively selective for the 5-hydroxytryptamine$_{1a}$ (5-HT$_{1a}$) autoreceptor. Because they are partial agonists, their activity depends on the initial state of this receptor. If there is low activity at the receptor they act as agonists. If there is high activity the net effect is antagonism. This flexibility may explain why this class of medications appear to be helpful in a variety of conditions, including anxiety, obsessive-compulsive disorder, premenstrual tension, and depression.

Although they were originally developed as anxiolytics, recent interest in these drugs as antidepressants has developed because of their activity in many of the animal models that predict antidepressant activity. In trials of anxious subjects it was also noted that depression and many of its associated symptoms improved. Several trials in patients with major depression, plus significant anxiety, have been completed. These suggest that the 5-HT$_{1a}$ partial agonists are effective in relieving the "core" symptoms of depression, such as lowered mood, psychomotor retardation, and disturbances in sleep and appetite.[5]

Several of the 5-HT$_{1a}$ partial agonists are either marketed in various countries or in various stages of development. The newer drugs appear even more selective than buspirone for 5-HT$_{1a}$ receptors. Therefore, they are probably less prone to produce unwanted effects.

Bupropion

Bupropion (Wellbutrin) is a trimethylated monocyclic phenylaminoketone. It is chemically and pharmacologically distinct from TCAs, MAOIs, and SSRIs. Like other antidepressants, it is active in animal models that predict antidepressant effects. Unlike other antidepressants, bupropion does not interact with neuroreceptors, inhibit monoamine oxidase, or significantly block the reuptake of serotonin or norepinephrine. Some evidence suggests its antidepressant effect may involve modification of noradrenergic function by means other than receptor blockade or uptake inhibition.[6]

Bupropion is a potent antidepressant.[7] It is valuable in many cases of otherwise refractory depression. It may be less likely than other antidepressants to precipitate mania and has very low toxicity in overdose.[8] Bupropion's main limitation is the need for divided dosing during the day. A single dose should not exceed more than 150 mg at a time because of an increased risk of seizures. Therefore it is possible that a sustained release form of bupropion or a bupropion analogue without this limitation may become available.

Reversible Monoamine Oxidase Inhibitors

Controlled data suggest that MAOIs are as effective as TCAs in major depression, but superior in atypical cases. Their use has been limited because of concerns about hypertensive episodes and other troublesome side effects. Conventional MAOIs bind irreversibly to MAO, which renders it inactive. The body must generate new MAO before one is again protected from pressor amines, such as tyramine. Reversible MAOIs bind competitively to the enzyme. In the presence of other substrates for MAO, such as tyramine, the drug molecule can be displaced. This allows the enzyme to inactivate the pressor amine. The reversible MAOIs therefore carry a considerably lower risk of hypertensive crises. This lowered risk has been substantiated in clinical studies as well as direct infusions of tyramine in volunteer subjects. Clinical efficacy has been shown in a number of trials of depression.[9–11] The reversible MAOIs include moclobemide, brofaromine, and toloxatone.

Benzodiazepines

Alprazolam is a triazolobenzodiazepine that has been shown to have antidepressant activity in several studies. Adinazolam is also a triazolobenzodiazepine with anxiolytic and antidepressant properties. Its effects on norepinephrine reuptake are more potent than those of alprazolam. Controlled trials have shown a significantly superior antidepressant effect compared to placebo, and comparable to TCAs.[12] Like other effective antidepressants, it has been reported to induce mania. The onset of action is often within the first week of treatment.

Because of its rapid onset, adinazolam could become useful as a short-term adjunctive antidepressant. Its advantages include lack of anticholinergic and cardiovascular side effects as well as low toxicity in overdose. Its main liability would likely be the potential for abuse and dependence that accompanies all benzodiazepines.

Neuroleptics

Phenothiazine and thioxanthene derivatives have been shown to have significant antidepressant properties in double-blind trials. However, the use of neuroleptics in depression is complicated by the risk of tardive dyskinesia. Patients with an affective disorder may also be at higher risk of tardive dyskinesia than those with nonaffective disorders. Currently neuroleptics are generally reserved for the treatment of psychotic or treatment-refractory depression. The role of neuroleptics in affective disorders may become more important with the advent of newer neuroleptics that carry less risk of tardive dyskinesia.

These newer neuroleptics are of two main types. The substituted benzamide derivatives, such as remoxipride, are highly selective for D_2 dopamine receptors. Blockade of these receptors produces antipsychotic effects with few extrapyramidal symptoms (EPS). Extrapyramidal symptoms are associated primarily with D_1 receptors.

Dibenzodiazepine and benzisoxazole derivatives, of which clozapine and risperidone are examples, respectively, have *relatively* weak activity at dopamine receptors but are fairly potent at serotonin receptor sites. This relatively weak activity at dopamine receptors produces a low risk of EPS. Both types of compounds have been noted to have mood-elevating effects in clinical trials.[13]

Triazalopyridine Derivatives

Trazodone is the prototype triazolopyridine derivative. Its primary action is thought to be due to its effects on serotonin. It lacks anticholinergic side effects and quinidine-like action on the heart. It appears to be relatively benign if taken in overdose. However, it also has moderate α-adrenergic receptor blocking properties. This probably accounts for the orthostatic hypotension that may occur with trazodone. Other problems with trazodone include excessive sedation, lethargy, hypotension, and a risk of priapism that may be higher than that for other psychotropics.

Two other triazolopyridine derivatives, nefazodone and etoperidone, are in an advanced stage of research. These compounds offer the potential advantages of trazodone with an improved side effect profile.[14]

Venlafaxine

Down-regulation of β-adrenergic receptors is hypothesized to underly the activity of many antidepressants. Venlafaxine is one of the fastest compounds to down-regulate these receptors. This often occurs within a matter of days rather than the weeks that are typical of many drugs. This rapid effect holds promise of rapid onset of action. Venlafaxine is also unique in that it inhibits uptake of serotonin, norepinephrine, and dopamine. Clinically it appears to have a stimulant profile, which may be related to its dopamine reuptake blockade. It may have special application in treatment-refractory depression.

Venlafaxine is currently under active study in the United States.[15]

S-Adenosylmethionine

S-adenosylmethionine (SAM) is an antidepressant compound with a unique mechanism of action, methyl group donation. It is active by both oral and intravenous administration. Several open and controlled studies suggest it has significant, rapid antidepressant effects.[16] It also has been reported to induce mania in susceptible individuals. Side effects are generally mild and well tolerated. S-Adenosylmethionine is already marketed in some countries for the treatment of other conditions, such as arthritis.

Other Possible Antidepressants

Clinical and research findings have stimulated interest in other possible mechanisms of antidepressant activity. These include mood-elevating effects of angiotensin-converting enzyme inhibitors, β_2-adrenergic agonists, phosphodiesterase inhibitors, gamma-aminobutyric acid mimetic agents, calcium channel blockers, metals such as rubidium and vanadium, and opiate derivatives. It is possible that antidepressant compounds that exploit one or several of these mechanisms may be developed in the near future.

CONCLUSION

A number of antidepressant compounds will become available over the next few years. This will provide more options for better quality treatment of depressed patients. A disadvantage is that it may become even harder to select the proper treatment for individual patients, leading to prolonged "trial and error." It is hoped that advances in diagnosis, laboratory tests, and genetics will offset this problem by making it easier to select specific treatments for particular types of depression. Older antidepressant compounds, which act on a variety of transmitter systems and therefore tend to cause more side effects, may also fall by the wayside.

Two main types of antidepressant compounds will be developed. One group represents a refinement of a preexisting drug. These are likely to act like the parent compound but cause fewer side effects. Examples include the SSRIs, $5-HT_{1a}$ partial agonists, and the analogues of trazodone. The other type are antidepressants that act by completely novel mechanisms. This second type will be most valuable, at least at first, in providing truly different options for treatment-refractory patients.

Currently electroconvulsive therapy and psychosurgery are the only established nonpharmacological somatic treatments for depression. Other modalities, such as sleep deprivation and bright light treatment, may expand this category. With advances in computer-aided studies of brain function, it may even become possible in the not too distant future to unlock some of the physiological foundations of pharmacological and nonpharmacological antidepressant treatments.

REFERENCES

1. Wehr TA: Manipulations of sleep and phototherapy: non-pharmacological alternatives in the treatment of depression. Clin Neuropharmacol 13(suppl 1):S54–S65, 1990.
2. Wu JC, Bunney WE: The biological basis of an antidepressant response to sleep deprivation and relapse: Review and hypothesis. Am J Psychiatry 147:14–21, 1990.
3. Feighner JP, Boyer WF: Selective Serotonin Reuptake Inhibitors. Chichester, England, John Wiley and Sons, 1991.
4. Fattaccini CM, Bolanos-Jimenez F, Gozlan H, et al: Tianeptine stimulates uptake of 5-hydroxytryptamine in vivo in the rat brain. Neuropharmacology 29:1–8, 1990.
5. Rickels K, Amsterdam JD, Clary C, et al: Buspirone in major depression: A controlled study. J Clin Psychiatry 52:34–38, 1991.
6. Golden RN, Rudorfer MV, Sherer MA, et al: Bupropion in depression. I. Biochemical effects and clinical response. Arch Gen Psychiatry 45:139–143, 1988.
7. Lineberry CG, Johnston JA, Raymond RN, et al: A fixed-dose (300 mg) efficacy study of bupropion and placebo in depressed outpatients. J Clin Psychiatry 51:197–199, 1990.
8. Haykal RF, Akiskal HS: Bupropion as a promising approach to rapid cycling bipolar II patients. J Clin Psychiatry 51:450–455, 1990.
9. Stabl M, Biziere K, Schmid-Burgk W, et al: Review of comparative clinical trials. Moclobemide vs tricyclic antidepressants and vs placebo in depressive states. J Neural Transm [Suppl] 28:77–89, 1989.
10. Zimmer R, Fischbach R, Breuel HP: Potentiation of the pressor effect of intravenously administered tyramine during moclobemide treatment. Acta Psychiatr Scand [Suppl] 360:76–77, 1990.
11. Zimmer R, Gieschke R, Fischbach R, et al: Interaction studies with moclobemide. Acta Psychiatr Scand [Suppl] 360:84–86, 1990.
12. Feighner JP, Boyer WF, Hendrickson GG, et al: A controlled trial of adinazolam versus desipramine in geriatric depression. Int Clin Psychopharmacol 5:227–232, 1990.
13. Tamminga CA, Gerlach J: New neuroleptics and experimental antipsychotics in schizophrenia. In Meltzer HY, ed. Psychopharmacology: The Third Generation of Progress. New York, Raven Press, 1987:1129–1140.
14. Feighner JP, Pambakian R, Fowler R, et al: A comparison of patients of nefazodone, imipramine and placebo in patients with moderate to severe depression. Psychopharmacol Bull 25(2):219–221, 1989.
15. Goldberg HL, Finnerty R: An open-label, variable-dose study of WY-45,030 (venlafexine) in depressed outpatients. Psychopharmacol Bull 24(1):198–199, 1988.
16. Kagan BL, Sultzer DL, Rosenlicht N, et al: Oral S-adenosyl methionine in the treatment of depression. In Stefanis CN, Rabavilas AD, Soldatos CR, eds. Psychiatry—A World Perspective. New York, Excerpta Medica, 1990:428–433.

87

FUTURE TRENDS IN THE PSYCHOPHARMACOLOGY OF ANXIETY DISORDERS

MICHAEL R. JOHNSON, M.D. and R. BRUCE LYDIARD, M.D., Ph.D.

There is an exciting future ahead for the pharmacological treatment of anxiety disorders. Advances in our understanding of the biological systems involved in anxiety have contributed to an unprecedented proliferation of new anxiolytic agents, many of which are currently under development. The vast majority of these newer agents act specifically at sites on gamma-aminobutyric acid (GABA) and serotonergic or adrenergic neurons. As a result of this increasing specificity, many of these drugs promise to be superior to those currently available, with both improved efficacy and more favorable side effects profiles. This new age of specificity will require,

however, a more sophisticated understanding of the unique biological activity of the new therapeutic agents. In this chapter we examine the biological sites of activity, side effect profiles, and current efficacy data for drugs that might soon be available for treatment of anxiety disorders.

GABAERGIC DRUGS

Our understanding of the GABA-benzodiazepine (BZ) receptor site has increased substantially over the last several years.[1] We have long known that agents active at the GABA receptor site, such as the BZs, are effective treatments for anxiety. Unfortunately, the high incidence of unwanted side effects such as ataxia, sedation, and cognitive disturbance has made these agents troublesome to use. Even more concerning have been the problems with the abuse potential of some agents and the frequent development of dependence and withdrawal syndromes. The future promises an abundance of new drugs that act at the BZ receptor and that may provide solutions to some of these problems. Table 87–1 lists the various compounds active at the BZ receptor.

Traditional BZs are full agonists acting at the BZ receptor site on the GABA-BZ complex. BZs facilitate binding of GABA to its receptor site, and this stimulates an influx of chloride ions through the chloride channel. The increased intracellular chloride concentration causes a decrease in the excitability of the neuron. This decrease in neuronal excitability appears to correlate with a decrease in anxiety. Other agents, such as β-carboline-3-carboxylate ethyl ester (βCCE) and diazepam binding inhibitor (DBI—a putative endogenous ligand for the BZ receptor), are inverse agonists at the BZ receptor and actually prevent flow of chloride ions through the channel, causing an increase in nerve excitability.

Compounds that bind to the BZ receptor, preventing the BZ molecules from acting but otherwise have no intrinsic activity at the site, are known as antagonists. One such agent, flumazenil, is currently available as a treatment for BZ overdose. The BZ partial agonists are a new class of agents that are active at the BZ receptor and have effects midway between full agonists and antagonists. Clinically they have been found to provide substantial anxiolytic effect while causing significantly fewer side effects than traditional BZs. Problems with sedation, cognitive disturbance, ataxia, and potentiation of alcohol effects all appear to be minimal. Additionally, the par-

tial agonists have demonstrated no significant problems with dependence or withdrawal syndromes and also appear to have minimal abuse liability.[2]

Alpidem is an imidazopyridine compound typical of the BZ partial agonists. It has been tested extensively in Europe[3] and has been found to be as effective as traditional BZs in the treatment of generalized or situational anxiety. There was no evidence of withdrawal symptoms or rebound anxiety following discontinuation even after extended use. Studies in the elderly[4] were particularly encouraging in demonstrating the lack of psychomotor or cognitive problems with use of alpidem.

In addition to alpidem, other partial agonists that may appear on the market within the next few years include abecarnil (ZK1120) and bretazenil. Abecarnil has been demonstrated in one study to be effective in generalized anxiety disorder (GAD)[5] and is currently being tested in panic disorder. Bretazenil has been demonstrated to be efficacious in both GAD and panic disorder.[2] Bretazenil has also been demonstrated to have surprising benefits in psychotic patients. In one report, bretazenil was found to ameliorate psychotic symptoms in 60 per cent of 73 psychotic patients with schizophrenia.[2] Flumazenil, a BZ antagonist that is currently marketed for use in BZ overdose, may also have some anxiolytic activity.[6] Inverse agonists such as βCCE have been demonstrated to produce anxiety[7] and currently are only of research interest.

In addition to exploiting differences in degree of receptor binding, we will soon be considering the additional dimension of degree of specificity for subtypes of BZ receptors. There is evidence now that there are at least two subtypes of BZ receptors that may have somewhat different distributions and actions.[1] Type 1 receptors have been suggested to mediate more of the anxiolytic effects and type 2 receptors more of the sedative effects of benzodiazepines.[8] Alpidem, which appears to have minimal sedative effect, has been reported to be relatively specific for the type 1 receptor, whereas quazepam (Doral), a newly available sedative-hypnotic, acts specifically at the type 2 receptor. This picture is already becoming more complicated, however, because zolpidem, which is currently marketed in Europe as a hypnotic, shows selectivity for type 1 receptors.[9]

SEROTONERGIC AGENTS

On the more immediate horizon are a group of new anxiolytic agents that are active at various sites within the central serotonin (5-hydroxytryptamine; 5-HT) system. There is good evidence to support the theory that serotonergic neurons play an important role in mediating anxiety.[10] Recent advances in our understanding of the serotonin system have allowed us to identify a large number of serotonin receptor subtypes (5-HT$_{1a}$, 5-HT$_2$, and 5-HT$_3$) and an even

TABLE 87–1.   DRUGS ACTIVE AT BENZODIAZEPINE RECEPTOR

Full agonists
    Traditional BZs
Partial agonists
    Alpidem
    Abecarnil
    Bretazenil
    Divaplon
Antagonists
    Flumazenil
Inverse agonists
    β-carboline-3-carboxylate ethyl ester (βCCE)
    Diazepam binding inhibitor (DBI)
Type 1 receptor specific
    Zolpidem
    Alpidem
    EGIS5278
    CL218872
Type 2 receptor specific
    Quazepam

larger number of drugs active at these sites. Many of the currently known receptor-specific drugs are listed in Table 87–2.

The selective serotonin reuptake inhibitors (SSRIs) are effective antidepressants with a much more tolerable side effect profile than traditional antidepressants. They have no anticholinergic or antihistaminic effects, minimal sedative and cardiovascular effects, and minimal lethality in overdose. They also are less prone to cause weight gain and have even been found to promote weight loss in some people. Negative effects include the development in some patients of nausea, insomnia, and a restlessness that has been likened to an akathisia. Their mechanism of antidepressant effect is likely to be related to the potent increase in serotonin function caused by reuptake inhibition.[11] In general, agents that stimulate serotonergic activity are anxiogenic,[10] and, in fact, SSRIs typically cause an initial elevation in the anxiety levels, which often results in premature discontinuation by patients prone to anxiety. The anxiolytic and antidepressant effect is delayed and may be related to gradual desensitization of postsynaptic serotonin receptors. Handled carefully, these agents appear to be of substantial value in the treatment of a variety of anxiety disorders.

Fluoxetine, the only highly selective SSRI currently available in the United States, has shown significant therapeutic potential in obsessive-compulsive disorder (OCD)[12–16] and in panic disorder,[17,18] and may possibly be useful in social phobia.[19] Many of the newer serotonin reuptake agents also appear to have promise in treatment of anxiety disorders. Fluvoxamine, which has been available in Europe since 1984, appears to be extremely effective in OCD[16,20] and in panic disorder.[21] Sertraline, another potent reuptake antagonist which has recently become available in the United States as an antidepressant, has also been demonstrated to be efficacious in OCD[22] and is now being evaluated for efficacy in panic disorder. Sertraline may be particularly useful for patients who have been unable to tolerate the restlessness that has often been associated with other SSRIs. Even newer SSRIs may be distinguished by an increasing degree of specificity for certain parts of the nervous system. One investigational SSRI, alaproclate, may have some selectivity for neurons in the hypothalamus and hippocampus.[23] The clinical implications of this specificity are not yet clear, but more specificity may confer unique advantages either in efficacy or in side effects profile.

Partial agonists at the 5-HT$_{1a}$ serotonin receptor site have also been demonstrated to be anxiolytic. While full agonists at the 5-HT$_{1a}$ site such as 8-OHDPAT are known to be anxiogenic,[24] the 5-HT$_{1a}$ partial agonists such as buspirone appear to be anxiolytic. This difference may be due to the fact that the azapirones, such as buspirone, act primarily at the presynaptic autoreceptor, which, when activated, inhibits neuronal firing and release of serotonin.[24] It may also be related to the partial agonist effects at the postsynaptic receptor, which may cause a relative antagonism of serotonin.[25] An alternative explanation more consistent with the delayed onset of action of these drugs would connect their anxiolytic effect to the gradual desensitization of presynaptic autoreceptors.[10] Whatever the explanation for their anxiolytic effects, these agents are sure to play an important role in the future treatment of anxiety. The 5-HT$_{1a}$ partial agonists have demonstrated significant advantages over the BZs in their lack of dependence and abuse potential as well as their relatively low incidence of significant side effects. Of particular note, they have a much lower incidence of sedation, depression, and motor or cognitive impairment than do the BZs.

Buspirone is the only one of these agents currently available on the U.S. market. It has been demonstrated in numerous studies to be effective in GAD[26,27] as well as being an effective adjunctive treatment in OCD.[28] One small open label study found it useful in treating social phobia,[29] and recently it has been found efficacious in depression.[30] The issue of buspirone's efficacy in panic disorder appears to be an open one, and studies to date have been inconclusive. Some have suggested that it may play a role in treating the anticipatory anxiety associated with panic disorder,[31] but certainly more study is needed.

There are several newer 5-HT$_{1a}$ partial agonists, including ipsapirone, gepirone, and enciprazine, that are poised to follow in the footsteps of buspirone. All of these agents maintain the benefits of buspirone, including lack of physical dependence or effects on cognitive or psychomotor processes. All have been demonstrated to be effective in GAD,[32–34] and ipsapirone and gepirone have been demonstrated to be effective in depression.[35,36] While they

TABLE 87–2. DRUGS SPECIFICALLY ACTIVE AT SEROTONIN RECEPTORS

Reuptake inhibitors
  Fluoxetine
  Sertraline
  Fluvoxamine
  Alaproclate
  Paroxetine
  Zimelidine
5-HT$_{1a}$ agonists
  Buspirone
  Gepirone
  Ipsapirone
  Enciprazine
5-HT$_2$ antagonists
  Ritanserin
  Kitanserin
  Nefazodone
  Mianserin
5-HT$_3$ antagonists
  Ondansetron
  Granisetron
  Zacopride

are very similar to buspirone in most ways, they may have some unique pharmacological actions. For example, gepirone may act in certain situations as a more potent serotonin agonist than buspirone or ipsapirone,[31] and enciprazine may have less activity at the dopamine receptor than buspirone.[34] It is not clear at this time, however, whether the different pharmacological profiles of the 5-HT$_{1a}$ agonists will be of clinical significance.

The 5-HT$_2$ antagonists are an intriguing new group of compounds that combine possible efficacy in multiple conditions, including depression, pain syndromes, migraine prophylaxis, and sleep disorders as well as anxiety disorders. Compounds in this class that are currently marketed either in the United States or abroad have been variously utilized for migraine prophylaxis (methysergide), for hypertension (ketanserin), and for rhinitis (cyproheptadine). More recently, interest has been focused on their efficacy in psychiatric disorders. Early studies demonstrating the efficacy of 5-HT$_2$ antagonists in animal models of anxiety[37] have been followed up with clinical studies in humans that have demonstrated the efficacy of one of these agents, ritanserin, in GAD.[38] Ritanserin has also been evaluated in panic disorder with mixed results,[39,40] but has been demonstrated to be an effective analgesic in treating chronic headaches,[41] has improved the sleep of chronic insomniacs,[42] and may be effective in depression as well.[11] Nefazodone and mianserin are two other 5-HT$_2$ antagonists that have been demonstrated to have efficacy in depression.[43-45] As of now we are not aware of any controlled data on the efficacy of nefazodone and mianserin in anxiety disorders, but the encouraging results with ritanserin suggest that these agents may be effective anxiolytics as well.

There are currently no 5-HT$_3$ receptor antagonists available on the American or European markets. The vast majority of studies on these agents have focused on their utility as antiemetics.[46] However, 5-HT$_3$ antagonists have also been demonstrated to be effective anxiolytics in many animal models of anxiety,[47] and, more recently, open label clinical trials with ondansetron, a selective 5-HT$_3$ receptor antagonist, have demonstrated efficacy in patients with general anxiety disorders. Moreover, these agents have typically been extremely well tolerated without evidence of sedation, tolerance, or withdrawal symptoms. Double-blind clinical trials studying the efficacy of 5-HT$_3$ antagonists in treating GAD are currently underway and should soon shed some light on their future potential as anxiolytics.

NORADRENERGIC AGENTS

Substantial evidence exists tying the noradrenergic system to anxiety disorders.[10] Agents with noradrenergic effects, such as tricyclic antidepressants and monoamine oxidase (MAO) inhibitors have become a mainstay in the treatment of panic disorder, agoraphobia, and social phobia. Despite the evidence for efficacy of these agents in treating anxiety, there appear to be no new anxiolytic agents that work specifically on the noradrenergic system. There are, however, agents being developed that combine efficacy in several systems, including the noradrenergic system.

Venlafaxine is a new bicyclic compound that acts as an uptake inhibitor of serotonin, noradrenaline, and dopamine in descending order of potency. It is unique in this combination of activity and has relatively few anticholinergic effects compared to more traditional tricyclic antidepressants. It has already been demonstrated to be effective in depression[48,49] and possibly in OCD.[50] It is currently under study in panic disorder.

Irreversible MAO inhibitors such as phenelzine have long been known to be particularly potent in treating a variety of anxiety disorders, including panic disorder[51,52] and social phobia.[53] Problems with dietary restrictions and potential for fatal hypertensive crises, however, have limited their utilization. With the discovery of the reversible MAO inhibitors, the value of these agents will have to be reconsidered. Moclobemide is a new reversible inhibitor of MAO type A that has been demonstrated to have substantially less potential for producing hypertensive responses to tyramine.[54] It has also been demonstrated to be effective in treating depression and to be better tolerated than tricyclic antidepressants.[55] There are currently no published data on the efficacy of moclobemide in anxiety disorders, but it is clear that moclobemide and similar-acting reversible inhibitors of type A MAO will likely have a place in treating anxiety disorders as well.

There is substantial evidence linking excessive noradrenergic activity in the locus ceruleus to the occurrence of anxiety disorders.[56] Clonidine, a potent α_2-adrenergic receptor agonist that decreases activity in the noradrenergic neurons of the locus ceruleus, primarily through α_2-autoreceptor stimulation, has been demonstrated to have some anxiolytic qualities, but these has been found to be short lived and complicated by hypotension.[57] Nevertheless, it makes sense that drugs active at these receptors may someday be found useful in the treatment of anxiety. Additionally, it has been suggested that drugs acting as postsynaptic α_2-antagonists may be of value in treating anxiety.[10] Mirtazapine is a new antidepressant that has been found to have α_2-antagonist effects as well as antiserotonin activity, and one study has found it to be an effective treatment for depression.[58] It will be important to investigate whether mirtazapine and other agents acting as postsynaptic α_2-antagonists will indeed have a place in the pharmacological treatment of anxiety disorders.

CONCLUSION

The introduction of anxiolytic agents acting with more specificity within the central nervous system has ushered in a new era in the treatment of anxiety disorders. In addition to the development of new serotonin reuptake inhibitors and new 5-HT$_{1a}$ partial agonists, the future availability of new classes of agents such as BZ partial agonists, 5-HT$_2$ and 5-HT$_3$ antagonists, and reversible MAO inhibitors is likely to improve our ability to treat our patients with anxiety more safely and effectively.

REFERENCES

1.* Zorumski CF, Isenberg KE: Insights into the structure and function of GABA-benzodiazepine receptors: Ion channels and psychiatry. Am J Psychiatry 148:162–173, 1991.

2.* Haefly W, Martin JR, Schoch P: Novel anxiolyotics that act as partial agonists at benzodiazepine receptors. TiPS 11:452–456, 1990.

3. Morselli PL: On the therapeutic action of alpidem in anxiety disorders: An overview of the European data. Pharmacopsychiatry 23:129–134, 1990.

4. Hindmarch I: Alpidem and psychological performance in elderly subjects. Pharmacopsychiatry 23:124–128, 1990.

5. Ballenger JC, McDonald S, Noyes R, et al: The first double-blind, placebo-controlled trial of a partial benzodiazepine agonist abecarnil (Zk 112–119) in generalized anxiety disorder. Psychopharmacol Bull 27:171–179, 1991.

6. Urbancic M, Gadek MA, Marczynski TJ: Chronic exposure to flumazenil: Anxiolytic effect and increased exploratory behavior. Pharmacol Biochem Behav 35:503–509, 1990.

7.* Breier A, Paul SM: The GABA-A/benzodiazepine receptor: Implications for the molecular basis of anxiety. J Psychiatr Res 24:91–104, 1990.

8. Hirsch JD, Garrett KM, Beer B: Heterogeneity of benzodiazepine binding sites: A review of recent research. Pharmacol Biochem Behav 23:681–685, 1985.

9. Evans SM, Funderburk FR, Griffiths RR: Zolpidem and triazolam in humans: Behavioral and subjective effects and abuse liability. J Pharmacol Exp Ther 255:1246–1255, 1990.

10.* Nutt DJ, Glue P, Lawson C: The neurochemistry of anxiety: An update. Prog Neuropsychopharmacol Biol Psychiatry 14:737–752, 1990.

11.* Charney DS, Krystal KH, Delgado PL, et al: Serotonin-specific drugs for anxiety and depressive disorders. Annu Rev Med 41:437–446, 1990.

12. Pigott TA, Pato MT, Bernstein SE, et al: Controlled comparisons of clomipramine and fluoxetine in the treatment of obsessive-compulsive disorder. Behavioral and biological results. Arch Gen Psychiatry 47:926–932, 1990.

13. Swerdlow NR, Andia AM: Trazodone-fluoxetine combination for treatment of obsessive-compulsive disorder [letter]. Am J Psychiatry 146:1637, 1989.

14. Liebowitz MR, Hollander E, Schneier F, et al: Fluoxetine treatment of obsessive-compulsive disorder: An open clinical trial. J Clin Psychopharmacol 9:423–427, 1989.

15. Jenike MA, Baer L, Greist JH: Clomipramine versus fluoxetine in obsessive-compulsive disorder: A retrospective comparison of side effects and efficacy. J Clin Psychopharmacol 10;122–124, 1990.

16. Murphy DL, Pato MT, Pigott TA: Obsessive-compulsive disorder: Treatment with serotonin-selective uptake inhibitors, azapirones, and other agents. J Clin Psychopharmacol 10:91S–100S, 1990.

17. Schneier FR, Liebowitz MR, Davies SO, et al: Fluoxetine in panic disorder. J Clin Psychopharmacol 10:119–121, 1990.

18. Brady K, Zarzar M, Lydiard RB: Fluoxetine in panic disorder patients with imipramine-associated weight gain. J Clin Psychopharmacol 9:66–67, 1989.

19. Sternbach H: Fluoxetine treatment of social phobia [letter]. J Clin Psychopharmacol 10:230–231, 1990.

20. Jenike MA, Hyman S, Baer L, et al: A controlled trial of fluvoxamine in obsessive-compulsive disorder: Implications for a serotonergic theory. Am J Psychiatry 147:1209–1215, 1990.

21. Den Boer J, Westenberg HG: Serotonin function in panic disorder: A double blind placebo controlled study with fluvoxamine and ritanserin. Psychopharmacology (Berlin) 102:85–94, 1990.

22. Chouinard G, Goodman W, Greist J, et al: Results of a double-blind placebo controlled trial of a new serotonin uptake inhibitor, sertraline, in the treatment of obsessive-compulsive disorder. Psychopharmacol Bull 26:279–284, 1990.

23. Price LH: Serotonin reuptake inhibitors in depression and anxiety. Ann Clin Psychiatry 2:165–172, 1990.

24. Marsden CA: The pharmacology of new anxiolytics acting on 5-HT neurones. Postgrad Med J 66:S2–S6, 1990.

25.* Eison MS: Serotonin: A common neurobiologic substrate for anxiety and depression. J Clin Psychopharmacol 10:26S–30S, 1990.

26. Petracca A, Nisita C, McNair D, et al: Treatment of generalized anxiety disorder: Preliminary clinical experience with buspirone. J Clin Psychiatry 51:31–39, 1990.

27. Strand M, Hetta J, Rosen A, et al: A double-blind, controlled trial in primary care patients with generalized anxiety: A comparison between buspirone and oxazepam. J Clin Psychiatry 51 (suppl):40–45 1990.

28. Markovitz PJ, Stagno SJ, Calabrese JR: Buspirone augmentation of fluoxetine in obsessive-compulsive disorder. Am J Psychiatry 147:798–800, 1990.

29. Munjack DJ, Bruns J, Baltazar PL, et al: A pilot study of buspirone in the treatment of social phobia. J Anxiety Disord 5:87–98, 1991.

30. Rickels K, Amsterdam J, Clary C, et al: Buspirone in depressed outpatients: A controlled study. Psychopharmacol Bull 26:163–167, 1990.

31. Robinson DS, Shrotriya RC, Alms DR, et al: Treatment of panic disorder: Nonbenzodiazepine anxiolytics, including buspirone. Psychopharmacol Bull 25:21–26, 1989.

32. Csanalosi I, Schweizer E, Case WG, et al: Gepirone in anxiety: A pilot study. J Clin Psychopharmacol 7:31–33, 1987.

33. Borison RL, Albrecht JW, Diamond BI: Efficacy and safety of a putative anxiolytic agent: Ipsapirone. Psychopharmacol Bull 26:207–210, 1990.

34. Schweizer E, Rickels K, Csanalosi I, et al: A placebo-controlled study of enciprazine in the treatment of generalized anxiety disorder: A preliminary report. Psychopharmacol Bull 26:215–217, 1990.

35. Heller AH, Beneke M, Kuemmel B, et al: Ipsapirone: Evidence for efficacy in depression. Psychopharmacol Bull 26:219–222, 1990.

36. Rausch JL, Ruegg R, Moeller FG: Gepirone as a 5-HT$_{1a}$ agonist in the treatment of major depression. Psychopharmacol Bull 26:169–171, 1990.

37. Chopin P, Briley M: Animal models of anxiety: The effect of compounds that modify 5-HT neurotransmission. Trends Pharmacol Sci 8:383–388, 1987.

38. Bressa GM, Marini S, Gregori S: Serotonin S2 receptor blockage and generalized anxiety disorders. A double-blind study on ritanserin and lorazepam. Int J Clin Pharmacol Res 7:111–119, 1987.

39. Griez E, Pols H, Lousberg H: Serotonin antagonism in panic disorder: An open trial with ritanserin. Acta Psychiatr Belg 88:372–377, 1988.

40. Westenberg GM, den Boer JA: Serotonin-influencing drugs in the treatment of panic disorder. Psychopathology 22:68–77, 1989.

41. Nappi G, Sandrini G, Granella F, et al: A new 5-HT$_2$ antagonist (ritanserin) in the treatment of chronic headache with depression. A double-blind study vs amitriptyline. Headache 30:439–444, 1990.

42. Adam K, Oswald I: Effects of repeated ritanserin on middle-

* Good general reference.

43. Altamura AC, Mauri MC, Rudas N, et al: Clinical activity and tolerability of trazodone, mianserin, and amitriptyline in elderly subjects with major depression: A controlled multicenter trial. Clin Neuropharmacol 12(suppl):25–37, 1989.
44. Mertens C, Pintens H: A double-blind, multicentre study of paroxetine and mianserin in depression. Acta Psychiatr Scand 350 (suppl): 140, 1989.
45. Feighner JP, Pambakian R, Fowler RC, et al: A comparison of nefazodone, imipramine, and placebo in patients with moderate to severe depression. Psychopharmacol Bull 25:219–221, 1989.
46. Gannon R, DeFusco P: Focus on ondansetron: An antiemetic with a unique mechanism of action. Hosp Formul 25:1209–1217, 1990.
47. Jones BJ, Costall B, Domeney AM, et al: The potential anxiolytic activity of GR38032F, a 5-HT$_3$-receptor antagonist. Br J Pharmacol 93:985–993, 1988.
48. Schweizer E, Weise C, Clary C, et al: Placebo-controlled trial of venlafaxine for the treatment of major depression. J Clin Psychopharmacol 11:233–236, 1991.
49. Khan A, Fabre LF, Rudolph R: Venlafaxine in depressed out patients. Psychopharmacol Bull 27:141–144, 1991.
50. Zajecka JM, Fawcett J, and Guy C: Coexisting major depression and obsessive compulsive disorder treated with venlafaxine. J Clin Psychopharmacol 10:152–153, 1990.
51.* Lydiard RB, Ballenger JC: Antidepressants in panic disorder and agoraphobia. J Affective Disord 13:153–168, 1987.
52. Sheehan DV, Ballenger JC, Jacobson G: Treatment of endogenous anxiety with phobic, hysterical, and hypochondriacal symptoms. Arch Gen Psychiatry 37:51–59, 1980.
53. Liebowitz MR, Fyer AJ, Gorman JM, et al: Phenelzine in social phobia. J Clin Psychopharmacol 6:93–98, 1986.
54. Korn A, Da PM, Raffesberg W, et al: Tyramine pressor effect in man: Studies with moclobemide, a novel, reversible monoamine oxidase inhibitor. J Neural Transm [Suppl] 26:57–71, 1988.
55. Stabl M, Biziere K, Schmid-Burgk W, et al: Review of comparative clinical trials. Moclobemide vs tricyclic antidepressants and vs placebo in depressive states. J Neural Transm [Suppl] 28:77–89, 1989.
56. Redmond DJ: The possible role of locus coeruleus noradrenergic activity in anxiety-panic. Clin Neuropharmacol 9:40–42, 1986.
57. Uhde TW, Stein MB, Vittone BJ, et al: Behavioral and physiological effects of short-term and long-term administration of clonidine in panic disorder. Arch Gen Psychiatry 46:170–177, 1989.
58. Smith WT, Glaudin V, Panagides J, et al: Mirtazapine vs. amitriptyline vs. placebo in the treatment of major depressive disorder. Psychopharmacol Bull 26:191–196, 1990.

88

FUTURE DIRECTIONS IN ANTIPSYCHOTIC DRUG TREATMENT

WILLIAM C. WIRSHING, M.D., STEPHEN R. MARDER, M.D., and THEODORE VAN PUTTEN, M.D.

The introduction of clozapine in 1990 represented an important milestone in the drug treatment of schizophrenia. Prior to this, all neuroleptic drugs were considered to be equally effective and all of them were associated with serious neurological side effects. Clozapine, in contrast, has been demonstrated to be more effective than conventional neuroleptics in studies of severely ill, treatment-refractory patients.[1] Moreover, clozapine is associated with negligible extrapyramidal symptoms (EPS) and has substantially less risk for tardive dyskinesia. Unfortunately, the relatively high rate of agranulocytosis with clozapine and the resultant requirement for frequent and costly complete blood cell counts will significantly limit its clinical use.

The advantages of clozapine—superior efficacy and reduced neurological side effects—have inspired an intense search for other antipsychotic drugs that have these same properties. A number of new strategies for developing antipsychotic drugs have been devised, and these have led to preclinical and clinical studies of several new compounds that have been designated as "atypical" or "clozapine-like" neuroleptics. At this point in time it is unclear which of these compounds will come to market. Nevertheless, it is safe to predict that, in the next several years, the drug treatment of schizophrenia will change substantially. This chapter reviews a number of new drugs that are being studied for schizophrenia as well as the putative biological mechanisms underlying their actions. Particular attention is devoted to the clinical use of clozapine, which is already available, and risperidone and remoxipride, which are likely to become available in the near future.

PUTATIVE MECHANISMS OF ACTION OF THE ATYPICAL NEUROLEPTICS

In the early 1960s it was noted that the conventional antipsychotic agents haloperidol and chlorpromazine increased the metabolites of dopamine in rat brains. This observation led to the speculation that the therapeutic efficacy of these drugs was mediated by blockade of dopamine receptors. The so-called dopamine theory of schizophrenia soon followed, and it remains among the most tested and enduring of all pathophysiological theories in biological psychiatry. The theory holds that schizophrenic symptomatology—particularly the positive psychotic symptoms such as auditory hallucinations, delusions, and conceptual disorganization—result from a hyperdopaminergic state in the limbic regions of the brain (e.g., nucleus accumbens, hippocampus, entorhinal cortex, and frontal lobe). While far from comprehensive, this theory has accurately predicted that the efficacy of antipsychotic compounds would be related to their ability to block dopamine. In fact, every agent, except clozapine, that has clearly and consistently demonstrated antipsychotic effect in humans blocks D_2 receptors (a particular subclass of dopamine receptors that is not adenylate cyclase linked) in direct proportion to its clinical potency (Fig. 88–1). Unfortunately, all conventional antipsychotic agents also block D_2 receptors in the striatum (caudate nucleus and putamen), and this results in a number of untoward EPS (e.g., parkinsonism, akathisia, dystonia, and tardive dyskinesia). Atypical agents, in contrast, are by definition antipsychotic but have little if any EPS liability.

A number of preclinical paradigms have been used to screen potential compounds for "atypical" activity. In the rat model, for example, inhibition of conditioned responses and apomorphine-induced hyperactivity is associated with antipsychotic efficacy in humans. Inhibition of oral stereotypies and the induction of catalepsy is believed to be due to blockade of striatal dopamine and consistently predicts EPS liability in humans. In general, atypical agents inhibit stereotypies and induce catalepsy only at three to ten times the dose necessary to inhibit hyperactivity.

The precise neurochemical mechanism responsible for these atypical properties is unknown. Schematic representations of the structures of some of the

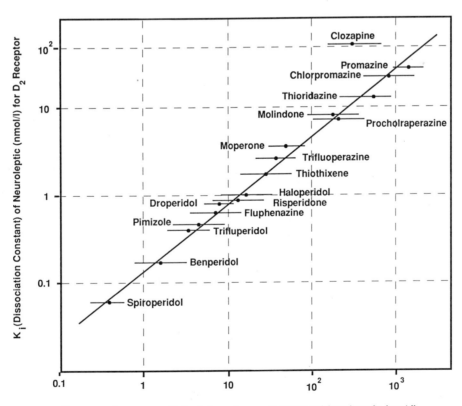

Range and average clinical dose for controlling schizophrenia (mg/d)

Figure 88–1. The dissociation constants for the D_2 receptor (ordinate) for various neuroleptics versus the range of clinical dosing used to treat schizophrenic patients (abscissa). (Adapted with permission from Seeman P, Lee T, Chau-Wong M, et al: Antipsychotic drug doses and neuroleptic/dopamine receptors. Nature 261:717–719, 1976.)

atypical and conventional compounds are shown in Figure 88–2. Some believe that differential affinity for striatal and limbic D_2 receptors could explain the activity of the atypicals. This has not, however, been convincingly demonstrated for any compound.[2]

Another theory is that some combination of receptor affinities underlies the atypical activity (Fig. 88–3). Clozapine, for example, blocks muscarinic receptors 20 to 50 times more potently than it blocks D_2 receptors. This simultaneous anticholinergic activity might counteract the striatal D_2 blockade. Likewise, clozapine blocks serotonin receptors (S_2) ten times more potently than does D_2. Because S_2 blockade by cyproheptadine or mianserin antagonizes the catalepsy of conventional neuroleptics,[3] this property, too, might explain clozapine's low EPS potential. Because serotonin is known to have an inhibitory effect on mesocortical dopamine neurons, S_2 blockade in this area would result in disinhibition and lead to enhanced dopamine function in the frontal lobes (the putative neuroanatomical locus of negative symptoms). Thus, clozapine's S_2 blockade might account for its apparent superior efficacy in the treatment of the negative symptoms.[1] Other receptors that have been implicated are the sigma opiate and N-methyl-D-aspartate glutamate receptors, but the data supporting a role for these receptors are scanty.

Endogenous dopamine can displace a drug from the D_2 receptor and thereby counteract its pharmacological effect.[4] Striatal concentration of dopamine is thought to be much higher than the concentration in limbic and prefrontal cortical areas.[5,6] The relatively weak D_2 affinity of some atypicals (e.g., clozapine and remoxipride) may allow them to be partially displaced in the striatum and give them the appearance of acting preferentially in the limbic areas. Such an explanation, though, would seem equally applicable to chlorpromazine—a conventional neuroleptic notorious for its EPS effects.

Finally, it has been reasoned that the atypical agents may in part act through the various linkages that are known to exist between some receptor subtypes. For example, D_1 receptors (a subclass of dopamine receptors that is linked to adenylate cyclase) can have either a facilitating or an augmenting effect on those D_2 receptors to which they are linked. This link clearly exists in the striatum but appears to be lacking between D_1 and D_2 receptors in the limbic forebrain (nucleus accumbens and olfactory tubercle).[7] Thus, it is conceivable that an atypical agent might, through its effect on striatal D_1 receptors, cause facilitation of linked D_2 receptors. This would result, then, in striatal D_2 receptors being relatively unblocked compared to their unlinked limbic counterparts (i.e., antipsychotic effect without EPS). There is little solid evidence, though, to support this hypothesis.

In summary, while many speculations have been advanced to explain the mechanism of action of the

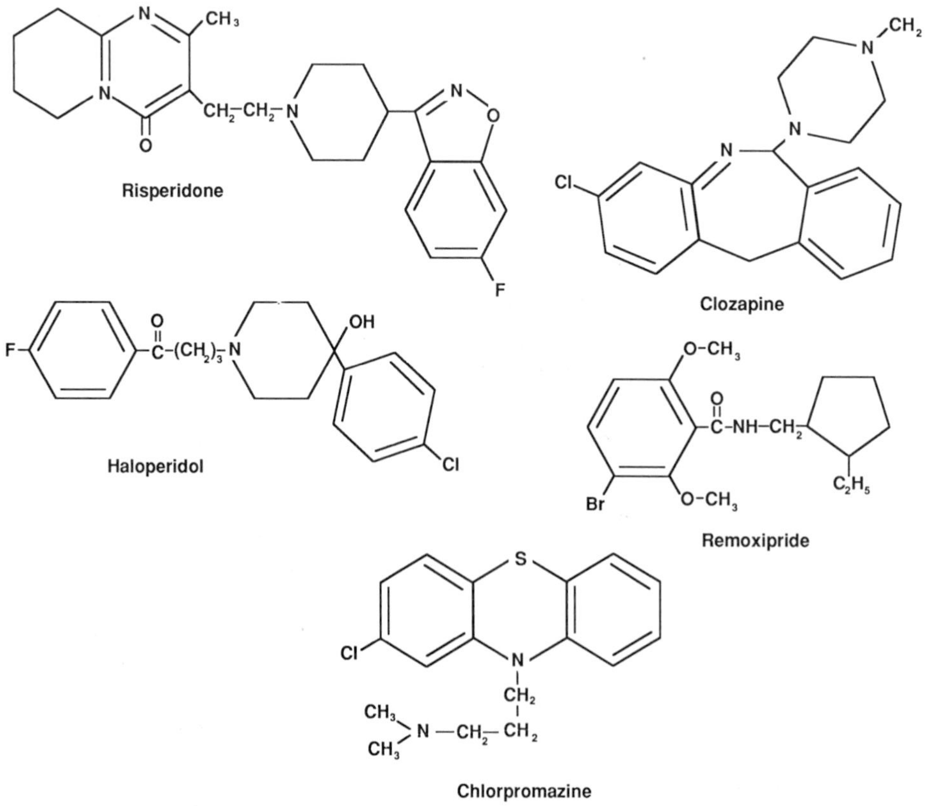

Figure 88–2. Schematic molecular structure for various atypical and conventional neuroleptic compounds.

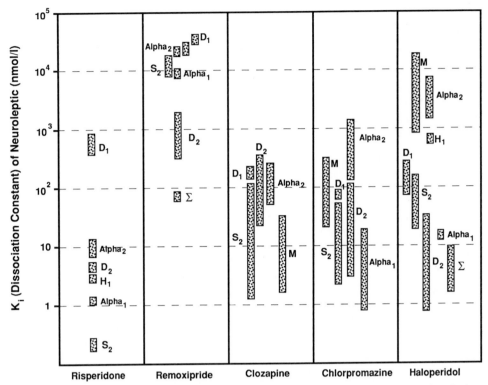

Figure 88–3. Dissociation constants for various neuroleptics at various receptors as reported in the literature. (Adapted with permission from Seeman P: Atypical neuroleptics: Role of multiple receptors, endogenous dopamine, and receptor linkage. Acta Psychiatr Scand (suppl) 358:14–20, 1990.)

atypical agents, none encompasses all of the available clinical and basic science data and all await further testing in both the laboratory and the clinic.

CLOZAPINE

The first atypical neuroleptic, clozapine, was introduced into clinical studies during the early 1970s. These early clinical trials indicated that the drug was highly effective and associated with negligible EPS. However, the early hopes that clozapine would significantly improve the treatment of schizophrenia were dashed when it was discovered that the drug was associated with a relatively high rate (1 to 2 per cent during the first year of exposure) of agranulocytosis. In 1975 it was reported that granulocytopenia developed in 16 patients in Finland, with agranulocytosis developing in 13. Eight patients died from secondary infection. As a result of these and other reports, the drug was removed from the market in most countries and clinical research on clozapine was stopped.

However, the agranulocytosis that developed with clozapine turned out to be reversible if the offending drug was discontinued. This finding allowed a series of studies in which clozapine was administered with careful monitoring of patients for agranulocytosis. In two European trials,[8,9] clozapine was found to be superior to chlorpromazine and haloperidol for patients with severe schizophrenic illnesses.

These findings led to a large multicenter trial[1] in the United States that was designed with consultation from the Food and Drug Administration. Patients selected for the study (N = 268) were individuals who remained severely psychotic despite prior trials with at least three conventional neuroleptics. Furthermore, these patients also failed to respond to a 6-week prospective, single-blind trial of haloperidol. These patients were then randomly assigned to 6 weeks of treatment with chlorpromazine plus benztropine mesylate or clozapine with a benztropine mesylate placebo. The results establish that, in a 6-week trial, clozapine is more effective than a conventional neuroleptic, chlorpromazine, in a group of treatment-resistant schizophrenic patients. The improvement in patients assigned to clozapine was consistent over the entire spectrum of positive and negative schizophrenic symptomatology. Among patients who were classified as having "improved" (by prospective criteria) to a clinically significant extent, 30 per cent of clozapine-treated patients improved versus only 4 per cent of chlorpromazine/benztropine-treated patients (p < .001).

The results from the Kane et al.[1] study probably underestimate the effectiveness of clozapine. The advantage of clozapine over chlorpromazine appeared to be growing at the end of the 6-week trial, suggesting that substantially more than 30 per cent of refractory patients would improve if they were treated with clozapine for longer than 6 weeks. Unfortunately, there are few data available from controlled trials to indicate the proportion of patients who will improve during a longer trial. In an uncontrolled study, Meltzer[10] reported that 70 per cent of clozapine-treated patients improved during 1 year of treatment. This suggests that an adequate trial of clozapine should last considerably longer than 6 weeks, perhaps 6 months to 1 year.

Clinicians who manage patients with clozapine will notice a range of clinical responses. In some cases, the improvements in both positive and negative symptoms will result in striking changes, with patients who appeared hopelessly lost in a psychotic world emerging as individuals who can be discharged from hospitals or participate meaningfully in rehabilitation programs. Other clozapine "responders" may not improve substantially in their positive symptoms, but will report that their mood and sense of well-being are much improved. For these individuals, the deficits associated with schizophrenia may not improve, but the quality of life is better.

Which Patients Should Receive Clozapine

The available data suggest that the patients who are most likely to benefit from clozapine treatment are those who have schizophrenic illnesses with severe positive symptoms such as hallucinations, delusions, and thought disturbances that are poorly responsive to conventional neuroleptic medications.[11] Clozapine is also a reasonable choice for patients who may have neuroleptic-responsive illnesses but suffer from severe EPS at drug doses that are needed to control the illness. As a result, the akathisia, parkinsonism, or other EPS may make the cure worse than the disease. Since clozapine has negligible EPS liability, many of these patients will feel considerably better.

Patients with severe tardive dyskinesia may also be candidates for clozapine treatment. A number of studies indicate that clozapine is associated with a substantially lower risk for tardive dyskinesia when compared with typical neuroleptics. Whether or not there is any risk at all associated with clozapine treatment will need to await further study. There is some indication that clozapine has direct effects in alleviating the abnormal movements that comprise tardive dyskinesia, and may be particularly effective in treating tardive dystonias. Therefore, clozapine represents a reasonable treatment alternative for patients who suffer from severe tardive dyskinesia since it will not promote the progression of the disorder and may decrease its severity. It is probably not a good alternative for the large population of patients who will do well on conventional neuroleptic medications and who have relatively mild movement disorders. This is because the usual course for tardive dyskinesia in the younger patient is one of decreasing severity over time even if neuroleptics are continued.

Monitoring For Agranulocytosis

Recent data indicate that the cumulative incidence of agranulocytosis with clozapine is approximately 1.6 per cent following 1 year of treatment.[1] This represents a substantial risk given that agranulocytosis can result in fatal infections if the disorder is not diagnosed early. Although the risk of agranulocytosis is greatest during the first 4 to 10 weeks of treatment, patients have developed agranulocytosis after more than 5 years of clozapine treatment.

Current guidelines for clozapine treatment require that a complete blood count be obtained weekly and repeated whenever the total white blood cell (WBC) count falls below 3500 per cu mm or if there is a substantial drop in WBCs. The drug should be discontinued if the WBCs drop below 3000 and the granulocyte count is below 1500. At that time, patients should be carefully monitored for evidence of infections. If the WBC and granulocyte counts rise above these levels, clozapine treatment may be resumed. However, if the WBCs drop below 2000 and the granulocyte count below 1000, patients should be carefully monitored by a hematologist and perhaps a specialist in infectious disease. Bone marrow aspiration and isolation should be seriously considered for these patients. Moreover, these individuals should not be rechallenged with clozapine.

Initiating Treatment with Clozapine

Clozapine should be started at a dose of 25 to 50 mg and gradually increased by 25 mg every 1 or 2 days until patients are receiving 300 mg daily. Because of the drug's side effects, particularly sedation and orthostatic hypotension, even this titration schedule may be too rapid for some. Since it may take some patients weeks to reach a therapeutic dose, it is reasonable to maintain most patients on their conventional neuroleptic until they have reached a therapeutic clozapine dose. Although the current practice in the United States is to treat most patients with 300 to 600 mg of clozapine daily, doses in the 200- to 300-mg range are commonly used in Europe. Patients who fail to respond may have their dose increased to 900 mg. This should be done cautiously since the risk of seizures with clozapine increases at doses above 600 mg.

Clozapine Side Effects

The most common side effect of clozapine is sedation. In our experience sedation is usually the limiting factor controlling both the rate at which the dose of clozapine can be increased and the maximum dose the patient can tolerate. Other commonly reported side effects include orthostatic hypotension, tachycardia, fever, constipation, nausea, vomiting, and sialorrhea. Clozapine has a higher likelihood of causing seizures than other neuroleptics, particularly at doses greater than 600 mg daily. Although this array of side-effects—along with the management of the risk for agranulocytosis—makes the treatment of patients with clozapine complex, it is common for patients to report a sense of relief from the dysphoric moods they reported on conventional drugs.

SULPIRIDE

Sulpiride—along with raclopride, remoxipride, and amisulpiride—is a member of the substituted benzamide group of neuroleptics. These four drugs have selective affinity for D_2 receptors, minimal D_1 activity, antipsychotic activity, and reduced EPS. Moreover, these drugs are relatively free of other troublesome side effects such as sedation and orthostatic hypotension. It has been suggested that the substituted benzamides, particularly sulpiride, may be associated with a reduced risk of tardive dyskinesia.[12] However, this theoretical claim has not yet been supported by adequate clinical studies.[13]

Sulpiride is the oldest and most studied drug of the substituted benzamides. Since this drug does not readily cross the blood-brain barrier, it is administered in relatively high doses (800 to 2300 mg daily). This results in the drug causing substantial elevations in plasma prolactin concentrations that can cause galactorrhea and amenorrhea in women and erectile incompetence, gynecomastia, or decreased libido in men.

In a number of double-blind studies (reviewed by Tamminga and Gerlach[13]), sulpiride was found to have antipsychotic efficacy comparable to conventional neuroleptics, including chlorpromazine, haloperidol, and trifluoperazine. Although sulpiride had less EPS in most reports, some patients receiving this drug developed parkinsonism and akathisia.[14]

REMOXIPRIDE

Remoxipride is likely to be the first benzamide to reach the market in the United States (see Fig. 88–2 for structure schematic). Since it more readily passes the blood-brain barrier than sulpiride, it can be administered in doses that are less likely to cause endocrinological dysfunction (150 to 600 mg daily). Otherwise, remoxipride shares sulpiride's property of providing antipsychotic activity with substantially fewer EPS than conventional neuroleptics.

The clinical activity of remoxipride has been demonstrated in nine different double-blind comparisons with haloperidol (reviewed by Lewander et al.[15]). These studies reveal a number of important guidelines for using the drug. A dose ranging study that used a low dose of 30 to 90 mg daily[16] found that this dose was less effective than a middle dose range of 120 to 240 mg or a high dose range of 300 to 600

mg. In contrast, a trial that used a dose of 100 to 300 mg daily[17] found that this dose was as effective as 10 to 30 mg daily of haloperidol and 200 to 600 mg daily of remoxipride. This suggests that the effective dose range of remoxipride has its lower limits at approximately 100 mg.

Lewander et al.'s review[15] revealed that the antipsychotic effectiveness of remoxipride and haloperidol were equal, although there were differences favoring haloperidol for positive symptoms such as suspiciousness and unusual thought content and remoxipride for negative symptoms such as motor retardation and blunted affect. Remoxipride had substantially fewer EPS than haloperidol in all of the trials. When the studies were summed, 20 per cent of remoxipride patients required antiparkinsonian medications compared to 51 per cent on haloperidol. Moreover, remoxipride was not associated with substantial amounts of sedation or cardiovascular side effects. This indicates that remoxipride is not a drug like thioridazine or chlorpromazine, which accomplish their low incidence of EPS through their relatively potent antimuscarinic properties (see Fig. 88–3) that in turn cause sedation, orthostatic hypotension, and anticholinergic effects.

In summary, remoxipride does appear to qualify as an effective atypical neuroleptic. At doses above 100 mg it combines antipsychotic activity with relatively few EPS or other side effects. Presently, there are a number of important questions that remain unanswered, including whether it has superior efficacy in any psychotic population and whether it has a lower tardive dyskinesia liability than conventional neuroleptics.

RISPERIDONE

Risperidone is a benzisoxizole derivative (see Fig. 88–2 for structure schematic) that is pharmacologically characterized by potent central antagonism of both serotonin (type 2 subclass; S_2) and D_2 receptors (Fig. 88–3). It has also demonstrated substantial antagonism of α_1, α_2, and histamine receptors. Preclinical animal experimentation has indicated that while it is 1.5 to 3.5 times as potent as haloperidol at D_2 antagonism, risperidone is several times less potent than haloperidol at inducing catalepsy.[18] Taken together, these data would predict that risperidone would have antipsychotic efficacy and reduced EPS liability in humans. The potent S_2 antagonism might theoretically be of utility in ameliorating the negative symptoms of schizophrenia, mirroring clozapine's enhanced efficacy in this spectrum of symptoms. The animal studies have also shown that risperidone readily elevates plasma prolactin and causes tachycardia and hypotension (presumably through its effects on D_2 and α-adrenergic receptors). These data suggest that it may have significant endocrinological and some cardiovascular liability in humans.

In Phase I trials (safety and pharmacology in healthy human volunteers) risperidone did cause tachycardia (average increase of 40 beats/min at 3-mg dose) and hypotension (average systolic drop of 20 mm at 3-mg dose) and a dose-dependent increase in plasma prolactin (up to five times the baseline). Other untoward effects included tiredness, headache, and dizziness at doses of 0.5 to 3 mg; it was otherwise well tolerated.

The short- and long-term open label studies with 5 to 25 mg/day of risperidone in chronically psychotic patients (over 2000 total subjects) have generally found antipsychotic efficacy and a low incidence of adverse intercurrent events (only 15 subjects had to discontinue the medication because of adverse experiences).

The double-blind studies (total of 260 subjects) have compared risperidone to haloperidol in the short-term treatment of psychotic patients. These studies indicated that risperidone has shown a trend toward superior antipsychotic efficacy,[19] has lower EPS liability (the consumption of antiparkinsonian medication was 10 times greater in the haloperidol group), fewer dropouts (20 per cent in the haloperidol group versus 5 per cent in the risperidone group), and an equivalent number of treatment-emergent adverse events. The average dose of risperidone in these double-blind studies ranged from 5 to 15 mg/day.

While more research is necessary, one would predict that risperidone will come into general use and prove itself to be well tolerated, relatively lacking in neurological toxicity, and free of serious adverse side effects.

OTHER POTENTIAL ATYPICAL AGENTS

There are literally dozens of compounds that have been synthesized and are currently undergoing testing for atypical activity. Among these agents are unusual D_2 blockers that cause little or no catalepsy (e.g., fluperlapine, melperone, and tefludazine); dopamine autoreceptor agonists [e.g., 3-(3-hydroxyphenyl)-N-n-propylpiperidine (3-PPP)]; partial dopamine agonists (e.g., HDC-912); selective D_1 antagonists (e.g., Sch 23390, Sch 39166); and selective S_2 antagonists (e.g., ritanserin). The road to ultimate clinical use, however, is long and difficult, and the vast majority of these agents will never be available to the average patient or clinician. The intensity of the current search, the great numbers of compounds being tested, and the realization in clozapine that such agents do exist would all predict that at least some of these drugs will see routine clinical use.

SUMMARY

The pharmacological treatment of the schizophrenic patient has remained substantively un-changed during the last 35 years. Conventional neuroleptics—the mainstay of antipsychotic treatment—have proven to be only partially effective, and their untoward side effects have led to notorious patient noncompliance and iatrogenic morbidity. However, the demonstration that clozapine possesses both increased efficacy and reduced neurotoxicity has forever altered the conventional wisdom that held all neuroleptics to be equally efficacious and uniformly neurotoxic. The pharmacological legacy of clozapine promises to provide clinicians with biological therapies that are at once safe, effective, and easy to administer. Likely early contenders for this role are remoxipride and risperidone.

ACKNOWLEDGMENTS

We are grateful to the Department of Veterans Affairs, the National Institute of Mental Health, and the National Alliance for Research on Schizophrenia and Depression for their continuing support of our research.

REFERENCES

1. Kane JM, Honigfeld G, Singer J, et al: Clozapine for the treatment-resistant schizophrenic: A double-blind comparison versus chlorpromazine/benztropine. Arch Gen Psychiatry 45:789–796, 1988.
2. Seeman P: Atypical neuroleptics: Role of multiple receptors, endogenous dopamine, and receptor linkage. Acta Psychiatr Scand (suppl) 358:14–20, 1990.
3. Costall B, Fortune DH, Naylor RJ, et al: Serotonergic involvement with neuroleptic catalepsy. Neuropharmacology 14:859–868, 1975.
4. Seeman P, Guan H-C, Niznik HB: Endogenous dopamine lowers the dopamine D_2 receptor density as measured by [^{3}H]raclopride: Implications for positron emission tomography of the human brain. Synapse 3:96–97, 1989.
5. Bowers MB Jr: Homovanillic acid in caudate and prefrontal cortex following neuroleptics. Eur J Pharmacol 99:103–105, 1984.
6. Anden N-E, Stock G: Effect of clozapine on the turnover of dopamine in the corpus striatum and in the limbic system. J Pharm Pharmacol 25:346–348, 1973.
7. Kelly E, Nahorski SR: Dopamine D_2-receptors inhibit D_1-stimulated cyclic AMP accumulation in striatum but not limbic forebrain. Naunyn-Schmiedebergs Arch Pharmacol 335:508–512, 1987.
8. Fischer-Cornelssen KA, Ferner UJ: An example of European multicenter trials: Multispectral analysis of clozapine. Psychopharmacol Bull 12:34–39, 1976.
9. Honigfeld G, Patin J, Singer J: Clozapine: Antipsychotic activity in treatment-resistant schizophrenics. Adv Ther 1:77–97, 1984.
10. Meltzer HY: Duration of a clozapine trial in neuroleptic-resistant schizophrenia. Arch Gen Psychiatry 46:672, 1989.
11. Marder SR, Van Putten T: Who should receive clozapine? Arch Gen Psychiatry 45:865–867, 1988.
12. Schwartz M, Moguillansky L, Lanyi G, et al: Sulpiride in tardive dyskinesia. J Neurol Neurosurg Psychiatry 53:800–802, 1990.
13. Tamminga CA, Gerlach J: New neuroleptics and experimental antipsychotics in schizophrenia. In Meltzer HY, ed. Psychopharmacology: The Third Generation of Progress. New York; Raven Press, 1987:1129–1140.
14. Gerlach J, Behnke K, Heltberg J, et al: Sulpiride and haloperi-

dol in schizophrenia: A double-blind cross-over study of therapeutic effect, side effects and plasma concentrations. Br J Psychiatry 147:283–288, 1985.

15. Lewander T, Westerbergh SE, Morrison D: Clinical profile of remoxipride—a combined analysis of a comparative double-blind multicenter trial programme. Acta Psychiatr Scand [Suppl] 358:92–98, 1990.

16. Lapierre YD, Nair NPV, Chouinard G, et al: A controlled dose-ranging study of remoxipride and haloperidol in schizophrenia: A Canadian multicentre trial. Acta Psychiatr Scand (suppl) 358:72–76, 1990.

17. Patris M, Agussol P, Alby JM, et al: A double-blind multicen-

tre comparison of remoxipride, at two dose levels, and haloperidol. Acta Psychiatr Scand (suppl) 358:78–82, 1990.

18. Janssen PAJ, Niemegeers CJE, Awouters F, et al: Risperidone (R 64 766), a new antipsychotic with serotonin-S_2 and dopamine-D_2 antagonist properties. J Pharmacol Exp Ther 244:685–693, 1988.

19. Meibach RC: Risperidone: Combined serotonin and dopamine receptor antagonism in the treatment of schizophrenia. In American College of Neuropsychopharmacology Abstracts of Panels and Posters, 29th Annual Meeting, December 10–14, 1990:79.

FUTURE PSYCHOPHARMACOLOGY FOR THE AGING PATIENT:
Treatment of Alzheimer's Disease

ALAN F. SCHATZBERG, M.D.

In recent years, Alzheimer's disease (AD) has become a major public health problem, in part reflecting growth in the elderly population in this country. Much research has been expended in defining the biological characteristics of AD, and considerable data have emerged that point to a major dysfunction in acetylcholine activity.[1,2] However, abnormalities involving several other neurotransmitter systems (e.g., dopamine and norepinephrine) have also been reported, and AD has come to be viewed as a complex cognitive-behavioral disorder or group of disorders.

Basic research has resulted not only in hypotheses regarding etiology but also in strategies for enhancing cognitive performance in AD patients. These have often proved of limited efficacy, although a number of approaches still hold promise, particularly for individual patients. Some of the approaches have been designed to increase activity of one or more neurotransmitters (e.g., acetylcholine). Others have been aimed at increasing general neuronal activity (e.g., oxiracetam). Still others have been based on attempts to increase blood supply to key brain regions (e.g., ergoloid mesylate or nimodipine); to decrease neurotoxicity due to calcium influx (nimodipine); to increase membrane fluidity (S-adenosyl-L-methionine); to increase memory by using peptide (e.g., vasopressin) analogues; or to decrease the neu-

rotoxic effects of free radicals (*Ginkgo biloba*). In this chapter, we review recent studies on the treatment of cognitive dysfunction in AD, with particular emphasis on possible future strategies. A large number of compounds are currently under study; however, because of space limitations, this chapter emphasizes only a representative sample of major approaches.

CHOLINERGIC AGENTS

Acetylcholine (ACh) plays a role in cognition and memory. Anticholinergic agents appear to cause confusion and memory impairment, and ACh activity in the nucleus basalis has been reported to be decreased in the brains of AD patients. Procholinergic agents, such as the cholinesterase inhibitor physostigmine, have been reported to increase cognitive performance in healthy controls. For all of these reasons, psychopharmacologists have attempted to treat AD patients by increasing central ACh activity.

Cholinesterase Inhibitors

One major approach to enhancing ACh activity has involved using agents that primarily inhibit the catabolic enzyme cholinesterase. In this regard, a shorter acting compound, physostigmine, has been tested, as has a longer acting compound, tetrahydroaminocridine. Two recent reports indicate that physostigmine has little effect on altering symptoms of AD. In one study, Jenike and colleagues[3] reported on 23 patients who were hospitalized in a general clinical research center. After determining the dose that produced maximum efficacy (dose-finding phase), patients were randomly assigned to receive either placebo or physostigmine, on a double-blind basis, for 1 week, at which point they were crossed over to the other "treatment" for an additional 7 days. Significant group differences were not observed between physostigmine and placebo on a number of neuropsychological measures.

In a study by Harrell et al.,[4] long-term physostigmine treatment was assessed in 20 AD patients. In this study, patients participated in a dose-finding study followed by a 2-week crossover design in which patients were randomly assigned to placebo or drug for 2 weeks each. Patients were rated as either physostigmine responders or nonresponders. Thereafter, patients were allowed to continue for rather extensive periods (mean ± S.D. time on drug for responders was 36 ± 5 months). A further crossover occurred at 18 months in which patients received drug or placebo for 2 weeks each. There was some suggestion that long-term physostigmine administration resulted in behavioral improvement in some patients, but meaningful changes overall in neuropsychological performance were not observed.

Since a major limitation of physostigmine revolves around its having a very short half-life, investigators have explored longer acting compounds. One, tetrahydroaminocridine or tacrine (THA), has received a great deal of attention in recent years since Summers and colleagues initially reported it to be effective in 17 patients with moderate to severe AD.[5] This report has spurred a great deal of heated debate not only about the methods used in the original report but also about the decision of the prestigious New England Journal of Medicine to publish an enthusiastic accompanying editorial.[6–8] The roller coaster hopes and disappointments of AD patients and their families regarding THA over the past 4 to 5 years have been unfortunate, but not unheard of for many proposed treatments for diseases without effective therapies.

A recent Canadian multicenter study[9] has explored the use of a THA-lecithin combination in intermediate-stage AD patients. In this study, the patient's maximum tolerated THA dose (up to 100 mg/day) was determined during an initial 8-week period. This was followed by a random assignment to 8 weeks of treatment with either THA or placebo with a subsequent crossover to the other treatment for an additional 8 weeks. Thirty-nine patients completed the double-blind phase. Although the Mini-Mental State scores were mildly (but significantly) improved after THA, the investigators concluded that THA failed to result in significant clinical im-

provement overall. Seventeen per cent of patients demonstrated elevations in liver transaminase levels to three times the upper limit of normal.

In another study, Molloy et al.[10] reported on a randomized double-blind crossover study of THA versus placebo. After a dose-finding study, patients received their optimal THA dose for two 3-week periods or placebo for one 3-week period. Ordering was assigned in a random fashion. Maximum THA dose was 100 mg/day. Thirty-four patients entered the study, of whom 22 completed the trial. In these 22 patients, THA failed to produce clinically or statistically significant effects on overall functional status, cognition, or behavior. A subgroup of THA responders was not identified. Fourteen of the 34 patients (41 per cent) experienced liver toxicity. The authors concluded that THA had little in the way of positive effects for AD patients but did exert considerable negative effects.

In the early study of Summers et al.,[5] a higher maximum dose of THA was used (200 mg/day) than has been used in the more recent studies, which, because of the risk of hepatotoxicity, have employed lower maximum daily doses (e.g., 100 mg/day). Of note, recent reports[8] have questioned the relative paucity of hepatotoxicity in the 1986 study by Summers et al.[5] Even though higher doses may increase THA efficacy in AD, hepatotoxicity may result in a relatively poor risk-benefit ratio vis-à-vis wide scale clinical application. Data from larger scale, multicenter studies on THA are currently being analyzed and should shed great light on the debate about the efficacy and safety of this compound.

Cholinergic Agonists

Another strategy for enhancing cholinergic activity has involved direct cholinergic agonists. Generally speaking, these strategies have also yielded little in the way of positive results. In one recent study, Tariot and colleagues[11] reported on 12 AD patients who received 1 mg, 2 mg, and 4 mg/hr infusions of arecoline or placebo. Each treatment was administered on a separate day at least 48 hours apart. Significant improvement was not observed in the vast majority of cognitive, memory, and learning tests, although a slight improvement in word finding and picture recognition was observed at lower doses. Dose-related behavioral effects were observed, with lower doses producing some degree of increased motor activity but higher doses causing psychomotor retardation.

In another study, Read and colleagues[12] explored the effects of bethanechol, administered intracerebroventricularly, to five male AD patients. Over a several-week period, dosage was adjusted upward until an optimal dose was obtained. Thereafter, patients were allowed to continue on their optimal dose. Three patients continued on bethanechol for more than 10 months. In these three, clinical status was reported to have been initially stable for 10 months but to have declined thereafter. There was great intersubject variability in optimal dose and in drug effect, limiting conclusions about efficacy. However, the investigators argued that this cholinergic agonist might produce limited clinical improvement in a subgroup of AD patients. The worsening of symptoms after a prolonged, initial stabilization period points to another, not uncommon, finding of studies on potential therapeutic agents for AD patients: their seeming effect on limiting further decline rather than reversing the disease itself. In this study, a placebo control was not included, making even more difficult any inferences about the drug's potential effects on AD progression. Some studies on other agents have included placebo controls. Some studies have reported positive (although often time-limited) effects of test agents on slowing cognitive decline but not on either reversing the disease permanently or dramatically improving memory or performance (see section "Calcium Channel Blockers" for further discussion).

Overall, cholinergic agents have not proven particularly effective in AD. This may reflect the irreversible nature of cholinergic denervation or the lack of "responsivity" of the remaining cholinergic neurons to the specific compounds used. Alternative, more indirect, modes of increasing cholinergic activity are being explored (see sections on "Oxiracetam" and "Ginkgo").

ERGOLOID MESYLATE

For many years, investigators and clinicians have been interested in the possible efficacy of vasodilators to treat AD patients. Considerable efforts have been expended in exploring the efficacy of ergoloid mesylates in AD. These compounds may increase neuronal oxygen utilization and increase alertness as well as act as vasodilators. One preparation, Hydergine, has been widely studied and commonly used in clinical practice. A recent report from Thompson et al.[13] on a new "liquid in a capsule" preparation (Hydergine LC) failed to find significant positive effects for this compound in comparison to placebo in 80 AD patients who were treated for up to 24 weeks. In fact, on two measures (one behavioral and one cognitive) placebo was associated with better scores at conclusion. The study used a maximum daily dose of 3 mg. Some investigators have argued the drug may be effective at much higher doses (e.g., 8 mg/day). Still, the results of this recent study are at best discouraging.

CALCIUM CHANNEL BLOCKERS

Calcium channel blockers have become widely used in medicine for their pronounced cardiovascular effects. One, nimodipine, has been studied in AD. This compound has been released in this country for the management of patients who have suffered a subarachnoid hemorrhage, in whom it is used to prevent brain damage resulting from reflex vasoconstriction. The mechanism of action for nimodipine exerting positive effects in AD is unclear, although its vasodilating effects may prove to be important. Other purported mechanisms of action for nimodipine are a decrease of the influx of calcium into damaged cells (thereby arresting further degeneration) and an increase in cholinergic activity. Further research is needed to determine how calcium channel blockers may actually work in AD.

In one multicenter, placebo-controlled study on 178 dementia patients carried out under double-blind conditions, Ban et al.[14] reported nimodipine was significantly more effective than placebo on a host of neuropsychological tests. The study involved a 12-week comparison trial of nimodipine (90 mg/day) and placebo after a 1-week placebo washout. Nimodipine was significantly more effective than placebo in improving scores on the Clinical Global Improvement Scale and the Hamilton Depression Rating Scale, although the degree of nimodipine-induced improvement on these two scales as well as on others was not dramatic. Using the Mini-Mental State Examination, nimodipine produced significantly greater improvement. Similar results were observed on a number of geriatric rating scales. On the Wechsler Memory Scale, nimodipine was again significantly more effective than placebo, with approximately 20 per cent improvement with nimodipine versus 6 per cent with placebo. In this study, some improvement on placebo was noted at conclusion, but positive effects had generally plateaued after 60 days; in contrast, nimodipine produced continued improvement between 60 and 90 days. Side effects of nimodipine were mild.

In another multicenter study, Tollefson[15] reported on a double-blind study comparing two doses of nimodipine (90 mg and 180 mg) and placebo in 227 patients. An initial placebo washout for 2 weeks was employed. Patients who were given placebo showed significant worsening on nine measures, behavioral as well as psychometric. In contrast, a number of psychometric measures were improved using 90 mg/day of nimodipine. The higher nimodipine dose (180 mg/day) produced more worsening on the Buschke Short-Term Recall test than was observed with placebo. These data are consistent with those of Ban et al. that 90 mg of nimodipine/day improves cognition. They also suggest a possible therapeutic window for nimodipine with poorer responses at higher doses.

VASOPRESSIN

Arginine vasopressin has been reported to exert a role in memory and learning, and deficiencies in this system have been reported in some AD patients. Synthetic vasopressin peptide analogues (without peripheral effects) have been developed as possible treatments for dementias. They are generally administered via a nasal spray.

In one study, Wolters et al.[16] reported that deglycinamide-arginine-vasopressin (DGAVP) was ineffective in reducing symptoms in AD. After a 2-week placebo washout, two doses of DGAVP were compared with placebo over 12 weeks in 115 patients with mild dementia. Positive effects for DGAVP were not observed on a variety of psychometric tests.

CATECHOLAMINERGIC AGENTS

Both the noradrenergic and dopaminergic systems have been postulated to play a role in the pathogenesis of AD, in part because they, too, play roles in attention and learning. Clonidine, an α_2-agonist used in the treatment of hypertension, was studied in eight AD patients who received three doses of clonidine (0.1 mg, 0.2 mg, and 0.4 mg/day) or placebo in a crossover design.[17] Significant effects on attention and psychometric performance were not observed.

Selegiline, an inhibitor of monoamine oxidase (MAO) B that degrades dopamine, has become an adjunctive treatment for parkinsonism. Several studies have pointed to selegiline exerting possible cognitive-enhancing effects in AD. In one recent trial, Monteverde et al.[18] compared 10 mg/day of selegiline to 200 mg/day of phosphatidylserine, under single-blind conditions. Twenty patients per cell were studied. Overall, daily living was improved in the selegiline group. In addition, cognition was significantly improved with selegiline as measured on specific psychometric tests. In contrast, phosphatidylserine did not result in similar, significant improvement. Progressive improvement with selegiline was observed across the 90 days; however, the maximal benefits appeared to occur within the first 60 days. The authors argued that enhanced memory with selegiline reflected improvement in encoding, storage, and retrieval, although they did note that improvement might have been due to effects on attention or alertness.

In other studies, selegiline at 10 mg/day has also been reported to improve cognition but at higher doses (e.g., 40 mg/day) it does not produce similar effects.[18,19] At such higher doses, selegiline becomes less specific in its MAO-inhibiting effects, inhibiting both MAO-A and MAO-B. (For further data on selegiline, see the section on "Oxiracetam".)

OXIRACETAM

Oxiracetam, a derivative of gamma-aminobutyric acid, has also been explored as a treatment for AD patients. It has been termed a nootropic,[2] reflecting its effects on enhancing general neuronal function. It appears to increase synaptic concentrations of ACh and to improve learning and memory deficits secondary to decreased cholinergic activity.

In one study, Maina et al.[20] reported on 289 patients with primary degenerative, multi-infarct, or mixed dementias treated with either oxiracetam (1600 mg/day) or placebo for 12 weeks. Oxiracetam was significantly more effective than placebo in improving both overall function and cognition. Differences in relative efficacy for oxiracetam were not observed among subtypes of dementias. Placebo produced some improvement in the first 4 weeks but not over the last 8 weeks. In contrast, oxiracetam produced steady improvement over the 12-week trial. Again, degree of improvement on oxiracetam was relatively small.

In another study, Falsaperla et al.[21] compared 1600 mg/day of oxiracetam with 10 mg/day of selegiline in 40 AD patients using a single-blind design. Selegiline produced significantly more improvement in daily living (as measured on various dementia scales), as well as on tests for memory, delayed recall, and acquisition, than did oxiracetam. However, both compounds produced significant improvement over baseline on most measures. Although a placebo control was not included in this study, data presented point to activity for both compounds.

S-ADENOSYL-L-METHIONINE

S-adenosyl-L-methionine (SAMe), a methyl donor compound, has been reported to increase the fluidity of membranes in various tissues. Since AD patients demonstrate decreased membrane fluidity in platelets, there has been some interest in the possible use of SAMe in AD patients. Cohen et al.[22] reported on SAMe in a small group of AD patients. No positive effects were observed, and the study was terminated early.

GINKGO

Extracts from the Ginkgo plant have become widely used in Europe for their purported effects on cognition. Originally, this regimen was developed in China, where it has been available for millennia. *Ginkgo biloba*, one extract, is currently being investigated in a large-scale multicenter study on AD and multi-infarct dementia in the United States. This compound has been reported in animal studies to bind free radicals and thus to decrease neurotoxicity, to protect central neurons against various insults, to increase muscarinic receptors, and to improve memory in healthy volunteers and cognition in neurological patients.[23] In the ongoing multicenter study, *Ginkgo biloba* is being compared under double-blind conditions to placebo for 6 months, with an additional extension for up to 5 years. Preliminary results of this interesting compound are not yet available. The strategy of using this natural plant derivative is intriguing, particularly because it has virtually no side effects and is apparently well tolerated.

DISCUSSION

Although some of the agents that are currently being tested offer considerable promise, available data to date suggest that these agents do not arrest the progression of the disease. To date, we have no agent that reverses AD. On the one hand, this could reflect the irreversible nature of the cholinergic denervation in AD. On the other, unsuccessful therapies may also reflect our limited knowledge of the pathophysiology of the disease.

Recently, a number of groups have been exploring various other aspects of the biology of AD. Such research has taken a variety of approaches. One such approach is to determine the processes involved in amyloid deposition in brain and other tissues, including its genetic control. Amyloid deposits are increased in the brains of AD patients as well as in other tissues. The behavioral and cognitive effects of such amyloid deposits are not clearly established, and some have argued these may be downstream from the key area of dysfunction. Still, however, determining the processes involved in amyloid formation may allow for the development of new treatments aimed at reversing such deposits or preventing them in individuals at risk. Such approaches offer great hope for therapy, but this is likely to be in the considerable future.

Another approach that has been elegantly articulated by Bowen[24] emphasizes dysfunction of excitatory amino acids, particularly glutamate, in AD. Glutamate acts as a neurotransmitter for cortical association fibers that link neurons within the cerebral cortex. Bowen has argued that degeneration of such glutamate-mediated neuronal connections may underlie AD and that partial glutamate agonists could have a beneficial effect on AD. Such approaches may prove more effective; however, considerable research will be required to develop and test potential compounds. At any rate, such efforts do reflect the current intense thinking and research regarding AD.

In summary, a number of agents for AD are currently under study in this country and abroad. Of particular immediate promise are nimodipine, selegiline, and oxiracetam, although none appears to produce dramatic reversal of the disease. The increase in interest and research in this increasingly prevalent disease is likely to yield new approaches over the next decade, and, it is hoped, more effective treatments.

REFERENCES

1. Bartus RT, Dean RL, Beer B, et al: The cholinergic hypothesis of geriatric memory dysfunction. Science 217:408–417, 1982.
2. Cooper JK: Drug treatment of Alzheimer's disease. Arch Intern Med 151:245–249, 1991.
3. Jenike MA, Albert MS, Heller H, et al: Oral physostigmine treatment for patients with presenile and senile dementia of the Alzheimer's type: A double-blind placebo-controlled trial. J Clin Psychiatry 51:3–8, 1990.
4. Harrell LE, Callaway R, Morere D, et al: The effect of long-term physostigmine administration in Alzheimer's disease. Neurology 40:1350–1354, 1990.
5. Summers WK, Majovski LV, Marsh GM, et al: Oral tetrahydroaminoacridine in long-term treatment of senile dementia. Alzheimer type. N Engl J Med 315:1241–1245, 1986.
6. Davis KL, Mohs RC: Cholinergic drugs in Alzheimer's disease. N Engl J Med 315:1286–1287, 1986.
7. Relman AS: Tacrine as a treatment for Alzheimer's dementia: Editor's note. N Engl J Med 324:349, 1991.
8. Division of Neuropharmacological Drug Products, Office of New Drug Evaluation (I), Food and Drug Administration: Tacrine as a treatment for Alzheimer's dementia: An interim report from the FDA. N Engl J Med 324:349–352, 1991.
9. Gauthier S, Bouchard R, Lamontagne A, et al: Tetrahydroaminoacridine-lecithin combination treatment in patients with intermediate-stage Alzheimer's disease: Results of a Canadian double-blind, crossover, multicenter study. N Engl J Med 322:1272–1276, 1990.
10. Molloy DW, Guyatt GH, Wilson DB, et al: Effect of tetrahydroaminocridine on cognition, function and behavior in Alzheimer's disease. Can Med Assoc J 144:29–34, 1991.
11. Tariot PN, Cohen R, Welkowitz JA, et al: Multiple-dose arecoline infusions in Alzheimer's disease. Arch Gen Psychiatry 45:901–905, 1988.
12. Read SL, Frazee J, Shapira J, et al: Intracerebroventricular bethanechol for Alzheimer's disease. Variable dose-related responses. Arch Neurol 47:1025–1030, 1990.
13. Thompson TL, Filley CM, Mitchell WD, et al: Lack of efficacy of hydergine in patients with Alzheimer's disease. N Engl J Med 323:445–448, 1990.
14. Ban TA, Morey L, Aguglia E, et al: Nimodipine in the treatment of old age dementias. Prog Neuropsychopharmacol Biol Psychiatry 14:525–551, 1990.
15. Tollefson G: Short-term effects of the calcium channel blocker nimodipine (Bay-e-9736) in the management of primary degenerative dementia. Biol Psychiatry 27:1133–1142, 1990.
16. Wolters EC, Riekkinen P, Lowenthal A, et al: DGAVP (Org 5667) in early Alzheimer's disease patients: An international double-blind, placebo-controlled, multicenter trial. Neurology 40:1099–1101, 1990.
17. Mohr E, Schlegel J, Fabbrini G, et al: Clonidine treatment of Alzheimer's disease. Arch Neurol 46:376–378, 1989.
18. Monteverde A, Gnemmi P, Rossi F, et al: Selegiline in the treatment of mild to moderate Alzheimer-type dementia. Clin Ther 12:315–322, 1990.
19. Piccinin G, Finali GC, Piccirilli M: Neuropsychological effects of L-deprenyl in Alzheimer's type dementia. Clin Neuropharmacol 13(2):147–163, 1990.
20. Maina G, Fiori L, Torta R, et al: Oxiracetam in the treatment of primary degenerative and multi-infarct dementia: A double-blind, placebo-controlled study. Neuropsychobiology 21:141–145, 1989.
21. Falsaperla A, Preti PAM, Oliani C: Selegiline versus oxiracetam in patients with Alzheimer-type dementia. Clin Ther 12:376–384, 1990.
22. Cohen BM, Satlin A, Zubenko GS: S-adenosyl-l-methionine in the treatment of Alzheimer's disease. J Clin Psychopharmacol 8:43–47, 1988.
23. Funfgeld EW: A natural and broad spectrum nootropic substance for treatment of SDAT—the Ginkgo biloba extract. Prog Clin Biol Res 314:1247–1260, 1989.
24. Bowen DM: Treatment of Alzheimer's disease: Molecular pathology versus neurotransmitter-based therapy. Br J Psychiatry 157:327–330, 1990.

APPENDIX I: CLASSIFICATION OF NEUROLEPTICS

Class	Example	Common Brands	Available Doses
Phenothiazine Alkylamino	Chlorpromazine	Thorazine	Tablets: 10 mg, 25 mg, 50 mg, 100 mg, 200 mg Oral concentrate: 30 mg/ml, 100 mg/ml IM injection: 25 mg/ml
Piperidine	Thioridazine	Mellaril	Tablets: 10 mg, 15 mg, 25 mg, 50 mg, 100 mg, 200 mg Oral concentrate: 30 mg/ml, 100 mg/ml
Piperazine	Fluphenazine	Prolixin Permital	Tablets: 1 mg, 2.5 mg, 5 mg, 10 mg Oral concentrate: 5 mg/ml IM injection: 2.5 mg/ml Enanthate depot injection: 25 mg/ml Decanoate depot injection: 25 mg/ml
Thiozanthenes	Thiothixene	Navane	Capsules: 1 mg, 2 mg, 5 mg, 10 mg, 20 mg Oral concentrate: 5 mg/ml Injection: 2 mg/ml, 5 mg/ml
Butyrophenones	Haloperidol	Haldol	Tablets: 0.5 mg, 1 mg, 2.5 mg, 10 mg, 20 mg Oral concentrate: 2 mg/ml Injection: 5 mg/ml Decanoate depot injection: 50 mg/ml
	Pimozide	ORAP	Tablet: 2 mg
Benzamides	Sulpiride		Not available in the United States
Dibenzoazepines	Clozapine	Clozaril	Tablets: 25 mg, 100 mg
	Loxapine	Loxitane	Oral concentrate: 25 mg/ml Injection: 50 mg/ml

Prepared by S. Potkin.

APPENDIX II: MEDICATION FOR EPS IN mg/day USUALLY PRESCRIBED b.i.d. or t.i.d. BECAUSE OF RELATIVELY SHORT HALF-LIVES

Medication	Brand Name	Dosage (mg/day)
Anticholinergic		
Benztropine	Cogentin	2–6
Trihexyphenidyl	Artane	4–15
Biperiden	Akineton	2–8
Diphenhydramine	Benadryl	50–300
(also potent H1 antagonist)		
Dopamine releasing		
Amantadine	Symmetrel[a]	100–300

Prepared by S. Potkin.
[a] Not available as parenteral formulations.

APPENDIX III: PHARMACOKINETICS OF COMMONLY PRESCRIBED BENZODIAZEPINES

Generic Name (Trade Name)	Dosage Equivalent (mg)	Lipid Solubility	Onset of Action	Elimination Half-Life (hours)[a]	Hepatic Metabolism
Alprazolam (Xanax)	0.5	0.54	Intermediate	6–20	Oxidation
Chlordiazepoxide (Librium and others)	10.0		Intermediate	5–100	Oxidation
Clonazepam (Klonopin)	0.25	0.28	Intermediate	18–50	Oxidation Nitroreduction
Clorazepate (Tranxene)	7.5	0.79	Fast	30–100	Oxidation
Diazepam (Valium and others)	5.0	1.00	Fast	30–100	Oxidation
Flurazepam (Dalmane)	30.0		Fast	50–100	Oxidation
Lorazepam (Ativan)	1.0	0.48	Intermediate	10–20	Conjugation
Oxazepam (Serax)	15.0	0.45	Slow	5–21	Conjugation
Temazepam (Restoril)	30.0		Slow	10–12	Conjugation
Triazolam (Halcion)	0.5		Fast	1.7–3.0	Conjugation

[a] Elimination half-life represents the total for all active metabolites.
Prepared by D. Cowley.

559

Drug (Generic and Trade Names)	Individual Variation in Metabolism	Elimination Half-Life, T½ (hours) Mean	Range	Starting Dosage[b] (mg/day)	Usual Daily Dose for Adults (mg)	Usual Dose Range (mg/day)	Projected[c] Optimal Therapeutic Plasma Range (ng/ml)
Tricyclic: tertiary amines							
Amitriptyline (Elavil, Endep)	10-fold	21	13–36	50	150–200	50–300	80–250[d]
Doxepin (Adapin, Sinequan)	10- to 15-fold	17	8–24	50	75–150	50–300	150–250[e]
Imipramine (Janimine, Tofranil)	30-fold	28	18–34	50	75–150	50–300	150–250[f]
Trimipramine (Surmontil)	—	13	—	50	100–200	50–300	150–250
Tricyclic: secondary amines							
Desipramine (Norpramin, Pertofrane)	10-fold	21	12–30	50	100–200	50–300	125–300
Nortriptyline (Pamelor)	30-fold	36	14–79	20	75–100	30–125	50–150
Protriptyline (Vivactil)	10- to 15-fold	78	55–127	10	15–40	10–60	70–260
Dibenzoxazepine							
Amoxapine (Asendin)	—	8	8–30[g]	50	200–300	50–400	200–600[h]
Tetracyclic							
Maprotiline (Ludiomil)	—	43	—	50	100–150	50–225	200–600
Triazolopyridine							
Trazodone (Desyrel)	—	7	3–16	50	150–400	50–600	800–1600
Benzenepropanamine							
Fluoxetine (Prozac)	—	87	26–220	20	20–80	20–80	—
Propiophenone							
Bupropion (Wellbutrin)	—	9.8	3.9–23.1	200[i]	300[j]	100–450[k]	—
Monoamine oxidase inhibitors							
Isocarboxazid (Marplan)	—	—	—	30	10–30	10–30[l]	—
Phenelzine (Nardil)	—	2.8	1.5–4	15	45–60	45–90[m]	—
Tranylcypromine (Parnate)	4-fold	2.4	1.5–3	10	30–40	30–60	—

[a] Modified and reproduced with permission from Richelson E: Antidepressants: Pharmacology and clinical use. *In* Karasu TB, ed. Treatments of Psychiatric Disorders. 1st ed. Washington, DC: American Psychiatric Association Press, 1989: Vol. 3, 1773.[36]

[b] Dosage should be divided initially for all listed drugs, and elderly persons should be treated with about half of the usual dosage for adults.

[c] Only amitriptyline, imipramine, nortriptyline, and desipramine have been significantly studied for blood level versus clinical response.[2]

[d] Amitriptyline + nortriptyline.

[e] Doxepin + desmethyldoxepin.

[f] Imipramine + desipramine.

[g] Amoxapine, 8 hours; 8-hydroxyamoxapine, 30 hours.

[h] Amoxapine + 8-hydroxyamoxapine; of total drug measured, amoxapine ≈ 20 per cent; 7-hydroxyamoxapine ≈ 15; and 8-hydroxyamoxapine ≈ 65 per cent.

[i] Dose should be divided, 100 mg b.i.d.

[j] Divided dose by fourth day of treatment.

[k] Maximum recommended divided dose achieved if no response after 3 weeks at the lower dosage.

[l] Dose should be reduced to a maintenance level of 10 to 20 mg daily (or less) once response begins because of the drug's cumulative effects.

[m] 1 mg/kg.[28]

INDEX

Note: Page numbers in *italics* refer to illustrations, page numbers followed by t refer to tables.